T0324044

Contemporary Research Methods in Pharmacy and Health Services

Contemporary Research Methods in Pharmacy and Health Services

Edited by

Shane P. Desselle
Professor of Social/Behavior Pharmacy, Touro University California, Vallejo, CA, United States

Victoria García-Cárdenas
Senior Lecturer in Pharmacy, University of Technology Sydney, Sydney, NSW, Australia

Claire Anderson
Professor of Social Pharmacy, School of Pharmacy, University of Nottingham, Nottingham, United Kingdom

Parisa Aslani
Professor in Medicines Use Optimisation, The University of Sydney, Sydney, NSW, Australia

Aleda M.H. Chen
Professor and Associate Dean, Cedarville University, Cedarville, OH, United States

Timothy F. Chen
Professor of Medication Management, The University of Sydney, Sydney, NSW, Australia

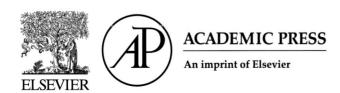

ACADEMIC PRESS
An imprint of Elsevier

ELSEVIER

Academic Press is an imprint of Elsevier
125 London Wall, London EC2Y 5AS, United Kingdom
525 B Street, Suite 1650, San Diego, CA 92101, United States
50 Hampshire Street, 5th Floor, Cambridge, MA 02139, United States
The Boulevard, Langford Lane, Kidlington, Oxford OX5 1GB, United Kingdom

Notices

Knowledge and best practice in this field are constantly changing. As new research and experience broaden our understanding, changes in research methods, professional practices, or medical treatment may become necessary.

Practitioners and researchers must always rely on their own experience and knowledge in evaluating and using any information, methods, compounds, or experiments described herein. In using such information or methods they should be mindful of their own safety and the safety of others, including parties for whom they have a professional responsibility.

To the fullest extent of the law, neither the Publisher nor the authors, contributors, or editors, assume any liability for any injury and/or damage to persons or property as a matter of products liability, negligence or otherwise, or from any use or operation of any methods, products, instructions, or ideas contained in the material herein.

ISBN: 978-0-323-91888-6

For information on all Academic Press publications
visit our website at https://www.elsevier.com/books-and-journals

Publisher: Stacy Masucci
Senior Acquisitions Editor: Andre G. Wolff
Editorial Project Manager: Tracy Tufaga
Production Project Manager: Punithavathy Govindaradjane
Cover Designer: Matthew Limbert

Typeset by STRAIVE, India

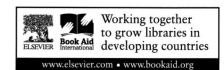

Dedication

This book is dedicated to the Social Pharmacy community.

Contents

Section I
Overarching Design and Reviews Considerations

1. Applying human factors and ergonomics methods to pharmaceutical health services research

Richard J. Holden, Ephrem Abebe, Alissa L. Russ-Jara, and Michelle A. Chui

2. Designing complex health interventions using experience-based co-design

Beth Fylan, Justine Tomlinson, D.K. Raynor, and Jonathan Silcock

3. Use of common models to inform and design pharmacy and health services research

Anandi V. Law and Marcia M. Worley

4. Implementation science to guide pharmacy and health services research

Victoria García-Cárdenas and Kenneth C. Hohmeier

5. CFIR framework in pharmacy and health services research

Sarah J. Shoemaker-Hunt, Ellen Childs, Holly Swan, and Geoffrey Curran

6. Principles and applications of metaresearch

Spencer E. Harpe

7. Best practices when conducting and reporting a meta-analysis

Fernanda S. Tonin, Aline F. Bonetti, and Fernando Fernandez-Llimos

8. Using methods from human-centered design in health research: An introduction for pharmacy and health services researchers

*Michelle Flood, Laura L. Gleeson,
Sarah Flynn, Mark Ennis, Aoife Ludlow,
Fabian F. Sweeney, Alice Holton,
Stephanie Morgan, Colleen Clarke,
Pádraig Carroll, Lisa Mellon, Fiona Boland,
Sarah Mohamed, Aoife De Brún,
Marcus Hanratty, Shaunna Kelly, and
Frank Moriarty*

Section II
Emerging Methodological Approaches and Updates

9. Applying action research in social pharmacy and health services research: An overview

Kritsanee Saramunee

10. Q methodology in pharmacy and health services research

*Robert Haua, Amanda Wolf, Jeff Harrison,
and Trudi Aspden*

11. Medicines optimization and illness management research using dyads

Dolly Sud

15. The draw and write technique to uncover nuance in pharmacy and health services delivery

Theresa J. Schindel, Christine A. Hughes, Tatiana Makhinova, and Jason S. Daniels

16. The use of art to analyze learning practices in pharmacy and to inform assessment and intervention practices

Ruth M. Edwards and John I'Anson

17. Evaluating benefits and harms of deprescribing using routinely collected data

Frank Moriarty, Wade Thompson, and Fiona Boland

18. Understanding and addressing the observer effect in observation studies

Sofia Kälvemark Sporrong, Birgitte Grøstad Kalleberg, Liv Mathiesen, Yvonne Andersson, Stine Eidhammer Rognan, and Karin Svensberg

37. Latent class and latent class regression

James B. Schreiber

38. Guidelines and standards in medication adherence research

Charlotte L. Bekker, Parisa Aslani, and Timothy F. Chen

39. Methodological and disciplinary competence and insecurity in qualitative research

Sofia Kälvemark Sporrong, Susanne Kaae, Lotte Stig Nørgaard, Mathias Møllebæk, Marit Waaseth, Lourdes Cantarero Arevalo, Christina Ljungberg Persson, Charlotte L. Bekker, Johanna Falby Lindell, and Louise C. Druedahl

40. Contemporary conceptualization of measurement validity

Michael J. Peeters and Spencer E. Harpe

Contributors

Numbers in parentheses indicate the pages on which the authors' contributions begin.

Ephrem Abebe (3), Department of Medicine, Indiana University School of Medicine, Indianapolis; Department of Pharmacy Practice, College of Pharmacy, Purdue University, West Lafayette, IN, United States

Enas Almanasreh (583), Faculty of Pharmacy, Mutah University, Al-Karak, Jordan; The University of Sydney School of Pharmacy, Faculty of Medicine and Health, The University of Sydney, Sydney, NSW, Australia

Yvonne Andersson (261), Hospital Pharmacies Enterprise, South Eastern Norway, Oslo, Norway

Rajender R. Aparasu (527), Department of Pharmaceutical Health Outcomes and Policy, College of Pharmacy, University of Houston, Texas Medical Center, Houston, TX, United States

Naoko Arakawa (447), School of Pharmacy, University of Nottingham, Nottingham, United Kingdom

Lourdes Cantarero Arevalo (201, 567), Department of Pharmacy, Social and Clinical Pharmacy Research Group, University of Copenhagen, Copenhagen, Denmark

Mohsen Askar (161), Department of Pharmacy, Faculty of Health Sciences, UiT The Arctic University of Norway, Tromsø, Norway

Parisa Aslani (553), The University of Sydney School of Pharmacy, Faculty of Medicine and Health, The University of Sydney, Sydney, NSW, Australia

Trudi Aspden (129), School of Pharmacy, Faculty of Medical and Health Sciences, University of Auckland, Auckland, New Zealand

Ahmed Awaisu (467), Department of Clinical Pharmacy and Practice, College of Pharmacy, QU Health, Qatar University, Doha, Qatar

Beata V. Bajorek (345), Discipline of Pharmacy, Graduate School of Health, University of Technology Sydney, Sydney, NSW, Australia

Mitchell J. Barnett (491, 617), Clinical Sciences, Touro University-College of Pharmacy, Vallejo, CA; Iowa Board of Pharmacy, Iowa Department of Public Health, Des Moines, IA, United States

Charlotte L. Bekker (553, 567), Department of Pharmacy, Radboud University Medical Center, Research Institute for Health Sciences, Nijmegen, The Netherlands

John P. Bentley (313), Department of Pharmacy Administration, University of Mississippi School of Pharmacy, University, MS, United States

Fiona Boland (103, 249), Data Science Centre, RCSI University of Medicine and Health Sciences, Dublin, Ireland

Aline F. Bonetti (85), Pharmaceutical Sciences Postgraduate Program, Federal University of Paraná, Curitiba, Brazil

Catriona Bradley (455), Irish Institute of Pharmacy, RCSI University of Medicine and Health Sciences, Dublin, Ireland

Pádraig Carroll (103), School of Pharmacy and Biomolecular Sciences, RCSI University of Medicine and Health Sciences, Dublin, Ireland

Stephen R. Carter (515), The University of Sydney School of Pharmacy, Faculty of Medicine and Health, The University of Sydney, Sydney, NSW, Australia

Timothy F. Chen (553, 583), The University of Sydney School of Pharmacy, Faculty of Medicine and Health, The University of Sydney, Sydney, NSW, Australia

Ellen Childs (57), Abt Associates, Inc., Cambridge, MA, United States

Wei Wen Chong (295), Centre of Quality Management of Medicines, Faculty of Pharmacy, The National University of Malaysia, Kuala Lumpur, Malaysia

Michelle A. Chui (3, 379), Social and Administrative Sciences Division; Sonderegger Research Center, University of Wisconsin-Madison School of Pharmacy, Madison, WI, United States

Colleen Clarke (103), Institute for Healthcare Delivery Design, Population Health Sciences Program, University of Illinois-Chicago, Chicago, IL, United States

Jack C. Collins (295), The University of Sydney School of Pharmacy, Faculty of Medicine and Health, The University of Sydney, Sydney, NSW, Australia

Geoffrey Curran (57), University of Arkansas for Medical Sciences, Center for Implementation Research, Little Rock, AR, United States

Jason S. Daniels (215), School of Public Health, University of Alberta, Edmonton, AB, Canada

Abilio C. de Almeida Neto (295), Neto Psychological Consulting, Pyrmont, NSW, Australia

Aoife De Brún (103), School of Nursing Midwifery and Health Systems, Health Sciences Centre, University College Dublin, Dublin, Ireland

Shadi Doroudgar (491, 617), Clinical Sciences, Touro University-College of Pharmacy, Vallejo; Department of Medicine-Primary Care and Population Health, Stanford University, Stanford, CA, United States

Ros Dowse (183), Faculty of Pharmacy, Rhodes University, Makhanda, South Africa

Louise C. Druedahl (567), Department of Pharmacy, Social and Clinical Pharmacy Research Group; Centre for Advanced Studies in Biomedical Innovation Law (CeBIL), University of Copenhagen, Copenhagen, Denmark

Sarah Drumm (455), Irish Institute of Pharmacy; School of Pharmacy and Biomolecular Sciences, RCSI University of Medicine and Health Sciences, Dublin, Ireland

Ruth M. Edwards (233), School of Pharmacy, University of Wolverhampton, Wolverhampton, United Kingdom

Stine Eidhammer Rognan (261), Department of Pharmacy, University of Oslo; Department of Pharmaceutical Services, Oslo Hospital Pharmacy, Oslo, Norway

Maguy Saffouh El Hajj (467), Department of Clinical Pharmacy and Practice, College of Pharmacy, QU Health, Qatar University, Doha, Qatar

Alla El-Awaisi (467), Department of Clinical Pharmacy and Practice, College of Pharmacy, QU Health, Qatar University, Doha, Qatar

Mark Ennis (103), TU Dublin School of Creative Arts, Technological University Dublin City Campus, Dublin, Ireland

Sadaf Faisal (369), University of Waterloo School of Pharmacy, Kitchener, ON, Canada

Fernando Fernandez-Llimos (85), Laboratory of Pharmacology, Faculty of Pharmacy, University of Porto, Porto, Portugal

Michelle Flood (103), School of Pharmacy and Biomolecular Sciences, RCSI University of Medicine and Health Sciences, Dublin, Ireland; Design Institute for Health, Dell Medical School, University of Texas at Austin, Austin, TX, United States

Sarah Flynn (103), School of Pharmacy and Biomolecular Sciences, RCSI University of Medicine and Health Sciences, Dublin, Ireland

Beth Fylan (21), University of Bradford, School of Pharmacy and Medical Sciences; Bradford Teaching Hospitals NHS Foundation Trust, Yorkshire Quality and Safety Research Group, Bradford, United Kingdom

Victoria García-Cárdenas (49), Graduate School of Health, Faculty of Health, University of Technology Sydney, Sydney, NSW, Australia

Aaron M. Gilson (379), Sonderegger Research Center, University of Wisconsin-Madison School of Pharmacy, Madison, WI, United States

Laura L. Gleeson (103), School of Pharmacy and Biomolecular Sciences, RCSI University of Medicine and Health Sciences, Dublin, Ireland

Birgitte Grøstad Kalleberg (261), Department of Pharmacy, University of Oslo, Oslo, Norway

Matthew Halliday (433), Division of Pharmacy, School of Allied Health, The University of Western Australia, Crawley, WA, Australia

Marcus Hanratty (103), Department of Product Design, National College of Art and Design, Dublin, Ireland

Spencer E. Harpe (73, 575), Department of Pharmacy Practice, Midwestern University College of Pharmacy, Downers Grove, IL, United States

Jeff Harrison (129), School of Pharmacy, Faculty of Medical and Health Sciences, University of Auckland, Auckland, New Zealand

Robert Haua (129), School of Pharmacy, Faculty of Medical and Health Sciences, University of Auckland, Auckland, New Zealand

Kenneth C. Hohmeier (49, 397), University of Tennessee Health Science Center, College of Pharmacy, Memphis, TN, United States

Richard J. Holden (3), Department of Health & Wellness Design, Indiana University School of Public Health, Bloomington; Center for Aging Research, Regenstrief Institute, Inc., Indianapolis; Center for Health Innovation and Implementation Science, Indiana Clinical and Translational Sciences Institute, Indianapolis; Department of Medicine, Indiana University School of Medicine, Indianapolis, IN, United States

Alice Holton (103), School of Pharmacy and Biomolecular Sciences, RCSI University of Medicine and Health Sciences, Dublin, Ireland

Su-Yin Hor (345), Centre for Health Services Management, Faculty of Health, University of Technology Sydney, Sydney, NSW, Australia

Christine A. Hughes (215), Faculty of Pharmacy and Pharmaceutical Sciences, University of Alberta, Edmonton, AB, Canada

John I'Anson (233), Faculty of Social Sciences, University of Stirling, Stirling, United Kingdom

Eric J. Ip (491, 617), Clinical Sciences, Touro University-College of Pharmacy, Vallejo; Department of Medicine-Primary Care and Population Health, Stanford University, Stanford; Internal Medicine, Kaiser Permanente Mountain View Medical Offices, Mountain View, CA, United States

Myriam Jaam (467), Department of Clinical Pharmacy and Practice, College of Pharmacy, QU Health, Qatar University, Doha, Qatar

Jacinta Johnson (433), Division of Pharmacy, UniSA Clinical & Health Sciences, University of South Australia; SA Pharmacy, SA Health, Adelaide, SA, Australia

Susanne Kaae (329, 567), Department of Pharmacy, Social and Clinical Pharmacy Research Group, University of Copenhagen, Copenhagen, Denmark

Sofia Kälvemark Sporrong (261, 329, 567), Department of Pharmacy, Uppsala University, Uppsala, Sweden; Department of Pharmacy, Social and Clinical Pharmacy Research Group, University of Copenhagen, Copenhagen, Denmark

Shaunna Kelly (103), School of Medicine, RCSI University of Medicine and Health Sciences, Dublin, Ireland

Vista Khosraviani (491, 617), Clinical Sciences, Touro University-College of Pharmacy, Vallejo, CA, United States

Sofie Rosenlund Lau (329), Department of Public Health, University of Copenhagen, Copenhagen, Denmark

Anandi V. Law (37), Department of Pharmacy Practice and Administration, College of Pharmacy, Western University of Health Sciences, Pomona, CA, United States

Kenneth Lee (433), Division of Pharmacy, School of Allied Health, The University of Western Australia, Crawley, WA, Australia

Johanna Falby Lindell (567), Department of Nordic Studies and Linguistics and University of Copenhagen Research Centre for Control of Antibiotic Resistance (UC-CARE), University of Copenhagen, Copenhagen, Denmark

Laura Lindsey (421), School of Pharmacy, Faculty of Medical Sciences, Newcastle University, Newcastle upon Tyne, United Kingdom

Aoife Ludlow (103), School of Pharmacy and Biomolecular Sciences, RCSI University of Medicine and Health Sciences, Dublin, Ireland

K. Luetsch (271), School of Pharmacy, The University of Queensland, St Lucia, QLD, Australia

I. Maidment (271), School of Life and Health Sciences, Aston University, Birmingham, United Kingdom

Tatiana Makhinova (215), Faculty of Pharmacy and Pharmaceutical Sciences, University of Alberta, Edmonton, AB, Canada

Liv Mathiesen (261), Department of Pharmacy, University of Oslo, Oslo, Norway

Colleen McMillan (369), School of Social Work, Renison University College, University of Waterloo, Waterloo, ON, Canada

Lisa Mellon (103), Division of Population Health Sciences, RCSI University of Medicine and Health Sciences, Dublin, Ireland

Deanna Mill (433), Division of Pharmacy, School of Allied Health, The University of Western Australia, Crawley, WA, Australia

Ardalan Mirzaei (515), The University of Sydney School of Pharmacy, Faculty of Medicine and Health, The University of Sydney, Sydney, NSW, Australia

Sarah Mohamed (103), School of Pharmacy and Biomolecular Sciences, RCSI University of Medicine and Health Sciences; School of Pharmacy and Pharmaceutical Sciences, Trinity College Dublin, Dublin, Ireland

Rebekah J. Moles (295, 583), The University of Sydney School of Pharmacy, Faculty of Medicine and Health, The University of Sydney, Sydney, NSW, Australia

Mathias Møllebæk (567), Department of Pharmacy, Social and Clinical Pharmacy Research Group, University of Copenhagen, Copenhagen, Denmark

Stephanie Morgan (103), Design Institute for Health, Dell Medical School, University of Texas at Austin, Austin, TX, United States

Frank Moriarty (103, 249, 455), School of Pharmacy and Biomolecular Sciences, RCSI University of Medicine and Health Sciences, Dublin, Ireland

Ashley O. Morris (379), Social and Administrative Sciences Division, University of Wisconsin-Madison School of Pharmacy, Madison, WI, United States

Lotte Stig Nørgaard (567), Department of Pharmacy, Social and Clinical Pharmacy Research Group, University of Copenhagen, Copenhagen, Denmark

Asad E. Patanwala (515), The University of Sydney School of Pharmacy, Faculty of Medicine and Health, The University of Sydney, Sydney, NSW, Australia

Michael J. Peeters (575), University of Toledo College of Pharmacy & Pharmaceutical Sciences, Toledo, OH, United States

Christina Ljungberg Persson (567), School of Public Health and Community Medicine, University of Gothenburg, Arvid Wallgrens Backe, Gothenburg, Sweden

Sujith Ramachandran (313), Department of Pharmacy Administration, University of Mississippi School of Pharmacy, University, MS, United States

Deepika Rao (407), Social and Administrative Sciences, School of Pharmacy, University of Wisconsin-Madison, Madison, WI, United States

Adam Pattison Rathbone (421), School of Pharmacy, Faculty of Medical Sciences, Newcastle University, Newcastle upon Tyne, United Kingdom

D.K. Raynor (21), University of Leeds, School of Healthcare, Leeds, United Kingdom

Sanika Rege (527), Department of Pharmaceutical Health Outcomes and Policy, College of Pharmacy, University of Houston, Texas Medical Center, Houston, TX, United States

Chelsea Phillips Renfro (397), University of Tennessee Health Science Center College of Pharmacy, Memphis, TN, United States

D. Rowett (271), Clinical & Health Sciences, University of South Australia, Adelaide, SA, Australia

Alissa L. Russ-Jara (3), Department of Pharmacy Practice, College of Pharmacy, Purdue University, West Lafayette, IN, United States

Teresa M. Salgado (313), Department of Pharmacotherapy & Outcomes Science, Virginia Commonwealth University School of Pharmacy, Richmond, VA, United States

Kritsanee Saramunee (117), Faculty of Pharmacy, Mahasarakham University, Maha Sarakham, Thailand

Theresa J. Schindel (215), Faculty of Pharmacy and Pharmaceutical Sciences, University of Alberta, Edmonton, AB, Canada

Carl R. Schneider (295, 515), The University of Sydney School of Pharmacy, Faculty of Medicine and Health, The University of Sydney, Sydney, NSW, Australia

James B. Schreiber (541, 601), School of Nursing, Duquesne University, Pittsburgh, PA, United States

Olayinka O. Shiyanbola (407), Social and Administrative Sciences, School of Pharmacy, University of Wisconsin-Madison, Madison, WI, United States

Sarah J. Shoemaker-Hunt (57), Abt Associates, Inc., Cambridge, MA, United States

Jonathan Silcock (21), University of Bradford, School of Pharmacy and Medical Sciences, Bradford, United Kingdom

Derek Stewart (467), Department of Clinical Pharmacy and Practice, College of Pharmacy, QU Health, Qatar University, Doha, Qatar

Dolly Sud (143), Pharmacy Department, Bradgate Site, Leicestershire Partnership NHS Trust, Leicestershire; College of Life and Health Sciences, Aston University, Birmingham, United Kingdom

Kristian Svendsen (161), Department of Pharmacy, Faculty of Health Sciences, UiT The Arctic University of Norway, Tromsø, Norway

Karin Svensberg (261), Department of Pharmacy, Uppsala University, Uppsala, Sweden

Holly Swan (57), Abt Associates, Inc., Cambridge, MA, United States

Fabian F. Sweeney (103), School of Pharmacy and Biomolecular Sciences, RCSI University of Medicine and Health Sciences, Dublin, Ireland

Wade Thompson (249), Women's College Hospital Research Institute, Toronto, ON, Canada

Justine Tomlinson (21), University of Bradford, School of Pharmacy and Medical Sciences, Bradford; Leeds Teaching Hospitals NHS Trust, Medicines Management and Pharmacy Services, Leeds, United Kingdom

Fernanda S. Tonin (85), Pharmaceutical Sciences Postgraduate Program, Federal University of Paraná, Curitiba, Brazil

Janine Marie Traulsen (329), Department of Pharmacy, Social and Clinical Pharmacy Research Group, University of Copenhagen, Copenhagen, Denmark

M.J. Twigg (271), School of Pharmacy, University of East Anglia, Norwich, United Kingdom

Marit Waaseth (567), Department of Pharmacy, The Arctic University of Norway, Tromsø, Norway

Amy Werremeyer (201), Department of Pharmacy Practice, North Dakota State University, Fargo, ND, United States

Amanda Wolf (129), Wellington School of Business and Government, Te Herenga Waka Victoria University of Wellington, Wellington, New Zealand

Phillip Woods (283), School of Pharmacy and Medical Sciences, Griffith University, Gold Coast Campus, QLD, Australia

Marcia M. Worley (37), Division of Outcomes and Translational Sciences, The Ohio State University, College of Pharmacy, Columbus, OH, United States

Faith R. Yong (345), Discipline of Pharmacy, Graduate School of Health, University of Technology Sydney, Sydney, NSW, Australia

About the Editors

Shane P. Desselle, RPh, PhD, FAPhA, is a Professor at Touro University California. He is founding Editor-in-Chief of *Research in Social and Administrative Pharmacy* (RSAP) and *Exploratory Research in Clinical and Social Pharmacy* (ERCSP). Additionally, he coedits the major text *Pharmacy Management: Essentials for All Settings*. He has published over 120 papers in peer-reviewed journals. In 2020, he coauthored a paper winning the Wiederholt Prize for the best paper published in *Journal of the American Pharmacists Association*, and in 2019, he won the American Association of Colleges of Pharmacy (AACP) Sustained Contribution Award for his teaching, scholarship, and service in social/administrative pharmacy. His research focuses on organizational culture, quality of work life, and advancing the roles of various professionals within the medication use and education systems.

Victoria García-Cárdenas, PhD, is a Senior Lecturer in Pharmacy at the University of Technology Sydney. Her teaching and research interests encompass different aspects of pharmacy practice such as medication adherence, the evaluation and implementation of professional pharmacy services, and practice change in community pharmacy. She has published over 40 papers in refereed journals and 6 major research reports and presented and coauthored 40 conference presentations. Victoria is currently involved in five national and international research projects for the evaluation and implementation of professional services in community pharmacy.

Claire Anderson, BPharm, PhD, FRPharmS, FFRPS, FFIP, FRSPH, is Professor of Social Pharmacy in the Division of Pharmacy Practice and Policy, School of Pharmacy, University of Nottingham. She is a global leader in pharmacy practice research, with significant national and international contributions to the development of evidence including developing and evaluating new professional roles for pharmacists, particularly in public health. She is also known internationally for research on pharmacy education and workforce development. She has extensive research leadership experience within pharmacy and across a number of health, education, and social science disciplines. She seeks to combine in-depth qualitative and ethnographic methodologies with the practical demands of producing timely and formative research outcomes that can inform and change practice and policy.

Parisa Aslani, BPharm(Hons), MSc, GradCertEdStud (Higher Ed), PhD, MPS, MRPharmS, FFIP, is a Professor in Medicines Use Optimisation, Director of Academic Career Development, and Deputy Head of School of Pharmacy at The University of Sydney, Australia. She is known internationally for her research in the areas of consumer medicines information and adherence to therapy. Her research has impacted policy and education in the healthcare sector, and at the Australian Government level, and has led to a global initiative on developing medicine information strategies for implementation at national and local levels. Her research skills range from qualitative techniques to survey design and randomized control trials.

Aleda M.H. Chen, PharmD, MS, PhD, FAPhA, is a Professor and Associate Dean at Cedarville University School of Pharmacy. Her teaching and research interests focus on health behavior change, motivational interviewing, and pharmacy education, leading to over 60 published papers in peer-reviewed journals and over 100 conference presentations. Methodological interests include instrument validation, survey research, and interventions. In the past decade, she has consistently engaged student pharmacists in research to build skills in research methodology and enthusiasm for research. She also oversees the Ohio Pharmacists Association's Ohio Research Forum, where pharmacists, graduate students, and student pharmacists can showcase their research.

Timothy F. Chen, BPharm, DipHPharm, PhD, FFIP, is Professor of Medication Management at The University of Sydney, Australia, where he is head of Pharmacy Practice and Health Services Research. Tim is nationally and internationally renowned for his research in medication review and strategies to reduce medication-related harm. His research has informed significant practice change, through the implementation of the Australian Commonwealth Government funded Home Medicines Review (HMR) program. He currently leads a large and productive postgraduate research team.

Preface

Historical underpinnings and growth of pharmacy and health services research

Pharmacy practice and social/administrative pharmacy have continued to gain momentum and recognition for their extraordinary contributions in advancing science, patient care, and the medication use process. One can argue that the disciplines are but a few decades old, at most. Work in organizational psychology in the broader sense on various disciplines and their scholarly progress can be dated back to the 1960s, even prior to the birth of social/administrative pharmacy, and for that matter, health services research. That work in organizational psychology produced, among many other things, a "hard-soft" continuum of various fields of study, where those in the "softer" or low-consensus disciplines have traditionally had a more difficult time establishing their scientific paradigms, which translates into greater hurdles for scientific breakthroughs, more difficulty in establishing the literature, coming to a consensus on research priorities, and greater challenges for publishing their scholarly work.

Pharmacy practice and social/administrative pharmacy apply concepts, theories, and models from social sciences and other disciplines that are a bit newer than others. There are many related terms used to describe the discipline of social pharmacy which include but are not limited to pharmacy practice, social and administrative pharmacy, social and behavioral pharmacy practice, and others. Although there may be different nuanced meanings between these terms, a distinction has not been made in this text, purely because we wish to be as broad as possible, the discipline is evolving rapidly, and many of the research methods have been adapted from other disciplines within the social, clinical, and health sciences. So for simplicity, the term social pharmacy has been adopted for this text.

While younger and borrowing from various disciplines, this does not make social pharmacy any less of a science. Research in social pharmacy adheres to very strict and rigorous scientific processes. As our research focus is on attitudes, opinions, beliefs, and behavioral intentions to explain patients' and the public's behaviors as well as the behavior of healthcare professionals and pharmacists, these methods are appropriate. However, use of these methods in social pharmacy varies from being in their infancy to becoming more established. Such methods are critical as we move forward to gather evidence and develop interventions to ultimately optimize patient-centered care by collaborative multidisciplinary healthcare teams within a healthcare system that is delivering such care that is culturally appropriate and at the person's health literacy, etc.

This book presents a range of such methods adapted by social pharmacy research. Given the relative nascence of these disciplines, there were relatively few outlets in which to publish scholarly work, and for a while, there were only a few "tried and true" methodological approaches and study design alternatives. The past 30 years or so, and especially the past decade, has seen extraordinary and exponential growth in the contributions of social pharmacy scientists and by other health services researchers. This growth has been enabled by wider availability of technology, such as statistical analysis software, as well as by availability of protected (and secured) medical records, records from governments and private sources of standardized, valid and reliable surveys, and increased collaboration and extramural funding opportunities for scientists in these fields. Likewise, leaders in social pharmacy and health services research in the early 2000s founded new peer-reviewed journals in which to publish theory-based research that could be used for later application and further trials among clinicians. This opened the door for the actuation of many more journals in the 2010s, which bears witness to even greater numbers of social pharmacy scientists collaborating with scientists in nursing, medicine, business, engineering, anthropology, organizational psychology, public health, public administration, and many other disciplines.

The compilation of methodological approaches and designs detailed in this text is testament to the growth of the social pharmacy and health services research disciplines, with many of them forging new approaches or very quickly adapting emerging approaches just recently founded in other disciplines and applying them toward pharmacy and health services research. Documentation of these methods for future researchers is especially salient given what we are increasingly becoming to know; that is, patient health outcomes are largely determined by psychosocial aspects of the medication use process, which often explain much greater variance in these outcomes than the biomedical model alone. These are important to consider to advance health equity. And, it is the research conducted by social pharmacy and health services researchers that addresses these, and many other related issues, head on.

Why we created this textbook

Given the importance of the research described above along with its proliferation, it is important to document emerging research approaches, while providing updates and offering best practices for those approaches that have been around a little longer. The numbers of doctoral students, postgraduates, and young researchers in the discipline likewise have grown considerably, along with researchers from a variety of countries engaging in this research. While primary literature exists on each of the designs and methodological approaches detailed herein, the text represents a large compendium and should serve as an excellent resource for research programs and the personnel (faculty, postgraduate students) who comprise them. Organization of these varied approaches into one source allows easy access for in-depth reading and even comparison of approaches among readers; the book's format of providing additional examples and other features described below guides readers more specifically into best practices, thus omitting any ambiguity that might exist from reading examples or application of the research in primary literature only.

How the book is organized and its contents

Each chapter in the book represents a methodological approach, study design, a consideration for ensuring validity and reliability in these approaches, and/or statistical analysis considerations that transcend many of the approaches discussed here and potentially others. The chapter is introduced with a brief summary, followed by learning objectives, the main body/text, questions for further consideration, and one or more application exercises. These additions should prove very helpful for research faculty reviewing these concepts along with postgraduate students; indeed, all researchers whose ideas can be stimulated from pondering these additional questions and exercises, thus making them even more aware of the challenges one faces and considerations one must contemplate when considering use of these methodological approaches.

The majority of chapters were born from themed issues in the peer-reviewed journal *Research in Social and Administrative Pharmacy* (RSAP), one of the most revered journals in pharmacy, having one of the highest impact factor scores among all pharmacy journals, and whose mission and scope place it as the foundational journal for theory-driven, methods-centered research in social pharmacy and health services research. The articles in that journal were enhanced for readers in this book and went through several quality control processes even in addition to having undergone peer review with the journal. Each chapter in the book stands on its own and is entirely independent of other chapters. However, the book has been organized into four overarching sections that group the various chapters together: Overarching Design and Reviews Considerations, Emerging Methodological Approaches and Updates, Qualitative, Hybrid, and Consensus-Gathering Approaches, and Quantitative Approaches and Analytical Considerations.

Overarching design and reviews considerations

The first chapter underscores the increasingly collaborative nature of social pharmacy and health services research, written by engineers, highlighting the collaborations with engineers and ergonomics scholars in the redesign of pharmaceutical care systems and interior designs of pharmacies to facilitate greater efficiency in the delivery of health services, with more engagement by patients and greater satisfaction by pharmacy and other healthcare personnel. This is followed by a chapter on codesign, a premise where designers and end users work together to tailor a product or service, in this case, interventions aimed at improving the medication use process. This section also includes an examination of models and theories that have and can be used to help guide research among social pharmacy and health services research, providing evidence and offering examples of how they might be further leveraged in the future. This segues into chapters on implementation science, an approach that emphasizes the sustainability of health services and interventions developed, rather than having seen their creation only to become insolvent or impractical once initial resources dedicated to their actuation have been expended. This is critical given the need to engage employees and patients in long-term programs that can evoke sincere and more permanent health change. One of the more commonly featured strategies within implementation science, the consolidated framework for implementation research (CFIR), has its own chapter, effectively describing its use to actuate programs. The section also includes a chapter on meta research, which is research on research, critical to evaluating quality of studies and gleaning important information from the literature, as well as advancing practice and these fields of study; an additional chapter provides key insights on performing systematic, narrative, and other types of reviews, which synthesize the literature, and proffers gaps in knowledge to be studied later as well as offers a critique of the strength of studies in an area to date, thus advising on future research approaches given any shortcomings of the research that had been conducted to that point. The section also includes a critical examination into the various study designs (inclusive of recruiting and sampling) often applied in social pharmacy and health services research.

Emerging methodological approaches and updates

The second major section of the book covers many emerging methods, or those that had not been used that frequently in social pharmacy and health services research, at least not until very recently. A chapter on action research describes how its principles concomitantly evaluate scientifically a new service or intervention along with taking initiative in the form of engagement, such as activating or attempting to evoke policy change. Another somewhat emancipatory approach is Q methodology, which combines qualitative and quantitative approaches. Unlike qualitative approaches (discussed later), which identify themes, Q methodology detects and interprets holistic and shared perspectives. Dyad models research examines or studies persons in dyads (e.g., a patient and a caregiver, two partners, even a practitioner and patient) in a manner that might provide key insights that focusing on the individual might not bring, given to some degree the interdependence of these individuals. On the other hand, network analysis is used to study a larger number of interconnected individuals or phenomena, with previous applications in social studies, ecological studies, genetics, and systems pharmacology. The chapter delves into how it might be effectively applied to study public health issues. The next three chapters are quite unique and compelling, lending yet further voice to approaches not previously seen much in pharmacy and health services literature. Pictograms can be highly useful for acquiring patients' reactions to illustrations, which may thus aid in marketing health interventions, creating compelling narratives to engage patients, and even substitute for words/text that might otherwise create obstacles for patients with marginal health literacy. Another chapter examines photovoice. Photovoice is a research method where people, through images (photography, drawings, or paintings), capture, represent, and communicate their experiences and perspectives about issues that are important to them with the final goal of raising awareness and triggering social change. Not entirely unrelated is the draw-and-write technique, where researchers contextualize drawings of patients to capture the richness and detail of their emotions and experiences through these drawings so as to better inform amendments to interventions and health services delivery. Still another chapter focuses on art, or more specifically the selection of artifacts by study participants that represented what learning is to them (i.e., pharmacy students). The chapter discusses this and its application for use in the evaluation of health services. The book also provides a couple chapters, each with different perspectives, on observation research, which can take any number of forms including unobtrusive examinations in person or on camera, or through disguised shoppers, and others. This type of research is very useful for discerning the actual behaviors of providers and/or patients rather than relying on self-report and can serve as an excellent foundation for educational interventions. Realist approaches to theory-driven evaluation consider these variations in programs, interventions, and the contexts of their implementation and establish theories on how they work best, for whom, and why. The chapter illustrates the practical application of the realist philosophy of science to pharmacy practice relevant areas of healthcare using case studies. On the other hand, the use of simulated patients (SPs) is also a potential boon to researchers aiming to improve knowledge retention and behaviors of practitioners and/or students, as SPs can simulate any number of persons or conditions when resources are scarce. Another chapter on process philosophy provides a comprehensive and unified perspective of reality, its character, and how we might understand ourselves in that reality. Process philosophy permits scope for exploring a variety of phenomena of the lived experience. It can deliver a different and complementary perspective, giving rise to new streams of inquiry that deliver novel and insightful explanatory forms of given phenomena.

Qualitative, hybrid, and consensus-gathering approaches

The third major section of the book concerns the use and application of various research approaches that are more qualitative in nature, or those which might be similar, such as consensus-gathering techniques that involve qualitative and similar input from participants to gather very rich data. The first chapter reports on proceedings of a workshop in social pharmacy research convened by social pharmacy faculty who discuss general challenges (and solutions) to conducting such research, including methodological and disciplinary competence and insecurity, reflections on the consequences of how many social pharmacy researchers come from a natural science background and how this (possibly) shapes the practice of qualitative research within the field. They discuss transparency and saturation, together with checklists and quality criteria, and offer suggestions for the discipline to take next steps in employing qualitative research approaches. There are chapters covering different topics under the auspices of ethnography research. Ethnography is a type of social research examining behavior of participants in a given social situation and understanding the group members' own interpretation of that behavior. One chapter provides a more general, yet comprehensive view of this approach. Another, on video-reflective ethnography, invites stakeholders (e.g., pharmacy staff) to participate in analyzing their everyday work practices as captured on video footage, which might be useful to engage a workforce with scarce amount of time to engage in research about themselves, a particular advantage with the research is not or cannot be present "in the field." Still another chapter explores the concept of reflexivity in ethnography research more specifically. The author, in this case, explores their journey from a practitioner to research with an ethnographic-informed study pertaining to patients with chronic disease and the medication-taking behaviors. The approach allowed the researcher to explore the lived experiences of participants using a smart medication adherence product. Through in-depth at home observations, photo-elicitation, and semistructured interviews, they gathered invisible meanings associated with their in-home medication intake process. Extensive field notes were written after each home visit in addition to a reflexive journal documenting inner thoughts, questions, and reflections. In contrast, rapid-turnaround qualitative analysis is a proven mechanism to gather rich data from interviews or from other content that allows for nuance and depth, but with the use of questions and coding that allow primary themes to be explicated without such a deep immersion into the data and that which can be used to provide data that can be leveraged for use in follow-up studies, such as with quantitative surveys. A different approach, cognitive task analysis, refers to a family of methods used in a variety of fields to understand decision-making in complex environments. The authors of this chapter take us through decision-making used by patients in categorizing, purchasing, and using over-the-counter (OTC) medications. A chapter on mixed-methods research describes the use of qualitative with quantitative approaches concomitantly to acquire rich data and data that might be generalizable to larger populations. The approach provides a wealth of varied types of information that can be used to triangulate or reinforce the veracity of the data gathered from the various methods employed. Another chapter discusses the ramifications for using qualitative approaches to study the content of existing data, sometimes present in larger swaths than we might be accustomed to when conducting a limited number of interviews or focus groups. The chapter employs three case studies analyzing data from boardroom meeting minutes, incident reports, and WhatsApp messages. Another chapter discusses the conduct of focus groups. While resources on conducting focus groups abound, the unique insights from this chapter address the art and science of conducting focus groups online, something likely to persist given the technology to do so that will extend well past the COVID-19 pandemic that struck the world in 2020. And speaking of art and science, perhaps nothing personifies the melding of these two concepts like the conduct of Delphi procedures. Delphis are used to gather consensus of persons, usually experts in a field, through a multiround iterative process to form an accurate and comprehensive "solution" to a problem or set of problems we face. One chapter focuses more on planning to prevent potential snags, while another offers best practices during data collection and analysis of data to ensure veracity and inspire confidence in the results.

Quantitative approaches and analytical considerations

The fourth major section of this book examines quantitative approaches to research as well as various statistical analysis considerations. A chapter on binary outcomes lends some assistance to analysis plans in this and other research approaches using moderation analysis, wherein binary outcomes can be more effectively determined by identifying which statistical models for binary outcomes lead to which measure of interaction. Thus, this has led to an increased focus on the fact that measures of interaction are scale-dependent. Another chapter focuses on the use of large, national (or other) databases to acquire substantial amounts of real-world data, primarily through patient records or through surveys conducted by federal government officials or some scientific body. This is a great asset for those conducting research in pharmacoepidemiology and/or attempting to evaluate medication use processes using validated data often in large sample sizes. A second chapter examines the need for making adjustments in data acquired from these and other sources, primarily diagnosis data, offering newer approaches more advantageous than previous approaches that adjusted for patient comorbidities when attempting to discern the effectiveness (and/or harm) in certain treatments. The next chapter discusses psychometric properties of various medication adherence measures. Medication adherence is one of the most important phenomena that challenge our health systems, our patients, and thus ourselves as pharmacy and health services researchers. Correspondingly, the importance of validity and reliability in the measures we use is paramount. Yet, psychometrics is critical to survey research in all matters of subject, and the discussion and examples used here can be employed to evaluate the psychometric properties of any instrument we might use in our research. Another chapter deals with missing data in surveys. Missing data are prevalent in almost any survey, even if not quite as problematic with the use of electronic survey distribution systems and forced-choice responses. How that missing data are handled has implications for sample size, thus power of the study, accuracy, precision, and even validity and reliability issues. Following that chapter is one on latent class analysis procedures. Researchers have an awareness that procedures like latent class analysis can be used to help discern the actual components of a particular, yet perhaps otherwise, nebulous construct or set of constructs in eventually creating a model for use in future inferential analysis and research approaches. The next chapters deal with validity and reliability, and this entire textbook utilizes these terms frequently. These concepts are hallmarks of the scientific method; that is, having valid and reliable data is one of the primary issues separating science from casual influence. One chapter in the text gets at validity and reliability, the relationship between the two, and their relationship with other aspects of your research. Another chapter examines in great detail the issue of content validity, the items comprising a survey method, and the extent to which they accurately reflect and measure the phenomenon of interest. The section concludes with a chapter discussing the need to make adjustments in post hoc statistical analyses (i.e., statistical corrections) to minimize Type-I errors. It discusses various adjustments, including the Bonferroni adjustment, including their advantages and risks involved with the application of these sometimes rigid types of corrections.

What we hope you will gain from this book

As described above, the book provides postgraduate students, their mentors, and even senior researchers with information on both emerging methodological approaches as well as updates and best practices on others that have been in longer use. We hope that the contents of the book will help the disciplines of social pharmacy and related health service research disciplines take another step forward in their respective scientific paradigms, help to enhance the quality of research undertaken, improve researchers' chances at getting funded and published, evoke new ideas to tackle age-old problems, and also provide a basis for provocative and edifying dialog between mentors and mentees in research. We are so very proud and excited to bring this resource to you.

Overarching Design and Reviews Considerations

Chapter 1

Applying human factors and ergonomics methods to pharmaceutical health services research

Richard J. Holden[a,b,c,d], Ephrem Abebe[d,e], Alissa L. Russ-Jara[e], and Michelle A. Chui[f,g]

[a]Department of Health & Wellness Design, Indiana University School of Public Health, Bloomington, IN, United States, [b]Center for Aging Research, Regenstrief Institute, Inc., Indianapolis, IN, United States, [c]Center for Health Innovation and Implementation Science, Indiana Clinical and Translational Sciences Institute, Indianapolis, IN, United States, [d]Department of Medicine, Indiana University School of Medicine, Indianapolis, IN, United States, [e]Department of Pharmacy Practice, College of Pharmacy, Purdue University, West Lafayette, IN, United States, [f]Social and Administrative Sciences Division, University of Wisconsin-Madison School of Pharmacy, Madison, WI, United States, [g]Sonderegger Research Center, University of Wisconsin-Madison School of Pharmacy, Madison, WI, United States

Objectives

- Define the field of human factors and ergonomics generally and specifically as it relates to pharmacy research and practice.
- Explain the major categories of human factors and ergonomics methods applicable to pharmacy, their uses, strengths, and limitations.
- Illustrate how projects have applied human factors and ergonomics methods in published pharmacy projects.
- Demonstrate how larger scale projects combine multiple human factors and ergonomics methods in practice.

Human factors and ergonomics (HFE) is a scientific and practical human-centered discipline that studies and improves human work performance and wellbeing in sociotechnical systems.[1,2] HFE in pharmacy involves the human-centered design of systems to support individuals and teams who perform medication-related work.[3]

HFE methods are effective[4] and therefore constitute standard practice in several industries, especially safety-critical arenas of aviation, surface transportation, military, and energy.[5,6] HFE methods are also routinely applied in office settings, service industries, leisure, consumer products, and medical devices.[7–10]

HFE first appeared in healthcare in 1960s studies of hospital medication safety.[11] Later that century, HFE grew in other inpatient settings such as anesthesiology and surgery.[12,13] Turn-of-the-century reports from the U.S. National Academy of Medicine (then the Institute of Medicine)[14–16] accelerated the application of HFE to patient safety and quality, particularly the discipline's incident analyses, team training, and aviation tools such as checklists.[17] Mass adoption of health information technology (IT) increased the demand for HFE methods for user-centered design and usability testing.[18,19] HFE methods have been used to study and improve the work and outcomes of healthcare professionals, nonprofessionals such as patients or families, and teams.[20] Applying HFE to study and improve the health-related work of patients, families, and other nonprofessionals is called *patient ergonomics*, simply defined as the science and engineering of patient work.[21] Patient ergonomics is a branch of HFE that has grown in parallel to paradigm shifts toward patient engagement and empowerment, consumer health IT, data democratization, and shared decision making.[22] There is also emerging interest in applying HFE to study and improve public health behaviors outside the context of illness and clinical care.[23]

Overall, HFE methods have gained penetration and success in healthcare[24–28] and are increasingly seen in pharmacy. This chapter reviews select HFE methods well suited to address pharmacy challenges and offers examples of how they have been applied in pharmacy.

Opportunities for HFE in pharmacy

HFE in pharmacy can be defined in two ways. First, it is the application of HFE in specific pharmacy settings, such as inpatient or community pharmacies. Second, it is the application of HFE to study or improve medication-related phenomena such as medication safety,[29] adherence,[30] or deprescribing.[31]

Many pharmacy settings can benefit from HFE methods, and there is growing realization that one such setting is the community pharmacy. HFE can be useful for community pharmacy research and design as community pharmacy practice evolves, expanding beyond dispensing to include immunization, medication therapy management, and point of care testing.[32,33] Roles in these settings are changing, as pharmacy technicians perform complex tasks traditionally assumed by pharmacists.[34–36] HFE is needed to address safety in community pharmacy settings, including to address an estimated medication error rate between 1.7% and 22%, of which 6.5% are clinically significant events.[37–39] Using the most conservative estimate, for a typical U.S. community pharmacy dispensing 250 prescriptions per day, this means approximately 4 errors per day, including 2 clinically significant errors per week—or 51.5 million dispensing errors annually nationwide. HFE offers tools to examine and address the systems factors contributing to errors in these complex environments.[40,41] Indeed, HFE methods have already been applied in community pharmacy settings to address e-prescribing workflow and cognitive needs,[42,43] medication safety,[44] stress and workload during dispensing,[45–47] and over-the-counter (OTC) medication decisions.[48,49]

HFE methods can address medication use and medication safety phenomena independent of settings and often across settings where professional care and self-care occur. Table 1 illustrates how studies using HFE methods have been performed across the medication use process,[50] to better understand or improve the medication-related performance of prescribers, pharmacy workers, nurses, and patients. Wherever medication-related work takes place, HFE can be used to redesign the system to be more human-centered and thus to improve the performance of the work and the wellbeing of those who perform it.[55]

TABLE 1 Examples of HFE methods applied at each step of the medication use process.

Medication use process step[50]	Example study objective	HFE method(s) used	Key findings
1. Prescribing	Identify factors contributing to prescribing errors in pediatric intensive care units.[51]	Hierarchical task analysis.	Identified 30 subtasks for pediatric intensive care prescribing; cognitive burden was the main contributory factor for errors.
2. Transcribing	Quantify pharmacists' workload for transcribing free-text patient directions from e-prescriptions and assess the quality of directions before and after transcription.[52]	Keystroke level modeling.	Pharmacy staff edited 83.8% of all e-prescription directions; readability increased by 68.6% after pharmacists' transcription.
3. Dispensing	Improve label design for 6 solid oral medications to increase accurate dispensing by retail pharmacists.[53]	Failure modes and effects analysis (FMEA), expert review by HFE specialists, and usability testing via simulations.	With the final label, no errors occurred among 450 filled prescriptions.
4. Administration	Apply HFE approach to explore medication administration in nursing homes and prevent adverse drug events.[54]	Direct observation and interviews using the SEIPS framework.	Identified 6 stages of medication administration in nursing homes and more than 60 associated facilitators and barriers.
5. Monitoring	Identify, describe, and analyze medication nonadherence events using HFE classification methods.[30]	Taxonomies and models for classifying and understanding the performance shaping factors contributing to errors and violations.	Identified 70 events, half classified as errors and half as violations, along with performance shaping factors related to person or team, task, tools and technologies, and organizational, physical, and social context.

HFE, human factors/ergonomics; *SEIPS*, systems engineering initiative for patient safety.

HFE methods for pharmacy research and clinical practice

HFE offers a broad toolkit of methods taught to HFE professionals and learnable by others.[56] At an introductory level, there are over 100 individual HFE methods, some with over 100 variations each.[57–59] This section describes seven categories of HFE methods that are well suited to widespread use for pharmacy research and clinical practice, with examples of how they have been used in published work on HFE in pharmacy.

Work system analysis methods

Work system analysis identifies, defines, and analyzes factors contributing to performance in sociotechnical systems.[60] Several models of work systems are available,[61] each depicting broad categories of interacting performance-shaping factors; for example, the Systems Engineering Initiative for Patient Safety (SEIPS) model's factors are persons, tasks, tools/technologies, organization, and environment.[62–64] These models are used to structure data collection or analyze data.[65] Work system analysis is also used to examine interactions between factors, such as the degree of alignment between a tool, its user, and the associated task. Work system analyses in pharmacy have primarily used interview or focus group data collection and applied deductive qualitative analysis to code findings using an existing work system model such as SEIPS,[62] SEIPS 2.0,[63] or others.[1,66,67] Quantitative analysis can be used, as in a nationwide survey of Australian community pharmacists[68] or a nursing home study correlating adverse drug events to clinicians' perceptions of work system factors assessed via surveys.[69] The method has been used to study factors affecting antipsychotic medication use by patients with serious mental illness,[70] barriers and facilitators to e-prescribing errors in community pharmacies,[71,72] barriers to providing safe OTC medication recommendations to older adults,[71] and performance of persons caring for patients with dementia.[73] Other applications in pharmacy include studying implementation (e.g., of collaborative practice agreements[74] or cognitive pharmaceutical services[75]) or developing interventions (e.g., for interruptions management in inpatient pediatric pharmacies[76] or medication use in nursing homes[77]). Holden and colleagues[66] also argue work system analysis can be leveraged "to better understand patient work systems and performance in a way that is comprehensive, theory-based, and methodologically rigorous."

To aid practitioners in the use of work system analysis methods, Holden and Carayon introduced SEIPS 101 and the seven simple SEIPS tools.[78] The SEIPS 101 model is a simplified depiction of the most critical components of the various SEIPS models; for example, it simplifies the work system component into the factors "People, Environments, Tools, and Tasks" or PETT. The seven tools, described in greater depth elsewhere[78] and summarized in Table 2, are designed to be used by both novices and experts.

Another type of work analysis, cognitive work analysis (CWA), is a comprehensive framework to identify requirements, constraints, and affordances for individuals' cognitive work within a system of interest, known as a "work domain."[79,80] CWA follows five phases, beginning with a high-level work domain analysis resembling the work system analysis above.[81,82] Subsequent analysis progressively narrows to characterize individual tasks (control task analysis), strategies used to perform tasks (strategies analysis), allocation of tasks across individuals (social organization and

TABLE 2 Seven simple SEIPS tools, based on Holden and Carayon.[78]

SEIPS tool	Purpose
PETT scan	describe or design the interacting parts of the entire sociotechnical system
People map	describe the people involved in a system and how they interact or relate to one another
Task and tools matrices	enumerate, describe, and evaluate tasks and tools in the system
Outcomes matrix	identify the relevant outcomes to consider
Journey map	depict a process over time and how work system conditions and outcomes change during the process
Interactions diagram	depict the relevant subset of work system factors whose interactions are meaningful or draw comparisons between two or more systems
Systems story	frame a story about how work systems, processes, and outcomes relate

SEIPS, systems engineering initiative for patient safety; *PETT*, people, environments, tools, tasks.

cooperation analysis), and cognitive requirements of workers (worker competencies analysis). As an example, researchers used CWA to model the medication management system in ambulatory care settings.[83,84]

An advantage of the CWA method is it allows system designers to focus on what is possible in terms of human performance to achieve system goals, given the constrains in the work domain (i.e., what can be done instead of what should be done). As a result, this method is ideally suited for the design of novel systems that do not yet exist. A fundamental principle of CWA is that users can achieve their end goals via different means and that there is no single path to doing so, thus promoting the adaptation and flexibility of workers.

Traditionally, CWA has mostly focused on the analytical stages (e.g., work domain analysis) and few instructive examples exist guiding analysts to translate CWA outputs into designs that benefit end users. In one example, combining CWA with user-centered design methods (reviewed below), researchers developed and tested a novel emergency department information system to serve as a decision-support tool for emergency care staff.[85] When combined with other methods (e.g., participatory design), the multilevel system analysis focus of CWA makes it ideal for designing novel systems with a transformative effect on how end users engage with and benefit from the new system.

Task analysis methods

Task analysis encompasses methods to deeply understand the tasks performed by individuals or teams. Task analysis can be used to model the work of pharmacy professionals, identify training needs, and formulate requirements for the design of work settings, processes, and job aids.

Cognitive task analysis (CTA) allows analysts to capture cognitive processes (e.g., information processing, decision making) underlying observable behaviors.[86] CTA has three aspects: knowledge elicitation; data analysis; and data representation. A popular knowledge elicitation approach is the critical incident technique or critical decision method, wherein interviewers ask probing questions to gather details about an incident: what happened, strategies used to detect problems, why a decision was made. A limitation of this method is reliance on individuals recalling past events, often spontaneously. To minimize recall bias, Russ et al. collected information about medication safety incidents prospectively from healthcare professionals.[87] They conducted follow-up critical decision method interviews with healthcare professionals, where healthcare professionals could access the electronic health record (EHR) to aid their recall as they responded to interview questions. This CTA adaptation was used to identify healthcare professionals' decision-making process for detecting and responding to medication safety incidents.[87,88] Similarly, Holden et al. developed a patient-centered CTA adapted for older adults, with whiteboard drawings to facilitate incident recall and interactive scenarios to simulate real-time decision making.[89,90] These studies analyzed elicited data to produce models of naturalistic decision making[88,90] and "personas" depicting different approaches to decision making.[89] Other common uses of CTA are comparing cognitive work of experts versus novices[91] and identifying which cognitive processes are involved in routine tasks such as medication adherence.[92]

Another popular task analysis is hierarchical task analysis (HTA). HTA is used to depict the hierarchy of tasks or goals, decomposing these into subtasks or subgoals until they are described at a level of resolution fit for the intended purpose, such as for training workers or designing decision-support tools.[93] Different data collection approaches can be used to inform HTA including observations, interviews, focus group discussions, and document reviews. For example, Lane et al. performed HTA to model inpatient medication administration errors.[94]

Link analysis is another specific type of task analysis used to examine how people interact with their physical environment. Lester and Chui used link analysis to describe the impact of the physical layout of a community pharmacy on pharmacists' task performance.[95] Using observation data, they developed a link diagram depicting movement of pharmacists between locations within a pharmacy.

Workload assessment methods

Workload is a multidimensional, multifaceted concept affecting performance outcomes such as error and healthcare professional outcomes such as stress and burnout.[96] Workload in healthcare has been defined as the ratio of demands to resources.[97,98] Workload thus depends on interactions of real or perceived work demands, the circumstances under which work is performed, and worker characteristics (e.g., pharmacist's years of experience, patient's skill level).[99]

Workload can be assessed at multiple levels, including organizational unit, job, and task levels.[98–100] At the organizational level, workload may be conceptualized as the amount or volume of work versus staffing resources, which may be directly related to the skill of pharmacists and technicians, or the perceived adequacy of technology. Job-level workload could be measured by the amount and kind of work required for a role (e.g., hospital pharmacist) relative to the training and tools provided. Job-related tasks may include monitoring and multitasking demands. The workload associated with these tasks might require reacting quickly to prevent problems or keeping track of more than one process at once. Task-level workload can be measured as the complexity, difficulty, and multitasking requirements of specific tasks relative to cognitive capacity or tools for the tasks.[47,98,100] Tasks may include activities such as reviewing a patient profile. The demands associated with that task may require concentration and mental effort or feeling rushed. Thus, HFE measures of workload can address the high fluctuation and unpredictability of the pharmacy work system and extend beyond the number of prescriptions dispensed at a pharmacy or medications prescribed to a patient. Both demands and resources, across all levels of analysis, can and should be assessed.[101]

Demands contributing to workload may be physical or cognitive (i.e., mental workload). Physical workload is measured using subjective and objective methods, the former including validated measures of self-reported exertion.[102] More objective measures of physical workload include assessing physiologic variables (e.g., oxygen consumption, heart rate), task outcomes (e.g., time to perform tasks), worker outcomes (e.g., fatigue), and the ratio of physical demands (e.g., task load, frequency, duration, distance) to available resources such as a person's work capacity, skill or fitness, or access to assistive equipment and tools.[103]

Increasingly, changes in pharmacy work such as new technologies and greater supervision have primarily increased cognitive demands. Cognitive (or mental) workload measures include the popular, validated NASA Task Load Index (TLX), one of several self-report approaches scholars have used to study pharmacy workload.[47,100,104,105] Other measures use physiological markers such as a person's pupillary dilation, brain activity, or heart rate;[106] task performance indicators used to infer workload;[107] or analytic modeling of demands inherent to known tasks.[108]

Medication safety and error analysis methods

Various HFE techniques inform the analysis of medication errors and safety incidents to generate interventions and sustainable safety solutions. Failure modes and effects analysis (FMEA) is one technique used to *prospectively* identify safety vulnerabilities and assess strengths of safety interventions, with the goal of preventing errors.[109] Other prospective HFE techniques applicable to healthcare include bowtie analysis,[110] probabilistic risk assessment, and proactive hazard analysis,[111] and some have applied these methods to medication safety.[112–114] Medication error reporting systems at national or local healthcare organizational levels provide essential data to help identify and analyze errors *retrospectively*. These data are especially useful to capture unexpected and rare medication errors. Data from medication error reports can be used for research on medication errors and combined with HFE techniques to further investigate incidents and generate solutions for implementation.

Root cause action and analysis (RCA^2) is used to retrospectively investigate an incident to identify all plausible causes and generate actionable solutions.[115,116] RCA^2, which is endorsed by the American Society of Health-System Pharmacists, was developed by HFE and clinical experts to explicitly overcome flaws in the traditional use of root cause analysis (RCA).[117]

Importantly, unlike traditional RCA methods, RCA^2 guidance includes these "Five Rules of Causation:"

- Rule 1. Clearly show the "cause and effect" relationship.
- Rule 2. Use specific and accurate descriptors for what occurred, rather than negative and vague.
- Rule 3. Human errors must have a preceding cause.
- Rule 4. Violations of procedure are not root causes, but must have a preceding cause.
- Rule 5. Failure to act is only causal when there is a preexisting duty to act.

The five rules are intended to shift analysts' focus away from inherent human shortcomings (e.g., "human error" as the primary cause) and instead direct their efforts to identifying and correcting the real, underlying system issues that facilitate errors. The five rules were first developed for the aviation industry and more recently adapted for healthcare. These rules are meant to guide analysts in the development of written causal statements, with the intent that one written statement is crafted for each underlying systems cause, and with each causal statement including a specific "cause," "effect," and "event."

To investigate or model past incidents or prospective risks, one could use task analysis methods described in a prior section. For example, one type of CTA, the critical decision method, can be used to retrospectively reconstruct a safety incident.[118] An interviewer and subject matter expert (e.g., healthcare professional involved in the incident) would create a basic timeline of events, then uncover goals, decision-making cues, cognitive challenges, and other factors that may have influenced the incident. These data can be subsequently used to elucidate decision-making requirements relevant to the incident type and to generate medication safety interventions.[87,88]

Once potential solutions are identified via RCA[2] or other HFE methods, the hierarchy of hazard control is a complementary tool that can be applied to evaluate the relative strengths of proposed safety solutions *prior to implementation*.[119] This hierarchy provides a broad view of whether a solution aligns with a relatively weak (e.g., training/policy changes), moderate (alerts/warnings), or strong (e.g., safeguards, designing out the possibility of an error) systems approach, with various degrees of effectiveness in between these levels. This hierarchy is a broad, generalizable tool that is independent from the context of the medication error, while the FMEA technique can once again be used prospectively at this stage of error mitigation to assess the strengths and weaknesses of a solution within the system context and constraints. Together, these two techniques can help inform which safety solutions warrant further investment of resources and time and are most promising as sustainable safety solutions.

User-centered and participatory design methods

Design-based approaches are increasingly adopted to address pressing healthcare quality and safety challenges. User-centered (or human-centered) and participatory design approaches are used to develop solutions that fit users' tasks, needs, and contexts.

With increasing demand for more accountability and public participation, several industries are turning to design-based approaches to develop systems that improve the experience of their customers. The design firm, IDEO, and Stanford University's d-school are among the organizations that have increased popularity of these approaches in recent years. IDEO has also created a human-centered design toolkit to increase accessibility of this methodology to a broader audience (www.ideo.org/tools). Interested readers can find free, openly accessible courses on human-centered design from IDEO and Massive Open Online Course websites such as Coursera and edX.

In typical user-centered design, designers and researchers conduct user needs assessment from observation, interviews, analysis of artifacts and documents, and secondary data analysis. It is best to derive needs from studying actual (or future) users doing actual work in actual settings.[120] Needs assessment forms the basis for iteratively developing a form of the design, progressing from early ideas and sketches to more interactive prototypes, which will be subsequently evaluated by target end users to ensure the product is usable and useful.[121] Other commonly used design tools are use-case scenarios, journey maps depicting the user journey over time and settings,[64] and personas—empirically derived archetypes of user types.[122]

In participatory design, end-user representatives codesign an intervention that meets the user population's unique needs.[123,124] That means end users take the role of designer and can be involved in different stages of the design process, often working in a team.[124] For example, Reddy et al. used participatory design with pharmacy staff and older adults to develop an OTC medication safety intervention in a community pharmacy setting.[123] The researchers employed an iterative, multistep process of problem identification, solution generation and convergence, prototyping, and evaluation. Siek et al. used participatory design to develop a digital personal health application to help older adults manage and share their medication regimens during care transitions.[125]

Despite slight variations in their approach, user-centered and participatory design methods both espouse the principle that the end users of the system must be the central focus of all design efforts. Thus, an important consideration during the design process is a deliberative effort to identify and engage the right mix of individuals and groups that will be affected by the planned system. Done the right way, these methods can create opportunities to design tools and services that promote health equity by removing barriers due to differential access to information, services, and decision-making power.

Design is close kin to innovation, or the introduction of novel concepts, tools, or techniques to solve problems. However, HFE methods for user-centered design are about systematically producing and testing design, not about the creative thinking that is often—erroneously—associated with innovation. Holden and colleagues[126] argue that innovation is not a light bulb event brought into being by creative disruptors; they introduce a systematic process of innovation based on user-centered design methods that can be implemented as an everyday approach to innovation. This Agile Innovation process, detailed elsewhere,[126,127] has the following eight steps:

- **Step 1. Confirm demand** for solving a particular problem.
- **Step 2. Study the problem** in need of solving.
- **Step 3. Scan for solutions** to similar or related problems.
- **Step 4. Plan for evaluation and termination** of future solutions.
- **Step 5. Ideate and select** candidate solutions.
- **Step 6. Run innovation development sprints** to iteratively produce minimum viable products (MVPs).
- **Step 7. Validate solutions** on user-centered outcomes.
- **Step 8. Package for launch**, so the solution can be implemented.

Usability evaluation methods

An important component of user-centered design is conducting usability evaluations of devices, technologies, software, and other solutions.[128] Usability is defined as the "measure of the quality of a user's experience when interacting with a product or system"[129] and refers to the degree to which a product or system "[supports] users [in their efforts] to achieve specified goals with effectiveness, efficiency, and satisfaction...."[130] Usability is vital for all healthcare devices, technologies, and tools, to ensure their effectiveness for healthcare delivery, efficiency for users, and safety for patients. To date, usability evaluations have been conducted on a range of pharmacy-related technologies, including computerized provider order entry,[131] hospital[132] and community pharmacy medication alerts,[133] and infusion pumps.[134] Usability evaluation can be accomplished through techniques such as heuristic evaluation,[135,136] cognitive walkthrough,[137] usability questionnaires,[138] and usability testing,[139,140] sometimes used in combination. These and additional usability techniques are further examined in other healthcare literature.[18,137–139,141]

Of these usability evaluations methods, formal usability testing is recognized as the most rigorous usability testing approach.[128] During usability testing, a moderator with usability expertise asks an end-user (e.g., pharmacist, technician) to complete realistic clinical tasks, without assistance, using one or more systems being tested. For example, usability testing might be conducted with a healthcare professional or patient to assess the usability of technology for medication ordering or refilling a medication, respectively. One example research study conducted usability testing with 20 prescribers in a head-to-head comparison of two different designs for EHR medication alerts, which each included a set of drug-allergy, drug–drug interaction, and renal-drug alerts.[132] Prescribers and their computer screen actions were recorded as they completed several realistic prescribing tasks. Usability outcomes from this study demonstrated that EHR alert designs incorporating known HFE design principles led to significant gains in prescribing efficiency *along with* a reduction in prescribing errors.

Guidance exists on selecting clinical task scenarios, as they are central to the quality of usability findings.[141] Performance is typically captured by video/screen recording.[139] Multiple usability measures are typically collected, and often assess usability errors (e.g., number and type of usability problems encountered); efficiency (e.g., time on task, number of mouse clicks); effectiveness (e.g., rate of successful task completion); and/or satisfaction (e.g., usability questionnaires, debrief interview with pharmacist). Examples of common usability questionnaires include the NASA Task Load Index,[142] which measures perceived workload; the 19-item Computer System Usability Questionnaire (CSUQ),[143] and the 10-item System Usability Scale (SUS).[144] For usability assessments where a goal is to examine visualization, eye-tracking technology can be used to estimate usability and cognitive load from gaze patterns.[145,146] Other usability techniques might include concurrent think aloud protocol (verbalizing reactions during use),[147] patient actors,[148] and safety probes.[149] As an example of safety probes, one study inserted artificial but realistic medication discrepancies into a medication reconciliation task for healthcare professionals and assessed the extent to which the software supported professionals' and patients' detection of discrepancies.[149] The probes for discrepancies included a missing medication, inappropriate medication, and incorrect dose. Usability testing can range from brief quality improvement projects in healthcare institutions[139,150] to sophisticated research studies.[132,151]

Usability evaluations and associated research are valuable throughout the product lifecycle, whether that be a health IT, medical device, or other medication-related tool. Usability evaluations are ideally first applied by manufacturers during product development and used in an iterative manner to improve product effectiveness and safety. Once a product becomes commercially available, healthcare administrators can coordinate with HFE professionals to apply usability testing with a small sample of end users to directly compare products and inform purchasing decisions. After implementation, usability evaluation methods can be a valuable way to further investigate product-related safety incidents and to identify opportunities to enhance product designs. Research can be conducted at any of these stages of the product lifecycle to provide knowledge for the scientific community and improve the delivery of healthcare.

Physical ergonomics methods

Physical ergonomics is the study and design of physical work, by attending to the interaction of human anatomical, anthropometric, physiological, and biomechanical characteristics with work system elements such as lighting, noise, vibration, layout, tools, furniture, forces, hazards, and climate. Many specific HFE theories, methods, and design guidelines are available, in service of improving physical safety (e.g., reducing falls or work-related musculoskeletal disorders), performance (e.g., increasing accuracy and speed of lifting or fine-motor tasks), and comfort.[152] In pharmacy work with a physical component—for instance, medication dispensing[153,154]—HFE methods can be used to *assess*:

- Lighting needed (vs. provided) for accurate label-reading under variable pace of work;
- Noise levels and other disruptive or interruptive conditions (e.g., overheard conversations) that might increase risk of error;
- Seated and standing work postures of pharmacists and technicians, including frequency and duration of each posture;
- Walking patterns and steps or distances traveled as a function of potentially modifiable conditions such as work processes, policies, layout, and storage design;
- Physical workload, fatigue, stress, strain, and worker physical complaints over a time (e.g., day, week, year) for various tasks or roles;
- Loads and other contributing factors (e.g., posture, distance, object shape) of supply lifting and carrying tasks;
- Available vs. used equipment for repeated physical tasks such as sitting, typing, screen (or paper) reading and navigation, or waste disposal;
- Visual angles and field of view between customers and staff, to identify any obstructions or other barriers to greeting, helping, or communicating with customers;
- Hazards in the environment such as vibration, spills, sharp objects, studied proactively or reactively (based on incidents or reports).

Just as important are HFE methods for the *design* of the physical workplace and other work system factors that shape the performance of physical work.[155] These methods address the design of physical tools and equipment (hardware, software, automation), workstations and workplace layout, the environment (e.g., changing temperature, vibration, noise, lighting, surface materials), tasks (e.g., to reduce repetition, fatigue, workload), processes (e.g., introducing break schedules or teamwork), and organizational programs (e.g., training, incentives, staffing levels). One example is supporting the physical work of pharmacists and technicians working in a hazardous drug compounding facility of a central pharmacy. Some institutions are redesigning their facilities to comply with the new USP 800 standards for handling hazardous drugs. HFE experts can collaborate with facility planners and designers to ensure that implementation of appropriate engineering controls and the workspace fully consider the physical work demands of these workers.

Comprehensive application of HFE methods in pharmacy research and practice

HFE methods are used in three broad phases of human-centered design and evaluation (Fig. 1).[156] They are used in the *study* phase to help understand the problem or situation to be addressed. For example, task analysis and cognitive workload assessment can be used to determine the cognitive tasks performed in an inpatient pharmacy and the demands of each task. Methods are used in the intervention *design* phase to create a solution or adapt existing solutions to the problem at hand. Methods in the *evaluation* phase are used to test a solution in a laboratory setting, through simulation, or when implemented in a clinical or patient setting, with measures often focusing on human-centered outcomes such as usability, use errors,

FIG. 1   The three phases of human-centered design.

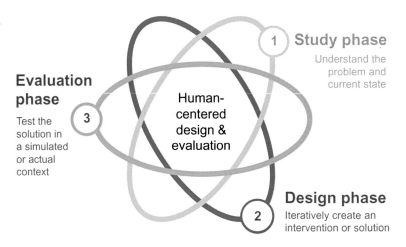

mental workload, and effect on workflow. HFE measures can be collected alongside traditional measures of clinical effectiveness, safety, and cost to comprehensively assess the intervention's consequences. The most robust applications of HFE involve the combination of methods across all three phases: study, design, and evaluation. Such comprehensive application of HFE involves both research and solution development,[126] as illustrated by the three cases below and elsewhere.[156–158]

Case 1: Medication package, label, and information design

HFE researchers have studied human processing of medication information to design and evaluate patient-centered instructions and labels.[159] Findings show, for instance, that designs matched with older and younger adults' mental schema for taking medications enhance their memory of medication information,[160–162] and consequently improve their medication adherence.[163] As another example, people prefer larger print and line spacing, additional white space, instructions organized as lists, and extended surface areas (pull-out labels) on medication containers.[164–167] Labels incorporating such designs led to an improvement in patients' response time and knowledge acquisition.[168–170] Pictorials and icons were found to be useful to those patients with low health literacy or inadequate reading skills.[171,172]

Researchers have also used eye tracking to evaluate how the design of medication labels may impact understanding and safety. One study focused on child resistant and product tampering warnings on OTC pain relievers.[173] Eye tracking was used in the study to quantify three measures related to the relative prominence and conspicuousness of the warnings: time spent examining the warnings compared to other areas of the label; recall of information from the OTCs viewed; and legibility of the warnings (how decipherable was the message) relative to the other label elements. Results showed less than 20% of participants registered any time in the product tampering warning zone and less than 50% of participants viewed the child resistant warning zone. Among all label information types, child resistant and product tampering warnings were least likely to be recalled and least legible. Therefore, despite legal requirements to highlight these warnings, the study demonstrated that the current design of OTC pain reliever packaging failed to effectively convey these important safety messages.

In a follow-up study, the team investigated how different OTC label designs attract attention to critical information, promote decision making, and facilitate rapid cross-product comparisons.[174] They sought to produce a medication label that successfully communicated critical drug information to at-risk older adults, thereby empowering them to make better medication selection decisions, and ultimately reducing adverse drug events. This study demonstrated improved patient attention to interactive and horizontal warning placements versus auxiliary labels placed vertically on prescription vials.[174]

Case 2: Human-centered design of a digital decision aid for medication safety

A multidisciplinary team, including HFE and pharmacy experts, sought to improve safety and brain health for older adults by addressing use of potentially unsafe prescription and OTC anticholinergic medications. In the study phase, interviews and observations of OTC shopping behaviors were conducted with older adults who take anticholinergic medications. This was complemented by a simulation study of OTC decision making using standard scenarios[175] and a realistic OTC aisle mockup.[49] The goal was to understand how older adults made decisions, barriers to making safe choices, and knowledge about anticholinergics. To study cognitive decision making, the contextual inquiry technique was employed as individuals made decisions in actual pharmacies or in scenario-based simulations; this entailed opportunistically asking questions about a person's thoughts while observing their behavior. In the simulation study, participants were also asked to rank order eight factors (e.g., cost, effectiveness, safety) influencing their OTC choices.

In the project's intervention design phase, data were analyzed to create personas and workflow maps depicting decision steps and barriers.[49] Using findings from this and a parallel study,[48,176] the team and its professional designers iteratively created multimedia content and mobile app software.[177] A prototype app was formatively tested with a sample of older adults ($n = 11$), iteratively refined over three design-test cycles, then programmed as working software.[177]

In the testing phase, the team performed summative usability testing on the Brain Buddy app with 23 older adult anticholinergic users and feasibility tested the app with a subset ($n = 17$) at medium or high risk of anticholinergic brain harm.[177] Usability testing combined task-based testing with observation of performance as well as a self-report questionnaire, Holden's Simplified SUS for Older and Cognitively Impaired Adults.[178] The Brain Buddy app performed well on usability, scoring in the "Good" to "Excellent" range for the SUS, while uncovering opportunities for further redesign. Feasibility findings showed 100% felt better informed, 94% indicated planning to talk to their physician about anticholinergic medication, and for 82% their physician confirmed having the conversation in an actual visit.[177] The app was further refined, rebranded as the Brain Safe app, and is being evaluated for efficacy and safety in an ongoing clinical trial, which

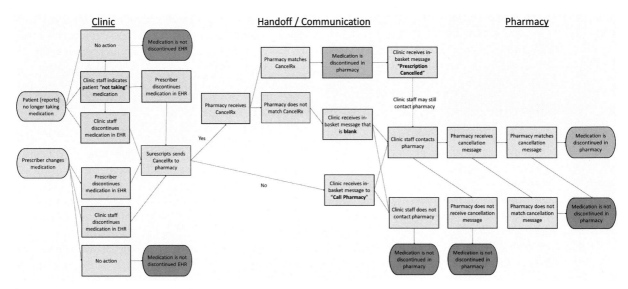

FIG. 2 Process map with identified vulnerabilities in clinic and pharmacy work systems.

also includes measures of self-reported usability and passively logged usage.[179] Developed multimedia content were also included in a clinical trial of a multicomponent intervention in a safety-net primary care system.[180]

Case 3: Clinic and pharmacy work system analysis of a medication cancellation health IT functionality

A multidisciplinary team partnered with a large health system in the Midwest United States to evaluate the implementation of CancelRx, a health IT functionality that sends a medication cancellation message from the clinic's EHR to the outpatient dispensing software. The team sought to describe the impact of CancelRx implementation on two work systems: the outpatient clinic and the community pharmacy.

A proactive risk assessment was conducted to identify vulnerabilities and consequences associated with each step of the CancelRx process.[181] Using the process map generated from the interviews and observations as a guide, 35 vulnerabilities that encompassed the clinic and pharmacy work systems were identified and organized into vulnerability themes (see Fig. 2). For example, an accurate clinic medication list was dependent upon the patient sharing information about which medications they were currently taking, clinic staff correctly documenting that information in the EHR, and proper interpretation of the medication list by the prescriber. Failure in any one of these steps could lead to the consequence of the medication list not being up to date or the patient continuing to take a medication that they should not be taking.

The fact that these consequences were not identified and addressed prior to CancelRx implementation may be due in part to the lack of transparency of the vulnerabilities across the clinic and pharmacy systems as well as a lack of diverse front-line users on the implementation team. While individual actors may understand the vulnerabilities that exist in their own sociotechnical system (i.e., in the clinic), they may not understand the vulnerabilities in other systems (i.e., the pharmacy) and the impact of their actions on one another.[182]

Conclusions and considerations

Pharmacy, including the places where pharmacy professionals work and the multistep process of medication use across people and settings, can benefit from HFE. This is because pharmacy is a human-centered sociotechnical system with an existing tradition of studying or analyzing the present state, designing solutions to problems, and evaluating those solutions in laboratory or practice settings. To put it simply, HFE fits pharmacy.

HFE can be implemented in pharmacy as a mindset or set of principles that drive research or clinical practice operations. HFE principles and underlying theories[183–185] can be usefully adopted as an operating system or culture, the way some organizations strive to become lean,[186] agile,[187] patient-centered,[188] or high-reliability[189] organizations.

HFE methods can be used to operationalize the HFE mindset or, importantly, as tools for individual projects. Several, but not all, of varieties of HFE methods suitable for studying and improving pharmacy phenomena were presented here.

Interested readers are encouraged to consult other comprehensive methods texts.[5,17,56,91,155,190–193] Training on HFE methods is also available, from webinars and workshops to short courses and degree-granting programs. In the United States, several health professional schools now offer HFE courses or degrees. In the UK, HFE education has been proposed as part of the pharmacy curriculum to address patient safety.[194] However, the best learning opportunities will likely come from hands-on experience, especially when applying the methods in field settings.[195,196] A few articles and books have been written specifically about practical considerations and uses of HFE and related methods in the field,[121,197] but most HFE textbooks assume the methods will be used in both laboratory research and practice settings.

Those considering HFE methods or using them for the first time often wonder whether their use requires an HFE professional's involvement, special training or certification, or a level of practical experience. When formal training or education is available, it is advisable to obtain it, because HFE methods are grounded in theories and mindsets that take time and tutelage to learn and internalize. We also believe collaborating with HFE professionals generally strengthens the quality of work. Moreover, many HFE professionals are available and motivated to partner with researchers, clinicians, administrators, and other pharmacy stakeholders to design, implement, or guide the use of HFE methods in pharmacy. These HFE professionals—and professionals from other human-centered disciplines or branches of HFE such as human-computer interaction—can also serve as consultants, mentors, and collaborators. Furthermore, the increasing community of pharmacy experts who have used HFE methods (some for decades!) can be the bridge for those just beginning to use HFE approaches. It is important to engage HFE professionals not only for the education they have but for the practical experiences they gathered modifying and implementing the methods across application areas. HFE experts can also help newer users select and customize "off-the-shelf" methods to fit the circumstances.[177]

At the same time, many HFE methods can be taught to and learned by novices or obtained in the form of tools.[198] One might be able to learn the rudiments of a method by reading about it and experimenting with its use (preferably with some input from more masterful users). Some HFE experts are also developing do-it-yourself (DIY) HFE method supports (e.g., software, tools, how-to books, video content) to help early-stage users adopt HFE methods without committing "malpractice."[199]

Whatever the path, HFE methods can be fruitfully adopted and used for pharmacy research and practice, toward improved medication-related outcomes and better health.

Questions for further discussion

1. In what ways are human factors and ergonomics methods distinct from other approaches?
2. Of the many human factors and ergonomics methods available, how does one select which one(s) to use in a particular situation? Are there times when some methods are not suitable?
3. How might one combine human factors and ergonomics methods in a multi-part project?
4. How does someone who does not have an advanced degree in human factors and ergonomics learn to use human factors and ergonomics methods?

Application exercise/scenario

You are working with a technology startup company launched to develop a medication-management application (app) for people with dementia and their family caregivers. Your team is committed to the general idea of the app, has a competent team of software developers, and just secured seed funding. However, your main investor is a former dementia caregiver herself and insists that the app be nothing short of "user-centered." The backer will give your team one year and an operating budget to apply the appropriate professional user-centered methodology. What methods might you use to deeply study the problem you are trying to solve, assess the current way medications are managed, and to characterize user needs? What methods will you choose and how will you apply them to design a truly user-centered prototype, before your software developers write their first line of code? How and when will you test the product to evaluate its user-centeredness? How will you organize your activities to ensure on-time, on-budget completion? How will you convince the investor that you used the appropriate professional methods and that your product is truly user-centered?

Acknowledgments

Funding: Dr. Abebe received support from the National Institutes of Health (NIH), National Center for Advancing Translational Sciences, Clinical and Translational Sciences Award, Grant Numbers, KL2TR002530 (PI: Carroll), and UL1TR002529 (PI: Shekhar). For some studies described in this article, Dr. Russ-Jara received funding support from the Department of Veterans Affairs (VA), Veterans Health Administration,

Health Services Research and Development Service (HSR&D), Center for Health Information and Communication CIN 13-416 (PI: Weiner) at the Richard L. Roudebush Veterans Affairs Medical Center in Indianapolis, IN and from a VA HSR&D Career Development Award 11-214 (PI: Russ-Jara). Work presented in Case Study 2 was supported by Agency for Healthcare Research and Quality (AHRQ) grants P30 HS024384 (PI: Callahan) and R18 HS024490 (PI: Chui) and NIH grant R01AG056926 (PI: Holden). Views expressed in this article are those of the authors and do not necessarily represent the views of the NIH, AHRQ, Department of Veterans Affairs, or the U.S. government.

References

1. Karsh B, Holden RJ, Alper SJ, Or CKL. A human factors engineering paradigm for patient safety – designing to support the performance of the health care professional. *Qual Saf Health Care*. 2006;15:i59–i65.
2. Dul J, Bruder R, Buckle P, et al. A strategy for human factors/ergonomics: developing the discipline and profession. *Ergonomics*. 2012;55:377–395.
3. Chui MA, Holden RJ, Russ AL, et al. Human factors in pharmacy. *Proc Hum Factors Ergon Soc Annu Meet*. 2017;61:666–670.
4. Stanton NA, Young MS. What price ergonomics? *Nature*. 1999;399:197–198.
5. Salvendy G. *Handbook of Human Factors and Ergonomics*. 4th ed. Hoboken, NJ: Wiley & Sons; 2012.
6. Proctor RW, Van Zandt T. *Human Factors in Simple and Complex Systems*. Boca Raton, FL: CRC Press; 2018.
7. IEC/ISO 62366:2007. *Medical devices – Application of Usability Engineering to Medical Devices 2007*; 2007.
8. ISO Standard 9241-210:2010. *Ergonomics of Human-System Interaction – Part 210: Human-Centred Design for Interactive Systems*. vol. ISO 9241-210:2010; 2010.
9. ISO/TR Standard 18529:2000. *Ergonomics – Ergonomics of Human-System Interaction – Human-Centred Lifecycle Process Descriptions*. vol. ISO/TR 18529:2000; 2000.
10. Weinger MB, Wiklund M, Gardner-Bonneau D. *Handbook of Human Factors in Medical Device Design*. Boca Raton, FL: CRC Press; 2011.
11. Chapanis A, Safrin MA. Of misses and medicines. *J Chronic Dis*. 1960;12:403–408.
12. Cohen T, Ley EJ, Gewertz BL. *Human Factors in Surgery: Enhancing Safety and Flow in Patient Care*. Boca Raton, FL: CRC Press; 2020.
13. Donchin Y, Gopher D. *Around the Patient Bed: Human Factors and Safety in Health Care*. Boca Raton, FL: CRC Press; 2013.
14. Institute of Medicine. *To Err Is Human: Building a Safer Health System. Institute of Medicine Report on Medical Errors*. Washington, DC: National Academies Press; 2000.
15. Institute of Medicine. *Crossing the Quality Chasm: A New Health System for the 21st Century*. Washington, DC: National Academies Press; 2001.
16. Institute of Medicine. *Patient Safety: Achieving a New Standard for Care*. Washington, DC: National Academies Press; 2004.
17. Carayon P. *Handbook of Human Factors and Ergonomics in Patient Safety*. 2nd ed. Mahwah, NJ: Lawrence Erlbaum; 2012.
18. Holden RJ, Voida S, Savoy A, Jones JF, Kulanthaivel A. Human factors engineering and human–computer interaction: supporting user performance and experience. In: Finnell J, Dixon BE, eds. *Clinical Informatics Study Guide*. New York: Springer; 2016:287–307.
19. Carayon P, Hoonakker P. Human factors and usability for health information technology: old and new challenges. *Yearb Med Inform*. 2019;28:71–77.
20. Hignett S, Carayon P, Buckle P, Catchpole K. State of science: human factors and ergonomics in healthcare. *Ergonomics*. 2013;56:1491–1503.
21. Holden RJ, Valdez RS. Patient ergonomics: the science (and engineering) of patient work. In: Holden RJ, Valdez RS, eds. *The Patient Factor: Theories and Methods for Patient Ergonomics*. Boca Raton, FL: CRC Press; 2021:3–18.
22. Holden RJ, Cornet VP, Valdez RS. Patient ergonomics: 10-year mapping review of patient-centered human factors. *Appl Ergon*. 2020;82, 102972.
23. Holden RJ, Valdez RS. Beyond disease: technologies for health promotion. *Proc Int Symp Hum Factors Ergon Health Care*. 2019;8:62–66.
24. Xie A, Carayon P. A systematic review of human factors and ergonomics (HFE)-based healthcare system redesign for quality of care and patient safety. *Ergonomics*. 2015;58:33–49.
25. Russ AL, Fairbanks RJ, Karsh B, Militello LG, Saleem JJ, Wears RL. The science of human factors: separating fact from fiction. *BMJ Qual Saf*. 2013;22(10):802–808. https://doi.org/10.1136/bmjqs-2012-001450.
26. Carayon P, Wooldridge A, Hose B-Z, Salwei M, Benneyan J. Challenges and opportunities for improving patient safety through human factors and systems engineering. *Health Aff*. 2018;37:1862–1869.
27. Waterson P, Catchpole K. Human factors in healthcare: welcome progress, but still scratching the surface. *BMJ Qual Saf*. 2016;25:480–484.
28. Gurses AP, Ozok AA, Pronovost PJ. Time to accelerate integration of human factors and ergonomics in patient safety. *BMJ Qual Saf*. 2012;21:347–351.
29. Carayon P, Wetterneck TB, Cartmill R, et al. Characterising the complexity of medication safety using a human factors approach: an observational study in two intensive care units. *BMJ Qual Saf*. 2014;23:56–65.
30. Mickelson RS, Holden RJ. Medication adherence: staying within the boundaries of safety. *Ergonomics*. 2018;61:82–103.
31. Holden RJ, Abebe E. Medication transitions: vulnerable periods of change in need of human factors and ergonomics. *Appl Ergon*. 2020;90, 103279.
32. Doucette WR, Rippe JJ, Gaither CA, Kreling DH, Mott DA, Schommer JC. Influences on the frequency and type of community pharmacy services. *J Am Pharm Assoc*. 2017;57:72–76.e71.
33. Trapskin K, Johnson C, Cory P, Sorum S, Decker C. Forging a novel provider and payer partnership in Wisconsin to compensate pharmacists for quality-driven pharmacy and medication therapy management services. *J Am Pharm Assoc*. 2009;49:642–651.
34. Gilmore V, Efird L, Fu D, LeBlanc Y, Nesbit T, Swarthout M. Implementation of transitions-of-care services through acute care and outpatient pharmacy collaboration. *Am J Health Syst Pharm*. 2015;72:737–744.
35. Evans JL, Gladd EM, Gonzalez AC, et al. Establishing a clinical pharmacy technician at a United States Army military treatment facility. *J Am Pharm Assoc*. 2016;56:573–579.e571.

36. Fleagle Miller R, Cesarz J, Rough S. Evaluation of community pharmacy tech-check-tech as a strategy for practice advancement. *J Am Pharm Assoc.* 2018;58:652–658.

37. Flynn EA, Barker KN, Carnahan BJ. National observational study of prescription dispensing accuracy and safety in 50 pharmacies. *J Am Pharm Assoc.* 2003;43:191–200.

38. Kessler DO, Arteaga G, Ching K, et al. Interns' success with clinical procedures in infants after simulation training. *Pediatrics.* 2013;131:e811–e820.

39. Allan EL, Barker KN, Malloy MJ, Heller WM. Dispensing errors and counseling in community practice. *Am Pharm.* 1995;NS35:25–33.

40. Flynn EA, Barker KN. Effect of an automated dispensing system on errors in two pharmacies. *J Am Pharm Assoc.* 2006;46:613–615.

41. Angelo LB, Christensen DB, Ferreri SP. Impact of community pharmacy automation on workflow, workload, and patient interaction. *J Am Pharm Assoc.* 2005;45:138–144.

42. Odukoya OK, Chui MA. E-prescribing: a focused review and new approach to addressing safety in pharmacies and primary care. *Res Soc Adm Pharm.* 2013;9:996–1003.

43. Odukoya OK, Stone JA, Chui MA. E-prescribing errors in community pharmacies: exploring consequences and contributing factors. *Int J Med Inform.* 2014;83:427–437.

44. Al Juffali L, Al-Aqeel S, Knapp P, Mearns K, Family H, Watson M. Using the human factors framework to understand the origins of medication safety problems in community pharmacy: a qualitative study. *Res Soc Adm Pharm.* 2019;15:558–567.

45. Reilley S, Grasha AF, Schafer J. Workload, error detection, and experienced stress in a simulated pharmacy verification task. *Percept Mot Skills.* 2002;95:27–46.

46. Johnson S, O'Connor E, Jacobs S, Hassell K, Ashcroft D. The relationships among work stress, strain and self-reported errors in UK community pharmacy. *Res Soc Adm Pharm.* 2014;10:885–895.

47. Chui MA, Mott DA. Community pharmacists' subjective workload and perceived task performance: a human factors approach. *J Am Pharm Assoc.* 2012;52:e153–e160.

48. Chui MA, Stone JA, Holden RJ. Improving over-the-counter medication safety for older adults: a study protocol for a demonstration and dissemination study. *Res Soc Adm Pharm.* 2017;13:930–937.

49. Holden RJ, Srinivas P, Campbell NL, et al. Understanding older adults' medication decision making and behavior: a study on over-the-counter (OTC) anticholinergic medications. *Res Soc Adm Pharm.* 2019;15:53–60.

50. Vest TA, Gazda NP, Schenkat DH, Eckel SF. Practice-enhancing publications about the medication use process in 2017. *Am J Health Syst Pharm.* 2019;76:667–676.

51. Sutherland A, Ashcroft DM, Phipps DL. Exploring the human factors of prescribing errors in paediatric intensive care units. *Arch Dis Child.* 2019;104:588–595.

52. Zheng Y, Jiang Y, Dorsch MP, Ding Y, Vydiswaran VV, Lester CA. Work effort, readability and quality of pharmacy transcription of patient directions from electronic prescriptions: a retrospective observational cohort analysis. *BMJ Qual Saf.* 2021;30:311–319.

53. Gerhart JM, Spriggs H, Hampton TW, et al. Applying human factors to develop an improved package design for (Rx) medication drug labels in a pharmacy setting. *J Saf Res.* 2015;55:177–184.

54. Odberg KR, Hansen BS, Aase K, Wangensteen S. A work system analysis of the medication administration process in a Norwegian nursing home ward. *Appl Ergon.* 2020;86, 103100.

55. Lee JD, Wickens CD, Liu Y, Boyle LN. *Designing for People: An Introduction to Human Factors Engineering.* 3rd ed. Charleston, SC: CreateSpace; 2017.

56. Stanton NA, Salmon PM, Rafferty LA, Walker GH, Baber C, Jenkins DP. *Human Factors Methods: A Practical Guide for Engineering and Design.* Surrey, UK: Ashgate; 2013.

57. Cooke NJ. Varieties of knowledge elicitation techniques. *Int J Hum Comput Stud.* 1994;41:801–849.

58. Carayon P, Cartmill R, Hoonakker P, et al. Human factors analysis of workflow in health information technology implementation. In: Carayon P, ed. *Handbook of Human Factors and Ergonomics in Patient Safety.* 2nd ed. Mahwah, NJ: Lawrence Erlbaum; 2012:507–521.

59. Helander M. *A Guide to Human Factors and Ergonomics.* Boca Raton, FL: CRC Press; 2005.

60. Carayon P, Wetterneck TB, Rivera-Rodriguez AJ, et al. Human factors systems approach to healthcare quality and patient safety. *Appl Ergon.* 2014;45:14–25.

61. Carayon P. Human factors of complex sociotechnical systems. *Appl Ergon.* 2006;37:525–535.

62. Carayon P, Schoofs Hundt A, Karsh B, et al. Work system design for patient safety: the SEIPS model. *Qual Saf Health Care.* 2006;15:i50–i58.

63. Holden RJ, Carayon P, Gurses AP, et al. SEIPS 2.0: a human factors framework for studying and improving the work of healthcare professionals and patients. *Ergonomics.* 2013;56:1669–1686.

64. Carayon P, Wooldridge A, Hoonakker P, Hundt AS, Kelly MM. SEIPS 3.0: human-centered design of the patient journey for patient safety. *Appl Ergon.* 2020;84:103033.

65. Werner NE, Ponnala S, Doutcheva N, Holden RJ. Human factors/ergonomics work system analysis of patient work: state of the science and future directions. *Int J Qual Health Care.* 2021;33:60–71.

66. Holden RJ, Schubert CC, Mickelson RS. The patient work system: an analysis of self-care performance barriers among elderly heart failure patients and their informal caregivers. *Appl Ergon.* 2015;47:133–150.

67. Holden RJ, Valdez RS, Schubert CC, Thompson MJ, Hundt AS. Macroergonomic factors in the patient work system: examining the context of patients with chronic illness. *Ergonomics.* 2017;60:26–43.

68. Saha SK, Kong DC, Thursky K, Mazza D. Antimicrobial stewardship by Australian community pharmacists: uptake, collaboration, challenges and needs. *J Am Pharm Assoc.* 2021;61:158–168.

69. Al-Jumaili AA, Doucette WR. A systems approach to identify factors influencing adverse drug events in nursing homes. *J Am Geriatr Soc.* 2018;66:1420–1427.

70. Abraham O, Myers MN, Brothers AL, Montgomery J, Norman BA, Fabian T. Assessing need for pharmacist involvement to improve care coordination for patients on LAI antipsychotics transitioning from hospital to home: a work system approach. *Res Soc Adm Pharm.* 2017;13:1004–1013.

71. Odukoya OK, Stone JA, Chui MA. Barriers and facilitators to recovering from e-prescribing errors in community pharmacies. *J Am Pharm Assoc.* 2015;55:52–58.

72. Odukoya OK, Chui MA. E-prescribing: characterisation of patient safety hazards in community pharmacies using a sociotechnical systems approach. *BMJ Qual Saf.* 2013;22:816–825.

73. Look KA, Stone JA. Medication management activities performed by informal caregivers of older adults. *Res Soc Adm Pharm.* 2018;14:418–426.

74. Bacci JL, Coley KC, McGrath K, Abraham O, Adams AJ, McGivney MS. Strategies to facilitate the implementation of collaborative practice agreements in chain community pharmacies. *J Am Pharm Assoc.* 2016;56:257–265.

75. Chui MA, Mott DA, Maxwell L. A qualitative assessment of a community pharmacy cognitive pharmaceutical services program, using a work system approach. *Res Soc Adm Pharm.* 2012;8:206–216.

76. Craig CM, Patzer B, Morris NL. Minimizing the impact of interruptions in a pediatric retail pharmacy. *Proc Hum Factors Ergon Soc Annu Meet.* 2018;62:480–484.

77. Strauven G, Vanhaecht K, Anrys P, De Lepeleire J, Spinewine A, Foulon V. Development of a process-oriented quality improvement strategy for the medicines pathway in nursing homes using the SEIPS model. *Res Soc Adm Pharm.* 2020;16:360–376.

78. Holden RJ, Carayon P. SEIPS 101 and seven simple SEIPS tools. *BMJ Qual Saf.* 2021. https://doi.org/10.1136/bmjqs-2020-012538.

79. Jiancaro T, Jamieson GA, Mihailidis A. Twenty years of cognitive work analysis in health care: a scoping review. *J Cogn Eng Decis Mak.* 2014;8:3–22.

80. Vicente KJ. *Cognitive Work Analysis: Toward Safe, Productive, and Healthy Computer-Based Work.* 1st ed. London: Lawrence Erlbaum Associates; 1999.

81. Naikar N. *Cognitive Work Analysis: Foundations, Extensions, and Challenges.* Fishermans Bend, Australia: Defence Science and Technology Organisation; 2012.

82. Naikar N. Beyond interface design: further applications of cognitive work analysis. *Int J Ind Ergon.* 2006;36:423–438.

83. Abebe E, Scanlon MC, Lee KJ, Chui MA. What do family caregivers do when managing medications for their children with medical complexity? *Appl Ergon.* 2020;87, 103108.

84. Baumgartner A, Kunkes T, Clark CM, et al. Opportunities and recommendations for improving medication safety: understanding the medication management system in primary care through an abstraction hierarchy. *JMIR Hum Factors.* 2020;7, e18103.

85. Clark LN, Benda NC, Hegde S, et al. Usability evaluation of an emergency department information system prototype designed using cognitive systems engineering techniques. *Appl Ergon.* 2017;60:356–365.

86. Crandall B, Hoffman RR. Cognitive task analysis. In: Lee J, Kirlik A, eds. *The Oxford Handbook of Cognitive Engineering.* Oxford: Oxford University Press; 2013:229–239.

87. Russ AL, Militello LG, Glassman PA, Arthur KJ, Zillich AJ, Weiner M. Adapting cognitive task analysis to investigate clinical decision making and medication safety incidents. *J Patient Saf.* 2019;15:191–197.

88. Elkhadragy N, Ifeachor AP, Diiulio JB, et al. Medication decision-making for patients with renal insufficiency in inpatient and outpatient care at a US veterans affairs medical centre: a qualitative, cognitive task analysis. *BMJ Open.* 2019;9, e027439.

89. Holden RJ, Daley CN, Mickelson RS, et al. Patient decision-making personas: an application of a patient-centered cognitive task analysis (P-CTA). *Appl Ergon.* 2020;87, 103107.

90. Daley CN, Cornet VP, Toscos TR, Bolchini DP, Mirro MJ, Holden RJ. Naturalistic decision making in everyday self-care among older adults with heart failure. *J Cardiovasc Nurs.* 2020. https://doi.org/10.1097/JCN.0000000000000778.

91. Crandall B, Klein G, Hoffman RR. *Working Minds: A Practitioner's Guide to Cognitive Task Analysis.* Cambridge, MA: MIT Press; 2006.

92. Mickelson RS, Unertl KM, Holden RJ. Medication management: the macrocognitive workflow of older adults with heart failure. *JMIR Hum Factors.* 2016;3:e27. https://humanfactors.jmir.org/2016/2012/e2027/.

93. Stanton NA. Hierarchical task analysis: developments, applications, and extensions. *Appl Ergon.* 2006;37:55–79.

94. Lane R, Stanton NA, Harrison D. Applying hierarchical task analysis to medication administration errors. *Appl Ergon.* 2006;37:669–679.

95. Lester CA, Chui MA. Using link analysis to explore the impact of the physical environment on pharmacist tasks. *Res Soc Adm Pharm.* 2016;12:627–632.

96. Vidulich MA, Tsang PS. Mental workload and situation awareness. In: Salvendy G, ed. *Handbook of Human Factors and Ergonomics.* 4th ed. Hoboken, NJ: Wiley & Sons; 2012:243–273.

97. Carayon P, Alvarado CJ. Workload and patient safety among critical care nurses. *Crit Care Nurs Clin North Am.* 2007;19:121–129.

98. Carayon P, Gurses AP. A human factors engineering conceptual framework of nursing workload and patient safety in intensive care units. *Intensive Crit Care Nurs.* 2005;21:284–301.

99. Holden RJ, Scanlon MC, Patel NR, et al. A human factors framework and study of the effect of nursing workload on patient safety and employee quality of working life. *BMJ Qual Saf.* 2011;20:15–24.

100. Holden RJ, Patel NR, Scanlon MC, Shalaby TM, Arnold JM, Karsh B. Effects of mental demands during dispensing on perceived medication safety and employee well being: a study of workload in pediatric hospital pharmacies. *Res Soc Adm Pharm.* 2010;6:293–306.

101. Grasha AF. Misconceptions about pharmacy workload. *Can Pharm J.* 2001;134:26–35.

102. Borg GAV. Psychophysical bases of perceived exertion. *Med Sci Sports Exerc.* 1982;14:377–381.

103. Lee JD, Wickens CD, Liu Y, Boyle LN. Work physiology. In: *Designing for People: An Introduction to Human Factors Engineering*; 2017:448–477.

104. Grasha AF, Schell K. Psychosocial factors, workload, and human error in a simulated pharmacy dispensing task. *Percept Mot Skills.* 2001;92:53–71.

105. Chui MA, Look KA, Mott DA. The association of subjective workload dimensions on quality of care and pharmacist quality of work life. *Res Soc Adm Pharm*. 2014;10:328–340.

106. Charles RL, Nixon J. Measuring mental workload using physiological measures: a systematic review. *Appl Ergon*. 2019;74:221–232.

107. Wickens CD. Multiple resources and mental workload. *Hum Factors*. 2008;50:449–455.

108. Xie B, Salvendy G. Review and reappraisal of modelling and predicting mental workload in single-and multi-task environments. *Work Stress*. 2000;14:74–99.

109. Vélez-Díaz-Pallarés M, Delgado-Silveira E, Carretero-Accame ME, Bermejo-Vicedo T. Using healthcare failure mode and effect analysis to reduce medication errors in the process of drug prescription, validation and dispensing in hospitalised patients. *BMJ Qual Saf*. 2013;22:42–52.

110. McLeod RW, Bowie P. Bowtie analysis as a prospective risk assessment technique in primary healthcare. *Policy Pract Health Saf*. 2018;16:177–193.

111. Marx DA, Slonim AD. Assessing patient safety risk before the injury occurs: an introduction to sociotechnical probabilistic risk modelling in health care. *Qual Saf Health Care*. 2003;12:ii33–ii38.

112. Karnon J, McIntosh A, Dean J, et al. A prospective hazard and improvement analytic approach to predicting the effectiveness of medication error interventions. *Saf Sci*. 2007;45:523–539.

113. Hovor C, O'Donnell LT. Probabilistic risk analysis of medication error. *Qual Manag Health Care*. 2007;16:349–353.

114. Hfaiedh N, Kabiche S, Delescluse C, et al. Performing a preliminary hazard analysis applied to administration of injectable drugs to infants. *J Eval Clin Pract*. 2017;23:875–881.

115. Kellogg KM, Hettinger Z, Shah M, et al. Our current approach to root cause analysis: is it contributing to our failure to improve patient safety? *BMJ Qual Saf*. 2016;26:381–387.

116. National Patient Safety Foundation. *RCA²: Improving Root Cause Analyses and Actions to Prevent Harm*. Boston, MA: National Patient Safety Foundation; 2015.

117. Peerally MF, Carr S, Waring J, Dixon-Woods M. The problem with root cause analysis. *BMJ Qual Saf*. 2017;26:417–422.

118. Klein GA, Calderwood R, Macgregor D. Critical decision method for eliciting knowledge. *IEEE Trans Syst Man Cybern B Cybern*. 1989;19:462–472.

119. Wickens CD, Lee JD, Liu Y, Gordon Becker SE. Safety and accident prevention. In: *An Introduction to Human Factors Engineering*. 2nd ed. Upper Saddle River, NJ: Pearson Prentice Hall; 2004:376–377.

120. Beyer H, Holtzblatt K. *Contextual Design: Defining Customer-Centered Systems*. San Francisco: Morgan Kaufmann; 1998.

121. Cornet VP, Toscos T, Bolchini D, et al. Untold stories in user-centered design of mobile health: practical challenges and strategies learned from the design and evaluation of an app for older adults with heart failure. *JMIR Mhealth Uhealth*. 2020;8, e17703.

122. Holden RJ, Kulanthaivel A, Purkayastha S, Goggins KM, Kripalani S. Know thy eHealth user: development of biopsychosocial personas from a study of older adults with heart failure. *Int J Med Inform*. 2017;108:158–167.

123. Reddy A, Lester CA, Stone JA, Holden RJ, Phelan CH, Chui MA. Applying participatory design to a pharmacy system intervention. *Res Soc Adm Pharm*. 2019;15:1358–1367.

124. Ahmed R, Toscos T, Rohani Ghahari R, et al. Visualization of cardiac implantable electronic device data for older adults using participatory design. *Appl Clin Inform*. 2019;10:707–718.

125. Siek KA, Ross SE, Khan DU, Haverhals LM, Cali SR, Meyers J. Colorado care tablet: the design of an interoperable personal health application to help older adults with multimorbidity manage their medications. *J Biomed Inform*. 2010;43:S22–S26.

126. Holden RJ, Boustani MA, Azar J. Agile innovation to transform healthcare: innovating in complex adaptive systems is an everyday process, not a light bulb event. *BMJ Innov*. 2021;7:499–505.

127. Boustani MA, Holden RJ, Azar J, Solid CA. *The Agile Network: A Model to Foster Innovation, Implementation, and Diffusion in Healthcare Settings*. St. Paul, MN: Beaver's Pond Press; 2020.

128. Hartson R, Pyla PS. *The UX Book: Process and Guidelines for Ensuring a Quality User Experience*. Hoboken, NJ: Elsevier; 2012.

129. US Department of Health and Human Services. The research-based web design & usability guidelines, enlarged/expanded edition. In: *Essentials of Research Methods in Psychology*. Washington, DC: US Government Printing Office; 2006.

130. ISO Standard 9241-11:1998. *Ergonomic Requirements for Office Work with Visual Display Terminals (VDTs). Part 11: Guidance on Usability*. International Organization for Standardization (ISO); 1998.

131. Chan J, Shojania KG, Easty AC, Etchells EE. Does user-centred design affect the efficiency, usability and safety of CPOE order sets? *J Am Med Inform Assoc*. 2011;18:276–281.

132. Russ AL, Zillich AJ, Melton BL, et al. Applying human factors principles to alert design increases efficiency and reduces prescribing errors in a scenario-based simulation. *J Am Med Inform Assoc*. 2014;21:e287–e296.

133. Snyder ME, Gernant SA, DiIulio J, Jaynes HA, Doucette WR, Russ-Jara AL. A user-centered evaluation of medication therapy management alerts for community pharmacists: recommendations to improve usability and usefulness. *Res Soc Adm Pharm*. 2020;17(8):1433–1443. https://doi.org/10.1016/j.sapharm.2020.1010.1015.

134. Miller KE, Arnold R, Capan M, et al. Improving infusion pump safety through usability testing. *J Nurs Care Qual*. 2017;32:141–149.

135. Savoy A, Patel H, Flanagan ME, Weiner M, Russ AL. Systematic heuristic evaluation of computerized consultation order templates: clinicians' and human factors engineers' perspectives. *J Med Syst*. 2017;41:129.

136. Zhang J, Johnson TR, Patel VL, Paige DL, Kubose T. Using usability heuristics to evaluate patient safety of medical devices. *J Biomed Inform*. 2003;36:23–30.

137. Kushniruk AW, Patel VL. Cognitive and usability engineering methods for the evaluation of clinical information systems. *J Biomed Inform*. 2004;37:56–76.

138. Johnson CM, Johnston D, Crowle PK. *EHR Usability Toolkit: A Background Report on Usability and Electronic Health Records.* Rockville, MD: Agency for Healthcare Research and Quality; 2011.
139. Russ AL, Baker DA, Fahner WJ, et al. A rapid usability evaluation (RUE) method for health information technology. *AMIA Ann Symp Proc.* 2010;2010:702–706.
140. Kushniruk AW, Borycki EM. Low-cost rapid usability engineering: designing and customizing usable healthcare information systems. *Healthc Q.* 2006;9(98–100):102.
141. Russ AL, Saleem JJ. Ten factors to consider when developing usability scenarios and tasks for health information technology. *J Biomed Inform.* 2018;78:123–133.
142. Hart SG, Staveland LE. Development of NASA-TLX (task load index): results of empirical and theoretical research. *Adv Psychol.* 1988;52:139–183.
143. Lewis JR. IBM computer usability satisfaction questionnaires: psychometric evaluation and instructions for use. *Int J Hum Comput Interact.* 1995;7:57–78.
144. Bangor A, Kortum PT, Miller JT. An empirical evaluation of the system usability scale. *Int J Hum Comput Interact.* 2008;24:574–594.
145. Peißl S, Wickens CD, Baruah R. Eye-tracking measures in aviation: a selective literature review. *Int J Aerospace Psychol.* 2018;28:98–112.
146. Poole A, Ball LJ. Eye tracking in HCI and usability research. In: *Encyclopedia of Human Computer Interaction.* IGI Global; 2006:211–219.
147. Jaspers MW, Steen T, Van Den Bos C, Geenen M. The think aloud method: a guide to user interface design. *Int J Med Inform.* 2004;73:781–795.
148. Li AC, Kannry JL, Kushniruk A, et al. Integrating usability testing and think-aloud protocol analysis with "near-live" clinical simulations in evaluating clinical decision support. *Int J Med Inform.* 2012;81:761–772.
149. Russ AL, Jahn MA, Patel H, et al. Usability evaluation of a medication reconciliation tool: embedding safety probes to assess users' detection of medication discrepancies. *J Biomed Inform.* 2018;82:178–186.
150. Holden RJ, Bodke K, Tambe R, Comer R, Clark D, Boustani M. Rapid translational field research approach for eHealth R&D. *Proc Int Symp Hum Factors Ergon Health Care.* 2016;5:25–27.
151. Russ AL, Chen S, Melton BL, et al. Design and evaluation of an electronic override mechanism for medication alerts to facilitate communication between prescribers and pharmacists. *Ann Pharmacother.* 2015;49:761–769.
152. Karwowski W, Marras WS. *The Occupational Ergonomics Handbook.* Boca Raton, FL: CRC Press; 1999.
153. Weir NM, Newham R, Bennie M. A literature review of human factors and ergonomics within the pharmacy dispensing process. *Res Soc Adm Pharm.* 2020;16:637–645.
154. James KL, Barlow D, McArtney R, Hiom S, Roberts D, Whittlesea C. Incidence, type and causes of dispensing errors: a review of the literature. *Int J Pharm Pract.* 2009;17:9–30.
155. Wilson JR, Sharples S. *Evaluation of Human Work.* Boca Raton, FL: CRC Press; 2015.
156. Srinivas P, Cornet V, Holden RJ. Human factors analysis, design, and testing of engage, a consumer health IT application for geriatric heart failure self-care. *Int J Hum Comput Interact.* 2017;33:298–312.
157. Cornet VP, Daley C, Cavalcanti LH, Parulekar A, Holden RJ. Design for self-care. In: Sethumadhavan A, Sasangohar F, eds. *Design for Health.* Amsterdam: Elsevier; 2020:277–302.
158. Siek KA, Khan DU, Ross SE, Haverhals LM, Meyers J, Cali SR. Designing a personal health application for older adults to manage medications: a comprehensive case study. *J Med Syst.* 2011;35:1099–1121.
159. Morrow DG, Weiner M, Young J, Steinley D, Deer M, Murray MD. Improving medication knowledge among older adults with heart failure: a patient-centered approach to instruction design. *Gerontologist.* 2005;45:545–552.
160. Morrow DG, Leirer VO, Andrassy JM, Tanke ED, Stine-Morrow EA. Medication instruction design: younger and older adult schemas for taking medication. *Hum Factors.* 1996;38:556–573.
161. Morrow D, Leirer VO, Andrassy JM. Designing medication instructions for older adults. *Proc Hum Factors Ergon Soc Annu Meet.* 1993;37:197–201.
162. Morrow D, Leirer V, Altieri P, Tanke E. Elders' schema for taking medication: implications for instruction design. *J Gerontol.* 1991;46:378–385.
163. Morrow D, Leirer V, Sheikh J. Adherence and medication instructions review and recommendations. *J Am Geriatr Soc.* 1988;36:1147–1160.
164. Wogalter MS. Enhancing information acquisition for over-the-counter medications by making better use of container surface space. *Exp Aging Res.* 1999;25:27–48.
165. Wogalter MS, Magurno AB, Scott KL, Dietrich DA. Facilitating information acquisition for over-the-counter drugs using supplemental labels. *Proc Hum Factors Ergon Soc Annu Meet.* 1996;40:732–736.
166. Vigilante Jr WJ, Wogalter MS. Over-the-counter (OTC) drug labeling: format preferences. *Proc Hum Factors Ergon Soc Annu Meet.* 1999;43:103–107.
167. Morrow D, Leirer V, Altieri P. List formats improve medication instructions for older adults. *Educ Gerontol.* 1995;21:151–166.
168. Wogalter MS, Vigilante WJJ. Effects of label format on knowledge acquisition and perceived readability by younger and older adults. *Ergonomics.* 2003;46:327–344.
169. Shaver EF, Wogalter MS. A comparison of older vs newer over-the-counter (OTC) nonprescription drug lables on search time accuracy. *Proc Hum Factors Ergon Soc Annu Meet.* 2003;47:826–830.
170. Mendat CC, Watson AM, Mayhorn CB, Wogalter MS. Age of differences in search time for two over-the-counter (OTC) drug label formats. *Proc Hum Factors Ergon Soc Annu Meet.* 2005;49:200–203.
171. Sojourner RJ, Wogalter MS. The influence of pictorials on evaluations of prescription medication instructions. *Drug Inf J.* 1997;31:963–972.
172. Morrow DG, Hier CM, Menard WE, Leirer VO. Icons improve older and younger adults' comprehension of medication information. *J Gerontol B Psychol Sci Soc Sci.* 1998;53:240–254.

173. Bix L, Bello NM, Auras R, Ranger J, Lapinski MK. Examining the conspicuousness and prominence of two required warnings on OTC pain relievers. *Proc Natl Acad Sci U S A.* 2009;106:6550–6555.

174. Bix L, Becker MW, Breslow R, Liu L, Harben A, Esfahanian S. Optimizing OTC labeling for use by older adults. *Innov Aging.* 2018;2:82.

175. Stone JA, Lester CA, Aboneh EA, Phelan CH, Welch LL, Chui MA. A preliminary examination of over-the-counter medication misuse rates in older adults. *Res Soc Adm Pharm.* 2017;13:187–192.

176. Stone JA, Phelan CH, Holden RJ, Jacobson N, Chui MA. A pilot study of decision factors influencing over-the-counter medication selection and use by older adults. *Res Soc Adm Pharm.* 2020;16:1117–1120.

177. Holden RJ, Campbell NL, Abebe E, et al. Usability and feasibility of consumer-facing technology to reduce unsafe medication use by older adults. *Res Soc Adm Pharm.* 2020;16:54–61.

178. Holden RJ. A simplified system usability scale (SUS) for cognitively impaired and older adults. *Proc Int Symp Hum Factors Ergon Health Care.* 2020;9:180–182.

179. Abebe E, Campbell NL, Clark DO, et al. Reducing anticholinergic medication exposure among older adults using consumer technology: protocol for a randomized clinical trial. *Res Soc Adm Pharm.* 2021;17:986–992.

180. Campbell NL, Holden RJ, Tang Q, et al. Multi-component behavioral intervention to reduce exposure to anticholinergics in primary care older adults. *J Am Geriatr Soc.* 2021;69(6):1490–1499. https://doi.org/10.1111/jgs.17121.

181. Watterson T, Xiong K, Stone J, et al. Implementing CancelRx: describing adoption barriers using a process map framework. In: *11th Annual Conference on the Science of Dissemination and Implementation.* Washington, DC: AcademyHealth; 2018.

182. Stone JA, Watterson T, Xiong KZ, et al. *Identifying Vulnerabilities in Health IT: A Case Study of CancelRx Implementation in Clinic and Pharmacy Sociotechnical Systems.* vol. 9. 1st ed. Los Angeles, CA: SAGE Publications; 2020:64–66.

183. Endsley MR. Toward a theory of situation awareness in dynamic systems. *Hum Factors.* 1995;37:32–64.

184. Wickens CD. Multiple resources and performance prediction. *Theor Issues Ergon Sci.* 2002;3:159–177.

185. Haines H, Wilson JR, Vink P, Koningsveld E. Validating a framework for participatory ergonomics (the PEF). *Ergonomics.* 2002;45:309–327.

186. Toussaint J, Berry LL. The promise of lean in health care. *Mayo Clin Proc.* 2013;88:74–82.

187. Holden RJ, Boustani M. The value of an 'Agile' mindset in times of crisis. *Mod Healthc.* 2020. May 11.

188. Bokhour BG, Fix GM, Mueller NM, et al. How can healthcare organizations implement patient-centered care? Examining a large-scale cultural transformation. *BMC Health Serv Res.* 2018;18:1–11.

189. Chassin MR, Loeb JM. High-reliability health care: getting there from here. *Milbank Q.* 2013;91:459–490.

190. Stanton NA, Hedge A, Brookhuis K, Salas E, Hendrick H. *Handbook of Human Factors and Ergonomics Methods.* Boca Raton, FL: CRC Press; 2005.

191. Nemeth CP. *Human Factors Methods for Design: Making Systems Human-Centered.* Boca Raton, FL: CRC Press; 2004.

192. Patterson ES, Miller JE. *Macrocognition Metrics and Scenarios: Design and Evaluation for Real-World Teams.* Surrey, UK: Ashgate; 2010.

193. Gawron VJ. *Human Performance, Workload, and Situational Awareness Measures Handbook.* 3rd ed. Boca Raton, FL: CRC Press; 2019.

194. Vosper H, Hignett S. A UK perspective on human factors and patient safety education in pharmacy curricula. *Am J Pharm Educ.* 2018;82:6184.

195. Holden RJ, Or CKL, Alper SJ, Rivera AJ, Karsh B. A change management framework for macroergonomic field research. *Appl Ergon.* 2008;39:459–474.

196. Holden RJ, McDougald Scott AM, Hoonakker PLT, Hundt AS, Carayon P. Data collection challenges in community settings: insights from two field studies of patients with chronic disease. *Qual Life Res.* 2015;24:1043–1055.

197. Blandford A, Furniss D, Makri S. *Qualitative HCI Research: Going Behind the Scenes.* Morgan & Claypool; 2016.

198. Stanton NA, Young MS. Giving ergonomics away? The application of ergonomics methods by novices. *Appl Ergon.* 2003;34:479–490.

199. Rayo MF, Fairbanks RJ, Parker SH, Wolf L, Kennedy R. Spreading the word: improving outcomes with human factors engineering (when common sense is not enough). *Proc Hum Factors Ergon Soc Annu Meet.* 2018;62:578–582.

Chapter 2

Designing complex health interventions using experience-based co-design

Beth Fylan[a,b], Justine Tomlinson[a,c], D.K. Raynor[d], and Jonathan Silcock[a]

[a]*University of Bradford, School of Pharmacy and Medical Sciences, Bradford, United Kingdom*, [b]*Bradford Teaching Hospitals NHS Foundation Trust, Yorkshire Quality and Safety Research Group, Bradford, United Kingdom*, [c]*Leeds Teaching Hospitals NHS Trust, Medicines Management and Pharmacy Services, Leeds, United Kingdom*, [d]*University of Leeds, School of Healthcare, Leeds, United Kingdom*

Objectives

- Outline the steps in EBCD when used as a method of health service improvement.
- Highlight the importance of listening to the patient voice when designing complex interventions for testing in pragmatic controlled trials.
- Explain the potential role of EBCD in the design of complex interventions for testing in controlled trials.
- Describe how experienced-based trial interventions can also be mapped to formal theory so that intervention fidelity and outcomes can be monitored.

Introduction

When problems are identified in the way care is delivered to or experienced by patients, researchers and healthcare staff often work together to design and implement "interventions" to improve care. An intervention can be a process, strategy, or tool that is specifically designed or developed to address the problem identified. Interventions are described as "complex" when they comprise several different components.[1] Implementation science can be divided into three aspects: process models for getting research into practice (e.g., the Knowledge-to-Action Framework or Plan-Do-Study-Act [PDSA] cycles); frameworks and theories for influencing behavior change (e.g., the Theory of Planned Behavior); and evaluation frameworks (e.g., economic evaluation, Consolidated Framework for Implementation Research or RE-AIM).[2] However, the starting point for implementation science is evidence for the effectiveness of interventions. This evidence is often gathered from clinical trials of simple interventions in ideal circumstances, for example, a commercially funded medication or device trial.

There is an increasing understanding that technological innovation alone will not necessarily lead to better and more efficient healthcare services. Complex interventions are often required, which combine technical and behavioral aspects. For example, treatment for coronary artery disease (CAD) may require: surgery, physiotherapy, lifestyle modification, and long-term pharmacotherapy. The management of common, complex, and chronic conditions should reflect the variability of patient pathways and engage patients in monitoring of safety or effectiveness. Interventions are required that can optimize both technical effectiveness (efficacy) and patient experience. Only then will real-world effectiveness be maximized.

Interventions to improve the safety of medication management

Medications are crucial to the management and prevention of health conditions and healthcare economies invest significantly in their provision. For example, in England, the National Health Service (NHS) spends approximately £17 billion a year on medication across primary and secondary care. Yet, while medications are frequently used, they are managed through systems that create risks to patient safety: there is potential for patient harm in the prescribing, dispensing and administering parts of the medication management system. In England alone, more than 237 million medication errors are made every year, 66 million of which are potentially clinically significant, at a cost of more than £98 million.[3] Therefore, interventions that can be implemented to improve the safety of medication management have the potential to reduce patient harm and optimize medication budgets.

To address this, numerous interventions have been developed to reduce harm from medications, targeting different stages in the management process.[4] Many of them are aimed at patients' use of medications, including the acquisition of skills to self-manage medications. However, it is difficult to discern if or how patients have been involved in intervention development. We also know that patients play a proactive and safety-critical role in managing their medications, undertaking tasks independently of healthcare professionals and without their guidance or support.[5–7] Indeed, there is a demonstrated link between improved patient experiences and both patient safety and clinical effectiveness in healthcare.[8]

There is an established United Kingdom (UK) guideline recommending the processes involved in complex intervention development and evaluation.[9] Different theories have been used in the literature to guide intervention design and implementation,[10,11] aiming to improve effectiveness and uptake. In this chapter, while we acknowledge there are many theoretical lenses that could underpin intervention design, we focus our attention on the example of behavior change theory. This is because an understanding of the likely behavioral mechanisms that will bring about change is instrumental when designing interventions to improve medication safety.

The process elements of the development guideline include understanding the theory of how the intervention will achieve its intended effect. There is also a recognition that behaviors and systems, such as medication management, are complex. There is limited detail in the guidance about intervention development. However, O'Caithan, Croot et al. (2019) have developed (from systematic review) a taxonomy of approaches to doing this, the first being the "partnership approach." Here, people who will use the intervention participate equally with the research team throughout intervention development.[12] When well-designed and managed, EBCD offers exactly such an approach. In the following sections we will outline how EBCD can be combined with the guidelines for intervention development and be underpinned by theory while still being grounded in and built from the experiences of the people it targets. We begin by offering an overview of co-design as a tool and of the methods involved in EBCD.

What is co-design?

Traditionally, industry has designed products for people or with people's needs in mind.[13] Methods where designers and end-users work together, as equal partners, to design new products, have been increasingly popular. Co-design, as one method of developing products and services, has been used in the fields of business marketing, design, IT, and architecture for decades.[14] It goes beyond basic stakeholder consultation, or observation, to encourage joint working aiming to create solutions. It is participatory in nature, where the basic principle is to bring stakeholders (researchers, designers, end users etc.) together to work collectively during a design process.[15] The value of co-design is the sharing of varied perspectives to understand both "demand" and "supply" in order to create successful outputs. Most importantly, by involving the end-user, more innovative ideas that better match users' needs are generated. In doing this, evidence demonstrates an overall improved customer satisfaction.[15]

The concept of co-design has been adopted within healthcare quality improvement practices. Here, staff and patients associated with a particular service work together to design different ways of working. Co-design has resulted in tangible improvements in, for example, breast services,[16] bedside handovers, and communication at hospital discharge.[17]

Co-design for healthcare involves engagement with, and empowerment of, those individuals (staff and patients) with lived experience. It aims to advance quality of life and health outcomes for all involved.[18] While co-design has notable benefits, it also has limitations. For example, it is important to plan stakeholder engagement carefully to ensure involvement is meaningful and beyond the tokenistic.

While co-design is increasing in popularity, its use has mainly been within quality or service improvement projects in a local area. There is, however, growing evidence of researchers using co-design within larger intervention development research projects. For example, Hahn-Goldberg et al. (2020) used participatory action research to inform the co-design of a patient-oriented discharge summary,[19] and Tsianakas et al. (2015) used EBCD to develop an intervention in a chemotherapy outpatients service to take forward to acceptability and feasibility research.[20]

In terms of understanding medication management routines and experiences, co-design offers the opportunity to build on the skills that many patients have, through involving them in developing interventions to enhance safety is crucial. Table 1 outlines the different areas of medication management where co-design approaches could be used to develop interventions to improve care.

TABLE 1 Examples of medication management which would benefit from co-designed interventions.

Area of focus	Co-design potential to make sure of patients' medication management expertise
Medication self-management	• Patient skills, strategies and tools to effectively and safely manage their own medications—including error mitigation and error management, supply management and support that can be leveraged.
Medication optimization at care transitions	• Interventions to optimize how patients can prepare for moving from hospital to home, managing ongoing supply ordering and collection, adapting routines to take into account changes made in hospital. • Ongoing communication with healthcare professionals, management of medications at care transitions—such as patient follow-up support with medications by community pharmacy after discharge from hospital.
Managing medications with regular dose changes	• Interventions to support patients after doses have changed, to understand how strategies and tools could help them check their prescriptions reflect those changes and manage their supplies.
Shared decision making for prescribing	• Interventions to support patients in their consultations with healthcare professionals about prescribing decisions—for example in the choice of medications or whether to discontinue a medication.

What is experience-based co-design?

One method of co-design increasingly used in healthcare is EBCD, originally known as Experience-Based Design (EBD). EBCD is a participatory design method which was originally developed and is still primarily used as a local healthcare quality improvement tool.[21] It is a multistage process involving patients, carers, and staff in identifying how healthcare services can deliver enhanced experiences to improve patient care. As an improvement tool it has combined four main underpinning approaches:

i. participatory action research,
ii. user-centered design,
iii. learning theory, and
iv. narrative-based approaches to change.[22]

While the method has been mainly used in single sites to improve experiences of local services, EBCD can be integrated into projects to develop complex interventions, which can then be tested more widely within the healthcare system. Indeed, the unrealized potential of EBCD to be used in developing complex healthcare interventions as part of a wider, multiphase research study has been highlighted; this would offer the dual benefits of ensuring person-centeredness and optimizing successful intervention uptake.[23]

Using EBCD, the experiences of those who use and deliver healthcare services are explored. Together, groups identify ways in which services can be adapted to improve those experiences. Traditionally, EBCD has been used as a service improvement technique focusing on the experiences and emotions of healthcare service users. It has done this through eliciting the points in the patient pathway where people's experiences of services are defined. These key points are variously referred to as "moments of truth" or "touchpoints," and those who developed the method emphasized its focus on designing experiences rather than processes.[24]

EBCD was first developed and piloted in 2005–2006 in a UK head and neck cancer service.[25] This work identified touchpoints related to the physical environment in which care was experienced, for example, a queuing system for clinical check-in confused and embarrassed patients. Other examples were weighing patients in a public place, and patients had problems reaching the bedside bell to attract attention when experiencing postoperative problems.[25] The language used and the style of conversation between staff and patients also featured as a touchpoint for patients in this project.

Since this first study, EBCD has been widely used: a 2013 survey found that 59 EBCD projects had been conducted or were underway in the UK, Australia, New Zealand, Canada, Sweden and the Netherlands for a range of services and conditions. These included palliative care, neonatal care, orthopedics, cancer, mental health, and diabetes.[26] At this time there were no EBCD studies focusing solely on the medication management system. A 2020 systematic review of published studies included one study focusing on multimorbid patients for whom managing polypharmacy was a priority.[27]

Harnessing EBCD in wider health research processes

Traditionally sited within single services or settings, EBCD has successfully yielded improvements through enhanced patient and staff involvement, grounded in the experiences of those delivering and receiving care in those places. The method has been adapted as part of a UK National Institute of Health Research Programme Grant for use in intervention development which is:

- embedded within a larger program of research,
- across multiple sites, and
- across transitions of care which form structural gaps in the safety and continuity of care.[28]

This research project adapted EBCD to provide a systematic way to prioritize the real-world problems experienced universally by patients in the management of their medications, which were common across the study sites. It included a range of stakeholders in intervention design, focusing on the parts of the system where change could help improve both patient experience and safety. The resulting intervention (the Medicines at Transitions Intervention) was mapped onto behavior change techniques[29] to understand its causal mechanisms. It then underwent feasibility testing,[30] and is now the subject of a national clinical cluster randomized control trial and process evaluation in 42 healthcare areas.[31]

The co-designed intervention included:

- patient-held information about their medications including a traffic light system of symptoms and a checklist of care that should take place while in hospital,
- a scripted introduction to the information by healthcare teams,
- transfer of discharge medications information to community pharmacy, and
- community pharmacy medications reconciliation and follow-up conversations.

Each component of the intervention was mapped onto the taxonomy of behavior change techniques to understand how those components could effect change, whether it be through helping patients understand changes to their medications, how they could identify problems such as incorrect prescriptions or if they started to become unwell, or to provide practical support in managing medications. The outcome measures of interest were all cause mortality and readmission to hospital, along with secondary outcomes of knowledge of medications.

What are the stages of EBCD?

There are several, well-documented stages to delivering EBCD which usually take up to one year to complete.[32] However, an accelerated version of EBCD exists to facilitate completing the process within a shorter timeframe.[33] Importantly, patients should be full partners in this process and be represented on the project steering group, and not just participants in the co-design stages. A full EBCD toolkit, is available online, which takes users through how EBCD works as a service improvement tool.[34]

In short, the main full EBCD stages comprise:

1. Project set-up, including establishing a steering group and training of staff and patient representatives.
2. Observations of service delivery. Observations can be conducted in different settings, for example in hospital, ward observations can shed light on the way care is delivered to patients. This could include the degree of patient involvement in conversations about medications, or how supplies are obtained by patients. In the community, observations can take place in clinics, in community pharmacies, or in GP practices.
3. Staff and patient interviews to understand experiences of giving and receiving care and to identify emotional touchpoints.
4. Patient interviews are filmed, and a short (20–30 min) trigger film is produced that communicates their experiences and the impacts of the emotional touchpoints on them. The trigger film is particularly effective at communicating aspects of the patient experience that are usually invisible to staff. For example, hospital staff may not be aware of how confused patients can be about their medications once they are at home after being discharged, or the errors that patients experience, such as mistakes in repeat prescriptions following an admission to hospital.
5. Group meetings with staff to review the evidence from observations and interviews and suggest priorities for change.
6. Group meetings with patients to view the trigger film, create an emotional map for their care experiences and suggest priorities for change.
7. A joint event during which staff and patients watch and discuss the trigger film and then agree priorities for service improvement.

8. Facilitated, co-design groups including patients and staff, work on creating tools or redesign services to address the agreed priorities.
9. A celebration event to reflect on the EBCD process and recognize the achievements of staff and patients who took part.

Adapting EBCD for intervention development and testing as part of a multiphase project

The MRC guideline for intervention development, evaluation and implementation process in healthcare comprises five main stages:

1. development,
2. piloting and feasibility,
3. evaluation,
4. reporting and
5. implementation.[35,36]

EBCD sits well within the development phase of the process, although it should be combined with essential steps of:

- identifying the evidence base in the relevant area (through conducting or identifying a systematic review), and
- conducting empirical research to inform the theory of change for the resulting intervention.

EBCD interviews with patients and healthcare staff plus observations can be deployed as empirical research with those the intervention will target and those who will deliver it. For example, in the early stages of a project to develop an intervention to support safe medications management at transitions of care for older people with frailty, Tomlinson et al. (2020) conducted a systematic review to establish the characteristics of effective interventions.[37] The team then used the interview stage of EBCD to conduct qualitative research in two healthcare areas with older people after discharge from hospital, analyzed using the Framework method.[38] Interviews generated an EBCD trigger film as well as a robust evidence base to support the process of change, which could then be mapped on to existing change theories (see *Combining EBCD with different theories and methods for intervention development* and Table 5 *for a case example*).

Methodological considerations

When designing research incorporating EBCD, methodological considerations need to be considered. These hallmark the project as research. For example, as a research project, the research settings need to be chosen so that they represent a wider population, rather than focusing on a local problem to initiate a quality improvement program. In this way, the transferability of the qualitative results can be optimized. To develop a medication management intervention that has the potential to be implementable for a wider population, selecting multiple sites so that different site characteristics that may influence service delivery and patient experiences may be important. For example, in our recent study, four different acute secondary care sites were selected to conduct the qualitative phase to capture variations in practice, local pathways and patient population.[6] Further to this, patient and staff sampling frames will need to represent the wider population, rather than just service users. The stages, purpose, and outputs of intervention development using EBCD are outlined in Fig. 1. The interviews that feed into the production of the trigger film are analyzed qualitatively to produce a research evidence base. As the project is research rather than local quality improvement, the necessary ethical opinions and approval must be sought.

Analysis of the interview data can be supported by appropriate methods, for example, Framework[38] or thematic analysis.[40] The interview data can also be combined and synthesized with data from observational research and routine data sources, such a local and national policies. This can be conducted across multiple settings to create a more robust research project and an intervention that can implemented in diverse environments. All the available data might be considered as forming a bounded case-study.[41] What range of data types are used and how it is combined will reflect the purpose of the research project and the ontological or epistemological assumptions of the various stakeholders.

The separate patient, staff, and joint events can bring together individuals associated with multiple healthcare organizations. This is beneficial when considering healthcare at transitions and where the patient pathway is complex.[42] However, the priorities agreed and potential solutions designed may reflect a particular context and local processes. In other words, the solutions designed may require further adaptation for implementation across a system of care or in different geographies.

Users and carers who experience the whole care pathway may easily appreciate the usefulness of multisite EBCD that brings together different parts of a system. The philosophy of bringing stakeholders from along the care pathway together fits with the concept of integrated care systems[43] and the smoothing out of transitions between levels of care. However,

FIG. 1 Stages, purpose and outputs of multisite intervention development using Experience Based Co-Design (EBCD).

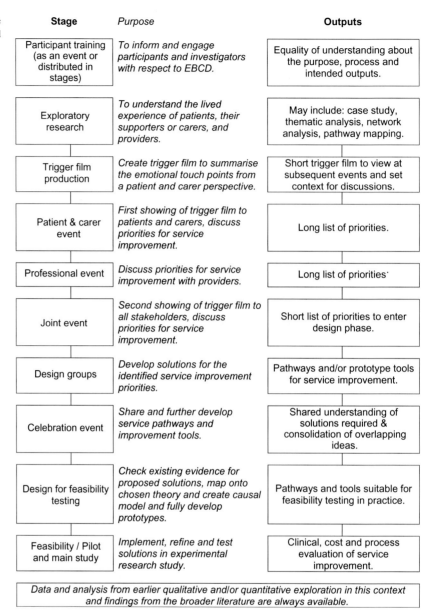

Stage	Purpose	Outputs
Participant training (as an event or distributed in stages)	To inform and engage participants and investigators with respect to EBCD.	Equality of understanding about the purpose, process and intended outputs.
Exploratory research	To understand the lived experience of patients, their supporters or carers, and providers.	May include: case study, thematic analysis, network analysis, pathway mapping.
Trigger film production	Create trigger film to summarise the emotional touch points from a patient and carer perspective.	Short trigger film to view at subsequent events and set context for discussions.
Patient & carer event	First showing of trigger film to patients and carers, discuss priorities for service improvement.	Long list of priorities.
Professional event	Discuss priorities for service improvement with providers.	Long list of priorities·
Joint event	Second showing of trigger film to all stakeholders, discuss priorities for service improvement.	Short list of priorities to enter design phase.
Design groups	Develop solutions for the identified service improvement priorities.	Pathways and/or prototype tools for service improvement.
Celebration event	Share and further develop service pathways and improvement tools.	Shared understanding of solutions required & consolidation of overlapping ideas.
Design for feasibility testing	Check existing evidence for proposed solutions, map onto chosen theory and create causal model and fully develop prototypes.	Pathways and tools suitable for feasibility testing in practice.
Feasibility / Pilot and main study	Implement, refine and test solutions in experimental research study.	Clinical, cost and process evaluation of service improvement.

Data and analysis from earlier qualitative and/or quantitative exploration in this context and findings from the broader literature are always available.

some may be more interested in local service improvement. Moreover, healthcare staff may be less invested in discussions that do not directly influence their immediate working environment or the parts of the pathway that they usually see. When adapting for a multisite research project with plans for a future large-scale evaluation, the scope to make local improvements as a result of EBCD should be agreed with each site. Changes to local practice may be deemed necessary after staff and patients view the trigger film and take part in co-design activities. However, changes made might preclude those sites from participating in future evaluations because their model of usual care may change to be too close to the intervention being trialed.

The success of multisite EBCD depends on the identification of willing volunteers with the time and experience to work for the common good. Clearly, some incentives and adaptations are required to cover stakeholder expenses and provide universal access to meeting locations.

Ethical considerations

Careful thought needs to be given to any ethical factors which will require approval before the study begins. It is, therefore, recommended to discuss the project's requirements with the study Sponsor.

As well as the typical considerations for conducting interviews and observations (e.g., how participants will be accessed for recruitment, consent procedures, data management, and storage), specific attention must be given to the trigger film (Step 4). Participants will need to be made aware that their involvement will potentially render them identifiable to those who view the film during the co-design. Researchers may like to suggest adjustments to maintain privacy if required and appropriate, e.g., filming from behind the individual so that their face cannot be seen. As with all other aspects of their involvement, participants must provide written consent to video record their interviews. They will also need to give their consent for its use within the EBCD sessions. It is also worth considering whether the film may be used within the public domain for other purposes outside of the research. For example, the film may have a value for education and training. Here, advice should be taken on how to appropriately seek permission to share audio-visual data from specialist organizations, such as the UK Data Service, which may include seeking approval from the participant to assign they copyright that they hold in the film to the researchers. Again, participants will need to provide written consent for this.

Finally, researchers need to consider the well-being of their participants and how their involvement in the EBCD events may impact on them. For example, discussing their personal experiences may cause some emotional distress, and facilitators will need to have a plan in place to ensure they can respond to and address any concerns, e.g., by signposting to additional support resources.

EBCD is a sequential process (Fig. 1). Each step has defined outputs which are reviewed and built on in the subsequent steps. EBCD is to an extent "self-healing" and incorporates reflection.

- This means participants have ample opportunities to suggest, create and refine ideas, whether these relate to problems (priorities) or solutions.
- It also carefully builds stakeholder consensus while privileging the views and experience of service users.
- It has the capacity to "bring along" divergent viewpoints and individuals.
- The entire process is conducted transparently, and participants can readily see if their suggestions influence the deliverables at each step.

In our experience, the trigger film is the key that unlocks common purpose and joint effort. This model of intervention development ensures that the overall objective of change (improved care for patients) is not lost and that, if needed, focus can easily be restored.

Accommodating local variation

When using EBCD as part of the process of development for complex interventions, some care is necessary to ensure that proposed solutions are realistic and tractable in multiple locations where they may need to adapt to local requirements. For example, the APEASE criteria (affordability, practicability, effectiveness and cost-effectiveness, acceptability, side-effects and safety, equity)[39] can be applied using consensus methods[44] and/or expert judgment. EBCD allows creative solutions to flow from service participants; however, research considerations require that these solutions are screened and validated. When EBCD is used for quality improvement in a single location any implementation issues can be easily resolved in the next rapid iteration, for example using PDSA cycles.[45] However, when a complex intervention is being developed for trial, the proposed interventions arising from EBCD will be fixed within the evaluation study protocol and fidelity to the intervention will be assessed during the trial phase. The intervention developed may, however, need to be flexible enough to be delivered in different sites and to allow for contextual factors, and here an implementation framework would be useful. The feasibility study stage consolidates knowledge of how the intervention can accommodate such local variation. These differences are highlighted in Table 2.

A useful step is the production of logic models[47,48] for all elements of the complex intervention and completion of a TIDieR checklist.[49] The logic model(s) will relate the practical aspects of the intervention to underpinning theories or mechanisms and outcomes that have previously been achieved. Intervention development will usually conclude with the production of an intervention manual to instruct those responsible for implementation.[50]

An overview of the materials necessary for implementing EBCD as a research project is shown in Table 3.

Face-to-face meetings can pose general difficulties for some of the populations who would most benefit from interventions to improve medication safety. For example, those who live with multimorbidities and frailty and people who may have recently been treated in hospital. Facilitators need adaptive skills in the online environment to ensure:

(a) everyone feels safe and respected and
(b) everyone has an equal opportunity to contribute.

TABLE 2 Differences in flexibility of interventions developed through EBCD for local improvement and for multisite evaluation.

EBCD for local quality improvement	EBCD for interventions for multisite evaluation
Changes can be made quickly, and differences observed.	Once the trial study protocol is set and patients are recruited, interventions cannot easily be changed.
Implementation can be managed locally.	Intervention may need to be flexible to adapt to local contexts, such as the type of staff involved in delivery. A multisite feasibility study can help understand the flexibility needed to implement the intervention more widely.
Local testing/feedback can offer an assessment of whether the intervention improves experiences.[46]	No assumptions are made about whether the intervention is effective in advance of the trial results.
The site may continue to deliver the improved service.	No sites will continue to deliver the intervention once trial data is collected.

TABLE 3 Stages to integrate EBCD into an intervention development and evaluation research project.

Stage	Adaptations and research methods needed
Research design phase	• Identify or conduct a literature review • Specify your research questions and objectives • Empirical research design including selecting the underpinning theories, selection of research sites to represent populations of interest and to capture different models of care delivery, sample design, data collection plan and analysis methods • Ethical and governance approvals
Non-participant observations	• Observations are performed by researchers rather than service providers • Information sheets and consent forms for observations • Observation schedule (based on the theoretical approach taken) • Field note booklets
Staff qualitative interviews	• Interview guide (informed by the theoretical approach taken) • Information sheets and consent forms • Audio recording devices
Patient/carer qualitative interviews	• Interview guide (informed by the theoretical approach taken) • Information sheets and consent forms • Audio and video recording devices
Synthesis and qualitative analysis	• Data collected from observations and interviews are analyzed using qualitative methods, such as Framework analysis,[38] or narrative analysis which can elicit meaning from patient and staff stories[51] • medication safety and continuity research programs have used qualitative research as the first stage of EBCD[6,52]
Trigger film editing	• The trigger film is edited from the video recordings of patient interviews focusing on emotional touch points • A patient representative should be involved in helping identify the relevant parts of the footage • This stage is managed separately from the synthesis and qualitative analysis of observations and patient and staff interviews. The film should tell the story of how patients experience the care they receive rather than the story of the data analysis

TABLE 3 Stages to integrate EBCD into an intervention development and evaluation research project—cont'd

Stage	Adaptations and research methods needed
Patient feedback event	• This event supports patients in an emotional mapping of their care journey and setting priorities for change • Taking careful notes of the emotional maps and priorities is essential • You may run more than one of these events depending on the number of sites
Staff feedback event	• This event offers feedback on research findings and support priority setting • You should document the priorities for change generated by staff
Joint event	• Document the agreed priorities and how they have been allocated
Co-design groups	• Participants are facilitated to develop prototypes or plans for change, which can be mapped onto the priorities generated. Teams can use a range of creative methods, such as character vignettes to aid their thinking, and craft materials or props can be used to help realize prototype interventions. Patients really want to be listened to and enjoy being practical, hands on, and seeing the results of their work • Prototypes from different groups can be broken down into components and compared against the evidence-base generated from qualitative research and systematic review
Building the intervention	• Components that will form the intervention can be agreed through stakeholder consensus, for example through an expert panel of patients and healthcare staff. Each component can be rated against specific criteria agreed by the wider research team and patient advisers. One such set of criteria to assess the components are the APEASE criteria: affordability; practicability; effectiveness and cost-effectiveness; acceptability; side-effects and safety; equity[39]
Intervention mapping	• Logic models[47] or a theory of change[48] can be developed using frameworks such as the Behavior Change Technique Taxonomy[29]
User-testing, feasibility study and intervention refinement	• User-testing of patient-facing tools such as medication information and a feasibility-testing phase will explore how your intervention will operate in a clinical environment • Sites should be chosen to reflect diversity in population and models of care delivery so that necessary adaptations can be identified for a multisite trial • Observations and qualitative research with patient and healthcare staff will uncover important barriers and facilitators to successful intervention implementation • A TIDieR checklist[49] can be used to describe the refined intervention and a user guide developed for implementation

These principles are broadly the same as in face-to-face meetings but operationalized differently online. If people do not have access to technology, then this can be provided or loaned, and Internet access can be supported. The costs of loans and network access (if necessary) remain lower than those associated with face-to-face methods, for example, the costs of room hire and transport.

Combining EBCD with behavior change theories and methods for intervention development

Researchers will often use underpinning theories to help them design their studies, interpret the data, and to help them understand phenomena.[53] Intervention development should be underpinned by a sound theoretical basis as this is more likely to result in effective design and implementation.[9] Many studies have used theory in this way to inform the design of their interventions by considering all influential factors. Some studies may choose to underpin their intervention design by implementation theory (e.g., the Consolidated Framework for Implementation Research),[54] which looks at system wide factors that can help with the uptake of new interventions. Others, such as ours, may choose to use behavior change theory to identify the behavioral barriers and enablers which the intervention can be designed to target.

TABLE 4 Synergistic use of EBCD and theories of behavior change.

Step of behavior change theory-informed intervention design	How EBCD can be used
Identify the key determinants of behavior	• EBCD participants review the trigger film and generate emotional touchpoints, which can also come from their own experiences. • Priorities for improvement are identified from the touchpoints that the researcher needs to then consider in terms of behavior.
Identify the techniques that target these determinants	• EBCD participants can select techniques (e.g., validated lists, literature search) they feel would be most efficacious in the given context, based on their personal experiences.
Model to fit the target population, culture and context	• Design of the intervention content closely involves those that will deliver (healthcare staff) and receive the service (staff or patients). • Event activities designed to elicit perspectives on acceptability, practicality and cost-effectiveness.

Kok et al. (2016) state that effective interventions will:

● target key determinants that predict the behavior that needs to change,
● use techniques that are able to modify key determinants, and
● fit the target population, culture and context.[55]

Clearly, co-design with patients and healthcare staff is beneficial and useful in achieving these ideals. EBCD, used as a research method for intervention design, rather than service improvement, is different as it will often first require the identification or development of appropriate theory. This can somewhat complicate the EBCD process as the researcher needs to find methods of synthesizing their chosen theory with EBCD output. The theory needs to underpin the methods of EBCD, as well as inform the design of the intervention. An example of the combination of theory and EBCD is presented in Table 4.

There are many theories which can be used to help make sense of intervention design and a discussion of them all is outside the scope of this chapter. The focus here is on the application of behavior change theory within EBCD, through the use of:

● the Theoretical Domains Framework (TDF),[56]
● the Behavior Change Technique Taxonomy (BCTT),[29] and
● the COM-B model[39]

We have chosen to underpin our intervention development of a care transition intervention for older people living with frailty with behavior change theory, namely because we want someone (a patient, family carer, or healthcare professional) to do something differently to promote medication safety. We have detailed the stages we undertook to develop the intervention in Table 5. Here, we have applied behavior change theory to help identify the barriers and facilitators to performing

TABLE 5 Case example—developing an intervention at transitions of care for older frail patients with diabetes.

Intervention development stage	Processes and outcomes
1: Systematic review and meta-analysis analysis	To establish the characteristics of effective interventions. The review demonstrated that interventions that bridged the care transition for up to 90 days were more likely to support successful care transitions for this population. The metaanalysis demonstrated that reduced hospital readmissions were associated with self-management activities, telephone follow up, and medication reconciliation.[37]
2: Qualitative research to understand patient experiences	Conducted with patients over 75 years of age living with frailty and with diabetes (n = 27) and their family carers (n = 9), admitted to one of two acute healthcare trusts.[7] Interviews took place at three time points: approximately two weeks after hospital discharge, then at two months, and finally six months after discharge. Interviews were audio and video recorded. Data were analyzed using the Framework method.[38]

TABLE 5 Case example—developing an intervention at transitions of care for older frail patients with diabetes—cont'd

Intervention development stage	Processes and outcomes
3: Creating the EBCD trigger film	Films made during the qualitative interviews were edited to make a 26-min EBCD trigger film presenting patient experiences with their medication during the care transition.
4: Patient and staff meetings	The trigger film was used in separate patient/carer and staff meetings, to generate discussion and to support emotional mapping and priority setting. A long list of key areas for improvement was generated. These meetings were held in the two healthcare regions in which the study was set.
5: Joint patient and staff meetings	Joint patient and staff meetings were held in the two healthcare regions to agree a shortlist of priorities from those discussed at the separate events. The trigger film was shown again at these meetings to help focus meeting activities. Priorities focused on better conversations about medication throughout the patient journey, more thorough assessment and person-centered resolution of any identified support needs and postdischarge follow up.
6: Identifying behavior change techniques	A pool of behavior change techniques likely to be effective for our study population and their corresponding target TDF domains were identified from analysis of behavioral determinants within our interviews. This pool was refined and agreed through expert consensus, guided by the APEASE criteria.[39] Experts were made aware of findings from Stage 1 during their consensus exercises. Eight potential behavior change techniques were identified.
7: Co-design meetings	Three co design meetings took place with patients, carers and staff. During the first meeting, each priority was reviewed in turn and participants suggested as many ideas as possible to help improve current practice. In the second meeting, these ideas were refined, thinking about the patients who would use the intervention and the staff who could deliver it. The final meeting further worked up these potential intervention components, identifying specifically who would need to do what and when. Throughout this process, the research team ensured that the meetings were guided by the findings from Stages 1 and 6. Three potential intervention components were designed, which were underpinned by all eight behavior change techniques and target TDF domains identified at Stage 6.

the chosen behavior (e.g., adherence, safe prescribing habits etc.) and prioritize suitable evidence-based intervention components that will promote your target behavior by overcoming the barriers and enhancing the facilitators. The TDF, BCTT, and COM-B are all potential tools that can be used to underpin EBCD methods. How we have applied these theories to our EBCD work is demonstrated in Table 6. By bringing theory into the EBCD process, participants are provided with an opportunity to interrogate academic processes of intervention design, and cognitively challenge what the theory tells us is the right course of action.

TABLE 6 Combining EBCD with behavior change theories to underpin intervention design.

Tool	Brief description	Suggestions for application	Considerations
Theoretical Domains Framework (TDF)[56]	A validated, broad framework of 14 (originally 12) theoretical constructs (e.g., skills, knowledge, emotion, etc.) relevant to behavior change determinants, identified from 33 theories.	• Researchers map the determinants of behavior arising from the qualitative interviews to the constructs of the TDF. • This is validated by EBCD participants, giving an understanding of the barriers and enablers to behavior change which can help prioritize the intervention mode of action and content.	• EBCD participants may need some training to help support this level of analysis. • Using the TDF allows participants to consider a wide range of factors that can affect behavior.
Behavior Change Technique Taxonomy[29]	A list of 93 behavior change techniques (BCTs), categorized into 16 clusters, linked to each theoretical construct of the TDF.	• Key determinants of behavior can be transparently and systematically mapped (via the TDF) to appropriate behavior change techniques that are likely to result in behavior change.	• The taxonomy is developed from public health interventions so some will not be relevant in your context.

Continued

TABLE 6 Combining EBCD with behavior change theories to underpin intervention design—cont'd

Tool	Brief description	Suggestions for application	Considerations
		• EBCD participants can then develop the intervention using these as a starting point.	• Some BCTs might be challenging to operationalize in real-life practice.
COM-B model[39]	Framework that considers the capability, opportunity and motivation that drives behavior. This is positioned within nine intervention functions and seven policy categories that could enable the intervention to occur.	• Participants can offer unique insights into capability, opportunity and motivation factors. • They are prompted to consider which functions and policy categories would be useful to promote behavior change based on their experiences of care.	• A broad model that considers the concepts and contexts necessary for intervention design. • Can be considered reductionist however, and therefore nuanced meaning can be lost.

TDF, theoretical domains framework; *COM-B*, capability, opportunity, motivation—behavior; *BCT*, behavior change technique; *EBCD*, experience-based co-design.

Skills needed for successful intervention development using EBCD

From our experience in delivering multiple EBCD research projects, we have developed a set of recommendations for the key skills needed in an EBCD research team. A highly collaborative, multidisciplinary team that includes patient/service user advisors is necessary. First of all, fieldwork skills are crucial to the initial drawing out of the experiences of patients and carers and to observe care environments. In these areas, the intersection between EBCD and traditional research methods is clear: qualitative interviewing skills, nonparticipant observation skills and the ability to manage, analyze, and synthesize data. Secondly, the ability to tell a story of the experience of care is crucial. This is done through exploring the emotional map of care with patients and through translating that story to the trigger film and to presentations at the EBCD joint event.

Facilitation at EBCD meetings is important to enable people to put forward their views of care and to make sure everyone's voices are heard. Good facilitation is needed to set priorities for improvement and during co-design sessions. It is necessary to consider the need to draw out the experiences of some patients who may be unwilling, in formal settings, to share their anxieties about how they can access services. Enabling staff to share their views honestly about the limitations of what they can provide is also a key skill.

Bringing on board an expert design team to help bring co-design groups' ideas to life is an essential step. We have found that both patients and staff are bounded by the horizons of what they feel the health service can achieve and by their own experiences of receiving and delivering care. For example, we have found that co-design groups have favored developing information booklets to support use of medication because they are used to giving or being given information, despite the evidence that this is not always effective. To help break though this, we think designers can bring ideas to life in unexpected ways, for example through helping co-design groups visualize solutions for medication management differently.

Engaging patients and service users from the planning stage of the project supports focusing the study on issues that are important to patients, developing study materials, advise on recruitment, coediting the trigger film, advising on recruitment, and interpretation of results. Patients have supported us throughout the lifecycle of several EBCD projects, one of which has developed an intervention for clinical trial. Patients in this group, all heart failure patients or carers, have also been coanalysts of data collected during the trial's qualitative process evaluation.

Finally, it is important to ensure the research team has access to collaborators with the appropriate skills to map the intervention onto the chosen theory or framework, understand the mechanisms with which it will effect change and how that change can be evaluated. Having a clearly documented and measurable outcome derived from the early empirical research, literature review and stakeholder conversations will aid this process.

Summary

EBCD has been recognized as being a collaborative approach to improving healthcare services that puts patients and healthcare staff at the heart of initiatives and potential changes and, as such, it is preferable to top-down service reorganization approaches. We have demonstrated how EBCD can be integrated into a research project that aims to develop and test an intervention to enhance the safety and continuity of medication management and suggested how existing research approaches can be assimilated into EBCD stages. We have also suggested where behavior change theories can be used to inform EBCD and to better understand intervention change mechanisms.

Questions for further discussion

1. What aspects of medication management in your local services would benefit from a co-design approach to intervention development?
2. Which organizations would need to work together to develop such an approach?
3. Who are your key stakeholders and how might you encourage them to take part in your EBCD project?
4. What do you consider to be the main ethical considerations for your study?

Application exercise/scenario

1. Consider older patients living with diabetes in your practice setting. What are the outcomes that patients care about and what clinical indicators are monitored? Are the outcomes and indicators currently optimized? Do you have reports or concerns about quality, safety or unexplained variations in care?
2. For your older patients with diabetes, what do the care pathways look like? Who is involved in routine care? How often are patients reviewed? Who are patients referred to when there are clinical problems? Who are the stakeholders that would provide information about service review and take part in service improvement?
3. Imagine that your stakeholders have met to review the care pathways for older patients with diabetes. What do you think the emotional touch points might be? How might they suggest the service is improved? What is your organization's capacity for change and collaboration?
4. At an individual level (professional and patient) what are the barriers to change? Consider aspects of capability, opportunity and motivation. Identify barriers that might be experienced by staff and by patients.
5. What types of information and resources would be needed to support change in your organization and along the care pathway? Are patients themselves considered to be part of the system? Are you committed to shared decision making?

Acknowledgments

We would like to thank Professor Peter Gardner for his help in commenting on the final draft. We also thank members of our patient steering group for their support through the study on which this article is based. We also thank Dr. Kate Karban and Mrs. Heather Smith for their expert advice.

This chapter presents work funded by the National Institute for Health Research (NIHR) under its Research for Patient Benefit (RfPB) Programme (Grants PB-PG-0317-20010 and NIHR201056). This work was also funded by the NIHR Yorkshire and Humber Patient Safety Translational Research Centre and by the NIHR Programme Grants for Applied Research (Grant RP-PG-0514-20009). The views expressed in this chapter are those of the authors and not necessarily those of the NIHR or the Department of Health and Social Care.

References

1. Campbell M, Fitzpatrick R, Haines A, et al. Framework for design and evaluation of complex interventions to improve health. *BMJ*. 2000;321:694. https://doi.org/10.1136/bmj.321.7262.694.
2. Nilsen P. Making sense of implementation theories, models and frameworks. *Implement Sci*. 2015;10:53. https://doi.org/10.1186/s13012-015-0242-0.
3. Elliott RA, Camacho E, Jankovic D, Sculpher MJ, Faria R. Economic analysis of the prevalence and clinical and economic burden of medication error in England. *BMJ Qual Saf*. 2021;30:96–105.
4. Ryan R, Santesso N, Lowe D, et al. Interventions to improve safe and effective medicines use by consumers: an overview of systematic reviews. *Cochrane Database Syst Rev*. 2014;(4). https://doi.org/10.1002/14651858.CD007768.pub3.
5. Fylan B, Armitage G, Naylor D, Blenkinsopp A. A qualitative study of patient involvement in medicines management after hospital discharge: an under-recognised source of systems resilience. *BMJ Qual Saf*. 2018;27(7):539–546. https://doi.org/10.1136/bmjqs-2017-006813.
6. Fylan B, Marques I, Ismail H, et al. Gaps, traps, bridges and props: a mixed-methods study of resilience in the medicines management system for patients with heart failure at hospital discharge. *BMJ Open*. 2019;9(2). https://doi.org/10.1136/bmjopen-2018-023440.
7. Tomlinson J, Silcock J, Smith H, Karban K, Fylan B. Post-discharge medicines management: the experiences, perceptions and roles of older people and their family carers. *Health Expect*. 2020;23:1603–1613. https://doi.org/10.1111/hex.13145.
8. Doyle C, Lennox L, Bell D. A systematic review of evidence on the links between patient experience and clinical safety and effectiveness. *BMJ Open*. 2013;3(1):1–18. https://doi.org/10.1136/bmjopen-2012-001570.

9. Skivington K, Matthews L, Simpson SA, et al. A new framework for developing and evaluating complex interventions: update of Medical Research Council guidance. *BMJ*. 2021;374:n2061. https://doi.org/10.1136/bmj.n2061.

10. Glidewell L, Willis TA, Petty D, et al. To what extent can behaviour change techniques be identified within an adaptable implementation package for primary care? A prospective directed content analysis. *Implement Sci*. 2018;13:32. https://doi.org/10.1186/s13012-017-0704-7.

11. Patton DE, Cadogan CA, Ryan C, et al. Improving adherence to multiple medications in older people in primary care: selecting intervention components to address patient-reported barriers and facilitators. *Health Expect*. 2018;21(1):138–148. https://doi.org/10.1111/hex.12595.

12. O'Cathain A, Croot L, Sworn K, et al. Taxonomy of approaches to developing interventions to improve health: a systematic methods overview. *Pilot Feasibility Stud*. 2019;5:41. https://doi.org/10.1186/s40814-019-0425-6.

13. Ward ME, De Brún A, Beirne D, et al. Using co-design to develop a collective leadership intervention for healthcare teams to improve safety culture. *Int J Environ Res Public Health*. 2018;15(6):1182. https://doi.org/10.3390/ijerph15061182.

14. Lee Y. Design participation tactics: the challenges and new roles for designers in the co-design process. *CoDesign*. 2008;4(1):31–50. https://doi.org/10.1080/15710880701875613.

15. Steen M, Manschot M, Koning ND. Benefits of co-design in service design projects. *Int J Des*. 2011;5(2):53–60.

16. Boyd H, McKernon S, Mullin B, Old A. Improving healthcare through the use of co-design. *N Z Med J*. 2012;125(1357):76–87.

17. Castro EM, Malfait S, Van Regenmortel T, Van Hecke A, Sermeus W, Vanhaecht K. Co-design for implementing patient participation in hospital services: a discussion paper. *Patient Educ Couns*. 2018;101(7):1302–1305. https://doi.org/10.1016/j.pec.2018.03.019.

18. Palmer VJ, Weavell W, Callander R, et al. The participatory zeitgeist: an explanatory theoretical model of change in an era of coproduction and codesign in healthcare improvement. *Med Humanit*. 2019;45:247–257. https://doi.org/10.1136/medhum-2017-011398.

19. Hahn-Goldberg S, Okrainec K, Huynh T, Zahr N, Abrams H. Co-creating patient-oriented discharge instructions with patients, caregivers, and healthcare providers. *J Hosp Med*. 2020;10(12):804–807. https://doi.org/10.1002/jhm.2444.

20. Tsianakas V, Robert G, Richardson A, et al. Enhancing the experience of carers in the chemotherapy outpatient setting: an exploratory randomised controlled trial to test impact, acceptability and feasibility of a complex intervention co-designed by carers and staff. *Support Care Cancer*. 2015;23(10):3069–3080. https://doi.org/10.1007/s00520-015-2677-x.

21. Bate P, Robert G. Experience-based design: from redesigning the system around the patient to co-designing services with the patient. *Qual Saf Health Care*. 2006;15(5):307–310. https://doi.org/10.1136/qshc.2005.016527.

22. Donetto S, Pierri P, Tsianakas V, Robert G. Experience-based co-design and healthcare improvement: realizing participatory design in the public sector. *Des J*. 2015;18(2):227–248. https://doi.org/10.2752/175630615x14212498964312.

23. Green T, Bonner A, Teleni L, et al. Use and reporting of experience-based codesign studies in the healthcare setting: a systematic review. *BMJ Qual Saf*. 2020;29:64–76. https://doi.org/10.1136/bmjqs-2019-009570.

24. Bate P, Robert G. *Bringing User Experience to Healthcare Improvement*. Abingdon: Radcliffe Publishing Ltd; 2007.

25. Bate P, Robert G. Toward more user-centric OD: lessons from the field of experience-based design and a case study. *J Appl Behav Sci*. 2007;43(1):41–66. https://doi.org/10.1177/0021886306297014.

26. Donetto S, Tsianakas V, Robert G. *Using Experience-Based co-Design to Improve the Quality of Healthcare: Mapping where we Are Now and Establishing Future Directions*. London: King's College London; 2014. https://www.kcl.ac.uk/nmpc/research/nnru/publications/reports/ebcd-where-are-we-now-report.pdf/. Accessed 20 November 2020.

27. Knowles S, Hays R, Senra H, et al. Empowering people to help speak up about safety in primary care: using codesign to involve patients and professionals in developing new interventions for patients with multimorbidity. *Health Expect*. 2018;21:539–548. https://doi.org/10.1111/hex.12648.

28. Raynor DK, Ismail H, Blenkinsopp A, Fylan B, Armitage G, Silcock J. Experience-based co-design-adapting the method for a researcher-initiated study in a multi-site setting. *Health Expect*. 2020;23:562–570. https://doi.org/10.1111/hex.13028.

29. Michie S, Richardson M, Johnston M, et al. The behavior change technique taxonomy (v1) of 93 hierarchically clustered techniques: building an international consensus for the reporting of behavior change interventions. *Ann Behav Med*. 2013;46(1):81–95. https://doi.org/10.1007/s12160-013-9486-6.

30. Fylan B, Ismail H, Hartley S, et al. A non-randomised feasibility study of an intervention to optimise medicines at transitions of care for patients with heart failure. *Pilot Feasibility Stud*. 2021;7:85. https://doi.org/10.1186/s40814-021-00819-x.

31. Powell C, Breen L, Fylan B, et al. Improving the safety and continuity of medicines management at transitions of care (ISCOMAT): protocol for a process evaluation of a cluster randomised control trial. *BMJ Open*. 2020;10. https://doi.org/10.1136/bmjopen-2020-040493, e040493.

32. Robert G, Cornwell J, Locock L, Purushotham A, Sturmey G, Gager M. Patients and staff as codesigners of healthcare services. *BMJ*. 2015;350. https://doi.org/10.1136/bmj.g7714, g7714.

33. Locock L, Robert G, Boaz A, et al. *Testing Accelerated Experience-Based Co-Design: A Qualitative Study of Using a National Archive of Patient Experience Narrative Interviews to Promote Rapid Patient-Centred Service Improvement*. Southampton, UK: NIHR Journals Library; 2014. https://www.ncbi.nlm.nih.gov/books/NBK259580/.

34. EBCD: Experience-based co-design toolkit. *The Point of Care Foundation*; 2020. https://www.pointofcarefoundation.org.uk/resource/experience-based-co-design-ebcd-toolkit/. Accessed 12 November 2020.

35. Craig P, Deippe P, Macintyre S, Michie S, Nazareth I, M.P. *Developing and Evaluating Complex Interventions New Guidance*. Medical Research Council; 2019. https://mrc.ukri.org/documents/pdf/developing-and-evaluating-complex-interventions/. Accessed 20 November 2020.

36. Craig P, Dieppe P, Macintyre S, et al. Developing and evaluating complex interventions: the new Medical Research Council guidance. *BMJ*. 2008;337. https://doi.org/10.1136/bmj.a1655, a1655.

37. Tomlinson J, Cheong V-L, Fylan B, et al. Successful care transitions for older people: a systematic review and meta-analysis of the effects of interventions that support medication continuity. *Age Ageing*. 2020;49(4):558–569. https://doi.org/10.1093/ageing/afaa002.

38. Gale NK, Heath G, Cameron E, Rashid S, Redwood S. Using the framework method for the analysis of qualitative data in multi-disciplinary health research. *BMC Med Res Methodol*. 2013;13(1):117. https://doi.org/10.1186/1471-2288-13-117.

39. Michie S, Atkins L, West R. *The Behaviour Change Wheel: A Guide to Designing Interventions*. London: Silverback Publishing; 2014.

40. Braun V, Clarke V. Using thematic analysis in psychology. *Qual Res Psychol*. 2006;3(2):77–101. https://doi.org/10.1191/1478088706qp063oa.

41. Harrison H, Birks M, Franklin R, Mills J. Case study research: foundations and methodological orientation. *Forum Qual Soc Res*. 2017;18(1): Art19. https://doi.org/10.17169/fqs-18.1.2655.

42. Fylan B, Tranmer M, Armitage G, Blenkinsopp A. Cardiology patients' medicines management networks after hospital discharge: a mixed methods analysis of a complex adaptive system. *Res Soc Adm Pharm*. 2019;15(5):505–513. https://doi.org/10.1016/j.sapharm.2018.06.016.

43. *Integrated Care Systems Explained. The King's Fund*; 2021. https://www.kingsfund.org.uk/publications/integrated-care-systems-explained;. Accessed 15 May 2021.

44. Jones J, Hunter D. Qualitative research: consensus methods for medical and health services research. *BMJ*. 1995;311:376–380. https://doi.org/10.1136/bmj.311.7001.376.

45. *Institute for Healthcare Improvement. How to Improve*; 2021. http://www.ihi.org/resources/Pages/HowtoImprove/ScienceofImprovementTesting Changes.aspx/;. Accessed 12 May 2021.

46. Springham N, Robert G. Experience based co-design reduces formal complaints on an acute mental health ward. *BMJ Open Qual*. 2015;4. https://doi.org/10.1136/bmjquality.u209153.w3970, u209153.w3970.

47. Mills T, Lawton R, Sheard L. Advancing complexity science in healthcare research: the logic of logic models. *BMC Med Res Methodol*. 2019;19:55. https://doi.org/10.1186/s12874-019-0701-4.

48. O'Cathain A, Croot L, Duncan E, et al. Guidance on how to develop complex interventions to improve health and healthcare. *BMJ Open*. 2019;9. https://doi.org/10.1136/bmjopen-2019-029954, e029954.

49. Hoffmann TC, Glasziou PP, Boutron I, et al. Better reporting of interventions: template for intervention description and replication (TIDieR) checklist and guide. *BMJ*. 2014;348. https://doi.org/10.1136/bmj.g1687, g1687.

50. Hoddinott P. A new era for intervention development studies. *Pilot Feasibility Stud*. 2015;1:36. https://doi.org/10.1186/s40814-015-0032-0.

51. Wong G, Breheny M. Narrative analysis in health psychology: a guide for analysis. *Health Psychol Behav Med*. 2018;6(1):245–261. https://doi.org/10.1080/21642850.2018.1515017.

52. Tomlinson J, Silcock J, Smith H, Karban K, Fylan B. Post-discharge medicines management: the experiences, perceptions and role of older people and their family carers. *Health Expect*. 2020;23:1603–1613. https://doi.org/10.1111/hex.13145.

53. Winit-Watjana W. Research philosophy in pharmacy practice: necessity and relevance. *Int J Pharm Pract*. 2016;24(6):428–436. https://doi.org/10.1111/ijpp.12281.

54. Damschroder LJ, Aron DC, Keith RE, et al. Fostering implementation of health services research findings into practice: a consolidated framework for advancing implementation science. *Implement Sci*. 2009;4:50. https://doi.org/10.1186/1748-5908-4-50.

55. Kok G, Gottlieb NH, Peters GJ, et al. A taxonomy of behaviour change methods: an intervention mapping approach. *Health Psychol Rev*. 2016;10 (3):297–312. https://doi.org/10.1080/17437199.2015.1077155.

56. Michie S, Johnston M, Abraham C, et al. Making psychological theory useful for implementing evidence based practice: a consensus approach. *Qual Saf Health Care*. 2005;14(1):26–33. https://doi.org/10.1136/qshc.2004.011155.

Chapter 3

Use of common models to inform and design pharmacy and health services research

Anandi V. Law[a] and Marcia M. Worley[b]

[a]*Department of Pharmacy Practice and Administration, College of Pharmacy, Western University of Health Sciences, Pomona, CA, United States,*
[b]*Division of Outcomes and Translational Sciences, The Ohio State University, College of Pharmacy, Columbus, OH, United States*

Objectives

- Define the terms theory, model, and framework within health care research.
- Describe common theories, models, and frameworks that have been used and tested in health care research.
- Describe the steps in developing an idea to operationalization, implementation, testing, and analyzing results; on the springboard of a theory, model, or framework.
- Explain the conversion of results into meaningful applications for patient care, behavioral change, practice advancement, policy, and future research.
- Describe common pitfalls during the process and pearls for success.

Experience by itself teaches nothing…Without theory, experience has no meaning. Without theory, one has no questions to ask. Hence without theory there is no learning.

W. Edwards Deming.

Define the terms theory, framework, and model within health care research

Most, if not all, pharmacy and health services researchers are familiar with terminology such as ***theory***, ***framework***, and ***model***. It is helpful, however, to start with a refresher to serve as a foundation for this chapter.

A ***theory*** is defined as "a plausible or scientifically acceptable general principle or body of principles offered to explain phenomena."[1] Shelby Hunt (1991) adds that a theory "must be capable of explaining and predicting real-world phenomena."[2] Theories can never be proven, but can be supported or refuted by a body of evidence generated from empirical testing.[2]

Researchers can use ***frameworks*** when they are trying to organize concepts that are relevant to their research question(s) and the purpose of their research project. This can be considered a ***conceptual framework***. Often, a theory, or set of theories, can be used as a method to organize and represent the concepts in a framework. In other words, theories can help explain the relationships among the concepts and serve as an underpinning in the framework, which is then described as a ***theoretical framework***. In this case, the theory can be helpful to develop the framework and ground the research project.[3] A useful way to think about this is while a **theory** might seem more abstract, ***frameworks*** (conceptual and/or theoretical) provide a more practical approach to connect the concepts in a logical and meaningful way. Whether you use a theory or framework, ***models*** can be used to visually depict relationships between and among study variables or constructs. Relationships in a model can be supported by empirical evidence in the literature and can also be supported by existing theory/theories. Researchers can test models statistically (e.g., path analysis, structural equation modeling) to see if study data fit the proposed model and can also propose new or alternative models based on their own study results.

In the beginning stages of a project, researchers often begin with an idea or concept that is spurred from reading the literature, from an observation in pharmacy practice, or through an experience. A thorough literature review should be the next step and will aid in developing these ideas and concepts into research question(s). The literature review also helps in identifying a framework or theory that relates to the research questions. The framework or theory serves as the "scaffolding" or "structure" around the research concepts and provides support for the research question(s) that the researcher is investigating. As the researcher reviews the possible relationships that can exist between the study concepts, variables (independent, dependent, preceding) and constructs can be identified in the literature. Models depicting directional relationships are then specified or hypothesized between these variables and/or constructs using support from the theory or framework. Oftentimes, the researcher can find an existing theory/framework/model in the literature to use in their project or can modify or adapt for use in their project. Thus, a theory or framework becomes the foundation for the project.

When a researcher conducts exploratory research, where the goal is to gain an initial understanding around an idea or concept, using a framework is still a good idea and again serves as a structure and grounds the researcher's work. Such grounding with a theory or framework helps the researcher interpret and give meaning to study results and helps avoid the trap of "fishing" for meaning in the results when data analysis is conducted.

Practical example: The authors of this chapter sought to develop a tool to identify and address barriers to patient medication adherence.[4] The authors and their research team began their project by conducting a literature review to better understand which theories/frameworks/models have been used by researchers in this domain. As the Health Belief Model has been widely applied to study medication adherence in a variety of conditions, the decision was made to use this model as a part of the research project.[5] However, the authors also wanted to understand if patient medication use expectations could help to predict medication adherence behavior. The work of Dolovich et al. was used, who developed a theoretical model that included patient expectations.[6] To develop the study model, constructs were used from both of these models. After substantial model testing and refinement, this work eventually resulted in the development of a patient-centered medication adherence tool called the Modified Drug Adherence Work-up (M-DRAW) Tool.[4]

Practical Example: When developing a health-related quality of life tool, the domains of health have been used as a framework to build items, including the core of Physical, Mental, and Social domains. For example, the PROMIS® (Patient-Reported Outcomes Measurement Information System) evaluates and monitors physical, mental, and social health in adults and children.[7]

Describe various theories, models, and frameworks that have been used and tested in health care research

This section focuses on the prominent and most commonly used theories, models and frameworks used in health care research, highlighting examples in pharmacy practice and patient care.

Health Belief Model (fondly known as HBM within the research community) by Irwin Rosenstock is perhaps among the oldest in origin and very widely known. It was initially developed in the early 1950s to help explain preventive health behavior and later utilized to understand and predict behavior change for a variety of health behaviors.[8]

As seen in Fig. 1, the model proposes that the likelihood of preventive health behavior or a change in behavior is based on the individual's *"Perceived Benefits"* of behavior modification and *"Perceived Threats"* from the condition, filtered through the information they have regarding the condition and its impact called *"Cues to Action"* and perceptions of their innate ability and control to change their behavior *(Self-efficacy)*. The concept of perceived threat itself is predicated by their *perceived susceptibility* of acquiring the disease and *perceived severity* of its impact on them. It encompasses environmental and individual factors in explaining behavioral change.

The HBM has been used in a variety of applications including screening preventive behavior in smoking cessation, HIV/AIDS, nutritional interventions, self-care with osteoporosis, and explaining sexual education, to name a few.[9–11] Evidence suggests its robustness and hence it has been used widely.[12]

The model itself has been modified by various researchers especially in placing cues to action and self-efficacy. These differences in placement of variables account for one of the limitations of this model. Another limitation cited is that it does not account for social factors impacting behavior.[13]

Practical example: A recent example of the use of this model has been in explaining the factors and barriers impacting the likelihood of getting vaccinated (influenza and COVID-19 vaccine). In this study, the authors found that the HBM helped in predicting vaccine intention for influenza and COVID-19. As seen below, results showed that modifying factors and cues to action significantly impacted individual perceptions of which perceived benefits and barriers influenced

Concept	Definition	Application
Perceived susceptibility	Belief about the chances of experiencing a risk or getting a condition or disease	Define population(s) at risk, risk levels
		Personailze risk based on a person's characteristics or behavior
		Make perceived susceptibiilty more consistent with individual's actual risk
Perceived severity	Belief about how serious a condition and its sequelae are	Specify consequences o risks and conditions
Perceived benefits	Belief in efficacy of the advised action to reduce risk or seriousness of impact	Define action to take: how, where, when; clarify the positive effects to be expected
Perceived barriers	Belief about the tangible and psychological costs of the advised action	Identify and reduce perceived barriers through reassurance, correction of misinformation, incentives, assistance
Cues to action	Strategies to activate "readiness"	Provide how-to information, promote awareness, use appropriate reminder systems
Self-efficacy	Confidence in one's ability to take action	Provide training and guidance in performing recommended action
		Use progressive goal setting
		Give verbal reinforcement
		Demonstrate desired behaviors
		Reduce anxiety

FIG. 1 Concepts of health belief model. *(Adapted from Glanz K, Rimer BK, Viswanath K, eds. Health Behavior and Health Education: Theory, Research, and Practice. 4th ed. p. 498.)*

intention but not perceived threats. The authors also proposed a new mediator (Decision-Making Determinant) that when tested, did not successfully impact the behavioral intention (Fig. 2).[14]

The Theory of Reasoned Action (TRA): This theory, developed by Martin Fishbein and Icek Ajzen, proposed that the intention to perform a behavior is a result of attitudes and subjective norms.[15] *Attitudes* are influenced by a combination of *Behavioral Beliefs* (whether the behavior will lead to an outcome) and *Evaluation of Outcomes* (whether the outcome will be positive or negative).[16] *Subjective norms* refer to the influence of social peers (family, friends, etc.) on the acceptability or approval of the behavior. It is impacted by *normative beliefs* of the group, and *motivation to comply* with these views of social peers. These two factors in turn are a result of external variables such as demographic and personality influences. The model differentiates between *intention to behave* and actual *behavior*, stating that the intention is based on the weights of attitude and subjective norms.[17,18]

TRA has been tested in various settings in consumer behavior and also in health behavior such as HPV vaccinations, condom use, etc.[19] Some of the challenges to the TRA have been in social norms playing a larger role in reality than suggested by the theory. This point is highlighted with the crosswalk between social and cultural norms impacting behavior. Other questions concern the weak correlation between intention and behavior that has been found in studies that use the theory.[20]

The Theory of Planned Behavior (TPB): This theory added to the TRA described above with a construct called *perceived control* seen in blue in the Fig. 3, which is preceded by *control beliefs* and *perceived power*.[21] The additions

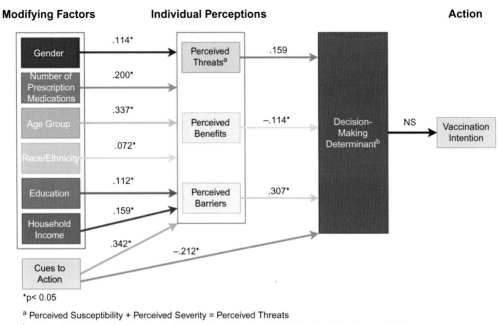

FIG. 2 Testing a modified health belief model for intention to vaccinate.[15]

were made to increase the predictive ability of the TRA. The TPB bases its model on the three beliefs impacting behavior: behavioral, norms and control. It posits that *behavioral beliefs* decide the attitude toward the behavior, i.e., if the behavior will produce a certain outcome. *Normative beliefs* relate to subjective norms or social norms which are societal expectations of behavior as perceived by an individual. Finally, *control beliefs* pertain to one's ability to have control in performing the behavior. *Perceived behavioral control* refers to the degree to which a person believes that they can

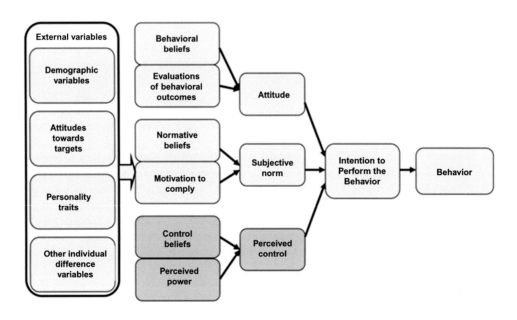

FIG. 3 Theory of reasoned action and theory of planned behavior. *(From Glanz K, Rimer BK, Viswanath K, eds. Health Behavior and Health Education: Theory, Research, and Practice. 4th ed.)*

perform a given behavior. This last concept is drawn from self-efficacy, introduced by Bandura's social cognitive theory.[22]

Practical example: Among the different applications of TPB is one centered on pharmacist intention to provide education on medication disposal. In this study, items were adopted from literature and customized to pharmacists and aspects of medication disposal. The survey of community pharmacists found that there was intention to provide such education to their patients. Reliability of this survey was moderate. Attitude, subjective norm, and perceived behavioral control were all significant predictors of the intention, totaling to 40% of explained variance in intention to provide education on medication disposal.

TPB has shown to have better predictability than TRA in health behavior such as condom use, weight loss, diet and exercise, to name a few.[19,23–26] However, it also struggles with the correlation between intention and behavior similar to TRA, perhaps due to its exclusion of factors such as the need to sometimes perform behavior even if there is little intention due social acceptability (an example is teenagers experimenting with street drugs to "fit in" even if they do not really intend to do drugs). Additional views propose that the relationships may not be unidirectional and may have some feedback mechanisms.

Social Cognitive Theory (SCT) was proposed by Bandura in the 1970s and derives from the Social Learning Theory he developed in the early 1960s.[22,27,28] Bandura's SCT proposes that humans learn through a variety of ways—cognitive factors, interactions with their environment, and in response to their own and other's behaviors, with reciprocal and dynamic interactions occurring among these areas which serve as a catalyst to change behavior. As depicted in Fig. 4, health behaviors can be predicted by the interaction of a patient's *self-efficacy expectations*, *outcome expectations*, an evaluation of *barriers and facilitators* to engaging in the behavior, as well as *goal setting*.[29]

Two prominent components of SCT include *outcome expectations* and *self-efficacy expectations*, which are important to optimize to change patient behaviors. *Outcome expectations* focus on the patient's beliefs that engaging in a particular activity or behavior will result in positive health outcomes. *Self-efficacy expectations* describe the patient's confidence in their abilities to engage in an activity or behavior, as well as overcoming perceived barriers.[22,27] According to Bandura's SCT, both *outcome* and *self-efficacy expectations* need to be considered to truly understand and optimize goal setting and behavior. An important point to consider is that outcome and self-efficacy expectations are specific to a given behavior. For example, if a person has high self-efficacy to use an inhaler for asthma, they might not have high self-efficacy to commit to an exercise program. Additionally, a person could have high outcome expectations (beliefs) but could have low self-efficacy expectations (confidence in their ability to perform a behavior). According to SCT, both types of expectations—outcome and self-efficacy—would need to be aligned to result in behavior change. For example, a person could believe that using their insulin will help them better control their diabetes and have better health outcomes (outcome expectations), but they might lack the confidence that they are able to give their insulin shots correctly (self-efficacy expectations). Therefore, they are not able to give themselves an insulin injection (behavior). A critical point is that researchers

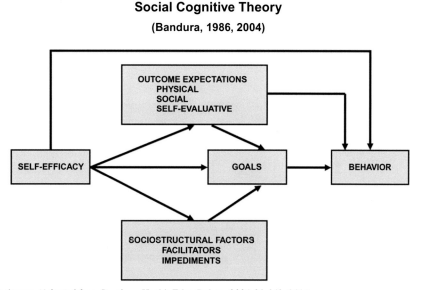

Social Cognitive Theory

(Bandura, 1986, 2004)

FIG. 4 Social cognitive theory. *(Adapted from Bandura.* Health Educ Behav. *2004;31:143–164.)*

should study both of these constructs to get a comprehensive understanding of how to change behavior. This will also help as results from studies are applied and used to design impactful tools and interventions to effect behavior change.

Through application of SCT, or using select components of SCT, researchers and practitioners have developed interventions and tools for use in health education programs to better understand, optimize, and change patient health behaviors. SCT, and in particular *self-efficacy expectations*, have been widely applied to a variety of disease states and conditions, such as weight loss, smoking cessation, contraceptive behavior, and medication use, to understand and design interventions in an attempt to modify patient behavior.[30]

Application of SCT in its entirety can be difficult, as the complexity of the theory can make it difficult to operationalize and develop measurement items for the constructs.[5] However, if a researcher only uses a part of SCT, for example *self-efficacy expectations*, this can result in an incomplete understanding of behavior change, which can be another criticism of SCT application to research projects.[28]

Practical example: In a study by Worley and Hermansen-Kobulnicky (2008), these authors used survey research methodology to examine how outcome and self-efficacy expectations for medication management and self-monitoring of patients with diabetes varied by different pharmacist-patient relationship indicators.[31] Results from their study support an association between self-efficacy expectations and stronger elements of the pharmacist-patient relationship. Although these authors only used two components of SCT in their study—outcome and self-efficacy expectations as they relate to a person's medication management, this was done purposefully in order to gain an initial understanding of how these constructs impact medication management, considering the impact of the pharmacist-patient relationship.

Other Models: Although there are many other theories, frameworks, and models that are used in health care research, the aforementioned appear more commonly in social administrative sciences research. The less commonly cited theories/frameworks/models are briefly described below.

Transtheoretical Model of Change (TTM): The TTM was proposed by Prochaska and colleagues in the 1970s where behavioral change was defined as a process involving progress through a series of stages.[32] These stages include *precontemplation, contemplation, preparation, action, maintenance,* and *termination*.[33] Although it is the most definitive and well known theory that details the proposed steps involved in behavior change, it has received criticism because it assumes that these stages are distinct and follow a chronology. For example, it has been used in explaining stress management, weight management, smoking cessation, and adherence to medication.[34–37] These processes are considered multidimensional and involve some overlapping stages in behavior. Assuming that they only occur sequentially in that order may not represent them accurately. In addition, the time intervals that the TTM suggests do not seem based on any strong evidence (Fig. 5).

PRECEDE-PROCEED: The PRECEDE-PROCEED model is a framework intended to help in health program planning, policy making and evaluation.[38] The acronym PRECEDE involves educational parameters and stands for *Predisposing Reinforcing* and *Enabling* Constructs in Educational Diagnosis and Evaluation. The PROCEED has an educational perspective and stands *for Policy, Regulatory and Organizational* Constructs in Educational and Environmental

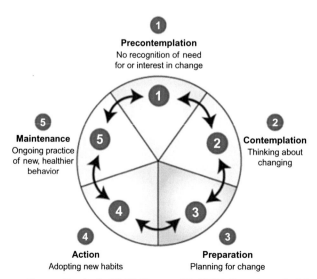

FIG. 5   Transtheoretical model of change. *(Source: Prochaska JO, Di Clemente CC. (1982). Transtheoretical therapy: toward a more integrative model of change. Psychother Theory Res Pract. 1982;19(3):276–288, Fig. 2, p. 283.)*

Development. This model has been used for creating community and public health interventions. It assumes that behavior change is voluntary and can be impacted by both environmental and individual factors.

Diffusion of Innovation: Diffusion of Innovation—This theory, proposed by Everett Rogers, presents the factors that determine the adoption of an innovation by individuals and organizations.[39] It names factors such as innovation, communication channels, time and a social system and accordingly categorizes consumers as *innovators, early adopters, early majority and laggards*. The theory suggests five stages that the adoption of innovation process goes through—knowledge/awareness, persuasion, decision, implementation, and confirmation/continuation. It has been used very widely in areas of communication, policy, technology and public health.[40–42] Although it has been used to understand the area, the theory faces a few criticisms; one is the assumption of a sequential nature of the process of diffusion, another is the one way communication approach of the theory within the proliferation of complex channels such as cultural and social media networks.[43]

Describe the steps in developing an idea to operationalization, implementation, testing, and analyzing results; on the springboard of a theory, framework, or model

It can be a daunting task to think about clearly defining and operationalizing research question(s), as well as a myriad of other elements to consider in terms of data collection, participant recruitment, statistical methods, and the list goes on! It is important to spend time at the beginning of a research project, particularly when you are thinking about the research question(s) and study objectives, to thoughtfully consider whether using a framework, theory, and/or model, is appropriate for the type of research you plan to conduct. A common question that researchers are often faced with is "How do I determine which framework, theory, or model is the best or most appropriate for my project? Some key FAQs listed below may help demystify the process.

FAQs
1. Where do I start?

A thorough literature review is key to understand what frameworks/theories/models exist in the literature that could be applicable to your project. Think of keywords and search terms to use in publication database search engines that are related to your research question(s) and keep a list of these terms so you can assess to see if you have completed a comprehensive literature review using a variety of databases. It is a good idea to explore literature domains outside of pharmacy and health care research. You might find frameworks/theories/models that you can apply to projects in pharmacy and health care (e.g., relationship marketing, psychology).

Once you have identified the framework/theory/model, your next step will be to think about how you will measure items in the variables or constructs. You might be able to use existing measurement items, or you might need to adapt them for use in your project. For example, you might need to modify the wording for your respondents, setting, or medication type, etc. Another option would be to design measurement items from "scratch," in which you will need to consider the resources (time, personnel, financial) if you decide to pursue this avenue. Whether adapting/modifying or developing measurement items from scratch in your study, pilot testing is necessary to assess the reliability and validity of multiitem constructs. The aim is to make the theory/framework/model parsimonious, elegant, tested, generalizable, and plausible in your discipline or research area.

2. Should I develop my own model or framework, or should I use an existing model/framework in the literature? What if the model(s) I find in the literature do not align with my research question(s)?

It is important to use your research question(s) to guide you as you are deciding which model and/or framework to use for your project. As you are working through the decision-making process, revisit your research question(s) often and ask yourself *"Do the variables/constructs and their proposed relationships in the model/framework align with what I need to measure to answer my research question(s)?"*

In general, it is better to adapt an existing model or framework for your research project, rather than build a new model. It is important to consider that developing and testing a new model takes a lot of time, effort, and resources. Also, an existing model/framework will most likely have information available about the psychometric properties (e.g., reliability and validity), which will be important for you to examine. If you are using or adapting a model or framework from the literature, remember to ask the authors for permission to use their work in your project and how they would like to be referenced and have their work attributed.

You might need to add additional variables/constructs that are germane to your study and research question(s) that necessitate you making adaptations to an existing model/framework. It is acceptable to tweak models and test them, and this could result in important new contributions to the scientific literature. On the flip side, you might adapt and test a model and find that the model constructs and relationships don't hold true or predict relationships as you hypothesized. This can also be an important contribution to the scientific literature! Sometimes only a portion of a model/framework is applicable to your project and the decision is made to use a portion of it in your project. Be sure to evaluate the pros/cons of this approach and justify such a decision. As seen in the earlier discussion about the creation of M-DRAW, the authors adopted an existing, well-established model (HBM) and added a new element (medication use expectations) from a theoretical framework, as they developed their patient-centered medication adherence tool.

3. How do I test the model?

As with any research project, start with a comprehensive and detailed data analysis plan. Analysis will begin with response rate or respondent participation, to ascertain (normal) distribution of respondents. Testing any survey or model begins with psychometrics, for example, determining reliability and validity of the survey scale and items. Model testing can then proceed using Exploratory factor analysis (EFA) if it is a newly developed or adapted model. Confirmatory Factor Analysis (CFA) helps with testing the model relationships in an already validated model. Path analysis can be used to test individual relationships, while Structural Equation Modeling (SEM) works for testing all model relationships and directionality at once. Exploratory Factor Analysis (EFA), Confirmatory Factor Analysis (CFA), and Structural Equation Modeling (SEM) are all statistical techniques that can be used to develop models and to test competing models. Having a theory or framework as part of your research project will serve as a "structure" and guide you during the decision-making process as models and/or alternative/competing models are developed and tested. Having this in place is critical to the research process and will help "guide" you as data are used along with the framework/theory to build alternative or competing models. This is key to avoiding the trap of "data fishing" or letting the data drive decision making at this stage.

Explain the conversion of results into meaningful applications for patient care, behavioral change, practice advancement, policy, and future research

The use of theories, frameworks and models are important in health care research in order to plan programs or protocols, implement action plans, study their impact and predict outcomes for future work. "Theories and models help explain behavior, as well as suggest more effective ways to influence and change behavior." Theories can be used to **inform** a study or intervention, to **apply** parts or the entirety of the theory, to **test,** evaluate and compare.[44]

In effect, the Plan, Do, Check, Act framework helps understand the usability of models. Models have applicability to patient care in terms of planning and implementing protocols. For example, HBM or TPB can be used to test if interventions such as increasing awareness about medication regimens or using motivational interviewing can help improve intention to adhere to medication.

Planning a program that has not had precedents, especially in a current institutional setting is facilitated if there is a model that can be adapted. For example, in the recent COVID-19 pandemic, planning for vaccine roll out may have been efficient and effective with a model visualization at the national, state, and local levels. Using normative social models and ecological, environmental and social factors, vaccine behaviors among different demographics could be predicted.[45]

As previously mentioned, behavioral models have been used in health care programs and policies for planning, implementing, evaluating, and predicting areas such as vaccine use, smoking cessation, weight and stress management. Similarly HBM, TTM, and SCT have been used in public health policy making.[46]

Describe common pitfalls during the process and pearls for success

Some key take-aways or tips for success can be helpful to beginning researchers, particularly student pharmacists or graduate students beginning to learn about the research process. Experienced researchers who are mentoring students about the research process might also benefit from the following tips in their mentoring and teaching.

Tip #1: Know your literature! Dig deep and do a comprehensive literature review to understand the types of theories/frameworks/models that could be applicable to your research project. Learn from other researchers who have used a particular theory/framework/model in their project—What were their challenges/barriers? What worked well in terms of measurement and study methods? What did they learn from their results?

Tip #2: When you are trying to choose the theory or framework for your project, use what you have learned from the literature and do a thoughtful comparison of the pros/cons of different theories/frameworks/models that you have identified. Write down your justification! This can not only help with the decision-making process but can also help when you are preparing manuscripts and presentations about your research project, as you will need to explain your choice of theory/framework/model.

Tip #3: Using a framework, theory, and/or model in a research project can help to organize concepts, and aid in meaningful interpretation of and application of results to advance pharmacy practice, patient care, policy, and education. This applies to exploratory research as well.

Tip #4: Having strong knowledge in research methods, as well as statistical techniques and programs is always a good start. It is also a good idea to continue to retool and hone your skills in these areas, whether or not you are a beginning or seasoned researcher.

Tip #5: Use what you learn from application of a theory/framework/model in one project, to help inform the application in a subsequent project. Incremental gains in understanding of a phenomena—either as you hypothesized or not as you hypothesized when you began the study—can still be meaningful and add to the body of scientific literature and make important advancements to practice, patient care, policy, and education.

Summary

Theoretical models and frameworks are needed in research to understand how behaviors or interventions can be planned, implemented, tested, and evaluated. In effect, theories inform, explain, and help predict behaviors of individuals and organizations. A solid research question precedes use of a theory and needs to be followed by good research practices. Although theories are often considered academic, conceptual, and not grounded in reality, evidence shows that interventions and strategies based in theory are often more effective and defensible than those without. Most commonly used models in social and administrative pharmacy research include the Health Belief Model, Theory of Planned Behavior/Reasoned Action and Social Cognitive Theory. The guidance offered by existing empirically tested, validated and generalizable theories find their applications in practice, education, patient care and policy.

Questions for further discussion

1. Why do you need a theory/model or framework for your research?
2. How would you decide if using a theory/model or framework would be most appropriate for your study?
3. What are some common pitfalls to be aware of during the research study process? How would you traverse some of these pitfalls to ensure success of your study?

Application exercise/scenario

One of your Pharmacy Practice faculty colleagues who practices at an ambulatory care clinic is struggling to convince the local population to get their COVID-19 vaccine. The clinic is in an underserved area with a minoritized population of Hmongs. The faculty member has approached you, given your passion for health care education and community engagement-based research, to help develop a plan to address this issue. As you explore reasons for this hesitancy, it becomes clear there is not a lot of information regarding the attitudes, beliefs, preferences and health care behavior of this particular population. How would you design a research study to address the issue? What theory/model or framework might you use?

References

1. Available from: https://www.merriam-webster.com/dictionary/theory.
2. Hunt SH. Chapter 6: The morphology of theory. In: *Modern Marketing Theory: Critical Issues in the Philosophy of Marketing Science*. Cincinnati, OH: South-Western Publishing Co.; 1991.
3. Varpio L, Paradis E, Uijtdehaage S, Young M. The distinctions between theory, theoretical framework, and conceptual framework. *Acad Med.* 2020;95(7):989–994.
4. Lee S, Bae Y, Worley M, Law A. Validating the modified drug adherence work-up (M-Draw) tool to identify and address barriers to medication adherence. *Pharmacy.* 2017;5(3):52.
5. Munro S, Lewin S, Swart T, Volmink J. A review of health behaviour theories: how useful are these for developing interventions to promote long-term medication adherence for TB and HIV/AIDS? *BMC Public Health.* 2007;7:104.
6. Dolovich L, Nair K, Sellors C, Lohfeld L, Lee A, Levine M. Do patients' expectations influence their use of medications? Qualitative study. *Can Fam Physician.* 2008;54(3):384–393.
7. PROMIS. Available from: https://www.healthmeasures.net/explore-measurement-systems/promis?AspxAutoDetectCookieSup.
8. Rosenstock IM. Historical origins of the health belief model. *Health Educ Monogr.* 1974;2:328–335.

9. Rosenstock IM, Strecher VJ, Becker MH. In: Diclemente RJ, Peterson JL, eds. *The Health Belief Model and HIV Risk Behavior Change in Preventing AIDS. AIDS Prevention and Mental Health.* Boston, MA: Springer; 1994.

10. Glanz KB, Donald B. The role of behavioral science theory in development and implementation of public health interventions. *Annu Rev Public Health.* 2010;31:399–418.

11. Schmiege SJ, Aiken LS, Sander JL, Gerend MA. Osteoporosis prevention among young women: psychological models of calcium consumption and weight bearing exercise. *Health Psychol.* 2007;26:577–587.

12. Janz NK, Becker MH. The health belief model: a decade later. *Health Educ Behav.* 1984;11(1):1–47.

13. Jones CLJJ, Scherr CL, Brown NR, Christy K. Weaver the health belief model as an explanatory framework in communication research: exploring parallel, serial, and moderated mediation. *J Health Commun.* 2015;30(6):566–576.

14. Mercadante AR, Law A. Will they, or Won't they? Examining patients' vaccine intention for flu and COVID-19 using the health belief model. *Res Soc Adm Pharm.* 2020;20:31240–31247.

15. Azjen I, Madden TJ. Prediction of goal-directed behavior: attitudes, intentions, and perceived behavioral control. *J Exp Soc Psychol.* 1986;22(5):453–474.

16. Fishbein M, Ajzen I. *Belief, Attitude, Intention And Behavior.* Addison-Wesley; 1975.

17. Ajzen I, Albarracín D. In: Ajzen I, Albarracin D, Hornik R, eds. *Predicting and Changing Behavior: A Reasoned Action Approach.* Mahwah, NJ: Lawrence Erlbaum Associates Publishers; 2007.

18. Fishbein M. A behavior theory approach to the relations between beliefs about an object and the attitude toward the object. In: Fishbein M, ed. *Readings in Attitude Theory and Measurement.* New York: John Wiley & Sons; 1967.

19. Albarracin DJ, Johnson BT, Fishbein M, Muellerleile PA. Theories of reasoned action and planned behavior as models of condom use: a meta-analysis. *Psychol Bull.* 2001;127(1):142–161.

20. Norberg PA, Horne DR, Horne DA. The pr paradox: personal information disclosure intentions versus behaviors. *J Consum Aff.* 2007;41(1):100–126.

21. Ajzen I. From intentions to actions: a theory of planned behavior. In: Kuhl J, Beckmann J, eds. *Action Control: From Cognition to Behavior.* Berlin, Heidelber, New York: Springer-Verlag; 1985.

22. Bandura A. *Self-Efficacy: The Exercise of Control.* New York, NY: WH Freeman; 1997.

23. Sheeran P, Taylor S. Predicting intentions to use condoms: a meta-analysis and comparison of the theories of reasoned action and planned behavior. *J Appl Soc Psychol.* 1999;29(8):1624–1675.

24. Nguyen MN, Potyin L, Otis J. Regular exercise in 30-to 60-year-old men: combining the stages-of-change model and the theory of planned behavior to identify determinants for targeting heart health interventions. *J Community Health.* 1997;22(4):233–246.

25. Conner MK, Kirk SFL, Cade JE, Barrett JH. Environmental influences: factors influencing a woman's decision to use dietary supplements. *J Nutr.* 2003;133(6):1978S–1982S.

26. McConnon A, Raats M, Astrup A, et al. Application of the theory of planned behavior to weight control in an overweight cohort. Results from a pan-European dietary intervention trial (DiOGenes). *Appetite.* 2012;58(1):313–318.

27. Bandura A. Self-efficacy: toward a unifying theory of behavioral change. *Psychol Rev.* 1977;84(2):191–215.

28. Baranowski T, Perry CL, Parcel GS. How individuals, environments, and health behavior interact. In: Glanz K, Lewis FM, Rimer BK, eds. *Health Behavior and Health Education.* San Francisco: Jossey-Bass Publishers; 2002.

29. Bandura A. Health promotion by social cognitive means. *Health Educ Behav.* 2004;31(2):143–164.

30. Strecher VJ, DeVellis BM, Becker MH, Rosenstock IM. The role of self-efficacy in achieving health behavior change. *Health Educ Q.* 1986;13(1):73–91.

31. Worley MM, Hermansen-Kobulnicky CJ. Outcome and self-efficacy expectations for medication management of patients with diabetes: influence of the pharmacist-patient relationship. *J Am Pharm Assoc.* 2008;48(5):621–631.

32. Prochaska JO, Norcross JC. *Systems of Psychotherapy: A Transtheoretical Analysis.* 8th ed. Australia/Stamford, CT: Cengage Learning; 2014.

33. Prochaska J, Velicer WF. The transtheoretical model of health behavior change. *Am J Health Promot.* 1997;12(1):38–48.

34. Johnson SS, Driskell MM, Johnson JL, et al. Transtheoretical model intervention for adherence to lipid-lowering drugs. *Dis Manag.* 2006;9(2):102–114.

35. Levesque DA, Van Marter DF, Schneider RJ, et al. Randomized trial of a computer-tailored intervention for patients with depression. *Am J Health Promot.* 2011;26(2):77–89.

36. Johnson SS, Paiva AL, Cummins CO, et al. Transtheoretical model-based multiple behavior intervention for weight management: effectiveness on a population basis. *Prev Med.* 2008;46(3):238–246.

37. Prochaska JO, DiClemente CC, Velicer WF, Rossi JS. Standardized, individualized, interactive, and personalized self-help programs for smoking cessation. *Health Psychol.* 1993;12(5):399–405.

38. Green L, Kreuter M. *Health Program Planning: An Educational and Ecological Approach.* 4th ed. New York, NY: McGrawHill; 2005.

39. Rogers E. *Diffusion of Innovations.* 5th ed. Simon and Schuster; 2003.

40. Jordana J. The global diffusion of regulatory agencies: channels of transfer and stages of diffusion. *Comp Pol Stud.* 2011;44(10):1343–1369.

41. Eveland JD. Diffusion, technology transfer, and implementation: thinking and talking about change. *Sci Commun.* 1986;8(2):303–322.

42. Muhiuddin H, Kreps GL. Forty years of diffusion of innovations: utility and value in public health. *J Health Commun.* 2004;3–11.

43. Lyytinen J, Damsgaard K. What's wrong with the diffusion of innovation theory. In: Ardis MA, Marcolin BL, eds. *Diffusing Software Product and Process Innovations*; 2001.

44. *Guidelines.* Available from: https://obssr.od.nih.gov/wp-content/uploads/2016/05/Social-and-Behavioral-Theories.pdf.

45. *COVID-19 Guidelines.* Available from: https://obssr.od.nih.gov/wp-content/uploads/2020/12/COVIDReport_Final.pdf.

46. *Social Behavioral Theories.* Available from: https://obssr.od.nih.gov/wp-content/uploads/2016/05/Social-and-Behavioral-Theories.pdf.

Bibliography for each model in social and administrative sciences research (in primary journals RSAP and JAPhA) in the past 5 years

Health Belief Model

Moses M, Olenik NL. Perceived impact of caregiver's participation in diabetes education classes on implementation of self-care behaviors. *J Am Pharm Assoc.* 2019;59(4S):S47–S51.e1. https://doi.org/10.1016/j.japh.2019.05.014. 31279837.

Mills AR, Arnett SJ, Shan M, Simmons C, Miller ML. Perception of immunizations and vaccine recommendation sources for persons living with HIV compared with persons without HIV. *J Am Pharm Assoc.* 2019;59(4S):S39–S46. https://doi.org/10.1016/j.japh.2019.05.008. 31248848.

Haggerty LC, Gatewood SS, JKR G. Public attitudes and beliefs about Virginia community pharmacists dispensing and administering naloxone. *J Am Pharm Assoc.* 2018;58(4S):S73–S77.e1. https://doi.org/10.1016/j.japh.2018.04.034. 30006189.

Kelly KR, Fernandez Marriott JR, Moses MG, Golembeski DM, Olenik NL. Exploring diabetes management behaviors among varying health literacy levels: a qualitative analysis. *J Am Pharm Assoc.* 2021. https://doi.org/10.1016/j.japh.2021.01.019. 33551254.

Theory of Planned Behavior

Gupchup GV, Abhyankar UL, Worley MM, Raisch DW, Marfatia AA, Namdar R. Relationships between hispanic ethnicity and attitudes and beliefs towards herbal medicine use. *Res Soc Adm Pharm.* 2006;2:266–279.

Carico Jr RR, Sheppard J, Thomas CB. Community pharmacists and communication in the time of COVID-19: Applying the health belief model. *Res Soc Adm Pharm.* 2021;17(1):1984–1987. https://doi.org/10.1016/j.sapharm.2020.03.017. 32247680.

Mercadante AR, Law AV. Will they, or Won't they? Examining patients' vaccine intention for flu and COVID-19 using the Health Belief Model. *Res Soc Adm Pharm.* 2020. https://doi.org/10.1016/j.sapharm.2020.12.012. 33431259.

Jonkman LJ, Tsuchihashi K, Liu E, et al. Patient experiences in managing non-communicable diseases in Namibia. *Res Soc Adm Pharm.* 2020;16 (11):1550–1557. https://doi.org/10.1016/j.sapharm.2020.08.004. 32919919.

Sedrak A, Glewis S, Alexander M, Lingaratnam MS, Chiang C, Luetsch K. Cancer patients' perspectives on participating in a community pharmacy-based hyperglycaemia screening service – a qualitative exploration of enablers and barriers. *Res Soc Adm Pharm.* 2021;17(3):613–618. https://doi.org/10.1016/j.sapharm.2020.05.023. 32563743.

Fathian-Dastgerdi Z, Khoshgoftar M, Tavakoli B, Jaleh M. Factors associated with preventive behaviors of COVID-19 among adolescents: applying the health belief model. *Res Soc Adm Pharm.* 2021. https://doi.org/10.1016/j.sapharm.2021.01.014. 33558153.

Gülpınar G, Keleş Ş, Yalım NY. Perspectives of community pharmacists on conscientious objection to provide pharmacy services: a theory informed qualitative study. *J Am Pharm Assoc.* 2021. https://doi.org/10.1016/j.japh.2021.03.014. 33895101.

Adeoye OA, Lake LM, Lourens SG, Morris RE, Snyder ME. What predicts medication therapy management completion rates? The role of community pharmacy staff characteristics and beliefs about medication therapy management. *J Am Pharm Assoc.* 2018;58(4S):S7–S15.e5. https://doi.org/10.1016/j.japh.2018.03.001. 29731422.

Mospan CM, Balenger SB, Gillette C. Student pharmacists' perceptions regarding pharmacist-prescribed hormonal contraceptives and their professional responsibility. *J Am Pharm Assoc.* 2021;61(2):e145–e152. https://doi.org/10.1016/j.japh.2020.11.020. 33359118.

Lauzier S, Guillaumie L, Humphries B, Grégoire JP, Moisan J, Villeneuve D. Psychosocial factors associated with pharmacists' antidepressant drug treatment monitoring. *J Am Pharm Assoc.* 2020;60(4):548–558. https://doi.org/10.1016/j.japh.2020.01.007. 32173335.

George DL, Smith MJ, Draugalis JR, Tolma EL, Keast SL, Wilson JB. Community pharmacists' beliefs regarding improvement of Star Ratings scores using the Theory of Planned Behavior. *J Am Pharm Assoc.* 2018;58(1):21–29. https://doi.org/10.1016/j.japh.2017.09.001. 29074146.

Theory of Reasoned Action

Fleming ML, Driver L, Sansgiry SS, et al. Physicians' intention to prescribe hydrocodone combination products after rescheduling: a theory of reasoned action approach. *Res Soc Adm Pharm.* 2017. https://doi.org/10.1016/j.sapharm.2016.07.001. 27567741.

Social Cognitive Theory

Worley MM, Hermansen-Kobulnicky CJ. Outcome and self-efficacy expectations for medication management of patients with diabetes: influence of the pharmacist-patient relationship. *J Am Pharm Assoc.* 2008;48(5):621–631. Cope LC, Tully MP, Hall J. An exploration of the perceptions of non-medical prescribers, regarding their self-efficacy when prescribing, and their willingness to take responsibility for prescribing decisions. *Res Soc Adm Pharm.* 2020;16(2):249–256. https://doi.org/10.1016/j.sapharm.2019.05.013.

Cope LC, Tully MP, Hall J. An exploration of the perceptions of non-medical prescribers, regarding their self-efficacy when prescribing, and their willingness to take responsibility for prescribing decisions. *Res Soc Adm Pharm.* 2020. https://doi.org/10.1016/j.sapharm.2019.05.013. 31151918.

PRECEED-PROCEED

Handyside L, Warren R, Devine S, Drovandi A. Utilisation of the PRECEDE-PROCEED model in community pharmacy for health needs assessment: a narrative review. *Res Soc Adm Pharm.* 2021;17(2):292–299. https://doi.org/10.1016/j.sapharm.2020.03.021. 32253124.

Handyside L, Warren R, Devine S, Drovandi A. Health needs assessment in a regional community pharmacy using the PRECEDE-PROCEED model. *Res Soc Adm Pharm.* 2020. https://doi.org/10.1016/j.sapharm.2020.08.023. 32912831.

Transtheoretical Model of Change

Emonds EE, Pietruszka BL, Hawley CE, Triantafylidis LK, Roefaro J, Driver JA. There's no place like home-Integrating a pharmacist into the hospital-in-home model. *J Am Pharm Assoc.* 2021. https://doi.org/10.1016/j.japh.2021.01.003. 33551255.

Chapter 4

Implementation science to guide pharmacy and health services research

Victoria García-Cárdenas[a] and Kenneth C. Hohmeier[b]

[a]Graduate School of Health, Faculty of Health, University of Technology Sydney, Sydney, NSW, Australia, [b]University of Tennessee Health Science Center, College of Pharmacy, Memphis, TN, United States

Objectives

- Describe the role of implementation science in health services research.
- Identify the moderators that influence the implementation of innovations in health care settings.
- Describe the stages involved in the implementation of innovations.
- Identify outcome indicators and main study designs used in implementation research.
- Discuss the role of implementation strategies in health services research.

Introduction

One of the main challenges faced by health systems is the effective integration of evidence-based innovations into routine practice. Many health services interventions which have been shown to be efficacious in controlled research environments are often not implemented in health care settings.[1] It has been suggested that the implementation of innovations takes on average 17 years and that less than 50% of them are finally put into practice,[1] highlighting the complexity around implementation. Implementation is a common challenge for many professions, such as pharmacy, and is largely due to the absence of evidence-based implementation programs. This lag or ultimate lack of implementation entails negative consequences, both for the patient and for health systems. As a consequence, the extensive resources invested in the design and evaluation of health service innovations may not make the health impact for which they were developed. Importantly, determining an innovation's effectiveness does not ensure its integration into routine practice.[1] Nowadays, no one doubts that the design and evaluation of new services are only the first steps to be able to transfer these benefits to the population in a generalized way. In fact, some have gone so far as to posit that researchers should routinely include implementation measures in the design of their prospective effectiveness research studies so as to plan for eventual implementation, scale, and spread of the intervention.[2]

This chapter aims to provide an overview of the different approaches used in implementation research. The chapter starts with presenting an overview of the moderators that influence the implementation of innovations in health care settings. The stages involved in the implementation of innovations, potential outcome indicators used to evaluate implementation programs and implementation strategies are discussed. The different types of implementation-hybrid designs commonly used in implementation research and recommendations for reporting implementation research are presented. Finally, general recommendations to conduct implementation research are provided.

An overview of implementation science

Before the emergence of implementation science in the mid-2000s, health services researchers often assumed that the adoption and widespread implementation of services could be achieved through the generation of evidence (i.e., efficacy or effectiveness of a given service) followed by dissemination of information. This mainly involved communicating the key elements of a given service and its benefits to the different stakeholders involved in its provision. Today, it is well known that the dissemination of information by itself or the use of isolated strategies is not enough to achieve and maintain a service's long-term implementation.[3] Instead, it has been recognized that evidence-based implementation programs and

Contemporary Research Methods in Pharmacy and Health Services. https://doi.org/10.1016/B978-0-323-91888-6.00046-6

FIG. 1 Implementation research.

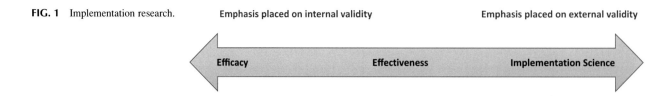

strategies are required for more rapid scale and spread.[3] For this reason, implementation science can be visualized as part of a spectrum of research modalities in which tightly controlled efficacy research experiments may be found on one side, and the more pragmatic, real-world implementation science research can be found on the opposite side (Fig. 1).[4]

It has been acknowledged that the incorporation and maintenance of innovations in any health care setting is a complex process, which requires implementation science for their effective integration. Although different definitions exist, a widely agreed definition for implementation science is "*the scientific study of methods to promote the systematic uptake of research findings and other evidence-based practice into routine practice and, hence, to improve the quality and effectiveness of health services.*"[5] Implementation science therefore embraces a wide range of research methods focused on improving the scaling up of effective behavioral, clinical, health care, public health, global health, and educational interventions with the ultimate objective of improving quality of care and health outcomes.[6] This requires the study of the different mechanisms through which knowledge and research outcomes (often generated in efficacy or effectiveness trials) can be translated into routine scenarios. Based on this need, a range of theoretical frameworks have been developed and tested with the ultimate objective to explain and facilitate the implementation of innovations in different settings. A widely cited narrative literature review identified different conceptual approaches for the implementation of innovations.[7] Authors classified these into different categories according to their main aim,[7] including *process models* (aimed at describing or guiding the implementation process through different stages), *evaluation frameworks* (whose main objective is to offer a guide for the evaluation of the implementation) and *determinants frameworks*, *classic theories*, and implementation *theories* (that aim to understand and explain what moderates implementation outcomes). How all these approaches are applied closely depends on the implementation research question. However, a range of criteria have been published to assist researchers in identifying an appropriate approach, instead of using theories that are convenient but not appropriate to meet the research objectives.[8,9] A summary of implementation frameworks alongside some examples is presented in Table 1.

Theories, models, and frameworks in implementation research

Factors that moderate the implementation of innovations in healthcare

There are three main categories used to describe the factors which influence implementation outcomes: *determinant frameworks*, *classic theories*, and *implementation theories*. These frameworks and theories aim to describe and explain the determinants (independent variables) that influence the implementation process and outcomes (dependent variables). These determinants (also called implementation factors or constructs) are elements that moderate an innovation's

TABLE 1 Summary of implementation theories, models, and frameworks.

Type	Objective	Examples
Determinants frameworks, classic theories, and implementation theories	To describe and explain what moderates implementation outcomes	Consolidated Framework for Implementation Research (CFIR),[10] Promoting Action on Research Implementation in Health Services (PARIHS),[11] Tailored Implementation for Chronic Diseases (TICD).[12]
Process models	To describe or guide the implementation process (usually through a number of stages)	Knowledge to action model, Quality implementation framework,[13] Exploration, Adoption/Preparation, Implementation, Sustainment model (EPIS),[a,14] and the Generic Implementation Framework (GIF).[15]
Evaluation frameworks	To guide the evaluation of the implementation	Reach Effectiveness Adoption Implementation Maintenance (RE-AIM),[16] Implementation outcomes framework.[17]

[a]*Some frameworks, models, or theories such as EPIS may fit in more than one category*
Adapted from Nilsen P. Making sense of implementation theories, models and frameworks. Implement Sci. 2015;10:1–13. doi:10.1186/s13012-015-0242-0.

implementation, either acting as barriers (exerting a negative moderation of the implementation), or as facilitators (exercising a positive moderation of the implementation of the service), interacting with each other through complex cause-effect mechanisms.[18]

Numerous implementation factors have been described in the literature.[10] These are usually distributed across different domains, which are generally related to: the intervention being implemented, the inner and outer setting or context, the individuals involved in the implementation or the implementation process.[10] However, it should be noted that these domains may vary between authors. The intervention domain encompasses implementation factors related to the innovation being implemented such as complexity or adaptability.[10] The inner context domain covers factors related to the specific setting in which the service is being implemented, such as the organization's culture, climate, or leadership.[10] The outer context refers to the characteristics of the specific context surrounding the setting in which the innovation is being implemented.[10] This domain includes the patient characteristics or the availability of funding or incentives, among others. The domain of the individuals involved in the implementation include factors like personal attributes or perceived self-efficacy to achieve implementation goals.[10] Finally, factors associated with the implementation process often include opinion leaders or external change facilitators.[10] Examples of factors alongside their definitions can be found in the CFIR (https://cfirguide.org) and EPIS (https://episframework.com) websites.

Implementation process: From exploration to sustainability

According to Nilsen,[7] process models are used to describe and guide the implementation of an innovation through different stages. Some authors[14,15] have suggested these stages do not have to be consecutive during the implementation process and therefore describe the stages in a nonlinear way. Some of these stages are described below.[14]

- *Exploration.* During the exploration stage, the organization in which the innovation is to be implemented (e.g., a community pharmacy implementing a professional service) and implementers or decision-makers (e.g., pharmacy owner or manager), evaluate the need to implement a certain evidence-based innovation aimed at addressing a local need. Implementation opportunities and barriers (e.g., the characteristics of the service to be implemented, the balance between the possible benefits and harms of the implementation, the associated costs, or the necessary resources, among others) are usually evaluated during this phase.[14] This phase ends with the decision to adopt or reject the service.
- *Preparation (also called installation).* During the preparation phase, implementers plan for integrating the evidence-based innovation into the organization. As part of this phase relevant implementation factors are evaluated and strategies are implemented accordingly. This process is usually undertaken by internal champions (e.g., who lead the implementation process) or external agents (e.g., practice change facilitators, change agents or coaches).
- *Trial (also called initial implementation).* During this phase, omitted in some models, the objective is to test the provision of the service in a limited sample. This allows for a preliminary evaluation of the strategies implemented during the preparation phase and whether alternative strategies or new interventions are required.
- *Implementation (also called full implementation).* During the implementation phase, the innovation is integrated into the daily practice of the organization. During this phase, relevant implementation factors continue to be monitored. Processes and implementation outcomes are also evaluated.
- *Sustainment (also called sustainability or maintenance).* During this phase, the innovation previously integrated in the organization is routinized and institutionalized over time. The objective is to maintain the expected results of the service for all the agents involved in it (e.g., patients, providers, policy-makers). However, some authors consider sustainment as an independent phase or even consider it as an implementation result.[19]

Implementation outcome indicators

It is essential to note that implementation outcomes are different outcomes to those used in determining the efficacy or effectiveness of the evidence-based practice itself. This is because in evidence-based practice research it is the outcome of the evidence-based practice which is being evaluated, whereas in implementation science research the strategy used to implement the evidence-based practice is the objective being evaluated. As previously mentioned, *evaluation frameworks* offer a guide for evaluating the implementation of an innovation or service.[7] Such evaluation can be undertaken using a range of outcome indicators, which have been defined in the literature as "*the effects of deliberate actions to implement new treatments, practices and services.*"[17] It should be noted that the core outcome set and definitions vary widely between frameworks. Nevertheless, it is imperative that outcome indicators be distinct from service and clinical outcomes. These indicators have been identified as essential elements in implementation programs, since they indicate the service

TABLE 2 Implementation outcome indicators according to Proctor et al.[17]

Outcome indicator	Definition
Acceptability	Perception among implementation stakeholders that a given evidence-based innovation is agreeable, palatable, or satisfactory
Adoption	Intention, initial decision, or action to try or employ an evidence-based innovation
Appropriateness	Perceived fit, relevance, or compatibility of the evidence-based innovation for a given practice setting, provider, or consumer; and/or perceived fit of the innovation to address a particular issue or problem
Feasibility	Extent to which an evidence-based innovation can be successfully used within a given setting
Fidelity	Degree to which an evidence-based innovation was implemented as described or as it was intended
Implementation cost	Cost of an implementation effort
Penetration	Integration of an evidence-based innovation within a service setting and its subsystems
Sustainability	Extent to which an implemented innovation is maintained or institutionalized

Adapted from Proctor E, Silmere H, Raghavan R, et al. Outcomes for implementation research: conceptual distinctions, measurement challenges, and research agenda. Adm Policy Ment Health Ment Health Serv Res. 2011;38:65–76. doi:10.1007/s10488-010-0319-7.

implementation's success or failure and can also be used as proxy indicators of the implementation process. The Implementation Outcomes Framework,[17] one of the most cited frameworks in the implementation science literature, identifies the following key indicators: acceptability, adoption, appropriateness, implementation cost, feasibility, fidelity, penetration and sustainability. The definition of each of these indicators can be found in Table 2. Nevertheless, authors of the Implementation Outcomes Framework suggest that the selection of specific implementation outcomes can be driven by the implementation stage and the unit of analysis of a given implementation program.

Implementation strategies in health services research

Implementation research may be most simply visualized as two related components (a) implementation context and (b) implementation strategies.[20] *Implementation context* is the barriers and facilitators (i.e., implementation factors or determinants) to the effective implementation of an evidence-based practice in a specific setting or settings. Identifying implementation context may be done through *contextual inquiry*, which may include both quantitative (e.g., existing software reporting functions, surveys) and qualitative (e.g., interviews, observations, focus groups) methodologies. Ideally, one begins with contextual inquiry prior to developing an *implementation strategy*.[21,22] Determinant frameworks, classic theories, and implementation theories are useful in understanding and explaining implementation context.

Implementation strategies are the "how to" of the implementation process.[21] Baker et al. define them as "…strategies to improve professional practice that are planned, taking account of prospectively identified determinants of practice…,"[23] which may be found through contextual inquiry. Historically, implementation strategies have been developed informally based on expert opinion or past experiences of those on an implementation team.[24] However, there are now several taxonomies which may be used to select and describe implementation strategies for a given study.[22,25–27] For example, using one such taxonomy, one may choose to "adapt and tailor" a new discharge medication reconciliation process to the context of the pharmacies and hospitals enrolled in the study (contextual adaptation) in addition to "supporting their clinicians" with an electronic relay of relevant clinical data on readmissions from which they can visualize process impact.

These implementation strategy taxonomies are useful for selection and description purposes. They also allow us to develop an evidence base for "discrete" (i.e., a single strategy) or "packaged" (i.e., multiple strategies) implementation strategies and subsequently generalize them across similar settings to aid in scale and spread.[28] Importantly, this involves the study of the implementation strategy itself as the intervention—and not the evidence-based practice being implemented. Using the example above, assuming there is established evidence for the value of discharge medication reconciliation, an implementation study would focus on strategies for the "contextual adaptation" and "supporting of clinicians" through a cluster randomized trial design. In some cases, it would be possible to study both implementation strategies and the desired healthcare practice to be implemented as the intervention. However, although linked, these are technically two separate research questions requiring two separate approaches to measurement. Instead, one should evaluate the implementation strategy itself through evaluation of the "contextual adaptation" and "support of clinicians" using a combination of quantitative and qualitative data collection strategies. One may wish to use an evaluation framework such as Proctor et al.[17] or RE-AIM.[16] For more information on this, please see the section on effectiveness-implementation hybrid designs within this chapter.

Selection of implementation strategies, even with supporting literature behind a discrete or packaged strategy, may still prove challenging. Several reviews have been published attempting to match "contextual inquiry" directly to "implementation strategies."[21,29,30] Waltz and colleagues have developed a Strategy Matching Tool which uses the Consolidated Framework for Implementation Research (CFIR) to map contextual factors to evidence based implementation strategies using the strategy taxonomy Expert Recommendations for Implementing Change compilation (ERIC).[24] A version of this context-strategy matching tool can be freely accessed on CFIR's website (www.cfirguide.org).

Although the study, development, and use in scale and spread of evidence-based implementation strategies are the ultimate endpoint of implementation research, the naming of the implementation strategy itself may not be enough to allow for generalizability and replication across diverse settings. Leeman and colleagues[31] argue that a more comprehensive view of such strategies must be taken and in addition to naming the strategy, they also suggest that the researcher specify the *actor* who enacts the strategy and the *target* of that strategy.

Implementation research designs

Originally described by Curran et al.,[2] effectiveness-implementation hybrid designs are widely used and reported in the implementation science literature. In these, design components of clinical effectiveness and implementation research are blended based on the study's main objective, allowing the assessment of both effectiveness and implementation outcomes in a given study. Three types of hybrid designs have been described, which are mainly driven by the balance between the effectiveness and implementation focus of the research. Although a detailed explanation of these designs has been reported elsewhere,[32] a brief overview is provided below and also presented in Fig. 2.

- Type 1 hybrid designs mainly focus on assessing the effectiveness of an evidence-based intervention or service, while gathering evidence on its implementability in a real-world context.[32] Type 1 hybrid designs usually involve an effectiveness assessment, combined with a process evaluation of the delivery and implementation of the intervention. Process evaluation can provide insights into implementation barriers and facilitators or inform the development of implementation strategies needed in future implementation research.
- Type 2 hybrid designs aim to assess both effectiveness and implementation outcomes, allowing a parallel evaluation of an intervention and associated implementation strategies. Hybrid 2 designs are therefore considered appropriate to evaluate a wide range of interventions such as professional pharmacy services and are optimal designs for certain ways of scaling-out interventions (i.e., those involving a full randomized hybrid trial).[33] Although there is no specific guidance on how much research focus should be allocated to each research component (e.g., 50% effectiveness and 50% implementation), type 2 hybrid designs should have a previously detailed implementation strategy and list of implementation outcomes to be assessed.[32]

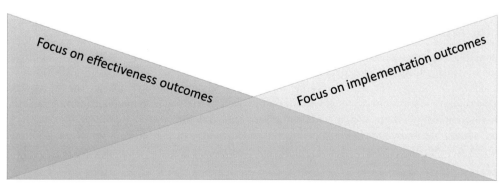

FIG. 2 Effectiveness-implementation hybrid designs.

Clusters							
	1	Control	Control	Control	Control	Control	Intervention
	2	Control	Control	Control	Control	Intervention	Intervention
	3	Control	Control	Control	Intervention	Intervention	Intervention
	4	Control	Control	Intervention	Intervention	Intervention	Intervention
	5	Control	Intervention	Intervention	Intervention	Intervention	Intervention
		1	2	3	5	5	6

"Steps" (Time Periods)

FIG. 3 Stepped-wedge design.

- Type 3 hybrid designs mainly focus on implementation outcomes but also gather some effectiveness outcomes of the intervention being implemented. These designs involve collecting clinical/patient outcomes (ideally through routinely collected data in clinical settings) alongside an implementation trial.

Although the randomized control trial (RCT) is considered the gold standard of experimental research study designs, it is often infeasible or impractical in implementation science research for a variety of reasons. The RCT has strong internal validity which is of high value in efficacy studies, but this comes at a cost as external validity is compromised. Given the need for high levels of external validity necessary in implementation science research, alternative research methods which prioritize external validity are preferred. Moreover, in nonacademic practice settings (e.g., community pharmacy chains, rural hospitals), random assignment of the evidence-based practice or intervention may not be possible. For instance, a pharmacists' intervention, which aims to improve vaccine recommendations, cannot be randomized at the patient level like a typical RCT due to reasons of contamination. Here, pharmacists who are asked to deliver the new vaccine recommendation to intervention patients but not to those in a control group are likely to still deliver components of the intervention even if they are asked to do so. In other circumstances, not delivering the evidence-based intervention to all patients may be unethical or unpreferred by the community partner. For example, a national community pharmacy chain may determine that the implementation of an evidence-based intervention proven to improve antiretroviral adherence must be implemented across all pharmacies nationwide as a prerequisite to their participation in the study for reasons of patient safety.

When a RCT or cluster RCT is not feasible, alternative experimental approaches can be considered. For these reasons, quasi-experimental designs (QED) have gained popularity in recent years as the study designs-of-choice among implementation scientists. For example, pragmatic designs such as stepped-wedge cluster randomized trials (Fig. 3), or sequential multiple assignment randomized trials (SMART) are expected to increase in the future.[34] Handley et al.[35] present a thorough review of reasons for selecting QEDs over RCTs, and each QED in detail. For the purposes of this chapter only a brief overview of each QED is covered, and readers can refer to the Handley et al.[35] article for further context.

Standards for reporting implementation research

It has been stated that implementation studies are often poorly reported, limiting their potential to improve health care.[6] With the aim of addressing this gap, The Standards for Reporting Implementation Studies (StaRI) initiative developed a guide to assist authors in the transparent and accurate reporting of implementation studies.[6] The StaRI was developed in 2015 based on the findings of a systematic review followed by a Delphi study, which included international implementation science experts. It comprises 27 items which guide authors on how to describe not only the strategies adopted to promote implementation, but also the innovation being implemented and how it is expected to improve overall healthcare or specific health outcomes. A strength of the StaRI is that it is applicable to the wide range of study designs commonly used in implementation science.

StaRI has been included in one of the numerous reporting guidelines of the EQUATOR (Enhancing the QUAlity and Transparency Of health Research) Network library, and it is accessible on their website (https://www.equator-network.org). Adoption of StaRI will potentially improve and standardize the reporting of implementation studies by researchers which may lead to the adoption and implementation of effective innovations into routine settings.

Overall recommendations for conducting implementation research

Considering the concepts discussed in this chapter, the following recommendations are made when conducting implementation research.

1. Clearly define the study objectives. Select the most appropriate research design to address the research questions and define the research methods accordingly.
2. Identify the most appropriate model to guide the implementation process. Researchers can use available tools to assist in the identification of an appropriate framework.[9,36]
3. Identify relevant implementation factors or determinants based on a relevant determinants framework, classic or implementation theory.
4. Identify and develop tailored implementation strategies according to the determinants identified in step 3.
5. Select relevant implementation outcomes (ideally based on a suitable evaluation framework) and appropriate evaluation tools.
6. Report the study protocol and findings in accordance with StaRI.

Questions for further discussion

1. What value does implementation science add to broader healthcare research efforts?
2. How is implementation science different from more traditional effectiveness and efficacy research? How is it similar?
3. What role does theory play in implementation science? What are the main classifications of theories used in implementation science?
4. What are implementation outcomes? How do they differ from traditional effectiveness or efficacy research outcomes?
5. What is an implementation strategy? How do these strategies relate to implementation context and evidence-based practices?
6. What are the advantages and disadvantages of effectiveness-implementation hybrid research designs?

Application exercise/scenario

You are the leader of an implementation research institute. Your research team has recently been approached by the CEO of a large group of community pharmacies to develop and evaluate a program for the implementation of a vaccination service in their pharmacies. Propose an implementation trial considering the following elements:

1. Research design.
2. Relevant implementation framework applicable to your research approach.
3. Potential implementation outcomes and associated evaluation tools.
4. Potential implementation strategies that could be applied at the different context levels.

References

1. Bauer MS, Kirchner JA. Implementation science: what is it and why should I care? *Psychiatry Res.* 2020;283(April). https://doi.org/10.1016/j.psychres.2019.04.025.
2. Curran GM, Bauer M, Mittman B, Pyne JM, Stetler C. Effectiveness-implementation hybrid designs: combining elements of clinical effectiveness and implementation research to enhance public health impact. *Med Care.* 2012;50(3):217–226. https://doi.org/10.1097/MLR.0b013e3182408812.
3. Bauer MS, Damschroder L, Hagedorn H, Smith J, Kilbourne AM. An introduction to implementation science for the non-specialist. *BMC Psychol.* 2015;1–12. https://doi.org/10.1186/s40359-015-0089-9.
4. Peters DH, Adam T, Alonge O, Agyepong IA, Tran N. Implementation research: what it is and how to do it. *BMJ.* 2013;347. https://doi.org/10.1136/bmj.f6753, f6753.
5. Eccles MP, Mittman BS. Welcome to implementation science. *Implement Sci.* 2006;1:1. https://doi.org/10.1186/1748-5908-1-1.
6. Pinnock H, Barwick M, Carpenter CR, et al. Standards for reporting implementation studies (StaRI) statement. *BMJ.* 2017;356(March):1–9. https://doi.org/10.1136/bmj.i6795.
7. Nilsen P. Making sense of implementation theories, models and frameworks. *Implement Sci.* 2015;10:1–13. https://doi.org/10.1186/s13012-015-0242-0.
8. Garcia-Cardenas V, Rossing CV, Fernandez-Llimos F, et al. Pharmacy practice research—a call to action. *Res Social Adm Pharm.* 2020;16(11):1602–1608. https://doi.org/10.1016/j.sapharm.2020.07.031.
9. Birken SA, Powell BJ, Shea CM, et al. Criteria for selecting implementation science theories and frameworks: results from an international survey. *Implement Sci.* 2017;1–9. https://doi.org/10.1186/s13012-017-0656-y.
10. Damschroder LJ, Aron DC, Keith RE, Kirsh SR, Alexander J, a, Lowery JC. Fostering implementation of health services research findings into practice: a consolidated framework for advancing implementation science. *Implement Sci.* 2009;4:50. https://doi.org/10.1186/1748-5908-4-50.

11. Harvey G, Kitson A. PARIHS revisited: from heuristic to integrated framework for the successful implementation of knowledge into practice. *Implement Sci.* 2016;11:33. https://doi.org/10.1186/s13012-016-0398-2.

12. Flottorp SA, Oxman AD, Krause J, et al. A checklist for identifying determinants of practice: a systematic review and synthesis of frameworks and taxonomies of factors that prevent or enable improvements in healthcare professional practice. *Implement Sci.* 2013;8(1):35. https://doi.org/10.1186/1748-5908-8-35.

13. Meyers DC, Durlak JA, Wandersman A. The quality implementation framework: a synthesis of critical steps in the implementation process. *Am J Community Psychol.* 2012;50(3–4):462–480. https://doi.org/10.1007/s10464-012-9522-x.

14. Aarons GA, Hurlburt M, Horwitz SM. Advancing a conceptual model of evidence-based practice implementation in public service sectors. *Adm Policy Ment Health Ment Heal Serv Res.* 2011;38:4–23. https://doi.org/10.1007/s10488-010-0327-7.

15. Moullin JC, Sabater-Hernández D, Fernandez-Llimos F, Benrimoj SI. A systematic review of implementation frameworks of innovations in healthcare and resulting generic implementation framework. *Heal Res Policy Syst.* 2015;13. https://doi.org/10.1186/s12961-015-0005-z.

16. Glasgow RE, Vogt TM, Boles SM. Evaluating the public health impact of health promotion interventions: the RE-AIM framework. *Am J Public Health.* 1999;89(9):1322–1327. https://doi.org/10.2105/AJPH.89.9.1322.

17. Proctor E, Silmere H, Raghavan R, et al. Outcomes for implementation research: conceptual distinctions, measurement challenges, and research agenda. *Adm Policy Ment Health Ment Health Serv Res.* 2011;38:65–76. https://doi.org/10.1007/s10488-010-0319-7.

18. Garcia-Cardenas V, Perez-Escamilla B, Fernandez-Llimos F, Benrimoj SI. The complexity of implementation factors in professional pharmacy services. *Res Social Adm Pharm.* 2018;14(5):498–500. https://doi.org/10.1016/j.sapharm.2017.05.016.

19. Crespo-Gonzalez C, Garcia-Cardenas V, Benrimoj SI. The next phase in professional services research: from implementation to sustainability. *Res Social Adm Pharm.* 2017. https://doi.org/10.1016/j.sapharm.2017.05.020.

20. Lane-Fall MB, Curran GM, Beidas RS. Scoping implementation science for the beginner: locating yourself on the "subway line" of translational research. *BMC Med Res Methodol.* 2019;19(1):1–5. https://doi.org/10.1186/s12874-019-0783-z.

21. Powell BJ, Beidas RS, Lewis CC, et al. Methods to improve the selection and tailoring of implementation strategies. *J Behav Health Serv Res.* 2017;44(2):177–194. https://doi.org/10.1007/s11414-015-9475-6.

22. Powell BJ, Waltz TJ, Chinman MJ, et al. A refined compilation of implementation strategies: results from the expert recommendations for implementing change (ERIC) project. *Implement Sci.* 2015;10(1):1–14. https://doi.org/10.1186/s13012-015-0209-1.

23. Baker R, Gillies C, Ej S, et al. Tailored interventions to address determinants of practice (review) summary of findings for the main comparison. *Cochrane Database Syst Rev.* 2015;(4). https://doi.org/10.1002/14651858.CD005470.pub3. www.cochranelibrary.com.

24. Waltz TJ, Powell BJ, Fernández ME, Abadie B, Damschroder LJ. Choosing implementation strategies to address contextual barriers: diversity in recommendations and future directions. *Implement Sci.* 2019;14(1):1–15. https://doi.org/10.1186/s13012-019-0892-4.

25. Mazza D, Bairstow P, Buchan H, et al. Refining a taxonomy for guideline implementation: results of an exercise in abstract classification. *Implement Sci.* 2013;8(1):1–10. https://doi.org/10.1186/1748-5908-8-32.

26. Michie S, Richardson M, Johnston M, et al. The behavior change technique taxonomy (v1) of 93 hierarchically clustered techniques: building an international consensus for the reporting of behavior change interventions. *Ann Behav Med.* 2013;46(1):81–95. https://doi.org/10.1007/s12160-013-9486-6.

27. Lokker C, McKibbon KA, Colquhoun H, Hempel S. A scoping review of classification schemes of interventions to promote and integrate evidence into practice in healthcare. *Implement Sci.* 2015;10(1). https://doi.org/10.1186/s13012-015-0220-6.

28. Proctor EK, Powell BJ, McMillen JC. Implementation strategies: recommendations for specifying and reporting. *Implement Sci.* 2013;8(1):1–11. https://doi.org/10.1186/1748-5908-8-139.

29. Colquhoun HL, Squires JE, Kolehmainen N, Fraser C, Grimshaw JM. Methods for designing interventions to change healthcare professionals' behaviour: a systematic review. *Implement Sci.* 2017;12(1):1–11. https://doi.org/10.1186/s13012-017-0560-5.

30. Lewis CC, Klasnja P, Powell BJ, et al. From classification to causality: advancing understanding of mechanisms of change in implementation science. *Front Public Health.* 2018;6(May). https://doi.org/10.3389/fpubh.2018.00136.

31. Leeman J, Birken SA, Powell BJ, Rohweder C, Shea CM. Beyond "implementation strategies": classifying the full range of strategies used in implementation science and practice. *Implement Sci.* 2017;12(1):125. https://doi.org/10.1186/s13012-017-0657-x.

32. Landes SJ, Mcbain SA, Curran GM. An introduction to effectiveness-implementation hybrid designs. *Psychiatry Res.* 2019 Oct;280. https://doi.org/10.1016/j.psychres.2019.112513, 112513.

33. Aarons GA, Sklar M, Mustanski B, Benbow N, Brown CH. "Scaling-out" evidence-based interventions to new populations or new health care delivery systems. *Implement Sci.* 2017;12(1):1–13. https://doi.org/10.1186/s13012-017-0640-6.

34. Grayling MJ, Wason JMS, Mander AP. Stepped wedge cluster randomized controlled trial designs: a review of reporting quality and design features. *Trials.* 2017;1–13. https://doi.org/10.1186/s13063-017-1783-0.

35. Handley MA, Lyles CR, McCulloch C, Cattamanchi A. Selecting and improving quasi-experimental designs in effectiveness and implementation research. *Annu Rev Public Health.* 2018;39:5–25. https://doi.org/10.1146/annurev-publhealth-040617-014128.

36. Birken SA, Rohweder CL, Powell BJ, et al. T-CaST: an implementation theory comparison and selection tool. *Implement Sci.* 2018;13(1):1–10. https://doi.org/10.1186/s13012-018-0836-4.

Chapter 5

CFIR framework in pharmacy and health services research

Sarah J. Shoemaker-Hunt[a], Ellen Childs[a], Holly Swan[a], and Geoffrey Curran[b]

[a]*Abt Associates, Inc., Cambridge, MA, United States,* [b]*University of Arkansas for Medical Sciences, Center for Implementation Research, Little Rock, AR, United States*

Objectives

- Provide an overview of the Consolidated Framework for Implementation Research (CFIR), how it should be used, and its strengths and limitations.
- Provide sample studies of pharmacy interventions using the CFIR.
- Provide examples of using CFIR to conduct reviews in pharmacy implementation research.

Introduction

The use of implementation science and research to understand and evaluate the implementation of pharmacy and other health services has been growing exponentially for over a decade, and has come to play a critical role in advancing these fields. This has been acknowledged by leading journals and professional organizations.[1–3] As discussed in the previous chapter, implementation science is a deep and broad field with much to contribute to health services research in pharmacy. The field of implementation science has seen a wide variation in terminology and considerable overlap across implementation theories, while also missing key constructs within any single theory.[4] In an attempt to develop a comprehensive framework which consolidated constructs found in the broad array of published theories, Damschroder et al. developed the Consolidated Framework for Implementation Research (CFIR).[4]

The consolidated framework for implementation research

The CFIR synthesizes constructs from existing theories (i.e., metatheoretical) "without depicting interrelationships, specific ecological levels, or specific hypotheses."[4] The CFIR offers an overarching typology—a list of constructs—from which researchers can select constructs that are most relevant for the study and setting. The CFIR consists of five domains: (I) intervention characteristics, (II) outer setting, (III) inner setting, (IV) characteristics of individuals, and (V) process. Within each of the domains there are several constructs (see https://cfirguide.org/).

Use of the consolidated framework for implementation research

The Consolidated Framework for Implementation Research (CFIR) offers an "overarching typology–a list of constructs to promote theory development and verification about what works where and why across multiple contexts. Researchers can select constructs from the CFIR that are most relevant for their particular study setting and use these to guide diagnostic assessments of implementation context, evaluate implementation progress, and help explain findings in research studies or quality improvement initiatives."[4] Since its publication in 2009, the CFIR has been widely used in implementation research in health care settings, including 831 articles (all types of articles) between 2009 and 2020 (Fig. 1). Similarly, there have been 66 articles referencing CFIR (Fig. 1).

Nilsen[5] described and analyzed how theories, models, and frameworks had been applied in implementation science, and proposed a taxonomy to distinguish different approaches and clarify common terminology to facilitate appropriate

Contemporary Research Methods in Pharmacy and Health Services. https://doi.org/10.1016/B978-0-323-91888-6.00045-4

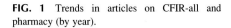

FIG. 1 Trends in articles on CFIR-all and pharmacy (by year).

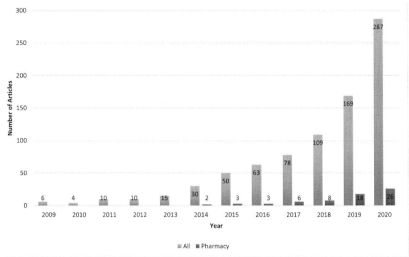

selection and application of relevant approaches in implementation research.[5] As Nilsen[5] explained, the CFIR is a determinant framework, which describes the:

> determinants that are hypothesized or have been found to influence implementation outcomes, e.g., health care professionals' behaviour change or adherence to a clinical guideline. Each type of determinant typically comprises a number of individual barriers (hinders, impediments) and/or enablers (facilitators), which are seen as independent variables that have an impact on implementation outcomes, i.e., the dependent variable.

A determinant framework, like CFIR, does not address how change occurs or explain causal mechanisms. Additionally, a determinant framework implies a systems approach to understanding implementation, accounting for multiple levels of influence and relationships within and across those levels for different determinants. Finally, context is a critical part of all determinant frameworks and "generally understood as the conditions or surroundings in which something exists or occurs, typically referring to an analytical unit that is higher than the phenomena directly under investigation."[5]

Following several years of CFIR use, Kirk et al.[6] conducted a systematic review to examine the extent to which CFIR had been used in implementation research to fulfill the goals set forth by Damschroder et al.[4] in terms of the breadth, depth, and contribution to implementation research.[6] Their systematic review of 26 studies found that CFIR had been used in a range of studies in terms of objectives, units of analysis, design, and methods, which suggested its applicability to a wide range of interventions, settings, and research designs. Kirk et al.'s[6] review of CFIR studies found wide variation in which CFIR constructs were chosen and little information on the logic for selecting specific constructs, which is inconsistent with the intent of the CFIR developers who recommended researchers report their decision and rationale for selecting and measuring specific constructs. Additionally, Kirk et al.[6] found that most studies used the CFIR only to guide data analysis, which was a reported limitation in many cases as the authors acknowledged they did not anticipate specific implementation factors. Thus, it is ideal to use the CFIR—like all theories and frameworks—a priori in study design including informing research questions and data collection protocols. Similarly, Kirk et al.[6] found that most studies used the CFIR during or postimplementation to understand barriers and facilitators, which they proffered is a missed opportunity given the studies that used CFIR prior to implementation were able to refine the strategy before implementation commenced.

Based on their review, Kirk et al.[6] developed recommendations to assist researchers in their application of the CFIR, which include:

1. Consider how to most meaningfully use the CFIR across different phases of implementation.
2. Report how CFIR constructs were selected, and which constructs were used.
3. Assess the association of CFIR constructs with outcomes.
4. Integrate the CFIR throughout the entire research process (e.g., to develop research questions and data collection materials, to refine CFIR constructs, and to promote theoretical development).

The recommendations of Kirk et al.[6] can help ensure that CFIR is used appropriately, as a determinant framework, when conducting research on health services, including pharmacy services.

Sample pharmacy studies using the consolidated framework for implementation research

The CFIR has been used in several studies of pharmacy interventions and services, examples of which are provided below. This section describes two recent empirical studies which have used the CFIR. To demonstrate versatility of the CFIR for studies with different methods and in different settings, these samples include a survey of community pharmacists and a mixed-methods study of site leaders at a hospital participating in a multicenter medication reconciliation quality improvement study.

Meyerson et al.[7] examined the feasibility and acceptability of a pharmacy-based harm reduction model intervention to reduce opioid overdose, HIV, and hepatitis C known as PharmNet.[7] The survey consisting of qualitative and quantitative response items was developed to align closely with the CFIR to measure intervention feasibility and acceptability. There were 303 pharmacist respondents with 215 providing detailed written comments. They found that in terms of *intervention characteristics*, 83.3% believed that PharmNet would benefit patients and that staff could deliver the intervention with adequate training (70.0%). For *inner setting*, over three-quarters believed their pharmacy culture supported practice change, yet over half of chain pharmacists believed their pharmacies would not have time for PharmNet. For *outer setting*, 73.0% of respondents believed additional addiction and overdose screening is needed in their community, and 79.5% believed that pharmacies should offer new services to help reduce opioid overdose and addiction among their patients. Ninety-seven percent were asked by patients in the past 2 years about syringe-related issues, and two-thirds were asked about syringes for nonprescription injection drug use.

Stolldorf and colleagues conducted a mixed-methods study of hospital site leaders who were participating in a multicenter medication reconciliation quality improvement study in the United States.[8] They used the CFIR to design survey and interview protocols and qualitatively analyze the data. The CFIR constructs, identified from the qualitative interviews included inner setting constructs: organizational culture, implementation climate, readiness for implementation, and structural systems; and process constructs: use of champions, engaging through use of external change agents, formally appointed internal implementation leaders, planning through process mapping, and reflecting and evaluation. They also identified barriers in four key categories, including: health information technology (e.g., functionality problems), resources (e.g., competing priorities, lack of physical space or staff), staff-related factors (e.g., limited clinician involvement in project, lack of initial project buy-in), and climate (e.g., limited experience with implementation, competing priorities).

Sample review applying and tailoring the CFIR framework to pharmacy services

Pharmacies have unique contextual features that may impact implementation (e.g., retail environment, incentive structures) and potentially unique staffing-related barriers compared to other health care professionals (e.g., not a recognized provider, dispensing workflow). Thus, given the unique features of community pharmacy compared to other health care settings, which are important for consideration in implementation research, Shoemaker et al.[3] conducted a critical review of 45 articles on professional services to provide a framework for implementation research for community pharmacy based on the Consolidated Framework for Implementation Research (CFIR).[3] The professional services included medication therapy management (MTM), immunizations, and rapid HIV testing. Most of the included studies did not use the CFIR or any implementation framework. However, study findings were mapped to CFIR constructs. This review synthesized the findings by specific services for each CFIR construct and then examined the findings from across all three services by CFIR domain. Key findings are presented in this chapter.

Findings

The review included 10 articles on MTM[9–18]; 26 articles on immunizations[19–43]; and 9 articles on rapid HIV testing[44–52] (Table 1). The findings are mapped to the five CFIR domains and the relevant constructs within each domain: intervention characteristics, outer setting, inner setting, characteristics of individuals, and process—to illustrate the application of CFIR to these pharmacy services in community pharmacy.

TABLE 1 Articles reviewed, the type of study employed, and CFIR domains represented in each.

First author (Year)	Type of study	Consolidated framework for implementation research (CFIR) domains				
		Intervention characteristics	Outer setting	Inner setting	Individual characteristics	Process
Medication therapy management (MTM)						
Blake and Madhavan[9]	Cross-sectional survey		X	X	X	
Blake et al.[10]	Survey of pharmacists-in-charge		X	X	X	
Chui et al.[11]	Qualitative; interviews with community pharmacists	X		X	X	
Herbert et al.[12]	Cross-sectional survey	X	X	X	X	
Lounsberry et al. (2009)[13]	Cross-sectional study	X	X	X	X	
MacIntosh et al.[14]	Cross-sectional descriptive study	X			X	
Mocyzgemba et al. (2008)[15]	Cross-sectional survey of pharmacists		X	X	X	
Rosenthal et al.[16]	Cross-sectional survey				X	
Smith et al.[17]	Qualitative; focus groups—pharmacists; interviews—health plan executives	X	X	X	X	
Trapskin et al.[18]	Descriptive	X	X		X	X
Immunizations						
Aderemi-Williams and Igwilo (2007)[19]	Cross-sectional survey	X		X		
Atkins et al.[20]	Program evaluation—time series, cross-sectional, cost analysis	X	X		X	
Brackett et al.[21]	Cross-sectional, descriptive	X				
Crawford et al.[22]	Cross-sectional survey		X	X	X	
Doucette et al.[23]	Financial analysis	X				
Duncan et al.[24]						
Edwards et al.[25]	Cross-sectional survey of pharmacists	X	X	X	X	X
Gardner[26]	Review	X	X	X		
Gatewood and Stanley (2009)[27]	Case study	X	X	X		

TABLE 1 Articles reviewed, the type of study employed, and CFIR domains represented in each—cont'd

First author (Year)	Type of study	Consolidated framework for implementation research (CFIR) domains				
		Intervention characteristics	*Outer setting*	*Inner setting*	*Individual characteristics*	*Process*
Goode et al.[28]	Longitudinal study	X				X
Kummer and Foushee (2008)[29]	Descriptive, nonexperimental, cross-sectional	X	X	X	X	
Murphy et al.[30]	Retrospective analysis	X	X			
Navarrete et al.[53]	Program evaluation utilizing multiple research designs	X	X	X	X	X
Ndiaye et al.[31]	Theory-guided exploratory study (qualitative) and confirmatory survey (quantitative)		X	X		
Neuhauser et al.[32]	Cross-sectional pilot study	X	X	X	X	
Pilisuk et al.[33]	Cross-sectional	X	X	X		
Usami et al.[34]	Cluster-randomized controlled trial	X				
Valiquette and Bédard (2015)[35]	Cross-sectional, descriptive	X	X	X	X	
Westrick et al. (2015)[42]	Cluster-randomized controlled trial	X	X	X	X	X
Westrick[37]	Nonexperimental multistage survey	X		X		
Westrick[38]	Nonexperimental multistage survey	X	X	X		
Westrick et al.[43]	Cross-sectional survey	X		X		X
Westrick et al.[43]	Nonexperimental multistage survey	X		X		
Westrick et al.[43]	Cross-sectional computer-assisted telephone interview (CATI)		X	X		
Westrick et al.[41]	Cross-sectional study		X	X		
Weitzel (2000)[36]	Case Study	X		X	X	X
Rapid HIV testing						
Amesty et al.[44]	Descriptive				X	
Amesty et al.[45]	Feasibility study; cross-sectional		X	X	X	
Calderon et al.[46]	Cross-sectional convenience	X	X	X		

Continued

TABLE 1 Articles reviewed, the type of study employed, and CFIR domains represented in each—cont'd

First author (Year)	Type of study	Consolidated framework for implementation research (CFIR) domains				
		Intervention characteristics	Outer setting	Inner setting	Individual characteristics	Process
Darin et al.[47]	Cross-sectional survey	X				
Dugdale et al.[48]	Descriptive	X	X			
Fernandez-Balbuena et al. (2015)[49]	Feasibility study		X	X	X	
Hammett TM et al. (2014)[50]	Feasibility mixed-methods study	X	X		X	
Lecher SL et al. (2015)[51]	Pilot study cost analysis	X		X		
Weidle PJ et al. (2014)[52]	Feasibility study		X	X		

Intervention characteristics

While *Intervention Characteristics* will ultimately depend on the specific service or intervention being implemented, we found relative advantage, adaptability, complexity and cost, of particular relevance to community pharmacy settings in 32 of the studies (Table 2).[11–14,17–21,23,25–30,32–40,42,46–48,50,51,53]

The relative advantage of the services examined included demonstrating pharmacists' value, potentially bringing in new patients, and better relationships with providers and other organizations (e.g., health departments). The services examined are often viewed as additive and a professional expansion for pharmacists, not as an alternative, per se, and often pose a cost–benefit challenge. All services require adaptability, at least in terms of determining how the new service will be incorporated into the existing workflow of a pharmacy. Complexity was particularly pronounced for MTM, which has limited standardization in terms of the services provided, payer documentation and reimbursement requirements, and the time and workload for pharmacists to provide MTM. On the other hand, immunizations, which require training to provide, were relatively simple to implement.

Because this review focused on services in pharmacy instead of interventions more broadly, there were several constructs within intervention characteristics that Shoemaker et al.[3] did not think appeared to be relevant. For example, intervention source does not readily apply to services like MTM, immunizations, and rapid HIV testing as they are a service vs a tool or resource developed by or authored by an organization or entity. Additionally, evidence strength and quality were only raised in one study conducted in 2009,[14] which may reflect an earlier period in MTM implementation. Additionally, design quality and packaging were only relevant to HIV testing as it is administered with additional documentation and engagement as compared to immunizations.

Outer setting

In terms of *Outer Setting*, there were 29 observations of these constructs in the literature (Table 3).[9,10,12,13,15,17,18,20,22,25–27,29–33,35,38,40–42,45,46,48–50,52,53] Patient needs and resources were factors for implementing these services in terms of if there was a demand, a need, or a willingness to receive these services by patients. Several external policies and incentives impacted pharmacists' provision of these services. The lack of standardization of MTM services, documentation requirements, billing systems and insufficient reimbursement were key challenges, in part due to numerous payers. Immunizations and HIV testing were impacted by certification and regulatory requirements. Cosmopolitanism was observed in immunizations and HIV testing when pharmacies were involved with health departments, for example. Finally, pharmacists' perceptions that peers also approved of a service or that pharmacists' roles were evolving were facilitators.

TABLE 2 CFIR constructs relevant to pharmacy—domain 1.

CFIR constructs	MTM	Immunizations	HIV testing	Description of observed CFIR constructs in literature
Evidence strength and quality	X			• Vast majority of studies did not refer to the evidence for strength of services, except one study on pharmacy managers' perspective on whether medication reviews will improve patient health
Relative advantage	X	X	X	• Relative advantage was not noted in most MTM studies reviewed, which may reflect the established notion that it is advantageous • Several areas of relative advantage were noted with respect to immunizations—e.g., bringing new patients into the pharmacy; enhanced relationships with providers, health departments, and organizations; improved patient heath; demonstrating new skills that pharmacists have to the public • Relative advantages cited regarding implementing HIV testing were bringing in new clients/patients; better relations with other community health organizations; improved patient health; demonstrating value of pharmacists' skills • New services can pose a cost–benefit challenge in light of the traditional dispensing role in community pharmacies. These services are often viewed as additive and a professional expansion for pharmacists, not as an alternative, per se
Adaptability	X	X	X	• Some documentation systems for MTM are prescriptive, and less adaptable, yet they facilitate use because they are less complex • Use of other staff to support delivery of MTM was helpful • All services require figuring out how to incorporate the service into the workflow and staffing of a community pharmacy • Providing an HIV test at no charge, a short wait time for results, or certainty of confidentiality were potential facilitators, all features that may be possible with pharmacy-based HIV screening
Trialability		X		• A common pattern among community pharmacies that adopted provision of immunizations was starting small (like flu shots) and then expanding over time
Complexity	X	X		• While pharmacists did need training and often certification to provide immunizations, the service *was not perceived to be overly complex*, which was a facilitator • There were several complexities with MTM services that posed challenges, including dealing with multiple payers and the lack of standardization in documentation requirements and payment across them. Additional challenges, included the time needed to provide MTM, pharmacists' workload, and the relationships to be built with providers • Less complex or multifaceted services seem to be more easily implemented than the more complex
Design quality and packaging			X	• The variety of testing kits available for HIV testing, such as over-the-counter and kits that can be used at home, was a facilitator
Cost	X	X	X	• Costs of buying vaccines and necessary supplies (e.g., refrigerator, band aids) can be prohibitive if reimbursement does not cover these costs • For HIV testing, the cost of staff time, testing kits; confirmatory testing for positive rapid test results were cited • MTM services were often viewed as being insufficiently reimbursed • Services presented opportunities for additional revenue; however, reimbursement was sometimes deemed insufficient

Intervention characteristics.

Inner setting

For *Inner Setting*, there were 31 studies that reflected these constructs.[9–13,15,17,19,22,25–27,29,31–33,35,37–43,45,46,49,51–53] Important structural characteristics for implementation included pharmacy type (e.g., chain, independent, safety net), pharmacy size, and the physical space to provide a service confidentially (Table 4). A culture of having the service align with the pharmacy's mission or priorities and a public health orientation were facilitative for immunizations and HIV testing.

In terms of implementation climate, a tension for change can be seen when pharmacists are faced with multiple clinical initiatives in their pharmacies. Compatibility was particularly key when pharmacists viewed a service as "what they do." Organizational incentives were not described in many studies, but viewed as a barrier when pharmacists were not incentivized, for example, to provide MTM.

For readiness for implementation, leadership engagement and access to knowledge and information were observed in a few studies; however, having available resources was observed as critical for all services on many fronts. Time and workload were among the most common barriers across services, particularly if dispensing responsibilities were not offset. No less, incorporating a new service into the community pharmacy workflow was important. Another key challenge was the availability of private space to ensure confidentiality of patients. There were several constructs that were not observed in the literature, including networks and communications, relative priority, goals and feedback, and learning climate.

TABLE 3 CFIR constructs relevant to pharmacy—domain 2.

CFIR constructs	MTM	Immunizations	HIV testing	Description of observed CFIR constructs in the literature
Patient needs and resources	X	X	X	• Patient demand for vaccinations helps drive adoption and sustainability • Providing HIV testing in pharmacies has the potential to increase health care access to high need areas • Patient acceptance and willingness to receive MTM was a facilitator
Cosmopolitanism		X	X	• Successful immunizing pharmacies were more networked with providers, health departments, and corporations (under contract) • Engagement with or partnering with local health departments can assist with overcoming negative testing norms and developing lists of HIV confirmatory testing sites and other HIV resources in the community
Peer pressure	X		X	• Increasing emphasis on shift from drug dispensers to active members of teams • Pharmacists had a stronger intent to provide MTM when they felt their peers approved
External policies and incentives	X	X	X	• The lack of standardization for MTM in terms of covered services, documentation requirements, payment levels and billing systems were key challenges, along with insufficient reimbursement for the service • Immunizations facilitated by policies that allow pharmacists to immunize and get reimbursed. Pharmacists need certification to immunize, which can be a barrier • Implementation of HIV testing is facilitated by government recommendations and mandates regarding HIV testing • Community norms around HIV could be a disincentive to implementing testing

Outer setting.

TABLE 4 CFIR constructs relevant to pharmacy—domain 3.

CFIR constructs	MTM	Immunizations	HIV testing	Description of observed CFIR constructs in literature
Structural characteristics	X	X	X	• When interns, pharmacy technicians, and clerks provide support for the services (scheduling, billing, etc.) it was an important facilitator of service implementation • Pharmacy type can affect implementation (e.g., chain, independent, safety net) • Key to implementing these services was space, particularly private space to ensure confidentiality, which was a challenge in many pharmacies • Size of the pharmacy and larger numbers of certified immunizers were facilitators for level of uptake (number of immunizations provided) and sustainability • Pharmacies, as less stigmatizing settings, was a facilitator for HIV testing
Culture	X		X	• Implementation was facilitated when pharmacy leadership perceived the intervention or service aligned with the pharmacy's mission/priorities (e.g., commitment to patient care) • Pharmacies that had a public health orientation and commitment to providing preventative services more readily implemented HIV testing
Implementation climate	X	X	X	• *Tension for change*: Pharmacists could be overwhelmed by the number of clinical initiatives • *Compatibility*: Immunizing pharmacists feel that service is *compatible* with their role as a pharmacist and fits with the mission of their organizations, and can fit with workflow if enough pharmacists are certified to immunize • *Compatibility*: Pharmacists viewing MTM as "what they do" was facilitative to implementation • *Compatibility*: Some pharmacies successfully providing HIV testing, had already been doing so in partnership with the health department. Also, HIV testing could be incorporated into pharmacies' existing services • *Organizational incentives and rewards*: It was a barrier for some pharmacists to provide MTM since they were not incentivized to do so
Readiness for implementation	X	X	X	• *Leadership engagement*: Leadership permitting time and resources and support were facilitative of implementation • *Available resources*: Time and workload was cited as the most common barrier to implementing a service into a community pharmacy, particularly if dispensing responsibilities were not offset • *Available resources*: incorporating a service into the pharmacy workflow was also an oft reported challenge • *Available resources*: Challenges to implementation also included available space, particularly private space to ensure confidentiality, and storage space for immunizations • *Available resources*: Training was often a key factor to successful implementation of any service • *Available resources*: Use of support staff was helpful • *Access to knowledge and information*: Was important in terms of pharmacists have the necessary skills or training to provide the professional service

Inner setting.

TABLE 5 CFIR constructs relevant to pharmacy—domain 4.

CFIR constructs	MTM	Immunizations	HIV testing	Description of observed CFIR constructs in literature
Knowledge and beliefs about the intervention	X	X	X	• Training programs for implementing services were often to expand knowledge and influence beliefs (immunizations, HIV testing) • Knowledge of and/or training on the services was often critical, but positive beliefs about the services were also important to implementation • Positive attitudes toward immunizations and pharmacists' beliefs that they "are part of the health care system" facilitate uptake and sustainability of immunization and HIV testing • Stigma of HIV and others (e.g., illicit drug use) was a barrier to uptake of HIV testing among pharmacists
Self-efficacy	X	X		• Self-efficacy was an observed factor in pharmacists' provision of MTM and immunizations
Other personal attributes	X			• Educational background was often important to provision of MTM, as well as other personal attributes • Providing immunizations was observed to improve job satisfaction

Characteristics of individuals.

Characteristics of individuals

Characteristics of Individuals constructs were identified in 23 studies.[9–18,20,22,29,32,35,36,42,44,45,49,50,53] Key *Characteristics of Individuals* included knowledge and self-efficacy of the pharmacist for providing new services (Table 5). Pharmacists' knowledge and skill with a service were crucial and often a driver of implementation, as were positive beliefs about the service. For example, pharmacists viewing themselves as part of the health care system were facilitative for immunizations and HIV testing. For HIV testing, pharmacists' beliefs about the stigma of HIV or illicit drug use affected uptake.

Few other characteristics were examined in the literature. The constructs of *individual stage of change* and *individual identification with organization* were not observed in the literature, which may be a function of the few formal implementation studies identified and reviewed.

Process

There were few observations of relevant constructs from the *Process* domain, which may reflect that studies informed by implementation science were uncommon at the time.. Only seven studies described a formal implementation process, approach to execution, or reflecting and evaluating the implementation.[18,25,28,36,39,42,53] The few studies that did address process were largely related to immunizations.[25,28,36,39,42,53] The constructs of note identified included the importance of engaging the appropriate individuals to facilitate implementation, usually within the pharmacy. Although few of the constructs were observed commonly, "opinion leaders" was the only construct that was not observed in the literature. See Table 6 for an overview of the relevant *Process* constructs observed in the literature.

A framework for implementation research on pharmacy services

The CFIR provides a comprehensive menu of implementation constructs from which to understand the implementation of professional services, like MTM, immunizations, and rapid HIV testing, into the community pharmacy setting. Table 7 provides a "Framework for Implementation Research on Pharmacy Services," a list and description of the constructs that appeared most salient to understanding determinants in the implementation of professional services in community pharmacy settings.

TABLE 6 CFIR constructs relevant to pharmacy—CFIR domain 5.

CFIR constructs	MTM	Immunizations	HIV testing	Description of observed CFIR constructs in literature
Planning	X	X		• There were few and limited descriptions of formal planning to implement services
Engaging		X		• *Formally appoint internal implementation leaders*: One study described a pharmacist was given the opportunity to lead immunization implementation • *Champions*: Successful adopters of immunization services often identified a *local champion* within the pharmacy to facilitate the process of implementation • *External change agents*: For immunizations, one study found external facilitators effective
Executing	X	X		• There was one study describing the follow-through on implementing MTM • One study of immunizations described an implementation checklist
Reflecting and evaluating		X		• There are select examples of evaluating and quality checking immunizations
Process.				

The review by Shoemaker et al.[3] offers a tailored version of the CFIR framework. It also expands the use of the CFIR, by examining its utility and application to a professional service and not just to a discrete intervention.[54] Focusing on a service, including a multifaceted service like MTM, highlighted differences in terms of the relevant constructs. For example, the CFIR's intervention characteristics, like *evidence strength* or *design quality and packaging* were far less applicable for understanding services like MTM, immunizations, and rapid HIV testing. In terms of *adaptability*, the desire for such might be limited, as there would need to be fidelity and a need to provide a service appropriately and consistently. *Complexity* of the service(s) can also be driven by *outer setting* and *inner setting* factors. There were few observations of the *process* domain in the literature, which may be a function of not identifying and having literature that actually studied implementation, but instead addressed experiences, barriers and facilitators, and sometimes attitudes or perceptions of barriers and facilitators. *Culture* was rarely observed in the literature; however, Rosenthal et al. have examined the culture of community pharmacy and concluded that the culture could be an important barrier to implementing change initiatives (e.g., professional services).[55]

In several examples, multiple CFIR constructs were interrelated for either promoting or barring successful implementation in community pharmacy settings. For example, the challenges with documentation systems for MTM could be applicable to *design quality and packaging* or to the *complexity* or *adaptability*—all under intervention characteristics. Similarly, when describing the use of interns, pharmacy technicians, or clerks to support the services, this was deemed reflective of *structural characteristics* and *available resources*. Additionally, the line between whether knowledge of a service was an *individual characteristic* or a function of the *inner setting* was often unclear. *Knowledge* or necessary training to provide the various services was critical and varied to the extent that additional training was needed, at the same time *beliefs* about a service might have been essential to implementation. Finally, the ability to be reimbursed for MTM *(cost)* is close to essential for implementation, and when combined with the limited *availability of resources* posed implementation challenges.

Shoemaker et al.[3] offers a framework for implementation research on pharmacy services that can be used to understand the determinants of success in implementing professional services in community pharmacy. Their paper highlights that there had been few studies that employed an implementation science approach to pharmacy research, yet the empirical studies provided insights reflective of the CFIR domains and constructs. To advance pharmacy research and the rigor of designing, studying or evaluating implementation, it is critical to employ a theory, model or framework drawn from implementation science. Thus, Shoemaker et al.[3] offer a framework applied to several complex pharmacy services that could inform the design and analysis of future implementation studies in pharmacy or of pharmacy and other health

TABLE 7 A framework for implementation research on pharmacy services.

Domains

Construct	Description
Pharmacy service characteristics	
Relative advantage	Pharmacy staff, providers, and patients' perception of the advantage or benefits of the service versus an alternative service or in addition to dispensing
Adaptability	The degree to which a service can be adapted, tailored, or refined to meet local needs of the pharmacy
Complexity	Perceived difficulty of implementing the service reflected by scope, radicalness, disruptiveness, incorporation into workflow, staff needed, and number of steps required to implement
Cost	Costs of providing a service, including implementing the service, investment, supplies and opportunity costs
Outer setting	
Patient needs and resources	The extent to which patient needs, as well as barriers and facilitators to meet those needs, are accurately known and prioritized by the pharmacy with the service
Cosmopolitanism	The degree to which a pharmacy is networked with other pharmacies and providers
Peer pressure	Competitive pressure to provide a service; typically because most or other key peers or competing pharmacies have already implemented these services
External policy and incentives	A broad construct that includes external strategies to spread a service, including policy and regulations (governmental or other central entity), external mandates, recommendations and guidelines, pay-for-performance, collaboratives, and public or benchmark reporting
Inner setting	
Structural Characteristics	The type of pharmacy, size, physical space, staffing and other structural characteristics
Culture	Norms, values, and basic assumptions of a pharmacy
Implementation climate	The absorptive capacity for change, shared receptivity of staff, and extent to which provision of the service will be rewarded, supported, and expected within the pharmacy
Tension for change	The degree to which pharmacy managers, pharmacists, and other pharmacy staff perceive the current situation as needing change and that a service should be provided
Compatibility	The degree of tangible fit between meaning and values attached to the service by pharmacy staff; how those align with pharmacists' own norms, values, and perceived risks and needs; and how the service fits with existing pharmacy workflows and systems
Organizational incentives and rewards	Incentives such as awards, performance reviews, promotions, and raises in salary, and less tangible incentives such as increased stature or respect
Readiness for Implementation	Tangible and immediate indicators of pharmacy commitment to its decision to implement a service
Leadership engagement	Commitment, involvement, and accountability of leaders and pharmacy managers with implementing and providing the service
Available resources	The level of resources dedicated for implementation and on-going provision, including money, training, education, physical space, and time, of the service
Access to knowledge and information	Ease of access to digestible information and knowledge about the service and how to incorporate it into workflow
Pharmacy staff characteristics	
Knowledge and beliefs about the service	Pharmacy staff's attitudes toward and value placed on the service as well as familiarity with service components, steps, documentation, care process, etc.
Self-efficacy	Pharmacy staff's belief in their own capabilities to provide the service
Other personal attributes	A broad construct to include other personal traits such as tolerance of ambiguity, intellectual ability, motivation, values, competence, capacity, and learning style

TABLE 7 A framework for implementation research on pharmacy services—cont'd

Domains *Construct*	Description
Process	
Planning	The degree to which a scheme or method of behavior and tasks for implementing a service are developed in advance, and the quality of those schemes or methods
Engaging	Attracting and involving appropriate individuals in the implementation and provision of the service through a combined strategy of education, role modeling, training, and other activities
Formally appointed internal implementation leaders	Individuals from within the pharmacy who have been formally appointed with responsibility for implementing and overseeing the service
Champions	Individuals who dedicate themselves to supporting, marketing, and "driving through" the implementation and provision of a service, overcoming indifference or resistance that the service may provoke in a pharmacy
External change agents	Individuals who are affiliated with an outside entity who formally influence or facilitate decisions in a desirable direction to provide a services like a professional pharmacy association or local pharmacy school
Executing	Carrying out or accomplishing the implementation according to plan
Reflecting and evaluating	Quantitative and qualitative feedback about the progress and quality of implementation and providing the service, with regular reflection about progress and experience

(Adapted from CFIR.)

services. Future research should empirically test implementation frameworks like this one, or utilize the CFIR in other studies or reviews like Weir et al.[56] did in a systematic review, which is described below.

Application of CFIR to a systematic review of factors influencing national implementation of innovations in community pharmacy

Weir et al.[56] conducted a systematic review of 39 qualitative, questionnaire design, and mixed-methods studies to identify facilitators and barriers to the national implementation of community pharmacy innovations.[56] From their review, Weir et al.[56] found 13 CFIR constructs cited by at least a quarter of the reviewed studies, which they grouped into the themes of pharmacy staff engagement, operationalization of the innovation, and external engagement. The specific CFIR constructs Weir et al.[56] identified within the three thematic areas were:

- *Pharmacy staff engagement*: The knowledge and beliefs of pharmacy staff [CFIR domain: characteristics of individuals] relating to an innovation, its compatibility [CFIR domain: inner setting] with their roles and values, whether it poses advantages or not [CFIR domain: innovation characteristics], and the incentives [CFIR domains: inner setting, outer setting] and strategies which engage community pharmacy staff [CFIR domain: process].
- *Operationalization of the innovation*: Innovation attributes (such as design and complexity) [CFIR domain: innovation characteristics] and surrounding factors including resources [CFIR domain: inner setting], compatibility with pharmacy systems [CFIR domain: inner setting], and pharmacy staff access to knowledge and information about the innovation [CFIR domain: inner setting].
- *External engagement*: The relationship with patients [CFIR domain: outer setting] and other healthcare professionals [CFIR domain: inner setting], their perceptions, and strategies to engage these stakeholders [CFIR domain: process].

As a result of their review, Weir et al.[56] presented a "preliminary theory of how salient factors influence national implementation in the community pharmacy setting" and acknowledged "further research is necessary to understand how the influence of these factors may differ within varying contexts."

Weir et al.[56] demonstrate another application of the CFIR to a review—this time in understanding the specific factors influencing national implementation of innovations in community pharmacy. Based on their review they also offered a preliminary theory and recommendations to facilitate the development of successful national implementation strategies.

Both Shoemaker et al.[3] and Weir et al.[56] used the CFIR as a framework to review published studies of pharmacy services implementation. While it is reasonable to use the CFIR and other implementation models and frameworks post hoc to analyze data, it is also in keeping with good science practices to consider the appropriate model or framework a priori in designing a study or evaluation. As a determinant framework, CFIR offers an overarching typology from which pharmacy researchers can select constructs that are most relevant or applicable to evaluate implementation progress, explain findings, or assess implementation context.

Conclusion

The Consolidated Framework for Implementation Research (CFIR) is a robust determinant framework that has been widely used in health services research, and growing use in pharmacy research. The CFIR has been adapted to pharmacy services[3] and used in a systematic review of national implementation of pharmacy services[56] and many studies of pharmacy interventions and services. The CFIR—as an implementation science framework—has a demonstrated utility in continuing to advance and understand the effective implementation of pharmacy and health services.

Questions for further discussion

1. How might you use CFIR to examine the implementation of a new pharmacy service?
2. Describe an example of when CFIR may not be an appropriate framework to use in pharmacy research.
3. How might you use CFIR to design a study on the implementation of a medication therapy management service in community pharmacy?

Application exercise/scenario

Identify at least two recent empirical studies published in a pharmacy journal on a specific pharmacy service (e.g., vaccine provision, naloxone for opioid overdose reversal, medication therapy management, pharmaceutical care) or intervention implemented in a community pharmacy, hospital pharmacy, ambulatory clinic or other setting. Conduct a post hoc analysis of the study findings by coding the determinants of success (i.e., barriers and facilitators) to implementing the service or intervention as described in the articles using the tailored CFIR framework (i.e., tailored domains and constructs provided by Ref. 3) in Table 7. Analyze and synthesize your coding and write a two-page summary of your findings.

References

1. Bacci JL, Chui MA, Farley J, et al. Implementation science to advance practice and curricular transformation: report of the 2019-2020 AACP research and graduate affairs committee. *Am J Pharm Educ.* 2020;84(10), ajpe848204.
2. Livet M, Haines ST, Curran GM, et al. Implementation science to advance care delivery: a primer for pharmacists and other health professionals. *Pharmacotherapy.* 2018;38(5):490–502.
3. Shoemaker SJ, Curran GM, Swan H, Teeter BS, Thomas J. Application of the consolidated framework for implementation research to community pharmacy: a framework for implementation research on pharmacy services. *Res Soc Adm Pharm.* 2017;13(5):905–913.
4. Damschroder LJ, Aron DC, Keith RE, Kirsh SR, Alexander JA, Lowery JC. Fostering implementation of health services research findings into practice: a consolidated framework for advancing implementation science. *Implement Sci.* 2009;4:50. https://doi.org/10.1186/1748-5908-4-50.
5. Nilsen P. Making sense of implementation theories, models and frameworks. *Implement Sci.* 2015;10(1):53. https://doi.org/10.1186/s13012-015-0242-0.
6. Kirk MA, Kelley C, Yankey N, Birken SA, Abadie B, Damschroder L. A systematic review of the use of the consolidated framework for implementation research. *Implement Sci.* 2016;11:72. https://doi.org/10.1186/s13012-016-0437-z.
7. Meyerson BE, Agley JD, Jayawardene W, et al. Feasibility and acceptability of a proposed pharmacy-based harm reduction intervention to reduce opioid overdose, HIV and hepatitis C. *Res Soc Adm Pharm.* 2020;16(5):699–709.
8. Stolldorf DP, Mixon AS, Auerbach AD, et al. Implementation and sustainability of a medication reconciliation toolkit: a mixed methods evaluation. *Am J Health Syst Pharm.* 2020;77(14):1135–1143.
9. Blake KB, Madhavan SS. Perceived barriers to provision of medication therapy management services (MTMS) and the likelihood of a pharmacist to work in a pharmacy that provides MTMS. *Ann Pharmacother.* 2010;44(3):424–431.
10. Blake KB, Madhavan SS, Scott VG, Elswick BLM. Medication therapy management services in West Virginia: pharmacists' perceptions of educational and training needs. *Res Soc Adm Pharm.* 2009;5(2):182–188.
11. Chui MA, Mott DA, Maxwell L. A qualitative assessment of a community pharmacy cognitive pharmaceutical services program, using a work system approach. *Res Soc Adm Pharm.* 2012;8(3):206–216.
12. Herbert KE, Urmie JM, Newland BA, Farris KB. Prediction of pharmacist intention to provide Medicare medication therapy management services using the theory of planned behavior. *Res Soc Adm Pharm.* 2006;2(3):299–314.

13. Lounsbery JL, Green CG, Bennett MS, Pedersen CA. Evaluation of pharmacists' barriers to the implementation of medication therapy management services. *J Am Pharm Assoc.* 2009;49(1):51–58.

14. MacIntosh C, Weiser C, Wassimi A, et al. Attitudes toward and factors affecting implementation of medication therapy management services by community pharmacists. *J Am Pharm Assoc.* 2009;49(1):26–30.

15. Moczygemba LR, Barner JC, Roberson K. Texas pharmacists' opinions about and plans for provision of medication therapy management services. *J Am Pharm Assoc.* 2008;48(1):38–55a.

16. Rosenthal M, Tsao NW, Tsuyuki RT, Marra CA. Identifying relationships between the professional culture of pharmacy, pharmacists' personality traits, and the provision of advanced pharmacy services. *Res Soc Adm Pharm.* 2016;12(1):56–67.

17. Smith MA, Spiggle S, McConnell B. Strategies for community-based medication management services in value-based health plans. *Res Soc Adm Pharm.* 2017;13(1):48–62.

18. Trapskin K, Johnson C, Cory P, Sorum S, Decker C. Forging a novel provider and payer partnership in Wisconsin to compensate pharmacists for quality-driven pharmacy and medication therapy management services. *J Am Pharm Assoc.* 2009;49(5):642–651.

19. Aderemi-Williams R, Igwilo C. Community pharmacies as possible centres for routine immunization. *Nig Q J Hosp Med.* 2007;17(4):131–133.

20. Atkins K, Van Hoek AJ, Watson C, et al. Seasonal influenza vaccination delivery through community pharmacists in England: evaluation of the London pilot. *BMJ Open.* 2016;6(2), e009739.

21. Brackett A, Butler M, Chapman L. Using motivational interviewing in the community pharmacy to increase adult immunization readiness: a pilot evaluation. *J Am Pharm Assoc.* 2015;55(2):182–186.

22. Crawford ND, Blaney S, Amesty S, et al. Individual-and neighborhood-level characteristics associated with support of in-pharmacy vaccination among ESAP-registered pharmacies: pharmacists' role in reducing racial/ethnic disparities in influenza vaccinations in New York City. *J Urban Health.* 2011;88(1):176–185.

23. Doucette WR, McDonough RP, Mormann MM, Vaschevici R, Urmie JM, Patterson BJ. Three-year financial analysis of pharmacy services at an independent community pharmacy. *J Am Pharm Assoc.* 2012;52(2):181–187.

24. Duncan IG, Taitel MS, Zhang J, Kirkham HS. Planning influenza vaccination programs: a cost benefit model. *Cost Eff Resour Alloc.* 2012;10(1):1–11.

25. Edwards N, Corsten EG, Kiberd M, et al. Pharmacists as immunizers: a survey of community pharmacists' willingness to administer adult immunizations. *Int J Clin Pharm.* 2015;37(2):292–295.

26. Gardner JS. A practical guide to establishing vaccine administration services in community pharmacies. *J Am Pharm Assoc.* 1997;37(6):683–693.

27. Gatewood SB, Stanley DD. Implementation of a comprehensive pretravel health program in a supermarket chain pharmacy. *J Am Pharm Assoc.* 2009;49(5):660–669.

28. Goode J-VR, Mott DA, Stanley DD. Assessment of an immunization program in a supermarket chain pharmacy. *J Am Pharm Assoc.* 2007; 47(4):495–498.

29. Kummer GL, Foushee LL. Description of the characteristics of pharmacist-based immunization services in North Carolina: results of a pharmacist survey. *J Am Pharm Assoc.* 2008;48(6):744–751.

30. Murphy PA, Frazee SG, Cantlin JP, Cohen E, Rosan JR, Harshburger DE. Pharmacy provision of influenza vaccinations in medically underserved communities. *J Am Pharm Assoc.* 2012;52(1):67–70.

31. Ndiaye S, Madhavan S, Washington M, et al. The use of pharmacy immunization services in rural communities. *Public Health.* 2003;117(2):88–97.

32. Neuhauser MM, Wiley D, Simpson L, Garey KW. Involvement of immunization-certified pharmacists with immunization activities. *Ann Pharmacother.* 2004;38(2):226–231.

33. Pilisuk T, Goad J, Backer H. Vaccination delivery by chain pharmacies in California: results of a 2007 survey. *J Am Pharm Assoc.* 2010; 50(2):134–139.

34. Usami T, Hashiguchi M, Kouhara T, Ishii A, Nagata T, Mochizuki M. Impact of community pharmacists advocating immunization on influenza vaccination rates among the elderly. *Yakugaku Zasshi.* 2009;129(9):1063–1068.

35. Valiquette JR, Bédard P. Community pharmacists' knowledge, beliefs and attitudes towards immunization in Quebec. *Can J Public Health.* 2015; 106(3):e89–e94.

36. Weitzel KW. Implementation of a pharmacy-based immunization program in a supermarket chain. *J Am Pharm Assoc.* 2000;40(2):252–256.

37. Westrick SC. Forward and backward transitions in pharmacy-based immunization services. *Res Soc Adm Pharm.* 2010;6(1):18–31.

38. Westrick SC. Pharmacy characteristics, vaccination service characteristics, and service expansion: an analysis of sustainers and new adopters. *J Am Pharm Assoc.* 2010;50(1):52–61.

39. Westrick SC, Breland ML. Sustainability of pharmacy-based innovations: the case of in-house immunization services. *J Am Pharm Assoc.* 2009; 49(4):500–508.

40. Westrick SC, Mount JK. Impact of perceived innovation characteristics on adoption of pharmacy-based in-house immunization services. *Int J Pharm Pract.* 2009;17(1):39–46.

41. Westrick SC, Mount JK, Watcharadamrongkun S, Breland ML. Pharmacy stages of involvement in pharmacy-based immunization services: results from a 17-state survey. *J Am Pharm Assoc.* 2008;48(6):764–773.

42. Westrick SC, Owen J, Hagel H, Owensby JK, Lertpichitkul T. Impact of the RxVaccinate program for pharmacy-based pneumococcal immunization: a cluster-randomized controlled trial. *J Am Pharm Assoc.* 2016;56(1):29–36.e21.

43. Westrick SC, Watcharadamrongkun S, Mount JK, Breland ML. Community pharmacy involvement in vaccine distribution and administration. *Vaccine.* 2009;27(21):2858–2863.

44. Amesty S, Blaney S, Crawford ND, Rivera AV, Fuller C. Pharmacy staff characteristics associated with support for pharmacy-based HIV testing. *J Am Pharm Assoc.* 2012;52(4):472–479.

45. Amesty S, Crawford ND, Nandi V, et al. Evaluation of pharmacy-based HIV testing in a high-risk New York City community. *AIDS Patient Care STDs.* 2015;29(8):437–444.

46. Calderon Y, Cowan E, Rhee JY, Brusalis C, Leider J. Counselor-based rapid HIV testing in community pharmacies. *AIDS Patient Care STDs.* 2013;27(8):467–473.

47. Darin KM, Scarsi KK, Klepser DG, et al. Consumer interest in community pharmacy HIV screening services. *J Am Pharm Assoc.* 2015;55(1):67–72.

48. Dugdale C, Zaller N, Bratberg J, Berk W, Flanigan T. Missed opportunities for HIV screening in pharmacies and retail clinics. *J Manag Care Pharm.* 2014;20(4):339–345.

49. Fernandez-Balbuena S, Belza MJ, Zulaica D, et al. Widening the access to HIV testing: the contribution of three in-pharmacy testing programmes in Spain. *PLoS One.* 2015;10(8), e0134631.

50. Hammett TM, Phan S, Gaggin J, et al. Pharmacies as providers of expanded health services for people who inject drugs: a review of laws, policies, and barriers in six countries. *BMC Health Serv Res.* 2014;14(1):1–11.

51. Lecher SL, Shrestha RK, Botts LW, et al. Cost analysis of a novel HIV testing strategy in community pharmacies and retail clinics. *J Am Pharm Assoc.* 2015;55(5):488–492.

52. Weidle PJ, Lecher S, Botts LW, et al. HIV testing in community pharmacies and retail clinics: a model to expand access to screening for HIV infection. *J Am Pharm Assoc.* 2014;54(5):486–492.

53. Navarrete JP, Padilla ME, Castro LP, Rivera JO. Development of a community pharmacy human papillomavirus vaccine program for underinsured university students along the United States/Mexico border. *J Am Pharm Assoc.* 2014;54(6):642–647.

54. Shoemaker SJ, Staub-DeLong L, Wasserman M, Spranca M. Factors affecting adoption and implementation of AHRQ health literacy tools in pharmacies. *Res Soc Adm Pharm.* 2013;9(5):553–563.

55. Rosenthal MM, Breault RR, Austin Z, Tsuyuki RT. Pharmacists' self-perception of their professional role: insights into community pharmacy culture. *J Am Pharm Assoc.* 2011;51(3):363–368a.

56. Weir NM, Newham R, Dunlop E, Bennie M. Factors influencing national implementation of innovations within community pharmacy: a systematic review applying the consolidated framework for implementation research. *Implement Sci.* 2019;14(1):1–16.

Chapter 6

Principles and applications of metaresearch

Spencer E. Harpe

Department of Pharmacy Practice, Midwestern University College of Pharmacy, Downers Grove, IL, United States

Objectives

- Define metaresearch.
- Describe common thematic areas or emphases within metaresearch.
- Identify common methods used in metaresearch.
- Describe the importance of metaresearch in pharmacy and health services research.

Introduction

Metaresearch seems quite simple at first glance—research on research. Unfortunately, this rather simplistic definition may not help researchers grasp the variety of topics that fall within the scope of this growing area. The definition of metaresearch proposed by Ioannidis provides a better sense of the discipline: "the study of research itself: its methods, reporting, reproducibility, evaluation, and incentives."[1] Taken together, metaresearch is concerned with the efficiency, quality, and bias within the entire scientific ecosystem.[2] When first hearing the term "metaresearch," many researchers may immediately think of metaanalysis. Research synthesis is one focus area within metaresearch, but there are many other areas to be explored. This chapter will introduce researchers to metaresearch, provide examples of metaresearch in pharmacy services research, and motivate the importance of sustained metaresearch.

Historical overview

Despite the recent emphasis on metaresearch in the modern research enterprise, it is far from new. The conceptual beginnings of metaresearch date back to the early 17th century when Sir Francis Bacon and Robert Boyle raised concerns about publication bias.[3] The mid-to-late 20th century saw an increased emphasis on the quality of science across a variety of disciplines[2] and changing structures for research funding.[4] In the early 2000s, scientists from diverse backgrounds began raising concerns about the lack of replication within science. Two fields of research that have received a great deal of attention from the perspective of replication are psychology[5,6] and medicine.[7–9] With increasing concerns about the credibility and utility of research, metaresearch has become more formalized as a discipline.[2]

Thematic areas within metaresearch

Ioannidis et al.[10] have proposed a categorization of metaresearch efforts using the following themes: methods, reporting, replicability and reproducibility, evaluation, and incentives. Organization has been added here as a sixth theme. These areas can also be viewed as a general framework for describing and coordinating metaresearch activities. Table 1 provides the six thematic areas of metaresearch and selected examples of specific topics of interest within each area. It is important to remember that these areas often interact with each other. For example, a metaresearch study examining the role of research in promotion and tenure criteria for faculty (Incentives) may also be concerned with the ways research impact and quality are evaluated (Evaluation). Examples from the literature are provided in the following subsections to highlight metaresearch within each thematic area.

Contemporary Research Methods in Pharmacy and Health Services. https://doi.org/10.1016/B978-0-323-91888-6.00038-7

TABLE 1 Metaresearch themes and selected examples.

Theme	Sample topics	Examples from the pharmacy literature
Methods (How is research performed?)	• Study designs and methods used • Analytical approaches used • Research synthesis methods • Research ethics and integrity	• Statistical methods used in the pharmacy literature[11] • Study designs used in pharmacy residency projects[12] • Staffing, research designs, and collaboration in US pharmacy practice research centers[13]
Reporting (How is research communicated?)	• Use of reporting standards • Study registration • Disclosure of conflicts of interests • Information sharing with stakeholders (e.g., patients, public, policymakers) • Publication ethics and integrity	• Publication rates of pharmacy residency projects[12] • Review of pharmacists' interventions in asthma management[14] • Registration of studies with pharmacist interventions[15] • Ghost and honorary authorship in pharmacy[16]
Replicability and Reproducibility (How is research verified or replicated? What happens when these efforts fail?)	• Methods for data sharing • Methods for promoting repeatability, replicability, and reproducibility • Efforts to repeat, replicate, or reproduce previous studies • Self-correction activities	• Replication of a successful case management program[17] • Retractions in the drug literature[18]
Evaluation (How is research evaluated?)	• Peer review processes (both pre- and postpublication) • Research funding criteria • Evaluating scientific quality • Measuring research impact • Examining issues related to equity and justice in research[a]	• Publications patterns of pharmacy practice faculty members[19] • Publication records of pharmacy school deans[20] • Relationship between altmetrics and 2-year citation counts[21] • Rating of health care administration journals[22] • Female authors in pharmacy[23] • Gender composition of health professions journals editorial boards[24] • Review of disparities intervention research[25]
Incentives (How is research rewarded or supported?)	• Role of research in promotion criteria • Use of rewards and/or penalties in research evaluation • Application of incentive structures across varying levels (individuals, teams, and institutions) • Methods to develop research capacity and support research engagement[a]	• Barriers to scholarship among pharmacy practice faculty[26] • Research productivity and training among junior pharmacy practice faculty[27]
Organization[a] (How is research organized or categorized?)	• Relationships between research topics or areas within a discipline • Interactions of disciplines in research efforts • Research collaboration[b] • Role of research categorization or classification in the discovery, use, or uptake of research	• Staffing, research designs, and collaboration in US pharmacy practice research centers[13] • Review of disparities intervention research[25] • Assignment of MeSH terms in pharmacy journals[28] • Mapping pharmacy journals[29]

[a] Not included in the original list of areas and topics proposed by Ioannidis et al.[10]

[b] Included under a different theme in the original list of areas and topics proposed by Ioannidis et al.[10]

Modified from Ioannidis JPA, Fanelli D, Dunne DD, Goodman SN. Meta-research: evaluation and improvement of research methods and practices. *PLoS Biol.* 2015;13(10):e1002264. doi:10.1371/journal.pbio.1002264.

Methods

When focusing on methods, metaresearch studies consider such issues as the types of study designs and analytical approaches used within a body of research, methods for research synthesis, and research collaboration. Lee et al.[11] reviewed articles published in six pharmacy journals in 2001 to characterize the type of statistical methods used. Their study reported that 28% of articles used only descriptive statistics with 69% using various forms of inferential statistics like t-tests or logistic regression. A similar study by McKelvey et al.[12] examined pharmacy residency project publication rates and study designs from 1981 to 2001. The authors found that the percentage of studies using experimental designs decreased over the period and quasiexperimental designs increased while observational studies stayed constant. Metaresearch need not be limited to individual publications. For example, Salgado et al.[13] characterized 20 pharmacy practice research centers across the United States with respect to staffing levels, funding, types of study designs frequently used, and collaboration.

Research synthesis is also a methods-related focus area within metaresearch. It is important to note the differences between research synthesis in a metaresearch context and traditional research synthesis approaches like systematic reviews, metaanalyses, or scoping reviews. Traditional, single topic synthesis approaches, such as a metaanalysis of the effects of value-based insurance design on medication adherence and healthcare costs, would not be the primary focus of research synthesis efforts in metaresearch. On the other hand, synthesis efforts that look across multiple reviews or metaanalyses and encompass a variety of methods, outcomes, or care settings would be a potential activity within metaresearch. This is not to say that single-topic and focused research synthesis methods are not important. They are extremely important and valuable. To describe this another way, research synthesis efforts in metaresearch may involve reviews of reviews or reviews of metaanalyses. The 2015 overview of systematic reviews of clinical pharmacy services by Rotta et al.[30] provides an example of a focus on research synthesis that fits within the framework of metaresearch in pharmacy.

Reporting

The dissemination and reporting of research findings is a key aspect of the research process. This may be viewed from two perspectives. The first is whether results were disseminated at all. The previously mentioned article by McKelvey et al.[12] noted an overall publication rate of 16% among pharmacy residency projects, but that decreased across the study period.

The second perspective relates to the quality of reporting. Speaking specifically to research on pharmacy services, these papers often lack sufficient quality to be included in systematic reviews or metaanalyses despite this body of literature being quite large.[31,32] As one example, Crespo-Gonzalez et al.[14] conducted a systematic review of pharmacists' interventions in asthma management and found that there was insufficient information about several elements of the pharmacists' activities, notably the core intervention components and intervention dose. Various reporting guidelines and tools, such as the updated version of the Descriptive Elements of Pharmacist Intervention Characterization Tool (DEPICT-2)[33] and the Pharmacist Patient Care Intervention Reporting (PaCIR) checklist,[34] have been developed to improve the quality of reporting and even reproducibility.

Registration of studies is another reporting-related element that provides a way to combat publication bias, promote transparency, and perhaps increase trust in biomedical research.[35–37] Dammo and Harpe[15] reviewed ClinicalTrials.gov to characterize registered studies involving pharmacists' services. Only 122 studies focused on pharmacists' services with an additional 29 where pharmacists' services were part of the study but not a focus. Compared to the size of the pharmacy services literature and the number of studies registered in ClinicalTrials.gov at the time of the review (almost 300,000), it appears there is room for substantial improvement in study registration in pharmacy research.

Publication practices representing questionable ethical decisions are another area of interest within reporting. Authorship is an issue fraught with potential misconduct. The International Committee of Medical Journal Editors (ICMJE) uses four criteria for authorship stating that "any individual not meeting all criteria should be acknowledged as a contributor rather than being listed as an author."[38] There are still instances of inappropriate authorship practices in the general biomedical literature. Two inappropriate practices of concern include ghost authorship and guest authorship. Ghost authorship, or ghostwriting, refers to situations where one or more individuals who meet authorship criteria are not included in the author list. Guest, or honorary, authorship can be thought of as the opposite of ghost authorship whereby individuals who do *not* meet authorship criteria are included as authors on a publication. For example, a paper from a study funded by a pharmaceutical company may be written by the company's employees or contracted medical writers. Not including those employees or medical writers in the author list would be an example of ghost authorship. To promote a sense of credibility, the company may offer authorship to a clinician leader in the field even though that individual did not serve as an author in any capacity (i.e., they are an honorary author).[39] Dotson and Slaughter[16] surveyed corresponding authors from three pharmacy journals. Their findings indicated that ghost authorship was extremely rare ($<1\%$), but honorary authorship was noted by 14% of respondents.

Replicability and reproducibility

Concerns have been raised about the inability to reproduce the results of previous studies. Explicit efforts to replicate pharmacy services studies in a similar fashion to large scale replication efforts in psychology are somewhat rare. The discussion in the previous section on Reporting about difficulties when including pharmacy services studies in systematic reviews and metaanalyses highlight potential struggles with reproducibility (i.e., finding similar results in two different settings) in pharmacy research. Admittedly, there are many factors that can affect the reproducibility of any research project, especially in practice-based research and health services research. It is, however, important to consider the benefit of these efforts to examine effects in different practice settings or locations with different sets of patients.

Despite sounding similar, the meanings of replicability and reproducibility vary across subject areas and can even be contradictory.[40] Barba[41] described the distinctions that biomedical research tends to make between replicability and reproducibility. Reproducibility relates to using the original data and same analytical methods to reproduce the results (i.e., different researchers, same methods, same data). Replicability involves repeating a study with the same or similar methods to see if the same or similar results are found (i.e., same or different researchers, same or similar methods, different data). Setting aside specific differences in definitions, the general concept is that studies are repeated to see if the original results still stand after repeated research efforts. Repeating, reproducing, or replicating studies requires clear and consistent reporting of methods and analytical techniques. In some cases, it requires posting the original data and computer code to facilitate analysis. Recent developments in the open science movement have promoted this increased level of transparency.[42,43]

Science has been said to be, at least in theory, self-correcting.[44] While peer review processes and scientific integrity policies provide some level of protection against fraud or other untoward actions, efforts to replicate or reproduce studies is another important mechanism to support this self-correction. Failed replication efforts may represent previously unexpected variability and highlight the importance of careful interpretation and extrapolation. For example, Peterson et al.[17] attempted to replicate a case management program. Their replication efforts were unsuccessful, and they offered reasons for this lack of replication in their discussion. Failed replication efforts may also uncover incorrect methods or even overt fraud. One way to examine the self-correction process is to consider retractions of publications. Samp et al.[18] identified 102 retractions among published drug therapy articles from 2000 to 2011 with 72% of those being retracted for reasons of scientific misconduct.

Evaluation

The evaluation of both the quality and impact of research has become a major effort for funders, researchers, and institutions. Funders depend on peer review processes to identify projects worthy of being supported. Researchers want indicators of their research quality or impact to support career advancement or additional funding. Institutions desire similar indicators for use in promotional material, as markers of prestige, or to garner additional support. Peer review is one of the most visible forms of evaluation, which has become an area of research emphasis on its own.[45,46]

Evaluation methods within metaresearch often rely on bibliometric or scientometric methods, which examine the extent and pattern of citations for various research outputs. Chisholm-Burns et al.[19] examined pharmacy practice faculty at US schools of pharmacy and identified an average of 0.51 publications per year over the 5-year study period. The authors also identified factors associated with increased publication rates (e.g., presence of a graduate program, affiliation with a health sciences campus, NIH funding). In a similar study of US pharmacy school deans, Thompson[20] used additional bibliometric parameters, such as average citations per paper and the h-index, and identified wide variation based on type of school, discipline, and training. Interestingly, Dixon and Baker[21] found no relationship between altmetric-based measures of research impact and 2-year citations to articles in the pharmacy literature. Other databases, such as the science-wide author databases of standardized citation indicators, exist to facilitate author-level analyses and even allow for comparison across scientific disciplines.[47,48] It is also possible to use bibliometric approaches to evaluate journals. For example, Dame and Wolinsky[22] used bibliometric methods to rank health care administration journals and compare them to previous ranking based on perceptions of program or department chairs.

Metaresearch can also support efforts to evaluate the extent to which equity and justice are considered in research, from the actual research processes to the researchers and even research participants or other stakeholders. One area that has been of interest in science is the extent to which authorship patterns and funding success is influenced by an individual's gender.[49,50] Gender differences in authorship and journal editorial board composition have both been examined in pharmacy. Dotson[23] found that female first authors in three pharmacy journals increased from 30% to 52% from 1989 to 2009; however, the percentage of females as last authors (considered an indication of senior author status) was considerably lower. Sarna et al.[24] considered the gender breakdown of journal editorial boards for selected medicine, nursing, and pharmacy journals from 1995 to 2016. Women were underrepresented among medicine and pharmacy journals while men were underrepresented in nursing journals. Across all journals, there were statistically significant increases for the minority gender over time. As another example of metaresearch being used to examine issues of equity, Clarke et al.[25] examined 30 years of research involving interventions to reduce racial and ethnic health disparities. Their work resulted in a proposed taxonomy of disparities interventions and highlighted areas that had not received adequate attention by researchers in the field.

Incentives

Various incentives are in place to promote research activities among both individuals and institutions. While these incentives are designed to promote and facilitate high quality research endeavors, this is not always the case as inappropriate or suboptimal behaviors may be incentivized. These incentives may be direct financial incentives (e.g., bonus pay for high research output) or part of career progression (e.g., promotion and tenure in academia). Metaresearch may examine the effect of these incentives on research efficiency, quality, and integrity.

Another important area to consider with incentives relates to how research is supported through nonfinancial means. There are known barriers to research productivity among health professionals in an academic setting where clinical practice activities are expected.[51–53] Various studies have examined research productivity of pharmacy practice faculty. Both Robles et al.[26] and Lee et al.[27] have described barriers to research, including lack of time, training, and support. This is despite faculty members' interest to engage in research.

Organization

With increasing efforts promoting interprofessional and transdisciplinary research, mapping or describing the relationships between disciplines is of increasing interest. Another aspect of organization is the way in which research is classified or categorized. Given the breadth of disciplines, research questions, and research methods, a single consistent ontology is difficult. One classification system with which pharmacy researchers may be familiar is the Medical Subject Heading (MeSH) vocabulary used by the United States National Library of Medicine to index, catalog, and search for biomedical research.[54] Despite its history and complexity, there are still shortcomings, especially within pharmacy practice research. Minguet et al.[28] described shortcomings of the use of pharmacy-specific MeSH terms in pharmacy journals indexed in MEDLINE. As one example, over half of the identified articles were published in a pharmacy journal without any pharmacy-specific MeSH terms assigned during indexing. In addition to the classification of articles within a journal, the classification of journals themselves can be of interest in metaresearch. Mendes et al.[29] used lexicographic analysis to map 285 journals relevant to pharmacy into six meaningful groups based on the use and distribution of words in the article texts. The previously mentioned study of disparities research by Clark et al.[25] could also fit into this thematic area of organization since their work proposed a taxonomy of disparities interventions.

Metaresearch methods and techniques

A particular metaresearch project may be descriptive, exploratory, or explanatory/predictive in nature. Metaresearch studies may use any of the traditional research design approaches: experimental, quasiexperimental, and observational. Additionally, metaresearch may involve quantitative, qualitative, or mixed methods. It is important to note these foundational similarities with other areas of research since pharmacy and health services researchers already have experience with the general approaches used in metaresearch.

Metaresearch frequently draws on secondary analysis of existing data. Most of the examples provided in the previous section involve the use of data gathered from published studies. This often requires the development and refinement of strategies to search databases such as MEDLINE. When possible, including a librarian on the project can be extremely helpful to optimize search strategies. Alternatively, it is possible to have search strategies formally peer reviewed by a colleague or librarian using the Peer Review of Electronic Search Strategies (PRESS) checklist.[55] Since database searches form a core part of data collection in metaresearch, clear descriptions of the search strategies are important. Researchers using literature searches as part of data collection are encouraged to follow the reporting guidelines in the PRISMA extension for literature searches (PRISMA-S).[56]

The extraction of data from the identified literature is an important second step when using published studies as a data source. Researchers should take care to identify the required data elements, ensure all individuals involved have been appropriately trained in the extraction process, and provide evidence of processes to ensure the reliability and validity of the data being extracted (e.g., dual extraction of data from a subset of articles with accompanying agreement statistics; audits of records by a research team member not involved in the original data extraction; description of the process whereby consensus is achieved should disagreements arise, especially when researcher judgment is involved). These are issues likely familiar to researchers who have used medical chart reviews in their previous work.

Although secondary data are arguably the most common data source in metaresearch, primary data can be used. For example, the previous example by Dotson and Slaughter[16] on authorship practices collected data through a survey of authors from three pharmacy journals. Guidance on the use of survey methods, interview techniques, and other primary data collection techniques has been described in detail in various research methods texts,[57–59] so additional discussion is beyond the scope of this chapter.

Given its diverse background, metaresearch involves techniques that may be more commonly used in other fields, such as information science, sociology, psychology, economics, and policy analysis. The techniques and principles applied in metaresearch from psychology, economics, and policy analysis may be somewhat familiar to pharmacy and health services researchers. Selected metaresearch techniques that may be less familiar are discussed here.

As noted earlier, the area of evaluation within metaresearch includes measuring research impact. One way to evaluate impact is through scientometrics, or the analysis of the use of the scientific outputs (e.g., published papers, books, and presentations). This is a subfield within bibliometrics, which is also a field within information science. Citation analysis is a common technique of scientometrics and bibliometrics. Citation analysis approaches range from a simple count of the total citations that a particular publication has received to examining more complex author-level metrics like the h-index.[60] Journal-level metrics (e.g., Clarivate's Journal Impact Factor, Elsevier's CiteScore) can also be used as part of citation analysis. It is important to mention that scientometric analyses can also be conducted at the research group or institutional level. Beyond bibliometric analyses, research funding and scientific outputs can be used to provide a broader evaluation of research at the university or institutional level and may even allow comparison across research areas, such as pharmacy. Some research rankings used for universities or institutions include QS World University Rankings, the *Times Higher Education* World University Rankings, and SCImago Institutions Rankings.

Thompson and Walker[61] provide an overview of bibliometric methods related to the medical sciences that may be useful for researchers interested in these sorts of analyses. As the communication of science has moved beyond traditional journal publication, alternative metrics, or altmetrics,[62] have been developed to examine impact through mentions in social media or the lay press. More recent advances in scientometrics draw on advanced text mining and natural language processing techniques to examine citation patterns.[63,64] Regardless of the specific type of analysis, Bornmann et al.[65] highlight important considerations and best practices when engaging in any sort of bibliometric or scientometric analysis.

As computer technology has expanded, the ability to mine text in existing documents has become more common. Text mining may be as simple as examining counts of words within a body of text to more advanced approaches looking at the cooccurrence of words or phrases to identify potentially meaningful groups, such as the lexicographic analysis of pharmacy journals conducted by Mendes et al.[29] More advanced techniques, such as natural language processing, have been developed to use artificial intelligence and machine learning approaches. As an example, Buljan et al.[66] conducted a linguistic analysis of over 470,000 peer review reports to examine the relationship between research area, type of peer review, and reviewer gender, and the length and analytical tone of the reviews submitted. The use of text mining on such a large data set offered views of important issues, such as bias in peer review (falling into the Evaluation area mentioned earlier), on a scale not readily possible without computer-aided analysis.

Network analysis is another technique that can be used in metaresearch. Originally developed in sociology, network analysis, or social network analysis, examines the relationships formed between a set of actors. In a metaresearch context, these networks may involve citation patterns among researchers, collaboration patterns, funding, and even the use of particular research methods. Furthermore, network analysis can be conducted at the individual level (e.g., researchers) or at the organizational level (e.g., research groups or institutions). Given the focus on interactions, network analysis has seen considerable use in organizational science.[67] Kjos et al.[68] provide a brief overview of social network analysis as applied to social pharmacy research. Network analysis has seen numerous applications in healthcare and health services research including coordination of healthcare services across agencies,[69] state-level tobacco control efforts,[70] and describing public health systems.[71] As an example within metaresearch, Li et al.[72] conducted a network analysis to examine global research collaboration of researchers conducting network metaanalyses.

Importance of metaresearch

Health services research, both in general and for pharmacy specifically, has reached a state of considerable depth and breadth. It may be time to take account of the types of research that have been conducted and ask some important questions of the research enterprise within pharmacy and health services research. Are there gaps in the knowledge being produced? Are there certain types of questions that have been ignored (if so why)? Are there inefficiencies due to unnecessarily duplicative research efforts? How is the research being used to improve patient and population health? Metaresearch allows researchers to answer these questions. Put another way, metaresearch allows for a healthy dose of reflection that can allow for continued improvement in pharmacy and health services research, which could facilitate increased uptake and use of the findings thereby resulting in increased impact.

Getting involved in metaresearch

For individuals interested in pursuing metaresearch, the six previously described thematic areas may be helpful to focus thinking about potential metaresearch studies. It may also be helpful to consider the translational framework proposed by Hardwicke et al.[2] As shown in Fig. 1, this framework involves a 4-step cycle that involves identifying problems, investigating problems, developing solutions, and evaluating those solutions. Those familiar with quality improvement will surely recognize similarities with the Plan-Do-Study-Act cycle. This again highlights that there are parts of metaresearch with which many pharmacy and health services researchers are already familiar. Drawing on this framework, metaresearch studies may begin with identifying and investigating problems within the body of pharmacy research using any of the six areas of metaresearch described in Table 1. When problems or challenges are sufficiently described, then potential solutions can be developed and evaluated.

Resources are an important consideration for any type of research. Fortunately, most pharmacy or health services researchers, particularly those at academic institutions, likely have many of the resources needed to engage in metaresearch (e.g., access to bibliographic databases, statistical software, bibliographic software). Selected databases are freely available (e.g., PubMed). For certain projects, specialized software may be needed (e.g., for network analysis or text analysis). The most important resource is a willingness to put forth the time and effort to learn new skills or adapt existing skills to engage in a new area of research. Most pharmacy and health services researchers have experience conducting literature searches and some may even have conducted systematic or scoping reviews. Adapting these skills for use in metaresearch projects is

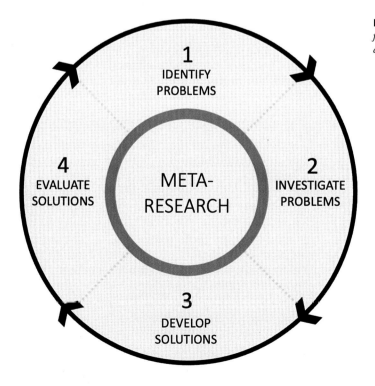

FIG. 1 Translational framework for metaresearch. *(Original figure by Tom Hardwicke. Available at: https://osf.io/cqrp8/ under a CC-BY 4.0 license.)*

TABLE 2 Additional resources.

Resource	Description
Methods in Research on Research (Project MIRoR) http://miror-ejd.eu/	• Multidisciplinary doctoral training program involving researchers and institutions from across Europe • Webinars and materials from past conferences and events archived on the website
Meta-Research Innovation Center at Stanford (METRICS) https://metrics.stanford.edu/	• Organization focused on promoting and developing metaresearch efforts • Supports postdoctoral fellows • Provides a list of training resources
Center for Open Science https://www.cos.io/	• Independent organization founded to promote the open science movement • Developed guidelines for ensuring transparency and openness in research • Supports the Open Science Framework (platform for sharing research; https://osf.io/) and Open Scholarship Knowledge Base (develops resources supporting education around open scholarship; https://www.oercommons.org/hubs/OSKB)
eLife Meta-Research Collection https://elifesciences.org/collections/8d233d47/meta-research-a-collection-of-articles	• Curated collection of articles on metaresearch published in the journal *eLife* • Covers a range of topics and disciplines • All articles are open access

relatively straightforward. As noted previously, the skills related to medical record abstracting can be readily translated into a metaresearch context. For those interested in pursuing metaresearch, Table 2 provides a brief list of informational resources that may be helpful.

Conclusion

Metaresearch, at least in the sense of a cohesive and formal line of inquiry, may still be relatively new to pharmacy and health services research. Most existing metaresearch studies have largely focused on descriptive or exploratory issues (i.e., identifying or investigating problems). These are important first steps; however, it will be important to continue beyond those early stages by developing ways to address problems or challenges in pharmacy research and evaluate whether improvement is occurring. Careful consideration of the training of future pharmacy and health services researchers may also be an important part of these metaresearch efforts. By considering the health services research ecosystem, pharmacy and health services researchers can be better positioned to improve healthcare services and outcomes for patients and populations.

Questions for further discussion

1. What are the six main thematic areas within metaresearch? Give an example of each.
2. Conducting a bibliometric analysis of the research output of an academic department and comparing it to peer departments at other universities would fit within which of the metaresearch thematic areas? Briefly explain. (More than one area is possible.)
3. Describe a situation where including a librarian in a metaresearch project would be helpful. Briefly explain why a librarian would be helpful.
4. Briefly explain how the translational metaresearch framework (by Hardwicke et al.[2]) aligns with the continuous quality improvement process (i.e., the PDSA cycle).

Application exercise/scenario

While conducting research on the health-related quality of life (HRQOL) of a particular condition, a colleague of yours has started to develop some concerns surrounding the types of instruments being used to measure HRQOL. Your colleague approaches you because he knows of your interest in HRQOL measurement. The two of you identify three concerns: the strength of the validity evidence supporting the use of the various HRQOL instruments, the apparent prefence for some instruments over others by research groups or in particular conditions, and whether there are any important concepts being excluded in the existing instruments, particular those relevant to the patient experience. Together, you determine that these concerns may lend themselves to a metaresearch project. Select one of these three concerns and briefly design two projects (one quantitative and one qualitative) to explore the concern. Be sure to state the thematic area that best aligns with your project (this need not be the same for both projects).

References

1. Ioannidis JPA. Meta-research: why research on research matters. *PLoS Biol.* 2018;16(3):e2005468. https://doi.org/10.1371/journal.pbio.2005468.
2. Hardwicke TE, Serghiou S, Janiaud P, et al. Calibrating the scientific ecosystem through meta-research. *Ann Rev Stat Appl.* 2020;7:11–37. https://doi.org/10.1146/annurev-statistics-031219-041104.
3. Dickersin K, Chalmers I. Recognizing, investigating and dealing with incomplete and biased reporting of clinical research: from Francis Bacon to the WHO. *J R Soc Med.* 2011;104(12):532–538. https://doi.org/10.1258/jrsm.2011.11k042.
4. Anderson J, Evered DC. Why do research on research? *Lancet.* 1986;2(8510):799–802.
5. Camerer CF, Dreber A, Holzmeister F, et al. Evaluating the replicability of social science experiments in nature and science between 2010 and 2015. *Nat Hum Behav.* 2018;2(9):637–644. https://doi.org/10.1038/s41562-018-0399-z.
6. Open Science Collaboration. Estimating the reproducibility of psychological science. *Science.* 2015;349(6251):aac4716. https://doi.org/10.1126/science.aac4716.
7. Ioannidis JPA. Contradicted and initially stronger effects in highly cited clinical research. *JAMA.* 2005;294(2):218–228. https://doi.org/10.1001/jama.294.2.218.
8. Ioannidis JPA. Why most clinical research is not useful. *PLoS Med.* 2016;13(6):e1002049. https://doi.org/10.1371/journal.pmed.1002049.
9. Mobley A, Linder SK, Braeuer R, Ellis LM, Zwelling L. A survey on data reproducibility in cancer research provides insights into our limited ability to translate findings from the laboratory to the clinic. *PLoS One.* 2013;8(5):e63221. https://doi.org/10.1371/journal.pone.0063221.
10. Ioannidis JPA, Fanelli D, Dunne DD, Goodman SN. Meta-research: evaluation and improvement of research methods and practices. *PLoS Biol.* 2015;13(10):e1002264. https://doi.org/10.1371/journal.pbio.1002264.
11. Lee CM, Soin HK, Einarson TR. Statistics in the pharmacy literature. *Ann Pharmacother.* 2004;38(9):1412–1418. https://doi.org/10.1345/aph.1D493.
12. McKelvey RP, Hatton RC, Kimberlin CA. Pharmacy resident project publication rates and study designs from 1981, 1991, and 2001. *Am J Health Syst Pharm.* 2010;67(10):830–836. https://doi.org/10.2146/ajhp090090.
13. Salgado TM, Patterson JA, Bajaj SK, et al. Characterization of pharmacy practice research centers across the United States. *Res Soc Adm Pharm.* 2020;16(2):230–237. https://doi.org/10.1016/j.sapharm.2019.05.009.
14. Crespo-Gonzalez C, Fernandez-Llimos F, Rotta I, Correr CJ, Benrimoj SI, Garcia-Cardenas V. Characterization of pharmacists' interventions in asthma management: a systematic review. *J Am Pharm Assoc.* 2018;58(2):210–219. https://doi.org/10.1016/j.japh.2017.12.009.
15. Dammo N, Harpe SE. Characteristics of studies of pharmacist services registered in ClinicalTrials.gov. *J Am Pharm Assoc.* 2020;60(4):609–617. https://doi.org/10.1016/j.japh.2019.12.001.
16. Dotson B, Slaughter RL. Prevalence of articles with honorary and ghost authors in three pharmacy journals. *Am J Health Syst Pharm.* 2011;68 (18):1730–1734. https://doi.org/10.2146/ajhp100583.
17. Peterson GG, Zurovac J, Brown RS, et al. Testing the replicability of a successful care management program: results from a randomized trial and likely explanations for why impacts did not replicate. *Health Serv Res.* 2016;51(6):2115–2139. https://doi.org/10.1111/1475-6773.12595.
18. Samp JC, Schumock GT, Pickard AS. Retracted publications in the drug literature. *Pharmacotherapy.* 2012;32(7):586–595. https://doi.org/10.1002/j.1875-9114.2012.01100.x.
19. Chisholm-Burns MA, Spivey C, Martin JR, Wyles C, Ehrman C, Schlesselman LS. A 5-year analysis of peer-reviewed journal article publications of pharmacy practice faculty members. *Am J Pharm Educ.* 2012;76(7):127. https://doi.org/10.5688/ajpe767127.
20. Thompson DF. Publication records and bibliometric indices of pharmacy school deans. *Am J Pharm Educ.* 2019;83(2):6513. https://doi.org/10.5688/ajpe6513.
21. Dixon DL, Baker WL. Short-term impact of altmetric attention scores on citation counts in selected major pharmacy journals. *J Am Coll Clin Pharm.* 2020;3(1):10–14. https://doi.org/10.1002/jac5.1141.
22. Dame MA, Wolinsky FD. Rating journals in health care administration. The use of bibliometric measures. *Med Care.* 1993;31(6):520–524. https://doi.org/10.1097/00005650-199306000-00005.
23. Dotson B. Women as authors in the pharmacy literature: 1989-2009. *Am J Health Syst Pharm.* 2011;68(18):1736–1739. https://doi.org/10.2146/ajhp100597.
24. Sarna KV, Griffin T, Tarlov E, Gerber BS, Gabay MP, Suda KJ. Trends in gender composition on editorial boards in leading medicine, nursing, and pharmacy journals. *J Am Pharm Assoc.* 2020;60(4):565–570. https://doi.org/10.1016/j.japh.2019.12.018.

25. Clarke AR, Goddu AP, Nocon RS, et al. Thirty years of disparities intervention research: what are we doing to close racial and ethnic gaps in health care? *Med Care.* 2013;51(11):1020–1026. https://doi.org/10.1097/MLR.0b013e3182a97ba3.

26. Robles JR, Youmans SL, Byrd DC, Polk RE. Perceived barriers to scholarship and research among pharmacy practice faculty: survey report from the AACP scholarship/research faculty development task force. *Am J Pharm Educ.* 2009;73(1):17. https://doi.org/10.5688/aj730117.

27. Lee KC, El-Ibiary SY, Hudmon KS. Evaluation of research training and productivity among junior pharmacy practice faculty in the United States. *J Pharm Pract.* 2010;23(6):553–559. https://doi.org/10.1177/0897190010373657.

28. Minguet F, Salgado TM, van den Boogerd L, Fernandez-Llimos F. Quality of pharmacy-specific medical subject headings (MeSH) assignment in pharmacy journals indexed in MEDLINE. *Res Soc Adm Pharm.* 2015;11(5):686–695. https://doi.org/10.1016/j.sapharm.2014.11.004.

29. Mendes AM, Tonin FS, Buzzi MF, Pontarolo R, Fernandez-Llimos F. Mapping pharmacy journals: a lexicographic analysis. *Res Soc Adm Pharm.* 2019;15(12):1464–1471. https://doi.org/10.1016/j.sapharm.2019.01.011.

30. Rotta I, Salgado TM, Silva ML, Correr CJ, Fernandez-Llimos F. Effectiveness of clinical pharmacy services: an overview of systematic reviews (2000–2010). *Int J Clin Pharm.* 2015;37(5):687–697. https://doi.org/10.1007/s11096-015-0137-9.

31. Viswanathan M, Kahwati LC, Golin CE, et al. Medication therapy management interventions in outpatient settings: a systematic review and meta-analysis. *JAMA Intern Med.* 2015;175(1):76–87. https://doi.org/10.1001/jamainternmed.2014.5841.

32. de Barra M, Scott CL, Scott NW, et al. Pharmacist services for non-hospitalised patients. *Cochrane Database Syst Rev.* 2018;9:CD013102. https://doi.org/10.1002/14651858.CD013102.

33. Rotta I, Salgado TM, Felix DC, Souza TT, Correr CJ, Fernandez-Llimos F. Ensuring consistent reporting of clinical pharmacy services to enhance reproducibility in practice: an improved version of DEPICT. *J Eval Clin Pract.* 2015;21(4):584–590. https://doi.org/10.1111/jep.12339.

34. Clay PG, Burns AL, Isetts BJ, Hirsch JD, Kliethermes MA, Planas LG. PaCIR: a tool to enhance pharmacist patient care intervention reporting. *J Am Pharm Assoc.* 2019;59(5). https://doi.org/10.1016/j.japh.2019.07.008.

35. Dickersin K, Rennie D. Registering clinical trials. *JAMA.* 2003;290(4):516–523. https://doi.org/10.1001/jama.290.4.516.

36. Sim I, Chan A-W, Gülmezoglu AM, Evans T, Pang T. Clinical trial registration: transparency is the watchword. *Lancet.* 2006;367(9523):1631–1633. https://doi.org/10.1016/S0140-6736(06)68708-4.

37. Zarin DA, Tse T. Medicine. Moving toward transparency of clinical trials. *Science.* 2008;319(5868):1340–1342. https://doi.org/10.1126/science.1153632.

38. *Recommendations for the Conduct, Reporting, Editing, and Publication of Scholarly Work in Medical Journals.* International Committee of Medical Journal Editors; December 2018. http://www.icmje.org/recommendations/. Accessed 17 February 2021.

39. Flaherty DK. Ghost- and guest-authored pharmaceutical industry-sponsored studies: abuse of academic integrity, the peer review system, and public trust. *Ann Pharmacother.* 2013;47(7–8):1081–1083. https://doi.org/10.1345/aph.1R691.

40. National Academies of Sciences, Engineering, and Medicine. *Reproducibility and Replicability in Science.* The National Academies Press; 2019. https://doi.org/10.17226/25303.

41. Barba LA. *Terminologies for Reproducible Research*; 2018. Preprint. arXiv;1802.03311 [cs] http://arxiv.org/abs/1802.03311. Accessed 20 November 2020.

42. Fecher B, Friesike S. Open science: one term, five schools of thought. In: Bartling S, Friesike S, eds. *Opening Science.* Springer; 2014:17–47.

43. McKiernan EC, Bourne PE, Brown CT, et al. How open science helps researchers succeed. *Elife.* 2016;5. https://doi.org/10.7554/eLife.16800.

44. Alberts B, Cicerone RJ, Fienberg SE, et al. Scientific integrity. Self-correction in science at work. *Science.* 2015;348(6242):1420–1422. https://doi.org/10.1126/science.aab3847.

45. Malički M, von Elm E, Marušić A. Study design, publication outcome, and funding of research presented at international congresses on peer review and biomedical publication. *JAMA.* 2014;311(10):1065–1067. https://doi.org/10.1001/jama.2014.143.

46. Rennie D, Flanagin A. Research on peer review and biomedical publication: furthering the quest to improve the quality of reporting. *JAMA.* 2014;311(10):1019–1020. https://doi.org/10.1001/jama.2014.1362.

47. Ioannidis JPA, Baas J, Klavans R, Boyack KW. A standardized citation metrics author database annotated for scientific field. *PLoS Biol.* 2019;17(8):e3000384. https://doi.org/10.1371/journal.pbio.3000384.

48. Ioannidis JPA, Boyack KW, Baas J. Updated science-wide author databases of standardized citation indicators. *PLoS Biol.* 2020;18(10):e3000918. https://doi.org/10.1371/journal.pbio.3000918.

49. Hankivsky O, Springer KW, Hunting G. Beyond sex and gender difference in funding and reporting of health research. *Res Integr Peer Rev.* 2018;3:6. https://doi.org/10.1186/s41073-018-0050-6.

50. Greider CW, Sheltzer JM, Cantalupo NC, et al. Increasing gender diversity in the STEM research workforce. *Science.* 2019;366(6466):692–695. https://doi.org/10.1126/science.aaz0649.

51. Jungnickel PW, Creswell JW. Workplace correlates and scholarly performance of clinical pharmacy faculty. *Res High Educ.* 1994;35(2):167–194.

52. Taylor GA. Impact of clinical volume on scholarly activity in an academic children's hospital: trends, implications, and possible solutions. *Pediatr Radiol.* 2001;31(11):786–789. https://doi.org/10.1007/s002470100543.

53. Ferrer RL, Katerndahl DA. Predictors of short-term and long-term scholarly activity by academic faculty: a departmental case study. *Fam Med.* 2002;34(6):455–461.

54. *Introduction: What is MeSH?* . https://www.nlm.nih.gov/bsd/disted/meshtutorial/introduction/index.html. [Accessed 23 November 2020].

55. McGowan J, Sampson M, Salzwedel DM, Cogo E, Foerster V, Lefebvre C. PRESS peer review of electronic search strategies: 2015 guideline statement. *J Clin Epidemiol.* 2016;75:40–46. https://doi.org/10.1016/j.jclinepi.2016.01.021.

56. Rethlefsen ML, Kirtley S, Waffenschmidt S, et al. PRISMA-S: an extension to the PRISMA statement for reporting literature searches in systematic reviews. *Syst Rev.* 2021;10(1):39. https://doi.org/10.1186/s13643-020-01542-z.

57. Groves RM, Fowlers Jr FJ, Couper MP, Lepkowski JM, Singer E, Tourangeau R. *Survey Methodology.* 2nd ed. John Wiley & Sons; 2009.

58. Dillman DA, Smyth JD, Christian LM. *Internet, Phone, Mail, and Mixed-Mode Surveys: The Tailored Design Method.* 4th ed. John Wiley & Sons; 2014.

59. Rea LM, Parker RA. *Designing and Conducting Survey Research: A Comprehensive Guide.* 4th ed. Jossey-Bass; 2014.

60. Hirsch JE. An index to quantify an individual's scientific research output. *Proc Natl Acad Sci USA.* 2005;102(46):16569–16572. https://doi.org/10.1073/pnas.0507655102.

61. Thompson DF, Walker CK. A descriptive and historical review of bibliometrics with applications to medical sciences. *Pharmacotherapy.* 2015;35(6):551–559. https://doi.org/10.1002/phar.1586.

62. Priem J, Taraborelli D, Groth P, Neylon C. *Altmetrics: A Manifesto*; October 26, 2010. http://altmetrics.org/manifesto/. Accessed 20 November 2020.

63. Jha R, Jbara A-A, Qazvinian V, Radev DR. NLP-driven citation analysis for scientometrics. *Nat Lang Eng.* 2017;23(1):93–130. https://doi.org/10.1017/S1351324915000443.

64. Atanassova I, Bertin M, Mayr P. Editorial: mining scientific papers: NLP-enhanced bibliometrics. *Front Res Metr Anal.* 2019;4. https://doi.org/10.3389/frma.2019.00002.

65. Bornmann L, Mutz R, Neuhaus C, Daniel H-D. Citation counts for research evaluation: standards of good practice for analyzing bibliometric data and presenting and interpreting results. *Ethics Sci Environ Polit.* 2008;8(1):93–102. https://doi.org/10.3354/esep00084.

66. Buljan I, Garcia-Costa D, Grimaldo F, Squazzoni F, Marušić A. Large-scale language analysis of peer review reports. *Elife.* 2020;9. https://doi.org/10.7554/eLife.53249.

67. Kilduff M, Brass DJ. Organizational social network research: core ideas and key debates. *Acad Manag Ann.* 2010;4(1):317–357. https://doi.org/10.1080/19416520.2010.494827.

68. Kjos AL, Worley MM, Schommer JC. The social network paradigm and applications in pharmacy. *Res Soc Adm Pharm.* 2013;9(4):353–369. https://doi.org/10.1016/j.sapharm.2012.05.015.

69. Provan KG, Sebastian JG. Networks within networks: service link overlap, organizational cliques, and network effectiveness. *Acad Manag J.* 1998;41(4):453–463. https://doi.org/10.2307/257084.

70. Luke DA, Harris JK, Shelton S, Allen P, Carothers BJ, Mueller NB. Systems analysis of collaboration in 5 national tobacco control networks. *Am J Public Health.* 2010;100(7):1290–1297. https://doi.org/10.2105/AJPH.2009.184358.

71. Wholey DR, Gregg W, Moscovice I. Public health systems: a social networks perspective. *Health Serv Res.* 2009;44(5 Pt 2):1842–1862. https://doi.org/10.1111/j.1475-6773.2009.01011.x.

72. Li L, Catalá-López F, Alonso-Arroyo A, et al. The global research collaboration of network meta-analysis: a social network analysis. *PLoS One.* 2016;11(9):e0163239. https://doi.org/10.1371/journal.pone.0163239.

Chapter 7

Best practices when conducting and reporting a meta-analysis

Fernanda S. Tonin[a], Aline F. Bonetti[a], and Fernando Fernandez-Llimos[b]

[a]*Pharmaceutical Sciences Postgraduate Program, Federal University of Paraná, Curitiba, Brazil,* [b]*Laboratory of Pharmacology, Faculty of Pharmacy, University of Porto, Porto, Portugal*

Objectives

- Identify the main guidelines which should be followed when performing and reporting a meta-analysis.
- Recognize the different components of a meta-analysis and how they are calculated.
- Interpret and critically evaluate the findings of a pairwise meta-analysis.
- Acknowledge the advantages and limitations of a pairwise meta-analysis.

Introduction

Since the 2010s, the expansion of an evidence-based healthcare culture among healthcare professionals, researchers, policy-makers, and other stakeholders has been driven by several factors such as patient-centered care, quality-linked incentives (i.e., performance-based payment models), and need to reduce costs.[1,2] Decisions grounded on the best and most up-to-date evidence are able to guide early interventions, better treatments and structured guidelines which work efficiently and reliably to produce the best possible clinical, humanistic, and economic outcomes.[3,4] The delivery of pharmaceutical care is no exception and should be informed by the best and most up-to-date evidence. This is particularly important given the advent of more tailored and specialized care provided by pharmacists, in both primary and secondary care settings.[5]

Pharmacy practice research is currently defined as a scientific discipline which studies the different aspects of the practice of pharmacy, and its impact on health care systems, medicine use, and patient care. The scope of this field encompasses clinical, behavioral, economic, and humanistic aspects of the practice of pharmacy, as well as practice change and implementation of healthcare innovations and patient-care services in daily practice. Innovations in pharmacy practice service are now recognized as a key resource for health systems for the promotion of safe and rational use of medicines, often via complex multidimensional interventions.[6] In fact, multiple studies have demonstrated the positive clinical outcomes associated with pharmacist-provided care for a wide array of condition, including diabetes, dyslipidemia, cardiovascular, respiratory, and mental health conditions.[7–13]

Nevertheless, the extensive body of evidence showing the effectiveness of pharmacist-led services is sometimes insufficient, unclear, or irreproducible to support a broader adoption and implementation of these services.[14,15] This occurs, among others reasons, because studies fail to undertake an adequate societal health needs assessment before the development of the professional pharmacy service; innovative research methods are not commonly explored; the use of terminology to describe the pharmacy service and its components is inconsistent; and because robust epidemiological research designs for evaluating pharmacist interventions and services are underused.[6]

The certainty of evidence, and hence the decisions based on it, relies on the quality of information and on the methods used to gather and synthesize it. Systematic reviews when carefully performed, are able to efficiently synthesize a body of evidence from an increasing stream of literature on a given topic, and to support healthcare decision-making. These studies are usually followed by additional approaches such as meta-synthesis or meta-analyses used to analyze qualitative and quantitative data, respectively. Studies using systematic methods to answer a specific healthcare-related question are, thus, placed on the top of the pyramid of evidence.[16]

A meta-analysis is a statistical technique able to quantitatively integrate the results of two or more independent epidemiological studies (e.g., randomized controlled trials, observational studies) on the same research topic, aiming at reducing

Contemporary Research Methods in Pharmacy and Health Services. https://doi.org/10.1016/B978-0-323-91888-6.00028-4

individual errors or biases. That is to say, a key benefit of this approach is the aggregation of information, leading to a higher statistical power and more robust point estimate than is possible from the measure derived from any individual study.[17] Pairwise meta-analyses, also called traditional or conventional meta-analyses, are those that directly compare the effects of two health technologies at a time (e.g., experimental vs control groups) reaching a final measure (i.e., effect size) that reflects the relationship between these two groups for a given outcome (i.e., clinical, economic, or humanistic) in a clinical setting.[16,18] A health technology (i.e., intervention) is defined as the application of organized knowledge and skills in the form of devices, medicines, vaccines, procedures, and systems developed to solve a health problem and improve the quality of life.[2] Thus, to be included in a meta-analysis, studies must share common interventions and comparators (e.g., studies on medication review led by the pharmacist vs usual care) and evaluation measures (e.g., reduction on hospital admission rate).[16]

The concept of network meta-analysis, also called indirect comparison or multiple or mixed treatment meta-analysis, is an extension of the pairwise meta-analysis,[19,20] and was introduced in the 2000s. This technique combines both direct (i.e., based on existing comparative studies in the literature) with indirect evidence (i.e., based on common comparators) to obtain pooled effects comparing each pair of treatments in the network. This approach has the advantage of providing a broader overview of all the technologies available for a clinical condition or setting in one single model.[19,20] Given the complexity of this model, this chapter will focus only on pairwise meta-analysis.

Nonetheless, the simple or multiple combination of the comparative results between interventions obtained from primary sources of information does not guarantee reliable evidence. This may be due to several reasons such as: the effects of the interventions are often multivariate rather than univariate; studies with low methodological quality may be included and lead to misleading conclusions; the data summarized may not be homogeneous; or grouping different causal factors may lead to meaningless estimates of effects.[3,21] In many fields, important pitfalls during the conduct and reporting of meta-analyses which threaten their quality, validity, and utility in practice have been documented.[22,23] In biomedical sciences—including pharmacy practice—about 20% of systematic reviews with meta-analyses present methodological flaws beyond repair caused by misapplication and misinterpretation of statistical methods.[24] This and other pitfalls in research performance can directly affect the decision-making process, patient care, and increase research waste.[25–28]

In science, "replicability" means obtaining consistent results with stated precision by a different research team using the same methods and data (i.e., different team, same experimental setup; "re-doing" the study). "Reproducibility" means obtaining the same results by a different team using different methods (i.e., different team, different experimental setup). That is to say, an analysis is reproducible when independent individuals are able to draw similar conclusions on the same data even when slightly different methods and conditions are used.[15,26,29] Because reproducibility and replicability are essential attributes in evidence-based healthcare literature, several guidelines for the conduct and reporting of meta-analyses have been proposed aiming at ensuring minimum standards of transparency and reliability.[27,29] International recommendations require the provision of thorough information of the study protocol and detailed description of all methodological steps of the study. Transparency of the metaanalytic data is essential for addressing readers' concerns about the possible presence of errors or bias and the degree to which the conclusions depend on subjective decisions (i.e., not grounded on robust data).[26] However, recent studies have shown that less than half published papers in biomedical sciences comply with these recommendations. This generic situation is similar in pharmacy practice literature, where lack of transparency and reproducibility of studies assessing clinical pharmacy services were frequently reported.[19,30,31] This significant variability among studies is also a consequence of the dynamic and evolving nature of pharmacy services (e.g., complex interventions, advances in research methods and increased number of reporting guidelines) and the important pitfalls of the studies conducted and reported in this field (e.g., lack of detailed description of the service, variability in the implementation of the service, inappropriateness of the evaluation measure).[6,32]

The quality appraisal of systematic reviews and meta-analyses should be a prerequisite before translating the findings into practice.[33] Readers should be aware of the basic components of a meta-analysis, understand how this type of analysis is performed and be able to properly interpret the results and appraise the final evidence. Thus, this chapter reviews the main methods for conducting and reporting pairwise meta-analyses and discusses the benefits and drawbacks of this statistical approach.

Meta-analysis: Main concepts

The term "meta-analysis" was introduced by the statistician Gene V. Glass in 1976 as a statistical procedure to reevaluate the published statistical results from a large number of independent studies on a specific topic aiming at integrating the findings in the context of educational research.[34] According to Glass, "meta-analysis refers to the analysis of analyses."

Researchers, when facing an abundance of information, should be able to extract the quantifiable information, group them in an orderly fashion according to categories, pool the data and summarize these results.[34,35]

Currently, meta-analysis is described as a statistical technique that combines or pools the results of several independent primary trials considered by the analyst to be "combinable," aiming at attaining an estimate of average effect size attributable to a certain intervention.[36,37] A meta-analysis is usually preceded by a systematic review, as this allows identification and critical appraisal of all the relevant evidence, thereby limiting the risk of bias in the overall estimates. Briefly, the main steps of this process according to the Cochrane Collaboration include[16]:

- Draw and publish the protocol of the systematic review and meta-analysis.
- Formulate the research question, typically entailing the PICOS acronym: population (e.g., patients/disease), the intervention (e.g., medicine, device, service under analysis), the comparator (e.g., placebo, standard care), the outcomes (e.g., efficacy, safety, costs), and the study design (e.g., randomized trials, observational studies).
- Systematically search the literature through electronic databases and manual searches.
- Select studies according to the previously established eligibility criteria.
- Extract data and critically appraise the information of the included studies.
- Synthetize the findings of quantitative data by means of a metasynthesis whenever possible.

Before formally performing a meta-analysis, researchers should consider the following questions:

1. Which pairwise comparisons should be made?
2. Which study results should be used in each comparison?
3. What is the best summary of effect (i.e., effect-size measure) for each comparison?
4. Are the results of studies similar within each comparison?
5. How reliable are the summarized findings of individual studies?

The first step in addressing these questions is to decide which pairwise comparisons to make and what sorts of data are appropriate for the outcomes of interest. The comparisons addressed in the review should relate clearly and directly to the questions or hypotheses that are posed when the review is formulated. Decisions about which studies are similar enough for their results to be grouped together require an understanding of the problem that the review addresses, the classification of the epidemiological studies (e.g., pyramid of evidence) and authors' judgments. The next step is to prepare tabular summaries of the characteristics and results of the primary studies that are included in each comparison. This allows estimates of effect to be derived across studies in a systematic way, to measure and investigate differences among studies and to interpret the findings.[16]

Thus, researchers should be familiar with the type of data (e.g., dichotomous, continuous) which result from measurement of an outcome in an individual study, and to select suitable effect-size measures for comparing intervention groups. Additionally, one should be aware of the different statistical methods and models that can be used to perform a meta-analysis. Most meta-analysis methods are variations on a weighted average of the effect estimates from the different studies. Variations across primary studies (i.e., between-study heterogeneity) must be considered by using, for instance, subgroup analysis or meta-regression. Sensitivity analyses should be conducted to examine whether overall findings are robust to potentially influence decisions.[21,38] These concepts are explained later in this chapter.

Guidelines for conducting and reporting a meta-analysis

The EQUATOR (Enhancing the QUAlity and Transparency Of health Research) Network is an international initiative that seeks to improve the reliability and value of published health research literature by promoting transparent and accurate reporting and wider use of robust reporting guidelines (https://www.equator-network.org/).

A reporting guideline is a simple, structured tool for healthcare researchers to use while writing their study. A reporting guideline provides a minimum list of items needed to ensure the work can be understood by a reader, replicated by another researcher, and used by other professionals to make clinical decisions. There are more than 30 freely available guidelines for reporting systematic reviews and meta-analyses that vary according to the type of study or research topic (e.g., diagnostic test accuracy studies; animal experiments; observational studies; individual patient data; interventional studies; protocols).[39]

The Preferred Reporting Items for Systematic Reviews and Meta-Analyses (PRISMA) statement, first published in 2009 and recently updated in 2020 is a gold-standard reporting guideline for systematic reviews of interventions.[40] It was designed to help systematic reviewers transparently report why the review was performed, what the authors did, and what they found. The PRISMA 2020 statement consists of a 27-item checklist, an expanded checklist that details reporting recommendations for each item, the PRISMA 2020 abstract checklist, and revised flow diagrams for original and updated reviews.[40] Similarly, the Meta-analysis of Observational Studies in Epidemiology (MOOSE) group developed and validated a checklist for reporting meta-analyses of observational studies in epidemiology (including background, search strategy, methods, results, discussion, and conclusion) that is widely used.[41,42] Formal guidance for conducting meta-analyses is also provided by the Cochrane Handbook for Systematic Reviews of Interventions (2020): https://training.cochrane.org/handbook/current.[16] Additional guidance especially referring to the systematic review process can also be found at:

- Joanna Briggs Institute, JBI Manual for Evidence Synthesis: https://wiki.jbi.global/display/MANUAL/JBI+Manual+for+Evidence+Synthesis.
- Center for Reviews and Dissemination at York: CRD's Guidance for Undertaking Reviews in Health Care: https://www.york.ac.uk/crd/SysRev/!SSL!/WebHelp/SysRev3.htm.
- Agency for Healthcare Research and Quality, AHRQ Methods Guide for Effectiveness and Comparative Effectiveness Reviews: https://effectivehealthcare.ahrq.gov/products/cer-methods-guide/overview.
- The Campbell Collaboration evidence synthesis tools: https://www.campbellcollaboration.org/research-resources/resources.html.

Regarding statistical synthesis methods, the above-mentioned statements and guidelines recommend that authors report, among others, the results of individual studies and syntheses along with details of the data presented. When a meta-analysis is performed, authors should specify the statistical model (i.e., fixed or random effects) and method (e.g., Mantel-Haenszel, inverse-variance) used, and provide the rationale for calculating and selecting these methods. The method used to identify and quantify statistical heterogeneity (e.g., visual inspection of results, formal statistical test for heterogeneity or inconsistency, prediction intervals) should also be disclosed. If authors have explored possible causes of statistical heterogeneity, then the methods used (e.g., subgroup analysis, meta-regression) should also be described. Authors should state which graphical methods were employed to visually display the results and the reference software/packages. These metaanalytical components are briefly described in the following sections.

Meta-analysis components

The visual results of a pairwise meta-analysis are commonly presented as a "forest plot" (see Fig. 1). The measures of individual effect (i.e., obtained by each primary study) are represented by a square whose area reflects the weight attributed

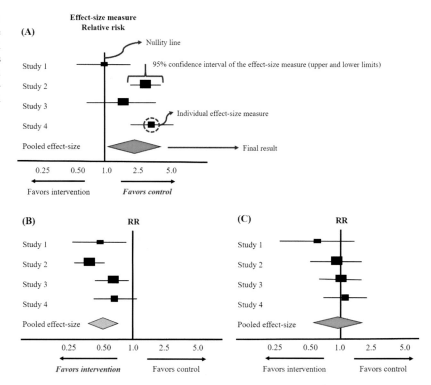

FIG. 1 Pairwise meta-analysis representation: forest plot. (A) Hypothetical model in which the results of an outcome/event favor the control group; (B) hypothetical model in which the results of an outcome/event favor the intervention group; (C) hypothetical model in which there are no statistical differences between intervention and control for a given outcome/event.

to it. That is to say, the larger the square (large sample size), the more it contributes to the overall position of the summary statistic when compared to a smaller square (small sample size). This measure of effect is accompanied by its confidence interval (CI)—usually 95%—which is represented by the horizontal lines in the graph. The evaluation of the lower and upper limits of the CI allows readers to conclude about the benefits or otherwise of an intervention when compared to a control group for a given outcome. The graph is divided by a vertical line which marks the null effect (called "nullity line"). When the CI of a study touches or crosses the vertical line of nullity, no statistical differences between the results of the experimental and control groups exists (Fig. 1C). If the results are placed on the left-side of the vertical line, the event is more likely to occur in one of the groups; conversely, results on the right-side of the graph demonstrate that the event has a greater likelihood to occur in the opposite group (Fig. 1A and B). The measure of the final or global effect common to all studies included in the meta-analysis is usually represented by the image of a rhombus or "diamond" at the end of the graph (i.e., pooled effect-size measure). Different software/packages can be used to build a meta-analysis; the most commonly used are: Review Manager (RevMan), Comprehensive Meta-analysis (CMA), R/R Studio (e.g., Metafor package), and Stata. Microsoft Excel add-ons (e.g., MetaEasy, MetaXL) can also be used.

Effect-size measures

Effect size is a statistical concept that measures the strength of the relationship between two variables on a numeric scale. Examples of effect sizes include the correlation between two variables, the regression coefficient in a regression, the mean difference, or the risk of a particular event (e.g., death) happening. Effect sizes complement statistical hypothesis testing, and play an important role in power analyses, sample size planning, and in meta-analyses.[16,43]

The term "effect-size" can refer to a standardized measure of effect (such as Cohen's d or the odds ratio), or to an unstandardized measure (e.g., the difference between group means). In meta-analyses, standardized effect sizes are used as a common measure that refers to the magnitude of the difference between two intervention groups. It can be calculated for different studies and then combined into an overall summary. These measures can be obtained by the division or subtraction of two frequency or occurrence measures observed in two different subgroups (e.g., intervention vs control) in the same population. Effect sizes can be measured in relative or absolute terms. In relative effect sizes, two groups are directly compared with each other (e.g., odds ratio or relative risk) by using statistical variations based on percentages. Measures of absolute effect-size employ numerical variations to determine the raw difference between average outcomes of groups. In this case, a larger absolute value always indicates a stronger effect. Many types of measurements can be expressed as either absolute or relative, and these can be used together because they convey different information.[44,45]

As in any statistical analysis of epidemiological studies, authors should acknowledge the type of data before calculating the effect size, which can be broadly divided into

- Continuous or quantitative data: the variable is a continuous number, i.e., it can assume any value in a given interval (e.g., patient' weight, height, mass index, temperature).
- Binary, also called dichotomous data: refers to variables that can be classified into categories (e.g., alive or dead; having the adverse event or not).
- Count data: corresponds to the number of events experienced by each individual in the study (e.g., number of fractures).
- Time-to-event data, also called survival data: refers to the time until the occurrence of a binary event (e.g., the time until death).

Continuous data can be broadly summarized with the "mean difference between groups (MD)" effect size. Some variations of this measure that can also be used are the standard mean difference or Cohen's d, Hedges' g, and Glass delta, among others. Dichotomous variables, which are the most used data in meta-analysis, can be combined into measures of effect such as relative risk or risk ratio (RR), odds ratio (OR), differences and risk reduction, and number needed to treat (NNT).[38,46] See Fig. 2 (part A and part B) for the main formula for calculating these effect-size measures. CI can be calculated for any of these measures. They are usually reported as upper and lower limits (95%) of the point estimate and account for the standard deviation and sample size.

"Risk" refers to the probability of an event occurring. It can be presented as a decimal number ranging from zero to one (0–1) or converted into a percentage (0%–100%). The RR is an asymmetric measure of likelihood that compares the risk of an event occurring between two groups: experimental (e.g., exposed group) vs control (e.g., unexposed group). From the RR, it is possible to calculate the relative risk reduction (RRR) using the formula "1 − RR" which is a measure for assessing the relative benefit of a given intervention. The absolute risk reduction (ARR) is the simple subtraction of risk in the control group minus the risk in the experimental group. The OR measures the chance (odds) of the event occurring in exposed individuals over the chance of the event occurring among the unexposed group. An RR (or OR) of 1.0 indicates that there

FIG. 2 Effect-size measures calculation. Part A: Contingency Table (2×2) of the relationships between experimental vs control group for a given outcome, whereas "A" refers to a patient with an outcome/event that is receiving a given intervention/exposure; "B" is a patient that also receives the intervention/exposure but does not present the outcome/event; "C" refers to a control group (without the intervention/exposure) that has the outcome/event; "D" does not receive the intervention/exposure and also does not present the outcome/event. Part B: Overall formula.

(Part A)

		Outcome/event		
		Yes	**No**	
Intervention or	**Yes**	A	B	A + B
exposure	**No**	C	D	C + D
		A + C	B + D	

(Part B)

Relative risk (RR)

$$RR = \frac{\left[A / (A+B) \right]}{\left[C / (C+D) \right]}$$

Relative risk reduction (RRR)

$$RRR = \left[\frac{C}{(C+D)} \right] - \frac{\left[A / (A+B) \right]}{\left[C / (C+D) \right]}$$

That is:

$$RRR = 1 - RR$$

Absolute risk reduction (ARR)

$$ARR = \left[\frac{C}{(C+D)} \right] - \left[\frac{A}{(A+B)} \right]$$

Odds ratio (OR)

$$OR = \frac{(A/B)}{(C/D)}$$

That is:

$$OR = \frac{AD}{CB}$$

Number needed to treat (NNT)

$$NNT = \frac{1}{ARR}$$

is no difference in risk (or odds) between the groups being compared. An RR (or OR) more than 1.0 indicates an increase in risk (or odds) among the exposed compared to the unexposed, whereas a RR (or OR) < 1.0 indicates a decrease in risk (or odds) in the exposed group[47,48] (see Fig. 2).

Though OR also indicates the nature of association between exposure and outcome, it is not identical to RR. The relationship of OR and RR is more complex. When there is no association between exposure and outcome, both OR and RR are identical and equal to 1.0. When there is an association between an exposure and an outcome, the OR exaggerates the estimate of their relationship (is farther from 1.0 than RR). Thus, when RR < 1.0, OR is lower than RR; by contrast, when RR is more than 1.0, OR is higher than the RR. When the outcome is rare (typically < 10%), the value of OR is not too dissimilar to that of RR, and the two can be used interchangeably irrespective of whether the risk is lower or higher in the exposed group as compared to the unexposed. As event rates increase the two ratios diverge and can no longer be used interchangeably. That is why RR is usually the preferred measure for longitudinal cohort studies and in clinical trials if the incidence of the event is > 10%. On the other hand, OR is usually used to interpret data from cross-sectional studies and case-controls. For rare cases/events (< 10%), both RR and OR are appropriate measures.[46,49]

The number needed to treat (NNT) or number needed to harm (NNH), although originally conceived to be used in randomized controlled trials,[50] are useful to express treatment differences in comparative studies including meta-analysis. These are intuitive measures that assist healthcare professionals in selecting therapeutic interventions, support benefit-risk assessments, and help decision-makers on medicine regulation.[51,52] The NNT is defined as the average number of patients who need to be treated to prevent one extra person from having an outcome. To better indicate the direction of the effect of this measures, Altman[53] suggested the terms "number needed to treat for an additional beneficial outcome" (NNTB) and "number needed to treat for an additional harmful outcome" (NNTH) instead of NNT and NNH, respectively. The NNTB and NNTH are calculated by taking the inverse of the risk difference, yet can also be calculated using other effect measures,

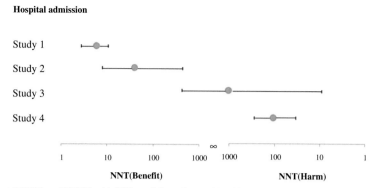

FIG. 3 Number needed to treat (NNTB and NNTH with 95% confidence intervals) with a given intervention for the outcome of hospital admission. The higher the NNTB value, the less effective the treatment will be; and, the higher the NNTH, the more safe a treatment is Study 1: the NNT for an additional beneficial outcome (i.e., reduce one hospital admission) is 10 [95% CI, 5–15]. Study 2: the NNT for an additional beneficial outcome (i.e., reduce one hospital admission) is 50 [95% CI, 5–900]. Study 3: the NNT for an additional harmful outcome (i.e., one hospital admission) is of 1000, varying between harm and benefit: 95% CI, 10 NNTH to 900 NNTB. This means that the effect of the intervention is unclear (varying from causing harm to benefit). Study 4: the NNT for an additional harmful outcome (i.e., one hospital admission) is of 100 [95% CI, 50–500].

such as the OR and RR, which are more commonly seen in the scientific literature. The higher the NNTB value, the less effective the treatment will be; and, the higher the NNTH, the more safe a treatment is. A NNTB of 100, for example, demonstrates that out of 100 treated patients, only one will benefit from the treatment.[53,54] Fig. 3 exemplifies the results of NNT values (with 95% CI) when comparing an intervention (e.g., medication review provided by the pharmacist) vs a control group (e.g., standard care) for the outcome of hospital admission. In Study 1, it is necessary to provide the pharmacy service to 10 patients (with a CI from 5 to 15) for one to have an additional benefit (reduce one hospital admission). In Study 3, the effect of the pharmacy service is unclear, so it varies from 10 NNTH to 900 NNTB. In Study 4, only one patient is admitted to the hospital after the review of the medication of 100 patients (CI, 50–500) (NNTH).

Metaanalytical methods

The main objective of any meta-analysis is to pool statistics from independent studies with a view to synthesizing them to calculate an estimate of the common effect-size. There are different ways of pooling statistics, depending on the type of weight used for individual studies in computing the pooled estimate.[38,48]

Conventionally, the inverse variance weights (IV) are commonly used in meta-analysis, both for continuous and dichotomous data. In this method, "weights" are given to each study according to the inverse of the variance of the effect estimate of the study (i.e., one over the square of its standard error). Thus, larger studies (with higher sample size and smaller standard errors) are given more weight than smaller studies, which have larger standard errors. This choice of weight minimizes the imprecision (uncertainty) of the pooled effect estimate.[16] However, it is important to know that the redistribution of weights varies significantly under various commonly used statistical models especially if there is significant heterogeneity among the studies.[47,55]

When data are sparse, either in terms of event rates being low or study size being small, the estimates of the standard errors of the effect estimates that are used in the IV methods may be poor. Therefore, alternative methods such as the Mantel-Haenszel should be used. This approach uses a different weighting scheme that depends upon which effect measure (e.g., RR, OR or risk difference of binary data) is being employed. Additionally, Peto's method is mostly recommended when events are sparse or null, as corrections for zero cells counts are not necessary when compared to other methods.[47,56]

Statistical models

One of the main points which differentiate meta-analysis from a simple pooled analysis is the weight attributed to each of the studies. Two statistical models can be used for weight assignment: the fixed-effect model and the random effect model. The main difference among the models is the way they allocate the IV weights to the individual studies. The objective of redistribution of weights among the studies is to find a more precise estimator of the common effect size to achieve a shorter CI.[57,58]

In the fixed-effect model, it is assumed that there is only a single effect common to all studies (i.e., the same effect); and any variation observed between individual studies is only due to random error (i.e., within-study variation). In practice, especially in clinical pharmacy and health services, this scenario is unusual as there is often variability in the conduct and reporting of studies, populations, type of technologies and their implementation. In the random effect model, the true effect can vary among studies, which is often a more realistic scenario. In this model, the weights are distributed to the individual studies in computing the pooled estimate of the common effect size using two sources of variation: within-study (i.e., random error) and between-study (i.e., variation of the true effect size, also known as "heterogeneity," and represented by the tau-squared [tau^2] parameter).[59]

Following these definitions on statistical models, studies with a larger sample size tend to receive a greater weight in fixed-effect models, since the global effect is unique and more accurate in larger studies. Conversely, the random effects model assumes that there is more than one true effect and, thus, the distribution of weights is more equal among studies.[16] Studies with a smaller sample size (more inaccurate) are given greater weight, which enlarges the CI (wider intervals), causing more uncertainty in the evidence.[60] The only exception is when tau^2 (heterogeneity) is null (zero); in this case, both fixed and random models will provide same results.[61] The DerSimonian and Laird approach[62] is commonly used for a random effects meta-analysis as the calculations are straightforward. This method incorporates an assumption in which the included studies are estimating different, yet related, intervention effects. The method is based on the IV approach, making an adjustment to the study weights according to the extent of variation, or heterogeneity, among the varying intervention effects.[16] However, the DerSimonian and Laird approach may lead to too many statistically significant results when the number of studies is small and there is moderate or substantial heterogeneity among studies.[16] In this case, the method described by Hartung and Knapp[63,64] and by Sidik and Jonkman[65] can be alternatively used, as it is claimed to be simple and robust especially when there is heterogeneity and the number of studies under analysis is small.[57,66] They modified the variance estimate to account for the fact that the weights are estimated and based the proposed test and CI on the t-distribution rather than the normal distribution.[57,66]

Between-study heterogeneity and prediction intervals

Since meta-analyses are based on the summary statistics of individual studies, the between-studies variation often plays a significant role in determining the estimate of the effect size. When the between-studies variation is not significant, the meta-analysis becomes simple and straightforward. However, as in many cases the studies are heterogeneous, authors should address this fact when computing the pooled effect size and the CI. If necessary, additional analyses to understand or minimize the source of heterogeneity (e.g., prediction intervals (PI) calculation, subgroup analyses, meta-regression) should be performed.[59,67,68]

If the CI for the results of individual studies (depicted graphically using horizontal lines in the forest plot, see Fig. 1) have poor overlap, this usually indicates the presence of statistical heterogeneity. The chi-squared (χ^2 or Chi^2) test can be performed to assess whether this heterogeneity is significant (i.e., considering the null hypothesis that all studies have the same effect estimate). If the value obtained is less than the defined α (e.g., $P = .1$) or a large chi-squared statistic relative to its degree of freedom, the null hypothesis is rejected. This provides evidence of heterogeneity of intervention effects (variation in effect estimates beyond chance). However, it is important to know that a $P > \alpha$ does not necessarily mean that the studies are homogeneous, since the lack of significance may be due to the lack of statistical power.[16,59]

The formal presence of between-studies variability (i.e., heterogeneity) is assessed by the Cochrane's Q-statistic or the I-squared (I^2) statistic.[16] The Q test is computed by summing the squared deviations of each study's effect estimate from the overall effect estimate, weighting the contribution of each study by its inverse variance. Under the hypothesis of homogeneity among the effect sizes, the Q-statistic follows a chi-square distribution with $k - 1$ degrees of freedom (k being the number of studies). Not rejecting the homogeneity hypothesis usually leads the metaanalyst to adopt a fixed-effects model because it is assumed that the estimated effect sizes only differ by sampling error. In contrast, rejecting the homogeneity assumption can lead to applying a random-effects model which includes both within- and between-studies variability.[69] The main limitation of the Q-statistic is that it only evaluates the presence or absence of heterogeneity, and not on the extent of heterogeneity. Additionally, its value increases as the number of studies in a meta-analysis increases, which means that a nonsignificant result for the Q test with a small number of studies can lead a reviewer to erroneously assume a fixed-effects model when there is true heterogeneity among the studies; and vice versa.[69] Thus, while it is useful to detect heterogeneity and inform on the degree of its statistical significance, it is unable to describe the extent of the presence of true heterogeneity.[16] An alternative method and most commonly used for assessing heterogeneity is the I^2 statistic or I^2 index, which should always be interpreted together with the CI. The I^2 index measures the extent of true heterogeneity dividing the difference between the result of the Q test and its degrees of freedom ($k - 1$) by the Q value itself, and multiplied by 100.[69] Therefore, the results of the I^2 statistic are depicted as percentage of the total variability that can be attributed to true degree of heterogeneity within a set of effect sizes. An I^2 statistic equaling 0% suggests that there is no between-study variability

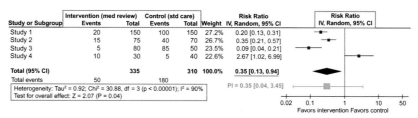

FIG. 4 Forest plot comparing an intervention (medication review) vs control (standard of care) for the outcome hospital admission (events). Meta-analysis performed using the inverse of variance (IV) method and random-effect model. Effect-size measure risk ratio (RR) reported with 95% confidence intervals (CI). Between-studies heterogeneity measured with I^2 statistics (software: Review Manager v.5.3). Prediction intervals (PI) additionally calculated and depicted on the forest plot.

and that all variation observed is a result of sampling error. Conversely, when I^2 approaches 100%, it suggests that the observed variation is the result of between-study variability rather than sampling error. According to the Cochrane, a rough guide for the interpretation of I^2 statistic is: 0%–40% might not be important; 30%–60% may represent moderate heterogeneity; 50%–90% may represent substantial heterogeneity; and 75%–100% is considerable heterogeneity.[16] Additionally, authors should consider that the importance of the observed value of I^2 also depends on the magnitude and direction of effect size (i.e., no differences between interventions or statistical differences favoring one of the interventions) and the strength of evidence for heterogeneity (e.g., P value from the chi-squared test, CI width).[16,67]

However, the clinical interpretation of these metrics is not straightforward and neither readily reveals the implications of the observed heterogeneity nor assist clinical decisions by means of an intuitive measure, especially if the statistical significance of the meta-analysis depends on the outcome of a few patients. Therefore, it is recommended that researchers should routinely report additional metrics which allow more informative inferences in meta-analysis.[66,70]

The prediction intervals (PI)—also called forecast intervals—can better predict the behavior of one randomly selected future measurement from a distribution of values especially when a high heterogeneity among studies exists (I^2 statistics different from null). The PI usually represents a wider dispersion than the CI, aiming at reflecting the true variation in treatment effects over different settings, including what effect is to be expected in future patients.[66,70]

Fig. 4 exemplifies a meta-analysis comparing the effect of an intervention (e.g., medication review performed by the pharmacist) vs a control group (e.g., standard or usual care) for the outcome hospital admission rates. Four randomized controlled trials were included. The meta-analysis was performed using the IV method and random effect model. The results are reported as RR with 95% CI for each study. Studies 1, 2 and 3 demonstrate higher risks for hospitalization in the control group (RR < 1.0; favoring the use of the intervention), while the opposite was found in study 4. In the original analysis, the pooled effect estimate was RR 0.35 [95% CI, 0.13–0.94], revealing significant differences between intervention and control for this outcome ($P = .04$). However, the between-studies heterogeneity is substantial and significant ($I^2 = 90\%$, $P < .00001$), probably caused by the difference estimated in study 4, which should be further investigated by the authors. The additional calculation of PI in this case (depicted in the forest plot as the green effect-size and CI estimates) demonstrates that, in fact, there are no significant differences between groups for this outcome as the upper and lower intervals are wider: PI 95% 0.04 to 3.45.

Subgroup analysis, meta-regression, and additional sensitivity analyses

One way to minimize the impact of heterogeneity in a meta-analysis is to group the studies based on the value of the individual study variance or their characteristics. Studies with similar characteristics (e.g., epidemiological design, patients' age or sex, studies' follow-up) can be subgrouped into a separate meta-analysis that should be reported along with the overall meta-analysis.[16,59]

Other approaches such as "sensitivity analyses" can also be performed to check the impact on the result of the estimate of the common effect size as a result of the inclusion of one particular study or a group of similar studies in a meta-analysis.[16] This can be done by the hypothetical removal of studies from the meta-analysis (so called "N-1 analysis" in which the results of a meta-analysis considering the removal of a given study are compared to those from the original meta-analysis including all studies) and by adjustments in the metaanalytical model and methods (e.g., change from fixed- to random-effect models and vice versa; compare the results of using IV or Mantel-Haenszel). The complete findings of both original analyses versus additional analyses should always be reported by authors. It is important to highlight that this is not a solution to the heterogeneity problem, but it provides some useful insight into the problem and how individual study effect size impacts on the meta-analysis.[15,21]

Meta-regression is a technique for performing a regression analysis to assess the relationship between the treatment effects and the study characteristics of interest (e.g., suture vs prosthesis) or factors concerning the execution of the study (e.g., allocation sequence concealment). meta-regression is an extension to subgroup analyses that allows the effect of continuous as well as categorical characteristics to be investigated in two or more groups. This approach is similar in essence to simple regression, in which an outcome variable is predicted according to the values of one or more explanatory variables. Here, the outcome variable is the effect estimate (e.g., mean difference, log OR, log RR) and the explanatory variables are characteristics of studies that might influence the size of intervention effect. The regression coefficient obtained from a meta-regression describes how the outcome variable (the intervention effect) changes with a unit increase in the explanatory variable (potential effect modifier). The statistical significance of the regression coefficient is a test of whether there is a linear relationship between intervention effect vs explanatory variable. It is not recommended to perform a meta-regression when there are less than 10 studies in a meta-analysis.[16]

The confidence we have in the conclusion of a meta-analysis depends on several factors (e.g., the methods used to produce the analysis, the quality of trials included, the number of trials, the heterogeneity of treatment effect estimates across trials, and the precision of each trial for estimating the treatment effect).[66,71] In the study of Atal et al.,[72] authors showed that for almost one-third of the evaluated meta-analyses, their statistical significance could be changed (i.e., significant to nonsignificant) with the modification of the event status (e.g., death vs alive) for five or fewer patients in at least one trial included in the meta-analysis. That is to say, in almost half of cases, the statistical significance depended on the event status of less than 1% of participants.

Grounded on this evidence that data are "fragile," researchers advocate the use of another metric, the fragility index (FI) to aid the interpretation of the meta-analysis.[72] The FI is another metric borrowed from the randomized controlled trials literature—as the NNT and corresponds to the minimum number of patients from one or more trials included in the meta-analysis for which a modification in the event status (i.e., changing an event to a nonevent or a nonevent to an event) would change the statistical significance of the pooled effect size to statistically nonsignificant. "Event" refers to the presence of an outcome or endpoint under assessment (e.g., patient with a given disease or health-related condition). The method used to evaluate the FI of meta-analyses is based on an iterative reevaluation of the statistical significance of the pooled treatment effect of "modified meta-analyses." These "modified meta-analyses" are derived from the original meta-analysis by performing single event-status modifications in each arm of each trial in turn.[71–73] Fig. 5 exemplifies a statistically significant meta-analysis with a FI = 2, which means that it was necessary to modify the event status of only 2 patients for the meta-

FIG. 5 Example of a statistically significant meta-analysis with a Fragility Index of 2. Meta-analysis performed using Mantel-Haenszel method and fixed-effect model. Effect-size measure risk ratio (RR) reported with 95% confidence intervals (CI). *Blue icons*: nonevent; *red icons*: event. 1st change: one event flipped to nonevent in a specific arm of a trial. 2nd change: one nonevent flipped to event in a specific arm of a trial. Changes are performed in sequence.

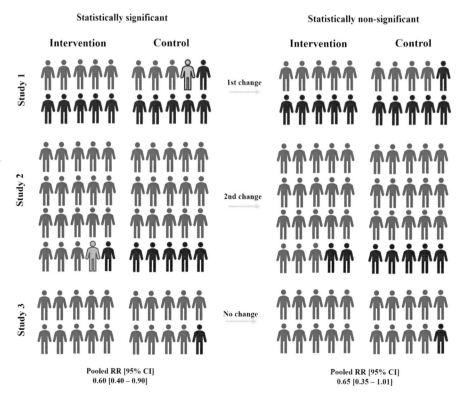

analysis to lose its significance (after changing one nonevent (e.g., healthy patient) to an event (e.g., patient with a disease) in a specific arm of a trial and one event to a nonevent in another specific arm of a trial, the meta-analysis resulted in statistical nonsignificance).

Bias in meta-analysis

A well-known threat to the reliability of meta-analysis is publication bias—a type of reporting bias, which occurs when studies with statistically significant or clinically favorable results are more likely to be published in international peer-reviewed journals than studies with nonsignificant or unfavorable results.[74] Other related biases such as time lag bias (where studies with unfavorable findings take longer to be published), language bias (i.e., non-English language articles are more likely to be rewritten in English if they report significant results), and selective outcome reporting (i.e., nonsignificant outcomes are entirely excluded from the study) also exist. When authors conduct a systematic review and specifically select the studies which will be included in the meta-analysis according to some characteristics such as studies' epidemiological design (e.g., only blinded randomized trials), methodological quality or risk of bias (e.g., only studies with low risk of bias), type of intervention or measure (e.g., only single component vs multicomponent complex interventions) without performing a sensitivity or subgroup analyses, they are also inserting a bias in the findings.[23,74]

These biases lead to meta-analyses which synthesize an incomplete set of the evidence and produce summary results potentially inaccurate toward favorable treatment effects. Thus, different statistical methods have been proposed to deal with these biases—especially for binary outcomes, such as test for the asymmetry of funnel plots and methods based on selection models.[74–76]

Funnel plots are the primary visual tool for investigation of publication bias in a meta-analysis. This approach is scatterplot of effect size (binary: logOR or logRR) against a measure of precision for each study included in the meta-analysis, such as the estimated standard error or sample size. Asymmetry in funnel plots indicates publication bias in meta-analysis, but the shape of the plot in the absence of bias depends on the choice of axes. There are at least two main sources that can contribute to asymmetry of a funnel plot: the publication bias (e.g., small and unfavorable treatment effects are more likely to be missing) and heterogeneity (e.g., smaller studies may select patients who are more likely to benefit from the intervention). However, although the funnel plot provides a graphical means to detect publication bias, it is open to subjective interpretation. Many statistical tests have been developed to detect asymmetry of funnel plots, such as rank correlation test (e.g., Begg's test, Schwarzer's test) and regression tests (e.g., Egger's test, Harbord test), but inappropriate interpretation and several controversies still exist, especially because these plots have a subjective interpretation.[77,78]

Selection models or weighted distributions are other ways to explicitly model publication bias. These methods are based on the assumptions that the P values or sample sizes of primary studies influence the probability of their publication: studies with smaller P values or large sample sizes are more likely to be published. Various weight functions and selection models, from parametric to nonparametric approaches, were developed including logistic weight function, Copas model and Bayesian framework.[77,79] However, due to the complexity of performing these methods and interpreting results, their use in clinical practice is limited.

Overall recommendations for reporting metaanalytical parameters

Every step in any meta-analysis must be scrutinized for potential bias, from the formulation of the research question to the interpretation and discussion of the results, to ensure the quality and value of the final product. Lakens et al.[26] proposed six practical recommendations to improve the overall conduct and reproducibility of meta-analyses:

- Disclose all metaanalytic data, such as effect sizes, sample sizes, test statistics and degrees of freedom, means, and standard deviations.
- Specify which effect size calculations are used and which assumptions are made for missing data.
- Adhere to reporting guidelines.
- Preregister the protocol.
- Provide completely reproducible scripts containing both the data and the reported analyses in free software.
- Recruit expertise.

Additionally, grounded on previous literature and considering the different metaanalytical elements,[15,18,19,26,80] further recommendations which would facilitate the replication of a meta-analysis for any researcher external to the original research team, and would increase their trustworthiness by increasing the robustness of the conclusions are available in

TABLE 1 Recommendations for conducting and reporting metaanalytical elements.[81]

Parameter	Brief description
1. Provide all data used to build the meta-analyses	Authors should make available in the main text, supplementary material or in an open data platform (e.g., Open Science Framework) a table with all the extracted information that was used for analysis (e.g., number of events for each intervention, total sample in each group)
2. Report the imputed data	Authors should report (together with the raw data used to build the meta-analysis) which variables were imputed or further recalculated and how this imputation was conducted (e.g., formulas and references used)
3. Report the data obtained from different sources	If any data was obtained by means of contact with primary studies' authors or from unpublished sources, this information, together with the collected data, should be disclosed
4. Perform sensitivity analyses when imputed or unpublished data are used	When data not available in primary studies are used, after imputing them or obtaining from unpublished sources, authors should repeat the meta-analyses omitting these unavailable data as a sensitivity analysis exercise
5. Report on the statistical method, models, and effect-size measure	Authors should report the mathematical methods (e.g., inverse of variance, Mantel-Haenszel, Peto), models (e.g., random or fixed-effect) and measures (e.g., RR, OR, mean difference) used to build each meta-analysis, including those obtained with the sensitivity or subgroup analyses
6. Provide the complete statistical results for each meta-analysis	Authors should report all the results and metaanalytical parameters obtained in their study for each meta-analysis, including data on: effect-size values, confidence intervals (lower and upper values), P value, heterogeneity parameters (tau^2, standard error)
7. Report the prediction intervals (PI)	PI analyses should be performed for all meta-analysis presenting heterogeneity (values of $I^2 > 0\%$). The final results should be reported alongside the CI
8. Report the number needed to treat	To allow further data interpretability and better decision-making process in practice, authors should perform NNTB or NNTH analyses (reported with a dispersion value—95% CI) for at least the primary outcome of the meta-analysis
9. Report the fragility index (FI)	To allow further data interpretability and a better decision-making process in practice, authors should perform FI analyses for all meta-analyses that present statistical significance (i.e., differences between interventions)

Data from: The authors (Bonetti AF, Tonin FS, Lucchetta RC, Pontarolo R, Fernandez-Llimos F. Methodological standards for conducting and reporting meta-analyses: ensuring the replicability of meta-analyses of pharmacist-led medication review. *Res Soc Adm Pharm* 2022;18(2):2259–2268).

Table 1.[81] Journal editors and peer reviewers should encourage authors to attend to these recommendations and produce transparent, reproducible, and reliable meta-analyses.

Benefits and limitations of meta-analyses

When well-performed, meta-analyses provide the highest level of evidence by controlling or reducing extraneous variation and biases of individual studies. The selection and implementation of the correct statistical model and method are able to produce reliable and reproducible findings, which can be used in clinical practice and for further decision-making processes. The results are accurate if the underlying model assumptions are met and there is no selection bias, and no error in the extraction of data.[3,21]

Nonetheless, the reliability of the results of a meta-analysis depends on the quality and design of the trials included in the synthesis and the presence of heterogeneity. This technique cannot be used if the measurement of outcome variables is not similar for all studies. The selection of inappropriate model and statistical method for performing the meta-analysis results in misleading conclusions. The validity of CI relies on the correct identification of the sampling distribution of the effect size estimator. In the presence of significant publication or reporting bias, the results of the meta-analysis will be inaccurate. Pairwise meta-analyses are able to compare the effect of only two technologies at a time; for multiple and simultaneous treatment comparisons, other approaches such as network meta-analyses should be considered.[20] Table 2 summarizes the main advantages and limitations of performing a meta-analysis.

TABLE 2 Advantages and limitations of a pairwise meta-analysis.

Advantages	Limitations
More precise estimate of the effect-size[a]	Is not completely free from bias
Allows for an objective appraisal of evidence	Uses summary data rather than individual data
Reduces the probability of bias	Depends on the quality of the included data
Helps explain the heterogeneity among studies	Compares only two technologies at the time[b]
Avoids Simpson's paradox[c]	Requires skilled human and technical resources
Increases the generalizability of the results of individual studies	Depends on the use of appropriate statistical methods[d]

[a]As it overcomes the limitation of small sample sizes of individual studies.
[b]For multiple treatment comparisons other approaches such as network meta-analyses can be used.
[c]Simpson's paradox[82] is a phenomenon in which a trend appears in several groups of data but disappears or reverses when the groups are combined. The paradox can be resolved when confounding variables and causal relations are appropriately addressed in the statistical modeling.
[d]Carelessness in abstracting and summarizing appropriate studies, failure to consider important covariates, bias on the part of the metaanalyst and overstatements of the strength and precision of the results contribute to invalid meta-analyses.

Meta-analyses on pharmacy services: Where do we stand?

The number of systematic reviews with meta-analyses published in recent years in the field of pharmacy practice has been steadily increasing as a result of the growth in the number of primary studies, as well as the desire to use accruing evidence as early as possible to improve healthcare decisions.[83] A recent overview showed that between 1989 and 2020 more than 100 meta-analyses (comprising more than 300 controlled trials) assessing the effect of pharmacists' interventions were published, most of them reporting positive conclusions.[84]

In fact, several studies have demonstrated clinical, humanistic, and economic benefits associated with pharmacist-provided care in a wide array of diseases.[5,10,11,13,85] The recent meta-analysis published by Al-Babtain et al. ($n = 12$ randomized controlled trials), for instance, showed that community pharmacist-led medication review programs significantly improved patients' outcomes, including blood pressure in patients with diabetes and hypertension, HbA1c in patients with diabetes and total cholesterol in patients with hyperlipidemia, when compared to usual care.[86] Another meta-analysis ($n = 49$ randomized controlled trials) revealed that pharmacist medication counseling vs no such counseling was associated with a statistically significant 30% increase in relative risk (RR) for medication adherence, a 24% RR reduction in 30-day hospital readmission (NNT = 4.2), and a 30% RR reduction in emergency department visits; yet RR reductions for primary care visits and mortality were not statistically significant ($P > .05$).[87] On the other hand, although the original meta-analysis of Bonetti et al. on the impact of pharmacist-led discharge counseling on hospital readmission ($n = 18$ trials) revealed a significant difference favoring the intervention vs usual care (RR = 0.864 [95% CI, 0.763–0.997], $P = .020$), the high heterogeneity among trials ($I^2 = 60\%$), and the wide PI (0.542–1.186) prevented further conclusions.[88] To exercise the interpretation of a meta-analysis on the effect of a pharmacy-led intervention, see Fig. 6. meta-analyses assessing clinical pharmacy services targeting specific conditions are usually more conclusive, given that the intervention is well defined, and the measured outcomes are unequivocal and tangible. Conversely, the results are mostly inconclusive for interventions with a broader target and with variability in established monitoring parameters. These findings emphasize the need to better define clinical pharmacy services and standardize methods for assessing the impact of these services on patient health outcomes.[83,89]

Intrinsic characteristics of the interventions used in pharmacy services alongside poor reporting practices may be the origin of the heterogeneity and inconclusive results identified in meta-analyses. Pharmacy services include complex interventions—usually with several components frequently provided through educational, attitudinal, or behavioral actions. Thus, standardizing the intensity and components of the intervention (i.e., the frequency) and ensuring the fidelity of the service is much more complex than ensuring administration of a certain dose of a medicine.[83] One way to overcome this issue is by means of standard and reliable tools such as the DEPICT (Descriptive Elements of Pharmacist Intervention Characterization Tool),[90] which was created in response to the frequently reported issue of poor intervention description across primary studies assessing the impact of clinical pharmacy activities. This tool has 146 items distributed in 11 domains aiming at characterizing components of clinical pharmacy services, which should be used to ensure consistent

FIG. 6 Forest plot comparing an intervention (medication therapy management—MTM) vs control (usual care) for the outcome mortality (event). Meta-analysis performed using the Mantel-Haenszel (M-H) method and random-effect model. Effect-size measure risk ratio (RR) reported with 95% confidence intervals (CI). Between-studies heterogeneity measured with I^2 statistics (software: Review Manager v.5.3).

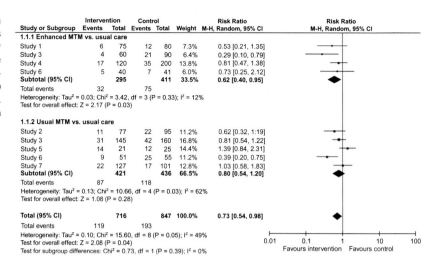

reporting of interventions in clinical trials to allow their reproducibility in practice, and comparability by means of a meta-analysis.[90]

The methodological quality and risk of bias of meta-analyses about pharmacy services has been explored by previous studies. An analysis of 151 systematic reviews showed that their quality varied from poor to moderate especially due to weak conduct and reporting of methods.[91] Lipovec et al.[92] performed an umbrella review to investigate the effects of pharmacist-led interventions and showed considerable heterogeneity between the studies. Authors additionally found that the effect on health resources use was inconsistent, with a significant variability among studies' quality. Similarly, MacLure et al.[93] and Bonetti et al.[84] identified common pitfalls, including the lack of a detailed protocol and focus on the research questions, bias and drift from the primary outcome, and errors in the metaanalytical process in at least one-third of the meta-analyses. Quality of the analyses, strength of evidence and data heterogeneity are rarely considered when synthetizing evidence and making recommendations in the field of pharmacy practice.[81,84] This highlights, once again, the need to strictly follow the guidelines for conducting and reporting meta-analyses in the biomedical field.

Conclusions

Potential benefits of meta-analyses include an increase in power, an improvement in precision, the ability to answer questions not posed by individual studies, and the opportunity to settle controversies arising from conflicting claims. However, they also have the potential to seriously mislead, particularly if specific study designs, within-study biases, variation across studies, and reporting biases are not carefully considered. Researchers and healthcare professionals should acknowledge the main approaches for performing and reporting a meta-analysis. Critical assessment and interpretation of the findings from these studies is essential for more assertive health decisions, including the provision of pharmacy services during the development of therapeutic guidelines and recommendations, and for implementing healthcare policies.

Questions for further discussion

1. The high growth of biomedical publications in the past years has led to the mass production of redundant, misleading, and conflicted meta-analyses. What can researchers and healthcare professionals do to enhance research quality, reliability, and transparency?
2. Extensions of pairwise meta-analyses, such as network meta-analysis and living meta-analysis, are being increasingly used in evidence-based practice. What are the challenges for conducting and reporting these new studies; and how are these challenges different from those encountered with pairwise meta-analyses?
3. What is the added value of using meta-analyses to ground pharmacy practice decisions?
4. How can the findings of a meta-analysis be used in pharmacy practice?

Application exercise/scenario

The forest plot in Fig. 6 refers to a meta-analysis that compared the effects of the intervention MTM (medication therapy management) performed by a pharmacist vs usual care in a hospital setting. The outcome of interest is mortality. The intervention was subgrouped into enhanced and usual MTM according to the characteristics of the service provided. Results are reported as risk ratio (RR) with 95% confidence intervals (CI).

1. What were the pooled effect estimates obtained for the overall and subgroup meta-analyses, and how should they be interpreted in practice?
2. What is the between-study heterogeneity for the overall and subgroup meta-analyses?
3. Which additional analyses could be performed to deal with heterogeneity?

References

1. Elliott RA, Putman K, Davies J, Annemans L. A review of the methodological challenges in assessing the cost effectiveness of pharmacist interventions. *PharmacoEconomics.* 2014;32:1185–1199.
2. Tonin FS, Aznar-Lou I, Pontinha VM, Pontarolo R, Fernandez-Llimos F. Principles of pharmacoeconomic analysis: the case of pharmacist-led interventions. *Pharm Pract (Granada).* 2021;19:2302.
3. Khan S, Memon B, Memon MA. Meta-analysis: a critical appraisal of the methodology, benefits and drawbacks. *Br J Hosp Med (Lond).* 2019;80:636–641.
4. Djulbegovic B, Guyatt GH. Progress in evidence-based medicine: a quarter century on. *Lancet.* 2017;390(10092):415–423.
5. Steed L, Sohanpal R, Todd A, et al. Community pharmacy interventions for health promotion: effects on professional practice and health outcomes. *Cochrane Database Syst Rev.* 2019;12:CD011207.
6. Garcia-Cardenas V, Rossing CV, Fernandez-Llimos F, et al. Pharmacy practice research—a call to action. *Res Soc Adm Pharm.* 2020;16:1602–1608.
7. Newman TV, San-Juan-Rodriguez A, Parekh N, et al. Impact of community pharmacist-led interventions in chronic disease management on clinical, utilization, and economic outcomes: an umbrella review. *Res Soc Adm Pharm.* 2020;16:1155–1165.
8. Schumock GT, Butler MG, Meek PD, et al. Evidence of the economic benefit of clinical pharmacy services: 1996-2000. *Pharmacotherapy.* 2003;23:113–132.
9. Abrahamsen B, Hansen RN, Rossing C. For which patient subgroups are there positive outcomes from a medication review? A systematic review. *Pharm Pract (Granada).* 2020;18:1976.
10. Rubio-Valera M, Bosmans J, Fernandez A, et al. Cost-effectiveness of a community pharmacist intervention in patients with depression: a randomized controlled trial (PRODEFAR study). *PLoS One.* 2013;8:e70588.
11. Martínez-Mardones F, Fernandez-Llimos F, Benrimoj SI, et al. Systematic review and meta-analysis of medication reviews conducted by pharmacists on cardiovascular diseases risk factors in ambulatory care. *J Am Heart Assoc.* 2019;8:e013627.
12. Sabater-Hernandez D, Sabater-Galindo M, Fernandez-Llimos F, et al. A systematic review of evidence-based community pharmacy services aimed at the prevention of cardiovascular disease. *J Manag Care Spec Pharm.* 2016;22:699–713.
13. Tan EC, Stewart K, Elliott RA, George J. Pharmacist services provided in general practice clinics: a systematic review and meta-analysis. *Res Soc Adm Pharm.* 2014;10:608–622.
14. Iqbal SA, Wallach JD, Khoury MJ, Schully SD, Ioannidis JP. Reproducible research practices and transparency across the biomedical literature. *PLoS Biol.* 2016;14:e1002333.
15. Page MJ, Altman DG, Shamseer L, et al. Reproducible research practices are underused in systematic reviews of biomedical interventions. *J Clin Epidemiol.* 2018;94:8–18.
16. Higgins J, Thomas J, Chandler J, et al. *Cochrane Handbook for Systematic Reviews of Interventions Version 6.1 (Updated September 2020).* Cochrane; 2020. Available from: www.training.cochrane.org/handbook.
17. Nagendrababu V, Dilokthornsakul P, Jinatongthai P, et al. Glossary for systematic reviews and meta-analyses. *Int Endod J.* 2020;53:232–249.
18. Ioannidis JP. Meta-analyses can be credible and useful: a new standard. *JAMA Psychiatry.* 2017;74:311–312.
19. Tonin FS, Borba HH, Leonart LP, et al. Methodological quality assessment of network meta-analysis of drug interventions: implications from a systematic review. *Int J Epidemiol.* 2019;48:620–632.
20. Tonin FS, Rotta I, Mendes AM, Pontarolo R. Network meta-analysis: a technique to gather evidence from direct and indirect comparisons. *Pharm Pract (Granada).* 2017;15:943.
21. Andrade C. Understanding the basics of meta-analysis and how to read a forest plot: as simple as it gets. *J Clin Psychiatry.* 2020;81:20f13698.
22. Schroll JB, Moustgaard R, Gøtzsche PC. Dealing with substantial heterogeneity in cochrane reviews. Cross-sectional study. *BMC Med Res Methodol.* 2011;11:22.
23. Every Palmer S, Howick J. How evidence-based medicine is failing due to biased trials and selective publication. *J Eval Clin Pract.* 2014;20:908–914.
24. Ioannidis JP. The mass production of redundant, misleading, and conflicted systematic reviews and meta-analyses. *Milbank Q.* 2016;94:485–514.
25. Ford AC, Guyatt GH, Talley NJ, Moayyedi P. Errors in the conduct of systematic reviews of pharmacological interventions for irritable bowel syndrome. *Am J Gastroenterol.* 2010;105:280–288.
26. Lakens D, Hilgard J, Staaks J. On the reproducibility of meta-analyses: six practical recommendations. *BMC Psychol.* 2016;4:24.

27. Rauh S, Torgerson T, Johnson AL, Pollard J, Tritz D, Vassar M. Reproducible and transparent research practices in published neurology research. *Res Integr Peer Rev*. 2020;5:5.

28. Wolfenden L, Grimshaw J, Williams CM, Yoong SL. Time to consider sharing data extracted from trials included in systematic reviews. *Syst Rev*. 2016;5:185.

29. Leichsenring F, Abbass A, Hilsenroth MJ, et al. Biases in research: risk factors for non-replicability in psychotherapy and pharmacotherapy research. *Psychol Med*. 2017;47:1000–1011.

30. Veroniki AA, Bender R, Glasziou P, Straus SE, Tricco AC. The number needed to treat in pairwise and network meta-analysis and its graphical representation. *J Clin Epidemiol*. 2019;111:11–22.

31. Alonso-Coello P, Carrasco-Labra A, Brignardello-Petersen R, et al. Systematic reviews experience major limitations in reporting absolute effects. *J Clin Epidemiol*. 2016;72:16–26.

32. Dautzenberg L, Bretagne L, Koek HL, et al. Medication review interventions to reduce hospital readmissions in older people. *J Am Geriatr Soc*. 2021;69:1646–1658.

33. Mittal N, Goyal M, Mittal PK. Understanding and appraising systematic reviews and meta-analysis. *J Clin Pediatr Dent*. 2017;41:317–326.

34. Glass G. Primary, secondary, and meta-analysis of research. *Educ Res*. 1976;5:3–8.

35. O'Rourke K. An historical perspective on meta-analysis: dealing quantitatively with varying study results. *J R Soc Med*. 2007;100:579–582.

36. Egger M, Smith GD. Meta-analysis. Potentials and promise. *BMJ*. 1997;315:1371–1374.

37. Davey Smith G, Egger M. Meta-analysis. Unresolved issues and future developments. *BMJ*. 1998;316:221–225.

38. Fleiss JL. The statistical basis of meta-analysis. *Stat Methods Med Res*. 1993;2:121–145.

39. Equator Network. Enhancing the Quality and Transparency of Health Research. EQUATOR Network. https://www.equator-network.org/.

40. Page MJ, McKenzie JE, Bossuyt PM, et al. The PRISMA 2020 statement: an updated guideline for reporting systematic reviews. *BMJ*. 2021;372:n71.

41. Briere JB, Bowrin K, Taieb V, Millier A, Toumi M, Coleman C. Meta-analyses using real-world data to generate clinical and epidemiological evidence: a systematic literature review of existing recommendations. *Curr Med Res Opin*. 2018;34:2125–2130.

42. Stroup DF, Berlin JA, Morton SC, et al. Meta-analysis of observational studies in epidemiology: a proposal for reporting. Meta-analysis of observational studies in epidemiology (MOOSE) group. *JAMA*. 2000;283:2008–2012.

43. Olejnik S, Algina J. Measures of effect size for comparative studies: applications, interpretations, and limitations. *Contemp Educ Psychol*. 2000;25:241–286.

44. Van Den Noortgate W, Onghena P. Estimating the mean effect size in meta-analysis: bias, precision, and mean squared error of different weighting methods. *Behav Res Methods Instrum Comput*. 2003;35:504–511.

45. Sullivan GM, Feinn R. Using effect size-or why the P value is not enough. *J Grad Med Educ*. 2012;4:279–282.

46. Spiegelman D, VanderWeele TJ. Evaluating public health interventions: 6. Modeling ratios or differences? Let the data tell us. *Am J Public Health*. 2017;107:1087–1091.

47. Chang BH, Waternaux C, Lipsitz S. Meta-analysis of binary data: which within study variance estimate to use? *Stat Med*. 2001;20:1947–1956.

48. Brockwell SE, Gordon IR. A comparison of statistical methods for meta-analysis. *Stat Med*. 2001;20:825–840.

49. Ranganathan P, Aggarwal R, Pramesh CS. Common pitfalls in statistical analysis: odds versus risk. *Perspect Clin Res*. 2015;6:222–224.

50. Laupacis A, Sackett DL, Roberts RS. An assessment of clinically useful measures of the consequences of treatment. *N Engl J Med*. 1988;318:1728–1733.

51. Mendes D, Alves C, Batel-Marques F. Number needed to treat (NNT) in clinical literature: an appraisal. *BMC Med*. 2017;15:112.

52. Mendes D, Alves C, Batel-Marques F. Benefit-risk of therapies for relapsing-remitting multiple sclerosis: testing the number needed to treat to benefit (NNTB), number needed to treat to harm (NNTH) and the likelihood to be helped or harmed (LHH): a systematic review and meta-analysis. *CNS Drugs*. 2016;30:909–929.

53. Altman DG. Confidence intervals for the number needed to treat. *BMJ*. 1998;317:1309–1312.

54. Altman DG, Deeks JJ. Meta-analysis, Simpson's paradox, and the number needed to treat. *BMC Med Res Methodol*. 2002;2:3.

55. Borestein MHL, Higgins JPT, Rothstein HR. Prediction intervals. In: *Introduction to Meta-Analysis*. 1st ed. Wiley; 2009:127–133. Chichester, England.

56. Longford NT. Estimation of the effect size in meta-analysis with few studies. *Stat Med*. 2010;29:421–430.

57. DerSimonian R, Kacker R. Random-effects model for meta-analysis of clinical trials: an update. *Contemp Clin Trials*. 2007;28:105–114.

58. Higgins JP, Thompson SG, Spiegelhalter DJ. A re-evaluation of random-effects meta-analysis. *J R Stat Soc Ser A Stat Soc*. 2009;172:137–159.

59. Borenstein M, Higgins JP, Hedges LV, Rothstein HR. Basics of meta-analysis: I(2) is not an absolute measure of heterogeneity. *Res Synth Methods*. 2017;8:5–18.

60. Riley RD, Higgins JP, Deeks JJ. Interpretation of random effects meta-analyses. *BMJ*. 2011;342:d549.

61. Schmidt FL, Oh IS, Hayes TL. Fixed- versus random-effects models in meta-analysis: model properties and an empirical comparison of differences in results. *Br J Math Stat Psychol*. 2009;62:97–128.

62. DerSimonian R, Laird N. Meta-analysis in clinical trials. *Control Clin Trials*. 1986;7:177–188.

63. Hartung J, Knapp G. A refined method for the meta-analysis of controlled clinical trials with binary outcome. *Stat Med*. 2001;20:3875–3889.

64. Hartung J, Knapp G. On tests of the overall treatment effect in meta-analysis with normally distributed responses. *Stat Med*. 2001;20:1771–1782.

65. Sidik K, Jonkman JN. A simple confidence interval for meta-analysis. *Stat Med*. 2002;21:3153–3159.

66. IntHout J, Ioannidis JP, Rovers MM, Goeman JJ. Plea for routinely presenting prediction intervals in meta-analysis. *BMJ Open*. 2016;6:e010247.

67. Dawson DV, Pihlstrom BL, Blanchette DR. Understanding and evaluating meta-analysis. *J Am Dent Assoc*. 2016;147:264–270.

68. Wang CC, Lee WC. A simple method to estimate prediction intervals and predictive distributions: summarizing meta-analyses beyond means and confidence intervals. *Res Synth Methods*. 2019;10:255–266.

69. Huedo-Medina TB, Sanchez-Meca J, Marin-Martinez F, Botella J. Assessing heterogeneity in meta-analysis: Q statistic or I2 index? *Psychol Methods*. 2006;11:193–206.

70. Spence JR, Stanley DJ. Prediction interval: what to expect when you're expecting .. a replication. *PLoS One*. 2016;11:e0162874.

71. Walsh M, Srinathan SK, McAuley DF, et al. The statistical significance of randomized controlled trial results is frequently fragile: a case for a fragility index. *J Clin Epidemiol*. 2014;67:622–628.

72. Atal I, Porcher R, Boutron I, Ravaud P. The statistical significance of meta-analyses is frequently fragile: definition of a fragility index for meta-analyses. *J Clin Epidemiol*. 2019;111:32–40.

73. Carter RE, McKie PM, Storlie CB. The fragility index: a P-value in sheep's clothing? *Eur Heart J*. 2017;38:346–348.

74. Ahmed I, Sutton AJ, Riley RD. Assessment of publication bias, selection bias, and unavailable data in meta-analyses using individual participant data: a database survey. *BMJ*. 2012;344:d7762.

75. Simes RJ. Publication bias: the case for an international registry of clinical trials. *J Clin Oncol*. 1986;4:1529–1541.

76. Ioannidis JP. Effect of the statistical significance of results on the time to completion and publication of randomized efficacy trials. *JAMA*. 1998;279:281–286.

77. Jin ZC, Zhou XH, He J. Statistical methods for dealing with publication bias in meta-analysis. *Stat Med*. 2015;34:343–360.

78. Sterne JA, Sutton AJ, Ioannidis JP, et al. Recommendations for examining and interpreting funnel plot asymmetry in meta-analyses of randomised controlled trials. *BMJ*. 2011;343:d4002.

79. Henmi M, Hattori S, Friede T. A confidence interval robust to publication bias for random-effects meta-analysis of few studies. *Res Synth Methods*. 2021;12(5):674–679. https://doi.org/10.1002/jrsm.1482.

80. Jones AP, Remmington T, Williamson PR, Ashby D, Smyth RL. High prevalence but low impact of data extraction and reporting errors were found in Cochrane systematic reviews. *J Clin Epidemiol*. 2005;58:741–742.

81. Bonetti AF, Tonin FS, Lucchetta RC, Pontarolo R, Fernandez-Llimos F. Methodological standards for conducting and reporting meta-analyses: ensuring the replicability of meta-analyses of pharmacist-led medication review. *Res Soc Adm Pharm*. 2022;18(2):2259–2268. https://doi.org/10.1016/j.sapharm.2021.06.002.

82. Simpson E. The interpretation of interaction in contingency tables. *J R Stat Soc*. 1951;13:238–241.

83. Bonetti AF, Della Rocca AM, Lucchetta RC, Tonin FS, Fernandez-Llimos F, Pontarolo R. Mapping the characteristics of meta-analyses of pharmacy services: a systematic review. *Int J Clin Pharm*. 2020;42(5):1252–1260.

84. Bonetti AF, Tonin FS, Della Rocca AM, Lucchetta RC, Fernandez-Llimos F, Pontarolo R. Methodological quality and risk of bias of meta-analyses of pharmacy services: a systematic review. *Res Soc Adm Pharm*. 2020. https://doi.org/10.1016/j.sapharm.2020.12.011. In press.

85. Presley B, Groot W, Pavlova M. Pharmacy-led interventions to improve medication adherence among adults with diabetes: a systematic review and meta-analysis. *Res Soc Adm Pharm*. 2019;15:1057–1067.

86. Al-Babtain B, Cheema E, Hadi MA. Impact of community-pharmacist-led medication review programmes on patient outcomes: a systematic review and meta-analysis of randomised controlled trials. *Res Soc Adm Pharm*. 2021. https://doi.org/10.1016/j.sapharm.2021.04.022. In press.

87. Kelly WN, Ho MJ, Bullers K, Klocksieben F, Kumar A. Association of pharmacist counseling with adherence, 30-day readmission, and mortality: a systematic review and meta-analysis of randomized trials. *J Am Pharm Assoc*. 2021;61:340–350.e345.

88. Bonetti AF, Reis WC, Mendes AM, et al. Impact of pharmacist-led discharge counseling on hospital readmission and emergency department visits: a systematic review and meta-analysis. *J Hosp Med*. 2020;15:52–59.

89. Rotta I, Salgado TM, Silva ML, Correr CJ, Fernandez-Llimos F. Effectiveness of clinical pharmacy services: an overview of systematic reviews (2000–2010). *Int J Clin Pharm*. 2015;37:687–697.

90. Rotta I, Salgado TM, Felix DC, Souza TT, Correr CJ, Fernandez-Llimos F. Ensuring consistent reporting of clinical pharmacy services to enhance reproducibility in practice: an improved version of DEPICT. *J Eval Clin Pract*. 2015;21:584–590.

91. Melchiors AC, Correr CJ, Venson R, Pontarolo R. An analysis of quality of systematic reviews on pharmacist health interventions. *Int J Clin Pharm*. 2012;34:32–42.

92. Lipovec N, Zerovnik S, Kos M. Pharmacy-supported interventions at transitions of care: an umbrella review. *Int J Clin Pharm*. 2019;41:831–852.

93. MacLure K, Paudyal V, Stewart D. Reviewing the literature, how systematic is systematic? *Int J Clin Pharm*. 2016;38:685–694.

Chapter 8

Using methods from human-centered design in health research: An introduction for pharmacy and health services researchers

Michelle Flood[a,b], Laura L. Gleeson[a], Sarah Flynn[a], Mark Ennis[c], Aoife Ludlow[a], Fabian F. Sweeney[a], Alice Holton[a], Stephanie Morgan[b], Colleen Clarke[d], Pádraig Carroll[a], Lisa Mellon[e], Fiona Boland[f], Sarah Mohamed[a,g], Aoife De Brún[h], Marcus Hanratty[i], Shaunna Kelly[j], and Frank Moriarty[a]

[a]*School of Pharmacy and Biomolecular Sciences, RCSI University of Medicine and Health Sciences, Dublin, Ireland,* [b]*Design Institute for Health, Dell Medical School, University of Texas at Austin, Austin, TX, United States,* [c]*TU Dublin School of Creative Arts, Technological University Dublin City Campus, Dublin, Ireland,* [d]*Institute for Healthcare Delivery Design, Population Health Sciences Program, University of Illinois-Chicago, Chicago, IL, United States,* [e]*Division of Population Health Sciences, RCSI University of Medicine and Health Sciences, Dublin, Ireland,* [f]*Data Science Centre, RCSI University of Medicine and Health Sciences, Dublin, Ireland,* [g]*School of Pharmacy and Pharmaceutical Sciences, Trinity College Dublin, Dublin, Ireland,* [h]*School of Nursing Midwifery and Health Systems, Health Sciences Centre, University College Dublin, Dublin, Ireland,* [i]*Department of Product Design, National College of Art and Design, Dublin, Ireland,* [j]*School of Medicine, RCSI University of Medicine and Health Sciences, Dublin, Ireland*

Objectives

- Define human-centered design.
- Explain why human-centered design methods may be useful in pharmacy and health services research.
- Describe key human-centered design methods that can be used in pharmacy and health services research.
- Five examples of how human-centered design methods have been used in pharmacy and health services research.
- Outline key challenges with including human-centered design approaches in health services research and discuss how they may be overcome.

Introduction

Health systems around the world are undergoing a process of reform and redesign based on the changing needs of the population and in response to new and increasingly complex health challenges, such as the growing burden of chronic disease, widening health inequalities, an increasing and aging population, and recently, the threat of global pandemics. These challenges are examples of "wicked problems," a concept coined by Rittel and Webber to describe those that are highly complex, systemic, interdependent, unpredictable, and resistant to solution through conventional interventions.[1] Addressing such problems requires an interdisciplinary, creative, and collaborative approach to problem solving, and sustained stakeholder engagement at all levels of the system. Within health services research, there has been an increasing interest in the potential for human-centered design—a discipline that involves an innovative, collaborative, and systemic approach to problem solving—as one approach that could help address "wicked problems" in healthcare systems.

Although applying human-centered design principles to pharmacy and health services research is still a relatively new concept, many leading international design consultancy firms such as IDEO (www.ideo.com), Frog (www.frogdesign.com), and Fjord (www.fjordnet.com) have leveraged designs to solve commercial healthcare projects for several years. Initially, these firms focused primarily on the design of medical devices, but have since expanded their focus to include challenges such as medication adherence and health literacy with several examples and case studies available on their websites. Designers have also been embedded in different ways around the world including centers in major healthcare

Contemporary Research Methods in Pharmacy and Health Services. https://doi.org/10.1016/B978-0-323-91888-6.00011-9

organizations (e.g., Kaiser Permanente), hospitals (e.g., the Centre for Innovation at the Mayo Clinic and the Helix Centre at St Mary's Hospital, London), and medical schools/universities (e.g., the Design Institute for Health, Dell Medical School, the University of Texas at Austin, the Health Design Lab at Jefferson University, and the Institute for Healthcare Delivery Design at the University of Illinois-Chicago).[2] Within the pharmacy and health services research literature, recent reviews report the application of human-centered design approaches across a broad range of medical specialties and health conditions, although the total number of peer-reviewed publications remains relatively small, with many projects reported only in gray literature.[3–5]

What is design?

In the broadest sense, design can be defined as a creative problem-solving process. This chapter focuses on human-centered design which is more specific, originally defined by the international standard ISO 9241-210 as the "use of techniques which communicate, interact, empathize and stimulate the people involved, obtaining an understanding of their needs, desires and experiences."[6] This definition, which emphasizes the technical aspects of human-centered design, reflects the fact that it was originally developed with reference to engineering disciplines including computer science and artificial intelligence. It is now generally interpreted in a broader sense emphasizing its focus on human behavior and experiences, with core features including understanding user needs, desires, and experiences.[7] Human-centered design is often operationalized by specific models or processes that can be used by multidisciplinary teams such as design thinking or the Design Council's Double Diamond Framework.[8,9] As well as focusing on users' needs, human-centered design also considers issues such as technology, available resources, and business requirements which ensures solutions generated to address problems are both desirable and feasible.[10]

There are many common misconceptions associated with human-centered design in pharmacy and health services research communities. For example, some people may think that design is focused primarily on esthetics or that it is only relevant when developing products or medical devices rather than having the potential for broad application across service delivery and patient experience.[4] These misconceptions often arise because of the lack of familiarity with human-centered design due to the historically limited overlap between the two disciplines.[5] Pharmacy and health services researchers may not know that designers generally complete formal undergraduate and often postgraduate training in one of a number of design disciplines. Just as healthcare professionals complete core clinical training followed by specialist training, designers possess core skills such as creative problem solving and visual thinking; they generally further specialize in one or more areas including visual design, interaction design, product design, service design, or strategic design. For health services researchers, this terminology is often unfamiliar and may initially prove challenging to interpret.[4] Examples of common design specialties are shown with a description and examples of their potential roles in pharmacy and health services research in Table 1. Of course, there are some overlapping elements in these definitions, and some designers may work across a number of specialties.

Key design approaches

Notwithstanding the specialty, a fundamental focus on engaging with and understanding the needs of all users of systems is common to all designers. This means that some methods and practices are commonly employed across all specialties.[5] Examples include the Design Council's four phase "Double Diamond" (discover, define, develop, deliver) and Stanford d.school's five modes (empathize, define, ideate, prototype, test).[9,11] All models allow for flexible movement back and forth between phases as the problem is addressed, encourage multidisciplinary working, and encourage active experimentation over thinking.[10] Three of the most common methods are journey mapping, prototyping, and formative evaluation. These three methods have direct applicability to pharmacy and health services research both as standalone methods and as complementary methods when combined with traditional health services research methods. An illustrative example in the form of a case study of a pharmacy-based project that employed each method is included for each method.

User research: Journey mapping

Driven by design's user-centered perspective, user research is considered the vital first step in any design research project. Sometimes termed "needfinding," it is an integral part of the design process.[8] Contrary to traditional health services research approaches which usually start with formal literature searches to synthesize existing evidence,[12] design approaches generally emphasize early engagement with users, prioritizing context-specific primary research which may be supplemented with some secondary research.[13] One user research method with particular applicability to health services

TABLE 1 Common design specialties and potential roles in pharmacy and health services research.

Design specialty	Description	Example of potential role in pharmacy/health services research
Visual design	The purposeful creation and organization of visual elements such as color, shapes, typography and images to improve usability, to lead the eye to important information, and ultimately to capture and hold attention	Wayfinding: Improving patient experience of hospital visits through using visual design to support navigation
Interaction design	The design of interaction between users and products and services, both digital and nondigital, with particular focus on the context of use and user needs	eHealth: Designing user-friendly interfaces for eHealth interventions such as electronic health records or electronic prescribing
Product design	The development of physical and digital products to fit better within people's lives by considering their needs and ergonomic principles when researching, ideating, conceptualizing, and building new products/devices	Medical devices: Designing inhalers or blood glucose monitors that are easy for patients to use, store, and handle
Service design	The (re)design of services to meet the needs of users, stakeholders, and organizations in a coherent, collaborative, efficient, and integrated manner	Mental health services: Redesigning patient pathways to improve access and clarity for patients who may need to engage with a range of health and social care professionals
Strategic design	The application of design principles and practices to systemic challenges to develop future-oriented innovative solutions	Health policy: Developing health reform strategies to inform policy and planning for future health services

research is journey mapping. Journey mapping enables visualization of the overall experience of a service user or staff member from their perspective, including feelings, motivations, and attitudes, as they move through various interactions or "touch points."[14] Unlike process mapping, which is usually focused on improving process efficiency or reducing waste using management principles such as lean thinking,[15] journey mapping facilitates a more holistic representation of the patient experience from the perspective of a particular user with a broader emphasis on both the physical and emotional journey thus promoting empathy for service users and/or staff members.[14]

Journey maps are useful in health services researchers in several ways. The visualization of complex data in a simple form that highlights a user's journey facilitates empathy development and allows diverse interdisciplinary teams to work efficiently and creatively using a service user's experience as a common denominator.[16] It helps teams to pinpoint distinct moments to redesign and improve while developing a shared vision. Journey mapping is a flexible tool that can be used to visualize current practice ("current state" or "as-is") or model potential future services ("future state" or "to be"). It can be used to map services from various perspectives (e.g., patient or health professional perspectives), to map journeys at various levels of detail (from seconds to decades), and to develop idealized journey maps in the form of service blueprints.[16] Service blueprints are an extension of journey maps that connect user experience with staff and other supporting processes that can be used as a tool during subsequent design steps.[16] Journey mapping has been used in research in a number of healthcare settings including mental health, social care, connected health, and exploring refugees' access to services.[17–20]

As with any map or model, the strength of a journey map depends on the quality of data used in its development. In many cases, data collection for a journey map will incorporate both primary and secondary research and the collection of quantitative and qualitative data from a number of sources. Before collecting any data, it is important to determine the user chosen for the map (e.g., patient, healthcare professional, other staff member), and the unit of analysis or level of "zoom" (e.g., at the level of an individual consultation or the entire service).[16] Qualitative data collection methods such as interviews, observations, focus groups, and document analysis are of particular importance and are ideally conducted over an extensive period of time to allow an in-depth analysis.[15,18] Visual data, including videos, photographs and screenshots, are valuable in enriching journey maps and enhancing credibility. Quantitative research data that may be of use include local metrics about service utilization, satisfaction surveys, cost analyses, and national/international metrics around population needs and priorities. In academic-design collaborations, formal literature reviews may be part of the initial project stages. Data gathered are generally pooled, and analyzed using either formal academic methods such as qualitative or quantitative content analysis[18] or similar but less formal qualitative techniques such as affinity mapping. Affinity mapping is a collaborative, visual approach to sense-making where relationships between concepts and ideas are made through arranging them in groups.[21] Participants generally use paper (or digital) sticky notes to share their ideas or observations on a particular topic with others, and these are then grouped based on perceived similarity. It is somewhat similar to thematic analysis, but is less structured and more collaborative, allowing designers greater flexibility to combine multiple data sources and make judgments. The data are then used by the project team to develop a visual representation that may include several "layers" seen from the perspective of the main actor, stages of the journey, specific steps, emotions, communication channels, stakeholders, and "backstage" or enabling processes.[14,18,22]

It is important for health services researchers to bear in mind that a journey map is a useful representative visualization to stimulate engagement, deeper understanding of challenges, and discussion to provide a basis for subsequent design steps rather than being exhaustive or a "truth."[18] Engaging services users using the journey mapping approach allows researchers to understand explicit and latent barriers, enablers, challenges, and opportunities, through developing empathy for users.[23] Leveraging tools such as journey maps ensures the focus remains on users and informs subsequent activities including the design of prototype interventions used in the next stages of the design process.[4]

Case study 1: Journey mapping in the HealthEir project

Context: A national project in Ireland conducted by the authors. It was funded by the Irish Government through the Sláintecare Integration Fund that supported the achievement of the Sláintecare goals for health system reform in Ireland, including to engage citizens in their own health and to support care delivery in the community.[24]

Goal: The HealthEir project aims to support the delivery of brief interventions for alcohol, drugs, healthy eating, smoking and physical activity in community pharmacy and primary care in line with national policy to improve preventative care in the community.[25] The potential for brief interventions to improve health are undisputed, but several complex systemic barriers to successful implementation are known including resources, training, and confidence.[26,27]

Application: For the HealthEir project, journey mapping was used to identify the existing patient journey in primary care pharmacy and general practitioner (family doctor) services as part of the project user research. Due to COVID-19 pandemic restrictions in 2020, direct observations were not possible so the team combined secondary research, document analysis, and semistructured telephone interviews with patients, community pharmacists, and general practitioners (GPs) to inform the development of the journey map. In this case, the unit of analysis was an initial and follow-up visit to a GP or community pharmacy. Documents including standard operating procedures and practice guidelines were analyzed to map what the patient journey "should be" which was then triangulated with the semistructured interview data to further enrich the initial map. Transcripts were analyzed to identify how stakeholders felt at each stage of the journey, any problems or deviations from guidelines, what interpersonal communication takes place, and what tools or resources were used at particular stages. This information was reviewed collaboratively by project team members and the journey map was developed (Fig. 1).

Outcome: This visualization allowed the project team to consider how brief interventions following the "5As" (Ask, Advise, Assess, Assist, Arrange) brief interventions approach could work best within the existing patient journey.[28] The team reviewed the existing patient journey using the journey map and the required activities relating to the 5As model and considered how to efficiently and effectively integrate the brief intervention into the existing workflows and interactions. This process unexpectedly highlighted the potential role for wider team (not pharmacists/doctors) in engaging with patients and introducing them to the service while patients waited to see the pharmacist or doctor, a potential solution that only became obvious when reviewing the journey maps. This informed the development of an innovative approach that blended human and technology elements to leverage waiting time. First, a member of the wider team invited the patient to participate using a standardized onboarding approach. Next, the patient completed the Ask, Advise, and Assess stages of brief interventions using a tablet device, before finally engaging with their health professional to complete the Assist and Arrange steps where they received tailored advice and referral to services if needed. The journey map was central to the development of the HealthEir intervention and was then used to develop a service blueprint to support implementation and staff training (Fig. 2).

Intervention development: Prototyping

When the user research data has been synthesized and potential solutions identified, the development of prototypes enables the design team to explore several potential solutions, before selecting the most suitable options(s) for further refinement.[23] Prototypes become physical manifestations of ideas or concepts, and give form to ideas arising from user research.[29] This stage is analogous to feasibility and pilot studies in health services research, but is approached with a more flexible approach and developmental intent.[30] From a design perspective, prototyping is vital to reducing risk and uncertainty as early and as cheaply as possible.[16] Prototypes are particularly helpful in making ideas tangible for service users and

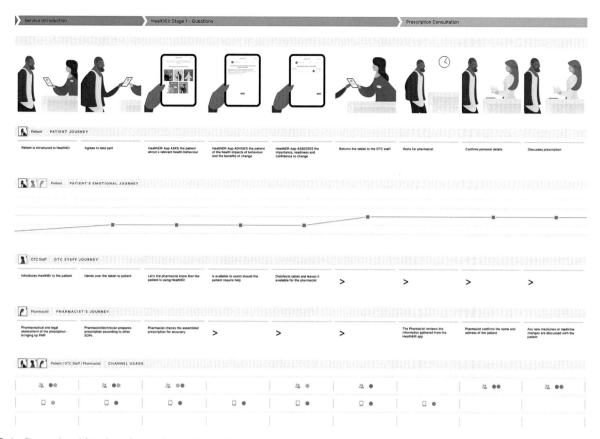

FIG. 1 Data gathered from interviews and secondary analysis were used to develop the journey map that modeled the stages in the patient (both physical and emotional) and stakeholder journeys using smaply.com software.

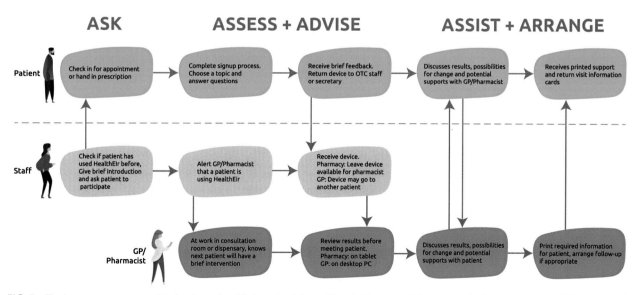

FIG. 2 The journey maps were used to develop a simplified service delivery blueprint that showed the stages in the intervention that could be included in training materials.

project teams and challenging their assumptions and opinions about a product or service because "the theory is not hidden in abstraction."[29] If done meaningfully, they help improve design quality and minimize challenges with implementation and sustainability, issues commonly encountered with health services research.[31] Prototyping is a structured and iterative process, usually completed after and driven by user research, but new questions or problems can also be uncovered at this stage, which may require more research to be conducted. The process can be viewed as "growing early conceptual designs through prototypes into mature products or services."[29] Prototyping can also be used earlier in the process as a research approach to enable stakeholders to externalize thoughts and ideas in the form of physical artifacts, which offer insights into possible futures.[32]

For health services projects, prototyping may include combinations of storyboards, physical models, walkthroughs, desktop walkthroughs, or process simulations.[16] Researchers may wish to prototype interactions, service processes, experiences, physical objects, environments, spaces, digital tools, or other elements of the service ecosystem. User research tools such as journey maps are helpful in identifying what should be included in prototyping. Decisions about how refined the prototype should be are important, with low-fidelity prototypes using paper or cardboard often used effectively initially, with the level of detail and quality of materials increasing as the project nears implementation.[33] Paper and cardboard can be used to prototype everything from desktop models to full-size physical spaces and furniture to digital tools in the initial stages, enabling rapid and low-cost representation of websites, Apps, and other digital interfaces. Using low-cost materials to prototype full-scale pharmacy services has been successful in assisting pharmacy teams to improve their patient care and secure funding for expanded service delivery.[34] Constantly refining or "iterating" the prototype(s) based on feedback is vital during the prototyping phase and a series of prototyping loops with set goals should be planned.

Case study 2: Prototyping in the Whittington hospital pharmacy project

Context: The Whittington Hospital Pharmacy team in the UK collaborated with the Design Council and two commercial design agencies to improve service delivery and patient experience.[34]

Goal: The Whittington Hospital Chief Pharmacist identified a need to improve the patient experience in their pharmacy service and sought help to do so from the Design Council in the United Kingdom. The interdisciplinary project team wanted to improve the experience for patients using their pharmacy services, increase opportunity for health promotion, and develop a commercial service to generate revenue to fund the intervention.

Application: The team used a codesign approach to develop innovative solutions to reconfigure the physical space and service delivery. Ideas were tested via a series of prototypes developed by the multidisciplinary team. This started with small low-fidelity paper and cardboard models generated during workshops that considered both the physical space and the services to be delivered, as well as patient and staff experience. Larger, low-fidelity cardboard prototypes were next developed and introduced to the pharmacy environment, allowing people not directly involved to provide feedback about the various prototypes introduced to the space. This included elements including cardboard signage, temporary barriers, and other physical elements that could support evaluation of a number of proposed solutions. The team then pooled feedback gathered and analyzed the feedback to understand and clarify what was needed from the space.

Outcome: The team used the prototypes and feedback to develop plans and costings for the space so that funding could be sought to implement the desired scheme.

Evaluation: Testing with users

Health services research methods frequently include formal structured evaluations at specific, predefined points in a project.[35] For example, an intervention may be evaluated initially as part of pilot and/or feasibility studies before moving on to a definitive randomized controlled trial.[30,36] These evaluations may include assessment against predetermined outcomes or standards that are considered important for academic research purposes, and for generalizability of the findings. Most evaluation in health services research is summative in nature, making judgments about a particular intervention at the conclusion of a specific activity or period. Efficacy, process, and economic evaluations are commonly conducted based on recommendations in frameworks such as the Medical Research Council (MRC) and National Institute for Health Research (NIHR) that promote use of conventional experimental designs with randomization and other traditional study designs.[35] The findings from these evaluations inform decisions about implementation and contribute to academic research on interventions as peer-reviewed publications. Of course, this approach has many strengths and is critical for evaluation of many intervention types such as medicines or medical procedures, but it reflects largely positivist, academic, and sometimes narrow view of what is important or can be known in terms of service delivery interventions and improving patient experience. Rather than prioritizing study design and "robustness," design research approaches tend to be more pragmatic and user-focused. They often engage in ongoing formative evaluations aiming to gather data to inform the continuous refinement of prototype services in a specific context, rather than add to a particular literature or evidence base.[37] As a new intervention is implemented, evaluation data is gathered using a variety of methods and used by the design team to make improvements before making a new improved version of the intervention or iteration. At the end of the design process, the aim is to have an intervention that can be readily implemented in a particular context rather than a context-independent intervention that moves to an implementation phase, which is commonly seen in traditional health services research frameworks.[35]

Evaluation methods used in design research often include qualitative and quantitative methods that may be familiar to health services researchers; however, it is important to note that they are often applied much more flexibly reflecting the focus on users in context rather than generalizability or academic publication. Interviews, observations, and focus groups are helpful to gather feedback about people's experiences and emotional responses to prototype services.[16] Surveys, time-in-motion studies, and other quasiexperimental quantitative methods such as A/B testing where two versions of a product or service are tested and compared are used to explore user experience preferences and issues. For digital interventions, heuristic evaluation, where principles of good design are compared with the digital interface, can be used to evaluate usability.[16] In many cases, designers use evaluation findings to inform iteration and development rather than publication in academic journals; however, for interdisciplinary projects involving academic researchers, formal evaluation leading to a peer-reviewed publication is more likely.

Case study: Evaluation of information design prototypes

Context: A study conducted in the United Kingdom on how to highlight and educate the public about antibiotic resistant infection in community pharmacies through effective information provision. This project was conducted by an interdisciplinary team of academics from design and pharmacy backgrounds in collaboration with a pharmacist working in a pharmacy chain.[38]

Goal (of evaluation): To evaluate two prototypes that had been installed in a community pharmacy.

Application: Several complementary approaches were used to gather information for the evaluation of the prototypes. Informal, opportunistic, semistructured interviews were conducted with visitors to the community pharmacy over a 3-week period. The interviewers asked open-ended questions aiming to explore participants' perceptions relating to the content and visual design of the materials. They also asked participants about what impact the content might have on their behavior and what about the prototypes didn't work from their perspective and why. Additional informal conversations between the research team, pharmacists and pharmacy staff allowed the team to identify their perspectives on people's responses to the materials. The prototypes were also displayed at an event held by the pharmacy chain and pharmacists and pharmacy workers were asked for their opinions.

Outcome: The evaluation process led to the development of a series of recommendations for both refining the prototypes and using space in community pharmacies effectively for health communication. Recommendations included considering how related information is displayed, using signs or notices to advise patients how to engage with the resources, developing additional supporting resources, keeping messaging brief and focused, and testing color schemes on site.

Human-centered design and health services research methods

Within health services research there has been increasing recognition that including current or potential health service users (individuals who access or use healthcare services, including patients, family members, or carers) in research may be an effective strategy to ensure that research develops interventions that would be acceptable to them and reflects their priorities.[39] Approaches taken range from "patient and public involvement" where service users participate in planning, conducting, overseeing, and/or disseminating research,[40] to participatory methodologies including coproduction or codesign which may focus more on intervention development and include other stakeholder groups.[41–43] These methods and approaches facilitate engagement with current or potential services users with the goal of incorporating their perspectives. Their use and application is increasingly evident in pharmacy and health services research publications. Coproduction methods have been previously employed by researchers in community pharmacy settings for specific reasons, e.g., to engage with marginalized communities and improve access to care.[44,45]

Similarly, patients have been increasingly consulted as part of quality improvement interventions. For example, Damschroder's Implementation Framework[46] involves eliciting stakeholders' needs as part of research development and implementation processes. However, such processes commonly use specific processes designed around an evidence-based healthcare perspective and models developed by healthcare professionals and researchers that invite patients/service users on their terms. Such frameworks are generally based on norms and assumptions arising from a largely positivist perspective including systematic reviews, scientific rigor, and rigid study protocols. This means that the consultation may be process-centered and linear with predetermined goals and outcomes rather than genuinely human-centered and responsive to the users' ideas, concerns, and expectations.

While it may seem that participatory and quality improvement approaches are very similar to human-centered design approaches, there are key differences in terms of how service users are engaged. Human-centered design approaches are unique in the depth and purpose of user engagement and the centrality of users rather than researchers and specific frameworks in the research process.[7] Engagement with user groups and stakeholders is intended to be collaborative rather than consultative, and go beyond the collection of feedback or perspectives on a particular topic. Such fundamentally collaboratively user-oriented approaches can harness diverse experiences and collective intelligence to promote interdisciplinary innovation and creativity in health systems research and design that is not seen with other commonly used approaches.[23] Design processes facilitate the "messy trajectories of engagement" needed to keep users' at the center of changing strategies and embrace iteration to ensure that solutions are really meeting the needs of users for whom they are intended to help.[47]

Working collaboratively

This chapter has provided an overview of three key design methods for health services researchers to consider alongside worked examples of pharmacy-based projects that employed design methods to address complex problems relating to brief interventions, pharmacy service delivery, and antibiotic resistance. However, it is important to emphasize that interdisciplinary collaboration and involving expert designers as part of the research team is needed to realize their full potential.[8] All of the projects described involved design professionals (practitioners and/or academics) rather than pharmacy or health services researchers simply using the methods. Design recognizes that no single discipline can solve complex health challenges as they exist across and between disciplinary boundaries rather than within them.[23] While health services researchers can learn and use design methods, designers bring unique perspectives, sensibilities, and skills to health services research projects that go beyond methodological and technical expertise.[48] Designers have extensive training and experience in working collaboratively at interfaces of people, complex services, and technology using participatory methodologies, often with further specialism in one area of design as previously discussed. Through this "radical" interdisciplinary collaboration, designers can help teams of pharmacy and health services researchers challenge tendency toward disciplinary groupthink and help researchers and practitioners become "un-stuck."[23] This has been of significant benefit within the authors' experience and is reflected in the outcomes of the case studies described in this chapter.

In promoting collaboration between designers and health services researchers, it is important to note that, as with any interdisciplinary working, there may be several challenges. For example, most healthcare researchers and practitioners simply remain unfamiliar with human-centered design as a discipline and its potential role in improving delivery of healthcare.[49] This can lead to challenges in communicating the value of design approaches, establishing rapport with stakeholders, managing relations, and building understanding about the differing goals and expectations of each discipline.[37] The most fundamental tensions arise from differences in disciplinary culture including methods, values, and theoretical approaches.[50] These differences extend to what can or should be studied or known (epistemological differences) and what is valuable to study or do (axiological differences). Design research most commonly involves highly contextual inquiry, purposive and convenience sampling with small numbers of participants, and the flexible use of multiple qualitative and quantitative research tools and methods in ways that differ from those used in health services research.[37] Some academic researchers may initially find this approach alien and may inappropriately conflate difference in approach with limitations in rigor or quality. However, it is important to note that academic considerations such as relationships to previous research, reliability, or generalizability are not always the primary concern of design, which prioritizes users' needs in a specific context, validity, and utility. Additionally, formal academic research procedures such as research ethical approval are not usually well equipped to deal with participatory approaches, and design researchers may be unfamiliar with their role and feel that they are overly restrictive.[51,52] Taking the time to explore and understand these key differences and come to a shared vision for projects is important to meaningful collaboration and avoiding disciplinary-based misunderstandings.

As the potential for productive collaborations between designers and health services researchers has been demonstrated through successful projects, findings from studies that combine the two fields are increasingly being published in peer-reviewed medical/health, design, and specialist journals rather than remaining as gray literature.[53] As there has been significant variation in reporting, it may be challenging for health services researchers to access and interpret design research as applied to healthcare settings. The thoughtful, collaborative development of proposed reporting guidelines for health research involving design that respect the traditions of both health services research and design will lead to improved transparency and accessibility for those wishing to learn more.[53]

Conclusion

Pharmacy and health services research involving design has enormous potential to contribute to addressing the challenges set out in the recent call to action for pharmacy practice research in human-centered and innovative ways.[36] Designers are uniquely skilled in identifying and responding to user needs and bring a creative and innovative perspective that complements the evidence-based perspectives and conventional research methods of pharmacy and health services researchers. Through inclusive collaboration, researchers and designers can maximize the potential of interdisciplinary research to address complex challenges, enhance practice and deliver benefits for service users, patients, and health systems.

Questions for further discussion

1. From your reading of the chapter, comment on the statement: "Human-centered design methods should be used by pharmacy and health services researchers in their work."
2. How might pharmacy and health services researchers and design professionals overcome potential challenges of interdisciplinary working?
3. What concerns might research ethics boards familiar with reviewing traditional health services research projects have reviewing a human-centered design based project for the first time?

Application exercise/scenario

Identify an unresolved complex challenge in your research or clinical practice.

1. Which design specialty could help address this?
2. Which conventional and human-centered design methods(s) could you combine to address it?
3. What challenges would you predict and how might you overcome them?

Funding

This work was supported by a Fulbright Irish-US Scholar Award from the Fulbright Commission in Ireland (MF); and the Government of Ireland's Sláintecare Integration Fund 2019 under Grant Agreement Number 252.

References

1. Camillus JC. Strategy as a wicked problem. *Harv Bus Rev.* 2008;86:98.
2. McCreary L. Kaiser Permanente's innovation on the front lines. *Harv Bus Rev.* 2010;88:92–97.
3. Oliveira M, Zancul E, Fleury ALJBI. Design thinking as an approach for innovation in healthcare: systematic review and research avenues. *BMJ Innov.* 2021;7. https://doi.org/10.1136/bmjinnov-2020-000428.
4. Altman M, Huang TT, Breland JY. Design thinking in health care. *Prev Chronic Dis.* 2018;15. https://doi.org/10.5888/pcd15.180128.
5. Bazzano AN, Martin J, Hicks E, Faughnan M, Murphy L. Human-centred design in global health: a scoping review of applications and contexts. *PLoS One.* 2017;12:e0186744. https://doi.org/10.1371/journal.pone.0186744.
6. International Organization for Standardization. *ISO 9241–210:2010—Ergonomics of Human-System Interaction—Part 210: Human-Centred Design for Interactive Systems.* Geneva: International Organization for Standardization; 2010.
7. Giacomin J. What is human centred design? *Des J.* 2014;17:606–623. https://doi.org/10.2752/175630614X14056185480186.
8. Seidel VP, Fixson SK. Adopting design thinking in novice multidisciplinary teams: the application and limits of design methods and reflexive practices. *J Prod Innov Manag.* 2013;30:19–33. https://doi.org/10.1111/jpim.12061.
9. Design Council. *What Is the Framework for Innovation? Design Council's Evolved Double Diamond;* 2019. https://www.designcouncil.org.uk/news-opinion/what-framework-innovation-design-councils-evolved-double-diamond. Accessed 26 November 2020.
10. Brown T, Wyatt J. Design thinking for social innovation. *Stanf Soc Innov Rev.* 2010;12:29–43.
11. Standord d:school. *Design Thinking Bootleg;* 2018. https://dschool.stanford.edu/resources/design-thinking-bootleg. Accessed 26 November 2020.
12. Craig P, Dieppe P, Macintyre S, Michie S, Nazareth I, Petticrew M. Developing and evaluating complex interventions: the new Medical Research Council guidance. *BMJ.* 2013;337. https://doi.org/10.1136/bmj.a1655.
13. Sanders EB-N, Stappers PJ. Co-creation and the new landscapes of design. *CoDesign.* 2008;4:5–18.
14. McCarthy S, O'Raghallaigh P, Woodworth S, Lim YL, Kenny LC, Adam F. An integrated patient journey mapping tool for embedding quality in healthcare service reform. *J Decis Syst.* 2016;25:354–368. https://doi.org/10.1080/12460125.2016.1187394.
15. Trebble TM, Hansi N, Hydes T, Smith MA, Baker M. Process mapping the patient journey: an introduction. *BMJ.* 2010;341:c4078. https://doi.org/10.1136/bmj.c4078.

16. Stickdorn M, Hormess ME, Lawrence A, Schneider J. *This Is Service Design Doing: Applying Service Design Thinking in the Real World.* O'Reilly Media; 2018.

17. Percival J, McGregor C. An evaluation of understandability of patient journey models in mental health. *JMIR Hum Factors.* 2016;3:e20. https://doi.org/10.2196/humanfactors.5640.

18. McCarthy S, O'Raghallaigh P, Woodworth S, Lim YY, Kenny LC, Adam F. Embedding the pillars of quality in health information technology solutions using "integrated patient journey mapping" (IPJM): case study. *JMIR Hum Factors.* 2020;7:e17416. https://doi.org/10.2196/17416.

19. Bartlett R, Robinson T, Anand J, et al. Empathy and journey mapping the healthcare experience: a community-based participatory approach to exploring women's access to primary health services within Melbourne's Arabic-speaking refugee communities. *Ethn Health.* 2020;1–17. https://doi.org/10.1080/13557858.2020.1734780.

20. Valentine L, Kroll T, Bruce F, Lim C, Mountain R. Design thinking for social innovation in health care. *Des J.* 2017;20:755–774. https://doi.org/10.1080/14606925.2017.1372926.

21. Kolko JJDi. Abductive thinking and sensemaking: the drivers of design synthesis. *Des Issues.* 2010;26:15–28. https://doi.org/10.1162/desi.2010.26.1.15.

22. Zomerdijk LG, Voss C. Service design for experience-centric services. *J Serv Res.* 2010;13:67–82. https://doi.org/10.1177/1094670509351960.

23. Roberts JP, Fisher TR, Trowbridge MJ, Bent C. A design thinking framework for healthcare management and innovation. *Healthc (Amst).* 2016;4:11–14. https://doi.org/10.1016/j.hjdsi.2015.12.002.

24. Burke S, Barry S, Siersbaek R, Johnston B, Fhallúin MN, Thomas SJHP. Sláintecare—a ten-year plan to achieve universal healthcare in Ireland. *Health Policy.* 2018;122:1278–1282. https://doi.org/10.1016/j.healthpol.2018.05.006.

25. Health Services Executive. *Making Every Contact Count: A Health and Behaviour Change Framework and Implementation for Health Professionals in the Irish Health Service*; 2016. https://www.hse.ie/eng/about/who/healthwellbeing/making-every-contact-count/framework/. Accessed 26 November 2020.

26. Johnson M, Jackson R, Guillaume L, Meier P, Goyder E. Barriers and facilitators to implementing screening and brief intervention for alcohol misuse: a systematic review of qualitative evidence. *J Public Health.* 2011;33:412–421. https://doi.org/10.1093/pubmed/fdq095.

27. Sinclair D, Savage E, O'Brien M, et al. Developing a national undergraduate standardized curriculum for future healthcare professionals on "Making Every Contact Count" for chronic disease prevention in the Republic of Ireland. *J Interprof Care.* 2020;34:561–565. https://doi.org/10.1080/13561820.2019.1684884.

28. Tobacco Use and Dependence Guideline Panel. *Treating Tobacco Use and Dependence: 2008 Update.* Rockville, MD: US Department of Health and Human Services; 2008. https://www.ncbi.nlm.nih.gov/books/NBK63952/.

29. Sanders EB-N, Stappers PJ. Probes, toolkits and prototypes: three approaches to making in codesigning. *CoDesign.* 2014;10:5–14. https://doi.org/10.1080/15710882.2014.888183.

30. Eldridge SM, Lancaster GA, Campbell MJ, et al. Defining feasibility and pilot studies in preparation for randomised controlled trials: development of a conceptual framework. *PLoS One.* 2016;11:e0150205. https://doi.org/10.1371/journal.pone.0150205.

31. Crespo-Gonzalez C, Garcia-Cardenas V, Benrimoj SI. The next phase in professional services research: from implementation to sustainability. *Res Soc Adm Pharm.* 2017;13:896–901. https://doi.org/10.1016/j.sapharm.2017.05.020.

32. Brodersen C, Dindler C, Iversen OS. Staging imaginative places for participatory prototyping. *CoDesign.* 2008;4:19–30. https://doi.org/10.1080/15710880701875043.

33. Hanrahan BV, Yuan CW, Rosson MB, Beck J, Carroll JM. Materializing interactions with paper prototyping: a case study of designing social, collaborative systems with older adults. *Des Stud.* 2019;64:1–26. https://doi.org/10.1016/j.destud.2019.06.002.

34. Design Council. *Whittington Hospital Pharmacy. Prototyping Improves Patient Experience*; 2014. https://www.designcouncil.org.uk/resources/case-study/whittington-hospital-pharmacy. Accessed 26 November 2020.

35. Skivington K, Matthews L, Craig P, Simpson S, Moore L. Developing and evaluating complex interventions: updating Medical Research Council guidance to take account of new methodological and theoretical approaches. *Lancet.* 2018;392:S2. https://doi.org/10.1016/S0140-6736(18)32865-4.

36. Garcia-Cardenas V, Rossing CV, Fernandez-Llimos F, et al. Pharmacy practice research—a call to action. *Res Soc Adm Pharm.* 2020;16:1602–1608. https://doi.org/10.1016/j.sapharm.2020.07.031.

37. Groeneveld B, Dekkers T, Boon B, D'Olivo P. Challenges for design researchers in healthcare. *Des Health.* 2018;2:305–326. https://doi.org/10.1080/24735132.2018.1541699.

38. Walker S, Hignett S, Lim R, Parkhurst C, Samuel FJ. Explaining drug-resistant infection in community pharmacies through effective information design. *Des Health.* 2020;4:82–104. https://doi.org/10.1080/24735132.2020.1731201.

39. Ocloo J, Matthews R. From tokenism to empowerment: progressing patient and public involvement in healthcare improvement. *BMJ Qual Saf.* 2016;25:626–632. https://doi.org/10.1136/bmjqs-2016-005476.

40. Brett J, Staniszewska S, Mockford C, et al. A systematic review of the impact of patient and public involvement on service users, researchers and communities. *Patient.* 2014;7:387–395. https://doi.org/10.1007/s40271-014-0065-0.

41. Bate P, Robert G. Experience-based design: from redesigning the system around the patient to co-designing services with the patient. *BMJ Qual Saf.* 2006;15:307–310. https://doi.org/10.1136/qshc.2005.016527.

42. Ward ME, De Brún A, Beirne D, et al. Using co-design to develop a collective leadership intervention for healthcare teams to improve safety culture. *Int J Environ Res Public Health.* 2018;15:1182. https://doi.org/10.3390/ijerph15061182.

43. Beaudry J, Consigli A, Clark C, Robinson KJ. Getting ready for adult healthcare: designing a chatbot to coach adolescents with special health needs through the transitions of care. *J Pediatr Nurs.* 2019;49:85–91. https://doi.org/10.1016/j.pedn.2019.09.004.

44. Latif A, Gulzar N, Gohil S, Ansong T. Quality improvement in community pharmacy: a qualitative investigation of the impact of a postgraduate quality improvement educational module on pharmacists understanding and practice. *Int J Pharm Pract*. 2021;29:84–89. https://doi.org/10.1111/ijpp.12663.

45. Latif A, Gulzar N, Lowe F, Ansong T, Gohil SJBOQ. Engaging community pharmacists in quality improvement (QI): a qualitative case study of a partnership between a higher education institute and local pharmaceutical committees. *BMJ Qual Saf*. 2021;10:e001047. https://doi.org/10.1136/bmjoq-2020-001047.

46. Damschroder LJ, Aron DC, Keith RE, Kirsh SR, Alexander JA, Lowery JC. Fostering implementation of health services research findings into practice: a consolidated framework for advancing implementation science. *Implement Sci*. 2009;4:1–15. https://doi.org/10.1186/1748-5908-4-50.

47. Adam MB, Minyenya-Njuguna J, Karuri Kamiru W, et al. Implementation research and human-centred design: how theory driven human-centred design can sustain trust in complex health systems, support measurement and drive sustained community health volunteer engagement. *Health Policy Plan*. 2020;35:ii150–ii162. https://doi.org/10.1093/heapol/czaa129.

48. Manzini E. *Design, When Everybody Designs: An Introduction to Design for Social Innovation*. Cambridge, MA: MIT Press; 2015.

49. Wildevuur S. Could health learn from design? *Des Health*. 2017;1:59–64. https://doi.org/10.1080/24735132.2017.1295707.

50. Reay SD, Collier G, Douglas R, et al. Prototyping collaborative relationships between design and healthcare experts: mapping the patient journey. *Des Health*. 2017;1:65–79. https://doi.org/10.1080/24735132.2017.1294845.

51. Goodyear-Smith F, Jackson C, Greenhalgh T. Co-design and implementation research: challenges and solutions for ethics committees. *BMC Med Ethics*. 2015;16:1–5. https://doi.org/10.1186/s12910-015-0072-2.

52. Godbold R, Lees A, Reay S. Ethical challenges for student design projects in health care settings in New Zealand. *J Art Des Educ*. 2019;38:182–192. https://doi.org/10.1111/jade.12170.

53. Bazzano AN, Yan SD, Martin J, et al. Improving the reporting of health research involving design: a proposed guideline. *BMJ Glob Health*. 2020;5. https://doi.org/10.1136/bmjgh-2019-002248.

Section II

Emerging Methodological Approaches and Updates

Chapter 9

Applying action research in social pharmacy and health services research: An overview

Kritsanee Saramunee

Faculty of Pharmacy, Mahasarakham University, Maha Sarakham, Thailand

Objectives

- Define action research, and discuss differences among various types of action research.
- List and explain key characteristics and quality criteria of action research.
- Describe methods that can be used for data collection in a spiral process.
- Identify and discuss common limitations of using action research.
- Construct a report based upon the findings of an action research project.

Introduction

Quality pharmacy and health care services cannot always be guaranteed in real-world practice because these services are normally delivered in a complex environment,[1] such as multisteps process, workload and time pressure, and other constraints.[1,2] Mistakes and medication errors can occur anytime, which can harm the patient and eventually result in the failure in maintaining quality. Medication errors are caused by several factors, such as health care providers and patients (e.g., inadequate knowledge of medicines), patients (e.g., multiple health conditions), work environment (e.g., workload and time pressures), or even organizational barriers (e.g., insufficient resources for service delivery).[2] To ensure quality, health care professionals must give careful attention when providing services to adhere to clinical guidelines and medication-related regulations. Since health care professionals and pharmacists are obligated to maintain patient safety, they are required to reconsider and modify their work process in order to minimize errors and preserve the quality of health services.

Patient safety is defined as *"the prevention of errors and adverse effects to patients associated with health care."*[3] Situations related to patient safety have been widely reported in the literature, with medication errors being the leading cause of injury in health care systems.[4] Prevalence of medication errors range from 2% to 94%,[5] and their annual cost is estimated to be approximately US$ 42 billion worldwide.[6] Patient safety and medication errors are closely associated, and both affect the quality of health care.[3] Health care practitioners and managers therefore play a key role in preventing such errors to enhance quality of healthcare.

Like other health services, the quality of pharmacy services is essential for the healthcare system to enhance patient safety. Quality of care is the key to promoting the strengths of health services and improving patient health outcomes for people. To ensure quality health service, stakeholders need to recognize the following three aspects: effectiveness, safety, and patient-centered approach.[7] Ideally, quality health services must be timely managed, equitable, integrated with all levels of care, and delivered efficiently.[7] Therefore, pharmacists and other practitioners must consider all these factors to ensure quality has been achieved.

It has been suggested that quality improvement approaches need to be incorporated into daily practice of health practitioners,[7] including pharmacists and pharmacy managers.[8] The World Health Organization defines quality improvement as *"the action of every person working to implement iterative, measurable changes, to make health services more effective, safe and people-centered."*[2] This approach provides practitioners an opportunity to identify service delivery gaps and configure solutions fitting within the context. The idea of quality improvement in healthcare was brought from the manufacturing management discipline. It focuses on organizational management, teamwork, work processes, and systems

Contemporary Research Methods in Pharmacy and Health Services. https://doi.org/10.1016/B978-0-323-91888-6.00004-1

thinking.[1,8] These factors can lead to changes in organizational structure and/or behavior and work protocol, and thus help in achieving favorable outcomes. Several models have been proposed to be used in quality improvement, with the Deming's cycle widely used in healthcare.[8] Deming's cycle is a managerial tool composed of four cyclical steps: Plan-Do-Study-Act, also called the *"PDSA model."* It starts by identifying problems, deciding what changes should be made, designing measurements, and evaluating the impact of the implemented changes.[1] Noticeably, this management paradigm is similar to the *"action research" (AR) approach.*

AR is a research approach that can be applied for quality improvement in the healthcare setting.[9,10] AR can assist in solving problems regarding service delivery by bringing healthcare providers, users, researchers, and other stakeholders to meet, rethink, plan, and evaluate strategies for service improvement.[11] Therefore, it is believed that AR leads to service initiatives and practice changes. A spiral process for developing services (plan, act, observe, and reflect) is the backbone of AR methodology.[12,13] Additionally, AR can be applied to any organization of any size: from a single small department to a larger complex organization.[11] In pharmacy practice, pharmacy services need regular modification or adaptation according to new environments, such as implementation barriers, updated guidelines, or new interventions. Therefore, AR has been seen as an appropriate approach that can be applied to pharmacy service improvement because of its ability to identify context-specific characteristic and make changes in practice.[12,14]

Since AR uses multiple methods, including a cyclical process, confusion may arise among practicing pharmacists, health care practitioners and novice researchers interested in using AR. Moreover, details about conducting AR in pharmacy practice and health services research are still scarce. Therefore, this chapter aims to describe key information about AR, including its definition, a brief history, spiral process and research methods used for data collection, key characteristics, and common limitations to help readers understand the AR approach.

Brief history

AR originated from several socialists and educational academics in the 1920s. Hart and Bond mentioned that AR was introduced in 1926 in the book titled, "Research for teachers" by Buckingham.[9] Master listed a few social reformists who used AR during the 1940–50s.[15] However, the AR concept proposed by Kurt Lewin, an American psychologist, is widely recognized as the origin of AR.[11] Lewin published a seminal paper titled "Action Research for Health and Social Care" explaining the way to figure methods for solving intergroup relations among minorities.[16] Lewin proposed that AR (referred to as rational social management) proceeds in a circle of planning, action, and fact-finding about the result of the action.[16] Later in 1986, Carr and Kemmis, highlighted two other components of AR in addition to Lewin's concept: The first is to give a group decision-making as a priority and the second is to carry a democratic approach.[11,17] This means that participants can influence decision-making based on their own circumstances related to work and life. Therefore, AR emphasizes raising awareness and empowers researchers and practitioners to work collaboratively.[11] A timeline showing major events of AR history is shown in Fig. 1.

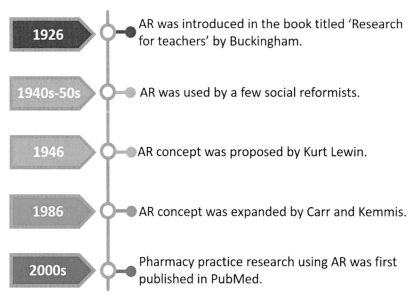

1926 — AR was introduced in the book titled 'Research for teachers' by Buckingham.

1940s-50s — AR was used by a few social reformists.

1946 — AR concept was proposed by Kurt Lewin.

1986 — AR concept was expanded by Carr and Kemmis.

2000s — Pharmacy practice research using AR was first published in PubMed.

FIG. 1 A timeline showing major events of action research history.

So far, AR has been applied in many disciplines such as organizational management, community development, education, and nursing.[11] In case of organizational issues, AR has been used to solve various industrial problems: industrial conflict, absenteeism, and intergroup relations. AR in community development emphasizes on diminishing poverty problems for people, and is conducted collaboratively by researchers and community workers. In education, AR is well-established, teachers and researchers have come together to observe school problems and refine teaching methods. Nursing research used AR to analyze and solve problems regarding nursing care and to devise an action plan to improve standard nursing practice.[11]

Clearly, AR has been widely applied in many disciplines,[11,13] but what about pharmacy practice? A quick literature search in PubMed using the two search terms ("action research") AND (pharmac*), revealed 13 AR articles (out of 140 results published until October 23, 2020) relevant to pharmacy practice. The mention of AR in pharmacy practice research commenced in the 2000s. In one of the two articles published in 2002, Gilberts and colleagues reported the use of a participatory AR to design a collaborative model for delivering and evaluating home medication reviews in Australia.[18] In the other, Haugbølle and colleagues from Denmark reported the use of AR to improve counseling practices for angina pectoris patients in community pharmacies.[19] According to the identified publications during the previous decades, researchers mainly used AR for developing or improving pharmacy services on the following topics: community pharmacy services,[19–21] home medication reviews,[18] medication management,[22,23] pharmacist roles in primary care,[24,25] regional collaborative service for benzodiazepine use,[26] medication safety behavior[27] and pharmacy education.[28] In addition, two commentary papers described the utilization and recommendations for conducting AR in pharmacy.[9,14] This preliminary search demonstrated an recent interest in AR among pharmacy practice researchers.

Definition

AR has been defined by several social scientists from various disciplines. Originally in social research, Lewin described AR as *"a comparative research on the conditions and effects of various forms of social action, and research leading to social action."* Lewin suggested that AR usually proceeds in spiral steps, composed of a circle of planning, action, and fact-finding about the result of the action.[16] Hart and Bond defined AR in health and social care as a research method in which *"problems are formulated and solutions are sought depending on the particular configurations of power and vested interests within a particular policy context."*[11] Waterman and colleagues conducted a systematic review and explained AR in health research as *"a period of inquiry that describes, interprets, and explains social situations while executing a change intervention aimed at improvement and involvement."*[13] AR has been founded on a partnership between action researchers and participants who are involved in the change process. It uses a dynamic approach that includes problem identification, planning, action, and evaluation.[13] Carr and Kemmis explained AR in education research as *"a form of self-reflective enquiry undertaken by participants in social situations in order to improve the rationality and justice of their own practices, their understanding of these practices, and the situations in which the practices are carried out."*[17] The authors added that AR often involves participants taking part in decision-making on work development. The AR spiral process proposed by Carr and Kemmis encompasses four steps: planning, acting, observing, and reflecting,[17] and has been cited widely.[13] In pharmacy practice, Nørgaard and Sørensen explained that AR is a research approach focusing on problem-solving through cooperation between researchers and related stakeholders.[12] AR aims at both solving a problem and generating new knowledge that leads to organizational changes. Significant characteristics include an organizational approach (context-specific), focus on the process and learning, and cooperation between researchers and practitioners.[12]

Based on these definitions of AR, it can be surmised that AR is a research approach that emphasizes solving problems related to practice or organizational issues. Researchers and practitioners work together to define problems and design solutions and methods for measuring outcomes and changes. AR involves several cyclical processes, normally each process divided in four steps: plan, act, observe, and reflect.[13,20,29] Researchers and practitioners are allowed to adjust the work solution (intervention) if the implementation of such a solution is found difficult to implement in practice. Additionally, researchers and practitioners can learn key factors from any failure and success that might occur in the meantime.

Regarding the use of specific terminology, this chapter will consistently use the terms practitioners and solutions, which may differ from other references. Practitioners are similar to clients or stakeholders, i.e., persons who work or are involved in the action research study setting. Solutions are referred to as work protocols, interventions or strategies, i.e., possible ways or methods to tackle identified problems.

Types of action research

Four types of AR have been proposed by Hart and Bond, namely, experimental, organizational, professionalizing, and empowering.[11] The *experimental type* is closely associated with the AR characterized by Lewin's experiment that

TABLE 1 Types of AR and their distinguished characteristics.

| | Research/outcome-focused ↔ Process-focused | | | |
| | Types of AR | | | |
Distinguished characteristics	Experimental	Organizational	Professionalizing	Empowering/ emancipatory
Educative base	Enhance social science, administrative control, and social change toward consensus	Enhance managerial control and organizational change toward consensus	Enhance professional control and individual's ability to control work situation	Enhance user-control and shifting balance of power; structural change toward pluralism
Focus	Researcher focused	Client focused	Practitioner focused	User/practitioner focused
Problem focus	Problems emerge from the interaction of social science/management interest	Problem defined by most powerful group and some workers	Problems emerge from professional practice and experience	Problems emerge from members' practice and experience
Change intervention	Experimental intervention to test theory	Top-down, directed change toward predetermined aims	Predefined, professional, process-led	Bottom-up, undetermined, process-led
Degree of collaboration between researcher and participants	Differentiated roles Outside researcher as an expert	Differentiated roles Client as a consultant work with researchers	Merged roles Practitioners and researchers as collaborators	Shared roles User and practitioners as coresearchers and cochange agent

Note: This table is summarized from Hart and Bond's handbook.[11]

discovered solutions for solving intergroup relations among minorities. The *organizational type* focuses on organizational problem-solving such as restriction of output, resistance to change practice/behavior, work relationship and absenteeism. The *professionalizing type* is informed by professional groups which intend to reflect current practice and enhance new professional roles. The *empowering type* is most closely associated with community development, appropriate when an explicit antioppressive stance or working with vulnerable groups in society. Table 1 illustrates the distinguished characteristics of each AR type, which can be read from left to right as representing a shift from a scientific approach (research- or practice-focused) to empowering social change (process-focused).

However, there is no single model that differentiates AR types.[30] Apart from the above typology, Hart and Bond also noted that other writers had classified them by using various terms; nonetheless, its core concepts are overlapped. For example, social scientists differentiate AR into several types: experimental, empirical, diagnostic, participative, and political.[11] While in nursing, it has been broken down into three approaches: technical collaborative, mutual collaboration, and enhancement.[11] Therefore, researchers should learn the concept of each AR type and realize the goal of their project before choosing the approach to use. Participatory action research (PAR) is another form of AR and frequently mentioned in pharmacy practice. PAR has been developed from sociology which aims to make a change in a social situation.[31,32] Van Buul and colleagues described that the change could be either improving practice or creating knowledge and theory.[33] Despite AR and PAR developed by the same paradigm, the level of participation seems slightly different.[12,31] In AR, although researchers and practitioners have to work collaboratively, the researcher might have a primary role in leading the group to identify the solution but does not necessarily engage in this solution. PAR requires researchers and practitioners to be engaged throughout the research process.[31]

Spiral process and research methods used for data collection

AR is a multiple-phase research approach in which an AR spiral is the core concept for researchers to follow. AR does not have its own methodology; but rather, it utilizes various research methods commonly used in pharmacy practice. Spiral (or cyclical) process is a pivotal characteristic of AR approach, initially mentioned by Lewin,[16] which means "*a continuously spreading and accelerating increase or decrease.*"[34] The spiral character has been given to AR approach as it is performed by four steps—plan, act, observe, and reflect. Following this approach for multiple rounds is believed to help improve health practice or service continuously—just like when the spiral spins. This section describes the objective of each step and suggests the research methods used for data collection. A summary of each spiral process is presented in Table 2; however, this spiral should be rotated several times (Fig. 2) to improve services and lead to change.

Planning. Planning is the step for finding facts or phenomena relevant to service quality. This step allows researchers and practitioners to explore the organizational context, identify problems, and propose possible solutions to tackle the identified problem. Various exploratory methods can be used simultaneously in this step.[13,32] Organizational context, client work experience, and perspective can be observed using a qualitative approach, such as observation, interview, working group meeting, and focus group. However, a quantitative method such as a survey can also be used if perspective from larger samples is deemed necessary. Evidence of work-related documents can be also reviewed to identify, for example, possible medication-related errors. These can include field notes, daily logs, work documents, and relevant databases. Data obtained from these multiple sources are used to identify pharmacy services-related problems, which can be brought over to the meeting with research partners for discussion and designation of possible solutions. The solution might be a new or modified work protocol or pharmacy intervention. Impacts of intervention should also be discussed in this meeting, especially regarding methods and indicators used for tracing outcomes. The following examples are action studies that use various methods for planning. Dollman and colleagues designed multiple strategies to reduce benzodiazepine use in

TABLE 2 Description of spiral process and methods used for data collection.

Spiral process	Description	Methods used for data collection
Planning	To explore organizational context, identify problems, and propose possible solutions to tackle the identified problem relevant to service quality	**Identify problem** *Qualitative methods*—observation, interview, working group meeting, and focus group *Quantitative methods*—survey *Review of work evidence*—field notes, daily logs, work documents, and relevant database **Design solution and outcome measurement** Steering group meeting
Action	To implement the proposed solution	**Kick off the solution** Agreement made by the steering group Official support from local health board/committee to help stimulate engagement from practitioners **Enhance understanding of practitioners** Training and workshop to ensure understanding among practitioners **Increase awareness of relevant stakeholders** *Advertising*—local newspaper, radio, poster
Observation	To monitor and measure the effects of the proposed protocol or intervention	**Observe practicability of the solution** Interview relevant practitioners and working group meeting **Measure effects of the solution** Monitor key outcomes—Review of patient medication; Review of drug related problems Survey satisfaction, opinion, knowledge of practitioners and patients. Pre- and postsolution comparison is also possible
Reflection	To obtain feedback and identify what practitioners have learned (learning) from being involved in the proposed solution and how it can change them in providing this service	Reflect can be done throughout the project or in the reflection step **Throughout the project** Individual interview Review of evidence-working group meetings, notes, and reflective diaries **In the reflection step** Steering group meeting

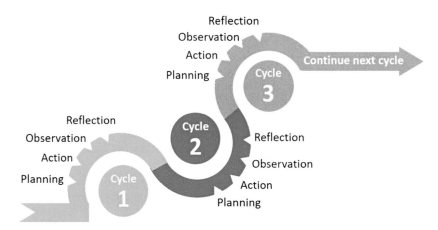

FIG. 2 Spiral process.

insomnia.[26] Methods used for gathering data before planning strategies included focus group, group meetings, interviews, and forums with various stakeholders.[26] Bakhshi and colleagues intended to develop medication safety behaviors among emergency staff.[27] The authors surveyed medication safety behaviors among medical and nursing staff as an initial phase, then held a working group meeting to identify problems and to plan possible strategies for enhancing good behavior to maintain patient safety.[27] Seeha and Saramunee developed a care process to enhance safety for warfarin patients in primary care.[35] Methods used before planning the care process included interviewing relevant stakeholders, retrospective review of patient medication records, and assessment of warfarin knowledge among primary care prescribers.[35]

Action. Action is the step for implementing the solution that has been agreed upon in the planning step. Training or workshops are often held prior to launching the solution. This strategy ensures that all practitioners understand the solution, particularly when the solution is complex. The methods used for implementation depend on the context of the study setting. Previously, two studies used an agreement of the steering group before proceeding with the solution,[20,27] while two other studies had official support from the local health board to help stimulate engagement from relevant practitioners to adhere to the proposed protocol.[18,35] Dollman and colleagues used advertising techniques (local newspaper, radio, poster) to promote interventions to increase awareness among relevant partners.[26]

Observation. Observation is a way to monitor and measure the effects or changes of the proposed solution. Researchers might select potential outcome indicators and relevant measurement methods to assess the impact of the solution. Applying quality improvement models in health care might be useful to design comprehensive indicators for measuring changes of interventions. For example, if researchers use Donabedian's model, they might propose some indicators that reflect process, structure, and outcome of care.[36] However, these indicators should have been considered by researchers and practitioners from the planning step onward. Observation can be undertaken in two alternatives, whether to follow the practicality of the solution or to measure its effects. Examples of indicators are key clinical outcomes, drug-related problems, stakeholder satisfaction, and practitioner behaviors that impact patients. Once the indicators have been set, tools and methods for data collection can be designed. Interviews with relevant practitioners and working group meetings are often used to observe the solution practicability. Elliott and colleagues observed qualitative data from various stakeholders to identify the applicability of the clinical pharmacy model in home nursing services, such as meeting minutes, notes, reflective diaries, interviews, and focus groups.[22] Descriptive research is frequently used to monitor effects of the solution, such as review of patient medication, survey of satisfaction, opinion, and knowledge. Moreover, if preferred, data can be collected in the preimplementation phase to perform a comparative analysis between pre and post action. Bakhshi and colleagues employed pre- and postintervention surveys to identify changes in medication safety behaviors among nursing and medical staff after the implementation of the intervention.[27]

Reflection. Reflection is the step to obtain feedback and identify what practitioners have learned (learning) from involvement in the proposed solution and how this involvement can change them (practitioners) in providing this service. Reflection can be traced and extracted by various pieces of evidence, such as working group meetings, notes, and reflective diaries. Researchers can also employ an independent interview with practitioners to share their learning experiences. A study by Blondal and colleagues used in-depth interviews, meetings, and research notes to collect data for evaluation and reflection among general practitioners of introducing pharmaceutical care in primary care.[37] Researchers can hold a group meeting to present findings from the observation step and ask practitioners to exchange their learning experiences. Learning may be reported with respect to many aspects, such as attitude, concern, and behavior. Irrespective of whether positive or negative effects are observed, it is believed that learning can lead to a change in routine practice.

Box 1 AR process and research methods used, learned from Blondal and colleagues' study.[36]

Title	Introducing pharmaceutical care to primary care in Iceland—an action research study	
Setting	Primary care clinic	
Participants	5 GPs and 125 patients received pharmaceutical care	
Cycle 1	**Goal**	**Methods used**
Planning 1	Understanding GPs' perspectives	In-depth interviews with GP
	Design the pharmaceutical care intervention	Group meeting with GP
Action 1	Participating researchers provided the designed intervention to involved patients	—
Observation 1	Obtain GPs' views about the designed intervention	In-depth interviews with GPs
Reflection 1	Summarize views of GPs toward the designed intervention and identify what should be improved	Data analysis from interviews and research notes
Cycle 2	**Goal**	**Methods used**
Planning 2	Find common ground to revise pharmaceutical care intervention	Group meeting with GPs
Action 2	Participating researchers provided the revised intervention to involved patients	—
Observation 2	Obtain GPs' views about the revised intervention	In-depth interviews with GPs
Reflection 2	Summarize views of GPs from interviews and research notes to identify what should be improved	Data analysis from interviews and research notes

---

To understand the AR process, the reader can refer to previously published studies. One good example is the AR work by Blondal and colleagues,[37] who used the AR approach to promote a pharmaceutical care service in Iceland. The researchers expected to gain more willingness to accept such a service among general practitioners (GPs). Two AR cycles were performed using in-depth interviews, group meetings, and research notes for data collection. In the beginning, the involved GPs had little knowledge about pharmacist clinical roles. They (GPs) thought that the pharmacists emphasized only medicines but not the patients. After involvement in this AR project, GPs acknowledged the usefulness of pharmaceutical care to clinical decision-making, especially management of medicine-related issues. GPs eventually agreed for the pharmacists to work at the primary care clinic as a part of the healthcare team. Box 1 shows the process and methods used in each spiral step.

Key characteristics

There are several points which the researchers need to consider when conducting AR, including partnership and participation, spiral process, and learning.

Partnership and participation

Research-practitioner partnership and participation are compulsory in AR. Since improving pharmacy services for a particular setting is context-oriented. Nørgaard and Sørensen recommended to gain the involvement of practitioners as soon as the research aim and questions are initiated.[12] Partnership and participation must be continued throughout the project; therefore, researchers and practitioners need to work and make decisions together in each step of the project. Collaborative researcher-practitioner work is driven on a democratic basis. If a well-designed solution is implemented but is difficult to apply in the study setting, then it needs to be reconsidered. It is important that researchers listen to practitioners' opinions and vice versa.

Spiral process

Being dynamic is an extraordinary characteristic of AR. The spiral process is an important core of this research approach that shows the movement of the development process during the research period.[12,13,17] It is necessary for action researchers to demonstrate their cycle of data collection to help readers understand how the solution is planned, implemented, and evaluated. However, sometimes it is difficult to adhere to the spiral process when reporting AR methodology and findings because the data from each step may be iterative and interlinked. Therefore, the pattern to present AR reports is not strictly fixed. Nonetheless, the spiral process should be reproduced and clearly seen. Another issue regarding the spiral process is how many loops of the spiral process are appropriate. Carr and Kemmis noted that a single cycle of the spiral process is called "arrested action research," which may be less likely to be regarded as AR. A single cycle AR is used only in the beginning of service development as a pilot study and might be able to solve only the problem, while the service may not be improved or the best solution may not be identified.[17] Ideally, several cycles are preferred, and thus a long timeframe is required for AR projects.[12] This may cause anxiety among investigators in a time-limited project, such as a Master's thesis. However, from the author's view, a single cycle AR seems possible and publishable as long as the key components of AR are comprehensively demonstrated.

Learning

Learning is a valuable asset that emerged in AR, and Waterman and colleagues termed this as "knowledge."[13] This signifies the tenets or experiences that AR partners gain from being involved in the AR project. Learning can be in various forms such as knowledge, skills, awareness, and behaviors that appear during the AR process. The advantages and disadvantages of the proposed solution are also counted as learning. Reflection is a way to extract learning,[12] which may be formally conducted in the reflect step or informally observed throughout the AR project. Learning encourages researchers and practitioners to understand the reasons underpinning success and failure, which will be used to redesign the solution and contribute to theory and other settings.

Quality criteria

Apart from the above characteristics, other criteria are also recommended to enhance AR quality: articulation of objective, partnership and participation, contribution to theory-practice, appropriate methods and process, actionability, reflexivity, and significance.[38] These criteria are considered for publication in the Journal of Action Research, which are described below:

1. *Articulation of objective*. AR should explicitly address its objectives.[38]
2. *Partnership and participation*. As mentioned in the key characteristics, AR should reflect participative characteristics by exhibiting collaboration between researchers and practitioners or clearly describing how the researcher-practitioner partnership has been established.[38]
3. *Contribution to action research theory-practice*. AR should create explicit links with or contribute to a broader body of practice knowledge and theory. Researchers should demonstrate the learning points gained from the project that can help narrow the theory-practice gap.[38]
4. *Appropriate methods and process*. AR process and methods should be clearly articulated and illustrated. Bradbury suggested that the AR paper must show the process of conducting AR and data analysis, including the participants' voices in the research.[38]
5. *Actionability*. Actionability (taking action) means the AR provides new ideas that guide action in response to need. Researchers should implement a new action, designed from new ideas, to build a positive impact.[38]
6. *Reflexivity*. Reflexivity (self-reflection)[31] means that action researchers are aware of their roles and context of the study. Consequently, they can reflect on how this awareness influences the situations of the AR project.[38]
7. *Significance*. Significance refers to ensure that the insights of action research are essential for the practice and wider community.[38]

Common limitations

Despite AR being accepted as a viable approach to empowering change, the context-specific and special characteristics of AR may result in some limitations.[12,13,39] First, findings from AR are useful only for a study setting, and thus generalizability may be limited by this research approach. However, transferability may still exist because lessons learned for delivering such services can be disseminated to others to learn.[29,39] Second, partnership and participation may somehow contribute to reluctance among action researchers. For example, if the researchers (as compared to the participants) have been dominating the project, this may lead to bias. Oppositely, if the practitioners have had greater input, the decision-making might be made based on work experience rather than scientific justification. Therefore, action researchers need to compromise, balance between theory and practice, and find the common ground among the working group. Third, ethical concerns might arise when AR is conducted by insider researcher, or called "insider AR." An insider has a role duality dealing with their own responsibilities in work, organizational politics, past and present relationships with coworkers, and ensuring research quality. These factors might interfere participant's willingness to join the project.[39] Therefore, freedom to accept or decline involvement in the research must be ensured.[40] Fourth, since the goal of AR is to find strategies to change practice that can improve pharmacy service quality, it is a long-run process. It is often difficult to predict the process and outcomes of AR; as such, the project timeline and budget are sometimes poorly estimated.[39] Fifth, involved key person could either facilitate or contribute negative impact on AR.[13] For example, a pharmacy manager would support it if they agreed with the project but might ignore it if they disagreed. In this case, Nørgaard and Sørensen recommended that the AR researcher should understand the organizational structure of the study setting, such as organizational leadership, work protocol, and staff competencies, then leverage these resources to support the project.[12] In spite of these limitations, a thorough understanding of the AR approach can minimize problems and be used to actuate effective projects.[41]

Recommendations to pharmacy practice and health service research

Pharmacy practice and health service research is an area of health discipline that normally deals with medication-related problems, which is influenced by multiple factors: patients, providers, and organizational culture. Medication-related mistakes and errors occur anytime during the pharmacy service provision and healthcare delivery. These errors can lead to degradation of the quality of services; and hence must be prevented. Previously, pharmaceutical or health interventions have been commonly designed from previous literature and theory, but impractical issues have been frequently detected—the so-called theory-practice gap in which AR has the ability to bridge this space. Pharmacists and health providers can choose to use AR to identify innovative pharmacy services or health interventions or devise solutions to improve the quality of health care. It can be applied in any setting, either hospital, community pharmacy, or primary care. Regarding AR implications, it is possible to apply AR in pharmacy practice and health service research in the same way as suggestions for use in healthcare practice[8] including monitoring the effectiveness of new interventions and policies, developing strategies that increase understanding among practitioners of new services, and improving awareness of poor-uptake pharmacy or health interventions and services. Moreover, AR can be used in combination with other methods. For example, researchers may use AR to develop an appropriate intervention before conducting a randomized controlled trial (RCT). Or, the researcher might start with an RCT to test effectiveness of the solution then follow by a professionalizing AR phase with practitioners to evaluate findings from the angle of practitioners.[11] Additional tips for conducting AR have been offered: begin the project at the right time (right for both research team and study site); compromise (something might be important to us but not to the others); identify motivation factors (i.e., what makes participants engaged and what does not); disseminate results through various platforms to share lessons learned from their experiences.[14,20,29]

Writing an action research report

Because of the spiral process and its repetitiveness, writing an AR report is a complex and challenging task. AR reports can be written in various styles, depending on the focus of such a project. For example, studies that attempted to improve pharmaceutical intervention in primary care, such as Blondal and colleagues,[37] Seeha and Saramunee,[35] described the methods and results following the AR spiral. Whereas Kolodziejak and colleagues provided thorough details of the guide for integrating a pharmacist into an established primary healthcare team.[25] Regarding the variety of AR reporting styles, Winter and Munn-Giddings recommended that the AR report should probably follow this sequence[42]:

1. *A brief statement of problem.* This component is required similarly to writing other types of research, justification underpinning the AR work should be described clearly.
2. *Background.* This component includes a description of the context, roles of participants, and the relevant literature which defines the current understanding of the problem.
3. *An explanation of the AR approach.* This component includes a general description of the AR concept and how it is appropriate to the project.
4. *A sequence of activities undertaken.* As mentioned in the spiral process, the pattern to present AR reports is not strictly fixed. However, at least, the spiral process should be traced and seen. Therefore, describing activities undertaken in AR should follow the spiral step.
5. *Data and data analysis.* It is suggested that examples of the data collected at different times should be given and detailed how to analyze them.
6. *A description of changes and evaluation.* Change is the goal of AR; it is important to describe what change observed during and after the project. Also, methods used for evaluating change should be enacted.
7. *Conclusions.* Conclusions should indicate whether there is any change (worse, no change, or improved) compared to the prestage of the AR intervention. Learnings should also be mentioned, particularly relevant findings. Finally, the conclusion should suggest what further research is required.

Summary

Pharmacy and health services researchers have demonstrated recent interest in using AR, considering its usefulness in improving quality of services provision. This research approach is systematic, dynamic, and complex, and can contribute new knowledge to practice. The spiral process is the backbone of AR that basically comprises four steps to be followed by the researchers: plan, act, observe, and reflect. Three special characteristics that distinguish AR from other research approaches include partnership and participation, spiral process, and learning. AR can be used in various pharmacy settings and can address various pharmacy related issues.

Questions for further discussion

1. Describe the similarities and differences between the four types of AR. Which types of AR do you think are mainly used in pharmacy practice?
2. Building research-practitioner partnership and participation in AR projects is challenging; what technique/strategies would you consider using to begin and continue this characteristic of AR?
3. What would you do if the intervention used in your AR project had unchanged the outcomes?
4. Locate an AR study published in a peer-reviewed journal. Identify the spiral process used in this study (as done in Box 1). Also, describe and discuss whether or not it has been conducted appropriately.

Application exercise/scenario

Imagine you are a full-time pharmacist working with three nonphysician practitioners in a primary care center. The primary care center, located close to the community, is a place where essential health services are provided to local people. Nonphysician practitioners include one registered nurse and two public health practitioners, they have already been trained to prescribe medicine for primary care. Generally, the primary care center is allowed to store approximately 150 drug items for potential use by patients. You (as the pharmacist) have kept recording medication errors (ME) for 3 months and have found that the number of such events has been rising. ME examples are such as:

- Diclofenac was prescribed to warfarin patients to help relieve his/her muscle pain.
- Amoxicillin dosing was incorrect for a child patient.
- Paracetamol was prescribed to a paracetamol-allergic patient.

As you recognize the importance of patient safety and quality of health care, you would like to start your own research to solve this problem. Would you consider using AR approach? Why or why not? How would you design this research project?

Acknowledgment

Author would like to thank Editage (www.editage.com) for English language editing.

References

1. Ronda H. Tools for quality improvement and patient safety. In: Hughes RG, ed. *Patient Safety and Quality: An Evidence-Based Handbook for Nurses.* Agency for Healthcare Research and Quality; 2008.
2. World Health Organization. *Medication Errors.* World Health Organization; 2016.
3. World Health Organization Regional Office for Europe. *Patient Safety.* https://www.euro.who.int/en/health-topics/Health-systems/patient-safety/patient-safety. Accessed 28 April 2021.
4. World Health Organization. *Patient Safety.* https://www.who.int/news-room/fact-sheets/detail/patient-safety. Accessed 28 April 2021.
5. Assiri GA, Shebl NA, Mahmoud MA, et al. What is the epidemiology of medication errors, error-related adverse events and risk factors for errors in adults managed in community care contexts? A systematic review of the international literature. *BMJ Open.* 2018;8(5). https://doi.org/10.1136/bmjopen-2017-019101.
6. IMS Institute for Healthcare Informatics. *Advancing the Responsible Use of Medicines: Applying Levers for Change*; 2012.
7. World Health Organization. *Improving the Quality of Health Services—Tools and Resources.* World Health Organization; 2018.
8. Bain A, Fowler D. Quality improvement methods in pharmacy practice research. In: Babar ZUD, ed. *Pharmacy Practice Research Methods.* Springer; 2020:75–91.
9. Tanna NK. Action research: a valuable research technique for service delivery development. *Pharm World Sci.* 2005;27(1):4–6.
10. Chenoweth L, Luck K. Quality improvement in discharge planning through action research. *Outcomes Manag.* 2003;7(2):68–73.
11. Hart E, Bond M. *Action Research for Health and Social Care: A Guide to Practice.* Open University Press; 1995.

12. Nørgaard LS, Sørensen EW. Action research in pharmacy practice. In: Babar Z-U-D, ed. *Pharmacy Practice Research Methods*. Springer International Publishing; 2015:69–90.

13. Waterman HA, Tillen D, Dickson R, de Koning K. Action research: a systematic review and guidance for assessment. *Health Technol Assess.* 2001;5(23):1–165. https://doi.org/10.1177/1524839914527591.

14. Nørgaard LS, Sørensen EW. Action research methodology in clinical pharmacy: how to involve and change. *Int J Clin Pharm.* 2016;38 (3):739–745. https://doi.org/10.1007/s11096-016-0310-9.

15. Masters J. The history of action research. In: Hughes I, ed. *Action Research Electronic Reader.* The University of Sydney; 1995. http://www.behs.cchs.usyd.edu.au/arow/Reader/rmasters.htm.

16. Lewin K. Action research and minority problems. *J Soc Issues.* 1946;2:34–46.

17. Carr W, Kemmis S. *Becoming Crititcal: Education, Knowledge and Action Research.* Taylor & Francis e-Library; 2004.

18. Gilbert AL, Roughead EE, Beilby J, Mott K, Barratt JD. Collaborative medication management services: improving patient care. *Med J Aust.* 2002;177(4):189–192.

19. Haugbølle LS, Sørensen EW, Gundersen B, Petersen KH, Lorentzen L. Basing pharmacy counselling on the perspective of the angina pectoris patient. *Pharm World Sci.* 2002;24(2):71–78. https://doi.org/10.1023/a:1015575731203.

20. Sørensen EW, Haugbølle LS. Using an action research process in pharmacy practice research—a cooperative project between university and internship pharmacies. *Res Soc Adm Pharm.* 2008;4(4):384–401. https://doi.org/10.1016/j.sapharm.2007.10.005.

21. Fonseca J, Violette R, Houle SK, Dolovich L, McCarthy LM, Waite NM. Helping unlock better care (HUB|C) using quality improvement science in community pharmacies—an implementation method. *Res Soc Adm Pharm.* 2020. https://doi.org/10.1016/j.sapharm.2020.05.006.

22. Elliott RA, Lee CY, Beanland C, et al. Development of a clinical pharmacy model within an Australian home nursing service using co-creation and participatory action research: the visiting pharmacist (ViP) study. *BMJ Open.* 2017;7(11):e018722. https://doi.org/10.1136/bmjopen-2017-018722.

23. Alagiakrishnan K, Wilson P, Sadowski CA, et al. Physicians' use of computerized clinical decision supports to improve medication management in the elderly—the seniors medication alert and review technology intervention. *Clin Interv Aging.* 2016;11:73–81. https://doi.org/10.2147/CIA.S94126.

24. Ramli AS, Selvarajah S, Daud MH, et al. Effectiveness of the EMPOWER-PAR intervention in improving clinical outcomes of type 2 diabetes mellitus in primary care: a pragmatic cluster randomised controlled trial. *BMC Fam Pract.* 2016;17(1):157. https://doi.org/10.1186/s12875-016-0557-1.

25. Kolodziejak L, Rémillard A, Neubauer S. Integration of a primary healthcare pharmacist. *J Interprof Care.* 2010;24(3):274–284. https://doi.org/10.3109/13561820903130149.

26. Dollman WB, Leblanc VT, Stevens L, O'Connor PJ, Roughead EE, Gilbert AL. Achieving a sustained reduction in benzodiazepine use through implementation of an area-wide multi-strategic approach. *J Clin Pharm Ther.* 2005;30(5):425–432. https://doi.org/10.1111/j.1365-2710.2005.00674.x.

27. Bakhshi F, Mitchell R, Nasrabadi AN, Varaei S, Hajimaghsoudi M. Behavioural changes in medication safety: consequent to an action research intervention. *J Nurs Manag.* 2020. https://doi.org/10.1111/jonm.13128.

28. Stupans I, McAllister S, Clifford R, et al. Nationwide collaborative development of learning outcomes and exemplar standards for Australian pharmacy programmes. *Int J Pharm Pract.* 2015;23(4):283–291. https://doi.org/10.1111/ijpp.12163.

29. Nørgaard LS, Sørensen EW. Action research in pharmacy practice. In: Babar ZUD, ed. *Pharmacy Practice Research Methods.* 2nd ed. Springer; 2020:55–73.

30. Hockley J, Stacpoole M. The use of action research healthcare research. *Eur J Palliat Care.* 2014;21(3):110–114.

31. Bradley H. Participatory action research in pharmacy practice. In: Babar ZUD, ed. *Pharmacy Practice Research Methods.* Springer International Publishing; 2015.

32. Mctaggart R. Principles for participatory action research. *Adult Educ Q.* 1991;41(3):168–187. https://doi.org/10.1177/0001848191041003003.

33. Van Buul LW, Sikkens JJ, Van Agtmael MA, Kramer MHH, Van der Steen JT, Hertogh CMPM. Participatory action research in antimicrobial stewardship: a novel approach to improving antimicrobial prescribing in hospitals and long-term care facilities. *J Antimicrob Chemother.* 2014;69(7):1734–1741. https://doi.org/10.1093/jac/dku068.

34. Merriam-Webster Dictionary. *Spiral Definitions.* https://www.merriam-webster.com/dictionary/spiral?src=search-dict-box. Accessed 13 September 2021.

35. Seeha A, Saramunee K. Development of a care process at sub-district health promotion hospitals in Kamalasai health district to enhance safety for warfarin patient. *Isan J Pharm Sci.* 2019;15(4):37–49.

36. Shroyer ALW, Carr BM, Grover FL. Data and measures in health services research. Springer science+business. *Media.* 2016. https://doi.org/10.1007/978-1-4899-7673-4.

37. Blondal A, Sporrong S, Almarsdottir A. Introducing pharmaceutical care to primary care in Iceland—an action research study. *Pharmacy.* 2017;5(4):23. https://doi.org/10.3390/pharmacy5020023.

38. Bradbury H. Introduction: how to situate and define action research. In: Bradbury H, ed. *The SAGE Handbook of Action Research.* 3rd ed. Sage Publications Ltd; 2015:8.

39. Whitehead D, Day J. Mixed-methods research. In: Schneider Z, Whitehead D, LoBiondo-Wood G, Haber J, eds. *Nursing and Midwifery Research: Methods and Appraisal for Evidence Based Practice.* 5th ed. Elsevier; 2016.

40. Rapoport RN. Three dilemmas in action research: with special reference to the Tavistock experience. *Hum Relat.* 1970;23(6):499–513. https://doi.org/10.1177/001872677002300601.

41. Holian R, Coghlan D. Ethical issues and role duality in insider action research: challenges for action research degree programmes. *Syst Pract Action Res.* 2013;26(5):399–415. https://doi.org/10.1007/s11213-012-9256-6.

42. Winter R, Munn-Giddings C. In: Winter R, Munn-Giddings C, eds. *A Handbook for Action Research in Health and Social Care.* Routledge; 2001.

Chapter 10

Q methodology in pharmacy and health services research

Robert Haua[a], Amanda Wolf[b], Jeff Harrison[a], and Trudi Aspden[a]

[a]School of Pharmacy, Faculty of Medical and Health Sciences, University of Auckland, Auckland, New Zealand, [b]Wellington School of Business and Government, Te Herenga Waka Victoria University of Wellington, Wellington, New Zealand

Objectives

- Identify pharmacy practice and health services research questions suitable for investigation using Q methodology.
- Explain how Q methodology differs from, and complements, semistructured interview and survey-based research.
- Describe the steps involved in completing a Q-methodology study and explain their rationale.
- Define operant subjectivity, concourse, and abduction, with reference to their roles in Q methodology.

Introduction

This chapter will describe Q methodology in an accessible manner to pharmacy and health services researchers, including postgraduate students. With attention to methodological fundamentals, it aims to equip and encourage researchers to explore complex phenomena within their own disciplines. Q methodology allows for the discovery and description of different, holistic viewpoints on any given topic.[1] In pharmacy practice research, Q methodology has been used to ascertain service user views and satisfaction with community pharmacy services,[2,3] understand how pharmacists prioritize clinical pharmacy services,[4] examine the factors influencing female community pharmacists' work patterns,[5] and establish views on integrating pharmacists into general practice.[6] More broadly, recent Q-methodological studies in the health services research sphere have investigated how staff prioritize care in residential aged care facilities,[7] the relative importance of different informational items in participant information leaflets for trials,[8] why pregnant women participate in clinical trials,[9] and the identification and categorization of key concepts and values about future health services.[10] Potential applications extend to any investigation of opinions or attitudes, such as adherence to medicines or other healthcare interventions, patients' experiences of medicines, views on innovative healthcare services, or the future of care. Unlike large sample surveys or in-depth qualitative interviews which privilege statistical and interpretive methods respectively, Q methodology combines the power of statistical technique with the richness of qualitative interpretation to find attitude or opinion profiles, typically using data from between 30 and 50 participants.

Procedurally, as described in greater detail in subsequent sections, participants arrange a sample of items (usually short statements) along a relevant dimension, for example, from most agree to most disagree, or most favorable to most unfavorable.[11] These "Q sorts" are then correlated and factor analyzed to reveal Q sorts that have been sorted similarly. These "shared and coherent points-of-view,"[1] which often privilege more marginalized voices,[12] are then compared to bring to light the diversity of participant views about the topic.[11] Characterizations of these views can then be used to design practices and services, communicate with patients and other stakeholders, or prompt follow-up research.

Understanding and capitalizing on the potential of Q methodology requires a short foray into its origins and underlying philosophical principles, which are discussed in the following sections. This is followed by an overview of the main steps of a Q-methodology study, supplemented by example data from a study that aimed to identify the different viewpoints present among New Zealand (NZ) stakeholders about how the concept of integrating pharmacists into general practice should or would be progressed. NZ stakeholders are generally very positive about this proposal, and the mathematical features of Q methodology helped to reveal and feature some of the more nuanced differences between participants that are often harder to identify when relying on manual or unaided observation by the researcher.

Origins

The origins of Q methodology lie in a 1935 letter to *Nature* written by William Stephenson (1902–1989).[13] It was developed over the following three to four years in a series of subsequent articles,[14–17] eventually culminating in a full exposition in *The study of behavior: Q-technique and its methodology*, published in 1953.[18]

Stephenson's methodological insight was initially premised on a simple adaptation of the quantitative technique known as factor analysis.[19] Factor analysis, invented by Charles Spearman at the turn of the 20th century, in its conventional form identifies associations between traits in a variable-by-variable correlation matrix.[20] Factor analysis operates on the idea that the associations between these observed traits are, at least in part, explained by a smaller number of underlying and unobserved factors.[21] Stephenson identified that the same techniques of factor analysis could be applied in a completely different framework so that people, rather than tests or traits, are the variables of interest. Thus, the groundwork was laid for Q methodology, using a "by-person" analysis to find a smaller number of factors, and thereby allowing a systematic study of subjectivity. Stephenson held PhDs in both physics and psychology, and his study in both disciplines influenced the principles and interpretive practices in Q methodology.

Principles

Q methodology is a complete methodology based upon a philosophical, ontological, and epistemological framework[22] centered on self-referent views,[23] or "subjectivity," and additional concepts. Taken together, the theoretical bases of Q methodology allow for a reliable study of subjectivity and the first-person perspective, "with full scientific sanction, satisfying every rule and procedure of scientific method."[18] Three of the most important concepts are briefly described in this section.

Operant subjectivity

Subjectivity in modern usage has been defined as "the unique perspective of an individual…that comprises their perceptions, beliefs, and expectations,"[24] and "the quality of existing in someone's mind rather than the external world."[25] The subjective arena is often thought of as psychical,[26] being associated with phenomenology and hermeneutics, and is contrasted with objectivity by positivists, who usually view subjectivity pejoratively on the basis that perspectives are inherently biased by personal values.[27] Consequently, subjectivity has nearly universally been treated as suited only to the domain of qualitative research, with its various methods designed to find what is "on people's minds," such as the meanings they ascribe to experiences.

Stephenson, however, rejected the mentalists' labeling of mind and consciousness as entities,[26] and the dualistic split between "events on the surface and an internal world,[28] such as body/mind, subjective/objective, and fact/value."[29] He claimed only one difference between the subjective and objective worlds: "It is … merely that only the individual himself can observe and measure [opinions], whereas it is [essential] of objectivity that everyone (or machines) can make the observations and measurements."[30] Typical measurement scales set meanings a priori through assumptions built into the tests,[31] whereas in Q methodology, the meaning of each statement is determined a posteriori by the sorters themselves.[32] In asking participants to speak for themselves, Q methodology provides the instrumental basis to reveal so-named *operant subjectivities*, in a natural setting, without confounding them with operational measurements.[31] To use a simple analogy: at a party, guests naturally gravitate to the garden, or the food table, or near the music. The Q researcher, having detected these revealed perspectives on the party, can then proceed to examine what comprises the choices of the various groups of guests, and seek to understand how they have come about.

Concourse

The volume of discussion that is possible about any topic is known as the *concourse*,[30] which is infinite in principle. Theoretically, all statements within a concourse are presumed to be equally possible a priori, and the same statement can hold different meanings for different people.[33] Participants operate on a representative sample of statements from a concourse, assigning relative salience to statements according to what is *psychologically significant* to them.[1] The result therefore creates meaningful and functional relationships among the statements.

While abstract in Q methodology, deriving from the "running together" of its etymology, concourse is directly analogous to its application to the great transit halls of a city train station. In the station, people of every description are coming and going without any immediately evident pattern, a single person no more or less likely than another to be there.

However, a variety of snapshots taken at different times and vantage points would readily reveal patterns—both predictable, such as the pathways of harried morning commuters, and less predictable, such as the locations favored by loitering teems.

Abduction

Deductive and inductive forms of logical inference are well known. Deduction begins with a formal theory and hypothesis, and an attempt is made to test and provide empirical support for the original hypothesis.[32] In contrast, induction approaches an object of enquiry on its own terms, through which observations are made and data gathered, so that probable generalizations and descriptions can be made about that instance.[32]

A third form of logical reasoning, abduction, begins with a surprising or unexpected event or observation, after which the investigator, guided by hunches and guesswork, examines the observations and data, to devise a plausible explanation of the event.[34] As described by Fann,[35] a researcher either selects a hypothesis, or creates one, drawing on both evidence and methodology (which some people see epitomized in the "method" of Sherlock Holmes). Abduction thus pertains to a particular way humans engage in a reasoning process leading to a hypothesis that is "likely in itself and renders the facts likely."[34]

It is the "unexpected event" that helps to best distinguish between induction and abduction. As a stylized example, consider an archeologist newly arrived on a site. The archeologist does not just dig 50 holes at random and then proceed to summarize and draw an initial conclusion about the site, following which the conclusion may be tested by digging another hole. Rather, initial forays guide an experienced scientist to notice features in the field that piques their interest, creating a feeling that digging in a particular spot could be rewarding. Thus, the seed of a testable hypothesis is in a hunch-triggering observation.

In the context of scientific inquiry, abduction is typically considered to be inference that leads to the discovery of new knowledge and the generation of theories or concepts to advance disciplines and science.[36] For example, early-career and highly experienced pharmacists may appear to agree on the core principles of ethical prescribing, but surprisingly differ about how those same principles are affected by a crisis such as a pandemic. A researcher may then generate theories that could plausibly explain this divergence.

Stephenson held that Q methodology provided the technical procedures to elucidate hypotheses de novo and make new discoveries possible, in contrast to other techniques used to test hypotheses.[37,38] The juxtapositions of statements and their scores in a factor, as well as comparisons between factors, are rich with the potential to explore plausible ideas, which is a hallmark of abduction. As will be elaborated in the discussion of factor analysis, insight often follows a shift in perspective. Hoffman, for example, cites the case of Aldo Leopold, who realized he had to "think like a mountain" and thereby achieved a "perceptual shift" in thinking about managing an ecosystem.[39]

Methodology

Q methodology has both qualitative and quantitative characteristics, with statistical procedures both aiding interpretation and ensuring the researcher stays true to participants' points of view. As a method of discovery, it does not suit investigation of the prevalence of views, nor does it seek demographic or other correlates of opinions. Q methodology instead reveals generalizations of perspective, pertaining to "substantive, rather than statistical, inference about a phenomenon."[22]

Unlike studies that privilege the detection of qualitative themes across all participants, the focus in Q methodology is the qualitative interpretations and comparisons of viewpoints *as wholes* that are present in the concourse for a given topic. The statistical features of Q methodology can also facilitate a better understanding of the more nuanced differences between viewpoints that may otherwise be missed by investigator observation. A further strength of the methodology is its reduced risk of interviewer or observer bias, since the viewpoints that emerge are solely the function of the Q sorters themselves and are "inextricably tied to and emerge from the concrete operations of the participants."[40]

Concerns about validity are moot in Q methodology. It is not appropriate to establish criteria that might be used to assign more or less validity to one person's opinion compared with another,[28,41] just as there is no sound basis to claim that one person's preference for blue is better reasoned than another's preference for green. Further, viewpoints are certainly subject to change over time, and so issues regarding reliability are equally as inconsequential.[42] For instance, a general practitioner (GP) completing a Q sort regarding views on pharmacist prescribing may have a negative outlook initially, but over time as they work more closely with prescribing pharmacists, this valence could potentially become more positive.

With Q methodology's focus on shared perspectives, one indicator in support of the trustworthiness of data is the finding of significant correlations between sorts. While it is possible that a person could concoct a false Q sort, such fakes would fall out of the analysis since they would not correlate closely with genuine data. At the same time, investigators should be mindful that a sort that does not correlate with others may also simply be a result of a study that has not included another person with a similar view, which would have otherwise established a correlation if included. Other potential quality indicators for a Q-methodology study include replicability, the acceptance of the findings by participants who recognize their points of view reflected in the interpretations, and the emergence of a "surprising" factor that suggests hypotheses worthy of further investigation.

Rationale for Q methodology

Q methodology provides a sound approach to help achieve the successful development, evaluation, and implementation of new healthcare policies,[43] with its ability to understand highly complex subject matters at a macroscopic level.[19] The example study presented throughout this chapter sought to identify what stakeholders think best represents a sustainable and practical model of pharmacist integration into general practice in New Zealand. The ways in which collaborative models of care between different health professionals are designed brings together a multitude of complex and intertwined principles, undoubtedly compounded by a range of different views on the best way to work in partnership. Questions around funding and employment, decision-making processes, role requirements, tasks and responsibilities, and so on, need to be answered. These questions can be seen to hold a policy- and future-orientated focus, and subjectivity is intrinsically involved in this process.

As Sir Geoffrey Vickers (1894–1982) said: "policy problems are by their nature unlike scientific or technological problems in that they admit of no solution which can be proved to be right or even to be the best."[44] Decision-makers are often faced with equally favorable or unfavorable options, and deciding on one route will "enhance the likelihood of achieving one desirable goal, but will lessen the likelihood of realising another."[45] Vickers labels this *multivalued choice* a part in the "policy-making process that chooses one among an indefinite number of possible mixes of value satisfaction, of which not more than a very few can be examined or even identified."[46]

One of the strengths of Q methodology is its ability to clarify areas of consensus and disagreement within stakeholder groups, which helps to reach decisions that are deemed legitimate by all contending parties.[47] As seen above, there are multiple facets to consider when designing a model that integrates pharmacists into general practice, and the relative importance of these dimensions varies among stakeholders. In contrast to a description of individual themes obtained via textual analyses, the value of Q methodology lies in its emphasis on holism, which facilitates a fuller understanding of how and why these elements relate and interconnect. Importantly, however, unlike survey methodology, the prevalence of any views that may emerge must be gauged by follow-up research. For example, one research team completed a Q-methodology study which identified five viewpoints on the principles involved in allocating resources to health care, and then surveyed over 30,000 people in a follow-up study to find the extent to which each of these viewpoints were held in nine countries.[48]

The factor analytic features in Q methodology also help to ensure a full and comprehensive engagement with what otherwise may be missed by unaided observation and manual coding of interview transcripts.[40,41] Further, the forced sorting distribution, which has become standard practice in Q-methodological studies, helps participants to make finer-grained distinctions around what is most important to them, which in turn helps investigators interpret that data. The results from the example study reveal a relatively high level of consensus among stakeholders about what would or should represent a practical and sustainable model of pharmacist integration into general practice. However, there remain nuanced, yet important, differences between these groups of stakeholders that require elucidation so that opportunities for collaboration are revealed.

Procedure

Q-set development

The Q set is a sample of items (usually statements, but images are used increasingly) from the concourse that participants are asked to sort. There is no single or correct way to create a Q set,[32] but it is necessary to first define the relevant concourse and extract a large number of items, from which a representative sample can be chosen.[45] Items are typically generated from interviews, participant observations, literature reviews, as well as the media and other popular texts. Q-set representativeness is essential, as this allows participants to respond to the research question effectively, and not feel constrained or limited by a Q set that is unbalanced and has insufficient coverage.[32]

It is therefore advised to structure the Q set by breaking down the subject matter into constituent themes or concepts.[32] One approach is based on a priori theoretical considerations (deductive design), with two or three dimensions comprising a

TABLE 1 Q set structure using the conceptual framework of access to health care by Levesque et al.

	Dimensions of accessibility	
Pathway to achieving access	Provider level	Service user level
1. Identify healthcare needs	Approachability	Ability to perceive
2. Seek healthcare services	Acceptability	Ability to seek
3. Reach healthcare resources	Availability and accommodation	Ability to reach
4. Obtain or use healthcare services	Affordability	Ability to pay
5. Offered appropriate services	Appropriateness	Ability to engage

sampling scheme.[31] In such cases, the Q set can be structured around theory or a conceptual framework.[49] For example, Levesque et al.'s conceptual framework of access to health care conceptualizes access as being influenced by five dimensions of provider accessibility and five corresponding abilities of persons to interact with these dimensions.[50] Table 1 exemplifies this as a potential schematic for a Q set that could be used for a Q-methodological study of patient experiences regarding access to health services. Given that the five aspects of the access pathway are influenced by dimensions at the provider and service user levels, there are $5 \times 2 = 10$ cells to which statements can be allocated. A statement such as "I would not use this service if there was a charge" fits under the "affordability" dimension. Once statements have been allocated, investigators operate on the *principle of heterogeneity*[49] to maximize the diversity of statements within each cell, to help ensure a representative and balanced Q set.

Table 1 also illustrates well the relationship between a topic, concourse, and subjectivity. Note that the "pathway" describes potentially observable activities in the context of research interests (a specific accessibility topic in this example). The two columns expressing "dimensions of accessibility" present themes that are amenable to health care stakeholders' subjective evaluations of those activities. In Q methodology, the elicitation of views is always with respect to a concourse, and the concourse in turn is the entire set of potential elements about some topic. It should be noted that the use of a conceptual framework and categorization of statements by investigators is only to help ensure representativeness. How individuals interpret and score each statement is an innately self-referent process that is independent of any sampling schemes developed by investigators.[49]

An alternative approach to Q set development is based on patterns that emerge as statements are collected (inductive design).[31] Items are then allocated approximately equally to each emergent theme from the data, with the aim of ensuring a representative sample for the topic at hand. The exact number of items included in the Q set is largely dictated by the subject matter; however, a typical study includes between 30 and 60 items.

P set

The sample of participants is known as the P set. Similar to Q-set design, the exact number of participants required for a particular Q-methodology study will depend on the nature and purpose of what is under investigation.[31] Variation exists in the literature regarding the number of people to include. For example, McKeown and Thomas[31] suggest 30 to 50, but more or fewer is not uncommon. The goal is to include participants who have a defined and pertinent viewpoint to express about the research topic, and to avoid an unduly homogenous group of participants.[32] This will help ensure that the positions of available viewpoints that structure subjectivity are uncovered.[1] Therefore, most Q-methodology studies use purposive sampling for participant recruitment,[11,51] meaning that investigators can justifiably approach individuals who are believed to hold interesting or pivotal viewpoints.[32] As participants sort the Q set independently, it is also important that the subject matter is understandable to participants, even if many items do not evoke strong opinions.[52]

Whilst it is useful to strive for representation and diversity in the P set, complete balance is rarely necessary,[40] because while participants are selected based on a priori assumptions that they will have pertinent viewpoints and define a factor, whether this eventuates or not is an empirical matter brought to light by factor analysis.[45] Therefore, although categories based on respondent characteristics can assist in participant selection, they are of little subsequent interest and rarely enter into ensuing analyses.[40]

Q sorting

Q sorting is, in essence, a modified rank-ordering technique whereby participants place stimulus items in an order that is significant from their own individual standpoint, while operating under specified conditions.[45] These conditions include instructions about the sorting task as well as an orientation to the task (see Fig. 1). Each Q sort represents a "single, holistic, and gestalt entity,"[32] and it is these distributions that are correlated and subjected to factor analysis.

To facilitate sorting, a quasi-normal distribution is most often used, with endpoints such as "most disagree" and "most agree," typically scaled from −5 or −4 to +5 or +4. For subject matters where participants are likely to be relatively uninformed or uninterested, a distribution approaching the normal curve of error is suitable, with more room provided in the middle to account for participants who might not hold opinions for some items.[45] For topics expected to be controversial and/or evoke strong emotions, or where the P set includes people that are subject experts, then a flattened distribution will allow for more fine-grained distinctions to be made at the extremes.[32] Fig. 1 illustrates the sorting distribution used in the study that asked participants what they thought would or should represent a sustainable and practical model of pharmacist integration into general practice in New Zealand. The middle score (zero column) is "a point neutral in meaning and without psychological significance."[31] Items that participants are ambivalent about or find problematic are placed in this column. However, during factor interpretation, because items are ranked relative to each other, items in the middle column may hold meaning when compared to items placed elsewhere in the configuration.

While a forced distribution is standard practice within Q-methodology studies, it is possible to use a free or nonstandardized distribution.[32] The shape and range of the distribution does not affect the existence of factors, and small variances have little to do with the final results, which derive from general patterns rather than where exact items have been placed.[45] However, where possible, participants should attempt to adhere to the forced distribution, because it encourages them to make distinctions between items that they are capable of separating, but otherwise would not volunteer.[45] An example of how this was of value in the example study is presented in the section on factor interpretation.

Procedurally, participants are presented with the set of statements, which they typically sort into three piles to help collate the statements that they view positively, negatively, or neutrally. They then take each pile sequentially and sort

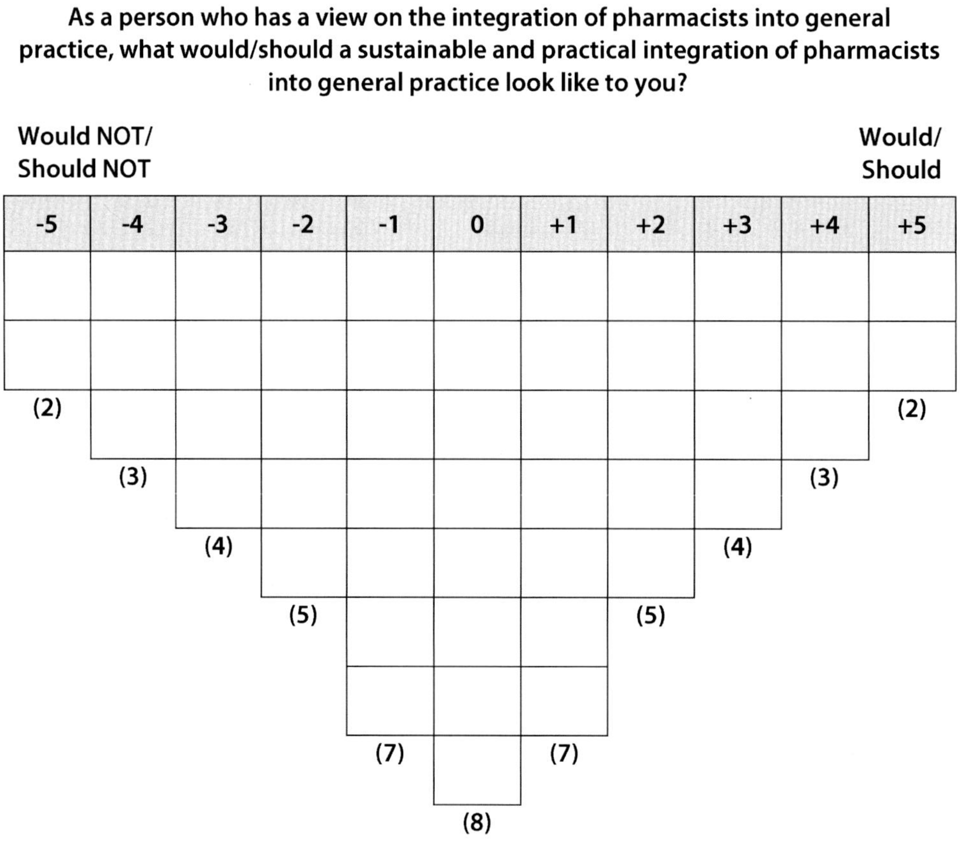

FIG. 1 Sorting distribution for the example study that contained 50 statements. The numbers at the top of each column represent the ranking value for statements assigned to each respective column. The numbers at the bottom of each column outline the number of statements that can be allocated to that ranking. Two statements can be sorted onto −5 and +5, three onto −4 and +4, and so on.

As a person who has a view on the integration of pharmacists into general practice, what would/should a sustainable and practical integration of pharmacists into general practice look like to you?

Would NOT/ Should NOT

Would/ Should

-5	-4	-3	-2	-1	0	+1	+2	+3	+4	+5
(2)	(3)	(4)	(5)	(7)	(8)	(7)	(5)	(4)	(3)	(2)

these onto the distribution. Once they have sorted all of the statements relative to each other, they can then review and edit the placing of statements, before their Q sort is captured for analysis.

A postsorting interview follows the sorting procedure. This interview assists in understanding why participants ranked the statements as they did,[40] clarifying seemingly obscure or contradictory points,[45] and ascertaining the participant's views and general understanding about the topic under investigation.[32] Particular focus is given to items at the extremes of the distribution, as well as other pertinent or interesting items upon which the researcher or participant wish to elaborate.

Factor analysis

Factor analysis reveals natural groupings of Q sorts.[45] A basic understanding of standard statistical terminology and factor analysis is useful, but researchers can rely on specialized software, such as Ken-Q Analysis and its desktop edition (KADE),[53] to perform the computations. Interested readers can refer to Brown's *Political Subjectivity*[45] (pages 204 to 247) for a complete breakdown of the mathematical steps and calculations.

To briefly elaborate, factor analysis includes the steps of factor extraction, factor rotation, and deciding on the number of factors to retain for interpretation. These steps are discussed below.

Factor extraction

Factor extraction begins with the correlation of each participant's Q sort with every other Q sort, by comparing how participants placed each item on the sorting grid. This results in a correlation matrix. Participants who sorted the statements similarly can be expected to have high positive correlations. Correlations approaching 0 indicate the Q sorts have comparably little in common, and those with high negative correlations have high levels of disagreement (statements sorted highly by one participant tend to be sorted low by the other, and vice versa). Factor extraction then identifies distinct portions of *what is common* between Q sorts, resulting in a set of factors.[32] This is illustrated as a matrix that shows the degree to which each Q sort loads on to (is correlated with) each factor.

In the general factor analytic community, factor extraction is most often achieved by principal component analysis (PCA), but many Q methodologists prefer the older, and less determinate, centroid factor analysis (CFA). Strictly speaking, PCA extracts components, while CFA extracts factors[21]; however, referring to components as factors is widespread in published Q-methodology studies. Preferences for the centroid method tend to be based around theoretical considerations rather than actual practicalities. In brief, PCA maximizes the variance extracted from each factor,[21] while centroid's indeterminacy offers an infinite number of possible solutions, meaning the researcher can be guided by their own inclinations and theories.[45] However, in practice, PCA and CFA results tend to vary little in terms of the initial factors extracted,[45] and both are used within the Q-methodology community.

Factor rotation

In order to improve interpretability, factors are most often rotated, which clarifies the relative positions of individual sorts on the factors. Two rotation options are typically available in Q-methodological software packages: varimax and judgmental (also known as theoretical, manual, or by-hand) rotation.

Varimax rotation operates statistically according to Thurstone's criterion of "simple structure,"[54] which maximizes the number of factor loadings with negligible (nonsignificant) values, while preserving a few values with high loadings.[55] Stephenson found it difficult to readily accept "one kind of geometrical substructure (i.e., simple structure) as, in principle, the only basis for inferences,"[18] because it is unlikely that a single algorithm irrespective of context and specificities would always lead to the best result. The varimax solution is often sufficient to capture factors that are operant, functional, and acceptable on theoretical grounds,[45,56] but this is not always the case, and the researcher is free to explore their own conceptions of the data as well. Along these lines, judgmental rotation involves the investigator examining the loadings in the factor space, and making decisions around how the factors should be rotated and be ultimately positioned, based on theory, prior knowledge, or expectations.[32] It is through the process of judgmental rotation that Peirce's abductory principles most saliently enter Q methodology, as the researcher is guided by "guesswork, intuition, [and] hunches … which are of such obvious importance to the growth of knowledge."[45]

Graphically, the results of a factor analysis can be illustrated in a n-dimensional space, where n represents the number of factors extracted and retained for rotation.[55] While this is easy enough to visualize when there are only two or three factors (i.e., two- or three-dimensional), it becomes increasingly complex and difficult to imagine as more dimensions (factors) are

FIG. 2   The factor space between Factors A and B in the example study investigating views on pharmacist integration into general practice in New Zealand.

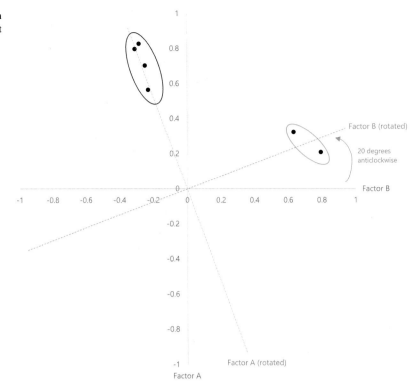

added to the factor space. As a consequence, investigators select two factors at a time for each rotation. Fig. 2 highlights the factor space between Factors A and B in the example study, using a selected sample of Q sorts. Two clusters of Q sorts are circled, highlighting two potential viewpoints. The factor axes have been rotated 20 degrees counter-clockwise to maximize the loadings of the Q sorts onto one factor and minimize the loadings onto the other. This will give a clearer picture when it comes to factor interpretation.

Prior to rotation, investigators will have to decide on how many factors to retain for rotation (explained in the following section). This is important if a varimax rotation is employed, because factor rotation will inevitably spread some of the variance from the first factors onto later ones.[57] If too many factors are retained for the rotation phase, then varimax will distribute the variance to them, such that previously unimportant factors become important by virtue of this statistical process.[55]

In contrast, some Q methodologists who use judgmental rotation will often keep more factors than that expected in the final solution, because "insignificant factors frequently contain small amounts of systematic variance that can help in improving the loadings on a major factor ... after rotation, insignificant residual factors are merely discarded."[45] During rotation, while Q-sort factor loadings change, their relationship to all other Q sorts is fixed. Rotation, therefore, is not some sleight of hand where the investigator changes the data to suit their needs, but simply a way of changing the vantage point.

Number of factors to extract and retain

The literature contains extensive discussion regarding the number of factors to extract and retain for rotation.[32,45] While in traditional factor analyses, various statistical criteria are used to determine the number of factors to extract, in Q methodology, "the significance of Q factors is not defined objectively (statistically), but theoretically in terms of the social–psychological situation to which the emergent factors are functionally related."[58] Exclusive use of statistical criteria in Q methodology may lead to investigators overlooking a factor that may be statistically insignificant in terms of the amount of variance explained, but nevertheless holds particular theoretical interest.[31]

Most of these statistical criteria revolve around eigenvalues, which are often taken as a measure of a factor's statistical strength and importance,[58] and are related to the amount of variance that each factor explains. For example, the Kaiser-Guttmann criterion, which extracts factors with eigenvalues greater than 1, is commonly used. However, this criterion is relatively insignificant in the Q context, because eigenvalues are influenced by the number of Q sorts in the study, and a large P set can lead to the inclusion of potentially spurious factors.[45] As a consequence of purposive sampling, a factor with a larger eigenvalue simply means that more people of that factor type happened to be included in the study,[58] and a factor with less explained variance can be equally or more interesting from a theoretical standpoint.

Accordingly, unless there is a strong theoretical basis for focusing on a single Q sort, Q methodologists rely on a rule of thumb to retain factors that, after rotation, have at least two (preferably three) defining sorts, that is, sorts that significantly load onto one factor and one factor alone.[32] A significant loading at the 0.01 level is calculated by the formula $2.58 \times (1 \div \sqrt{\text{no. of items in Q set}})$.[45] Thus, a final decision on how many factors to retain for rotation is only made *after* the researcher examines several preliminary analyses with a sequential series of retained and rotated factors, to determine at what point in the process a factor does not meet this criterion. Factor extraction should also operate according to the principle of parsimony, that is, if something can be described equally well in simpler terms, then it should be.[59] This means that no more factors should be extracted than necessary to explain the data, because while each retained factor increases the amount of variance explained, it also increases the complexity of the solution. Thus, if an additional factor only accounts for one or two more Q sorts than the prior solution, it may not be worthwhile retaining that factor.

Regardless of statistical aids, it is always important to qualitatively examine the final factor arrays to ensure they make sense, are substantive, and theoretically sound. There is no guarantee that *any* of the solutions will include factors that make substantive sense. This can result from poor design of the Q set or P set, poor sorting instructions, or faulty decisions in the statistical analysis. If there is no clear distinction between some of the final factors (the software generates a table of factor intercorrelations that can assist with this), then perhaps fewer factors should be extracted. On the other hand, if there is a factor that is statistically insignificant in terms of the amount of variance it explains or in the number of significant loaders it has, but it is theoretically significant, then its interpretation is valuable.

Factor interpretation

To prepare for interpretation, factor estimates (or factor arrays) are derived from a weighted averaging of all the Q sorts that were flagged as being defining for each respective factor.[11] The term "flagging" refers to choosing which sorts to include in the final factor arrays. Each factor array depicts the contributing sorts as a single, amalgamated set of statement scores, thus representing the factor viewpoint. Q-methodological software packages come with a preflagging option that identifies defining Q sorts based on statistical principles; however, investigators are also at liberty to manually select which sorts are included based on their own understandings of the data. Table 2 illustrates a sample of Q sorts that have been purposively selected from the example study to highlight groups of Q sorts that are defining for each factor, that is, load significantly onto a single factor only. These Q sorts will inform the final factor array for each of their respective factors.

Researchers have developed a range of strategies for undertaking factor interpretation. All make use of the data holistically, typically examining statements at the extremes of the composite factor arrays, as well as any distinguishing and

TABLE 2 Excerpt of the rotated factor matrix from the example study investigating views on pharmacist integration into general practice in New Zealand.

Q Sort	Factor A	Factor B	Factor C
1	**0.53**	0.00	0.25
2	**0.55**	0.18	0.25
3	**0.64**	0.28	0.35
4	0.20	**0.45**	−0.01
5	−0.13	**0.61**	0.04
6	0.17	0.14	**0.68**
7	0.24	0.09	**0.66**
8	0.33	0.17	**0.68**

The bolded numbers are to highlight that these Q Sorts (i.e., 1, 2, and 3 for Factor A; 4 and 5 for Factor B; and 6, 7, and 8 for Factor C) significantly load onto that factor, and not onto the other factors.

consensus statements for the factor, as they gradually refine an overall sense of the factor as a whole, in relation to the full statement set.

Again, an abductive, insight-pursuing lens is recommended. Each time a statement is examined, the researcher needs to consider what it adds to the overall picture, and if it confirms or otherwise changes the story thus far.[32] Throughout interpretation, it is important to refer to any postsorting interview data, as well as the demographic information collected, because these can help make sense of the factor. Cross-factor comparisons aid in interpreting and distinguishing factors.

Q-methodology research reports full and holistic interpretations of each factor, which typically present a range of interconnecting themes and the evidence for them using statements and statement scores. However, for illustration purposes, brief summaries of the three factors identified in the example study are presented in Fig. 3, noting that more comprehensive expositions are standard in Q-methodology studies.

Throughout this chapter, reference has been made to Q methodology's strength of identifying and exploring the sometimes nuanced differences between people's viewpoints. To exemplify this point, participant views from the example study concerning how community pharmacy would be impacted if pharmacists were integrated into general practice will be explored in more detail. Table 3 highlights several statements from the Q set around this topic, and how these have been ranked in the final factor arrays for the three example study factors.

A quick glance at the ranking of statements in each factor array illustrates a clear point of difference between Factor B and the other two factors when it comes to the perceived impact on community pharmacy. Statements that Factor B sorted positively tended to be sorted negatively by the other factors, and vice versa.

Factor A
Value undisputable, role is a necessity

- The value of practice pharmacists is clearly evident, and funding should be promptly earmarked
- A fundamental reform to primary care funding would likely be required
- A centralised funding model would help ensure equitable access across the country
- Role is predominantly patient-facing with a clinical focus, superseding the traditional supply function of pharmacists
- Physical co-location within the practice would enable the development of relationships and trust, facilitating pharmacists working collaboratively, but independently, with GPs
- Community pharmacists continue to have an important, but distinct, role from practice pharmacists

Factor B
Cautious approval with checks and balances

- Acceptance and success of practice pharmacists would be contingent on having clear guidelines and role specifications
- Advanced training or certification would be mandatory to ensure pharmacists are appropriately skilled
- The role would be primarily supportive, focusing on services to improve medicines adherence rather than optimising pharmacological outcomes
- Overall clinical responsibility remains at all times with GP
- The proposed roles for practice pharmacists should not be performed by community pharmacists
- Scope for community pharmacy would likely diminish

Factor C
Community pharmacy takes precedence

- Practice pharmacists would add significant value to patient care, however their introduction must not result in the marginalisation of community pharmacy
- Community pharmacy remains integral to primary care
- Successful integration does not necessarily require physical co-location
- Medicines management services could be just as effectively delivered from community pharmacies, especially in rural or provincial areas where access is an issue

FIG. 3   Summaries for the three factors identified in the example study that investigated stakeholder views on pharmacist integration into general practice in New Zealand.

TABLE 3 Excerpt of the final factor arrays for the three example study factors, illustrating statements related to views on community pharmacy and their rankings.

		Factor arrays		
Statement		A	B	C
8	Reduce the need for DHBs to invest in community pharmacy services	−2	2	−5
13	Have funded pharmacist-led medicines management services being concurrently provided by both community pharmacists and pharmacists working in general practice	0	−4	4
17	Reduce the clinical component of community pharmacy	−3	3	−5
23	Reduce the need for patients to interact with community pharmacists	−3	3	−3
24	Contract a community pharmacist to work in a general practice for a specified length of time each week	0	−2	1

Both Factors A and C clearly still see value in community pharmacy if pharmacists were to be integrated into general practice. However, the forced sorting distribution has uncovered a difference in the relative importance of this view between the two factors. Factor C has ranked statements around community pharmacy more negatively than Factor A, with statements 8 and 17 taking the most negative spots in the composite Q sort of Factor C. The difference in the strength of the feeling would likely be missed in thematic coding, as each instance of a transcript in which respondents expressed rejection of claims such as those in 8 and 17 would be simply aggregated in a category. Moreover, this illustration is a small extract, concerning only one dimension of the findings. The full picture of each factor incorporates the relative views on community pharmacy in the context of other patterns in the data, and additional data from the postsort interviews, which would further distinguish between the factors.

Recall that participants assign relative salience to statements according to what is *psychologically significant* to them,[1] and the meaning of each statement is determined a posteriori by the sorters.[32] Reference to the postsorting interview data revealed that Factors A and C saw community pharmacy as being important for different reasons. Those aligned with Factor A recognize the value of community pharmacists. However, they believe that community pharmacists have a different role than practice pharmacists, for example, advising on minor ailments, health system navigation, and public health matters. On the other hand, Factor C reveals a viewpoint that more prominently sees community pharmacists as being able to perform the same medicines management roles as practice pharmacists. In stark contrast to the other two factors, participants associated with Factor B think that community pharmacists should not be performing the medicines management roles proposed for practice pharmacists, and the role for community pharmacy would likely diminish if pharmacists were to work more prominently in general practice.

Although brief, the factor summaries presented in Fig. 3, alongside the subsequent discussion about a particularly important and distinguishing subject matter, reinforces that Q methodology is able to discover and elucidate distinct viewpoints about any given subject matter, at all times prioritizing participants' own voices.

Conclusion

This chapter was designed to introduce Q methodology to pharmacy and health services researchers, rather than provide a complete description of all its concepts and procedures. Readers are encouraged to learn more about Q methodology by consulting the guide to completing a Q-methodological study by Watts and Stenner.[32] Brown[28] offers a thorough overview of Q methodology's concepts, and his 1980 book[45] comprehensively describes its principles and methods. Readers may also discover that there are lively methodological debates in the literature, and indeed find published studies that follow practices seemingly inconsistent with our presentation.

As with many less common methodologies, lack of prevalence in the literature may itself be a reason for researchers to bypass Q methodology. At the same time, peer-reviewed Q-methodology papers are becoming ever more numerous, and as methodologically sound studies proliferate, we might expect to see more applications pertinent to health and pharmacy research. Q methodology is not well-suited to studies investigating the prevalence of views or that aim to correlate these with various demographic profiles. Its benefit lies in addressing matters of curiosity concerning the nature of people's varied opinions about a topic—an objective that complements both opinion surveys and strictly qualitative approaches. In particular, we see value in potential applications with a degree of both consensus and conflict, whereby the mechanics of the structured sorting exercise provides participants with a stimulus to more deeply reflect on the components of their views, and when composite associations between elements of an opinion are of interest rather than disaggregate themes.

Potential applications in health services and pharmacy practice research are wide-reaching. Gauging stakeholder acceptability of services, uncovering the lived experiences of consumers, and understanding pharmacists' views of their own profession are all valuable considerations for a Q-methodology study. Q methodology can also give voice to marginalized groups and perspectives, which is useful when aiming to uncover the views and experiences of indigenous peoples or minority populations on topics such as reasons for pursuing a particular health career pathway, or the role and influence of pharmacists or others in their use of medicines and utilization of health services. Q methodology is also well-placed to help the successful development, implementation, and evaluation of new health services. With its focus on shared perspectives, the ability to investigate complex and contested issues, and emphasis on the centrality of self, Q methodology offers a valuable addition to health services and pharmacy practice research.

Questions for further discussion

1. Why does Q methodology often reveal both expected and unexpected perspectives on a topic?
2. What are the similarities and differences between the analysis of Q-sort data and interview data?
3. What does a sampling scheme contribute to the quality of data collection via Q sorts?
4. Can Q methodology be used with statements representing factual claims, such as "the number of children relying on daily medication is increasing," instead of opinions, such as "I worry about increasing numbers of children on daily medication." Why or why not?

Application exercise/scenario

A number of possible topics for Q-methodology research are indicated in the final paragraph in the main part of the chapter above. Choose one of these, or a similar one of interest to you. Write a research question that would guide your investigation and sketch the main steps you would follow to answer the question using Q methodology. Before you can proceed with your study, as is the normal expectation, you would require clearance from a research ethics committee. With persuading this committee in mind, create an explanatory information sheet suitable for gaining informed consent from participants. Your explanation needs to be complete and accurate regarding the purpose of the study, and the explanation of the method, but written in a way that is understandable to participants.

References

1. Stenner P, Watts S, Worrell M. Q methodology. In: Willig C, Stainton-Rogers W, eds. *The SAGE Handbook of Qualitative Research in Psychology.* 2nd ed. London: SAGE Publications; 2017:212–235.
2. Renberg T, Wichman Törnqvist K, Kälvemark Sporrong S, Kettis Lindblad Å, Tully MP. Pharmacy users' expectations of pharmacy encounters: a Q-methodological study. *Health Expect.* 2011;14:361–373.
3. De Tran V, Dorofeeva VV. Applying Q-methodology to study customer satisfaction with quality of community pharmacy services in Vietnam. *Trop J Pharm Res.* 2018;17:2281–2289.
4. Van De Pol JM, Koster ES, Hövels AM, Bouvy ML. How community pharmacists prioritize cognitive pharmaceutical services. *Res Social Adm Pharm.* 2019;15:1088–1094.
5. Gidman W, Day J, Hassell K, Payne K. Delivering health care through community pharmacies: are working conditions deterring female pharmacists' participation? *J Health Serv Res Policy.* 2009;14:141–149.
6. Hazen AC, Van Der Wal AW, Sloeserwij VM, et al. Controversy and consensus on a clinical pharmacist in primary care in the Netherlands. *Int J Clin Pharmacol.* 2016;38:1250–1260.
7. Ludlow K, Churruca K, Mumford V, Ellis LA, Braithwaite J. Staff members' prioritisation of care in residential aged care facilities: a Q methodology study. *BMC Health Serv Res.* 2020;20:1–14.
8. Innes K, Cotton S, Campbell MK, Elliott J, Gillies K. Relative importance of informational items in participant information leaflets for trials: a Q-methodology approach. *BMJ Open.* 2018;8, e023303.
9. Meshaka R, Jeffares S, Sadrudin F, Huisman N, Saravanan P. Why do pregnant women participate in research? A patient participation investigation using Q-Methodology. *Health Expect.* 2017;20:188–197.
10. Kim J, Piao M, Byun A, Lee J. A typology of future health services by exploring core concepts and values: a Q-methodology approach. *Comput Inform Nurs.* 2019;37:107–115.

11. Stainton RR. Q methodology. In: Smith JA, Harré R, Van Langenhove L, eds. *Rethinking Methods in Psychology*. London: SAGE Publications; 1995.

12. Brown SR. A match made in heaven: a marginalized methodology for studying the marginalized. *Qual Quant*. 2006;40:361–382.

13. Stephenson W. Technique of factor analysis. *Nature*. 1935;136:297.

14. Burt C, Stephenson W. Alternative views on correlations between persons. *Psychometrika*. 1939;4:269–281.

15. Stephenson W. The inverted factor technique. *Br J Psychol*. 1936;26:344.

16. Stephenson W. The foundations of psychometry: four factor systems. *Psychometrika*. 1936;1:195–209.

17. Stephenson W. Correlating persons instead of tests. *J Pers*. 1935;4:17–24.

18. Stephenson W. *The Study of Behavior: Q-Technique and its Methodology*. Chicago, IL: University of Chicago Press; 1953.

19. Watts S, Stenner P. Doing Q methodology: theory, method and interpretation. *Qual Res Psychol*. 2005;2:67–91.

20. Mulaik SA. *Foundations of Factor Analysis*. 2nd ed. Boca Raton, FL: CRC Press; 2009.

21. Kline P. *An Easy Guide to Factor Analysis*. Abingdon, England: Routledge; 1994.

22. Ramlo S. Theoretical significance in Q methodology: a qualitative approach to a mixed method. *Res Sch*. 2015;22:73–87.

23. Stephenson W. Scientific creed-1961: the centrality of self. *Psychol Rec*. 1961;11:18–25.

24. Subjectivity. *Dictionary of Organizational Behaviour*. Oxford: Oxford University Press; 2019.

25. Subjectivity. *Oxford Dictionary of English*. 3rd ed. Oxford: Oxford University Press; 2015.

26. Stephenson W. Perspectives in psychology: XXVI consciousness out—subjectivity in. *Psychol Rec*. 1968;18:499–501.

27. Subjectivity. *Dictionary of Media and Communication*. 3rd ed. Oxford: Oxford University Press; 2011.

28. Brown SR. Subjectivity in the human sciences. *Psychol Rec*. 2019;69:565–579.

29. Good JM. Introduction to William Stephenson's quest for a science of subjectivity. *Psychoanal Hist*. 2010;12:211–243.

30. Stephenson W. Protoconcursus: the concourse theory of communication. *Operant Subjectivity*. 1986;9:37–58.

31. McKeown B, Thomas DB. *Q methodology*. vol. 66. SAGE Publications; 2013.

32. Watts S, Stenner P. *Doing Q Methodological Research: Theory, Method & Interpretation*. SAGE Publications; 2012.

33. Stephenson W. Newton's fifth rule and Q methodology: application to educational psychology. *Am Psychol*. 1980;35:882.

34. Peirce CS. In: Hartshorne C, Wieiss P, Burks A, eds. *Collected Papers of Charles Sanders Peirce (8 Vols)*. Cambridge: Harvard University Press; 1931-1958.

35. Fann K. *Peirce's Theory of Abduction*. The Hague: Martinus Nijhoff; 1970.

36. Minnameier G. Peirce-suit of truth–why inference to the best explanation and abduction ought not to be confused. *Erkenntnis*. 2004;60:75–105.

37. Stephenson W. Scientific creed-1961: Abductory principles. *Psychol Rec*. 1961;11:9.

38. Stephenson W. Scientific creed-1961: philosophical credo. *Psychol Rec*. 1961;11:1.

39. Hoffmann MH. "Theoric transformations" and a new classification of abductive inferences. *Trans Charles S Peirce Soc: Quart J Am Philos*. 2010;46:570–590.

40. Brown SR. Q methodology. In: Given LM, ed. *The SAGE Encyclopedia of Qualitative Research Methods*. Thousand Oaks, CA: SAGE Publications; 2008.

41. Brown SR. A primer on Q methodology. *Operant Subjectivity*. 1993;16:91–138.

42. Cross RM. Exploring attitudes: the case for Q methodology. *Health Educ Res*. 2005;20:206–213.

43. Alderson S, Foy R, Bryant L, Ahmed S, House A. Using Q-methodology to guide the implementation of new healthcare policies. *BMJ Qual Saf*. 2018;27:737–742.

44. Vickers G. Commonly ignored elements in policymaking. *Pol Sci*. 1972;3:265.

45. Brown SR. *Political Subjectivity: Applications of Q Methodology in Political Science*. Yale University Press; 1980.

46. Vickers G. Management and the new specialists. *Organ Dyn*. 1972;1:3–11.

47. Brown SR. Q methodology in research on political decision making. In: Redlawsk DP, ed. *The Oxford Research Encyclopedia of Political Decision Making*. New York, NY: Oxford University Press; 2019.

48. Mason H, van Exel J, Baker R, et al. From representing views to representativeness of views: illustrating a new (Q2S) approach in the context of health care priority setting in nine European countries. *Soc Sci Med*. 2016;166:205–213.

49. Brown S, Baltrinic E, Jencius M. From concourse to Q sample to testing theory. *Operant Subjectivity*. 2019;41:1–17.

50. Levesque J-F, Harris MF, Russell G. Patient-centred access to health care: conceptualising access at the interface of health systems and populations. *Int J Equity Health*. 2013;12:1–9.

51. Watts S. Develop a Q methodological study. *Educ Prim Care*. 2015;26:435–437.

52. Rhoads J. Q Methodology. In: *SAGE Research Methods Cases [Internet]*. London: SAGE Publications; 2014. Available from: https://methods.sagepub.com/case/q-methodology.

53. Banasick S. *Ken-Q Analysis (Version 1.0.6) [Software]*; 2019. Available from: https://shawnbanasick.github.io/ken-q-analysis/.

54. Thurstone LL. *Multiple-Factor Analysis*. Chicago: University of Chicago Press; 1947.

55. Bennett S, Bowers D. *An Introduction to Multivariate Techniques for Social and Behavioural Sciences*. London and Basingstoke: Palgrave Macmillan UK; 1976.

56. Stephenson W. General theory of communication. *Operant Subjectivity*. 2014;37:38–56.

57. Goldberg LR. Doing it all bass-ackwards: the development of hierarchical factor structures from the top down. *J Res Pers*. 2006;40:347–358.

58. Brown SR. The importance of factors in Q methodology: statistical and theoretical considerations. *Operant Subjectivity*. 1978;1:117–124.

59. Epstein R. The principle of parsimony and some applications in psychology. *J Mind Behav*. 1984;5:119–130.

Chapter 11

Medicines optimization and illness management research using dyads

Dolly Sud[a,b]

[a]Pharmacy Department, Bradgate Site, Leicestershire Partnership NHS Trust, Leicestershire, United Kingdom, [b]College of Life and Health Sciences, Aston University, Birmingham, United Kingdom

Objectives

- Describe dyadic study designs used in health research.
- Discuss some of the challenges faced in dyadic studies with regards recruitment and data collection and identify strategies that can be used to overcome them.
- Describe some methodological and substantive considerations that require consideration when using dyadic data analysis.

Introduction

There has been much growth in the interest in and use of family-level and dyadic-level theories and methodologies to explore the influence of social relationships on health[1-3] and the influence of health on social relationships.[4,5] Social relationships include those with romantic partners, friends, siblings, children, and care professionals. These individuals play a significant role in the physical health, mental health, and well-being of a patient. An important part of this relationship includes medicines optimization and illness management. Individuals who occupy these roles may themselves experience changes in their own physical health, mental health, and well-being.

Studying health and well-being and consideration of both partners in the context of these close, social relationships is clearly important in health research. As such, both partners become the unit of study—also known as a dyad. Dyadic research approaches can be utilized in qualitative,[6,7] quantitative[8] and mixed methods studies.[9] Illness experience occurs within the contexts of relationships, which underscores the need for dyadic perspectives in research methods and design. Previous literature on chronic illness and stages of illness has highlighted the need to study dyads in health care.[10-13] Dyadic approaches can be utilized during participant recruitment, data collection, data analysis, and as an important target for interventions in both research and in clinical practice.

Studies designed to capture the interdependent complexities of relationships utilizing dyads can provide researchers with new and significant insights that cannot be fully realized with individualistic study designs. This is evident in studies where outcomes have been studied in dyads and then compared to outcomes studied in individuals.[14] Lyons and Lee[15] suggested that the management of illness is a dyadic phenomenon. This is the core tenet of the Theory of Dyadic Illness Management which is expounded in their paper.[15] Further, the way in which dyads appraise illness as a unit influences the ways in which they engage in behaviors to manage illness. Furthermore, there is a bidirectional relationship between this and the "health" of the dyad (Fig. 1). Research can help elucidate contextual factors that are important in this dyadic illness management such as severity of symptoms, age, or type of relationship.

The Theory of Dyadic Illness Management is enhanced by the incorporation of these contextual factors that are considered as risk or protective influences on dyadic appraisal and management behaviors. Contextual factors may be stable or dynamic in their influence over time (Fig. 2). Risk factors are those that contribute to greater incongruence in illness appraisal and less collaboration in dyadic illness management behaviors. Protective factors, on the other hand, are those that impact positively on illness appraisal and lead to more collaborative illness management behaviors. Furthermore, contextual factors are categorized at individual, dyad, family, social or cultural level to represent the various contexts within which the patient and informal carer are situated.

Contemporary Research Methods in Pharmacy and Health Services. https://doi.org/10.1016/B978-0-323-91888-6.00021-1

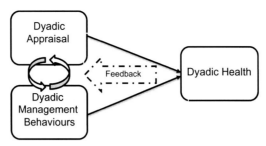

FIG. 1   Central elements of the theory of dyadic illness management. *(Adapted from Lyons KS, Lee CS. The theory of dyadic illness management.* J Fam Nurs. *2018;24(1):8–28. https://doi.org/10.1177/1074840717745669.)*

FIG. 2   Theory of dyadic illness management with predictors. *(Adapted from Lyons KS, Lee CS. The theory of dyadic illness management.* J Fam Nurs. *2018;24(1):8–28. https://doi.org/10.1177/1074840717745669.)*

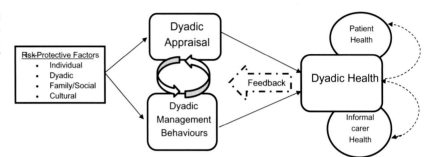

The degree of congruence or incongruence in appraisal of care values and preferences between a patient and their informal carer illustrates very clearly the value of utilizing dyads. For example, in dementia care it is important to ensure that decisions and care planning are made in accordance with wishes and desires of the patient while at the same time empowering their informal carer to be able to make those critical decisions when needed.[16] One study found that incongruence for preferences relating to socioemotional care was a predictor of greater relationship strain and worse mood for the patient with dementia.[17] On the other hand, perceived incongruence for preferences relating to socioemotional care was related to worse mood and a lower quality of life for the informal carer.

Although dyadic research is gaining traction in providing important insights into the interdependence of health within dyads and the transactional nature of how each individual influences the other's health, there is a distinct lack of evidence regarding medicines optimization, illness management and the health of the dyad as a unit. Conceptualization of dyadic health is relatively new but builds upon the second-order dyadic data described by Thompson and Walker.[8] Dyadic factors are important in medicines optimization and health, this may include modifiable individual, dyadic and familial factors associated with optimal versus poor dyadic health. Identification of these factors has enormous potential to inform how interventions in research and clinical practice are tailored to the dyad as a unit. Importantly, in a way that not possible with "one size fits all" or individual approaches.

This chapter is broken down into five main sections.

(1) Dyadic study configurations used in health research
(2) Challenges faced in dyadic research that can occur during recruitment and data collection, and strategies that can be used to overcome them
(3) Dyadic data collection and analysis
(4) Methodological and substantive considerations that require consideration when using dyadic study designs
(5) Medicines optimization and illness management research which utilize dyads

(1) Dyadic study configurations used in health research

There are potentially four different configurations with each individual within the dyad either diagnosed (D) with an illness/disease/ailment or undiagnosed (U)[18–22]:

● Diagnosed/Undiagnosed (DU) studies: one individual is diagnosed and the other member of the dyad is undiagnosed.
● Undiagnosed/Undiagnosed (UU) studies: for example, in health prevention or health promotion studies.

- Diagnosed/Diagnosed (DD) studies: for example, the diagnosis is couple-level, e.g., infertility.
- A blend of DU, DD, and UU couples all within the same study, such that one, both, or neither of the members is diagnosed.

The most frequently used configuration in the current published literature is diagnosed/undiagnosed (DU). In these studies, the individual who is undiagnosed is commonly referred to as an informal carer, carer, caregiver or someone who provides support. Table 1 provides some examples of dyadic study configurations.

(2) Challenges that can be faced in dyadic research that can occur during recruitment and data collection, and strategies that can be used to overcome them

Although dyadic research is a significant approach to understand different perspectives on relationships, it is accompanied by a unique set of methodological challenges. These challenges center around participant recruitment, participant retention, and data collection.[23–26] Thoughtful study design and planning can help overcome many of these. Table 2 provides an in depth description of the challenges and potential strategies to overcome them.

The terminology and language used during the recruitment process can be important. For example, considering sensitivities around the use of the terms "informal carer," "carer," or "caregiver" when asking a patient to identify someone to participate in a study as their dyad. Patients may be reluctant to acknowledge their need for informal carers and may not think of family members or persons helping them as informal carers. Similarly, individuals who are informal carers may not see themselves in this role. Instead, a patient could be asked to identify someone who is not a care professional but provides a significant amount of support for them.

Consideration and monitoring for informal carer burden when planning the study intervention and data collection scheme, including measures of informal carer burden as a study outcome can be useful. Eligibility criteria for informal carers must be clearly thought through, clearly defining the dyad-specific protocol as criteria might limit the participation of the informal carer and prevent completion of the study protocol of studies applying these dyadic configurations. Finally, during budget planning the need to provide clear and separate incentives for informal carer depending on the extent of participation in the study is important. Table 2 provides more detail.

(3) Dyadic data collection and analysis

Methods used to analyze data will depend on whether the study is qualitative or quantitative. Analytical methods used in these studies will thus be driven by how the data are collected. For example, in qualitative studies if separate interviews are undertaken, then data analysis will involve a process of contrasting and comparing data obtained from each individual to identify contrasts and overlaps. With regards quantitative approaches, there are three main methods: Actor-Partner Interdependence Model, One-with-many design, and the Social Relations Model.

- **Methods used to collect and analyze qualitative dyadic data**

There are different approaches to collecting qualitative data from dyads. These include:

- Separate (individual) interviews.
- Separate interviews performed simultaneously by different interviewers.
- Joint interviews.
- Both separate and joint interviews with same individuals.
- Separate interviews with some informants and joint interviews with others.

Although interviews are specified here, this approach might equally apply to the use of other qualitative data collection methods (e.g., observation, document studies such as personal diaries).

Each of these approaches has its own benefits and drawbacks and may be applicable or more suitable in particular circumstances. Table 3 provides a detailed comparison of the different data collection approaches.[27] For example, benefits of conducting separate interviews simultaneously by different interviewers include: the research interviewer is not influenced by the previously interviewed individual and individuals taking part in the research may feel this as an additional safeguard of confidentiality. A potential drawback of this approach is that each research interviewer comes with a slightly different and unique worldview on phenomenon, with unique way of constructing the interview situation. Therefore, it may be preferable then to use this when the two interviewers have similar worldviews on the phenomenon under study.

Approaches to dyadic data analysis are no different to those used qualitative studies involving individuals, which can for example involve a thematic analysis or a grounded theory approach. What is unique to dyadic data analysis is the process by which themes are identified. This is performed by contrasting and comparing data obtained from each individual involved

TABLE 1 Dyadic study configurations and examples.

Design—dyad	Type of study	Brief summary of study objective	Country, number and description of dyad and data analysis approach	Outcomes and results
Diagnosed/ Undiagnosed (DU)	Quantitative	To examine the influence of racial/ ethnic concordance between participants and research staff on respiratory study attrition.[19]	USA. 509 dyads. Data were pooled from participants and clinical research coordinators in six longitudinal studies of respiratory illness. Multilevel modeling examined the effect of racial/ ethnic concordance on attrition at the first and one-year follow-ups	Reported that Spanish language, lower education, and greater depressive symptoms predicted greater attrition, but these effects disappeared in adjusted models. Race/ethnicity, age, gender, and health literacy did not predict attrition. Contrary to hypotheses, attrition was greater among concordant than discordant dyads: attrition was almost five times greater at first follow-up for Black and Hispanic participants in concordant dyads, and almost four times greater at one year.
Undiagnosed/ Undiagnosed (UU)	Quantitative	To assess the role of adolescent romantic partners on the expression of health behavior.[20]	USA. 80 romantic dyads. A longitudinal multilevel analysis was conducted.	The study found evidence for partner similarity and partner influence with the majority of health-harming behaviors. Specifically, partner influence was evident for smoking and alcohol use with partner influence approaching significance for marijuana use. Limited evidence was found for partner similarity and partner influence for health-protective behaviors.
Diagnosed/ Diagnosed (DD) There is a paucity of data using this approach	Quantitative	Explore the transmission of depressive symptoms among spouses undergoing assisted reproduction treatment.[21]	Germany. 82 romantic dyads. Both partners' stress appraisals and depressive symptoms were assessed at three measurement points throughout assisted-reproduction treatment. Relations among partners' variables were tested using the actor-partner interdependence model.	Findings indicated positive transmission effects of depressive symptoms from men to women across both measurement intervals. A positive transmission effect of stress appraisals from men to women was observed from before until after the pregnancy test. Women's stress appraisals mediated part of the transmission of depressive symptoms from men to women. Men's stress appraisals, however, were unrelated to women's earlier depressive symptoms. Men's earlier depressive symptoms might have operated as cues for women's adjustment of their own stress appraisals, which then predicted women's increased depressive symptoms.

TABLE 1 Dyadic study configurations and examples—cont'd

Design—dyad	Type of study	Brief summary of study objective	Country, number and description of dyad and data analysis approach	Outcomes and results
A blend of DU, DD, and UU couples all within the same study, such that one, both, or neither of the members is diagnosed.	Quantitative	Weight status and weight concerns were examined[22]	USA. 208 romantic dyads. Romantic partners' weight status and weight concerns were examined using the Actor—Partner Interdependence Model.	Results indicated that participants' weight concerns were associated with their weight status. Men and women who were relatively heavy and who had relatively thin romantic partners were most likely to express weight concerns.

in the dyad, to identify contrasts and overlaps. Analysis of data following this process can lead to reconstruction of existing themes and generation of new themes. Eiskovits and Koren[27] provide an excellent review on approaches to dyadic interview analysis. Perspectives acquired from contrasting and comparing views of each individual within the dyad provides insights on particular issues, such as the impact of the dynamic of the relationship on health. As such, this analysis generates a dyadic version that is greater than the sum of the two individual parts.[27] This dyadic version is produced by the researcher while simultaneously keeping individuals' data intact.

- **Methods used to collect and analyze quantitative dyadic data**

Data collection methods are no different to those used to collect data in individualistic study designs (e.g., questionnaires, rating scales) and will be driven by the research question. A wide range of models have been developed to study dyads, with three approaches being the most common: Actor-Partner Interdependence Model (APIM), One-with-many design, and the Social Relations Model (SRM).

Actor-partner interdependence model (APIM)

The actor-partner interdependence model is the most widely used standard dyadic model for quantitative data analysis.[28] It simultaneously estimates the effects of individuals' characteristics on an outcome variable. As such, it requires variables, X and Y, where X causes or predicts Y. It is important to note that because the APIM assesses both actor and partner effects, both X and Y must be measured within both members of the dyad.

For example, consider the effect of coping with a diagnosis of schizophrenia on informal carers' quality of life. It may be that the patient's coping with their diagnosis of schizophrenia impacts both their own and their informal carer's quality of life. The effect of the patient coping with their diagnosis on his/her own quality of life is called an actor effect, and the effect of the patient's coping with their diagnosis on informal carer's quality of life is called a partner effect (see Fig. 3).

One-with-many design

Here, each person is paired with many other dyadic individuals, but these are not paired with any other individuals.[28] For example, a pharmacist might be paired with many patients. The patients may rate their satisfaction with the quality of care provided by this one pharmacist. As such, there are multiple patients rating the same pharmacist. In this design, patients are not linked to each other in any way, and they do not interact with each other.

Social relations model

In a social relations model (SRM), each individual is a dyad with multiple other individuals and each of these individuals is also paired with multiple other individuals. There are two types of SRMs,[28] the first is a round-robin design in which a group of individuals rate or interact with each other, meaning that all individuals are linked to everyone else in the group. For example, in a random group of third year pharmacy students each individual rates the ability of each of the other students in

TABLE 2 Common challenges that can arise in recruitment and data collection in dyadic research, and strategies that can be used to overcome them.[23]

	Potential challenges	Possible strategies
Recruitment and sampling Dyads can be accessed from many settings: e.g., secondary care (inpatient, outpatient), primary care (GP, clinics). Each setting requires carefully developed recruitment strategies.	**Terminology** Patients may be reluctant to acknowledge the need for informal carers and may not think of family members or persons helping them as informal carers. Individuals who are informal carers may not see themselves in this role.	Asking the patient to identify a person who(m): - is spending the most time with them, - is providing the most support or care for them, - is a family member with whom they discuss their health concerns with most of the time, - they turn to for assistance with medication or illness management. These are suggested examples, the decision as to how this is phrased will ultimately be driven by the need to identify of the most appropriate informal carer for the study.
	Approach to recruitment—who to recruit first Informal carer may be recruited via the patient or vice-versa or both. In other words, recruit the patient first and then recruit the informal carer via them or recruit the informal carer and then recruit the patient via them. This may depend on, for example, the setting.	Be clear in recruitment strategies as to which approach has been chosen taking account of contextual factors such as setting. Using both approaches may maximize the number of dyads recruited.
	Approach to recruitment—medium Recruitment using postal methods only has been shown to yield varying results[24]	Consider combining different methods, e.g., face-to-face contact followed up by a phone call.[25] A phone call will also provide an opportunity to discuss the study in more detail and answer any questions.
	Attrition of either member of the dyad due to details of study not being clear Reliance on either member of the dyad to explain the purpose and expected involvement may not be effective.	Develop materials and strategies to ensure each member of the dyad clearly understands the study, e.g., "script" for telephone call, easy to read leaflet (using lay language). This material should also explain why the involvement of both individuals is helpful.
	Timing of recruitment Each individual within the dyad may have their own commitments that may need accommodating (e.g., other caring responsibilities).	Inquire as to when might be an appropriate time for either or both to be involved in the study will help the patient and their informal carer plan and be prepared and will minimize the risk of attrition. Be flexible and accommodating in your approach.
	Eligibility criteria for informal carers Criteria might limit the participation of the informal carer and prevent completion of the study protocol. On the other hand, the protocol may necessitate recruiting dyads where both members have an illness.	Specific and clear eligibility criteria must be stated in the research protocol. This may depend on the study aims and objectives.
	Participation may be dependent upon discussion between individuals within the dyad Even if one individual is interested in participating, they may not be willing to agree until they have had the opportunity to discuss the study with the other member of the dyad and obtained their agreement. In addition, patients may be reluctant to ask informal carers to participate if they feel that that individual is already doing too much for them and participating in the study might be viewed as another burden they are adding.	Obtain permission from one individual within the dyad then calling the other individual and explain the study to them. Accommodate for potential refusals, e.g., time, resources

	Both individuals have the same diagnosis During the recruitment process it may be revealed that both individuals have the same diagnosis.	This may serve as part of the exclusion criteria (see above). Develop clear guidance ahead of study commencement to accommodate for this, e.g., the individual who has been most recently diagnosed will be assigned as the patient. Alternatively, randomly select one individual from the dyad who will be assigned as the patient.
	Sample size Consider the statistical power needed to answer the research question taking into account the potential attrition of either or both individuals	Estimation of sample size must be based on patient and informal carer attrition rates described in the existing literature or obtained in preliminary studies.
Consent Individual separate written consent forms are usually required for patients and informal carers before study-related activities.	**Each member of the dyad** Individual separate written consent forms will be required for each member of the dyad.	Seek advice from your ethics committees and research teams for further details.
	Consent forms—content It is important to reduce family members' perceptions of coercion to participate.	Consent forms need to include comment that indicates that the data will be used together. Informal carers are not receiving care, so the language in the consent needs to indicate that, if the family member declines, the patient will still receive all entitled care.
Retention Personal contact and development of a good rapport between the researcher and participant have been identified as crucial strategies for recruitment and retention into any study.[26]	**Effective communication skills** Each individual within the dyad may have their own and different concerns about the study. They must be in an environment that they feel comfortable in and may express to do this with the other member of the dyad or separately or both.	During the first conversation allow each participant an opportunity to share concerns about the study or about his or her own life situation facilitates trust They may want to do this at their own home rather than in a healthcare setting. If this is done at their own home then, take care to ensure privacy is observed if they express concern, e.g., other member of the dyad within earshot.
Attrition Careful tracking is required.	**One member of the dyad may want to drop out** Plans and decisions need to made well in advance at the start of the study as how this will be dealt with, e.g., will the patient or informal carer continue in the study if the other dyad member drops out? The decision should be based on the potential contributions of the retained individual from the dyad to the knowledge development, study results and available study resources. Including an "incomplete dyad" in the study could add costs unless the data collected are useful.	If the patient drops out and continuing to follow the informal carer will not contribute to the study aims, the research staff can thank the informal carer for his or her contribution and time thus far and provide any incentive, e.g., gift voucher due the person. Depending on the questionnaires used in the study, the researcher can also explain that it might be difficult to respond to the study questions because the situation with the original dyad has changed.
Data collection and delivery of study. Intervention	**Collection of data—together, separately, or both** This will influence the proximity of participants to each other.	Whether or not the data collection takes place together or separately will be driven by the underlying purpose, framework, and design of the study. However, consider how this might affect the quality and accuracy of the data and incorporate that into the final decision.

Continued

TABLE 2 Common challenges that can arise in recruitment and data collection in dyadic research, and strategies that can be used to overcome them—cont'd

Potential challenges	Possible strategies
	Depending on the study and if the protocol allows then participants may be asked to give express their preference. But bear in mind this could introduce a bias in responses due to one individual exerting an influence on the other individual's responses. If the data collection occurs at home, then separate rooms out of earshot of others may be necessary (e.g., sensitive data are being collected).
	If collecting information from the dyad (two individuals together) then the protocol needs to include specific instructions for research staff to give to dyads about responding, e.g., the importance of gaining each individual's different perspective and asking them not to confer.
	If the decision is made to collect the data from each individual separately then, before separating them, each person should be assured of confidentiality regarding his or her responses.
Confidentiality Researchers collecting data need to be careful that they do not share data about an individual in the dyad with the other individual.	Depending on the purpose of the study, researchers should reinforce that the information gained will not be shared by study staff with either individual in the dyad without his or her permission. To keep patient and partner information confidential, the research protocol may require separate data collectors. If only one data collector is available, the dyad should be given the choice of having the researcher work with one participant at a time. This allows each participant the opportunity to address concerns or questions separately. Thus, if there is only one data collector, the additional burden of time on the participants and researcher for data collection must be accounted for in the planning of the study.
Intervention delivery Consider the potential effect of the intervention on not only the patient but also the informal carer, e.g., the informal carer may need to take on additional responsibilities.	Different parts of the study intervention may need to be delivered together to the dyad as a unit and separately to each individual. Separating may cause some concern for either individual in the dyad; thus, the research staff need to be trained adequately to address concerns and provide explanations. Consider including measures of burden or distress to ensure that interventions to improve patient outcomes do not also have unintended negative effects on the informal carer.

Data collection at different time points from individuals	If collecting data from individuals within the dyad at different time points then the individual who participates first may discuss the study with the other individual within the dyad and this may impact on the data collected.	Request to the first participant that they avoid discussing the study with the other dyad member. This may be difficult to fully account for and unavoidable. However, it must be acknowledged as a limitation
Budgeting	**Costs to be considered** Travel, incentives, additional caring responsibilities.	If individuals travel separately then account for the travel needs of each individual. If the study requires both individuals to be present to take part at the same time then ensure that the time is scheduled to account for the fact that they may be traveling from different places. Each individual within the dyad should receive an incentive to take part. A greater number of research staff may be needed (see above) as well as office space and computers and this will also need to be accounted for Informal carers may have other caring responsibilities, e.g., children.

Although much of the focus is on the patient-informal carer dyad a lot of what has been discussed could apply to other types of dyads (different types of relationships).

TABLE 3 Comparison between five modes of dyadic analysis for qualitative data.

Mode	Benefits	Drawbacks	Contextual information that should be considered
Separate interviews	Each individual within the dyad can provide information from their own perspective. They capture the individual within the dyad, without forgoing the dyadic perspective. The dyadic view (a third version) provided by the researcher(s) enriches the perspective on the phenomenon. Trustworthiness is increased (by triangulation.	The partner is virtually present in the research space. It can limit the perception of the phenomenon, as restricted by what partner said. The dyadic version provided by the researcher (s) is largely interpretive and distant from the descriptive level. There is an ethical problem of revealing information to partner when presenting quotes of each partner alongside each other	This mode is particularly useful when researching sensitive topics. Most couples have topics that remain private and are not discussed or shared with each other. Interviewer as stranger makes it easier to reveal and discuss issues, e.g., coercive behaviors.
Separate interviews performed simultaneously by different interviewers	All of the advantages stated above. Interviewer will not be influenced by the previously interviewed participant; participants feel additional safeguard.	Each interviewer comes with a slightly different and unique worldview.	This mode is preferable when two interviewers have similar worldviews on the phenomenon.
Joint interviews	Allows for a view of a joint picture and shared narrative. Enables learning from the way partner interact, dominate, or are subdued about their role in the relationship.	This mode does not allow for the development individual versions. Reduces imbalances (which are desirable in dyadic research) between versions because partners are witness to each other and this decreases the material for analysis	Is useful for analyzing interactions between individuals with the dyad.
Both separate and joint interviews with same participants	Carries the benefits of separate and joint interviews.	Impact of what each individual is witness to in the joint interview may impact on versions presented and vice versa.	When topic is not too sensitive. When interaction analysis is a required part of the research study.
Separate interviews with some informants and joint interviews with others.	Facilitates comparisons, cross-checking, and is a form of triangulation.	Triangulation only possible when large sample sizes are used.	When large samples and budgets available.

Adapted from Eisikovits Z, Koren C. Approaches to and outcomes of dyadic interview analysis. *Qual Health Res.* 2010;20(12):1642–1655. https://doi.org/10.1177/1049732310376520.

the group to communicate information about a prescribed medication or health condition (reciprocal measurement). In round robin designs, all individuals in the group are engaged in interactions in all possible pairs. This allows researchers to study the whole group and to gather dyadic interaction data.

The second is known as block design. In block design, a group of individuals is divided into two subgroups, and members of each subgroup rate or interact with members of the other subgroup. All the individuals of one group interact with all individuals of another group and vice versa. There are two types of block design: in symmetric block design: the two groups are indistinguishable (e.g., both groups are made up of students from the same school of pharmacy) and asymmetric block design: the two groups are distinguishable (each group is made up of students from different schools of pharmacy). Data are collected on the interactions of individuals from one group with individuals of the other group.

(4) Methodological and substantive considerations that require consideration when using dyadic study designs

There are a range of important issues that researchers should consider when utilizing dyadic data designs in health research. Study findings are more robust if these issues are properly addressed. Given that this is still a growing area of research,

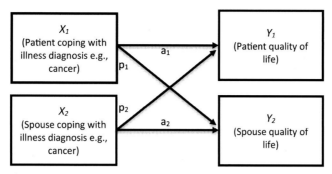

FIG. 3 The Actor-Partner Interdependence Model (APIM). An actor effect, denoted as "a," occurs when an individual's score on the predictor variable (X_1) predicts that same individual's score on the outcome variable (Y_1). A partner effect, denoted as "p," occurs when an individual's score on a predictor variable (X_1) predicts her partner's score on an outcome variable (Y_2). Both members of the dyad have an actor effect and a partner effect. *(Adapted from Reed RG, Butler EA, Kenny DA. Dyadic models for the study of health. Soc Personal Psychol Compass. 2013;7(4):228–245. doi:10.1111/spc3.12022.)*

this is even more important as it will ensure that the growing body of literature being formed further informs our understanding in the field of dyadic research. Most of the discussion around methodological considerations in dyadic research will focus on the diagnosed/undiagnosed (DU) configuration, as this has been the most frequently adopted dyadic configuration to date.

- **Impact of partner effects**

The presence of partner effects is important as they traverse individualistic thinking and allow for analysis of interdependent mechanisms that impact on health. An example of a partner effect might be where the mental health of a patient affects their informal carers mental health. A study of 341 parent-adolescent dyads conducted over five years in the United States of America (USA)[29] aimed to examine how discrimination changes over time, how discrimination is related to health and substance use, and whether discrimination spills over to affect the health of family members. One of the outcomes explored was the association between an individual's experiences of discrimination and their family member's mental health. One of the findings of this study was that increases in parents' reports of discrimination were related to increases in adolescents' levels of depressive symptoms. Partner effects are useful, as they reveal the role that partners may have in promoting others' health above and beyond the effect that individuals have on promoting their own health.

Role as a moderator of actor and partner effects

Frequently, in diagnosed/undiagnosed (DU) configuration studies a key question is whether actor or partner effects for diagnosed and undiagnosed partners can reveal differences intra-person versus inter-person.[28] To test for asymmetry of effects by role (i.e., "diagnosed" vs. "undiagnosed"), one can undertake tests of interactions between the distinguishing feature (e.g., the role, such as "diagnosed" vs. "undiagnosed") and the predictor variables (e.g., coping). The aim here is to elucidate if any of the interactions by role predicts the outcome. One example of asymmetry in actor effects can be seen in a diagnosed/undiagnosed (DU) configuration study in which fear of cancer recurrence in survivors and their informal carers was examined.[30] Dyadic individuals (both survivors and informal carers) who reported less positive meaning of the illness had more fear of recurrence, but this relation was stronger for survivors than for informal carers.

Testing interactions with role helps elucidate factors that might have a greater or lesser importance to diagnosed and undiagnosed individuals, and therefore to their well-being. Identifying asymmetric effects by testing interactions with role provides useful information that could potentially facilitate focus intervention efforts for both diagnosed and undiagnosed partners.

Bidirectional influence

The concept of bidirectionality represents a process of influence between individuals within a dyad whereby each influences the other as well as the dyadic relationship. It represents the idea of mutual influence and cocreation of dyadic outcomes including health outcomes. Bidirectional influence can be tested using two hypotheses.[28] Bidirectionality is supported only if both partner effects are present (e.g., if X_1 predicts Y_2 and X_2 predicts Y_1, or in other words the diagnosed partner's X predicts the undiagnosed partner's Y and vice versa). Bidirectional effects can either be symmetric (the two effects are both either positive or negative predictors of the outcome) or asymmetric (both are present, but with opposite signs). In a longitudinal study of grandparent-grandchild well-being,[31] grandchild and grandparent well-being were found to be related in a bidirectional manner, but grandchild difficulties have a greater impact on grandparent distress than do grandparent difficulties on grandchild distress.

Identification of specific bidirectional processes which are conserved, and which are diminished by a diagnosis can inform about which relational processes could be maximized, versus those that may need extra attention when dyads are making adjustments (e.g., taking a newly prescribed medication) as the result of a new diagnosis or a different stage within a diagnosis.

Asymmetry in Y intercepts

A question that is of particular relevance to diagnosed/undiagnosed (DU) studies is whether or not asymmetry exists in the Y intercepts, or the predicted average score on the outcome variable, when comparing diagnosed partner with an undiagnosed partner.[28] For example, mothers with cancer may report higher, lower, or the same quality of life as their adult informal carer daughters.[32] Frequently, there are mean differences on Y between the diagnosed and undiagnosed members of the dyad. As the outcome variable is often related to physical and/or mental health then this is likely. Additionally, it can be assumed that health scores may differ between the diagnosed and undiagnosed member of the dyad. Further, undiagnosed and diagnosed individuals within a dyad may also be different in outcome measures related to physical health and this may of particular interest; in such instances physical health would need to be controlled during the data analysis process to demonstrate that individuals differ on these outcomes after controlling for differences in their health.

Including an undiagnosed-undiagnosed group

Researchers might want to consider including an undiagnosed/undiagnosed (UU) group as a control in diagnosed/diagnosed (DD) or diagnosed/undiagnosed (DU) studies.[28] In a DD study, this would allow for an exploration of the strength of impact of actor and partner effects. In a DU study, this would allow an understanding of how undiagnosed partners in DU couples, compare to individuals in couples completely free of the diagnosis and would provide important information about whether undiagnosed individuals in DU couples have poorer health than those in couples without a diagnosis. Studies conducted with couples in which both smoked reported increased positive emotion and emotional synchrony when smoking together. On the other hand, couples where only one person smoked reported decreased positive emotion and synchrony when their partner lit up.[33,34] These findings illustrate that those experiencing dissonance in relationships (e.g., one member smokes and the other does not) may be at greater risk for experiencing relationship- or health-oriented concerns.

Examining mediation

Mediation in its simplest sense consists of three variables X (the causal variable), M (the mediator) and Y (the outcome).[28] For example, positive communication between a mother and child where the child has asthma may reduce distress due to greater closeness. For this example, maternal communication is X, closeness is M, and distress is Y. The idea being that mediation explains the association between X and Y. A more advanced topic involves moderated mediation, and readers should consult additional resources for examples and further explanation.[35–37] Moderation is usually examined by looking at the interaction between the causal variable (X) and another variable called the moderator; if mediation is moderated, then mediation is stronger for one individual (e.g., diagnosed) than another (e.g., undiagnosed). This method is useful if there is an interest in understanding causal processes that occur when studying dyads and the impact of disease.

Including time

Longitudinal research is a growing field within dyadic studies that involve multiple time points per variable or per person.[28] Longitudinal studies have the potential to address the dynamic aspects of health and social relationships. Similar to studies with individuals, these can take the form of daily-diary studies (e.g., exploring the impact of pain from metastatic breast cancer on spousal relationships[38]), intervention studies (e.g., the influence of a "warm touch" intervention in married couples on blood pressure, oxytocin, alpha amylase, and cortisol[39]) or repeated mental or physical health assessments (e.g., measurements of cortisol levels and mood states in romantic partners[40]).

This type of study might be useful if, for example, researchers want to explore the impact of baseline characteristics over time or to assess if an intervention's effects were maintained over time. Introducing time in dyadic research allows researchers to assess partners' health change and flexibility (or inflexibility) over a specified duration.

(5) Medicines optimization and illness management research which utilize dyads

This section discussed specific examples of medicines optimization research that utilize approaches and methods outlined previously. The results of studies using these approaches can inform clinical practice.

- **A dyadic approach to understanding the medication dialogue in patient–provider relationships.**[41]

  The objectives of the study were to describe typologies of dyadic communication between healthcare professionals and their hypertensive patients about prescribed antihypertensive medications in primary care settings. The dyads were (i) nurses and patients (ii) doctors and patients.

  Qualitative data analysis of 94 audiotaped encounters between individuals in each dyad was carried out using grounded theory. In this study, four types of dyadic exchanges were identified: interactive (53% of interactions), divergent-traditional (24% of interactions), convergent-traditional (17% of interactions), and disconnected (6% of interactions). In the interactive and convergent-traditional types, healthcare professionals adopted a patient-centered approach and used communication behaviors to engage patients. The divergent-traditional type was characterized by provider verbal dominance, which had a negative impact on patients' abilities to interact. In the disconnected type, healthcare professionals used closed-ended questions and terse conversation, which was frequently disregarded by patients who diverted the conversation to psychosocial issues.

  Examining the processes that underpin communication in patient–healthcare professional interactions can provide useful information toward improve conversations about medication.

- **A qualitative analysis of a dyad approach to health-related quality of life measurement in children with asthma.**[42]

  The objective of this research was to observe and describe the interaction between the parent and the child in a dyad interview. Specifically, this study sought to understand how parent and child perspectives are used and where the parent may expand the child's cognitive abilities to create a more meaningful description of the child's health-related quality of life (HRQOL). The dyad was a child with a clinical diagnosis of asthma and their parent (primary informal carer).

  Qualitative data analysis of 16 audiotaped interactions between individuals in each dyad was carried out using grounded theory. Eleven themes relating to dyad interaction were identified: (1) recall difficulty (e.g., recall of frequency of medication use), (2) respondent bias (e.g., social desirability), (3) interviewer bias (e.g., cultural bias), (4) frustration (e.g., irrelevant questions), (5) coercion/parental influence (e.g., answering questions for children), (6) inter-relational conflict (e.g., conflict aversion), (7) psychic discomfort for health states (e.g., concerns about past, present and future health and ability), (8) emotional sensitivity (e.g., physical burden of illness), (9) parent as advocate (e.g., providing interviewer with additional relevant information about child), (10) parent as enabler (e.g., discussing and negotiating answer with child), and (11) comprehension (e.g., difficulty understanding the meaning of a particular word).

  The study resulted in the creation of an interview guide to accompany the administration of standardized HRQOL questionnaires to parent child dyads. This guide could help facilitate discussion between parent and child and enhance the consistency during research and clinical practice. The authors reported that parents were a valuable resource in overcoming issues associated with inaccurate recall of medication for example. Parents often enhanced their child's ability to remember by providing examples of past activities as chronological "bookmarks" to aid recall of medication use and asthma-related difficulties.

- **Long-term antidepressant use: A qualitative study on perspectives of patients and general practitioners in primary care.**[43]

  The objective in this study was to understand the motivations of patients and GPs related to long-term antidepressant use and to gain insight into possibilities to prevent unnecessary long-term use. The dyad was a patient and their general practitioner (GP), 30 dyads were included in the study. Patient in the study had anxiety and/or depressive disorder. Semistructured interviews were undertaken separately with the patient and their GP.

  Data analysis was carried out based using the constant comparative method. This method allows for updates to topic guides in the light of themes identified during interview conduct. Through identification of new and discussion of a priori understandings, this method is both inductive and deductive in its approach. Interviews were analysed using computer-assisted data analysis (MAXQDA®) software. The motives and barriers to continue or discontinue antidepressants were related to availability of supportive guidance during discontinuation, personal circumstances of the patient, and considerations of the patient or GP.

  This study adds information about an aspect of care that could benefit from a shared decision-making process. The authors of the study reported large variation in policies of general practices around long-term use and continuation or discontinuation of antidepressants in dyads. Patients and GPs appeared to be unaware of each other's [mismatching] expectations regarding responsibility to start discussions around discontinuation or continuation. The findings of this study highlight the importance of the need for discussion between patients and GPs about antidepressant use and continuation and that this may help clarify mutual expectations and opinions. Agreements between a patient and their GP can be included in a person-centered treatment plan.

- **Differential patient—Informal carer opinions of treatment and care for advanced lung cancer patients.**[44]

  This study sought to find out two therapeutic questions. First, what the major differences are in opinions regarding treatment and care decisions between patients and their informal carers. Second, how differences of opinion regarding treatment and care decisions in the family affect the psychological well-being of patients and informal carers. Cancer patients and their informal carers (dyads) were recruited. Data was collected using questionnaires undertaken separately with each individual within 171 dyads about healthcare decisions such as where, when, and how to receive treatment; decisions on trade-off treatment benefits and side effects; and decisions about hospice care.

  Quantitative data analysis was carried out using nonparametric tests and regression analysis. Significant disagreement occurred about three issues: trade-off between treatment side effects and benefits; reporting adverse effects of medication to clinicians, and hospice care. Informal carers were more concerned about patient's quality of life and more willing to discuss hospice issues than were patients. Perceived family disagreement is associated with depression in both informal carers and patients.

  The study provided empirical evidence for patient-informal carer disagreement about treatment and care decisions and its significant adverse impact on both patients and informal carers.

- **Patient and physician beliefs about control over health: Association of symmetrical beliefs with medication regimen adherence.**[45]

  The objective of this study was to examine the extent to which patient and doctor (dyad) symmetry in health locus of control (HLOC) beliefs was associated with objectively derived measure of medication adherence in patients with diabetes mellitus and hypertension. A total of 224 dyads were included in the study. Data was collected using questionnaires undertaken separately with the patient and their doctor.

  Quantitative data analysis was conducted using linear modeling to account for clustering of patients within doctors. In dyads in which there were congruent beliefs about the degree of personal control that individual patients have over health outcomes the patients significantly higher overall and cardiovascular medication adherence ($p = 0.03$) and lower diastolic blood pressure ($p = 0.02$) when compared to dyads in which the patient had a stronger belief in their own personal control than did their doctor. Dyads in which patients held a weaker belief in their own personal control than did their doctor did not differ significantly from symmetrical dyads.

  This study demonstrated the importance of attitudinal symmetry on medication adherence and suggested that a brief assessment of patient HLOC may be useful for tailoring the doctors' approach in clinical interactions or for matching patients to doctors with similar attitudes toward care.

- **Factors associated with intensification of oral diabetes medications in primary care provider-patient dyads: A cohort study.**[46]

  The objective of this study was to identify previously unidentified visit-based factors associated with intensification of oral diabetes medications in diabetes. The dyad in this study was an adult who had a diagnosis of diabetes and their healthcare professional. Data was collected from two main sources. First, electronic files (enrolment, utilization, laboratory results, and pharmacy use). Second, from handwritten medical records (data on medical history and visit-based clinical factors).

  Analysis of clinician-patient interactions were carried out using generalized estimating equations with an exchangeable correlation structure to construct unadjusted and partially adjusted (for patient age, race, sex, comorbidity using resource utilization bands, and glycemic control using HbA_1c) logistic regression models for each of these variables. Data analysis was carried out for 574 hyperglycemic patient visits.

  Clinician-patient dyads intensified oral diabetes treatment in 128 (22%) of 574 hyperglycemic visits by patients. Worse glycaemia was an important predictor of intensification. Treatment was more likely to be intensified for patients who attended for a "routine" visit, patients taking two or more oral antidiabetic drugs, or for patients with longer intervals between visits. Treatment was less likely to be intensified in the presence of the following: patients with less recent HbA_{1c} measurements, patients with a higher number of prior visits, and patients identified as African American.

  This study reported that many patients with poor glycemic control, despite treatment do not receive timely and appropriate intensification of therapy.[47] This study highlights aspects of practice that could be the focus of quality improvement measures in the management of type 2 diabetes: overcoming inertia, improving continuity of care, and reducing racial disparities.

Key considerations when utilizing dyads in medicines optimization and illness management research

- Although dyadic research is a significant approach to achieve perspectives on relationships, it is accompanied by a unique set of methodological challenges. These challenges center around recruitment, retention, and data collection.[23–26] Thoughtful study design and planning ahead can help overcome many of these.
- Methods used to analyze data will depend on whether the study is qualitative or quantitative, in all cases will be driven by how the data is collected. Method chosen will also depend on the research question being asked.
- Partner effects are useful as they reveal the role that partners may have in promoting the others' heath above and beyond the effect that individuals have on promoting their own health.
- Identifying asymmetric effects by testing interactions with role provides useful information about factors that could potentially facilitate the focus of intervention efforts for both diagnosed and undiagnosed partners.
- Identification of bidirectional processes can provide information about which relational processes could be maximized, versus those that may need extra attention when dyads are making adjustments, such as taking a new medication, as the result of a new diagnosis or a different stage within a diagnosis.
- Including undiagnosed-undiagnosed dyads in research aids in understanding of the impact of concordant and discordant relationships on risk for experiencing more relationship- or health-oriented concerns due to diagnosis.
- Examining the effect of mediation is useful if there is an interest in understanding causal process that occurs when studying dyads and the impact of disease.
- Including time (longitudinal research) has the potential to address dynamic aspects of health and social relationships. For example, in research if the effects or implementation of interventions are maintained over time.

Conclusion

Individuals' physical and mental health can impact on their social relationships and vice versa. Partners, parents, children, friends, and care professionals all play a critical role in supporting the health of patients; utilizing dyads in research has great potential. An important, unique, and valuable perspective is obtained on the complex interactions that underpin the management of illness and medicines optimization by situating experiences of these within the dyad. The purpose of this chapter was to provide a gentle introduction to this growing field and to clarify some of the main issues with regards the research process and possible implications for clinical practice. Additionally, shedding light on some important methodological and substantive considerations that researchers may want to focus on. This chapter should provide a starting point to inform researchers who wish to pursue this within their own work. The provision of specific examples in relation to medicines optimization and illness management should also further excite readers to consider dyadic research. It would appear, that this is yet relatively untouched but potentially vast area for researchers who have an interest in medicines optimization and illness management.

Questions for further discussion

1. How does dyadic appraisal of illness and medication change over time with the course of illness and treatment, and what is the recursive association of this with dyadic management?
2. Mention has been made of the important role that research using dyads might play in driving future interventions to improve patient-informal carer dyadic health. What is the distinction between such interventions being dyad based versus interventions that are dyad focused?
3. Is it possible to have a healthcare system that can provide dyad focused interventions and what might the long term benefits be, e.g., for the healthcare system itself?

Application exercise/scenario

Think about a patient or a person you provide care for or who you know has a long-term condition (e.g., schizophrenia, autism, arthritis, asthma, diabetes, epilepsy). Consider the different relationships they have that are important in their care and choose one of these to focus on. Think about specific contextual factors that are important within those relationships that might impact on medicines optimization or illness management. Then think about the most appropriate methods that might be used to research that dyad relationship to explore those contextual factors. Finally, consider how might the findings of such a research project inform or be important for provision of healthcare services or guidelines and policy.

References

1. Reblin M, Uchino BN. Social and emotional support and its implication for health. *Int J Behav Healthc Res.* 2008;21(2):201–205. https://doi.org/10.1097/YCO.0b013e3282f3ad89.Social.

2. Harandi TF, Taghinasab MM, Nayeri TD. The correlation of social support with mental health: a meta-analysis. *Electron Physician.* 2017;(September):5212–5222. https://doi.org/10.19082/5212.

3. Wallston B, Alagna S, DeVellis B, DeVellis R. Social support and physical health. *Health Psychol.* 1983;2(4):267–391.

4. Rolland J. In sickness and in health: the impact of illness on couples' relationships. *J Marital Fam Ther.* 2007;20(4):327–347.

5. Martire L, Helgeson V. Close relationships and the management of chronic illness: associations and interventions. *Am Psychol.* 2017;72(6):601–612.

6. Allan G. A note on interviewing spouses together. *J Marriage Fam.* 1980;42(1):205–210.

7. Morgan DL, Ataie J, Carder P, Hoffman K. Introducing dyadic interviews as a method for collecting qualitative data. *Qual Health Res.* 2013;23(9):1276–1284. https://doi.org/10.1177/1049732313501889.

8. Thompson L, Walker AJ. The dyad as the unit of analysis: conceptual and methodological issues. *J Marriage Fam.* 1982;44(4):889–900. https://doi.org/10.2307/351453.

9. Habermann B, Shin JY, Shearer G. Dyadic decision-making in advanced Parkinson's disease: a mixed methods study. *West J Nurs Res.* 2020;42(5):348–355. https://doi.org/10.1177/0193945919864429.

10. Whitlatch C, Judge K, Zarit S, Femia E. Dyadic intervention for family caregivers and care-receivers in early-stage dementia. *Gerontologist.* 2006;46(5):688–694.

11. Menne H, Tucke S, Whitlach C, Feinberg L. Decision-making involvement scale for individuals with dementia and family caregivers. *Am J Alzheimers Dis Other Demen.* 2008;23(1):23–29.

12. Schmid B, Allen R, Haley P, DeCoster J. Family matters: dyadic agreement in end of life medical decision making. *Gerontologist.* 2010;50(2):226–237.

13. Badr H, Acitelli LLKL. Rethinking dyadic coping in the context of chronic illness. *Curr Opin Psychol.* 2017;13(13):44–48. https://doi.org/10.1016/j.copsyc.2016.03.001.

14. Maroufizadeh S, Hosseini M, Rahimi Foroushani A, Omani-Samani R, Amini P. Application of the dyadic data analysis in behavioral medicine research: marital satisfaction and anxiety in infertile couples. *BMC Med Res Methodol.* 2018;18(1):1–10. https://doi.org/10.1186/s12874-018-0582-y.

15. Lyons KS, Lee CS. The theory of dyadic illness management. *J Fam Nurs.* 2018;24(1):8–28. https://doi.org/10.1177/1074840717745669.

16. Orsulic-Jeras S, Whitlatch CJ, Szabo SM, Shelton EG, Johnson J. The SHARE program for dementia: implementation of an early-stage dyadic care-planning intervention. *Dementia.* 2019;18(1):360–379. https://doi.org/10.1177/1471301216673455.

17. Shelton EG, Orsulic-Jeras S, Whitlatch CJ, Szabo SM. Does it matter if we disagree? The impact of incongruent care preferences on persons with dementia and their care partners. *Gerontologist.* 2018;58:556–566.

18. Reed RG, Butler EA, Kenny DA. Dyadic models for the study of health. *Soc Personal Psychol Compass.* 2013;7(4):228–245. https://doi.org/10.1111/spc3.12022.

19. Mindlis I, Livert D, Federman AD, Wisnivesky JP, Revenson TA. Racial/ethnic concordance between patients and researchers as a predictor of study attrition. *Soc Sci Med.* 2020;255(April). https://doi.org/10.1016/j.socscimed.2020.113009, 113009.

20. Aalsma MC, Carpentier MY, Azzouz F, Fortenberry JD. Longitudinal effects of health-harming and health-protective behaviors within adolescent romantic dyads. *Soc Sci Med.* 2012;74(9):1444–1451. https://doi.org/10.1016/j.socscimed.2012.01.014.

21. Knoll N, Schwarzer R, Pfüller B, Kienle R. A study with couples undergoing assisted-reproduction treatment. *Eur Psychol.* 2009;14(1):7–17. https://doi.org/10.1027/1016-9040.14.1.7.

22. Markey C, Markey P. Romantic partners, weight status, and weight concerns: an examination using the actor-partner interdependence model. *J Health Psychol.* 2011;16(2):217–225. https://doi.org/10.1177/1359105310375636.

23. Quinn C. Challenges and strategies of dyad research. *Appl Nurs Res.* 2010;23(2):1–9. https://doi.org/10.1016/j.apnr.2008.10.001.Challenges.

24. Kurylo M, Elliott T, DeVivo L, Dreer L. Caregiver social problem solving abilities and family member adjustment following congestive heart failure. *J Clin Psychol Med Settings.* 2004;11:151–157.

25. Clark P, Dunbar S, Aycock D, Blanton S, Wolf S. Pros and woes of interdisciplinary collaboration with a national clinical trial. *J Prof Nurs.* 2009;25(2):93–100.

26. Steinhauser KE, Clipp EC, Hays JC, et al. Identifying, recruiting, and retaining seriously-ill patients and their caregivers in longitudinal research. *Palliat Med.* 2006;20(8):745–754. https://doi.org/10.1177/0269216306073112.

27. Eisikovits Z, Koren C. Approaches to and outcomes of dyadic interview analysis. *Qual Health Res.* 2010;20(12):1642–1655. https://doi.org/10.1177/1049732310376520.

28. Kenny D, Kashy D, Cook W. *Dyadic Data Analysis.* Guilford Press; 2006.

29. Huynh VW, Rahal D, Mercado E, et al. Discrimination and health: a dyadic approach. *J Health Psychol.* 2019. https://doi.org/10.1177/1359105319857171.

30. Mellon S, Kershaw TS, Northouse LL, Freeman-Gibb L. A family-based model to predict fear of recurrence for cancer survivors and their caregivers. *Psychooncology.* 2007;16:214–223.

31. Hayslip B, Heidemaire B, Garner A. Health and grandparent–grandchild wellbeing: one-year longitudinal findings for custodial grandfamilies. *J Aging Health.* 2014;26(4):559–582.

32. Kim Y, Wellisch DK, Spillers RL. Effects of psychological distress on quality of life of adult daughters and their mothers with cancer. *Psychooncology*. 2008;17(11):1129–1136. https://doi.org/10.1002/pon.1328.

33. Rohrbaugh MJ, Shoham V, Butler EA, Hasler BP, Berman JS. Affective synchrony in dual- and single-smoker couples: further evidence of "symptom-system fit"? *Fam Process*. 2009;48(1):55–67. https://doi.org/10.1111/j.1545-5300.2009.01267.x.

34. Shoham V, Butler EA, Rohrbaugh MJ, Trost SE. Symptom-system fit in couples: emotion regulation when one or both partners smoke. *J Abnorm Psychol*. 2007;116(4):848–853. https://doi.org/10.1037/0021-843X.116.4.848.

35. Bauer DJ, Preacher KJ, Gil KM. Conceptualizing and testing random indirect effects and moderated mediation in multilevel models: new procedures and recommendations. *Psychol Methods*. 2006;11(2):142–163. https://doi.org/10.1037/1082-989X.11.2.142.

36. Edwards JR, Lambert LS. Methods for integrating moderation and mediation: a general analytical framework using moderated path analysis. *Psychol Methods*. 2007;12(1):1–22. https://doi.org/10.1037/1082-989X.12.1.1.

37. Muller D, Judd CM, Yzerbyt VY. When moderation is mediated and mediation is moderated. *J Pers Soc Psychol*. 2005;89(6):852–863. https://doi.org/10.1037/0022-3514.89.6.852.

38. Badr H, Laurenceau JP, Schart L, Basen-Engquist K, Turk D. The daily impact of pain from metastatic breast cancer on spousal relationships: a dyadic electronic diary study. *Pain*. 2010;151(3):644–654. https://doi.org/10.1016/j.pain.2010.08.022.

39. Holt-Lunstad J, Birmingham WA, Light KC. Influence of a "warm touch" support enhancement intervention among married couples on ambulatory blood pressure, oxytocin, alpha amylase, and cortisol. *Psychosom Med*. 2008;70(9):976–985. https://doi.org/10.1097/PSY.0b013e318187aef7.

40. Saxbe D, Repetti RL. For better or worse? Coregulation of couples' cortisol levels and mood states. *J Pers Soc Psychol*. 2010;98(1):92–103. https://doi.org/10.1037/a0016959.

41. Schoenthaler A, Basile M, West TV, Kalet A. It takes two to tango: a dyadic approach to understanding the medication dialogue in patient-provider relationships. *Patient Educ Couns*. 2018;101(8):1500–1505. https://doi.org/10.1016/j.pec.2018.02.009.

42. Ungar WJ, Mirabelli C, Cousins M, Boydell KM. A qualitative analysis of a dyad approach to health-related quality of life measurement in children with asthma. *Soc Sci Med*. 2006;63(9):2354–2366. https://doi.org/10.1016/j.socscimed.2006.06.016.

43. Bosman RC, Huijbregts KM, Verhaak PFM, et al. Long-term antidepressant use: a qualitative study on perspectives of patients and GPs in primary care. *Br J Gen Pract*. 2016;66(651):e708–e719. https://doi.org/10.3399/bjgp16X686641.

44. Zhang AY, Zyzanski SJ, Siminoff LA. Differential patient—caregiver opinions of treatment and care for advanced lung cancer patients. *Soc Sci Med*. 2010;70(8):1155–1158. https://doi.org/10.1016/j.socscimed.2009.12.023.

45. Christensen A, Howren M, Hillis S, et al. Patient and physician beliefs about control over health: association of symmetrical beliefs with medication regimen adherence. *J Gen Intern Med*. 2010;25:397–402.

46. Bolen SD, Bricker E, Samuels TA, et al. Factors associated with intensification of oral Diabetes medications in primary care provider-patient dyads: a cohort study. *Diabetes Care*. 2009;32(1):25–31. https://doi.org/10.2337/dc08-1297.

47. Reach G, Pechtner V, Gentilella R, Corcos A, Ceriello A. Clinical inertia and its impact on treatment intensification in people with type 2 diabetes mellitus. *Diabetes Metab*. 2017;43(6):501–511. https://doi.org/10.1016/j.diabet.2017.06.003.

Chapter 12

Using network analysis in pharmacy and health services research

Mohsen Askar and Kristian Svendsen

Department of Pharmacy, Faculty of Health Sciences, UiT The Arctic University of Norway, Tromsø, Norway

Objectives

- Introduce the theoretical background of network analysis.
- Describe the terminology commonly used in network analysis.
- Highlight the potential usefulness of network analysis in medication use studies.
- Provide a description of how to create medication use networks from raw medical data.
- Demonstrate how to use network analysis in medication use studies using some real-life examples.

Electronic sources of information about medication use are growing increasingly common. Using these sources, research into drug utilization as well as the effectiveness and safety of medicines is also on the rise. Within this research field, pharmacoepidemiology, statistical methods for testing causal relationships is frequently used. However, explorative methods are often also useful. One such method is the topic of this chapter, Network Analysis.

What is a network?

A network is a graph that represents a set of interacting actors. The network consists of two components. The actor, which is represented by a *node*, and a relationship that is represented by an *edge* (i.e., connection) between two nodes.[1] A network can represent a description of a real-world system, a mathematical model, or a simulation among others.

As seen in Fig. 1, a network can be undirected (a and b), which means the relationship between nodes does not have a specific direction. In directed networks (c and d), the edges (i.e., arrows) go in a specific direction. Networks are either weighted or unweighted. In an unweighted network (a and c), the two nodes either have a relationship or not, while a weighted network (b and d) considers how many times these two nodes were connected by a sort of relationship (also called edge thickness or tie strength). In other words, it shows the intensity of the relationship between two given nodes.

A network can be uni- or multipartite. Fig. 2 shows a unipartite network (a) that only has one set of nodes, while in bipartite networks (b) the nodes belong to two disjointed sets (such as prescribers and patients). In a bipartite network, edges connect the nodes from different sets.[2,3]

What is network analysis (NA)?

How a network is described can vary according to the research discipline and the context. In general, NA is a mathematical representation method to study the pattern or the regularities in relationships among interacting units.[4]

The principal types of data used in quantitative studies in social pharmacy and pharmacoepidemiology are Attribute data and Relational data. Attribute data includes the characteristics of the studied objects, for example, sex, education, income, etc., while relational data concerns the connections between the data objects. Various epidemiological methods are used to study data attributes and relationships among them, whereas, in the case of relational data, NA is an appropriate

Contemporary Research Methods in Pharmacy and Health Services. https://doi.org/10.1016/B978-0-323-91888-6.00042-9

FIG. 1 Different types of networks, (A) undirected and unweighted network, (B) undirected and weighted network, (C) directed and unweighted, and (D) directed and weighted.

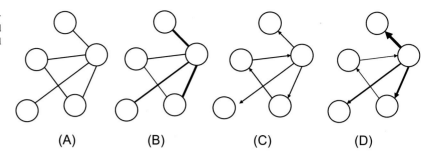

(A)   (B)   (C)   (D)

FIG. 2 (A) Unipartite network consisting of one type of nodes; (B) bipartite network consisting of two different types of nodes *(circles and squares)* in which the edges link between nodes from different types.

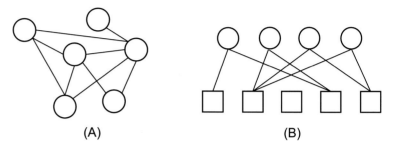

(A)   (B)

approach to analyzing the relationship between data objects.[5] What makes NA unique is its ability to plot an entire dataset into one graph. This all-in-one-place representation allows researchers to explore and discover patterns in the dataset.

A brief introduction to the historical background of networks and network analysis

The history of the development of NA is complex and has its roots in different research disciplines.[6] Perhaps the very first attempt of using networks was in the description of the food chain from *Al-Jāḥiẓ* in the 8th century, which aimed to illustrate the interaction between different species.[7] Despite the complexity of NA development history, researchers from different fields of study agree that the development of networks as a tool to study patterns began properly in the 18th century with graph theory. Leonhard Euler (1707–1783) created graph theory to solve a famous problem. The problem questioned whether it was possible to walk around the town of *Königsberg*, (now Kaliningrad, Russia) crossing each of its seven bridges only once and return to the starting point.

By using a network of nodes and links, Euler showed that it was impossible to walk through the city crossing all its seven bridges only once.[8]

$$G = (V, E)$$

Graph theory is considered the heart of NA,[9] in which a graph (G) consists of two elements, vertices (V) or nodes, which are the actors in a network and edges (E), which represent the links or the connections between these actors. The mathematical background of NA will not be covered in this chapter, but it is summarized elsewhere for interested readers.[10,11]

Another early use of networks took place in the 19th century by the Norwegian ethnologist Eilert Sundt (1817–1875), who noticed a formation of social circles among rural Norwegian farmers. Sundt wrote about what he called "*bedelag*" or an "invitation group," which means in the old Norwegian traditions that neighbors who live nearby invite each other to their special occasions, such as weddings, and hence forming a sort of isolated circles.[12]

Sociologists Auguste Comte (1798–1857) and Georg Simmel (1858–1918) and their contributions in sociology provided many ideas in developing social networks. In 1932, Jacob Moreno used what he called "*sociometry*" to study the problem of students from Hudson School in New York skipping school.[13] This technique allowed him to elaborate on how the social influence and ideas flow among students.[14]

There are two salient, landmark studies from the 1950s. The first was led by James S. Coleman (1926–95) and colleagues, who in 1957 showed that the social relations between physicians had influenced their adoption of a new drug.[15] The second study was done by Paul Erdős (1913–1996) and Alfréd Rényi (1921–1970) who in 1959 introduced a random network model suggesting that the number of connections between the networks' actors becomes lower as the network grows.[16]

Since the 1970s, sociologists, psychologists, and mathematicians have continued to use and develop network measures, structures and models. Over the past decades, applications of NA have greatly increased in a variety of fields. In 1977, Berry Wellman founded the "International Network for Social Network Analysis" (INSNA),[17] a nonprofit professional association that focuses on NA development, discussions and publishing.

Additional reading on network analysis history can be found in a book by L. Freeman who demonstrated in detail, the history of the development of social networks [17], and an article by E. Delmas et al., who summarized various milestones in the ecological network development.[18]

How has network analysis been used in public health?

Public health is an empiric and multidisciplinary field that aims at maintaining and promoting health on the population level.[19] Using NA in this field is not a new approach. *Transmission networks* have been used to examine the risk of disease transmission by investigating the relations between infected people and healthy ones.[20–22] Another form of transmission networks is the *information transmission networks*, which helps to show the dissemination of health-related information between different organizations and consumers. Some network characteristics reveal the pattern and the main actors contributing the most to information spread. A famous example of this type of networks mentioned previously explains the diffusion of information among physicians regarding a new drug.[15] Researchers have developed simulation networks that describe diffusion properties and predict how the information could be spread faster or more efficient.[23]

Significant effort went into studying health workers' behavior using social NA as well.[24] Different themes have been studied in this area including diffusion of information and innovation, prescribing behavior, social influence and decision-making.[25] Studying social interaction networks helped to expose how health workers' professional and personal behavior impact health services.[26] For further reading, Douglas A. Luke and Jenine K. Harris give a thorough explanation of the use of NA in Public Health.[6]

The introduction of network analysis in drug utilization studies

Drug utilization studies are a relatively new application of NA. To our knowledge, Cavallo et al. were the first to study a drug prescription network in 2013. They used medications as the nodes and the number of patients being prescribed these medications as weighted edges. They aimed mainly at describing the topology of the coprescription network to demonstrate which drug classes are most coprescribed. They also compared the male/female networks and networks from different age strata and found that women in general were coprescribed more drug classes.[27]

Bazzoni et al. were likely the first to use the term Drug Prescription Networks (DPNs) in their paper published in 2015. They described the DPNs as dense, highly clustered and modular, and assortative. In this specific study, density reflected frequent coprescribing. Modularity suggested that the network could be subdivided into clusters corresponding to various patient groups such as patients with musculoskeletal inflammation, obstructive airway diseases and cardiovascular diseases. The study also showed that it is possible to highlight spatial and temporal changes by comparing different networks.[28]

How to create a medication use network?

In order to create a medication use network it is necessary to define the nodes and edges as well as managing the data to make a data set that can be used. In this paragraph is an example of how this can be done. A precise definition of the edges allows the researcher to extract the correct information. Medical data is often represented in a long format including patients' attributes such as sex, age and dispensed medications. To create a network, this data needs to be reshaped. The first step is to create a file with only the medications that are comedicated sorted by a unique patient's identifier (ID). The comedicated drugs can vary according to the comedication definition used.[29] The comedication definition we used is described in the next section. Secondly, the file needs to be aggregated to create an edge list. The edge list contains 2 variables defining the pairs of drugs (nodes) and one variable with the number of users comedicating each pair of drugs (edge weight). An edge list is the data format that can be used by various software to create the network. The process is summarized in Fig. 3. The Stata syntax for creating the edge list can be downloaded here: https://github.com/MohsenAskar/NA-in-medication-study. The edge lists for the created networks are openly available at the UiT The Arctic University of Norway open data repository here: https://doi.org/10.18710/1OUTYI.

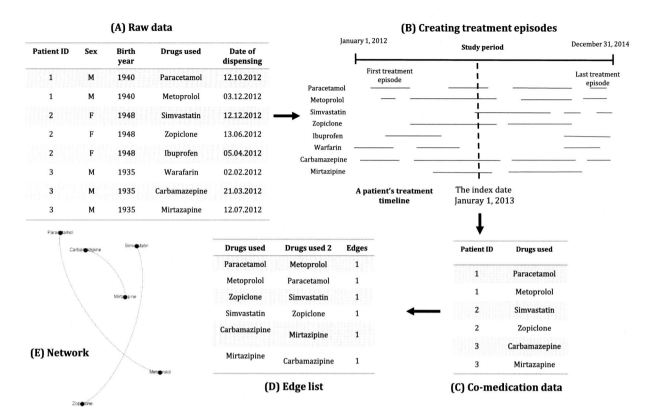

FIG. 3 Data preparation process. (A) Raw clinical data in the long format. (B) Creating treatment episodes, a line indicates an episode. Gaps between lines indicate a medication-free period of more than 14 days. (C) Data including only medications used at the index date (D) Creating the edge list including 3 variables; two variables represent the nodes (Drug used, Drug used 2) and the third variable is the edge weight between the pair of nodes. (E) Using the software to generate the network.

Example data sources and the created networks

After creating the edge lists as described above, they were used to create a network of comedication in elderly persons in Norway. In addition, a network representing severe drug–drug interactions (DDIs) was also created. Finally, these two networks were combined into a network representing the actual use of medications with severe DDIs.

The first network: Comedication network

The dataset used comes from the Norwegian Prescription Database (NorPD). It covers all dispensed prescriptions to elderly persons ($\geq$65 years) in Norway between 2012 and 2014. The NorPD collects data from all pharmacies in Norway and covers all outpatient dispensing for the entire Norwegian population. Details on the NorPD are published elsewhere.[30] In total, the dataset included 765,383 patients, 344,285 men (45%), and 421,098 women (55%) with 75 years as mean patient age. Edges in this network represented the number of patients who combined pairs of medications. To define the comedication, we created treatment episodes using the Proportion of Days Covered (PDC) approach.[31] It was assumed that patients used one Defined Daily Dose (DDD)[32] per day and 20% additional time was added to each prescription duration to account for imperfect adherence. Furthermore a medication-free gap of 14 days before ending a treatment episode and starting another was allowed. This means that if the patient exceeds 14 days without the medication, the treatment episode for this medication ends and a new episode starts if the patient picks up a new prescription. Finally, comedication was defined as the overlapping drug treatment episodes at the index date, January 1, 2013.

For each pair of nodes (drugs), we summed up the number of comedication occurrences (i.e., number of patients who combined these two drugs) to create a weighted and undirected network.

Any medications that had no defined DDD such as the medications for topical use, vaccines, and ophthalmologicals was excluded. This was in total 357 medications (217 local and 140 systematic drugs). The resulting comedication network can be accessed on the following link: https://mohsenaskar.github.io/co-medication/network/. The network is searchable by active ingredient. Some network measures and all the nodes connected to this node will appear on the right side of the web page.

The second network: Severe drug-drug interactions network

To create this network, a dataset derived from the Norwegian Electronic Prescription Support System (FEST) was used. FEST is a national information service that provides common pharmaceutical data to the IT systems that are involved in the drug prescribing process including systems used by physicians, hospitals and pharmacies.[33] Drug-drug interactions are a part of the FEST database. In FEST, the DDIs are divided into 3 categories; interactions that should be avoided (i.e., severe), interactions where precautions should be taken and interactions that do not require any action. Only severe DDIs were included in the study. There were 57.151 unique severe interactions. The edges in this network represent the presence of a severe interaction between the two nodes. The network is undirected and unweighted. The severe DDIs network can be accessed on the following link: https://mohsenaskar.github.io/DDI/network/.

The third network: Combining comedication and DDIs networks

Both the DDI and comedication network had drugs as nodes. When the two networks were combined only edges that existed in both networks were included (only edges with any users combining the medications and where there was a severe DDI). The number of users for each edge from the comedication network became the weight of the edges in the combined network. As in the comedication network, the edges are weighted and represent the number of patients comedicating. This resulting network is shown here: https://mohsenaskar.github.io/DDI-in-co-medication-network/network/.

Examples of software to use for creating and studying networks

There are many available tools and softwares for NA. Here the focus will be on how to use the *nwcommands* package in *Stata* and the *igraph* package in *R* as well as visualization in *Gephi*. Other packages like "*igraph*" or "*NetworkX*" for *Python* are popular as well. All these packages can be used for visualizing and computing different network measures with differences in their integrated features and performance.[34,35]

a. *Stata (nwcommands, nwANND)*

Nwcommands is a suite of commands that can be installed in Stata to create and analyze network data. Using an edge list, *nwcommands* will create an adjacency matrix.[36] The adjacency matrix is a square matrix that contains the relationships between each pair of nodes in the network. The adjacency matrix can be saved as *Pajek* format that can be later imported and used by *Gephi*. In addition, *nwcommands* can display some network measures on both the network and node-level. *NwANND* is used for calculating the assortativity coefficient.[37] The syntax can be found here https://github.com/MohsenAskar/NA-in-medication-study.

b. *R (igraph)*

Igraph (https://igraph.org/) is a library for creating and analyze graphs. It is widely used by network researchers to analyze graphs and networks. It is currently available for *C, C++, Python, R* and *Mathematica*.

One of the strengths of *igraph* is that it can be programmed with a high-level programming language and still be very efficient when handling large networks. In an *R* context, *igraph* integrates well with the visualization package (ggplot2) via the *ggraph* library.

Igraph uses an edge list and can link it with attribute data for each node as well. An example of code for visualization using *Igraph* and *ggraph*, is shown here https://github.com/MohsenAskar/NA-in-medication-study.

c. *Gephi*

Gephi is an open-source and free standalone software. The software can handle small to medium-sized networks (up to 150,000 nodes). *Gephi* is user-friendly and requires no programming experience.[35] With many visualizing layouts and network measures, *Gephi* can provide a good starting point for a drug network study.[38] After importing the adjacency matrix to *Gephi*, the network can be processed by applying different visualizing layouts, adding filters and colors. The structure of most drug networks can be complex and the unprocessed form of the network is often uninformative. By using different attributes (e.g., sex, modularity, etc.) networks can become more easily interpretable.[39]

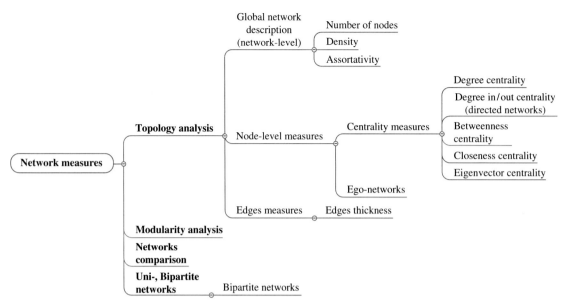

FIG. 4 Summarizing some of the Network Analysis measures that can be useful in the studies of medication use.

Terminology of network analysis and examples of applied measures

Network analysis has a wide variety of measures that can be useful in the medication use context. This section will introduce the terminology of some network analysis measures followed by examples of applying these measures in drug prescription data. The key measures can be organized under 4 main categories: (1) Topology analysis (2) Modularity analysis (3) Network comparison (4) Uni- and multipartite networks[40](Fig. 4).

1. Topology analysis:

    Network topological features refer to a group of characteristics, which either describe the network as a whole unit (network-level) or define some parts/positions/actors of the network (node-level). There are many topological measures and each of them gives information about a specific network attribute, which then may warrant further investigation. Table 1 provides a comparison of topological measures between the comedication network and the drug-drug interactions network. The text later in this section has more information about each measure in the table.

a. *Global network description (network-level)*: A group of measures that describes the network as a whole.
    - *The number of nodes*: the total number of drugs in the network,
    - *Density:* the density of a network is the number of actual edges divided by the total edge number of edges that would exist if all the nodes in the network were connected. This theoretical number can be calculated by the formula:

$$\frac{n \times (n-1)}{2}$$

where $n =$ number of nodes. Density will always have a value between 0 and 1.

    The density of the comedication and the DDIs networks was low because most possible comedication/interactions do not occur. The density of the comedication network is 0.26 while the DDIs network density is 0.04. Density can be useful in terms of comparison between different networks that describe the same context in different populations.

- *Assortativity:* a network is assortative when the nodes that share a similar trait tend to connect. This trait can be many characteristics such as the nodes' degree. In this case, the assortativity means that nodes with a high number of edges tend to connect. Assortativity can be examined in terms of other common characteristics between the nodes as well. The assortativity coefficient is the same as the Pearson coefficient of degrees at either side of an edge, over the set of all edges. The assortativity coefficient is a scale between -1 and 1, where 1 is most assortative.[41] The assortativity coefficient shows that the comedication network is nonassortative in terms of degree similarity, while the severe DDIs network is more assortative.

The assortativity coefficient of the entire comedication network was -0.26. This means that the network is not assortative in terms of nodes degree (i.e., correlation between nodes of different degrees). Bazzoni et al. found the DPN assortative by Anatomical Therapeutic Chemical (ATC) classes, which means that drugs that share either the anatomical (first level),

TABLE 1 The topological measures of comedication and severe DDIs networks.

Outcome	Comedication network	DDIs network	Interpretation
1. Topology analysis			
(a) Network-level measures			
Number of nodes	762	1699	The number of drugs present in the network.
Number of edges	75,052	57,151	Number of connections between the network nodes
Density	0.26	0.04	The extent of connections between the network's nodes
Average degree	99	34	The average number of connections that each node has.
Assortativity coefficient	−0.26	0.4	To what extent drugs with a higher degree tend to cluster.
(b) Node-level measures			
Centrality measures			
Nodes with the **highest Degree** centrality scores	Acetylsalicylic acid Simvastatin Zopiclone Paracetamol Metoprolol	Typhoid vaccine Erythromycin Hypericum (St John's-wort) Clarithromycin Moxifloxacin	Combining these centrality measures can be used to assign the importance of each drug in the network. The same five drugs have the highest centrality in the comedication network while there is some more variation among the different measures for the DDI network
Nodes with the **highest Betweenness** centrality scores	Acetylsalicylic acid Zopiclone Simvastatin Paracetamol Metoprolol	Typhoid vaccine Padeliporfin Hypericum(St John's-wort) Tuberculosis vaccine Ginkgo leaves	
Nodes with the **highest Closeness** centrality scores	Acetylsalicylic acid Simvastatin Zopiclone Paracetamol Metoprolol	Bromelains Telbivudine Peg interferon alfa-2a Diazepam Oxazepam	
Nodes with the **highest Eigenvector** centrality scores	Acetylsalicylic acid Simvastatin Zopiclone Metoprolol Paracetamol	Typhoid vaccine Erythromycin Clarithromycin Chloramphenicol Moxifloxacin	

Continued

TABLE 1 The topological measures of comedication and severe DDIs networks—cont'd

Outcome	Comedication network	DDIs network	Interpretation
(c) Edge-level measures			
Average path length	1.77	3.09	The average shortest path between two nodes.
Largest edge weight	82,948	1	For the weighted comedication network the edge weight reflects the number of patients comedicating for the DDI network edges are not weighted
Edges weight range	1–82,948	0–1	
2. Modularity			
Modularity	0.088	0.54	Indicates the presence of communities in the network.
Number of modules (communities)	4	11	Number of communities in the two networks
Number of nodes in largest module	530 (module 0)	372 (module 4)	Number of drugs in each largest community in each network.

therapeutic (second level) or pharmacologic (third level) class tend to connect to each other more than to other classes. The assortativity of the drugs from the same anatomical group connected to each other was examined. A searchable version of the complete ATC index is available below at the World Health Organization (WHO) Collaboration Centre for Drug Statistics Methodology website https://www.whocc.no/atc_ddd_index/. We calculated the ratio between the densities in-between drugs from the same anatomical class to the density of the general network, which was 0.26 (Table 2). If the ratio was higher than 1, it implied a higher density between these drugs than the network density and indicated a tendency to correlate. This means that the drugs from the same anatomical group tend to be more coprescribed.

Fig. 5 shows that the majority of anatomical drug classes were assortative. This means that the drugs from the same anatomical group tend to be more coprescribed. It is also possible to investigate the assortativity of the drugs on the pharmacological group level (3rd level ATC classification). Table 3 shows the assortativity score (ratio density) of the 20 most assortative pharmacological groups. Fig. 6 represents the assortativity of all pharmacological groups showing which groups are assortative and which are not.

b. *Node-level measures*

Node-level measures describe the role of the different nodes across the network.

TABLE 2 Assortativity of anatomical groups by ATC codes similarity sorted by higher assortativity.

Anatomical group	No. of ATC codes in each group	Potential no. of edges[a]	Actual no. of edges	Density between ATCs of the same anatomical group[b]	Ratio density (group/network density)
S Sensory organs	14	91	81	0.890	3.42
C Cardiovascular system	98	4753	2544	0.535	2.06
M Musculoskeletal system	32	496	226	0.456	1.75
R Respiratory system	69	2346	1066	0.454	1.75
B Blood and blood forming organs	35	595	245	0.412	1.58
V Various	4	6	2	0.333	1.28
A Alimentary tract and metabolism	108	5778	1802	0.312	1.20
N Nervous system	166	13,695	3653	0.267	1.03
H Sys. Hormonal prep, excl. Sex hormones, insulin	27	351	75	0.214	0.82
G Genitourinary system and sex hormones	49	1176	209	0.178	0.68
J Antiinfectives for systemic use	75	2775	305	0.110	0.42
L Antineoplastic and immunomodulation agents	70	2415	170	0.070	0.27
D Dermatologicals	6	15	0	0.000	0.00
P Antiparasitic products	9	36	0	0.000	0.00

[a]*Expected number of edges if all nodes were connected. Calculated as N*(N − 1)/2.*
[b]*Calculated as actual number edges/theoretical number of edges.*

FIG. 5 Assortativity of network nodes in terms of similarity by the anatomical group. Squares above 1 represent a drug group with a higher density than the general density of the network (0.26). The S (Sensory organs) anatomical group had the highest assortativity. D (Dermatologicals) and P (Antiparasitic products) groups had no edges because these drug classes were excluded from the study.

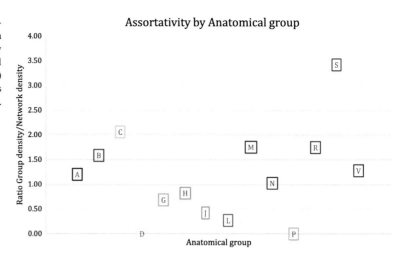

TABLE 3 The most 20 assortative pharmacological groups in the comedication network.

ATC pharmacological group	Group name	Ratio density (pharmacological group/ network density)
A01A	Stomatological preparations	3.84
A03A	Drugs for functional gastrointestinal disorders	3.84
A09A	Digestives, incl. enzymes	3.84
A12B	Mineral supplements, Potassium	3.84
C01A	Cardiac glycosides	3.84
C01D	Vasodilators used in cardiac diseases	3.84
C03A	Low-Ceiling diuretics, Thiazides	3.84
C08D	Selective calcium channel blockers with direct cardiac effects	3.84
G04C	Drugs used in benign prostatic hypertrophy	3.84
H01C	Hypothalamic hormones	3.84
H03A	Thyroid preparations	3.84
H03B	Antithyroid preparations	3.84
J01E	Sulfonamides and trimethoprim	3.84
N06D	Antidementia drugs	3.84
B03B	Vitamin B12 and folic acid	3.46
S01E	Antiglaucoma preparations and Miotics	3.42
A10A	Insulins and analogues	3.41
M04A	Antigout preparations	3.2
C08C	Selective calcium channel blockers with mainly vascular effects	3.08
R03A	Adrenergics, inhalants	2.99

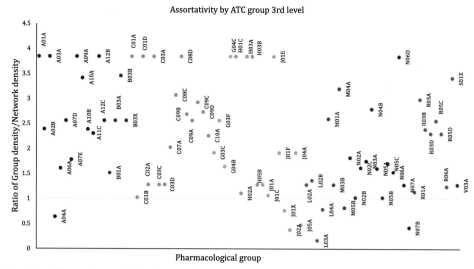

FIG. 6 Assortativity of the different pharmacological groups. Groups above 1 indicate a higher density between them than the density of the general network. Most of the groups lie above 1 in the figure indicating a tendency to be comedicated together.

Centrality measures:

Centrality measures indicate the importance of network nodes by assigning a score to each of them. Centrality measures are many and each of them examines a specific type of importance. By comparing the different centrality measures of a node, we can understand how a node is influential to the network. This chapter discusses four of the most common types of centrality measures: degree, betweenness, closeness, and eigenvector centrality. The mathematical explanations of these measures have been described elsewhere[42,43].

Degree centrality (C_D)

Degree centrality is the number of edges that are connected to a node. A higher score indicates that the node is connected to many other nodes. Node A in Fig. 7 has a degree score of 4. In a directed network, the degree is split into in-degree, which is the number of edges that direct to a node and out-degree, which is the number of edges that originate from the node. In and out degrees will therefore show the directions of relationships in a directed network. In Fig. 7, nodes C and D have an in-degree score of 3, while nodes A and G have an out-degree score of 3.

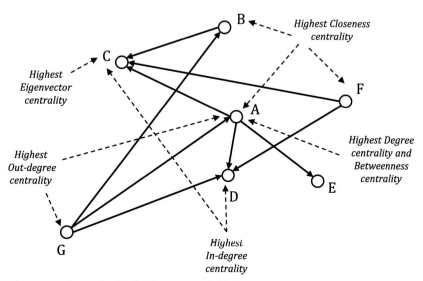

FIG. 7 Illustrating the different types of centrality. Node (A) represents the highest score of Degree and Betweenness centralities. The highest Eigenvector centrality score is assigned to the node (C). Nodes (A, B, F) have similar closeness Centrality. Nodes with the most in-degree edges are (C, D), while (A, G) have the most out-degree edges.

Betweenness centrality (C_B)

The betweenness centrality of a node indicates how many times this node was used to connect two other nodes by the shortest possible path. Increasing the number of shortest paths increases the betweenness centrality score.[42] In Fig. 7, node A has the highest betweenness centrality score of 1.5.

Closeness centrality (C_C)

It is a measure of the average distance between the node and all other nodes in the network. Nodes with the highest closeness score have the shortest distances to all other network nodes. The nodes A, B and F have the highest closeness centrality score of 1.

Eigenvector centrality (C_E)

It is a measure of the importance of a node in a network based on the node's connections with other *vital* nodes. Relative scores are given to all nodes in the network based on the concept that connections to high-scored nodes give a higher score to the node than equal connections to low-scored nodes. In other words, a high eigenvector score means that a node is connected to many nodes, which themselves are connected to important nodes in the network and have high scores of eigenvector centrality. This means that a node with a high eigenvector centrality score is not necessarily connected to the highest number of nodes in the network but is connected to the nodes with a high number of edges.[44] Node C in Fig. 7 has the highest eigenvector centrality score of 1.

As shown in Table 1, centrality measures in the comedication network revealed that the same 5 drugs are the most central in all measures; while in the severe DDIs network, there was more variation in the top 5 drugs in each centrality measure. As mentioned, centrality measures show how influential each node is in the network. It is possible to have high centrality of one type and a low of another for the same node.[18] To study the importance of the nodes, it is necessary to use more than one measure of centrality.

Employing centrality measures in the drug study introduced an opportunity to observe the influence of the different drugs prescribed in real-world settings from another perspective. Determining this influence can be useful for both clinicians and decision-makers. Furthermore, recent studies suggest using centrality measures as an alternative approach for variable selection for multivariable and multivariate analyses. Lutz et al. used the centrality measures to identify four additional variables contributing to the prediction of treatment dropout in patients with anxiety disorders.[45] Valenzuela et al. described a methodology based on degree and centrality measures to obtain the most representative variables to create an index for predicting "successful aging."[46] These approaches are interesting and represent an alternative method to other variable selection methods. Assigning the centrality of each node in the network may help to visualize the network from a single specific important node perspective; this is called an *Ego network*.

Ego networks

An ego network is a visualization of a part of the network, which consists of a node of interest and any other nodes that are directly connected to it. This concept can be important in terms of representing all the connections related to an important node. For example, the coprescribed drugs with the drug subject of study. Ego networks as a measure can be seen by accessing the online networks we created and selecting individual nodes.

c. *Edge-level measures:*

Edge weight: in a weighted network, edge weight represents a quantitative measure of how many times two nodes were connected. This representation is unique for NA and can answer many research questions. The top 10 edge weights for the severe DDIs in the comedication network and comedication only network are shown in Tables 4 and 5 respectively. As shown in Table 4, the number of patients using drugs causing severe DDIs are relatively low (less than 1000 users for all) while the most commonly comedicated drugs seen in Table 5 is much higher, with acetylsalicylic acid (aspirin) and simvastatin having around 83.000 users and representing nearly 11% of the population. In this context, larger edge weights represent more frequently used medication pairs.

2. Modularity analysis (Community detection)

After studying the network as a whole and its individual nodes, the next step is to study the structure of the network. One key feature of network structure is its modularity. A module or community is a group of nodes that have more connections

TABLE 4 The top 10 clinically relevant severe DDIs in the comedication network.

	The severe DDI drug pair		No. of patients comedicating
1	Codeine and paracetamol	Tramadol	855
2	Esomeprazole	Clopidogrel	823
3	Simvastatin	Carbamazepine	480
4	Metoprolol	Paroxetine	454
5	Metoprolol	Verapamil	380
6	Lansoprazole	Clopidogrel	308
7	Diclofenac	Ibuprofen	305
8	Diazepam	Oxazepam	300
9	Carbamazepine	Zopiclone	280
10	Omeprazole	Clopidogrel	277

between each other and fewer connections to the other modules in the network.[47] There are many techniques of detecting modules including density-based, centrality-based, partition-based and hierarchical clustering techniques.[40,48]

There were four modules in the comedication network, including one large module and three other smaller ones. A description of the algorithm we used for modularity detection is illustrated here.[49] The number of medications (nodes) under each module is shown in Table 6.

Identifying these modules did not only highlight the often coprescribed medicines but also shed light on the comorbidities pattern by assigning each drug group to its corresponding diagnosis. Collapsing the ATC codes to the therapeutic level (2nd level), allowed us to group the ATC codes under their corresponding therapeutic group and reduce the number of studied objects in each module (Table 7). The number of users of each therapeutic group was added to assign a measure of the importance of each therapeutic group to the modules if these therapeutic groups were common between more than one modules.

Further work could be done to identify smaller groups by detecting the sub-clusters inside each module. For example, Nervous and Respiratory system groups (N- and R- groups) drugs are found only in module 0, while Cardiac-, Alimentary- and Blood groups (C-, A- and B- groups) are common groups between modules 1 and 2. By considering

TABLE 5 The top 10 combined drugs in the comedication network.

	Most combined drugs		No. of patients comedicated
1	Acetylsalicylic acid	Simvastatin	82,948
2	Acetylsalicylic acid	Metoprolol	52,577
3	Acetylsalicylic acid	Atorvastatin	42,753
4	Metoprolol	Simvastatin	36,792
5	Acetylsalicylic acid	Amlodipine	32,628
6	Acetylsalicylic acid	Zopiclone	29,173
7	Amlodipine	Simvastatin	22,554
8	Acetylsalicylic acid	Ramipril	19,660
9	Simvastatin	Zopiclone	18,845
10	Metformin	Acetylsalicylic acid	18,507

TABLE 6 The four modules found in the comedication network.

Module	Number of nodes	Percent
0	530	68%
1	49	24%
2	167	6%
3	16	2%

TABLE 7 The four modularity classes obtained from our comedication network.

Group	No. of users	Therapeutic indications
Modularity class 0		
N05[a]	149,142	Hypnotics and sedatives
R03[a]	125,913	Drugs for obstructive airway diseases
A02	107,657	Acid disorders
N02[a]	87,051	Antimigraine preparations
N06[a]	78,403	Psychoanaleptics
M01[a]	60,442	Antiinflammatory and antirheumatic products
B03	57,100	Antianemic preparations
H03[a]	56,354	Iodine therapy
R06[a]	53,993	Antihistamines for systemic use
J01[a]	40,218	Antibacterials for systemic use
M05	35,792	Bone diseases
H02[a]	35,343	Corticosteroids for systemic use
G04	23,622	Urologicals (prostatic hypertrophy)
R01[a]	21,306	Nasal preparations
G03[a]	20,842	Sex hormones
N03[a]	17,032	Antiepileptics
R05+	16,266	Cough and cold preparations
C03	14,703	Diuretics
L04	12,827	Immunosuppressants
N04[a]	10,016	Anti-Parkinson drugs
A06	7932	Drugs for constipation
A07	6774	Antidiarrheals, intestinal antiinflammatory/antiinfective agents
L02	5189	Endocrine therapy (hormones related)
A11	5113	Vitamins
B01	4793	Antithrombotic agents
A03	4159	Drugs for functional gastrointestinal disorders

TABLE 7 The four modularity classes obtained from our comedication network—cont'd

Group	No. of users	Therapeutic indications
C07	3349	Beta blocking agents
C10	3309	Lipid modifying agents
N07[a]	1823	Other nervous system drugs
A12	1631	Mineral supplements
A09	1519	Digestives, incl. enzymes
P01[a]	1342	Antiprotozoals
D01	1262	Antifungals for dermatological use
H01[a]	804	Pituitary and hypothalamic hormones and analogs
M03	742	Muscle relaxants
A04	735	Antiemetics and antinauseants
A05	595	Bile and liver therapy
A08	516	Antiobesity preparations, excl. diet products
L01	476	Antineoplastic agents
J05	392	Antivirals for systemic use
L03	288	Immunostimulants
J04	269	Antimycobacterials
D05	247	Antipsoriatics
J02	188	Antimycotics for systemic use
A01	185	Stomatological preparations
H05	131	Calcium homeostasis
G02	115	Other gynecologicals
B02	113	Antihemorrhagics
Modularity class 1		
A11	1635	Vitamins
C03	70,736	Diuretics
B01	52,433	Antithrombotic agents
M04[a]	15,650	Antigout preparations
C01	15,616	Cardiac therapy
C07	13,343	Beta blocking agents
C08	7445	Calcium channel blockers
A12	5858	Mineral supplements
B03	1282	Antianemic preparations
V03	487	All other therapeutic products
H05	240	Calcium homeostasis
A02	194	Drugs for acid related disorders
C02	163	Antihypertensives
L04	161	Immunosuppressants

Continued

TABLE 7 The four modularity classes obtained from our comedication network—cont'd

Group	No. of users	Therapeutic indications
Modularity class 2		
C09	293,008	Agents acting on the renin-angiotensin system
B01	260,482	Antithrombotic agents
C10	258,050	Lipid modifying agents
C07	128,165	Beta blocking agents
C08	126,834	Calcium channel blockers
A10[a]	96,241	Drugs used in diabetes
S01[a]	67,468	Ophthalmologicals
G04	45,302	Urologicals (prostatic hypertrophy)
C01	26,825	Cardiac therapy
C03	22,963	Diuretics
L02	11,148	Endocrine therapy
C02	10,313	Antihypertensives
L01	708	Antineoplastic agents
C04[a]	467	Peripheral vasodilators
A07	171	Antidiarrheals, intestinal antiinflammatory/antiinfective agents
Modularity class 3		
J05[a]	237	Antivirals for systemic use

[a]Unique drug group for this module.

the number of users in each module could be possible to allocate to which module these therapeutic groups has the most importance. Drugs used for diabetes, (A10) group, only exist in module 2.

In the DDIs network, there were 11 modules (Fig. 8). Modules in the DDI network could be connected to pharmacological data to see the importance of pharmacokinetic interactions through systems such as the cytochrome P450 system. This has not explored, but there is great potential in using modularity analyses in order to understand the mechanisms that are behind these interactions.

3. Network comparison

It is possible to compare two or more networks to show the changes over time (temporal), between different areas (spatial), or between different groups of patients. These comparisons can be done by comparing the characteristics of the networks to highlight the differences in numbers and influences of the nodes. Another way to compare different networks is to subtract or divide the values of the edges between two networks. This will create edges representing the differences between the networks. By comparing many networks, dynamic graphs can be created to show the topological changes from a network to the next. Nodes will appear, disappear, or change their locations as the dynamic graph moves through the different networks.[39]

As an example of temporal comparison, another comedication network representing the medication use on January 1, 2014 was created and compared with the original comedication network that represented the medication use on January 1, 2013.

By using these two networks a new network was created that showed the difference between 2013 and 2014 comedication networks. This was done by dividing the weight of each edge (number of patients who used these pairs of medications) in 2013 with the 2014 network. This resulted in some unmatched edges, that are unique for each network, which were excluded, while the new weights of the matched edges, which represent the ratio of users in the 2013 network compared to

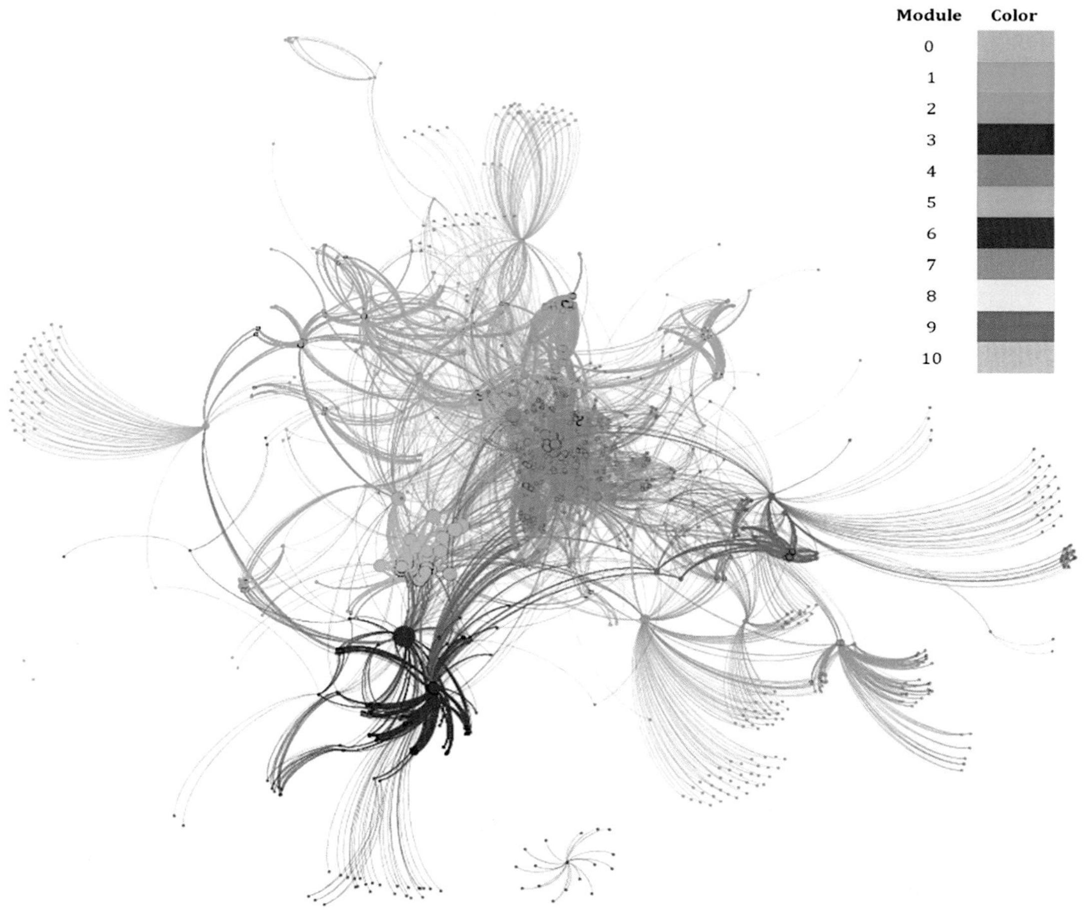

FIG. 8 The 11 modules that were detected in the severe DDIs network. Different colors indicate different modules.

the 2014 network. For example, a pair of medicines used by 20 patients in the 2013 network and by 10 patients in the 2014 network, the new edge weight in the generated network would be 2, meaning that this combination was used twice as many times in 2013. In total, 84% of the edges were common between the two networks, while 16% of edges were unique in each. Only 19% of edges did not change between years (edge weight = 1), while 31% of edges had increased use in 2014 and 50% showed increased use in 2013 (Table 8).

Table 9 represents the most used drug pairs in 2013 compared to 2014 and vice versa in Table 10. There are many possible reasons for increasing or decreasing use. These include withdrawal of medicines from the drug market, e.g., digitoxin or approval of others, e.g., dapagliflozin and apixaban. More changes are expected to take place if the time gap between the two networks compared is longer.

TABLE 8 Drug-combination frequency comparison (2013–2014).

	Frequency	Percent
Edges with lower frequency of combining in 2013 than in 2014	19,381	31%
No change	11,861	19%
Edges with higher frequency of combining in 2013 than in 2014	31,567	50%
Total	62,809	100%

TABLE 9 Top combinations used with higher frequency in 2013 compared to 2014.

ATC 1	Medication 1	ATC 2	Medication 2	Ratio users 2013/2014
C01AA04	Digitoxin	L04AX03	Methotrexate	21
B01AB04	Deltaparin (Fragmin®)	M01AB55	Diclofenac combinations	19
C01AA04	Digitoxin	R03BA02	Budesonide	17
A11CC01	Ergocalciferol (AFI-D2 forte®)	J01CA04	Amoxicillin	16
C01AA04	Digitoxin	C09AA01	Captopril	16
M01AB05	Diclofenac	N02AB01	Ketobemidone (Ketorax®)	16
A04AA01	Ondansetron (Zofran®)	J01EE01	Sulfamethoxazole and Trimethoprim	15
C01AA04	Digitoxin	N06AA09	Amitriptyline	15
C01DA08	Isosorbide dinitrate	J01CE02	Phenoxymethylpenicillin	15
C03EA01	HCT/Pot. sparing agents	P01AB01	Metronidazole	15
G04CA01	Alfuzosin (Xatral®)	G04CA02	Tamsulosin	15

TABLE 10 Top combinations used with higher frequency in 2014 compared to 2013.

ATC 1	Medication 1	ATC 2	Medication 2	Ratio users 2014/2013
A10BK01	Dapagliflozin (Forxiga®)	C10AA05	Atorvastatin	143
B01AF02	Apixaban (Xarelto®)	C07AB07	Bisoprolol	102
C09DA04	Irebsartan/HCT (CoAprovel®)	G04BD12	Mirabegron (Betmiga®)	74
A10BA02	Metformin	A10BK01	Dapagliflozin (Forxiga®)	73
A10BK01	Dapagliflozin (Forxiga®)	B01AC06	Acetyl salicylic acid	71
B01AF02	Apixaban (Xarelto®)	C01DA14	Isosorbide mononitrate	71
A10BK01	Dapagliflozin (Forxiga®)	C10AA01	Simvastatin	70
A02BC02	Pantoprazole	B01AF02	Apixaban (Xarelto®)	68
B01AF02	Apixaban (Xarelto®)	C09CA01	Losartan	64
A10BD08	Metformin/Vildagliptin (Eucreas®)	A10BK01	Dapagliflozin (Forxiga®)	62

4. Bipartite networks

For this measure, two examples from the literature had to be used as the comedication and DDI networks do not have more than one type of nodes.. The first example of a useful application of using bipartite networks is to study the relationship between patients and prescribers or to study the relations between drugs and diseases. Hu et al. studied the prescribing of some opioids by creating a network of patients and prescribers and using the network to analyze the relationship between patients and prescribers and detect the "doctor shopping" and suspicious network nodes.[50] An example of such networks is redrawn from the mentioned paper (Fig. 9). The second example of the possible use of the bipartite networks is creating a drug-disease network to study the interactions between drugs and comorbidities as was shown by Dasgupta and Chawla.[51]

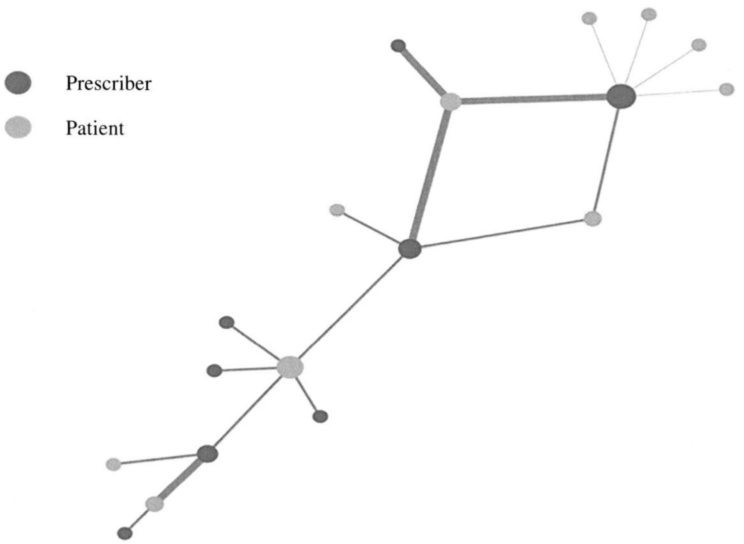

FIG. 9 An example of a bipartite network representing a sub-graph of two types of nodes (i.e., prescribers and patients) linked by the number of Fentanyl® patches prescriptions. The bigger nodes indicate more number of connections. The thicker edges indicate a higher number of prescriptions. *(Redrawn from Hu X, Gallagher M, Loveday W, Dev A, Connor JP. Network analysis and visualisation of opioid prescribing data.* IEEE J Biomed Heal Inform. *2020;24:1447–1455. doi:10.1109/JBHI.2019.2939028.)*

Conclusion

The main purpose of this chapter was to demystify network analysis as a method to use in studies of medication use. It provided a brief introduction to networks as well as a concise description of network analysis development history. The chapter guided the reader through to the process of creating medication use networks and how to use different network measures efficiently, using real-world examples from data and from the literature. Network analysis is a descriptive approach with a unique ability to represent relational datasets in one graph. Network analysis is suitable for generating hypotheses that arise while exploring the different networks. The approach has many different descriptive measures that can fit with many research questions. Modularity analysis of groupings within a network represents one of the most important measures of network analysis. Further investigation of the existing modules is necessary to justify their presence. Using network comparisons can reveal the pattern of change temporally, spatially, and in different populations. Although a variety of network measures were discussed, other measures can be tested in the future to evaluate their benefits for medication study. It is important to remember that NA also has its limitations. It can be challenging to interpret results from some networks, especially larger ones. This is why NA is primarily suited for hypothesis generation as opposed to hypothesis testing. Network analysis cannot explore many sets of relationships between variables at the same time.

The data and results presented herein also have some limitations. Defining drug exposure can be challenging, and such comedication relationships are highly dependent on the choice of method that defines the exposure. Using DDD to create treatment episodes and, using 1 DDD per day as the daily dose will work less well for the drugs that have a wide dose range such as prednisolone. It is important that researchers spend enough effort to create good exposure measurements if NA is to be useful in the medication studies. The future will likely see many new applications of NA and interesting results for researchers in social pharmacy and pharmacoepidemiology.

Questions for further discussion

1. In this chapter, network analysis was used to represent two drug-drug relationships (i.e., comedication and severe drug-drug interactions). What other drug-drug relationship(s) can be studied by network analysis? What are the expected benefits of studying these relationships?

2. Network analysis is a descriptive approach that is suitable for framing hypotheses. However, to test these framed hypotheses we need creative methods. What method(s)/approach(es) can we use to test/explain the results found in our modularity analysis for both comedication and DDIs modules?

3. From the provided references in this chapter and your own readings, what other network outcomes you think will be beneficial to investigate in the medication use context?

4. Integration of drugs and health workers in a bipartite network highlights many useful patterns. This chapter presented an example of the literature to physicians/patient bipartite network. What other forms of bipartite networks can be thought of as useful in medication use research?

Application exercise/scenario

Use the dataset provided at the repository (https://doi.org/10.18710/1OUTYI) to reproduce the severe DDIs network, apply the betweenness centrality measure to the network. What are the drugs with the highest betweenness centrality score? How do you interpret this in terms of the role these drugs play in the network? What happens if these nodes (drugs) are removed from the network?

Acknowledgments

We thank Lars Småbrekke and Elin Lehnbom for their useful feedback on the chapter. We also thank Raphael Nozal Cañadas for creating the R network syntax.

References

1. Prell C. *Social Network Analysis: History, Theory & Methodology*. Sage; 2012.
2. Asratian AS, Häggkvist R, Denley TMJ, eds. Introduction to bipartite graphs. In: *Bipartite Graphs and their Applications. Cambridge Tracts in Mathematics*. Cambridge University Press; 1998:7–22. https://doi.org/10.1017/CBO9780511984068.004.
3. Guillaume J-L, Latapy M. Bipartite structure of all complex networks. *Inf Process Lett*. 2004;90:215–221. https://doi.org/10.1016/j.ipl.2004.03.007.
4. Wasserman S, Faust K. *Social Network Analysis*. Cambridge University Press; 1994. https://doi.org/10.1017/CBO9780511815478.
5. Scott J. *Social Network Analysis*. SAGE Publications Ltd; 2017. https://doi.org/10.4135/9781529716597.
6. Luke DA, Harris JK. Network analysis in public health: history, methods, and applications. *Annu Rev Public Health*. 2007;28:69–93. https://doi.org/10.1146/annurev.publhealth.28.021406.144132.
7. Egerton FN. A history of the ecological sciences, part 6: Arabic language science: origins and zoological writings. *Bull Ecol Soc Am*. 2002;83:142–146. http://www.jstor.org/stable/20168700.
8. Hopkins B, Wilson R. The truth about königsberg. *Stud Hist Philos Math*. 2007;5:409–420. https://doi.org/10.1016/S0928-2017(07)80022-3.
9. Scott J. *Social Network Analysis : A Handbook*. 2nd ed. Sage; 2000.
10. Newman M. *Networks*. Vol. 1. 2nd ed. Oxford University Press; 2018. https://doi.org/10.1093/oso/9780198805090.001.0001.
11. Newman MEJ. Mathematics of networks. In: *The New Palgrave Dictionary of Economics*. Palgrave Macmillan UK; 2018:8525–8533. https://doi.org/10.1057/978-1-349-95189-5_2565.
12. Lundby K. Closed circles. An essay on culture and pietism in Norway. *Sociol Compass*. 1988;35:57. https://doi.org/10.1177/0037/6868803500105.
13. Moreno JL. *Who Shall Survive?: A New Approach to the Problem of Human Interrelations*. Nervous and Mental Disease Publishing Co; 1934. https://doi.org/10.1037/10648-000.
14. Borgatti SP, Mehra A, Brass DJ, Labianca G. Network analysis in the social sciences. *Science*. 2009;323:892–895. https://doi.org/10.1126/science.1165821.
15. Coleman J, Katz E, Menzel H. The diffusion of an innovation among physicians. *Sociometry*. 1957;20:253–270. https://doi.org/10.2307/2785979.
16. Bollobás B. *Random Graphs*. Vol. 73. Cambridge, GBR: Cambridge University Press; 2001. https://doi.org/10.1017/CBO9780511814068.
17. Freeman L. *The Development of Social Network Analysis, A Study in the Sociology of Science*. Vancouver, BC, Canada: ΣP Empirical Press; 2004.
18. Delmas E, Besson M, Brice M-H, et al. Analysing ecological networks of species interactions. *Biol Rev*. 2019;94:16–36. https://doi.org/10.1111/brv.12433.
19. Schmitt J. In: Schmitt NM, Kirch W, eds. *Definition of Public HealthDefinition of Public Health BT—Encyclopedia of Public Health*. Springer Netherlands; 2008:222–233. https://doi.org/10.1007/978-1-4020-5614-7_723.
20. Ken TDE, Matt JK. Modeling dynamic and network heterogeneities in the spread of sexually transmitted diseases. *Proc Natl Acad Sci U S A*. 2002;99:13330. https://doi.org/10.1073/pnas.202244299.
21. Keeling MJ, Eames KTD. Networks and epidemic models. *J R Soc Interface*. 2005;2:295–307. https://doi.org/10.1098/rsif.2005.0051.
22. Grande KM, Stanley M, Redo C, Wergin A, Guilfoyle S, Gasiorowicz M. Social network diagramming as an applied tool for public health: lessons learned from an HCV cluster. *Am J Public Health*. 2015;105:1611–1616. https://doi.org/10.2105/AJPH.2014.302193.
23. Valente TW, Davis RL. Accelerating the diffusion of innovations using opinion leaders. *Ann Am Acad Pol Soc Sci*. 1999;566:55–67. https://doi.org/10.1177/0002716299566001005.
24. Poghosyan L, Lucero RJ, Knutson AR, Friedberg MW, Poghosyan H. Social networks in health care teams: evidence from the United States. *J Health Organ Manag*. 2016;30:1119–1139. https://doi.org/10.1108/JHOM-12-2015-0201.
25. Chambers D, Wilson P, Thompson C, Harden M. Social network analysis in healthcare settings: a systematic scoping review. *PLoS One*. 2012;7. https://doi.org/10.1371/journal.pone.0041911, e41911.

26. Scott J, Tallia A, Crosson JC, et al. Social network analysis as an analytic tool for interaction patterns in primary care practices. *Ann Fam Med.* 2005;3:443. https://doi.org/10.1370/afm.344.

27. Cavallo P, Pagano S, Boccia G, De Caro F, De Santis M, Capunzo M. Network analysis of drug prescriptions. *Pharmacoepidemiol Drug Saf.* 2013;22:130–137. https://doi.org/10.1002/pds.3384.

28. Bazzoni G, Marengoni A, Tettamanti M, et al. The drug prescription network: a system-level view of drug co-prescription in community-dwelling elderly people. *Rejuvenation Res.* 2015;18:153–161. https://doi.org/10.1089/rej.2014.1628.

29. Tobi H, Faber A, van den Berg PB, Drane JW, de Jong-van den Berg LT. Studying co-medication patterns: the impact of definitions. *Pharmacoepidemiol Drug Saf.* 2007;16:405–411. https://doi.org/10.1002/pds.1304.

30. Furu K. Establishment of the nationwide Norwegian Prescription Database (NorPD); new opportunities for research in pharmacoepidemiology in Norway. *Nor Epidemiol.* 2008;18:129–136. https://doi.org/10.5324/nje.v18i2.23.

31. Raebel AM, Schmittdiel JJ, Karter LA, Konieczny FJ, Steiner FJ. Standardizing terminology and definitions of medication adherence and persistence in research employing electronic databases. *Med Care.* 2013;51(Suppl. 8):S11–S21. https://doi.org/10.1097/MLR.0b013e31829b1d2a.

32. Üstün TB. International classification systems for health. In: *International Encyclopedia of Public Health.* Elsevier; 2017:304–311. https://doi.org/10.1016/B978-0-12-803678-5.00237-X.

33. Norwegian Medicines Agency. *Fest Implementation Guidelines*; 2019. Published https://legemiddelverket.no/Documents/Andretemaer/FEST/Hvordan bruke FEST/Implementation guide FEST v3.0.pdf.

34. Pavlopoulos GA, Paez-Espino D, Kyrpides NC, Iliopoulos I. Empirical comparison of visualization tools for larger-scale network analysis. *Adv Bioinfma.* 2017;2017:1–8. https://doi.org/10.1155/2017/1278932.

35. Akhtar N. Social network analysis tools. In: *2014 Fourth International Conference on Communication Systems and Network Technologies.* IEEE; 2014:388–392. https://doi.org/10.1109/CSNT.2014.83.

36. Grund T. *Network Analysis Using Stata*; 2015. https://nwcommands.wordpress.com/tutorials-and-slides/.

37. Joyez C. NWANND: Stata module to compute ANND (average nearest neighbor degree) and related measures. In: *Stat Softw Components*; 2016. https://ideas.repec.org/c/boc/bocode/s458261.html. Accessed 29 October 2020.

38. Bastian M, Heymann S, Jacomy M. *Gephi: An Open Source Software for Exploring and Manipulating Networks*; 2009. https://doi.org/10.13140/2.1.1341.1520.

39. Cherven K. *Mastering Gephi Network Visualization Produce Advanced Network Graphs in Gephi and Gain Valuable Insights Into Your Network Datasets*; 2015.

40. Kim E-Y. Knowledge-based bioinformatics: from analysis to interpretation. *Healthc Inform Res.* 2010;16:312. https://doi.org/10.4258/hir.2010.16.4.312.

41. Barrenas F, Chavali S, Holme P, Mobini R, Benson M. Network properties of complex human disease genes identified through genome-wide association studies. *PLoS One.* 2009;4. https://doi.org/10.1371/journal.pone.0008090, e8090.

42. Freeman L, Freeman L. A set of measures of centrality based on betweenness. *Sociometry.* 1977;40:35–41. https://doi.org/10.2307/3033543.

43. Bonacich P. Power and centrality: a family of measures. *Am J Sociol.* 1987;92:1170–1182. https://doi.org/10.1086/228631.

44. Ruhnau B. Eigenvector-centrality—a node-centrality? *Soc Netw.* 2000;22:357–365. https://doi.org/10.1016/S0378-8733(00)00031-9.

45. Lutz W, Schwartz B, Hofmann SG, Fisher AJ, Husen K, Rubel JA. Using network analysis for the prediction of treatment dropout in patients with mood and anxiety disorders: a methodological proof-of-concept study. *Sci Rep.* 2018;8:7819. https://doi.org/10.1038/s41598-018-25953-0.

46. Valenzuela JFB, Monterola C, Tong VJC, Fülöp T, Ng TP, Larbi A. Degree and centrality-based approaches in network-based variable selection: insights from the Singapore Longitudinal Aging Study. *PLoS One.* 2019;14. https://doi.org/10.1371/journal.pone.0219186, e0219186.

47. Ji X, Machiraju R, Ritter A, Yen PY. Examining the distribution, modularity, and community structure in article networks for systematic reviews. In: *AMIA. Annu Symp proceedings AMIA Symp. 2015*; 2015:1927–1936.

48. Zhang M, Lu LJ. Modules in networks, algorithms and methods. In: *Encyclopedia of Systems Biology.* Springer New York; 2013:1447–1450. https://doi.org/10.1007/978-1-4419-9863-7_557.

49. Blondel VD, Guillaume J-L, Lambiotte R, Lefebvre E. Fast unfolding of communities in large networks. *J Stat Mech: Theory Exp.* 2008;2008:P10008. https://doi.org/10.1088/1742-5468/2008/10/P10008.

50. Hu X, Gallagher M, Loveday W, Dev A, Connor JP. Network analysis and visualisation of opioid prescribing data. *IEEE J Biomed Heal Inform.* 2020;24:1447–1455. https://doi.org/10.1109/JBHI.2019.2939028.

51. Dasgupta D, Chawla NV. Disease and medication networks: an insight into disease-drug interactions. In: *2nd Int. Conf. Big Data Analytics Healthcare*; 2014:157–168.

Chapter 13

Designing, evaluating and applying pictograms in pharmacy practice research

Ros Dowse

Faculty of Pharmacy, Rhodes University, Makhanda, South Africa

Objectives

- Provide an overview of health-related pictograms and their application.
- Consider the current status of pictogram-related research and offer suggestions for improving the quality and reporting of pictogram studies.
- Present considerations and general guidance for designing and modifying pictograms.
- Discuss methods of evaluating pictograms.
- Consider future research direction in the context of improving overall research quality.

Overview of health-related pictograms

In our daily lives where we are inundated with information from our fast-moving world, visuals are increasingly being used to summarize information, make it more accessible, and enhance its appeal. Many of us have learnt how to interpret symbols, icons, emojis, emoticons, infographics, etc. and to use them for personal communication. Although this boon to communication is expanding to many areas of our lives, its uptake in the all-important and often challenging area of health information and health communication practice has been slow.[1,2]

The literature is replete with reports of the high literacy demands and inadequate quality of written health and medicines information resulting in a perceived lack of usefulness and poor uptake by patients.[3,4] Health websites are frequently populated with text written at an unacceptably high reading level.[5] Groups particularly at risk of encountering problems with comprehending health information are those with low health literacy, poor reading skills and limited education, along with ethnic minorities, refugees or immigrants in countries where only information written in English is available,[6–9] as well as older patients with a higher comorbidity burden, complex medication regimens and possible cognitive decline.[10] Information communicated verbally by health providers has its limitations, as it is known to be poorly retained, with up to 80% of the information being forgotten almost immediately.[11] Within this context, a strong case can be made for the inclusion of visual images to mitigate these challenges as they offer distinct advantages; visual content is more rapidly recognized than text and is more easily processed by the brain, with memory for visuals being superior to that for words (the pictorial superiority effect). Visuals outperform text in prompting recall of information,[12,13] whereas a combination of visuals and words is superior to use of either visuals or words alone.[14]

Pictograms, which are also referred to as signs, symbols, or icons, are widely used as public information symbols appearing on traffic signs, in airports, in hospitals, as safety labeling on chemicals, or in the workplace. A pictogram can be described as a figurative/metaphorical two-dimensional drawing intended to attract attention and convey information about an object or express an idea.[15,16] In the healthcare context, a significant body of literature has shown the benefits of pictograms. Studies have explored their successful application when combined with text, and when used to supplement verbal health communication. Including visual content or pictograms in information materials enhances its readability and attractiveness and has a positive impact on patient satisfaction.[17–21] Pictograms have been shown to improve comprehension of information related to medicines use, improve knowledge of disease states and health maintenance and are particularly valuable in enhancing recall of information.[17,22–37] Pictograms can also have a positive impact on health behaviors such as medicines adherence and self-efficacy.[24,28,38–47]

Contemporary Research Methods in Pharmacy and Health Services. https://doi.org/10.1016/B978-0-323-91888-6.00024-7

Current status of pictogram-related research

Communication is an essential element in patient-centered care and is key to developing a meaningful relationship with the patient. Although the core role of pharmacists is aligned with medicines and medicine-taking behavior, allied to this is a broad spectrum of activities involving educating and informing patients about disease states, disease prevention, self-care, improving heath literacy, offering advice on diet and lifestyle, and providing input into public health campaigns. All involve communication with patients/clients, but to be effective the information must be communicated in a way that allows easy comprehension, particularly for at-risk populations. Pictograms, if well-designed and robustly evaluated, have the potential to be a valuable communication tool.

The most common application of health pictograms is in medicines and their use, and this accounts for roughly 80% of the health pictogram literature. However, a pharmacist appeared as lead author in less than half of these. Other diverse applications for pictograms have been addressed, many of which could involve pharmacist input: asthma action plan, prevention and treatment,[48-50] injury prevention,[51] discharge instructions,[21] breast healthcare,[52] decision aid for breast cancer,[53] dyspepsia,[54] pediatric anaphylaxis plan,[55] burn injury in children,[56] organ and body donation,[57] CT scan risks and benefits,[58] medicines and driving risks,[59] safety symbols,[60] cannabis health warning,[61] rheumatoid arthritis patient-reported outcomes dashboard,[62] HIV and TB,[31,37,63-65] gout,[66] diabetes,[67] oral rehydration,[36] and health promotion activities.[68]

Reviews of the pictogram literature from 2016 and earlier tend to support the use of pictures in health communication to improve patient knowledge.[22,29,30,69-71] However, more recent reviews are generally less positive and more critical, noting questionable quality evident in all stages of the pictogram research cycle. The inadequacy of the pictogram design process was noted by Lühnen et al.,[72] which, according to Pedersen,[73] contributes to the poor quality of current pharmaceutical pictograms. Pedersen advises that pictograms should incorporate additional elements and details to make their meaning more understandable for a variety of people across age groups, literacy, language and culture, and must meet certain legibility criteria. Van Beusekom et al.[74] identified a lack of consistency in the methods used to evaluate pictograms with the evaluation process often being inadequate, as is the lack of reported criteria to guide scoring of pictogram interpretation as either correct or incorrect.

Intervention studies based on pictograms also received criticism in three reviews.[22,26,74] They noted considerable heterogeneity between studies in terms of study design and quality, the design of the interventions and the outcomes measured. This precluded the inclusion of many studies which, according to Lühnen et al.[72] prevented them from asserting that pictograms are effective in improving adherence and concluding that "the overall effect of using pictures in health information remains unclear." These considered criticisms send a clear message to researchers working with pictograms to improve the quality of the design for all study stages and to ensure more detailed reporting of the overall study.

Aspects of health pictogram research and their use includes the following:

- designing new pictograms or modifying existing ones
- testing pictogram comprehension
- comparing comprehension of pictograms from different sources/in different populations
- assessing end-user pictogram preferences and opinions
- evaluating the impact of pictograms on comprehension and recall of health or medicines information compared with only text and/or verbal communication
- assessing the influence of pictograms on health behavior and health outcomes.

Insight into pictograms and their interpretation

Visual literacy refers to the abilities to understand (read), and use (write) images, as well as to think and learn in terms of images.[75] Although visual literacy is a cognitive ability, it also draws on the affective domain by evoking feeling and attitudes. Visual "language" (in this case, a pictogram) requires learning. Children in school are formally taught the alphabet, learn the shapes of each letter, and the sound each represents and then progress to combining letters to form words and thereafter begin developing reading literacy skills. However, the ability to "read" visuals is not typically taught in homes or at schools but is a more passively acquired skill developed from informal exposure to a variety of visual sources. The level and extent of exposure differs, affecting visual literacy skills and resulting in significant variations in visual literacy. This variation is particularly evident when comparing visual literacy in typical high-income country (HIC) versus low-to-middle-income country (LMIC) populations.

Table 1 offers definitions to clarify the meanings of words used in relation to pictogram characteristics, pictogram design and pictogram evaluation. Pictograms are a complex combination of visual/graphic elements, which complicates

TABLE 1 Definitions of words used in relation to pictogram characteristics, design and evaluation.

Word	Definition
Comprehension	The process of interpreting the meaning of words or pictures to understand their collective meaning
Recall	The ability to remember the meaning of each pictogram after a period of time has elapsed
Referent	An idea or object that a graphical symbol is intended to represent
Concreteness	The degree of abstraction of symbol to its referent (concrete signs depict objects which have obvious connection to the world)
Complexity	The degree of simplicity of the image or design
Meaningfulness	The extent of the relationship of a symbol to its function
Familiarity	The frequency with which symbols/signs have been encountered
Semantic distance	A measure of closeness between a symbol and its referent
Transparency	The "guessability" of the meaning of the pictogram/picture/image when its meaning is unknown
Translucency	A measure of the strength of the relationship between a pictogram and its intended meaning
Legibility	The ease with which the viewer is able to see and to identify elements of the pictogram

the interpretation of pictograms, with some being more easily understood than others. These may be analogous (or concrete), abstract, or abstract analogous (metaphorical).

- Analogous/concrete element appears "realistic" and similar to an object in the real world. They depict people (pregnant woman), places (hospital), and objects (box of tablets) all of which can be directly observed, are familiar and are therefore more easily understood.
- Abstract elements bear no direct relation to reality and represent information using graphic conventions such as arrows, shapes, symbols (symbols for male and female, mathematical + plus and minus signs). They do not exist in the real world, cannot be observed, so have be learnt.
- An abstract analogous element reflects a metaphor (circles and stars above the head reflecting dizziness, a thought balloon, a cross (or "X") superimposed over an image to suggest "do not" or prohibition.). Again, they do not actually exist but are metaphors for situations, experiences, etc., and they require learning.

This complex mix of elements and essential contextual clues imposes a heavy cognitive load on the viewer, who has to recognize the function of these individual elements, attribute relevant roles to them in the depicted scene, and then integrate this information to derive the intended meaning of the message.[76]

There is a common assumption that pictograms can be universally understood, but it is now well established that successful interpretation of the intended meaning of a visual message depends on numerous factors such as its overall design, differences in education levels, visual literacy skills, lifestyle, culture, and age, as well as viewer familiarity with the subject matter. Pictograms are open to misinterpretation which can have serious consequences for health outcomes if, for example, a medicine is taken incorrectly. Accordingly, pictograms should never be used as the sole source of information but should always be combined with verbal or written communication modes.[7]

Many examples of poor comprehensibility and misinterpretation are reported in the literature, even with well-designed pictograms. Studies have revealed significant differences in comprehension between high- versus low-literacy groups, with the difference growing as the elements become increasingly abstract and less concrete or realistic.[76] Table 2 shows misinterpretations of two sets of pictograms tested in the same population; the well-known United States Pharmacopeia (USP) pictograms[78] versus comparable pictograms designed in South Africa, an LMIC. Comprehension was evaluated in eight African language groups, with 304 participants having a maximum of 7 years of formal education.[77] The results clearly highlight the importance of evaluating the appropriateness of the original design even when using a widely applied, internationally renowned source of pictograms such as those from the USP. The impact of limited education and a totally different culture resulted in many seemingly "familiar," "simple," and "obvious" visuals appearing as overwhelmingly complex and unfamiliar to the South African viewers.

TABLE 2 Misinterpretation of two different sets of pictograms in a limited literacy study population.[77]

USP pictograms		South African pictograms	
Comprehension	Misinterpretations	Comprehension	Misinterpretations

Do not store near heat or in the sunlight

(10%)	• Take half the medicine • Take/do not take when there are clouds/smoke/in the mountains • Do not smoke when taking medicine • Do not drink water/milk with medicine • Medicine is poisonous/dangerous/expired • A rubbish bin/empty tin/bucket	(52%)	• Do not take medicine and sit near the fire/in the sun • Put the tablets next to the fire • Do not eat oranges/bananas/pineapples with medicine • Medicine will burn you/make you warm • Fire was seen as a hand/ herbal medicine/flowers/leaf

Do not drink alcohol while taking medicine

(51%)	• Take one tablet with three glasses of water • Take/do not take with water/milk/milkshake • Drink the milk, water or juice • Take medicine before you drink alcohol • Jug with cotton wool inside it	(84%)	• Take/do not take medicine with milk/any liquids • Medicine for person who drinks a lot of alcohol • Drink alcohol first then take medicine • Do not drink milk

Take this medicine on an empty stomach

(62%)	• Take the medicine with food • Take medicine before eating meat/with food/after drinking tea • Cut the tablet with the knife and fork/"these things" • Do not take tablets with a knife and fork/spoon • The plate is empty, there should be food on the plate	(87%)	• Slash means a pair of scissors • Take three tablets before meals • Take tablets after eating food • Eat a lot of food before taking tablets • Do not take the tablets

Place drops in the ear

(53%)	• Put medicine in the mouth/eye/nose/vagina • Medicine for the lungs/headache • An injection • A shoe/upper leg/head/eye/stomach/womb/vagina • Person has a sore on his lips	(95%)	• Put medicine in the eye • The man put medicine into his nose as he has a sore ear

Insert into the vagina

(42%)	• Take medicine and lie on your back • Inject yourself in the leg • Rub medicine onto thigh/in the leg • Medicine for aborting baby • Person with sore knee/hip/sore on thigh • Woman giving birth • Washing private parts	(63%)	• Take medicine if you are pregnant/have periods/sore stomach/bladder infection • Take medicine to help you fall pregnant • Medicine makes you urinate • Rub medicine on stomach • Have an injection for contraception • Woman is naked/healthy/has painful leg

Designing and/or modifying pictograms and reporting the process

This section offers a general overview of the requirements and basic guidelines for designing and/or modifying pictograms. It is not within the remit of this chapter to provide in-depth, step-by-step guidelines for this complex process. A range of design processes for generating health-related pictograms have been reported in the literature with papers emanating from various parts of the globe, from both HICs and LMICs involving highly diverse populations. Examples of papers are offered here.[32,38,40,53,64,67,76,79–100] Other texts to refer to include *Teaching Patients with Low Literacy Skills*, a 1996 book from Doak et al.[7] and a highly cited 2016 paper by Houts et al.[68]

A useful paper by Montagne[101] reviews the theoretical and taxonomic foundations of symbol (pictogram) meaning and comprehension and, drawing on a review of previously published research, proposes a model for pictogram development, testing and utility. Other sources of design information and insight into the characteristics of visuals are visual design or ergonomics journals.[73,90,102] As is evident from the diversity of methods employed in all these papers, there is no established "gold standard" for designing pictograms intended for use in healthcare and health promotion.

Target population and study setting

The target population for which new pictograms are to be designed must be clearly defined in terms of education levels, literacy, potential visual literacy skills, culture, local customs, diet, leisure activities, general lifestyle and living conditions. This insight should guide the design team in generating images that contain visual elements that are familiar and reflect local content. As pictogram research often focuses on groups who have some difficulty accessing and comprehending written or verbal health information, contextualizing their place within the more general population of the study country is essential, i.e., do they reflect a majority of the population or are they an ethnic minority/refugee/immigrant population?[103]

Educational status must be noted, as the ability to comprehend pictograms is associated with education.[84] Level of formal education must be noted in generic terms that can be universally understood by global readers, avoiding locally used terminology such as "matric," "General Certificate of Secondary Education (GCSE)," and "middle school." For example, the word "school" in the United States is often used to describe tertiary education/university, rather than the 12-year basic schooling more broadly understood by others. Descriptions of education level should be clarified in terms of the number of years required for each phase, such as "primary"/"junior," "middle" or "senior"/"high."

The descriptive term "low/limited literacy" is open to varying interpretation and can create a confounding issue in reporting education level. For example, research conducted in a HIC with almost universal literacy may stratify participants by education level into two groups—participants who completed 12 years of schooling and participants also having tertiary education, with the implication of lower literacy being associated with the former. However, in many LMICs, "lower literacy" often applies to a majority population, with many people typically having only primary school ($\sim$7 years). In this case, stratification of education level would typically be primary versus secondary school. Those with tertiary education (usually only a small percentage in LMICs) would usually be excluded. This inconsistent lens through which literacy is viewed and interpreted confounds the findings of the impact of pictograms in a "true" limited literacy population—a term for which no universally agreed-upon definition exists. Conducting a health literacy test would offer valuable insight in identifying participants who should possibly be excluded from the study, versus those who constitute a more vulnerable population in terms of access to, and understanding of, health information.[103]

Collaboration is key

Pictograms should be tailor-designed for different populations, incorporating visual images that are culturally appropriate and reflect local lifestyle and customs[7,84] Designers and researchers from many disciplines have been involved in researching aspects of health pictogram design and generation, with each team approaching it from their unique perspective.

Best practice for designing new pictograms is to adopt a collaborative approach, working with a design team consisting of the researcher(s), communication/graphic designer, health professionals and end-users. Incorporating and integrating different perspectives is essential as each team member will visualize the pictogram from an entirely different perspective and offer their unique expert opinion. This hopefully avoids assumptions of "what 'they' need to know is…" and "of course 'they' will understand that image…." Particularly important is codesign with end-users to understand local context and ensure that the end result satisfies their needs. End-users should be involved not only in an informative role but also, if possible, in a participatory role in all phases of the design process. A recent visual studies paper concluded "it is essential to place a population with a low-literacy level at the heart of [the] visual information."[102] In a systematic review investigating the extent and effects of patient involvement in pictogram design,[74] only a few studies describing this participatory approach were identified. It also found that repeatedly involving the target group in an iterative design-evaluation-redesign process was successful in developing pictograms that were more easily understood, valued and had a positive effect on end-user perception.

Generating design ideas and designing successive versions

The success of pictograms in communicating their message demands a rigorous, multistage, consultative design-test-redesign process (Fig. 1). This is time-consuming and resource-intensive but is the only approach likely to generate high quality pictograms, or to improve existing pictograms by modification.[67,73,84,93,101] Poor pictogram design and overall complexity and legibility is known to contribute to poor comprehensibility and misinterpretation.[68,104–106]

Although visuals may appear to be simple, they impose a heavy cognitive load, particularly on unskilled viewers, as the process of "reading" a visual requires recognition of individual elements, attributing relevant roles to these elements in relation to the whole picture, and finally integrating them to derive the intended meaning of the visual message. Skilled and unskilled viewers differ in their visual processing.[7] Unskilled lower literacy viewers have greater difficulty identifying the central focus or starting point; instead, their eyes tend to wander randomly, often honing in on a minor but familiar detail for comment, while ignoring the main element. The ability to integrate the elements to create overall meaning is frequently lacking. Skilled viewers, however, rapidly scan the entire image to locate the principal feature, separate core detail from background detail, and rapidly interpret the information to make meaning.[7]

Various methods have been adopted for this initial idea-generating stage including focus group discussions, workshops, semistructured interviews or application of the Delphi technique. A number of other studies have used convenient, easily accessible nonpatient groups in the early stages of idea generation, design and testing such as university students or staff members within an organization that are an easily accessible convenient sample. Others have used an online approach which has its advantages, but which therefore more or less excludes many who do not have online access.

The ideas and concepts generated from these interactions inform the initial design version and would be communicated to the graphic artist/designer who would generate the first version of the pictogram. Alternatively, the graphic artist/designer could be required to generate a draft pictogram for further discussion; in this case early input from end-users is advised. Guidelines for designing pictograms have been summarized from a number of papers and are shown in Table 3.

Initial versions are likely to require many minor, interim modifications as opinions a collected using either formal (focus group discussion) or informal means (convenience approach, e.g., asking anyone of the target population who may work in the organization). Once pictograms have been deemed acceptable by the design team, they must be pretested for comprehension in a pilot study with representative of the target population. End-user comments and misinterpretations noted during this stage are invaluable in informing further modifications prior to the final evaluation stage. In some cases, reconceptualization of the pictogram may be required. End-user acceptability of the final pictogram(s) should be assessed in all studies.

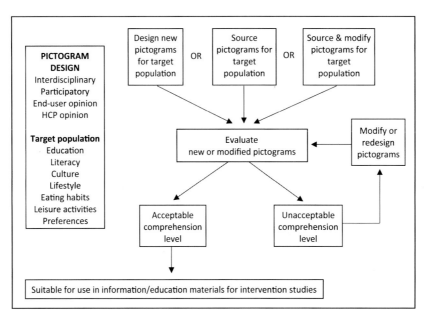

FIG. 1 Pictogram design-test-redesign cycle.

TABLE 3 Considerations in designing health pictograms for diverse populations.[7,16,80,84,101,105]

Recommendations	Notes and examples
General design	
Design simple pictures with a clear, central focus	Avoid highly complex images as they have a high cognitive load
Ensure appropriate complexity to maximize visibility and offer contextual clues	Contextual clues increase comprehension. Increased complexity can have a negative impact on legibility, and hence on comprehension
Minimize distracting details	For example, shading, texture lines, fold lines in clothes
Represent objects in a realistic manner	Restrict stylized/cartoon visuals for viewers familiar with these styles
Use familiar images if possible	Familiarity improves comprehension
Contextualize setting with familiar images	Show local clothing, hairstyles, food, eating habits, transport, etc.
Consider cultural and religious norms	Avoid potential offensive images, or those absent from the target culture
Depict the human body in an accurate, proportionally correct lifelike manner	Expanding one part of the body for emphasis is often literally and incorrectly interpreted
Use the expressive power of the body to suggest emotions, fatigue, pain	For example, body posture (upright, bending forward), knitted eyebrows (worry, pain), facial expressions (happy, sad), etc.
Display elements that are bold and large enough	Pay attention to line thickness which is linked to legibility
Maximize separation between visual elements	Elements can "merge" on size reduction and lose their legibility which can influence overall comprehension
Include adequate white space	Avoid a "busy" cluttered look and nonessential detail which can distract from the central message
Ensure words in visuals are carefully positioned and are bold and large enough to easily read	A word becomes another visual element requiring attention to its design (font and size) and positioning
Elements to avoid if possible/use with caution	
Isolated body parts	For example, only displaying an ear without attachment to the head
Internal anatomical images	Unfamiliar to many viewers
Abstract visuals using graphical conventions	For example, symbols for male and female, + and − symbols, prohibition slash or cross, arrows to show direction, thought balloon with text shown above a head
Pictograms with different border shapes	Often ignored during interpreting and may promote confusion
Challenging to represent visually	
Sequential representation of visuals denoting an activity	For example, take medicine until course completed; swilling medicine in the mouth then swallowing/spitting out
Movement	Often represented by lines and/or arrows, both graphic conventions that require learning
Behaviors, emotions, states of being, feelings	For example, depressed, confused, feeling ill, low energy, drowsiness, no appetite, hungry, dizziness, fever
Continue taking medicine for a stated number of weeks/months	Depicting passage of time on a calendar can be unfamiliar to some viewers
Remember to take medicine at a certain time	Metaphorical representation of a clock or watch to represent time
Do not share your medicines	Difficult to depict

Modification of existing pictograms

Researchers may choose to source existing pictograms and adapt them for use and evaluation in their local population. The following databases of downloadable health-related pictograms are available online or by request:

- USP pictograms: first globally accessible database, offers 81 pictograms that can be freely downloaded.[78]
- FIP pictograms (International Pharmaceutical Federation): comprehensive resource of pictograms showing variations in design for different populations.[107] Also includes pictogram-based storyboards, medication labels, drug information sheets, medication calendars, action plans for asthma, diabetes, eczema, and anaphylaxis. Associated text is available in 13 languages.
- Royal Dutch Pharmacist Association: has developed their own set of pictograms (icons) which can be accessed from their website.[108]
- Rhodes University (RU) health pictograms: South African collection of around 100 pictograms designed and tested with low health literacy end-users includes disease-based pictograms designed for HIV and TB.[109]

Many other sources of images, icons, pictograms, etc. are available online which may better suit your unique needs. However, it is essential to note differences between the original target population for which these were designed versus your study population; if they differ significantly in terms of education, culture, socioeconomic status or lifestyle, comprehension may be affected and the pictograms may require modification. From the literature it is evident that the USP pictograms are the most widely used and tested pictograms and have been evaluated in both HICs and LMICs. It should be noted, however, that results often indicate poor comprehensibility in populations outside of the United States, most particularly in LMICs.

Pictograms may be modified to improve their cultural and contextual relevance. This may require including visuals that are more familiar and reflect local context such as images of hair, faces and clothing. Modification may also aim at modifying previously tested pictograms that were poorly comprehended and did not comply with standard criteria. Minor modifications may be done to improve visual clarity and legibility, particularly, for example, if the pictograms are to be reduced in size to use on a medicine box. Some examples of modification studies are described in these papers.[80,84,95,97]

The process for modifying existing pictograms should follow the same iterative cycle as that for designing new pictograms (Fig. 1). An example of a long-term multistage design and modification process for the indication pictogram for "fever" is presented in Table 4. The target population was African first language (isiXhosa) with limited literacy. The first designs were generated as part of a 2009 Masters study.[110] In designing this pictogram, we drew on our experience gained from two prior intensive design workshops with pharmacy students aimed at generating ideas and rough images for six particularly challenging side effects of antiretrovirals, e.g., peripheral neuropathy and nightmares. We regarded fever as a simpler concept to communicate visually given its familiarity to most people. The following discussion relates to the numbered pictograms in Table 4:

#1: The graphic artist generated the initial hand-drawn image showing a person in distress, feeling his head for a temperature, with perspiration running down the forehead and throat. The hand position was changed for subsequent computer-generated versions.

#2–7: During this developmental design stage, opinions were garnered via two sources: an informal approach where a few university employees were asked who represented the target population for opinions, and a formal focus group discussion with five target population members to elicit their interpretation and opinions (of 23 pictograms, including fever). #2 was considered to contain inadequate detail and context, so a variety of symbols were added in an attempt to suggest heat (#3–5).The lightning bolts (#3) were added for emphasis and to suggest heat but were seen to represent pain. Shorter wavy lines (#4) were then added to suggest heat radiating from the head. The sweat droplets were either overlooked or taken be a rash so were removed. Three further designs that were attempted showed a corkscrew-like symbol (#5), a single layer of wavy lines interspersed with wavy lines radiating out from the head (#6) and, finally, two layers of wavy, irregular lines circling the head (#7). Informal feedback identified #7 as the favorite.

#7 Testing (2008): This version was formally tested in 40 participants, resulting in 72.5% correct interpretation. Misinterpretations included "checking for pain," "checking for headache," "person praying for better health," and "person thinking."

#7–8 Testing (2012): In an unpublished study on indication pictograms, a new attempt (#8) shows the back of the hand rather than the palm side touching the forehead. This was discarded in the pilot as most chose #7. Testing of #7 showed an extremely low comprehension of 17.5%. As for the 2008 study, the most common problem was perceiving headache to be the major focus, rather than fever.

TABLE 4 An example of the design and modification process showing successive versions of a pictogram depicting fever.

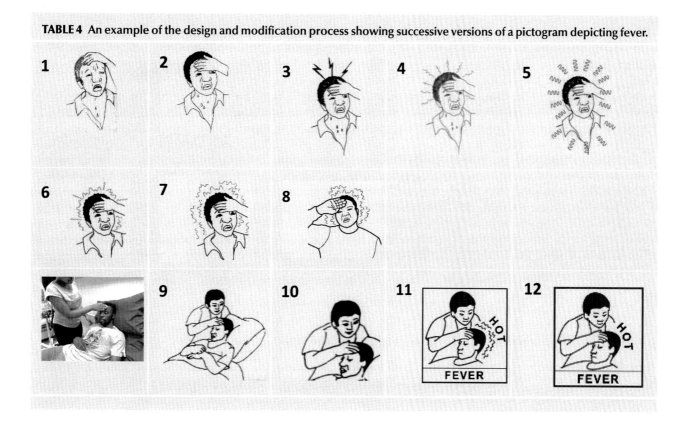

#9–13: Redesign and testing (2019): This study aimed to improve previous poorly interpreted indication pictograms and test them for comprehension. Initially, a contextual element to #7 was added—a thermometer—but it was not easily recognized and did prevent misinterpretation as "headache." The "fever" pictogram was completely reconceptualized during 2 workshops: one with 3 members of the target population, and one with 5 university students. The concept of a carer checking for a high temperature in a sick person who was lying down was adopted. A posed photograph (Table 4) was used to generate #9. In #10, unnecessary details were eliminated and the overall visual simplified by honing in on the core elements—carer, patient, hand on forehead. However, this version still caused confusion. It was decided to introduce some text into the pictogram which is not often done. Two very simple, common words, "hot" and "fever" were added, along with health waves around the head (#11). In pilot testing, the heat lines were ignored, but otherwise this version appeared promising. The heat lines were removed for the final version (#12) and this achieved a high 85.6% which achieves compliance with the ANSI 85% correct standard. This pictogram was considered to be acceptable for inclusion in health information materials, and of an appropriate quality to use in further pictogram-based intervention studies.

The above summarized description falls far short of a complete documentation of the myriad of interim minor alterations made, the multiple back-and-forth interactions within the team and with the graphic artist, and the frequent informal garnering of visual content opinion. Hopefully it reflects the multistage, intensive nature of the design process which facilitates in generating a good quality pictogram that is well comprehended and acceptable to the end-user. But no pictogram is perfect. There is always the potential for misinterpretation which should be acknowledged in terms of how it is ultimately used—never as the sole source of information, but always with verbal or written information and an explanation. Failure to follow a rigorous, multistage design process could result in inadequate and poorly comprehended visual content in pictograms, bias in reported outcomes and a possible false-negative outcome of the influence of pictograms. This shortcoming is, unfortunately, evident in the current pictogram literature.

Methods used to evaluate pictogram comprehension and recall

Several approaches to evaluating pictograms have been described in the literature. The most commonly used method directly evaluates comprehension or interpretation of the pictogram in a face-to-face interview. A number of authors have adopted an approach that includes evaluation of a selection of constructs: guessability, translucency, transparency, visibility, legibility, concreteness, complexity, meaningfulness, familiarity, and semantic distance. These appear to relate to the literature around symbols, notably public safety symbols, with their origins from around 40 years ago. The original citations emanate from a wide-ranging literature base spanning visual design, visual language, engineering, the human-computer interface, cognitive psychology, mining, air transport, human factors (ergonomics), and others.

Symbols were regarded as being easily recognized and could be used quickly to rapidly communicate safety information in public spaces. The application of these constructs to health pictogram evaluation has not been adequately supported by design theory or with a conceptual framework. Unfortunately, in many pictogram-related papers using these constructs, referencing is inadequate and, in many cases, overtly incorrect, with most authors merely citing previous pictogram studies by other health researchers. This practice compounds inappropriate and incorrect referencing. However, for researchers aiming to investigate visual design in greater depth and detail in order to contribute to design theory as it applies to health pictograms, these constructs offer a range of visual properties to explore.

The term "guessability" was initially used in the context of safety symbols for public use where the goal was to elicit a rapid response from the viewer in order to avoid imminent danger, with the response time to "guess" the meaning of the symbol being highly relevant. However, our intention in using pictograms is to enhance comprehension and retention of information. With medicines and health applications, the speed of interpreting visual images is of little relevance. Rather than rapidly attempting to "guess" the meaning of a pictogram, what is preferable is for viewers to closely scrutinize the overall pictogram, "read" and interpret the various visual elements and integrate them to derive the intended meaning of the message, which can then be applied to a health-related issue such as medicine usage.

Criteria and global standards for pictogram acceptability

There is no global standard formally assessing the acceptability of health-related pictograms. However, most authors tend to use either one of two standards. The International Organization for Standardization (ISO) publishes standards for graphical symbols. The ISO 9186-1:2014 requires that graphical symbols (pictograms) should be understood by a minimum of 67% of users when no explanatory text is offered.[111] The other is the ANSI Z535.3 standard from the American National Standards Institute which specifies a minimum 85% correct interpretation, and a maximum 5% critical confusion.[112]

Context, familiarization and comprehension evaluation

The context of the research and the role of pictograms must be well established. To allay participant anxiety about what is expected from them, a useful strategy is to show the participant a sample pictogram and to guide them through the interpretation process. It alerts them to the need to look at all visual elements, rather than focusing on one easily recognizable aspect while ignoring the rest (common with low visual literacy skills). This can serve to reassure and build confidence for what may, for some, be a particularly daunting process.

During the evaluation process, gentle prompting can serve to encourage participants to persevere in their attempts to identify individual aspects of the pictograms and work out the overall message. An example of a prompt to refocus the attention of a viewer who is only offering general vague comments could be: "What do you think this is trying to tell you about taking your medicine?". The interviewer's challenge is to walk the line between helpful general prompting as opposed to more focused prompting that might inappropriately reveal the solution. This skill has to be developed during formal interviewer training with guidance from a skilled interviewer who should sit in on pilot and early interviews to guide the research assistant.

Methods of evaluation include the following:

Correct/incorrect: The response can be categorized as either "correct or incorrect." Additional response options reported by various authors have included "partially correct," "no response," "critically confused," "opposite answer," and "I don't know/I can't guess." This process is open to bias, as opinions of what can be considered fully "correct" are likely to differ. Score allocation criteria must be clearly defined, and the calculation of the overall score described, for example: 0—incorrect, I—partially correct, 2—correct.

Fixed choice: Methods may include multiple choice tests requiring the participant to choose the correct answer from a limited set of alternative options, or may ask, for example, "which one of these four meanings is the closest to what the pictogram is trying to convey?" This type of test is invariably open to guessing and may mask incorrect comprehension.

Ranking method: Participants are asked to sort different symbols/pictograms into an order from the easiest to the hardest to understand. The problem here may be that the highest-ranked symbol of a set of poor symbols will remain a poor symbol, so this method does not reflect best practice.

Ideally, the same interviewer should collect all data to ensure consistency in the evaluation of responses. However, in cases where multiple interviewers collect data face to face, or where participants record their responses and comments online, an evaluation protocol should be developed to ensure harmonization in assessing responses relating to comprehension. All responses should be collated and evaluated by a team of assessors. Failure to formalize such a process could introduce an unacceptable degree of bias and uncertainty in the findings; this has been reported as a study limitation.[113]

Calculating an overall comprehensibility score for each participant provides useful data, as it enables investigation of statistical associations with a variety of sociodemographic and other characteristics. An average comprehensibility score for each pictogram can be calculated which can then be tested for compliance with either ANSI (85% correct) or ISO (67% correct) criteria to deem the pictogram acceptable. Pictograms deemed unacceptable or that do not comply with established criteria should, ideally, undergo further rounds of revision and retesting.

Assessing memory and the ability to recall the meaning of a pictogram has been done both short- and long-term. Short-term may, for example, be a 20-min period after pictogram testing during which some distraction is offered to participants before retesting. Long-term recall of pictogram meaning should allow for a significant time lapse between initial and follow-up testing. Papers have typically described intervals ranging from 2 weeks to a month or more.

Comments on pictogram-based intervention studies

The National Academies of Sciences, Engineering and Medicine consensus study report urges researchers to ensure reproducibility and replicability of their studies by offering "… a clear description of all methods, instruments, materials, procedures, measurements, and other variables involved in the study; a clear description of the analysis of data and decisions for exclusion of some data or inclusion of other; and discussion of the uncertainty of the measurements, results, and inferences."[114] Contrary to these recommendations, a recurring theme in all reviews in the pictogram literature is the lack of detail and incomplete description in the reporting of all stages of pictogram research. Complying with the requirements noted above is an essential step in improving the current quality of the pictogram literature and this is particularly important in intervention studies as their results provide the foundation for creating a body of literature that establishes an evidence base for the role of pictograms in healthcare.

In designing and developing information and including visual content, the overall attractiveness and readability of the message is determined by content (words and visuals) as well as by presentation. Legibility of the message depends on the technical design of words, text and visuals to ensure optimal clarity and result in information being as clear, simple, unambiguous and transparent as possible. There is a significant body of literature informing this information design process, as well as many examples of designing illustrated health and medicines information (see some examples in "Current status of pictogram-related research" section).

A recent paper offering comprehensive guidance on reporting health interventions is a useful resource.[115] In practice settings where the intervention may be delivered by a number of on-site practice staff, the challenge is to ensure that all those involved in data collection are trained to ensure consistent application of the intervention and are fully conversant with study criteria and processes. A detailed account of how the delivery of the intervention was standardized for all participants must be included when reporting the study.

Comprehensive details of the intervention must be reported. Merely offering "... the interviewer educated the participants ..." does little to enable replication of a complex pictogram intervention study. Researchers can refer to checklists such as the Template for Intervention Description and Replication (TIDieR) checklist and guide developed by an international group of experts and stakeholders to promote improvement in the completeness of reporting interventions and in their replicability.[116] The intervention tools, be they individual pictograms, illustrated written or online information, a visual tool for use in practice, or an illustrated research scale, must be pretested in a pilot study and should be fully described in the text and be displayed in the paper.

Study details often inadequately reported/absent[103]

- **Study setting and site**: The study country and the region/province/town should be named. This communicates either an HIC or LMIC status, which affords valuable insight into **general** literacy and levels of formal education, accessibility of healthcare, availability of and access to health information, use of digital media, and socioeconomic status (SES). Other descriptors could include site information (inner-city urban clinic, rural primary care clinic, tertiary/primary hospital). For LMICs, it is useful to note average education/literacy levels, mean income, primary language(s), employment and access to healthcare. All this detail affords insight into the place and potential role of pictograms in that unique healthcare setting and system and is particularly relevant as the vast divide between conditions in HICs and many LMICs is often not fully appreciated.

- **Number of pictograms to be tested**: Population characteristics should guide this decision as the cognitive load associated with interpreting pictograms is significantly higher for lower literacy individuals who are more likely to encounter viewer fatigue and disengagement with the process. A personal recommendation for limited literacy groups is between 15 and 30 pictograms. Number of pictograms tested must be stated.
- **Interview duration**: The average duration of the interview should be noted when reporting studies as if it is too long, it negatively influences sustained attention and responses become less considered. Personal experience has identified 1 h as being too long to sustain continued cognitive engagement of lower literate individuals when attempting to interpret pictograms. A maximum of 45 min or less per interview is recommended.
- **Different size pictograms for testing**: Pictogram size can affect comprehension, particularly for limited literacy viewers.[117] Best practice is to have both the original large size as well as a smaller version tested for comprehension, as reducing the size can negatively affect legibility. In practice, using pictograms on labels or in patient information leaflets dispensed with the product demands smaller sizes.
- **Randomization of pictograms**: This detail is seldom reported but is essential to implement to avoid a familiarity effect with the pictograms shown late in the testing, as they tend to be better comprehended. Pictograms should be randomized/shuffled between each testing session.
- **Visual materials not displayed in an article**: Visual material used in the study usually comprises the core component of the study and should therefore be displayed either in its entirety or at least a sample thereof. Their absence is surprisingly common in the literature, and prevents others learning from both the successes and the mistakes made. If allocated space is inadequate, the materials should be appended as supplementary information to make them available to other researchers.

Aspects to consider in future research

The inclusion of graphic designers in research teams is essential to produce visuals that have been developed according to best practice design principles. Future research should focus on the features of legibility and visibility, such as color, size, shape, line thickness, figure-background contrast, crowding, viewing distance and print quality, as well as the type of information to be communicated. A design-oriented approach could contribute new knowledge about the use of these different components and how to isolate these variables when designing test material, as well as investigating how they influence legibility. Multistage pictogram design studies are needed to improve understanding of the factors influencing comprehension, as unsatisfactory pictograms can be modified and retested in successive follow-ups until an acceptable visual is achieved.

The impact of pictograms has been shown in numerous once-off, cross-sectional studies, but there is a gap in evidence of their sustained use in practice and whether the pictogram superiority effect is sustained. Well-designed longitudinal randomized controlled trials are essential in establishing the long-term effectiveness of pictogram interventions in educating patients, influencing health behavior and contributing to health outcomes.

Lack of consensus on standard guidelines for pictogram design, modification and assessment seems to be reflected in the overall inadequate quality of health pictogram research. A collaborative global initiative should be initiated to consider guidelines informing best practice in all these areas. This could inform the generation of a more reliable, reproducible body of evidence for highlighting the role and impact of pictograms in health communication.

Questions for further discussion

1. Medicine-taking behavior is influenced by the ability to understand medicines information communicated verbally and in writing. If pictograms are used to illustrate selected medicine information, current practice is to use the ISO or ANSI standards to determine their acceptability; however, these standards apply to public signs and symbols intended as the sole source of communication and for rapid response. How do we as researchers and health professionals address the need for a more appropriate approach to determining the acceptability of a pictogram so that we can use it with confidence on a label, in written information or with verbal communication?
2. Although validation criteria are applied broadly in research, there are currently no specific standard methods for the validation of health-related pictograms. Apart from identifying a predetermined level of comprehension as representing acceptability, what other validation criteria should be applied to visual content?

3. Literature clearly shows the absence of a "gold standard" method for assessing comprehension of pictograms despite this process being significantly more complex than evaluating a response offered verbally or in writing. What might some considerations be in establishing a rigorous method for assessing the extent of comprehension and recording the responses?

Application exercise/scenario

You are interested in initiating a project to address problems with medicines administration to pediatric patients, as you have noted frequent errors by parents/grandparents/carers in the administration of certain liquid medicines. Two particular problems have been identified: (1) errors in measuring the correct volume in a syringe to administer oral medication, and (2) incorrectly administering skin lotion intended for external application via the oral route. You want to develop information for these two scenarios and include pictograms to help with comprehension as many of the older population in the area have limited literacy. You recently saw the USP pictograms and know there is a pictogram showing a syringe. Is it suitable for you to use or does it require modification? Why—what needs changing? Are there any USP pictograms that illustrate "apply lotion on the skin" and "do not take by mouth"? if not, what will some of your initial steps be to gather information and assistance? Would you be happy with working alone? If you felt it better practice to include other members, who would you try to include in your team? What are the various aspects to consider in designing and evaluating new and modified pictograms?

References

1. Entwistle V, Williams B. Health literacy: the need to consider images as well as words. *Health Expect.* 2008;11(2):99–101. https://doi.org/10.1111/j.1369-7625.2008.00509.x.
2. Dowse R. Pharmacists, are words enough? The case for pictograms as a valuable communication tool. *Res Soc Admin Pharm.* 2021;17(8):1518–1522. https://doi.org/10.1016/j.sapharm.2020.10.013.
3. Protheroe J, Estacio EV, Saidy-Khan S. Patient information materials in general practices and promotion of health literacy: an observational study of their effectiveness. *Br J Gen Pract.* 2015;65(632):e192–e197. https://doi.org/10.3399/bjgp15X684013.
4. Grime J, Blenkinsopp A, Raynor DK, Pollock K, Knapp P. The role and value of written information for patients about individual medicines: a systematic review. *Health Expect.* 2007;10(3):286–298. https://doi.org/10.1111/j.1369-7625.2007.00454.x.
5. Mcinnes N, Haglund BJA. Readability of online health information: implications for health literacy. *Inform Health Soc Care.* 2011;36(4):173–189. https://doi.org/10.3109/17538157.2010.542529.
6. Bellamy K, Ostini R, Martini N, Kairuz T. Access to medication and pharmacy services for resettled refugees: a systematic review. *Aust J Prim Health.* 2015;21(3):273–278. https://doi.org/10.1071/PY14121.
7. Doak CC, Doak LG, Root JH. *Teaching Patients With Low Literacy Skills.* 2nd ed. J.B. Lippincott; 1996.
8. Institute of Medicine. *Health Literacy: A Prescription to End Confusion.* The National Academies Press; 2004. https://doi.org/10.17226/10883.
9. Williams MV, Parker RM, Baker DW, et al. Inadequate functional health literacy among patients at two public hospitals. *JAMA.* 1995;274(21):1677–1682. https://doi.org/10.1001/jama.1995.03530210031026.
10. Baker DW, Gazmararian JA, Sudano J, Patterson M. The association between age and health literacy among elderly persons. *J Gerontol B Psychol Sci Soc Sci.* 2000;55(6):S368–S374. https://doi.org/10.1093/geronb/55.6.S368.
11. Kessels RPC. Patients' memory for medical information. *J R Soc Med.* 2003;96:219–222.
12. Paivio A, Rogers TB, Smythe PC. Why are pictures easier to recall than words? *Psychon Sci.* 1968;11(4):137–138. https://doi.org/10.3758/BF03331011.
13. Mayer RE. *Multimedia Learning.* Cambridge University Press; 2009.
14. Haber RN, Myers BL. Memory for pictograms, pictures, and words separately and all mixed up. *Perception.* 1982;11(1):57–64. https://doi.org/10.1068/p110057.
15. Abdullah R, Hübner R, Cziwerny R. *Pictograms, Icons & Signs: A Guide to Information Graphics.* Thames & Hudson; 2006.
16. Tijus C, Barcenilla J, de Lavalette BC, Meunier J-G. The design, understanding and usage of pictograms. In: *Written Documents in the Workplace.* Brill; 2007:17–31. [chapter 2] https://brill.com/view/book/edcoll/9789004253254/B9789004253254-s003.xml. Accessed 27 May 2020.
17. Houts PS, Doak CC, Doak LG, Loscalzo MJ. The role of pictures in improving health communication: a review of research on attention, comprehension, recall, and adherence. *Patient Educ Couns.* 2006;61(2):173–190. https://doi.org/10.1016/j.pec.2005.05.004.
18. Mansoor L, Dowse R. Written medicines information for South African HIV/AIDS patients: does it enhance understanding of co-trimoxazole therapy? *Health Educ Res.* 2006;22(1):37–48. https://doi.org/10.1093/her/cyl039.
19. Sansgiry SS, Cady PS, Adamcik BA. Consumer comprehension of information on over-the-counter medication labels: effects of picture superiority and individual differences based on age. *J Pharm Mark Manage.* 1997;11(3):63–76. https://doi.org/10.3109/J058v11n03_05.
20. Bernardini C, Ambrogi V, Perioli LC, Tiralti MC, Fardella G. Comprehensibility of the package leaflets of all medicinal products for human use: a questionnaire survey about the use of symbols and pictograms. *Pharmacol Res.* 2000;41(6):679–688. https://doi.org/10.1006/phrs.1999.0639.

21. Hill B, Perri-Moore S, Kuang J, et al. Automated pictographic illustration of discharge instructions with glyph: impact on patient recall and satisfaction. *J Am Med Inform Assoc.* 2016;23(6):1136–1142. https://doi.org/10.1093/jamia/ocw019.

22. Park J, Zuniga J. Effectiveness of using picture-based health education for people with low health literacy: an integrative review. In: Lee A, ed. *Cogent Med.* 3; 2016. https://doi.org/10.1080/2331205X.2016.1264679 [1].

23. Browne SH, Barford K, Ramela T, Dowse R. The impact of illustrated side effect information on understanding and sustained retention of antiretroviral side effect knowledge. *Res Social Adm Pharm.* 2019;15(4):469–473. https://doi.org/10.1016/j.sapharm.2018.05.012.

24. Dowse R, Ehlers M. Medicine labels incorporating pictograms: do they influence understanding and adherence? *Patient Educ Couns.* 2005;58(1): 63–70. https://doi.org/10.1016/j.pec.2004.06.012.

25. Dowse R, Ehlers MS. The evaluation of pharmaceutical pictograms in a low-literate South African population. *Patient Educ Couns.* 2001;45(2): 87–99. https://doi.org/10.1016/S0738-3991(00)00197-X.

26. Sletvold H, Sagmo LAB, Torheim EA. Impact of pictograms on medication adherence: a systematic literature review. *Patient Educ Couns.* 2020; 103(6):1095–1103. https://doi.org/10.1016/j.pec.2019.12.018. Published online December.

27. Garcia-Retamero R, Okan Y, Cokely ET. Using visual aids to improve communication of risks about health: a review. *Scientific World Journal.* 2012;2012:1–10. https://doi.org/10.1100/2012/562637.

28. Chan H-K, Hassali MA. Modified labels for long-term medications: influences on adherence, comprehension and preferences in Malaysia. *Int J Clin Pharmacol.* 2014;36(5):904–913. https://doi.org/10.1007/s11096-014-0003-1.

29. Barros IMC, Alcântara TS, Mesquita AR, Santos ACO, Paixão FP, Lyra DP. The use of pictograms in the health care: a literature review. *Res Soc Admin Pharm.* 2014;10(5):704–719. https://doi.org/10.1016/j.sapharm.2013.11.002.

30. Katz MG, Kripalani S, Weiss BD. Use of pictorial aids in medication instructions: a review of the literature. *Am J Health Syst Pharm.* 2006;63 (23):2391–2397. https://doi.org/10.2146/ajhp060162.

31. Mansoor LE, Dowse R. Effect of pictograms on readability of patient information materials. *Ann Pharmacother.* 2003;37(7–8):1003–1009. https://doi.org/10.1345/aph.1C449.

32. Zeng-Treitler Q, Perri S, Nakamura C, et al. Evaluation of a pictograph enhancement system for patient instruction: a recall study. *J Am Med Inform Assoc.* 2014;21(6):1026–1031. https://doi.org/10.1136/amiajnl-2013-002330.

33. Yin HS, Mendelsohn AL, Fierman A, van Schaick L, Bazan IS, Dreyer BP. Use of a pictographic diagram to decrease parent dosing errors with infant acetaminophen: a health literacy perspective. *Acad Pediatr.* 2011;11(1):50–57. https://doi.org/10.1016/j.acap.2010.12.007.

34. Sorfleet C, Vaillancourt R, Groves S, Dawson J. Design, development and evaluation of pictographic instructions for medications used during humanitarian missions. *Can Pharm J.* 2009;142(2):82–88. https://doi.org/10.3821/1913-701X-142.2.82.

35. Wolf MS, Davis TC, Bass PF, et al. Improving prescription drug warnings to promote patient comprehension. *Arch Intern Med.* 2010;170(1): 50–56. https://doi.org/10.1001/archinternmed.2009.454.

36. Heyns J, van Huyssteen M, Bheekie A. The effectiveness of using text and pictograms on oral rehydration, dry-mixture sachet labels. *Afr J Prim Health Care Fam Med.* 2021;13(1). https://doi.org/10.4102/phcfm.v13i1.2646.

37. Dowse R, Barford K, Browne SH. Simple, illustrated medicines information improves ARV knowledge and patient self-efficacy in limited literacy South African HIV patients. *AIDS Care.* 2014;26(11):1400–1406. https://doi.org/10.1080/09540121.2014.931559.

38. Ngoh LN, Shepherd MD. Design, development, and evaluation of visual aids for communicating prescription drug instructions to nonliterate patients in rural Cameroon. *Patient Educ Couns.* 1997;31(3):245–261. https://doi.org/10.1016/s0738-3991(97)89866-7.

39. Yin HS, Dreyer BP, van Schaick L, Foltin GL, Dinglas C, Mendelsohn AL. Randomized controlled trial of a pictogram-based intervention to reduce liquid medication dosing errors and improve adherence among caregivers of young children. *Arch Pediatr Adolesc Med.* 2008;162(9):814. https://doi.org/10.1001/archpedi.162.9.814.

40. Braich PS, Almeida DR, Hollands S, Coleman MT. Effects of pictograms in educating 3 distinct low-literacy populations on the use of postoperative cataract medication. *Can J Ophthalmol.* 2011;46(3):276–281. https://doi.org/10.1016/j.jcjo.2011.05.004.

41. Zerafa N, Adami MZ, Galea J. Impact of drugs counselling by an undergraduate pharmacist on cardiac surgical patient's compliance to medicines. *Pharm Pract (Granada).* 2011;9(3):156–161.

42. Kripalani S, Schmotzer B, Jacobson TA. Improving medication adherence through graphically enhanced interventions in coronary heart disease (IMAGE-CHD): a randomized controlled trial. *J Gen Intern Med.* 2012;27(12):1609–1617. https://doi.org/10.1007/s11606-012-2136-z.

43. Negarandeh R, Mahmoodi H, Noktehdan H, Heshmat R, Shakibazadeh E. Teach back and pictorial image educational strategies on knowledge about diabetes and medication/dietary adherence among low health literate patients with type 2 diabetes. *Prim Care Diabetes.* 2013;7(2):111–118. https://doi.org/10.1016/j.pcd.2012.11.001.

44. Kalichman SC, Cherry C, Kalichman MO, et al. Randomized clinical trial of HIV treatment adherence counseling interventions for people living with HIV and limited health literacy. *J Acquir Immune Defic Syndr.* 2013;63(1):42–50. https://doi.org/10.1097/QAI.0b013e318286ce49.

45. Mohan A, Riley MB, Schmotzer B, Boyington DR, Kripalani S. Improving medication understanding among Latinos through illustrated medication lists. *Am J Manag Care.* 2014;20(12):9.

46. Monroe AK, Pena JS, Moore RD, et al. Randomized controlled trial of a pictorial aid intervention for medication adherence among HIV-positive patients with comorbid diabetes or hypertension. *AIDS Care.* 2018;30(2):199–206. https://doi.org/10.1080/09540121.2017.1360993.

47. Avarebeel S, Nikita N, Pereira P. Study on impact of pictorial drug labelling on medication compliance among elderly. *AGEMS.* 2020;7(1): 32–38. https://doi.org/10.18231/j.agems.2020.005.

48. Wrench W, Van Dyk L, Srinivas S, Dowse R. Outcome of illustrated information leaflet on correct usage of asthma-metered dose inhaler. *Afr J Prim Health Care Fam Med.* 2019;11(1). https://doi.org/10.4102/phcfm.v11i1.2079.

49. Tulloch J, Vaillancourt R, Irwin D, Pascuet E. Evaluation, modification and validation of a set of asthma illustrations in children with chronic asthma in the emergency department. *Can Respir J.* 2012;19(1):26–31. https://doi.org/10.1155/2012/367487.

50. Yin HS, Gupta RS, Tomopoulos S, et al. A low-literacy asthma action plan to improve provider asthma counseling: a randomized study. *Pediatrics.* 2016;137(1):e20150468. https://doi.org/10.1542/peds.2015-0468.

51. Powell EC, Tanz RR, Uyeda A, Gaffney MB, Sheehan KM. Injury prevention education using pictorial information. *Pediatrics.* 2000;105(1):e16. https://doi.org/10.1542/peds.105.1.e16.

52. Choi J. Development and pilot test of pictograph-enhanced breast health-care instructions for community-residing immigrant women: pictograph-based breast care instruction. *Int J Nurs Pract.* 2012;18(4):373–378. https://doi.org/10.1111/j.1440-172X.2012.02051.x.

53. Durand M-A, Alam S, Grande SW, Elwyn G. 'Much clearer with pictures': using community-based participatory research to design and test a picture option grid for underserved patients with breast cancer. *BMJ Open.* 2016;6(2):e010008. https://doi.org/10.1136/bmjopen-2015-010008.

54. Tack J, Carbone F, Holvoet L, Vanheel H, Vanuytsel T, Vandenberghe A. The use of pictograms improves symptom evaluation by patients with functional dyspepsia. *Aliment Pharmacol Ther.* 2014;40(5):523–530. https://doi.org/10.1111/apt.12855.

55. Mok G, Vaillancourt R, Irwin D, Wong A, Zemek R, Alqurashi W. Design and validation of pictograms in a pediatric anaphylaxis action plan. *Pediatr Allergy Immunol.* 2015;26(3):223–233. https://doi.org/10.1111/pai.12349.

56. Liu H-F, Lin F-S, Chang C-J. The effectiveness of using pictures in teaching young children about burn injury accidents. *Appl Ergon.* 2015;51:60–68. https://doi.org/10.1016/j.apergo.2015.04.013.

57. Irwin J, Roughley M, Smith K. 'To donate or not to donate? That is the question!': an organ and body donation comic. *J Vis Commun Med.* 2020;43(3):103–118. https://doi.org/10.1080/17453054.2020.1770059.

58. Dowling S, Hair H, Boudreau D, et al. A patient-focused information design intervention to support the minor traumatic brain injuries (mTBI) choosing wisely Canada recommendation. *Cureus.* 2019;11(10):e5877. https://doi.org/10.7759/cureus.5877.

59. Emich B, van Dijk L, Monteiro SP, de Gier JJ. A study comparing the effectiveness of three warning labels on the package of driving-impairing medicines. *Int J Clin Pharmacol.* 2014;36(6):1152–1159. https://doi.org/10.1007/s11096-014-0010-2.

60. Handcock HE, Rogers WA, Schroeder D, Fisk AD. Safety symbol comprehension: effects of symbol type, familiarity, and age. *Hum Factors.* 2004;46(2):183–195. https://doi.org/10.1518/hfes.46.2.183.37344.

61. Leos-Toro C, Fong GT, Meyer SB, Hammond D. Perceptions of effectiveness and believability of pictorial and text-only health warning labels for cannabis products among Canadian youth. *Int J Drug Policy.* 2019;73:24–31. https://doi.org/10.1016/j.drugpo.2019.07.001.

62. Ragouzeos D, Gandrup J, Berrean B, et al. "Am I OK?" using human centered design to empower rheumatoid arthritis patients through patient reported outcomes. *Patient Educ Couns.* 2019;102(3):503–510. https://doi.org/10.1016/j.pec.2018.10.016.

63. Okeyo I, Dowse R. An illustrated booklet for reinforcing community health worker knowledge of tuberculosis and facilitating patient counselling. *Afr J Primary Health Care Family Med.* 2018;10(1):1687.

64. McDonald J, Vaillancourt R, Mishra P, Pouliot A. HIV-TB treatment pictogram tool designed from semiotic analysis for community pharmacists in India. *Indian J Pharm Sci.* 2019;81(2):373–379. https://doi.org/10.36468/pharmaceutical-sciences.519.

65. Stonbraker S, Flynn G, George M, et al. Feasibility and acceptability of using information visualizations to improve HIV-related communication in a limited-resource setting: a short report. *AIDS Care.* 2021;10:1–7. https://doi.org/10.1080/09540121.2021.1883517. Published online February.

66. Krasnoryadtseva A, Dalbeth N, Petrie KJ. The effect of different styles of medical illustration on information comprehension, the perception of educational material and illness beliefs. *Patient Educ Couns.* 2020;103(3):556–562. https://doi.org/10.1016/j.pec.2019.09.026.

67. Cloutier M, Vaillancourt R, Pynn D, et al. Design and development of culture-specific pictograms for type 2 diabetes mellitus education and counselling. *Can J Diabetes.* 2014;38(6):379–392. https://doi.org/10.1016/j.jcjd.2014.03.010.

68. Houts PS, Shankar S, Klassen AC, Robinson EB. Use of pictures to facilitate nutrition education for low-income African American women. *J Nutr Educ Behav.* 2006;38(5):317–318. https://doi.org/10.1016/j.jneb.2006.06.002.

69. Ray D, Louis VDR, Villarreal DG, Pouliot DA. Pictograms: can they help patients recall medication safety instructions? *Visible Language.* 2016;50(1):13.

70. Mansukhani S. The effect of using pictograms on comprehension of medical information- a meta-analysis. *J Pharm Pharm Sci.* 2015;1(1):22–32. https://doi.org/10.24218/vjpps.2015.05.

71. Chan HK, Hassali MA, Lim CJ, Saleem F, Tan WL. Using pictograms to assist caregivers in liquid medication administration: a systematic review. *J Clin Pharm Ther.* 2015;40(3):266–272. https://doi.org/10.1111/jcpt.12272.

72. Lühnen J, Steckelberg A, Buhse S. Pictures in health information and their pitfalls: focus group study and systematic review. *Z Evid Fortbild Qual Gesundhwes.* 2018;137–138:77–89. https://doi.org/10.1016/j.zefq.2018.08.002.

73. Pedersen P. Legibility of pharmaceutical pictograms: towards defining a paradigm. *Visible Language.* 2019;52(2):37–99.

74. van Beusekom MM, Kerkhoven AH, Bos MJW, Guchelaar H-J, van den Broek JM. The extent and effects of patient involvement in pictogram design for written drug information: a short systematic review. *Drug Discov Today.* 2018;23(6):1312–1318. https://doi.org/10.1016/j.drudis.2018.05.013.

75. Avgerinou MD, Pettersson R. Toward a cohesive theory of visual literacy. *J Visual Literacy.* 2011;30(2):1–19. https://doi.org/10.1080/23796529.2011.11674687.

76. Carstens A, Maes A, Gangla-Birir L. Understanding visuals in HIV/AIDS education in South Africa: differences between literate and low-literate audiences. *Afr J AIDS Res.* 2006;5(3):221–232. https://doi.org/10.2989/16085900609490383.

77. Dowse R, Ehlers M. Pictograms for conveying medicine instructions: comprehension in various south African language groups. *S Afr J Sci.* 2004;100(11–12):687–693.

78. USP. *Download USP Pictograms.* USP. U.S. Pharmacopeia. https://www.usp.org/download-pictograms (Accessed 7 May 2020).

79. Wolff JS, Wogalter MS. Test and development of pharmaceutical pictorials. *Interface*. 1993;93:187–192.

80. Mansoor LE, Dowse R. Design and evaluation of a new pharmaceutical pictogram sequence to convey medicine usage. *Ergonomics SA*. 2004; 16:29–41.

81. Kassam R, Vaillancourt R, Collins JB. Pictographic instructions for medications: do different cultures interpret them accurately? *Int J Pharm Pract*. 2010;12(4):199–209. https://doi.org/10.1211/0022357044698.

82. Zeng-Treitler Q, Kim H, Hunter M. Improving patient comprehension and recall of discharge instructions by supplementing free texts with pictographs. *AMIA Annu Symp Proc*. 2008;2008:849–853.

83. Ruland CM, Starren J, Vatne TM. Participatory design with children in the development of a support system for patient-centered care in pediatric oncology. *J Biomed Inform*. 2008;41(4):624–635. https://doi.org/10.1016/j.jbi.2007.10.004.

84. Dowse R, Ramela T, Barford K-L, Browne S. Developing visual images for communicating information about antiretroviral side effects to a low-literate population. *Afr J AIDS Res*. 2010;9(3):213–224. https://doi.org/10.2989/16085906.2010.530172.

85. Chuang M-H, Lin C-L, Wang Y-F, Cham T-M. Development of pictographs depicting medication use instructions for low-literacy medical clinic ambulatory patients. *JMCP*. 2010;16(5):337–345. https://doi.org/10.18553/jmcp.2010.16.5.337.

86. Grenier S, Vaillancourt R, Pynn D, et al. Design and development of culture-specific pictograms for the labelling of medication for first nation communities. *J Commun Healthc*. 2011;4(4):238–245. https://doi.org/10.1179/1753807611Y.0000000007.

87. Park M. Effects of interactive pictorial education on community dwelling older adult's self efficacy and knowledge for safe medication. *J Korean Acad Nurs*. 2011;41(6):795. https://doi.org/10.4040/jkan.2011.41.6.795.

88. Rajesh R, Vidyasagar S, Varma DM, Sharma S. Design and evaluation of pictograms for communicating information about adverse drug reactions to antiretroviral therapy in Indian human immunodeficiency virus positive patients. *J Pharm Biomed Sci*. 2012;16(16):11.

89. Wilson EAH, Vaillancourt R, Pascuet E, Besançon LJR, Wolf MS. Seeking international consensus in the use of icons for medication instructions. *J Commun Healthc*. 2012;5(1):67–72. https://doi.org/10.1179/1753807611Y.0000000014.

90. Zender M, Mejia GM. Improving icon design: through focus on the role of individual symbols in the construction of meaning. *Visible Language*. 2013;47(1):2–25.

91. Stones C, Knapp P, Malmgren L. The interpretation of triangular borders to indicate warning in medicines pictograms and the potential influence of being a driver. *IDJ*. 2013;20(2):161–170. https://doi.org/10.1075/idj.20.2.06sto.

92. Kheir N, Awaisu A, Radoui A, El Badawi A, Jean L, Dowse R. Development and evaluation of pictograms on medication labels for patients with limited literacy skills in a culturally diverse multiethnic population. *Res Soc Admin Pharm*. 2014;10(5):720–730. https://doi.org/10.1016/j.sapharm.2013.11.003.

93. van Beusekom M, Bos M, Wolterbeek R, Guchelaar H-J, van den Broek J. Patients' preferences for visuals: differences in the preferred level of detail, type of background and type of frame of icons depicting organs between literate and low-literate people. *Patient Educ Couns*. 2015;98(2): 226–233. https://doi.org/10.1016/j.pec.2014.10.023.

94. Berthenet M, Vaillancourt R, Pouliot A. Evaluation, modification, and validation of pictograms depicting medication instructions in the elderly. *J Health Commun*. 2016;21(Sup 1):27–33. https://doi.org/10.1080/10810730.2015.1133737.

95. Wolpin SE, Nguyen JK, Parks JJ, et al. Redesigning pictographs for patients with low health literacy and establishing preliminary steps for delivery via smart phones. *Pharm Pract (Granada)*. 2016;14(2):686. https://doi.org/10.18549/PharmPract.2016.02.686.

96. Vaillancourt R, Khoury C, Pouliot A. Pictograms for safer medication management by health care workers. *Can J Hosp Pharm*. 2016;71:258–266.

97. Merks P, Świeczkowski D, Balcerzak M, et al. The evaluation of pharmaceutical pictograms among elderly patients in community pharmacy settings: a multicenter pilot study. *PPA*. 2018;12:257–266. https://doi.org/10.2147/PPA.S150113.

98. Phimarn W, Ritthiya L, Rungsoongnoen R, Pattaradulpithuk W, Saramunee K. Development and evaluation of a pictogram for thai patients with low literate skills. *Indian J Pharm Sci*. 2019;81(1):89–98. https://doi.org/10.4172/pharmaceutical-sciences.1000483.

99. Vaillancourt R, Zender MP, Coulon L, Pouliot A. Development of pictograms to enhance medication safety practices of health care workers and international preferences. *Can J Hosp Pharm*. 2018;71(4):243–257. https://doi.org/10.4212/cjhp.v71i4.2834.

100. Haragi M, Ishikawa H, Kiuchi T. Investigation of suitable illustrations in medical care. *J Vis Commun Med*. 2019;42(4):158–168. https://doi.org/10.1080/17453054.2019.1633237.

101. Montagne M. Pharmaceutical pictograms: a model for development and testing for comprehension and utility. *Res Soc Admin Pharm*. 2013;9 (5):609–620. https://doi.org/10.1016/j.sapharm.2013.04.003.

102. Cohen G, Moliner P. Analogic and symbolic dimensions in graphic representations associated with patient information leaflets for medicines. *Visual Studies*. 2021;30:1–11. https://doi.org/10.1080/1472586X.2021.1900745. Published online March.

103. Dowse R. Designing and reporting pictogram research: problems, pitfalls and lessons learnt. *Res Soc Admin Pharm*. 2021;17(6):1208–1215. https://doi.org/10.1016/j.sapharm.2020.08.013.

104. Lesch MF, Powell WR, Horrey WJ, Wogalter MS. The use of contextual cues to improve warning symbol comprehension: making the connection for older adults. *Ergonomics*. 2013;56(8):1264–1279. https://doi.org/10.1080/00140139.2013.802019.

105. van Beusekom MM, Land-Zandstra AM, Bos MJW, van den Broek JM, Guchelaar H-J. Pharmaceutical pictograms for low-literate patients: understanding, risk of false confidence, and evidence-based design strategies. *Patient Educ Couns*. 2017;100(5):966–973. https://doi.org/10.1016/j.pec.2016.12.015.

106. Wogalter MS, Conzola VC, Smith-Jackson TL. Research-based guidelines for warning design and evaluation. *Appl Ergon*. 2002;33(3): 219–230. https://doi.org/10.1016/S0003-6870(02)00009-1.

107. FIP Foundation for Education and Research. *Pictogram Software—FIP Foundation. Pictograms Support. Pictogram Software*; 2017. https://www.fipfoundation.org/pictograms-support/pictogram-software/. Accessed 7 May 2020.

108. Uitleg in beeld. *Wat betekenen de iconen?*. Apotheek.nl. https://www.apotheek.nl/kunt-u-dat-even-uitleggen/beelden (Accessed 2 July 2020).

109. Dowse R, RU Health Pictograms. Available at: http://rupictogramsdowse.co.za/. Accessed November 21, 2021.

110. Ramela T. *An Illustrated Information Leaflet for Low-Literate HIV/AIDS Patients on Antiretroviral Therapy: Design, Development and Evaluation*; 2009. http://hdl.handle.net/10962/d1007563.

111. ISO 9186-1:2014. *Graphical Symbols—Test Methods—Part 1: Method for Testing Comprehensibility*. ISO; 2014. https://www.iso.org/cms/render/live/en/sites/isoorg/contents/data/standard/05/92/59226.html. Accessed 1 July 2020.

112. American National Standard for Criteria for Safety Symbols. *NEMA National Electrical Manufacturers Association*; 2017. https://www.nema.org/Standards/Pages/American-National-Standard-Criteria-for-Safety-Symbols.aspx#:~:text=Provides%20general%20criteria%20for%20the,information%20to%20avoid%20personal%20injury. Accessed 1 July 2020.

113. Vaillancourt R, Truong Y, Karmali S, et al. Instructions for masking the taste of medication for children: validation of a pictogram tool. *Can Pharm J*. 2017;150(1):52–59. https://doi.org/10.1177/1715163516669383.

114. Consensus Study Report. *Reproducibility and Replicability in Science*. The National Academies Press; 2019. https://www.nap.edu/catalog/25303/reproducibility-and-replicability-in-science. Accessed 1 July 2020.

115. Duncan E, O'Cathain A, Rousseau N, et al. Guidance for reporting intervention development studies in health research (GUIDED): an evidence-based consensus study. *BMJ Open*. 2020;10(4):e033516. https://doi.org/10.1136/bmjopen-2019-033516.

116. Hoffmann TC, Glasziou PP, Boutron I, et al. Better reporting of interventions: template for intervention description and replication (TIDieR) checklist and guide. *BMJ*. 2014;348(mar07 3):g1687. https://doi.org/10.1136/bmj.g1687.

117. Knapp P, Raynor DK, Jebar AH, Price SJ. Interpretation of medication pictograms by adults in the UK. *Ann Pharmacother*. 2005;39(7–8):1227–1233. https://doi.org/10.1345/aph.1E483.

Chapter 14

Application of photovoice in pharmacy and health services research

Lourdes Cantarero Arevalo[a] and Amy Werremeyer[b]

[a]Department of Pharmacy, Social and Clinical Pharmacy Research Group, University of Copenhagen, Copenhagen, Denmark, [b]Department of Pharmacy Practice, North Dakota State University, Fargo, ND, United States

Objectives

- Describe attributes of the Photovoice Method that make it useful for studying topics of interest in pharmacy and health services research.
- List steps that are helpful for implementation of Photovoice in pharmacy and health services research.
- Describe ethical challenges in the Photovoice implementation process.
- Describe considerations for data analysis when utilizing the Photovoice method.

What is photovoice?

Photovoice is a qualitative research method where people, through images (photography, drawings, or paintings), capture, represent, and communicate their experiences and perspectives about issues that are important to them, with the final goal of raising awareness and triggering social change.[1] Though Photovoice has been used solely as a means of gathering qualitative data, when applied in its truest form and according to its original intent, development of a shared vision for social change and a shared method for promoting and carrying out that social change between the researchers and the participants is the ultimate goal. Photovoice is informed by participatory action research approaches, feminist theory, Paulo Freire's critical pedagogy, and theory of photography.[2] Freire emphasized the importance of people speaking from their own experience, critically analyzing current situations to develop deeper understanding, and formulating solutions.[3] Feminist theory posits that power accrues to those who have a voice, make history, and participate in decisions.[4,5] Community-based documentary photography approaches emphasize a grassroots approach to representation of present realities and the use of photography as a personal voice.[4,6,7] Photovoice combines these theoretical perspectives to empower individuals and groups who traditionally do not have a voice by placing a camera in their hands and asking them to share their reality on their terms while giving them a platform to share this perspective.[8] When employing Photovoice, the researcher hands over control to the participants who choose the aspects of the topic that will be focused on and further explored as they highlight them with their photographs and reflections. This lends itself to an authentic discovery of the topic and its nuances and a collective voice from those who know it best. Photovoice was developed with the explicit purpose of gathering voices to advocate for structural social change in the early 1990s.[9]

The application of Photovoice to pharmacy and medicines use began in the early part of this century in a sub-discipline known as social pharmacy. Social pharmacy has been defined as "The endeavour to integrate drugs into a broader perspective and to include legal, ethical, economic, political, social, communicative, and psychological aspects into their evaluation in order to contribute to the safe and rational use of drugs."[10] Social pharmacy incorporates and evaluates the social implications associated with the therapeutic and nontherapeutic uses of pharmaceutical preparations as examined from the perspective of individual and group behavior and the social systems that exist between them.[10] The first social pharmacy Photovoice studies principally aimed to understand patients' experiences with their medications,[11–13] thus informing the social and broader health services context associated with medications in people's lives. Photovoice has also been integrated with interventions focused on enhancing adherence to pharmacologic treatments.[12–14] As such, there are opportunities for researchers in pharmacy and health services to employ Photovoice for a variety of applications and projects.

Contemporary Research Methods in Pharmacy and Health Services. https://doi.org/10.1016/B978-0-323-91888-6.00010-7

Photovoice is a research method not only with the potential to unmute patients' voices, but also to enhance community engagement and raise awareness of the social injustices linked to the development, access, and use of medicines. For example, a project developed by Mohammed et al. in Karachi, Pakistan, utilized Photovoice to understand the experiences of people affected by tuberculosis (TB).[14] In addition to elucidating information about the weakness and side effects of medications used in treatment of TB, photographs, stories, and a Call for Action developed by the participants' committee in this project were shared at a gallery event held at a hospital with patients, practitioners, and policy-makers in attendance. This study elucidated the complexities surrounding TB, emphasized the need for holistic interventions that address all aspects of the disease, including its social determinants, and highlighted the intersection of those social determinants with medications. It also illustrated the potential of Photovoice as an effective means to bring much-needed attention to TB.

The purpose of this chapter is to describe the Photovoice method and practical approaches to its use, as well as the attributes that make it useful for studying topics of interest to social pharmacists and for furthering health promotion at its intersection with medication use.

Background

Wang and Burris developed Photovoice as a component of their work with women living in rural farming communities of Yunnan province in China to assess women's health and socioeconomic needs, with the intention to improve reproductive health outcomes.[9] Wang and Burris explained that the purpose of Photovoice "was to promote a process of women's participation that would be analytical, proactive, and empowering."[9] Photovoice as a community-based participatory action research (CBPR) expresses the idea that "power is held by those who have voice, set language, make history, and participate in decision-making processes."[15] Perhaps because of its empowering nature, Photovoice has gained popularity in healthcare and social work in the last twenty years.[16] As Liebenberg argues, the popularity of this method has been driven by the benefits it provides to researchers, participants, communities, service providers and policy makers.[2]

As a research method, Photovoice is accessible to people of most ages and abilities, and it has the capacity to facilitate communication across cultural and linguistic barriers, as well as power hierarchies.[1] Photovoice has three main goals:

1. to enable people to record and reflect their community's strengths and concerns,
2. to promote critical dialogue and knowledge about personal and community issues through large and small group discussion of their photographs, and.
3. to reach policymakers with an agenda that is framed by the collective input of the people that policies effect.[17]

The potential of Photovoice to engage marginalized and disenfranchised groups has long been recognized. Research suggests that the process of Photovoice can contribute to the self-development of the participants by fostering recognition of the need for change, improved self-awareness, personal worthiness and confidence, as well as awareness of social resources and problem-solving abilities.[1,18] To understand the emancipatory and empowering traits of this method, the theories behind Photovoice are described in Table 1.

Guidelines to implement photovoice within pharmacy and health services research

Because of the high level of involvement of the community of participants, and the combination of narratives and images, Photovoice is a demanding research process, requiring significant time and resource commitments. Researchers and facilitators need to be strong in interpersonal skills, preferably have previous experiences with participatory action research methods, and have in-depth knowledge of Photovoice. Together with social pharmacists and community participants, experts in social movements and in theory of photography will add great value to a project. To bring the project to its full potential, a strong advisory team should consist of members of the community of participants, local policy makers, healthcare professionals and other significant figures of the larger community who can trigger a change. Engaging with local governments, patients' organizations or health and/or medicines authorities enhances the possibilities of engagement and eventual receptivity by the community, which can increase the chances of actually triggering social change. Table 2 shows an overview of fifteen recommended steps when applying Photovoice in pharmacy and health services research, based on the pioneering work of the first Photovoice researchers and others who have applied the method.[1,2,9,29–31]

Vaughan argues that reflection and critical thinking develop over time—and that it takes time to develop the group relationships that can support action and effective dissemination to address the issues identified through photography.[32] It is thus crucial to plan with ample time to develop a good collaboration between researchers and the community. A preparatory step for pharmacist and health services researchers should therefore be to get acquainted with the community of

TABLE 1 The original theories behind photovoice.

Community-based Participatory Research (CBPR) or Participatory Action Research (PAR)

- Concerned with the democratization of knowledge development as a component of social justice.[2]
- Involves community members throughout the research process to produce data that are authentic to community experience and create appropriate and meaningful intervention.[19]
- It is a response to elitist forms of science together with policy and service structuring, driven by outside "experts," that are failing individuals and communities.[20]
- Concerned with reconnecting science with society for the purpose of social transformation.[21]
- Action and research converge to inform theory in ways that effectively support community advocacy for change.[22]
- It has four essential components: participation, action, research, and social change for social justice.

Feminist theory

- Enables The private, the daily, and the apparently trivial in women's activities to be understood as shared rather than individual experiences, and as socially and politically constructed.[9]
- Collaboratively identifies the taken-for-granted and explores the positioning of women within dominant and marginalizing social discourses, as well as historical, economic, and political structures to promote social change.
- It echoes various critical theories, cultural studies, postcolonial studies, queer theory, and the new sociology of childhood among others.
- To achieve comprehensive awareness and understanding of the taken-for-granted requires elevated levels of group engagement.
- Asserts that power accrues to those who have voice, set language, make history, and participate in decisions.[23]

Paulo Freire's critical pedagogy

- PAR has the potential to empower people to become aware of the factors that affect them, and to give them the confidence to either demand change or, through their own initiative, take action.
- Enhanced awareness of self-in-context can inform social change. To do this, Freire made use of photographs, which function as a mirror to communities, reflecting everyday social and political realities that impact people's lives.
- In discussing the content of images, people are able to step back from their lives and engage more readily with the abstract.
- Meaning is established via a process of naming through dialogue. "Only dialogue is capable of generating critical thinking. Without dialogue there is no communication, and without communication there can be no true education," as Freire explained.[3]
- Through a collective process of reflection, introspection, and discussion of images, communities are able to uncover the social and political constructions that maintain their marginalization and thus achieve a level of consciousness need to trigger social change.

The principles of photography

- Community values shape what individuals choose to photograph, when, and how they would like to reflect on their lives.
- Interpreting images is subjective and informed by personal meaning making frameworks and the social contexts that shape them.[24]
- Images prompt a different kind of reflection on lived experiences, as they are able to prompt emotions and thoughts about experiences in ways that narrative alone cannot.[25]
- Interpreting an image creates a slower and more critically reflective space within the research process. This may begin with the making of an image: "why is it that I made that photograph, in that moment?".[26]
- Reflection also happens while participants think about the meaning they attach to images: "what am I seeing in this image?", "why is it important?", and "how do I understand or interpret what I am seeing?".[27]
- Images introduced into narrative research create important links that participants can use to reflect critically on their lived experiences and to discuss and share these experiences with others.[28]

patients they would like to work with. It can be either through patients' organizations, nongovernmental organizations or through healthcare professionals closely working with the community of interest.

Though the fifteen steps in Table 2 below may appear daunting to a researcher who is interested in beginning a Photovoice study, it is often the case that several of the steps may happen in tandem, and thus getting the process started, implemented, and carried out need not be intimidating or done with total perfection as the goal. In general, a researcher who is interested in beginning a Photovoice project may think first about what topic they wish to explore and why. For example, author Werremeyer, in her clinical pharmacy practice experience noted that patients taking psychotropic medications often dealt with many issues in relation to their medications that weren't discussed with their prescribers and these issues sometimes led to nonadherence to or general distaste for medications, or to extreme affection for a particular medication. Werremeyer and colleagues wanted to explore more about what led to these issues and how they were experienced by patients in order to make them known to other healthcare team members who can improve care provision.[33,34] This topic and motivation for studying it fit with the spirit and intent of the Photovoice method, which fulfilled steps 1 and 2 (Table 2). From

TABLE 2 Fifteen steps to implement photovoice in social pharmacy research.

1	Choosing potential research areas	• Examples of Action Steps:
		  ◦ Enhancing patients' participation in medicines development and regulatory approval
		  ◦ Exploring and representing barriers and inequities in access to medicines, including pricing of medicines, sharing the stigma, discrimination and shame associated with the need for use of medicines chronically with society
		  ◦ Sharing the burden and daily implications of living with side effects of medicines

2	Checking the feasibility of Photovoice	• Is the community of participants willing to take a proactive role in most/all phases of the research process? • Does the research project include the intention to trigger social change or revert a social injustice related to the development, access or use of medicines? • Is there a receptive audience open to consider the desired change? • Are facilitators in photography as a research method part of the team? (This is the ideal, but if unavailable, should not prevent a Photovoice study from proceeding) • Are advocacy actions included as part of the research project?
3	Working on the project aim	• Photovoice participants should lead, or at a minimum, influence the process of deciding on the research focus, and on what to explore through narratives and photographs. • The project aim should include a component of awareness raising that can eventually lead to a social change. • It is recommended to run sessions to harmonize aims and expectations among the Photovoice participants with the help of an experienced facilitator. • If the community is a virtual community (e.g., Facebook closed group), it is recommended to include in the facilitation workshop activities that can help the Photovoice participants perceive each other as a community who share a common aim.
4	Setting up your teams	• Recommended types of teams: management, advisory, and advocacy, dissemination teams with multidisciplinary backgrounds. • It is important to include in the advisory team individual patients or patient representatives—children or adolescents if relevant for the project—, experts in pharmacy, social pharmacy and/or use of medicines under investigation, researchers with previous experience in qualitative analysis, and local decision makers. • The advocacy and dissemination team should ensure that the participants' voices are heard by the intended audiences and meets its social justice intent. The support of experts in outreach can substantially increase the impact of the project.
5	Selection of participants	• Selection of participants interested in active involvement • It is recommended to work with patients' organizations in the recruitment of participants. • Participants should give their informed consent to participate in the research after all relevant risks and benefits are presented to them. • Caution should be used when recruiting participants via social media. It is important to clarify that Photovoice may imply meeting and working physically with others, if the study is not being conducted through remote means. • Consider oversampling. As photovoice can take a lot of time, expect some participants to drop out during the process.
6	Preparing the community and the participants' environment.	• Define the community to which the project is being targeted to influence and impact (e.g., hospital, community pharmacists, regulators, etc.). • Present the project to the chosen community target. • There will likely be a need to obtain permission, as the Photovoice participants might be walking around taking pictures.

TABLE 2 Fifteen steps to implement photovoice in social pharmacy research—cont'd

7	Creating a space of trust between participants and facilitators	<ul><li>It is recommended to run "get-to-know-each-other" workshops with participants and researchers</li><li>Build a sense of togetherness among the participants.</li><li>Mingling activities such as visiting a photography museum, a healthcare event, or other activity that facilitators and participants find interesting and can attend together. Meals are often provided.</li></ul>
8	Refining the research question together	<ul><li>Jointly crafting a research question and a thus an aim, can provide Photovoice participants with a sense of purpose[1].</li><li>Consider starting with listing objectives and agreeing on them.</li><li>If the Photovoice participants feel stuck, the researchers might share some examples of research questions such as: what are the barriers that prevent young men from adhering to a given treatment? How do participants living with mental conditions like to be heard and well-received by community pharmacists?</li></ul>
9	Learning how to answer the research questions via images and photographs	<ul><li>Participants develop and agree on a set of questions that can guide their photography and storytelling to answer the research question.</li><li>At all times, the project team has to bear in mind the ethical nature of the questions, especially when working with highly vulnerable groups. Certain questions, for example, inductively negative questions, can trigger vulnerability and thus create stress among participants.</li></ul>
10	Checking and enhancing photography literacy	<ul><li>With the abundance of smartphones, taking pictures has become one of the easiest and most common activities. However, awareness of elements of good photography is rare.</li><li>It is recommended to run a photography workshop together with the Photovoice participants and an expert in theory of photography to get the basics of good photography (framing, light, movement, symbolism, visual metaphors). In contrast, some studies have touted the benefits of unrefined and raw photography approaches when a photography workshop was not held.</li><li>It is important to discuss the power and ethics of camera use and the "ground rules" agreed upon by the Photovoice participants</li></ul>
11	Speaking through photography and images	<ul><li>Taking pictures can take from a couple of weeks to six months. When periods are long, participants and researchers should meet once a month to reflect on the photographs taken. Castleden and Garvin[29] argue that such arrangements can lead to greater reflection and empowerment of the participants.</li><li>It is important to remove the pressure of suddenly becoming a photographer and make it an activity based more on sensitive observation rather than on performance.</li><li>It is not about the amount of pictures, but of taking pictures when something "calls" or resonates with the participant.</li></ul>
12	Building the story	<ul><li>Each one of the participants chooses five or six of their favorite photographs and has the opportunity to share with the group the significance of the photos chosen.</li><li>Wilson et al.[30] proposed the SHOWeD method, a set of questions that can help to open up the discussion around photographs. What do you See here? What's really Happening here? How does this relate to Our lives? Why does this situation, concern, or strength exist? What can we Do about it?.</li></ul>
13	Analyzing stories and pictures	<ul><li>Photographs and stories gathered by the Photovoice participants should be grouped in higher-order themes.</li><li>Participants and researcher together engage in the condensing of data into more interpretative themes. In depth, qualitative analysis of photograph reflections may also be conducted.</li></ul>

Continued

TABLE 2 Fifteen steps to implement photovoice in social pharmacy research—cont'd

14	Exhibition development	• Key step of Photovoice: The team develops a strategy for displaying the photographs and their accompanying reflections.[31] • Work toward agreement on the goal to be reached with the exhibition, defining the target audience, and the action to trigger. • Working together with patients' organizations and sensitized healthcare professionals with insight into how community leaders can be reached. • Together with experts in photography and storytellers, build a story around your case. • Format can be digital and shared through YouTube and similar platforms • Most importantly organize a physical event to have a dialogue with the audience. • Circulate a press statement and a policy brief to continue the impact of the exhibition through different channels for six months or more. • If the participants are open to it, a documentary is a strong communication tool.
15	Medium- and long-term advocacy endeavors	• Core step of Photovoice: engage each key stakeholder that can contribute to make a change to discuss the issues at stake. • Social pharmacist researchers work together with advocates who can echo and amplify the voice of the participants. • Recurrent outreach activities should be organized during at least 6 months to 1 year to sustain the impact. These activities can be linked to an international day (UN days) or to national events. • Use social media wisely and with a social communication expert, in order to avoid the work being drowned in the abundance of images, messages and digital stories.

Table structured with insights from Blackman and Fairey,[31] Castleden and Garvin,[29] Liebenberg,[2] Skovdal and Cordish,[1] and Wilson et al.[30]

this point, the researcher can then strategize how to get in contact with and begin to meet with the population of people who are in a position to know about what the researcher seeks to learn about. Werremeyer and colleagues started by recruiting a pilot group of 5 participants who were prescribed at least 1 psychotropic medication. Werremeyer and colleagues met with the participants to introduce the idea of studying their experiences with psychotropic medications. Participants were enthused about this idea and helped to shape the research focus. Werremeyer and colleagues presented a PowerPoint to these pilot participants with information about the study rules, risks and benefits of participating in a Photovoice study, and some examples of what the outputs (i.e., photos and reflections) from previous Photovoice studies on other topics were like. This all took place over a shared meal and a two hour discussion, and it essentially fulfilled steps 3, 5–9, and 11 to some degree. Steps 11 to 15 were carried out in partnership with the participants at subsequent group and individual study meetings over the ensuing 3 months.[34] Step 10 was not an area of emphasis for this study and was not fulfilled, yet the study still proceeded successfully.

The ethics of photovoice

Ethical challenges linked to research aims and expectations

Because Photovoice has the embedded capacity to trigger social change, it is a research method with the potential for shaking the status quo within a community. Facilitating some to speak up, or "give" disenfranchised groups of populations a voice, is not free from potential disturbance in the larger society. It might also be that, even though a change is expected, it might just not happen, causing frustration and a sense of being let down among the participants. In both cases, the researchers should carefully study the participants' context and honestly start by explaining to them the different scenarios that might occur, not hiding the possibility that the impact of the project in the wider community may not happen right away or happen at all. Some authors have pointed out this risk and propose considering Photovoice more like a policy-informing method rather than a policy-changing one.[35] However, it is preferred to respect the potential transformative value of Photovoice with prerequisites of performing a socio-political mapping of participants' context and the need for transparency vis-à-vis the participants throughout the whole process. It is also highly recommended that pharmacist and health services researchers work closely with experts in social movements and with strong insight into the community's contextual characteristics.

Active participation of the community members or patient groups is at the core of Photovoice. In some cases, because of the degree of self-efficacy, health literacy, or simply due to the vulnerability inherent in the participants, their engagement might not be as active as the researcher desires. Researchers may need to comply with a calendar or reporting to donors and thus keep up with deadlines, while participants might experience the need to withdraw, take a pause, or simply disengage from the process. Confronted with such a challenging situation, researchers experience the dilemma between respecting the tempo and need of the participants or going on with the process, complying with the project plan but leaving some participants behind. If, however, one of the goals was actually to empower the community, the decision cannot be made to proceed without the community of participants' agreement. In general, it is best to be generous with time when planning the different phases, especially when working with highly vulnerable populations such as patients living with severe mental conditions or communities in situations of high socioeconomic vulnerability.

Ethical challenges during the implementation process

Because of the use of images and photographs, Photovoice can potentially be an ethically loaded research method. This implies not only asking permission and obtaining informed consent of the person(s) appearing in the photograph, but also respecting his or her privacy, intimacy, and vulnerability. It is also important to raise awareness about how to take pictures in a noninvasive and discreet way, and in all cases ensure that the larger community has been properly informed of the research project in a transparent and honest way. Participants should be reminded not to take pictures of embarrassing situations that might incriminate or shame the persons appearing in the pictures, including themselves.[1] Below are some recommendations to overcome ethical dilemmas.

Training on photography ethics

It is highly recommended to run a workshop with the help of experts and with the participants who will be taking pictures on basic principles of ethics and, whenever possible, work with concrete questions and specific cases. For example, what to do when the participants would like to tell a story of end-of-life treatments. Or what to do in case of wanting to document minors' experiences with unsanctioned use of medicines for enhancement of academic performance (e.g., stimulants). Here different options might be possible. Participants might be encouraged to take symbolic pictures of objects, colors or environments evoking the experiences they wish to draw, or use excerpts of a movie or a book. Creative options can be enhanced during the workshop. To make sure that participants have fully understood the potential and the risk of taking pictures, it is recommended to conduct a pilot and go through the images from an ethical point of view. Time and financial constraints may make a workshop infeasible. In this case, simply providing examples of ethical and unethical pictures accompanied by discussion of each is recommended.

Informed consent

There are several types of informed consent that should be obtained when running a Photovoice project. The first is from the Photovoice participants. The informed consent form should contain the aims, objectives and potential risks and benefits of participating in the study, including whether and how anonymity and confidentiality will be maintained. It should also include whether or not photo reflection discussions will be audio-recorded and/or transcribed and how they will be analyzed. Most importantly, it should contain the rights of the participants to withdraw from the project at any point they wish without providing any further explanation to the researchers. In case of not being able to consent due to age or mental condition, a guardian should provide the consent. Whenever possible the minors or the participants living with mental conditions should be informed and involved during the process of consent and in some cases, may give their assent to participate.

Persons appearing in the pictures should also consent. Here, the form is an agreement between the Photovoice participant (the photographer) and the person(s) who appears in the photograph (the "model(s)"). The agreement seeks permission from the "model" to take their picture and use it for a particular and declared purpose. Again, special attention should be paid to "models" who are minors or who are living with a mental condition. In all cases, it is important to first obtain permission before taking pictures and obtain informed consent with the pictures at hand. The "model" should provide consent for the pictures, not of the act of taking pictures.

Finally, a photo release consent should also be obtained. This third and final form is primarily used to give permission to the project to use the photographs for the purpose of research and advocacy. A form clarifies copyrights and whether the participant's real name or a pseudonym will be used to credit the photographs. The form also acts as a backup to fully disclose the purpose and use of the photograph to both the photographer and the "models." This is particularly important if the photographs are likely to go on the internet or be used to advocate for a particular issue.[1]

Considerations for data analysis

Wang and Burris[36] recommend a three-stage approach to participatory group analysis of Photovoice data. The three stages are: (1) selecting photographs that most accurately reflect the participants' views, (2) contextualizing the photographs, and (3) codifying issues, themes, or theories that emerge. For the participants to effectively lead and properly influence the collection of and emphasis upon the data that comes from the Photovoice work, it is imperative that they, not the researchers, select the photographs that will be analyzed, discussed, and shared. This can be done simply by asking the participants to choose the photographs that, for them, are of greatest significance to inform the topic under study. The use of the SHOWeD technique (Table 3), a set of guided reflection questions applied to each photo, is recommended in Photovoice studies to assist with carrying out stage 2, contextualizing the photographs.[2,9,30] The SHOWeD technique allows the participants to give meaning to the image(s) depicted and to express what the photo's message is. Note, some Photovoice studies have modified one of the technique's questions and thus operated under the SHOWED pneumonic (Table 3).[37] Group discussion around each photo adds further context to the photo from the perspective of the community. Typically, reflections by individual participants as well as group discussions are transcribed into a collective narrative pertaining to each photo; however, there may be situations or populations for which group discussion is less appropriate and use of individual photo reflection is preferred.[38] Stage 3 can be carried out in multiple ways and with emphasis on different aspects of the data that has been collected. Wang and Burris[36] posited that analyzing photographs alone, outside the context of the participant's own voice, is contradictory to the essence of Photovoice. Instead, the reflective narrative must accompany the photograph in the analysis process. Most Photovoice studies have focused on qualitative analysis of narratives and journal entries of participants,[39] resulting in issues, themes or theories that are grounded in the data and the collective voice of the participants.[36] These issues, themes and/or theories can then be articulated and shared in many ways including, but not limited to photographic and narrative exhibits, advocacy initiatives, and development of models and further change-oriented research approaches.[12,16]

Best practices for reporting research studies that implemented photovoice

With the increase in use of Photovoice as a method in pharmacy and health services research, there is the need to develop a tool for reporting of studies and their associated results. The development of this list of best practices for reporting Photovoice research studies is based on the steps and ethical challenges embedded in Photovoice as a research method. The best practices included in this checklist can help researchers to report important aspects of Photovoice, from the criteria to choose potential research areas, to long-term advocacy endeavors (Table 4).

TABLE 3 SHOWeD[9,30] and SHOWED[36] techniques.

SHOWeD	SHOWED
What is **SEEN** here?	What is **SEEN** here?
What is really **HAPPENING** here?	What is really **HAPPENING** here?
How does this relate to **OUR**/your lives?	How does this relate to **OUR**/your lives?
Why does this problem, concern, or strength **EXIST**? OR How can we become **EMPOWERED** through our new understanding?	How could this image **EDUCATE** people?
What can we **DO** about it?	

TABLE 4 Best practices for disseminating results gained from the conduct of photovoice studies.

	Criteria	Guiding statement
A	Relevance	1. The research project included the intention to trigger social change or revert a social injustice related to the development, access or use of medicines. 2. The research question(s) were susceptible to be answered via the use images and photographs. 3. The aim and research question have been crafted jointly with the participants.
B	Feasibility	4. The community of participants were willing to take a proactive role in most/all phases of the research process. 5. The receptive audience was open to consider the desired change. 6. Facilitators in photography as a research method were part of the team. 7. Advocacy actions were included as part of the research project. 8. Workshops and team-building action to enhance trust among participants were included. 9. A method that helped to open up the discussion around photographs was included and described.
C	Empowerment	10. Photovoice participants influenced the process of deciding on the research focus. 11. Medicine users, patients or patients representatives took part in the advisory group/committee. 12. An outreach strategy was designed together with participants to ensure that advocacy actions would reached the intended audience(s). 13. Participants and researcher together engaged in the condensing of data into more interpretative themes.
D	Ethics	14. Permissions to take photos in the community were obtained. 15. A workshop on the ethics of photography was implemented. 16. Photographs were taken in a respectful, noninvasive way.
E	Impact	17. There was a clear definition of the community to which the project was targeted to influence 18. The project was presented to the chosen community target. 19. The team developed a strategy for displaying the photographs and their accompanying reflections. 20. Social pharmacist researchers worked together with advocates to echo and amplify the voice of the participants.

Examples of photovoice projects relevant for pharmacy and health services research

Three inspiring studies illustrating how Photovoice was used in pharmacy research are presented below. For an additional review of the literature available on Photovoice in the field, please see a review of Photovoice published in Research in Social and Administrative Pharmacy.[40]

Using photovoice to document living with mental illness on a college campus[13]

Background and aim

Mental illnesses commonly begin in late adolescence or early adulthood; thus, they may first manifest among college students. The purpose of this study was to allow college students living with mental illness to document and communicate their realities with peers and university stakeholders through Photovoice. Seventeen college students who were prescribed at least one medication used to treat mental illness participated in an 8-week Photovoice study in which they were asked to take photographs reflecting their realities of living with mental illness on campus. The purpose of the study was to put forth student-generated observations on current practices and experiences to improve the lived experiences of others like them.

Key results

Photographs and accompanying reflections using the SHOWED technique resulted in four over-arching themes: (1) Insights into campus services, (2) Increasing awareness and educating others, (3) Support, and (4) Barriers to getting better. Student participants praised campus services designed to help students affected by mental health concerns and also shed light on utility of campus services that were not originally intended for the purpose of benefitting mental health nor previously identified as such by the general campus community. One example is the image of the campus bike-share program (Fig. 1).

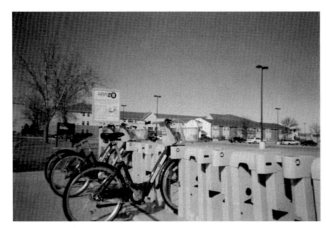

FIG. 1   When I get stressed, I get on a bike and bike around. It really helps me. It helps me to release stress and anxiety. You know that exercise has good effect on your mind.[13]

Implications for practice

College campuses can better serve their students' needs when students are given the opportunity to speak and share their experiences living with a mental illness on campus. Photographs help to point out key issues and problems while also highlighting helpful approaches that can be amplified and supported. Student participants also felt connected with one another and with caring figures among the campus community as a result of participating in the Photovoice project.

Outreach

Campus stakeholders attended a presentation of photos and narratives lead by the researchers and student participants. Participant sharing of their lived experiences resulted in policy change and additional support toward mental illness awareness initiatives on the college campus. Furthermore, a campaign was begun with collaboration across university disciplines to promote awareness and stigma reduction and resulted in an online conversation and sharing forum known as Snap the Stigma (Snapthestigma.com).

Through our eyes: A photovoice intervention for adolescents on active cancer treatment[41]

Background and aim

Photovoice was used as an intervention for eliciting and addressing the psychosocial needs of adolescents on active cancer treatment. Six adolescents, aged thirteen to seventeen years old, who were on active treatment or had completed treatment in the three months prior to recruitment participated in a seven-week photovoice group that took place from March to May 2017 at The Hospital for Sick Children (SickKids) under the oncology program organized by social workers. The goals of the group were to (i) provide an environment for peer support; (ii) bring a stronger voice to the experiences of teens; (iii) facilitate better communication between teens and their health care team; and (iv) influence changes in how healthcare teams and hospital environments interface with teenagers.

Key results

The framework categorized the themes into six domains: (i) physical changes and symptoms associated with the treatment (hair loss, surgery, amputations), (ii) psychosocial impacts of the diagnosis (fears of death, loss of normalcy, and feelings of isolation), (iii) short-term social impacts (disruption in family roles, often with unexpected challenges and rewards), (iv) long-term social impacts (changes in social network, school life and extracurricular activities and contact with peers), (v) impacts on holistic well-being (use their experiences for posttraumatic growth), and (vi) informational needs (relationships with healthcare professionals) (Fig. 2).

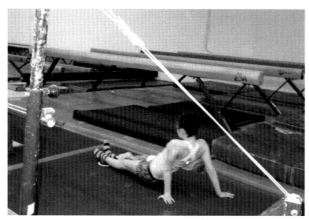

FIG. 2 Participant photo of them returning to sports activities they did prior to diagnosis.[41]

Despite their struggles, many participants found meaning in their physical changes, often through their involvement in arts, sports, and camps:

> *P1: I heard about this other girl in the States who dances and has the surgery.... And I also wanted the surgery, because I know it's very functional, and you can basically do whatever a normal person can do.... I feel like I just wouldn't be able to stand it for the rest of my life [not choosing surgery], not being able to dance or run or anything like that.*[41]

Implication for practice

When teenagers' informational needs are met and they are provided opportunities to advocate for themselves, they are more empowered, better able to cope with stress, and have improved treatment outcomes—an important consideration for clinical interventions.

Outreach

The Photovoice participants provided an important avenue to discuss the ways that clinicians, teachers, and peers helped or hindered participants' psychosocial well-being. They also explored ways that clinicians and teachers could better meet their informational needs, either by involving them in decisions around what to share and with whom or respecting when they do not want to know something. The insights that teenagers provided formed the basis of many important practice and policy changes to be implemented within the oncology department.

Photovoice as a promising public engagement approach: Capturing and communicating ethnic minority people's lived experiences of severe mental illness and its treatment[42]

Background and aim

Mental health-related stigma, resulting in widespread discrimination and exclusion, inhibits many from seeking help. Moreover, conventional therapeutic methods relying on the spoken word, only, may not elucidate the full range and nuances of lived experiences.

Key results

Seven workshops were hosted over 6 months, with three subsequent exhibitions at community centers and two public exhibitions split between London and Manchester. Twenty-one people participated in the project. Post-it notes provided a simple, unstructured and anonymous feedback method after each workshop/exhibition, revealing how photography was seen as an accessible and creative means to communicate priorities, while exhibition delegates overwhelmingly agreed that photos and captions were well displayed to communicate mental health narratives.

Implication for practice

The use of photography alongside narratives (Photovoice) can provide a powerful means for ethnic minority service users and their carers to communicate these experiences, with photographic displays to a broader audience contributing toward destigmatizing mental illness and its treatments.

Outreach

Public exhibition attendees represented a broad range of stakeholders, including service users, carers, charity representatives, healthcare professionals, journalists, and policymakers. Many participants considered how photography provided an empowering platform from which to communicate sensitive issues. This was consistent across a diverse sample of ethnic minority people and mental illness diagnoses. The exhibitions then enabled their visual testimonies of common humanity and creative potentials to further destigmatize the issue publicly.

Conclusion

Photovoice is a participatory action research method with nearly limitless possibilities for expansion and exploration. The researcher can find the method to be a highly useful tool when it is used in partnership with communities or individuals to give voice to practice areas or treatment approaches that are poorly understood. The exploration and sharing of the perspective of persons with lived experience through photos and images via Photovoice is an opportunity to open doors and create changes. However, the researcher must also be diligent in taking careful and recommended steps in conducting Photovoice research in order to preserve the spirit of the method and integrity of the message of the participants. The researcher employing Photovoice should seek a delicate balance of guiding their participants' actions while handing over much of the control in directing the project, trusting that their participants' experience will shape the project into what it needs to be, so as to share meaningful and impactful messages to those who need to hear and/or see them.

Questions for further discussion

1. What are the pros and cons of using Photovoice to study topics of interest to pharmacy and health services researchers?
2. Which of the ethical implications associated with use of Photovoice is/are most concerning? Which are the most difficult to appropriately address? Which are easiest to appropriately address?
3. Why is it important to understand social pharmacy phenomena from the experience of a patient participant?
4. What are the implications of studying social pharmacy phenomena from the patient's/participant's perspective rather than from the healthcare provider's or researcher's perspective?

Application exercise/scenario

You are a pharmacy researcher who has heard and read about stigma experienced by persons with schizophrenia. You would like to know more about how persons with schizophrenia are affected by stigma around them, specifically stigma from healthcare providers. You would like to consider utilizing the Photovoice method to explore this topic. Create an initial plan and timeline summarizing the steps you'll take to begin and carry out this project. Ensure that at a minimum you've included what your research team's make-up will be, which stakeholders you wish to connect with and what you want to talk with them about, where and how you will recruit potential participants, and approximately how much funding you will require to execute the project effectively.

References

1. Skovdal M, Cornish F. *Qualitative Research for Development*. Rugby, UK: Practical Action Publishing; 2015.
2. Liebenberg L. Thinking critically about Photovoice: achieving empowerment and social change. *Int J Qual Methods*. 2018;17(1). 1609406918757631.
3. Freire P. *Pedagogy of the Oppressed*. New York: Penguin Books; 1972.
4. Peters JS, Wolper A. *Women's Rights, Human Rights: International Feminist Perspectives*. Routledge; 2018.
5. Allen A. *The Power of Feminist Theory*. Routledge; 2018.
6. Coemans S, Hannes K. Researchers under the spell of the arts: two decades of using arts-based methods in community-based inquiry with vulnerable populations. *Educ Res Rev*. 2017;22:34–49.
7. Wolper A. Making art, reclaiming lives: the artist and homeless collaborative. In: *But Is It Art*; 1995:251–282.
8. Milne E, Muir R. Photovoice: a critical introduction. In: *The SAGE Handbook of Visual Research Methods*; 2019:282.

9. Wang C, Burris MA. Empowerment through photo novella: portraits of participation. *Health Educ Q.* 1994;21(2):171–186.

10. Harding G, Taylor K. Defining social pharmacy: it needs its own distinct identity. *Int J Pharm Pract.* 1993;2(2):62–63.

11. Baker TA, Wang CC. Photovoice: use of a participatory action research method to explore the chronic pain experience in older adults. *Qual Health Res.* 2006;16(10):1405–1413.

12. Werremeyer A, Skoy E, Aalgaard KG. Use of photovoice to understand the experience of taking psychotropic medications. *Qual Health Res.* 2017;27 (13):1959–1969.

13. Skoy E, Werremeyer A. Using photovoice to document living with mental illness on a college campus. *Clin Med Insights Psychiatry.* 2019;10. 1179557318821095.

14. Mohammed S, Sajun SZ, Khan FS. Harnessing photovoice for tuberculosis advocacy in Karachi, Pakistan. *Health Promot Int.* 2013;30(2):262–269.

15. Schneider B. *Hearing (our) Boices: Participatory Research in Mental Health.* University of Toronto Press; 2010.

16. Catalani C, Minkler M. Photovoice: a review of the literature in health and public health. *Health Educ Behav.* 2010;37(3):424–451.

17. Wang C, Burris MA. Photovoice: concept, methodology, and use for participatory needs assessment. *Health Educ Behav.* 1997;24(3):369–387.

18. Teti M, Majee W, Cheak-Zamora N, Maurer-Batjer A. Understanding health through a different lens: Photovoice method. In: Liamputtong P, ed. *Handbook of Research Methods in Health Social Sciences.* Singapore: Springer Singapore; 2017:1–20.

19. Hergenrather KC, Rhodes SD, Cowan CA, Bardhoshi G, Pula S. Photovoice as community-based participatory research: a qualitative review. *Am J Health Behav.* 2009;33(6):686–698.

20. Green LW. From research to "best practices" in other settings and populations. *Am J Health Behav.* 2001;25(3):165–178.

21. Chevalier J, Buckles D. *Participatory Action Research.* London: Routledge; 2019.

22. Kemmis S, McTaggart R. Participatory action research: communicative action and the public sphere. In: *The Sage Handbook of Qualitative Research.* 3rd ed. Thousand Oaks, CA: Sage Publications Ltd; 2005:559–603.

23. Wang CC, Pies CA. Family, maternal, and child health through photovoice. *Matern Child Health J.* 2004;8(2):95–102.

24. Dicks B, Soyinka B, Coffey A. Multimodal ethnography. *Qual Res.* 2006;6(1):77–96.

25. Harper D. Talking about pictures: a case for photo elicitation. *Vis Stud.* 2002;17(1):13–26.

26. Liebenberg L. The visual image as discussion point: increasing validity in boundary crossing research. *Qual Res.* 2009;9(4):441–467.

27. Grimshaw A. *The Ethnographer's Eye: Ways of Seeing in Anthropology.* Cambridge: Cambridge University Press; 2001.

28. Liebenberg L, Ungar M, Theron L. Using video observation and photo elicitation interviews to understand obscured processes in the lives of youth resilience. *Childhood.* 2014;21(4):532–547.

29. Castleden H, Garvin T. Modifying photovoice for community-based participatory indigenous research. *Soc Sci Med.* 2008;66(6):1393–1405.

30. Wilson N, Dasho S, Martin AC, Wallerstein N, Wang CC, Minkler M. Engaging young adolescents in social action through photovoice. The youth empowerment strategies (YES!) project. *J Early Adolesc.* 2007;27(2):241–261.

31. Blackman A, Fairey T. *The Photovoice Manual: A Guide to Designing and Running Participatory Photography Projects.* London, United Kingdom: Photo Voice Publications; 2007.

32. Vaughan C. Participatory research with youth: idealising safe social spaces or building transformative links in difficult environments? *J Health Psychol.* 2014;19(1):184–192.

33. Werrremeyer A, Aalgaard-Kelly G, Skoy E. Living with my medication: using photovoice to explore patients' experiences with mental health medication. *Ment Health Clin.* 2016;6(3):142–153.

34. Werremeyer A, Skoy E. Using photovoice to study patient experience with psychotropic medications. In: *SAGE Research Methods Cases*; 2020. https://doi.org/10.4135/9781529711219.

35. Johnston G. Champions for social change: photovoice ethics in practice and 'false hopes' for policy and social change. *Glob Public Health.* 2016;11(5–6):799–811.

36. Wang C, Burris MA. Photovoice: concept, methodology, and use for participatory needs assessment. *Health Educ Behav.* 1997;24(3):369–387.

37. National Association of County & City Health Officials. *Photovoice Hamilton Manual and Resource Kit*; 2007. Retrieved from https://www.naccho.org/uploads/downloadable-resources/Programs/Public-Health-Infrastructure/Photovoice-Manual.pdf.

38. Nykiforuk CI, Vallianatos H, Nieuwendyk LM. Photovoice as a method for revealing community perceptions of the built and social environment. *Int J Qual Methods.* 2011;10(2):103–124.

39. Wang Q, Hannes K. Toward a more comprehensive type of analysis in photovoice research: the development and illustration of supportive question matrices for research teams. *Int J Qual Methods.* 2020;19. 1609406920914712.

40. Cantarero Arevalo L, Werremeyer A. Community involvement and awareness raising for better development, access and use of medicines: the transformative potential of photovoice. *Res Soc Admin Pharm.* 2021;17(12):2062–2069. https://doi.org/10.1016/j.sapharm.2021.05.017.

41. Georgievski G, Shama W, Lucchetta S, Niepage M. Through our eyes: a photovoice intervention for adolescents on active cancer treatment. *J Psychosoc Oncol.* 2018;36(6):700–716.

42. Halvorsrud K, Rhodes J, Webster GM, et al. Photovoice as a promising public engagement approach: capturing and communicating ethnic minority people's lived experiences of severe mental illness and its treatment. *BMJ Open Qual.* 2019;8(4), e000665.

Chapter 15

The draw and write technique to uncover nuance in pharmacy and health services delivery

Theresa J. Schindel[a], Christine A. Hughes[a], Tatiana Makhinova[a], and Jason S. Daniels[b]

[a]Faculty of Pharmacy and Pharmaceutical Sciences, University of Alberta, Edmonton, AB, Canada, [b]School of Public Health, University of Alberta, Edmonton, AB, Canada

Objectives

- Discuss the aims of arts-informed research and its applicability to pharmacy and health services research.
- Describe the draw and write technique as well as its recent adaptations.
- Discuss the advantages and limitations to using the draw and write technique in combination with focus group interviews.
- Identify potential ethical issues related to the draw and write technique.
- Discuss potential applications of the draw and write technique in pharmacy education.

Arts-informed research

The arts have been used in health research to communicate ideas, to reflect on experiences, and as a form of therapy.[1,2] Arts-informed research aims to enhance understanding of the human condition and to make scholarship more accessible by connecting the work of the researcher with the community, including audiences outside of academia.[3,4] Research incorporating art forms enhances public knowledge of issues and affects health care policy and practice.[3] Completing an art-based activity allows study participants to express ideas and experiences that are difficult to convey in words alone.[5,6] It also provides opportunities to realize changes in their own perspectives. It allows researchers to access, retrieve information about, and communicate on a diverse range of experiences. Researchers may seek opportunities to collaborate with artists to realize the potential of art as a catalyst for ideas, theories, and concepts as well as an aid in designing methods and analyzing data.[6,7] Visual methods involving photography, painting, or drawing are commonly used in combination with other qualitative research methods such as individual or focus group interviews.[1,5,6,8,9]

In *Art as Experience*, Dewey asserts that drawing is a form of self-expression—"drawing is drawing out" what an individual has to say about matters of everyday life.[10 (p96)] Qualitative research methods that include drawings have been used to collect rich data and gain insight into how people make sense of their experiences in the world.[8,9] Drawing allows expression of thoughts, feelings, and experiences.[8] In health services research, drawings have provided an authentic, insider view of patients' perceptions and experiences with illness and treatment.[11] Participant drawings have been used to study experiences and perceptions of health and illness,[8,11] elicit feedback about health care services,[11] and, more recently, in pharmacy education to understand pharmacy students'[12] and educators' experiences.[13,14]

Draw and write technique

The draw and write technique is an arts-informed research method that has been used since the 1980s to explore a range of social and health-related topics, initially with children.[15–18] The concept emerged from Wetton's work in the 1970s to capture the language of children's emotions.[19,20] The method involved asking children to create a drawing and prompting them to write or speak about their drawing, often in combination with individual or focus group interviews.[15] The draw and write technique begins with a question, for example, "what makes you healthy?" and usually incorporates discussion.[17]

Contemporary Research Methods in Pharmacy and Health Services. https://doi.org/10.1016/B978-0-323-91888-6.00002-8

The original intent of the drawing portion of the technique was to incorporate a task that resembled a classroom activity so that children would feel comfortable performing an activity that was familiar to them.[17,20] In some of the early studies, only the written words or verbal accounts were analyzed while the drawings were used to elicit the child's understanding of an abstract idea.[17] Studies using the draw and write technique have guided teachers and researchers to develop curriculum and transform health education.[17]

Researchers tailor their approach by selecting materials and strategies appropriate for the research question, context, and participants. Pridmore et al. studied Botswanan children's beliefs regarding health, illness, and death.[15] In a classroom setting, they gave each child a blank sheet of white paper and a pencil and asked them to draw as many things as possible that made them healthy on one side of the paper and to write about what was happening in each of their drawings. After 20 min, the children were asked to turn over their papers and repeat the activity, this time depicting what makes them unhealthy.[15] Similarly, Horstman et al. explored opinions toward their hospital care of children diagnosed with cancer.[18] In this study, children were given a blank white paper and a pencil and invited to create a drawing and write words in response to a question adapted to their stage of cancer treatment. The researchers combined this draw and write activity with individual interviews conducted in either the hospital or home setting. The drawings, words and notes from the interviews were included in the analysis.

Variations of the draw and write technique have also been used to study adults in academic contexts[6] and information science education.[21] The draw, write, reflect approach was developed to explore academics career progression.[6] It combines drawing and writing activities with individual interviews. In one study, researchers provided participants with several pieces of A4 white paper and black fine-liner pens and gave them the option of either drawing or writing, or both, to capture the progression of their academic careers. Another adaptation, the iSquare protocol, was developed for implementation in classrooms of university-level students.[7] The protocol employs a standardized data collection instrument, a 4×4 in. piece of white art paper, and a traditional black pen. Researchers using the iSquare protocol invited students to answer the question, "what is information?" in the form of a drawing on one side and words about the drawing on the other side.[21]

Users of the draw and write technique contrast the relative ease of data collection with the often time-intensive and more difficult task of analyzing visual data.[16] Challenges associated with the method include participants experiencing unease or expressing reluctance to draw, having difficulty determining what to depict, drawing what is easy to depict rather than what they might actually feel, and feeling influenced by other participants in close proximity.[22] Researchers use a variety of approaches to analyze drawings. Visual analysis methods used in conjunction with the iSquare protocol include thematic analysis, compositional analysis, pictorial metaphor analysis, and content analysis.[23] Other research incorporating drawings has included participants' interpretations of their own drawings in the analysis.[11]

Five decades following its introduction, the draw and write technique offers a flexible and creative method to explore individuals' perceptions and gain insight into how they interpret experiences and make sense of the world around them. This method brings together art, research, and education. An adaptation of the draw and write technique, incorporating aspects of draw, write, reflect[6] approach and the iSquare protocol,[7] was applied to explore a new context: public perceptions and experiences with community pharmacy services. The use of an arts-informed method offers the opportunity to contribute a more nuanced understanding of pharmacy and health service delivery.

In the following sections of this chapter, details are presented of the arts-informed qualitative research method based on the draw and write technique that was used to explore the public's experiences and perceptions of community pharmacy services in Alberta. First, context for the study is provided; this is followed by methods, results, discussion of those results, and discussion of the researchers' experience with this approach, and suggestions for its potential application to pharmacy education.

Public perceptions of community pharmacy services

In many countries around the world, people go to community pharmacies to receive health care services.[24,25] Community pharmacies offer a range of services from products to professional pharmacy services. Professional pharmacy services include drug therapy (e.g., prescribing, medication reviews), health promotion (e.g., influenza vaccines, smoking cessation), and primary care (e.g., care planning services, blood pressure monitoring).[26] Understanding public views and experiences may help to identify barriers, needs, and opportunities for greater uptake of professional pharmacy services provided by pharmacists in community pharmacies.

Research has examined public awareness and attitudes toward professional pharmacy services in the United Kingdom,[27,28] Netherlands,[29] Australia,[30] and the United States.[31] In Canada, research exploring the public's views and experiences with professional pharmacy services is limited. Results of a national online survey reported that most Canadians were aware of services such as provision of influenza vaccinations but less aware of other services such as prescribing for minor ailments, smoking cessation, medication reviews, and administration of other vaccines.[32] In the Canadian provinces of British Columbia,[33] Saskatchewan,[34] Nova Scotia,[35] and Newfoundland,[35] public views toward the profession were generally positive. In Nova Scotia, patients who regularly interact with their pharmacists and who already feel comfortable communicating with them, are more likely to utilize professional pharmacy services.[36] This research reinforces the importance of understanding the public's perceptions as well as their experiences in order to meet their health care needs.

Pharmacists in Alberta have had authority to access patient health information,[37] administer drugs by injection, and prescribe medications since 2007.[38] In 2012, a publicly-funded compensation plan was introduced to remunerate community pharmacies for providing some professional pharmacy services.[39,40] However, after more than a decade of access to professional pharmacy services in the province of Alberta and other parts of Canada, public awareness of many services provided in community pharmacies remains low.[41] Understanding the public's views on the roles of pharmacists and their awareness of pharmacy services is important during this time of transformation in the professional work of pharmacists.[42]

In 2017, the pharmacy regulatory organization in Alberta identified a strategic goal to improve understanding of individuals' health care experiences.[43] The new vision included an accessible and supportive environment for community-based care and more meaningful experiences for individual patients.[43] Understanding current and past experiences can inform future policy and initiatives in service provision, enabling transformation of primary health care and greater awareness of what pharmacists have to offer. This study was undertaken to explore public perceptions and experiences with community pharmacy services.

Methods

The methods developed to explore public perceptions and experiences with community pharmacy services were informed by two adaptations of the draw and write technique developed for adults: draw, write, reflect approach, which was created to study academics[6] and the iSquare protocol, which was developed for implementation in the classroom.[7] Table 1 highlights

TABLE 1 Examples of variations of the draw and write technique.

	Draw, write, reflect[6]	iSquare protocol[21]	Adapted draw and write technique
Focus of research question	Career progression of adults engaging in academic careers	Concept of information	Public perceptions and experiences with community pharmacy services
Context	Tertiary education institution, Australia	Tertiary education institution, Canada	Community and public venues, Canada
Data collection setting	Private office or room	Classroom	Meeting rooms
Participants	Adults, academics	Adults, graduate students in a Master of Information degree program	Adults
Researcher's relationship to participants	Peer	Research assistant	Researcher, research assistant
Drawing materials	Blank white papers (A4), black fine-liner pens	iSquare—Smooth heavy white art paper (4 × 4 in.), black pen	iSquare—Textured white heavy art paper (4.25 × 4.25 in.), black gel ink pen
Activity	Draw and/or write, reflect	Draw and write	Draw and write
Time for activity	10–15 min	7 min	5–20 min
Combined with another research method	Interview: Verbal elicitation to reflect on the activity	No	Focus group interview: Verbal elicitation on the drawing plus group discussion
Data analyzed	Drawings and/or writing, interview transcript	Drawings, words	Drawings, words, focus group transcript

these adaptations as well as the approach developed to study members of the public. Further details of the method are outlined in the following sections, on sampling and recruiting, data collection using the iSquare protocol combined with focus group interviews, and data analysis.

Sampling and recruiting

The context for this study was the province of Alberta in western Canada. Members of the public, including users and nonusers of community pharmacy services, were recruited to provide information about their experiences and share their perspectives. Through purposeful sampling, recruitment efforts targeted participants who fulfilled a variety of criteria, ensuring that the research question would be thoroughly addressed.[44] Criteria were based on variables associated with community pharmacy services such as chronic health conditions, medication use, caregiving, and location. The study team aimed for a maximally varied sample with respect to gender, culture, income, education, and experience with pharmacies and the health care system. Three population segments were identified: young adults, adults with young children, and older adults. Sampling was conducted in different locations and population centres[45] situated within 25 km of Edmonton, a large population center in Alberta.

Information about the study was posted in public places, universities, community leagues, day cares, and community social media pages.[46] Members of the research team personally contacted individuals representing community organizations to obtain permission to advertise the study. Recruitment materials and posters included tailored information for specific population segments outlining eligibility criteria such as, for example, parents with young children. A $25 gift card was offered to all participants in addition to reimbursement for parking or public transit, if required. Individuals interested in the study were directed to the e-mail address created for the study. They were contacted by a research team member and provided with detailed information about the study. They were then contacted again to confirm dates and venues for attending a specific focus group interview at a specific time. Participants were eligible for the study if they were at least 18 years old, capable of speaking English, and provided written informed consent. The University of Alberta Research Ethics Board approved the study (Pro00081946).

Data collection

At least two research team members were scheduled to attend each focus group interview. One member facilitated the focus group interviews. The other team members in attendance took field notes and observed the process. Materials, including consent forms and a one-page questionnaire to collect demographic data, were prepared and placed in strategic locations prior to the start of the interviews. The drawing materials, as specified in the iSquare protocol, included a square piece of white art paper (4.25 × 4.25 in.) and a black gel ink pen.[7]

Participants did the following at the focus group interviews: (1) completed a demographic questionnaire, (2) described and drew their view of community pharmacy services, and (3) engaged in a focus group discussion. The facilitator started the focus group interviews with an overview of the process, introducing the members of the research team in attendance and presenting information to facilitate obtaining of informed consent. At this point participants were given time to complete the paperwork before the drawing started. Verbal instructions were given to invite participants to create a drawing using the materials provided. The facilitator began as follows:

> *Please answer the question, "What do community pharmacy services mean to you?" in the form of a drawing on one side of the square. Please also write 6 to 10 words in answer to this question on the other side of the square.*

Participants were given approximately 5 min to complete the drawing and writing tasks. Once participants put their pens down, the facilitator prompted them to describe their drawings to clarify what they represented. Participants were encouraged to speak about their drawings but were assured that they were not obligated to do so. The postdrawing discussion was conducted on a volunteer basis. Participants were free to comment on other individuals' drawings. The facilitator encouraged open discussion and provided opportunities for all study participants to contribute but did not offer interpretation of the drawings. The discussion was guided initially by topics and issues introduced by the participants themselves, based on their drawings or the words they wrote to describe their drawings, and then by questions corresponding to the interview topic guide developed for this study (Table 2). The interview topic guide was not pilot tested.

At the end of the focus group interviews, a member of the research team collected the drawings and other materials. Drawings were assigned an identifying number related to the relevant focus group, photocopied front and back, and digitally scanned. Focus group interviews were digitally audio-recorded and transcribed verbatim, checked for accuracy, and anonymized to ensure that names or phrases that could reveal the identity of the speaker were removed. Participants were

TABLE 2 Focus group interview topic guide.

Topics

Draw and write: Participants were invited to answer:

- "What do community pharmacy services mean to you?"

Discuss: Participants were invited to discuss their drawings and words.

- Tell us about your drawing.

Focus group questions: The facilitator asked questions about the following topics:

- Experiences with community pharmacy
- Services sought, received, valued
- Environment of a community pharmacy
- Role of the community pharmacist

not offered a copy of the transcripts. Following each focus group session, the facilitator prepared a written summary including the number of participants, room set up, content areas discussed, and reflections on the research procedures. This summary was shared and reviewed with other research team members who were encouraged to add observations and reflections and to identify new questions or directions to discuss at the regularly scheduled research team meetings. This process of writing, reviewing, and discussing the summaries facilitated reflexivity as the researchers considered their own involvement and role in the process.

Data analysis

The drawings and associated text were considered the primary source of data while the focus group interviews provided verbal elucidation of the drawings for the researchers. An inductive approach was used to analyze data thematically.[23,47] Data analysis was accomplished in phases. The drawings were analyzed using a combination of manual sorting and coding using NVivo 12. First, the drawings were sorted to identify overall thematic categories; then, the words and phrases associated with the drawings were coded based on those themes. The approach used in this study incorporated the participants' interpretation of their drawings as well as their accounts of their experiences and perspectives captured in the focus group interview transcripts. The first phase of transcript analysis involved perusal of the transcripts by all members of the research team to generate initial codes following the first three focus group interviews. In the second phase, data with codes that were identified as most significant and frequent were analyzed further for all transcripts. In the final phase of analysis, data interpretation and synthesis were performed by all research team members in face-to-face meetings. Data, codes, and themes from each focus group were compared to those from subsequent focus groups. Sampling continued until saturation was achieved, as agreed by the research team; this occurred after 15 focus group interviews. NVivo 12 was used for coding and data management.

Results

Seventy-four study participants took part in a series of focus group interviews ($n = 15$) conducted between October 2018 and February 2019 at 10 different venues in a variety of population centers (Table 3). Demographic characteristics of study participants are outlined in Table 4. The average number of participants in the focus group sessions was 5 (range: 2 to 11 participants). Focus group discussions ranged in length from 22 to 106 min, with an average of 57 min, resulting in 918 min of recorded data. It was not uncommon for some participants to cancel their registration for a focus group interview. Several cancellations were experienced with one focus group resulting in 2 individuals participating in a session concluding after 22 min. The proportion of the focus group time devoted to discussion arising from the draw and write exercise was approximately 20%, ranging from 5 to 20 min. In total, 69 drawings were collected for the data set. Analysis of the drawings, words, and focus group interview transcripts identified 4 themes: accessibility, services, environment, and caring

TABLE 3 Details of focus group (FG) interviews.

FG	Venue	Segment	Participants (Drawings)	[a]Population centre[45]
1	University	Young adults	6 (6)	Large
2	University	Young adults	3 (3)	Large
3	Public Library	Adults with young children	4 (4)	Large
4	University	Young adults	4 (4)	Large
5	Community Senior Centre	Older adults	6 (6)	Large
6	Private Senior Residence	Older adults	9 (8)	Medium
7	Community Senior Centre	Older adults	2 (1)	Large
8	Community Religious Housing	Young adults	2 (2)	Large
9	Supportive Living Senior Residence	Older adults	5 (5)	Large
10	Supportive Living Senior Residence	Older adults	7 (4)	Large
11	Public Library	Adults with young children	3 (3)	Small
12	Public Library	Adults with young children	7 (7)	Small
13	University	Young adults	2 (2)	Large
14	Community Church Hall	Older adults	11 (11)	Large
15	Public Library	Adults with young children	3 (3)	Large

[a]*Population Centers defined:*
Small—population between 1000 and 29,999.
Medium—population between 30,000 and 99,999.
Large—population 100,000 and over.

relationship. Data, including examples of drawings, are presented for each theme in the sections below. Quotes representing participants' descriptions of their drawings are provided in Table 5.

Accessibility

Participants' experiences and perceptions of community pharmacy services emphasized accessibility. This theme included access to community pharmacies, services, and pharmacists' expertise. The drawings in Fig. 1 and corresponding explanations (Table 5) are examples of initial representations of accessibility by participants. Discussions with participants in the focus group interviews revealed details of their perceptions of accessibility, including hours of operation, services outside of the pharmacy such as delivery, options to speak directly with a pharmacist on the telephone, and the convenience of being able to consult with a pharmacist without having to make an appointment. Participants compared access to pharmacists and physicians; generally, there was a perception of easier access to pharmacists. They felt that the public could access community pharmacy services when needed. Participants describing their experiences expressed a sense of relief and deep appreciation for access to care through community pharmacies.

Services

Experiences with community pharmacy services varied among the participants. Drawings created by participants depicted a range of services related to products, information, and professional pharmacy services. Many participants' drawings featured either medications alone (Fig. 2), medications and pharmacists situated in a dispensary (Fig. 3), or interactions with pharmacists (Fig. 4). Discussions elicited explanations of the drawings and exploration of participants' varied experiences with community pharmacy services.

As the discussion at the focus group interviews evolved, participants revealed more detail about their experiences with community pharmacy services. From their pharmacists, they received information; they also had consultations about self-

TABLE 4 Demographic characteristics of participants (*n* = 74).

Characteristics	Number
Gender	
Female	54
Male	19
Nonbinary	1
Age	
≤30	17
31–50	9
51–70	15
>71	33
Education	
No high school	4
High school	24
Apprentice/trade	4
Community college	15
University	27
Annual income	
<20,000	9
20,000–49,999	17
50,000–100,000	22
>100,000	10
Prefer not to say	10
No response	4
Visits to a pharmacy	
Never	12
1 time/month	43
2–4 times/month	16
>5 times/month	1
Chronic conditions	
Yes	37
Medications, taking >4	
Yes	18

medication and utilized professional pharmacy services such as prescribing for existing or new conditions. Some participants described experiencing positive emotions, including feelings of relief, gratitude, and satisfaction, in response to services or information received, or having their medication needs addressed. Other participants expressed negative emotions related to experiences with services provided by community pharmacists. In a discussion with participants from Focus Group 10 (Older Adults), 1 participant voiced dissatisfaction with receiving an unexpected comprehensive annual care plan service.[40]

TABLE 5 Participants' descriptions of their drawings.

Theme	Figure	Quote describing drawing
Accessibility		
	1	"You have easy access to the building, to the pharmacist. They're always available. They're teaching, they're giving information, and they're helping me. And they're always open to do that." (Focus Group 5/Older Adult)
	1	"I tried to depict a pharmacist coming and delivering medications to someone's home… I've had a lot of interactions with pharmacy services for people pretty much home bound in a way or they can't go out and get their own things… Having that delivery part for some pharmacies is a big part that I see." (Focus Group 1/Young Adult)
	1	"I just found them very, very helpful. And [I can get] information on the phone, too… You can't get through and talk to a doctor the way you can talk to a pharmacist." (Focus Group 7/Older Adult)
Services		
	2	"I don't really think anything of pharmacy except for medication, that's the only reason why I go there, so that's the only reason why I use it." (Focus Group 4/ Young Adult)
	2	"First thing I thought of was just a pill, stereotypical pharmacy thing. That's just what I thought of." (Focus Group 11/ Adult with young children)
	2	"On mine I just have one, I don't know what it's called, pill bottles. A pill bottle full of pills. And it means to me that, like, when I go to the pharmacy, I expect them to help me get better… they're willing to hear me out and hear my concerns and my concerns for that pill, facilitate helping me get better soon." (Focus Group 4/ Young Adult)
	3	"Mine is much more literal. That's the local pharmacy that I always use. I'm very familiar with them. And I'm there frequently. So that is supposed to be probably one of the assistants working at the register, that was my impression because I'm there a lot." (Focus Group 3/ Adult with young children)
	3	"I just drew a picture of someone standing behind a desk with the shelves of other medications, so you can put a number on the back, a place to pick up prescriptions or other medications, like, over the counter and stuff like that. Helpful staff." (Focus Group 1/ Young Adult)
	4	"I drew a pharmacist working behind the counter and this person approaching the pharmacist… I go there and come with a question… They advise you on all the surrounding things and potential side effects and when you take other medication how they could interact with each other… I haven't actually made use of the app, but apparently there's also an app you can even just order your refill." (Focus Group 13/ Young Adult)
	4	"I drew me holding a prescription, and he's helping me. And he's very friendly and nice. I [wrote] informative, caring, and they know me because it's a small town." (Focus Group 11/ Adult with young children)
	4	"I drew a person behind a counter and a person at the counter, and they're having a discussion over a medication prescription that the pharmacist is educating the other person on, I guess. They're talking about their health needs. And so basically that's what I described on the back is when I think of pharmacy. I think of a place where I can go to receive consultation about my health needs, more often if it's something that involves medication. So, if it's something that I think cannot be dealt with in other ways, then that's where I would go." (Focus Group 7/ Young Adult)
	5	"When your doctor's at the end of his or her tether because they've tried all these things on you, and in the end a pharmacist came from the hospital and then she had other suggestions that, you know, that might be helpful. So, I think the doctors really rely on them… And I think that's a great service." (Focus Group 9/ Older Adult)
	5	"We brought the kids for a flu shot, so that brought us there. I wanted more information about pharmacists being able to prescribe medications as well as doctors and other professionals. So, I talked to [named a pharmacist] about that." (Focus Group 3/ Adult with young children)
	5	"Well, I have my [drawing of an] eyeball, and it's the observant pharmacist catching small things and making sure…. So, it's catching little things." (Focus Group 14/ Older Adult)
Environment		
	6	"I feel like the pharmacy is a completely separate part of that building or structure, because you look back there and it's more like a doctor's office. That kind of makes me more comfortable, I would say, because it's organized, it's clean, they have a way that they want to do things, so that it gets done properly. And still being able to see back there, and see like that open space, makes me believe that they're not like trying to hide anything." (Focus Group 2 / Young Adult)

TABLE 5 Participants' descriptions of their drawings—cont'd

Theme	Figure	Quote describing drawing
	6	"I'm 18 and my mom picks up all my prescriptions. So, I rarely go in [to the pharmacy]. But I don't like going in. When I do sometimes… it's not really welcom[ing]. My pharmacy in [large chain] is at the back of the store, and it just seems like the scary corner. I just I don't like going there. Usually everyone has lab coats on or something. So, it's like drugs. Scary." (Focus Group 4/ Young Adult)
	6	"I did go to pharmacists in a larger setting, and they were fine. And now I'm going to an independent, and these are really great… So, it depends on the pharmacy. It's pharmacists themselves, in my experience." (Focus Group 7/ Older Adult)
	7	"When I've gone to the pharmacy, I get kind of frustrated that he's actually giving more than five minutes to the person in the line-up ahead of me. I understand why now. I want to be up there first. And that's not me being selfish. But the pharmacist is giving undivided attention to that person right in front of him and listening to whatever they have to say." (Focus Group 12/ Adult with young children)
	7	"Sometimes I go in there and the pharmacist is dealing with someone else, and he or she is explaining everything. And I either have to wait or I come back. But I'm happy with that because it shows that the pharmacist is also caring about everybody, not just one person. But they're caring, they're devoting that kind of time to everybody. And that means a lot." (Focus Group 7/ Older Adult)
	7	"I would suggest a modification on the environment… because I think if they can have more private rooms that they can drop off prescription and get more information later, that would be more helpful. It would not take that much time, maybe each person two or three minutes." (Focus Group 4/ Older Adult)
Caring relationship		
	8	"I'm no Picasso, so [the drawing is] very simple. Just two-way conversations. For me conversation was my number one. Being able to be open." (Focus Group 11/ Adult with young children)
	8	"I expect to walk into a pharmacy full of love and caring spirit." (Focus Group 3/ Adult with young children)
	8	"I did little stick people holding hands … it's like a cooperative thing. It's a good relationship. And then I kind of did like the caring aspect." (Focus Group 11/ Adult with young children)

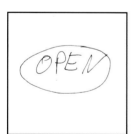 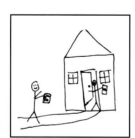 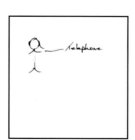

FIG. 1 Examples of drawings that express the theme of accessibility.

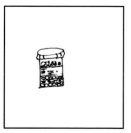 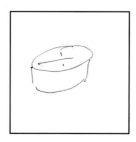 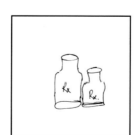

FIG. 2 Examples of drawings that depict medications.

FIG. 3 Examples of drawings that depict medications and pharmacy staff situated in a dispensary.

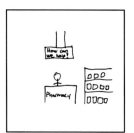 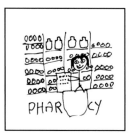 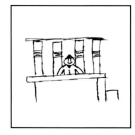

FIG. 4 Examples of drawings that depict interaction with a pharmacist.

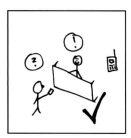 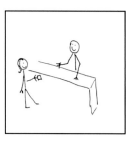 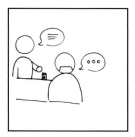

Awareness of professional pharmacy services ranged considerably within the three participant segments included in this study. Overall, participants in the young adult segment described having limited exposure to pharmacists and community pharmacy services. Some had never personally accessed the care of a pharmacist. Their needs were expressed in terms of issues relevant to their stage in life; for example, they were interested in services related to mental health and sexual and reproductive health. In contrast, participants in the older adult segment expressed greater awareness and made more frequent use of community pharmacy services. They had multiple experiences associated with their care including utilizing services to address chronic diseases and conditions.

Some participants had experienced professional pharmacy services, such as prescribing by pharmacists. However, other participants were unaware of the ability of pharmacists to prescribe or the range of available services at community pharmacies such as comprehensive annual care plans. Participants offered a variety of approaches to increase awareness of professional pharmacy services (Table 6). Many felt that the best method to disseminate information about community pharmacy services was through personal communication from their pharmacists. Drawings in Fig. 5 highlight aspects of professional pharmacy services and collaboration with physicians, with pharmacists providing influenza vaccines and monitoring medication therapy.

Some participants in this study valued collaboration, teamwork, and information sharing among patients, physicians, and pharmacists. There was awareness that collaboration between pharmacists and physicians is important for quality patient care and a recognition that pharmacists should be a part of the health care team.

Participants in this study acknowledged pharmacists' changing roles and the expansion of community pharmacy services. They described pharmacists as being more professional than in the past, spending more time talking with patients and providing information. Participants noted, however, that not all services are provided by all pharmacists. Some participants were cautious about whether a full range of professional pharmacy services should be expected from all pharmacies. They mentioned the boundaries between pharmacists' and physicians' roles and wondered about the ability of all pharmacists to provide the same level of service.

Environment

The pharmacy environment influenced how participants in this study experienced community pharmacy services. Drawings in Fig. 6 feature varied environments. Some participants preferred the convenience of large pharmacies located within larger stores, while other participants appreciated independent pharmacies. Participants emphasized the importance of a professional environment with private areas for consultation. They also expressed loyalty toward the pharmacies in their communities. Some perceived that pharmacies located in small population centers are more welcoming and that medicine-only pharmacies exhibit a desired level of professionalism in terms of providing health care services. However,

TABLE 6 Increasing public awareness about community pharmacy services.

Advertising

- Billboards
- Local and national campaign
- Public transit

Community events

- Pharmacist presentations and attendance

Media

- Radio
- Television
- Print newspapers and magazines
- Social media

Personal communication

- Pharmacist
- Physician
- Friends

Pharmacy

- Posters
- Post cards
- Bag stuffer

Physician office

- Referral to pharmacist
- Posters

Public spaces

- Public libraries

School curricula

- Elementary schools
- High schools
- Universities

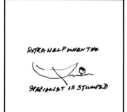 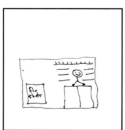 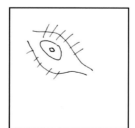

FIG. 5 Examples of drawings that depict aspects of professional pharmacy services.

FIG. 6   Examples of drawings that express the theme of environment.

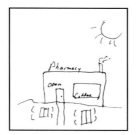 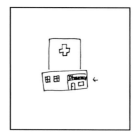 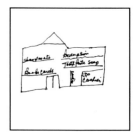

FIG. 7   Examples of drawings that illustrate frustration with line-ups.

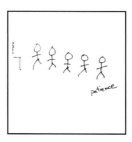 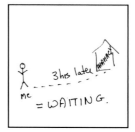 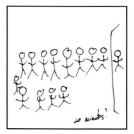

participants accessing services at chain pharmacies in large population centers expressed similar views, saying that their pharmacies were both welcoming and professional. As a result of their experiences, participants felt different levels of comfort with community pharmacies. One vital aspect of the environment was related to the pharmacists themselves, who ultimately created the welcoming environment.

Experience with community pharmacy services was described in terms of time, specifically, time waiting to consult with a pharmacist and the time pharmacists spent with people. Participants talked about pharmacists taking time to listen to them, time to educate them and provide information. There was thus an acknowledgement that community pharmacy services take time. Many participants noted that pharmacists appeared to make time for them no matter how busy they were. Wait times for community pharmacy services were frustrating yet tolerated; an individualized approach and time devoted to patients were appreciated (Fig. 7).

Caring relationships

Participants perceived having a caring relationship to be an important aspect of community pharmacy services. Relationships were created through conversations, pharmacists knowing the patient's name, building trust, and taking a genuine interest in people and their family members. Caring was experienced when pharmacists took time to make eye contact, give their full attention to the patient, shift their focus from other tasks or computers, acknowledge patients by name, listen, and engage in conversation. While most participants shared positive experiences in this regard, some participants felt an absence of caring when a pharmacist or pharmacy staff member did not acknowledge or greet them when they arrived at the pharmacy. Participants described the experience of engaging with pharmacists as part of building caring relationships. This involved sharing information about themselves and asking questions about health and medications. Drawings that represent caring relationships depicted conversation, caring emotions, and human touch (Fig. 8).

FIG. 8   Examples of drawings that express the theme of caring relationship.

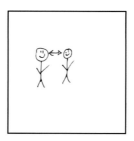  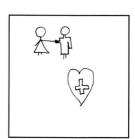

Discussion

This study employed an arts-informed approach to explore public perceptions and experiences with community pharmacy services using an adapted version of the draw and write technique combined with focus group interviews. Members of the public created drawings and shared descriptions of what community pharmacy services meant to them in focus group interviews. Analysis of drawings and focus group data revealed four themes related to participants' individual and varied experiences: accessibility, services, environment, and caring relationships. In this section, the results are discussed with consideration of previous research in the area and applications of an arts-informed approach using the draw and write technique.

In many ways, the results of this study echo those of previous research highlighting the value of access, convenience, and the ability to consult a community pharmacist without an appointment.[27–31] Access to a pharmacist for services and developing a relationship with the pharmacist were as important as other factors, such as location or type of pharmacy. Participants expressed loyalty to pharmacies close to where they live and a desire for private consultation rooms. As in other studies, there were differing opinions regarding service provision by small independent versus large chain pharmacies.[27,28,48] In Canada, accessibility and established relationships have been recognized as factors supporting uptake of professional pharmacy services.[34–36]

Similar to other research, there were differences in awareness of community pharmacy services.[27,28] In this study, most participants had experience with services related to medications and some were familiar with injection and prescribing services. In the Alberta context, there may be growing awareness and utilization of professional pharmacy services as many pharmacists there have authorization to administer drugs by injection (80%) and prescribe medications (51%).[49] However, not all participants had had these experiences. Consistent with the findings of other studies, participants in the segment representing younger individuals described having little exposure to services; their perspectives differed from those of older individuals and those having more experience with community pharmacy services.[30,35,36] In a previously mentioned study of public and patient perceptions in the United Kingdom, Hindi et al.[27] identified two themes of public cognizance and attitudes toward services characterizing perceptions that reflect expectations and experiences of using community pharmacy services. The results of this current study point to connections between needs, awareness, perceptions, and experience. If patients are aware of and have a need for health care services, there is a better chance that they will seek and experience those services and perceive them as helpful.

Despite the recent increase in the range of professional pharmacy services provided by community pharmacies[50–52] and the number of pharmacy services covered by compensation plans[40,53] the need to increase awareness of professional pharmacy services persists.[27–29,48,54] Given the highly variable perspectives and experiences reported by participants in this study, engaging pharmacists in an awareness campaign aimed to inform the patients in their communities personally about the professional pharmacy services they offer may impact the public's experience of the community pharmacy environment, service delivery, and caring relationships. Other mechanisms to inform the public of community pharmacy services aimed at different demographic groups, as suggested by participants in this study (Table 6), also warrant consideration.

This study adds to what is known about the public's experience with community pharmacy services. The results of this study differ from those of other research with respect to participants' disclosure of the emotions they experience related to pharmacy services; the arts-informed approach utilized here revealed a depth, richness, and complexity of experience not reported in other studies. The arts, even everyday activities such as drawing, allow people to express themselves and represent their experiences[10] in a more emotional way[55] than simply providing statement or completing questionnaires. For example, participants visually depicted how they experienced community pharmacy services, emphasizing their emotions and feelings. They expressed a range of complex emotions in response to community pharmacy environments such as tolerance or frustration, feeling accommodated or inconvenienced, comfortable or uncomfortable. Their drawings and the text describing them indicated that openness, conversation, reciprocity, connection, touch, and love were part of the caring relationships that characterized their experiences with pharmacists. Participants shared both the positive effects of being acknowledged and treated "as a real person" as well as their negative emotions when acknowledgement and individualized treatment were absent from their encounters in community pharmacies. Meaningful experiences arose from accessing a variety of services, visiting various community pharmacy environments, and developing caring relationships with pharmacists. It is possible that the arts-informed approach used in this study encouraged greater disclosure of experiences and feelings by participants than they would have provided otherwise. It is also possible that participants in other studies experienced similar emotions and shared them in the research process. Overall, the arts-informed approach utilized in this study allowed the researchers to access a very diverse range of experiences and perspectives.

The adapted version of the draw and write technique used in this study, with the addition of the specific data collection instrument based on the iSquare[7] protocol, was easy to prepare and administer. Asking participants to respond through drawing and writing to the question, "What do community pharmacy services mean to you?" elicited fresh perspectives about community pharmacy services; each participant was offered an opportunity to express his or her views individually prior to discussion with all participants.[46,56] In this study, showing each other the drawings and reading the accompanying written text was an effective way to start the focus group interviews, drawing participants into the discussion and encouraging interaction.[44] Lively discussion flowed from participants' explanations of their drawings. The additional question asked in the focus group interviews promoted interactions between participants and allowed them to refine, reinforce, or challenge their understanding of experiences with community pharmacy services. However, one limitation of the focus group method is the possibility that participants may not disclose the intended meaning of their drawings or may be influenced by others in the group.[44] Combining drawing with individual interviews may produce different results.

Further limitations of this approach relate to the time and materials provided for data collection. Approximately 5 min was allocated for participants to complete the drawing portion of the draw and write activity. This may not have been sufficient for all participants to think about their responses to the questions and engage fully in the drawing activity. With future applications of this technique, scheduling at least 10 min and providing additional information presented as background to the instructions may benefit participants and draw out more of their experiences.[7] Participants in this study were provided with one piece of art paper and a black pen. These materials may have limited creativity and influenced the drawings. In a study to understand public perceptions of healing, Rahtz et al.[57] found that using crayons and paper facilitated a playful and instinctive approach to the drawing activity. In some studies, participants can choose from an array of art materials that inspire creative expression.[11,20]

Most participants in this study contributed a drawing. There were no instances where participants verbally indicated refusal to draw. Reasons for the nonparticipation of 5 individuals in this aspect of the study are unknown. Incorporating questions about their experience of the draw and write technique in a future study would add another dimension to the results. Potential issues associated with this technique include unease with the activity, reluctance to draw, drawing what is easy to depict, or being influenced by others' drawings, all of which pertain to the validity of the results.[9,22] In addition, the presence of research team members while participants made drawings may have introduced bias; drawing in a more isolated setting may have produced different results. In this study, many participants drew stereotypical depictions of community pharmacy experiences and interactions. In addition, the drawings included in Fig. 7 were all created in the same focus group interview. Their similarity suggests that some participants may have been influenced by others in the group. Potential ethical issues associated with the draw and write technique relate to the making of a drawing, the image itself, and its reception.[9,16] Other concerns with the technique are associated with consent and use of images during and after the study.[7] In this study, the intended use of their images was outlined to participants as part of the informed consent process.

Other limitations associated with the draw and write technique relate to methods of data analysis and interpretation.[7–9] The adapted version of the draw and write technique used here, specifically combining it with focus group interviews, helped to mitigate issues of interpretation. Linking data from drawings and focus groups prevented the data from becoming fractured during the analysis.[20] Involvement of all team members in the data collection and analysis, as well as incorporating participants' own interpretations of their drawings, contributed to the trustworthiness of the results. Other approaches give priority to the art work, placing emphasis on the process of drawing and engaging participants in the interpretation of the data.[57] There are also sophisticated models of analysis based on multiple possible reactions to art, and encompassing emotional, physiological, and evaluative factors.[58] The themes identified through this analysis represent one possible interpretation of the data. Other methods used to analyze iSquare data, such as compositional analysis, pictorial metaphor, or content analysis, could produce alternate interpretations.[23]

In arts-informed research, various dissemination methods may facilitate the translation of knowledge into practice. The research team of this study endeavored to make this arts-informed research accessible to community stakeholders through written reports, discussions, and presentations that highlight the drawings and individuals' own interpretations of their experiences. Its results were disseminated to community groups that provided venues for the research such as community public libraries and seniors' centers. An arts-informed approach is an impactful way to engage with the public and bolster awareness of community pharmacy and other primary health care services. For example, art exhibits featuring drawings of health care professionals help them enter into the experience of their patients.[59] Future projects similar to the iSquare project could add to the dataset and incorporate art shows to display visual data.[7]

Arts-informed research may also be extended to pharmacy education. The draw and write technique blends art with education and research and has roots in curriculum development.[19] Educators have previously incorporated drawing as a learning activity.[12,14] Drawing has been used to develop health care students' knowledge and skills, improving their appreciation of the patient's perspective, encouraging critical thinking, and reflecting on humanistic aspects of health care.[14] Future opportunities to blend scholarship and art in Doctor of Pharmacy programs might include incorporating the draw and write technique as a classroom activity to gain insight into students' understanding of concepts, identify learning needs, and inform curriculum development projects using art.

Another educational application relates to using the draw and write data set as a resource for learning. Insights from this study can be incorporated into pharmacy curricula to deepen students' understanding of the public's perceptions and experiences with provision of primary health care by pharmacists. Learning activities that incorporate interaction with the actual iSquares may tap into different ways of thinking by students. Practical matters, such as how to create a welcoming environment by acknowledging individuals when they arrive at the pharmacy, may be addressed and observed through interaction with the data set. Including research using art-informed methods in pharmacy education will provide insight into patients' experiences with illness and treatment, aid in developing relationships with patients, and facilitate a patient-centered approach to care.[11]

The draw and write technique also has potential as a research method to explore pharmacy students' insights into how they perceive pharmacists' roles and the profession. The iSquare protocol is one of the methods used to explore pharmacy student's professional role formation in conjunction with a student-led program to explore pharmacy careers.[60] Hartel's iSquare research program with students has expanded to include information from schools worldwide, creating a large data set with potential for greater understanding of the field as well as opportunities for interdisciplinary research. The iSquare protocol offers a mechanism to build a large data set that can be used in research to address novel questions and disseminate information through creative mechanisms, ways such as art exhibits, to the broader pharmacy community.

Conclusion

Arts-informed research provides researchers with an approach to gain further insight into how individuals interpret experiences and make sense of the world around them. The adapted version of the draw and write technique combined with focus group interviews was a creative approach to explore public perceptions of community pharmacy services. This approach allowed the researchers to access a diverse range of experiences and perspectives. This study elucidates both personal and emotional aspects of experience with community pharmacy services. Research illuminating public perceptions and experiences can be used to educate and inform students, practicing pharmacists, and pharmacy organizations about barriers, needs, and opportunities for greater uptake of health care services provided by pharmacists. Arts-informed research methods facilitate making scholarship more accessible by connecting the work of the researcher with the broader community.

Questions for further discussion

1. What research topics of interest to you might benefit from use of an arts-informed approach, even if it were to address only a facet or component of that research?
2. How would the use of different drawing materials, such as paper of different sizes, paints, colored pens, or pencils affect participants' experiences with the draw and write technique? How might data collection, analysis, and results be affected by using different materials? How might issues of validity and reliability intersect with these variations in methodological tools?
3. What are some considerations when adapting the draw and write technique to incorporate reflection activities, individual interviews, or focus groups?
4. How might researchers share arts-informed research with community stakeholders?

Application exercise/scenario

Your research team is embarking on a qualitative research study to explore peoples' experiences with health care services in your region during the COVID-19 pandemic. There are several qualitative research methodologies that would address your research question. However, your team opted for an arts-informed approach to draw out the affective nature of peoples' experiences. How will you design this arts-informed study? What are some considerations you will use to determine details of the sampling, data collection, and data analysis phases of the study?

References

1. Fraser KD, Al Sayah F. Arts-based methods in health research: a systematic review of the literature. *Arts Health.* 2011;3:110–145. https://doi.org/10.1080/17533015.2011.561357.

2. Finley S. Arts-based research. In: Knowles JG, Cole AL, eds. *Handbook of the Arts in Qualitative Research: Perspectives, Methodologies, Examples, and Issues.* Thousand Oaks, CA: SAGE Publications, Inc; 2008.

3. Boydell KM, Gladstone BM, Volpe T, Allemang B, Stasiulis E. The production and dissemination of knowledge: a scoping review of arts-based health research. *Forum Qual Soc Res.* 2012;13:32.

4. Cole AL, Knowles JG. Arts-informed research. In: Knowles JG, Cole AL, eds. *Handbook of the Arts in Qualitative Research: Perspectives, Methodologies, Examples, and Issues.* Thousand Oaks, CA: SAGE Publications Inc; 2008:55–71.

5. Bagnoli A. Beyond the standard interview: the use of graphic elicitation and arts-based methods. *Qual Res.* 2009;9:547–570. https://doi.org/10.1177/1468794109343625.

6. Sharafizad F, Brown K, Jogulu U, Omari M. Letting a picture speak a thousand words: arts-based research in a study of the careers of female academics. *Sociol Methods Res.* 2021. https://doi.org/10.1177/0049124120926206.

7. Hartel J, Noone R, Oh C, Power S, Danzanov P, Kelly B. The iSquare protocol: combining research, art, and pedagogy through the draw-and-write technique. *Qual Res.* 2018;18:433–450. https://doi.org/10.1177/1468794117722193.

8. Guillemin M. Understanding illness: using drawings as a research method. *Qual Health Res.* 2004;14:272–289. https://doi.org/10.1177/1049732303260445.

9. Umoquit MJ, Tso P, Burchett HED, Dobrow MJ. A multidisciplinary systematic review of the use of diagrams as a means of collecting data from research subjects: application, benefits and recommendations. *BMC Med Res Methodol.* 2011;11:11. https://doi.org/10.1186/1471-2288-11-11.

10. Dewey J. *Art as Experience.* New York, NY: Penguin Putnam; 1934.

11. Cheung MMY, Saini B, Smith L. Using drawings to explore patients' perceptions of their illness: a scoping review. *J Multidiscip Healthc.* 2016;9:631–646. https://doi.org/10.2147/JMDH.S120300.

12. Armstrong J, Ward KL. Applying visual research methods in pharmacy education. *Am J Pharm Educ.* 2020;84:95–105. https://doi.org/10.5688/ajpe7123.

13. Cheung MMY, Saini B, Smith L. 'It's a powerful message': a qualitative study of Australian healthcare professionals' perceptions of asthma through the medium of drawings. *BMJ Open.* 2019;9. https://doi.org/10.1136/bmjopen-2018-027699.

14. Cheung MMY, Saini B, Smith L. Integrating drawings into health curricula: university educators' perspectives. *Med Humanit.* 2020;46:394–402. https://doi.org/10.1136/medhum-2019-011775.

15. Pridmore P, Bendelow G. Images of health: exploring beliefs of children using the 'draw-and-write' technique. *Health Educ J.* 1995;54:473–488. https://doi.org/10.1177/001789699505400410.

16. Hartel J. Draw-and-write techniques. In: Atkinson P, Delamont S, Cernat A, Sakshaug JW, Williams RA, eds. *SAGE Research Methods Foundations.* Thousand Oaks, CA: SAGE Publications Inc; 2019.

17. McWhirter J. The draw and write technique as a versatile tool for researching children's understanding of health and well-being. *Int J Health Promot Educ.* 2014;52:250–259. https://doi.org/10.1080/14635240.2014.912123.

18. Horstman M, Aldiss S, Richardson A, Gibson F. Methodological issues when using the draw and write technique with children aged 6 to 12 years. *Qual Health Res.* 2008;18:1001–1011. https://doi.org/10.1177/1049732308318230.

19. Wetton NM, McWhirter J. Images and curriculum development in health education. In: Prosser J, ed. *Image-Based Research: A Sourcebook for Qualitative Researchers.* New York, NY: Routledge; 2005:235–254.

20. Angell C, Alexander J, Hunt JA. 'Draw, write and tell': a literature review and methodological development on the 'draw and write' research method. *J Early Child Res.* 2014;13:17–28. https://doi.org/10.1177/1476718X14538592.

21. Hartel J. An arts-informed study of information using the draw-and-write technique. *J Assoc Inf Sci Technol.* 2014;65:1349–1367. https://doi.org/10.1002/asi.23121.

22. Backett-Milburn K, McKie L. A critical appraisal of the draw and write technique. *Health Educ Res.* 1999;14:387–398. https://doi.org/10.1093/her/14.3.387.

23. Hartel J. Adventures in visual analysis. *Vis Methodol.* 2017;5:80–91.

24. Feehan M, Walsh M, Godin J, Sundwall D, Munger MA. Patient preferences for healthcare delivery through community pharmacy settings in the USA: a discrete choice study. *J Clin Pharm Ther.* 2017;42:738–749. https://doi.org/10.1111/jcpt.12574.

25. Policarpo V, Romano S, António JHC, Correia TS, Costa S. A new model for pharmacies? Insights from a quantitative study regarding the public's perceptions. *BMC Health Serv Res.* 2019;19. https://doi.org/10.1186/s12913-019-3987-3.

26. Moullin JC, Sabater-Hernández D, Fernandez-Llimos F, Benrimoj SI. Defining professional pharmacy services in community pharmacy. *Res Social Adm Pharm.* 2013;9:989–995. https://doi.org/10.1016/j.sapharm.2013.02.005.

27. Hindi AMK, Schafheutle EI, Jacobs S. Patient and public perspectives of community pharmacies in the United Kingdom: a systematic review. *Health Expect.* 2018;21:409–428. https://doi.org/10.1111/hex.12639.

28. Kember J, Hodson K, James DH. The public's perception of the role of community pharmacists in Wales. *Int J Pharm Pract.* 2018;26:120–128. https://doi.org/10.1111/ijpp.12375.

29. van de Pol JM, van Dijk L, Koster ES, de Jong J, Bouvy ML. How does the general public balance convenience and cognitive pharmaceutical services in community pharmacy practice. *Res Social Adm Pharm.* 2021;17:606–6120. https://doi.org/10.1016/j.sapharm.2020.05.014.

30. Taylor S, Cairns A, Glass B. Consumer perspectives of expanded practice in rural community pharmacy. *Res Social Adm Pharm.* 2021;17:362–367. https://doi.org/10.1016/j.sapharm.2020.03.022.

31. Steckowych K, Smith M, Spiggle S, Stevens A, Li H. Building the case: changing consumer perceptions of the value of expanded community pharmacist services. *J Pharm Pract.* 2019;32:637–647. https://doi.org/10.1177/0897190018771521.

32. AbacusData. *Pharmacists in Canada: A National Survey of Canadians on Their Perceptions and Attitudes Towards Pharmacists in Canada.* Canadian Pharmacists Association; 2015. http://www.pharmacists.ca/cpha-ca/assets/File/news-events/PAM2015-Poll.pdf;. Accessed 21 November 2020.

33. Tsao NW, Khakban A, Gastonguay L, Li K, Lynd LD, Marra CA. Perceptions of British Columbia residents and their willingness to pay for medication management services provided by pharmacists. *Can Pharm J.* 2015;148:263–273. https://doi.org/10.1177/1715163515597244.

34. Perepelkin J. Public opinion of pharmacists and pharmacist prescribing. *Can Pharm J.* 2011;144:86–93. https://doi.org/10.3821/1913-701X-144.2.86.

35. Kelly DV, Young S, Phillips L, Clark D. Patient attitudes regarding the role of the pharmacist and interest in expanded pharmacist services. *Can Pharm J.* 2014;147:239–247. https://doi.org/10.1177/1715163514535731.

36. Bishop AC, Boyle TA, Morrison B, et al. Public perceptions of pharmacist expanded scope of practice services in Nova Scotia. *Can Pharm J.* 2015;148:274–283. https://doi.org/10.1177/1715163515596757.

37. Hughes CA, Guirguis LM, Wong T, Ng K, Ing L, Fisher K. Influence of pharmacy practice on community pharmacists' integration of medication and lab value information from electronic health records. *J Am Pharm Assoc.* 2011;51:591–598. https://doi.org/10.1331/JAPhA.2011.10085.

38. Yuksel N, Eberhart G, Bungard TJ. Prescribing by pharmacists in Alberta. *Am J Health Syst Pharm.* 2008;65:2126–2132. https://doi.org/10.2146/ajhp080247.

39. Breault RR, Schindel TJ, Whissell JG, Hughes CA. Updates to the compensation plan for pharmacy services in Alberta, Canada. *J Am Pharm Assoc.* 2018;58:597–598. https://doi.org/10.1016/j.japh.2018.08.005.

40. Breault RR, Whissell JG, Hughes CA, Schindel TJ. Development and implementation of the compensation plan for pharmacy services in Alberta, Canada. *J Am Pharm Assoc.* 2017;57:532–541. https://doi.org/10.1016/j.japh.2017.05.004.

41. Henry M. *Rxa Benchmark Study.* Edmonton, Alberta: ThinkHQ Public Affairs Inc; 2015. October 13.

42. Schindel TJ, Yuksel N, Breault R, Daniels J, Varnhagen S, Hughes CA. Perceptions of pharmacists' roles in the era of expanding scopes of practice. *Res Social Adm Pharm.* 2017;13:148–161. https://doi.org/10.1016/j.sapharm.2016.02.007.

43. Alberta College of Pharmacists. *Setting the Pace for Pharmacy Excellence in Person-Centered Care*; 2017. https://abpharmacy.ca/sites/default/files/ACP%20Business%20Plan%202017-19%20-%20final.pdf;. Accessed 23 November 2020.

44. Rosenthal M. Qualitative research methods: why, when, and how to conduct interviews and focus groups in pharmacy research. *Curr Pharm Teach Learn.* 2016;8:509–516. https://doi.org/10.1016/j.cptl.2016.03.021.

45. Statistics Canada. *Population Centre and Rural Area Classification*; 2021. https://www.statcan.gc.ca/eng/subjects/standard/pcrac/2016/introduction;. Accessed 27 November 2020.

46. Ferguson SD. *Researching the Public Opinion Environment: Theories and Methods.* Thousand Oaks, CA: SAGE Publications Inc; 2000.

47. Charmaz K. *Constructing Grounded Theory.* 2nd ed. London: SAGE Publications Ltd; 2014.

48. Wood K, Gibson F, Radley A, Williams B. Pharmaceutical care of older people: what do older people want from community pharmacy? *Int J Pharm Pract.* 2015;23:121–130. https://doi.org/10.1111/ijpp.12127.

49. Alberta College o fPharmacy. *2019–2020 Annual Report*; 2020. https://abpharmacy.ca/sites/default/files/ACP_2019-20_Annual_Report.pdf;. Accessed 3 December 2020.

50. Sim TF, Wright B, Hattingh L, Parsons R, Sunderland B, Czarniak P. A cross-sectional survey of enhanced and extended professional services in community pharmacies: a pharmacy perspective. *Res Social Adm Pharm.* 2020;16:511–521. https://doi.org/10.1016/j.sapharm.2019.07.001.

51. Schindel TJ, Yuksel N, Breault R, Daniels J, Varnhagen S, Hughes CA. Perceptions of pharmacists' roles in the era of expanding scopes of practice. *Res Social Adm Pharm.* 2017;13:148–161. https://doi.org/10.1016/j.sapharm.2016.02.007.

52. Goode J-V, Owen J, Page A, Gatewood S. Community-based pharmacy practice innovation and the role of the community-based pharmacist practitioner in the United States. *Pharmacy.* 2019;7. https://doi.org/10.3390/pharmacy7030106.

53. Houle SKD, Carter CA, Tsuyuki RT, Grindrod KA. Remunerated patient care services and injections by pharmacists: an international update. *Can Pharm J.* 2019;152:92–108. https://doi.org/10.1177/1715163518811065.

54. McMillan SS, Kelly F, Sav A, King MA, Whitty JA, Wheeler AJ. Consumer and carer views of Australian community pharmacy practice: awareness, experiences and expectations. *J Pharm Health Serv Res.* 2014;5:29–36. https://doi.org/10.1111/jphs.12043.

55. Eisner E. Art and knowledge. In: Knowles JG, Cole AL, eds. *Handbook of the Arts in Qualitative Research: Perspectives, Methodologies, Examples, and Issues.* Thousand Oaks, CA: SAGE Publications Inc; 2008:3–13.

56. Morgan DL. *Focus Groups as Qualitative Research.* 2nd ed. Thousand Oaks, CA: SAGE Publications Inc; 1997.

57. Rahtz E, Warber SL, Dieppe P. Understanding public perceptions of healing: an arts-based qualitative study. *Complement Ther Med.* 2019;45:25–32. https://doi.org/10.1016/j.ctim.2019.05.013.

58. Pelowski M, Markey PS, Forster M, Gerger G, Leder H. Move me, astonish me… delight my eyes and brain: the Vienna integrated model of top-down and bottom-up processes in art perception (VIMAP) and corresponding affective, evaluative, and neurophysiological correlates. *Phys Life Rev.* 2017;21:80–125. https://doi.org/10.1016/j.plrev.2017.02.003.

59. Lapum J, Church K, Yau T, David AM, Ruttonsha P. Arts-informed research dissemination: Patients' perioperative experiences of open-heart surgery. *Heart Lung.* 2012;41:e4–e14. https://doi.org/10.1016/j.hrtlng.2012.04.012.

60. Schindel TJ, Chahade J. What is your story? Student-initiated program to support pharmacy students' professional identity formation. *Pharm Educ.* 2021;21(4):9. https://doi.org/10.46542/pe.2021.214.186.

Chapter 16

The use of art to analyze learning practices in pharmacy and to inform assessment and intervention practices

Ruth M. Edwards[a] and John I'Anson[b]

[a]School of Pharmacy, University of Wolverhampton, Wolverhampton, United Kingdom, [b]Faculty of Social Sciences, University of Stirling, Stirling, United Kingdom

Objectives

- Explore the use of fine art as a lens to make sense of thematic data.
- Review pharmacy students' assessment and feedback practices, and how they influence their learning practices.
- Identify the impact of the affective dimension on pharmacy students' learning.

Introduction

It has been argued in the literature that pharmacy is an integration of art and science[1] with, for example, authors describing the "art and science" of counseling patients.[2] Similar wide-ranging discussion exists in the literature around other health professions, including medicine and nursing, with debate extending back for decades.[3–10] Authors argue that successful practice as a health professional requires an entwining of both the "so-called 'soft,' co-creative, relationship-building art, and 'hard,' linear, controlling science"[3] which have been separated in health care recently. Panda[4] posits that the doctor needs to be "an artist armed with basic scientific knowledge in medicine," which requires a combination of emotion and intuition alongside employing rational analysis. Convention tries to distinguish between the "artist" and the "scientist," and it is argued that there is a "confused notion that one uses emotion and intuition, drawing support from inward genius, achieving great effects without knowing how or why, but that the other, employing rational analysis, is cold and precise, analytical and detached, surrounded by highly complex instruments that baffle the lay mind."[8]

Thomas,[3] in his discussion of combining art and science in healthcare argues that both are required and makes the case for researchers to use multiple methods of inquiry more often to counter the limitations of "naïve positivism," including using traditions such as constructivism.[11] This chapter describes the methodological process of using carefully chosen fine art (paintings) as a lens[12] or an alternative way, through which to view thematic data about a "scientific" concept, a method which currently appears to be unique in the literature.

The research was conducted using a constructivist socio-material approach[13] with artifacts used to explore pharmacy students' learning and assessment practices.[14] The idea for using art in the analysis came partly from a desire to use a creative method of analysis, and also from a serendipitous visit to the Tate Modern gallery in London. While conducting the interviews there was a realization that, in keeping with using a visual and creative method of data collection, the researcher had a desire to analyze the data in a similarly creative way. There was an attempt to juxtapose the ordered, structured and "scientific" concept of assessment with fine art by comparing the experiences recounted by participants with specific paintings by the early 20th century artist, Pierre Bonnard.

During a visit to the Tate Modern Gallery in London, the author was inspired by a painting by Bonnard called The Bowl of Milk.[15] The curator's commentary on Bonnard's technique of painting was striking; he did not paint in front of his subject or "before the motif"[16] but instead allowed his reflections on, and his memory of, a scene to influence how he portrayed it. He painted entirely from memory; he wanted his works to reflect his subjective response to the subject[17] and attempted to translate the "first possession of a moment"[18] in his work. His art is "based on deeply felt experiences, filtered through memory and expressed by relationships between colour, light and composition."[16]

Contemporary Research Methods in Pharmacy and Health Services. https://doi.org/10.1016/B978-0-323-91888-6.00040-5

This idea of Bonnard's representations being filtered through his memory triggered a connection to the data in this study. The conception that what participants represented and articulated was filtered through their memory was one that had been reflected on by the researcher, hence the decision to use some of Bonnard's paintings and their associated commentaries make sense of the data relating to participants assessment practices and their implications. In addition, student assessment usually evokes a strong emotional response,[19] and similarly art can stimulate the affective or emotional dimension of our being. Art evokes emotion via use of color, form, and composition, drawing people in both cognitively and emotionally.[20] There is a language of neutrality associated with how we write about and speak about assessment in academia and by attending to a different perspective that art brings, we may be able to understand better how assessment practices impact on pharmacy students' learning. Taking this approach appeared to be untried and innovative in educational research so following a robust discussion within the research team, the decision was made to "give it a try."

Qualification as a pharmacist within the United Kingdom involves obtaining a General Pharmaceutical Council (GPhC) accredited Master of Pharmacy (MPharm) degree followed by 1 year of preregistration training, during which a trainee demonstrates competence under the supervision of a preregistration tutor. Passing the GPhC registration assessment and meeting fitness to practice requirements complete these necessary stages.[21] The MPharm is a 4 year, undergraduate masters' degree which integrates the science and practice of pharmacy,[22] a key component of the curriculum under study. The majority of entrants to the program come from high school; however, some enter having completed a previous degree or other qualification. In the MPharm curriculum at the time of this study, professional development was a key focus in teaching and learning with an emphasis on "soft skills" for example, empathy, communication, reflexivity and adaptability.[23,24] Although the program assessment strategy had incorporated OSCEs and other skills-based assessments,[25,26] at the time of the study, traditional end-of-semester examinations were used in throughout the course, balanced with other types of assessment which in many cases contributed as much to the final module grade as the examination.

The findings presented in this chapter related to pharmacy students' assessment practices. The data were collected in qualitative interviews in which the focus was investigating how pharmacy students negotiate[27] the pedagogical demands of a pharmacy curriculum.[14] The specific research questions addressed in this chapter are

- What are pharmacy students' assessment practices, and how do these influence their learning practices?
- How does feedback influence pharmacy students' learning practices?
- How does the affective dimension impact on pharmacy students' learning?
- Can fine art be used as a lens to make sense of thematic data?

The findings and the methods used may stimulate researchers in pharmacy education and health services research to consider different approaches to viewing data.

Methods

Data collection was qualitative in nature and took the form of individual semistructured interviews with undergraduate pharmacy students in a UK Pharmacy School. The methodological position taken in the study was interpretivist,[28] which is underpinned by constructivist ontology,[29] and is principally concerned with meaning, understanding and insight.

Participants were asked to select three artifacts (a photograph, an object, a song, a picture or something else) that represented what learning as a pharmacy student meant to them and bring that along to an interview.[30] The interviews were conducted using both the artifacts and a semistructured interview plan constructed as a mind map. In conducting the interview, flexibility was applied to changing the sequence of themes and additional probing questions were used in response to the stories told by the participants. Data were analyzed thematically using mind-mapping[31] and subsequently, theoretical constructs were applied to make sense of the analysis.

Analysis of data for this study involved exploring the themes relating to assessment. Initially, thematic analysis of the data was carried out using an inductive approach and mind-mapping. Mind-mapping is a thinking tool underpinned by the concept of "radiant thinking"[32] where associative thought processes radiate from a central idea, allowing concepts to be integrated and connections to be made.[14] For the data on assessment practices, an electronic mind map was created (Appendix), then a selection of Pierre Bonnard's art was used as a "lens"[12] through which to view the themes. Tepper[20] argues that art can enhance learning in a number of ways including making connections in all directions, enhancing higher-order thinking skills and creating epistemic curiosity and these were the aims of using art as the theoretical construct in this way.

In choosing to use art, a number of questions were explored including what art might add to the analysis, whether it was possible to use this as a method and would it work? In being reflexive about the data analysis, the researcher also had perspectives of being a pharmacist and artist (as well as educator and researcher) with a strong desire to integrate these multiple "selves" in the project. Peshkin[33] challenges researchers to be aware of their own subjectivity and to have an increased awareness of my own professional stance. He discusses the different is that affect subjectivity in research and argues that subjectivity is inevitable and that researchers should systematically seek out their own subjectivity while the research is actively in progress and be aware of how subjectivity may be shaping inquiry and outcomes. This was an important part of the process of using art but in the end, the decision was made to just try it and see what happened.

In choosing Bonnard's art, there was a combination of the researcher's passion for impressionist and postimpressionist art alongside the chance encounter with Pierre Bonnard's work and his way of working, described in the introduction. For this reason, using other artists' work was not explored. If the researchers had used different artists or genres of work as the inspiration, there may have been different outcomes to the project. The method used below could potentially be adapted to any project using the arts, for example fine art, music, theater, or poetry.

The first stage of analysis was generation of inductive themes relating to assessment practices, derived thematically from the student interviews using mind-mapping. These were conceptions of assessment, the impact of the nature of assessment on learning practices, feedback, strategies used in assessment practices, the affective dimension of assessment and assessment constrains free-thinking.

Following the inductive analysis, the first step in using art was identifying something that "spoke to" the project and the researcher, in this case the inspiration was the Bonnard painting and the curator's description. Then an overview of Bonnard's prolific work and his techniques were explored using a textbook catalog of a 1998 Tate Gallery exhibition[34] while considering the inductive themes. Other exhibitions will have similar publications or online catalogs which could be used by researchers trying this technique. Following this a review of the history genre of Bonnard's art (postimpressionist) was completed, using textbooks and articles.[16–18] One of Bonnard's most famous paintings is called Coffee,[35] which was also an artifact which featured heavily in student interviews, and this consolidated the decision to use Bonnard's work in this way.

Once the decision was made to select Bonnard's work to compare with the data, a painting was chosen for each inductive theme. This was a major part of the process and was done using Whitfield and Elderfield's catalog as well as curator descriptions, along with the researchers' own reaction to the paintings. Some choices were straightforward, for example, the use of Coffee[35] and Nude in a Mirror[36]; however, other choices required more reflection and analysis. The choice of painting is explained in more detail in the results and discussion.

In using art to make sense of the data, six of Bonnard's works were compared to the specific themes relating to participants' assessment practices. In doing so, Bonnard's composition, subject, use of color, technique and, where documented, the ideas behind the painting were considered. Alongside this, commentators' analysis of the piece along with the researcher's and others' impressions of the paintings and the ideas that each stimulated. In most cases, the author was unable to view the original work and used the internet and art textbooks but wherever possible took the opportunity to view the original painting.

Ethical approval was received for the study from the ethical review panel of two higher education institutions. The ethical issues involved in the study are discussed in detail elsewhere[14] but included informed consent, consideration of power in the researcher-participant relationship and the location of the interview. Pseudonyms are used for the participants throughout.

Results and discussion

Eighteen students were interviewed over a 6-week period with interviews lasting between 45 and 80 min. Each participant was given a pseudonym to protect their confidentiality. Table 1 gives the breakdown of participants' pseudonym, sex, stage, age, previous educational experience and the artifacts chosen.

In the interviews, some themes emerged from the objects that participants brought, in other cases these relate to particular questions asked around assessment during the interview. This paper focuses on the themes relating to assessment practices: conceptions of assessment, the impact of the nature of assessment on learning practices, feedback, strategies used in assessment practices, the affective dimension of assessment and assessment constrains free-thinking and each of these has been explored using a different Bonnard painting.

Coffee—Conceptions of assessment

The first painting chosen was Coffee,[5] and this has been used to explore the theme "conceptions of assessment." This painting was chosen firstly because many participants brought coffee as one of their artifacts but also because of the composition that Bonnard has used in this work. Using composition, Bonnard succeeds in making the viewer feel part of a normal or routine event but yet, at the same time, separate to it. This echoes with the researcher's experience in listening

TABLE 1 Participant characteristics.

Year of course	Pseudonym	Sex	Age	Educational background prior to MPharm	Artifacts
1	Gordon	Male	51	Science degree	Calculator, Royal Society of Chemistry (RSC) membership card
2	Jessica	Female	19	School leaver	iPod, "achievements" folder, stress man
3	Peter	Male	19	School leaver	Song, desk and nuts, study notes
3	Dave	Male	29	Engineering degree	Mind map, book on the "cosmos," photo (him and partner)
4	Debra	Female	26	Science degree	Mind map, British National Formulary (BNF), photo (family)
4	Gavin	Male	21	School leaver	Wallet, rugby ball/ champagne, Facebook page
4	Kat	Female	22	School leaver	BNF, spider's web, bath
4	Emily	Female	21	School leaver	Sticky notes, photo (family), coffee cup
4	Helen	Female	28	Arts and humanities degree	USB stick, diary, results transcript
4	Donna	Female	26	Science degree	Mind map, BNF, colored notes
4	Ewen	Male	21	School leaver	Colored pens, iPod, coffee
4	Lisa	Female	21	School leaver	Coffee cup, diary, iPod
4	Karen	Female	22	School leaver	Photo (friends), study notes, library silent study area
4	Diane	Female	27	Science degree	Assessment criteria, photo (family), highlighter pen
4	Victoria	Female	24	Science degree	Green pen, mobile phone, mints
4	Jill	Female	25	Science degree	Paper/highlighter pens, photo (family), ear plugs
4	Georgia	Female	23	School leaver (overseas) and Further Education College (United Kingdom)	Music, highlighter pens, body language picture
4	James	Male	24	Science degree	BNF, external hard drive, study notes

to participants' narrative around assessment. Assessments in pharmacy education are a normal and routine event and by participants sharing their reflections, the researcher felt part of the experience, but at the same time separate.

This idea of being part of but yet separate also echoes with the finding that participants appear to conceive assessments as end of semester examinations; a routine event but separate to their learning rather than part of it. Peter used different study strategies before end of semester exams compared to coursework assessments and only used his desk when studying for exams.

[For an essay] I'll take my laptop through to the kitchen and I'll sit with my mum or dad or whoever's through. I'll sit and read through there but if it's for an exam, I am in my bedroom by myself, sort of at that desk.

Emily described end of semester exams as her main goal while learning and pictured herself sitting the exam.

Crossman,[37] in a qualitative analysis of the role of relationships and emotions in student perceptions of learning and assessment, describes how past experiences of assessment influences current perceptions and this aligns with participants' experiences in this study. Their emphasis on written exams in their past experience (perhaps through the assessment driven culture in secondary school education[38]) may be leading them to overemphasize the importance of exams. This conception of assessment as the end of semester exam also appears to have an impact on participants views on feedback which will be discuss later.

The MPharm curriculum is designed as a progression, with assessments intended to move students along the journey to becoming a pharmacist; however, participants did not perceive assessments in that way. They appeared to conceive them as events in and of themselves, as intense moments in their journey, creating a break (or punctuation) in their learning. Participants gave the impression of assessments as "hurdles to clear" rather than as an integral part of their learning process. Despite a global pedagogic move toward assessment for learning[39] and visible learning,[40] participants in this study still viewed assessments as separate to the learning process, raising questions for pharmacy curriculum design and pharmacy student assessment literacy. Returning to Coffee, observing the painting, we can see that Bonnard draws attention to a moment captured over a cup of coffee portraying this ordinary event as an intense moment because of his dramatic use of color and unusual composition. This intensity echoes how participants viewed assessments in this study.

In Coffee, Bonnard challenges convention in the way he composes the painting by not adhering to traditional rules of perspective and by framing the picture in an unusual way. Part of one of the subjects is "cut off" and the table and the items on the table form the main foreground rather than the people meaning that Bonnard draws attention to the normally unnoticed aspects of the moment. In the same way, the findings of this study have highlighted what is normally in the background (their conceptions of assessment) and has been brought to the foreground. In the spirit of Bonnard's challenge to the convention of composition, in designing assessment for a pharmacy curriculum, a similar challenge to convention is worth considering. A growing emphasis on innovative assessment methods appear to challenge students to learn for understanding and to develop as professionals.[41] It appears, however, that we need to engage students' fundamental conception of the end-of-semester written examination being the important assessment.

Dining room in the country—The impact of the nature of assessment on learning practices

The Dining Room in the Country[42] is the second painting chosen, as it represented the researcher's role in looking through the window on participants' learning and assessment practices. This painting was used to explore the theme of "the impact of the nature of assessment on learning practices."

For a period of Bonnard's work, he was preoccupied with the window as a metaphor: "a window, like a painting, is both an opening and a barrier, a three dimensional view and two dimensional object."[7] In this picture, the door and the window are open and the subject is looking in from the outside; "the open door and windows invite the spectator into the composition and at the same time flatten form in an interwoven network of abstract colour patterns across the surface."[16] The researcher felt that participants had invited her in to their reflections on assessment but at the same time she remained looking in from the outside. This is not to say that these assessment practices formed an independent reality (an "outthereness" to use Law's[43] terminology) but that, similar to the discussions around Coffee, the researcher's role as tutor and researcher kept her part of, but yet separate from these practices. She felt slightly distant from the practices she was trying to make sense of and was aware of a gap; however, the researcher's own practices around using artifacts and engaging with students in data generation happened within that gap, analogous with the effect that Bonnard achieves of evoking a "strong feeling that we are 'in' the space of the represented image."[18] This allowed the researcher to construct a sense of the practices being explored and enabled her to construe participants' practices in a novel way.

In "looking through the window" on participants' assessment practices it emerged that the nature of assessments affected their learning practices. Debra discussed multiple choice questions (MCQs) and how she felt that these did not motivate her to understand a subject;

> I find when you are studying for an MCQ, it's just like trying to memorise as much as you possibly can ... I mightn't always understand what I'm learning and I'm just learning to reach that goal of passing that MCQ. So you're just ... surface learning, you're not learning to understand.

Others discussed using this type of rote learning prior to exams, perceiving this as "not a very good kind of learning" (Kat) and as a poor strategy especially when this included "spotting" (predicting what will be in the exam and revising those subjects only). Gavin described an example of this practice:

so on countless occasions we've sat and gone ... right there's eight parts to this course, there's five questions, that lecture had those two questions last year, you work it out and you can get down to four or five topics out of say eight or nine and you can discard ... a few topics.

Gavin acknowledged the practice occurred but expressed concern about how it would impact on his future practice as a pharmacist;

... I remember last year ... it was majorly hinted at that oncology wouldn't be an essay question, and I know a lot of people just didn't learn oncology because it was such a huge chunk ... if you knew it wasn't an essay question you could sacrifice those five marks and give yourself so much time to learn other stuff, which everyone knows, in the back of their head, is bad because you can't be a pharmacist who doesn't know a thing about cancer ... but you need to pass the exam.

Hargreaves[44] argues that "conventional assessment practices do not encourage lifelong learning, critical thinking, or a deep understanding of the subject matter." Barnett[45] similarly asserts that if students "sense that the forms of assessment are calling for factual knowledge or for descriptive accounts of situations, the students will mirror these perceptions in their knowing accomplishments." Entwistle and Entwistle[46] describe a distinction between learning as "reproduction of information presented" or as "transformation of that information in the process of coming to understand it for oneself" and the assessment practices described by Gavin, Kat and Debra appear to fit with their categorization as the reproduction of information. Participants appeared to be adopting this approach without feeling comfortable with it and reflected on the potential negative impact on their professional knowledge in the future.

Participants also described assessment practices which align more with transformative learning.[47] Jill described how the final year assessments were about integration:

Assessments this year is just for me, is actually bringing everything together. I think that's happening in fourth year that everything that you've learned ... not everything, but quite like the majority of things you've learned in first to third year has been pulled together and you're realising why these things are actually important whereas at the time, you would be like, what's the point in this? what's the point in learning that? it's always hard to see the relevance to pharmacy ... I'm going to do the bare minimum to pass the exam ... you could rote learn it whereas ... the assessments this year are bringing nearly everything together, and it's kind of putting a common thread through everything.

Jill described how the learning in early years started as rote learning but how in final year, in integrating this knowledge, the learning became transformational and part of her development as a professional. Georgia also described how she looked back and saw the relevance of assessments later and how these had contributed to her development:

first and second year ... lab reports. At that time I didn't know the purpose, I just thought "oh it's just, you know they want to give us lot of work," you know ... but looking back, I realise that it was actually the beginning. They wanted to ... build us, you know, through first year, second year, to teach us and how to write and how to, you know, erm ... how to erm ... kind of reflect back what we've done in the lab ... every time when I looked back and realised "oh yeah, yeah, that was the point."

The "strategic approach" suggested by Entwistle and others,[47–49] where students aim to achieve good grades by using organized study methods and are alert to assessment requirements, appears to link with the practices of Gavin and others. Boud[50] refers to a number of connections between assessment and learning which link directly with the practices described by Gavin and others. Not only does Boud argue that the nature of the assessment task influences the learning but also that students tend to focus on the topics being assessed at the expense of those which are not. Gibbs[51] cites course characteristics which he argues are associated with a "surface approach" to study such as a heavy workload, high class contact hours, an excessive amount of course material, a lack of opportunity to pursue subjects in depth and a lack of choice over subjects or method of study and a threatening or anxiety provoking assessment system. At the time that this study was conducted, the curriculum possessed many of these characteristics, and therefore, it is perhaps unsurprising that participants in this study describe the assessment practices above.

The perception of relevance to the future was raised by a number of participants and appeared to have an influence on both their learning practices and on their assessment practices. Debra described how assessments that "examine the subject as a whole" and that she would use in the future meant that she was "not memorising as such for those because I need to have an ultimate understanding to sit those exams so I find those much more beneficial." Karen likewise expressed that she took a different approach to assessments in clinical based modules which she perceived as being important for the future.

Continuous assessment was discussed by a number of participants in this study. This can be defined as the evaluation of students' progress throughout the course of study, as well as, or instead of, end of term examinations.[52] Hernandez[53] has studied the extent to which continuous assessment practices facilitate student learning and asserts that there is a tension between assessment as grading students' progress and supporting students in learning, i.e., the summative and formative purposes of assessment. Georgia described how deadlines and continuous assessment allowed her to be disciplined;

I need to have you know, deadlines you know, I need to have, you know a time that things, when things are going to be tested you know, so if erm, so for me it's very important in my learning, it makes me do it, it kind of disciplines me, it makes me to actually study and go back and try to revise.

Lisa described the "healthy stress" associated with continuous assessment.

Continuous assessment is, I think, a really good way of learning, but also with, it just takes the pressure off the ... final exam a bit more as well, because that's when people crack and that's when people are like "oh I can't, I don't care if I've got a re-sit," you know. Because there's too much going on, but if they learned to adapt it all during the year, they might be stressed all through the year, but it might be like a healthy type of stress—a motivational type of stress.

She appeared to find the continuous deadlines she had experienced in final year as motivational. Students in Hernandez's study also associated continuous assessment with their increased motivation to learn on an ongoing basis.[53]

James had positive and negative views of continuous assessment and its impact on his learning.

Erm ... I guess it does, in good, I suppose good ways and bad ways, erm ... the good ways; obviously ... assessment ... it strengthens your knowledge in a particular subject and I guess the wider the question or the broader the question, like the more, probably, knowledge that you gain about it, and I think, like as you do more and more assessments, like, if you do an assessment and then you do an assessment after that; the assessment that you do after, I guess, like you had more experience in how to do things ... assessment is sometimes a pressure that, if you have multiple assessment at the same time it's a kind of, it puts you under that undue pressure.

Boud[50] argues that it is a commonly held view that assessment measures learning but does not influence it and in "looking through the window" on these participants' assessment practices it would appear that this view is not supported here.

Nude in a Mirror—Feedback

The third painting chosen was Nude in a Mirror.[35] Bonnard used mirrors in many of his paintings, and this picture has been linked to the theme of feedback because of the link between a mirror, reflection, and therefore feedback.

Participants expressed a number of views on feedback on assessment and on how and whether it impacts on their learning. The quantity of feedback received was commonly commented on as were the participants' feelings when receiving feedback. Crisp[54] argues that recent research has emphasized that, rather than the feedback itself, it is how students make sense of this and whether they actively engage with the feedback, which is important. Some participants in this study saw feedback as having a "benchmarking" purpose and others spoke about how they used it to improve future work.

Many of the participants started by saying they never get feedback:

I couldn't understand where I had gone wrong in the actual written paper and you never find out 'cos no one ever gives you feedback.

(Debra)

When probed further it became clear they were talking about summative written examinations:

say the final exams before the summer you don't really get any feedback on them because you just get your certificate through, you've passed, and then you start next year, so you get your percentage, but that's it, you obviously don't know where you fell down.

(Gavin)

Gavin also explained he had received feedback when he had failed an exam:

obviously the feedback on the subjects that I failed first time round was massively important because you know where you fell down.

Most who started by saying they did not get feedback then went on to comment on receiving feedback on other types of assignments:

when you pass the OSCEs and stuff that you do during the term you get feedback on them.

(Gavin)

Price et al.[55] argue that students are dissatisfied and staff frustrated about the way the feedback process is working and this appears to be echoed by participants in this study where dissatisfaction about the quantity and nature of feedback was expressed. Linking back to participants' conceptions of assessment as being the summative written examination, it is perhaps unsurprising that participants in this study perceive that they "never" receive feedback. Hanna et al.[56] explored the reasons for low student satisfaction with feedback. Their findings show general dissatisfaction with feedback especially with examination feedback and they subsequently implemented a "mandatory requirement" for more detailed examination feedback across all modules. They reflect on the difficulties in establishing the correct level of detail in examination feedback but found that student satisfaction improved.

Participants in this study expressed feelings in response to feedback; on receiving a low mark, Kat felt she wanted to do better. Helen and Debra felt, although disappointing, it was motivation to improve;

it's kinda really disheartening when you get a low mark and you think you've done really well … erm … so definitely it makes you work harder the next time … because you ultimately wanna achieve that higher grade.

(Debra)

On receiving a high mark, Lisa felt proud. The emotional aspects of assessment and feedback are discussed in more depth below.

In terms of how participants used feedback, some indicated they used it as a way of benchmarking themselves. Gordon felt it was "nice to know where you are at" and Kat tended to compare herself with her peers; "You measure yourself against your friends, of course you do" (Kat). Debra, Helen and Karen explained that they would use formative feedback in their next assignment;

if it's a formative … a formative exam you get feedback, you know. Then for the summative I'll look at it quite a lot and I'll see what I need to do, need to improve on.

(Karen)

Lisa felt that she concentrated on "could do better" comments:

I don't sit down and analyse it completely just because I know myself just how much work I put in or like how well I thought I knew it … I concentrate on, like if they've said "could have done something better" or if there's something that's been ticked and you're only at like a six compared to like the seven to ten box … then look like "what could I have done … to make that better this time?"

(Lisa)

Karen explained that she only really looked at feedback if she did not do well in an assignment and Jill felt that by time she had reached fourth year she was set in ways and feedback was less useful to her;

I think in fourth year you've already got your own style of answering exam questions, so if it's like feedback on whether you're writing an essay or something, I think it would be hard for me to kind of change the way.

(Jill)

In Hernandez's study,[53] 21% of students took no action as a result of feedback, 63% intended to use the feedback to inform future work, and 16% provided evidence that they had acted on recommendations. Brockbank and McGill[57] argue that the impact of feedback may be limited if it is vague and nonspecific; however, participants in this study made no comment on the nature of their feedback. Hernandez also argues that the practices of feedback that include a grade have less impact on students' learning. In this study, other than Lisa's previous comment, participants did not refer to the impact of feedback with or without grades, possibly as most formal feedback at the time of the study was associated with a grade.

In Nude in the Mirror, Bonnard has created an interesting illusion with the reflection in the mirror seen by the viewer being different to the one seen by the subject. In considering practices and sense-making, Haraway[58] discusses the metaphor of optical diffraction and how this differs to reflection:

Diffraction does not produce "the same" displaced, as reflection and refraction do. Diffraction is a mapping of interference, not of replication, reflection, or reproduction. A diffraction pattern does not map where differences appear, but rather maps where the effects of difference appear.[58]

If we use Haraway's definition of diffraction to consider feedback in pharmacy education, we could reconceptualize feedback as diffraction rather than reflection and reconsider the way that we construct feedback. Crisp[54] reflects negatively on "unilateral pronouncements by assessors rather than dialogue with students" and perhaps by creating Haraway's "mapping of interference"[58] in the way that we construct feedback to students allowing disruption of ideas to take place, academics could open up a conversation to support students in knowledge creation rather than making a judgment on successful achievement of propositional knowledge. With large numbers of students on pharmacy programs however, this may be challenging to operationalize.

The French Window—Strategies used in assessment practices

The fourth painting chosen was The French Window[59] to represent the strategies and techniques used by participants in their assessment practices, many of which relate to the study practices discussed elsewhere.[14] Practices recounted by participants were using assessment criteria, visualizing notes, "loading and dumping," repetition, peer support, study/life balance, past papers,

In The French Window, Bonnard uses a number of artistic techniques to create the effect he is aiming for[18]; the mirror in the background has the artist himself reflected in it, the use of pencil marks etched into the paint around the hands gives vitality and he uses charcoal marks to define the head's tilt. For participants in this study, their learning was enacted in a number of techniques and strategies described within their assessment practices.

Diane used published assessment criteria to direct her learning. In his review of the impact of assessment on student learning, Rust[60] raises the issue of ensuring active engagement with assessment criteria, challenging the assumption that giving explicit criteria automatically results in better performance. In Diane's case, there appears to be active engagement with published criteria as a strategy in her quest for success. Other participants did not articulate this, and other unpublished research conducted with pharmacy students at the same institution indicates that active engagement with published criteria is not a widespread practice.

Others (Georgia and Donna) described the strategy of visualizing their notes during exams:

yeah, [in an exam] I always picture things so much, and … if for example if there was a diagram even in what I've been studying it really helps me, you know, to remember the actual, you know erm, the context.

(Georgia)

Dave, as a mature student, felt that he had well established assessment practices which involved a number of strategies such as the "ritual" of locking himself away before exams and in some cases a "load and dump" strategy for subjects he perceived as less relevant;

I do a lot of loading and dumping, which is really shocking though, which is why I try and avoid that with the subjects that … I find are … going to be more functional to me as a pharmacist after University … I understand why I'm doing it and I see the function in terms of getting me through the course and getting a really good broader understanding of everything that's going on, but I don't see it as being really useful towards me, like postuniversity, so for that reason I do load and dump quite a lot of that information which is probably not that ideal but ….

Donna found that repetitive practice alleviated her nerves before exams and Jessica likewise found that being prepared helped with stress: "I'm one of the few that has to be overly prepared, I don't like going into something blind." Jessica described a situation where she went away on holiday just before an exam: "having that distraction was a little bit frustrating going into the exam, because I did fail it," and she perceived that this loss of focus and deviation from her usual practice caused her to fail.

Peer support in preparing for assessment was important for a number of participants; Karen discussed working with her friend in preparing for assessment. Dave likewise discussed his support strategies during assessments; "my phone bill normally goes up during exam time as well, 'cos I'm always ringing some of the guys." Victoria also used feedback from her peers as she prepared for assessment;

even last time we were practising for the OSCE. There were things that you wouldn't consider even mentioning it in the patient interview … I would never have thought of and there were things I would have thought of that they wouldn't have thought of, and that's where we just kind of pick up from each other.

Karen described how having a balance between study and other aspects of her life was a strategy which helped her not "get stressed out" about assessments;

I have a lot of extracurricular stuff going on and I said "I'm going to apply myself as much as I can, still have a good time". I don't know, you have to just enjoy it as well and erm … I think the people who just really, really stress about it, they just work themselves up and they just don't … I don't know … maybe they … get enjoyment out of their stress and stuff, but I personally wouldn't.

Langley et al.[61] noted that female pharmacy students are more socially oriented and think ahead to the work life balance they want to make.

Gavin described how he used past papers to help build his confidence for examinations and be clear about the expectations;

everyone kept saying 'why wasn't there a model answer up on Moodle [virtual learning environment]?' … that would have been a massive help, because then you would … you wouldn't … it felt like you were going into that exam quite blind in terms of … how much depth do they want us to go in to … I felt … some exams you go into and you've seen past papers, maybe two or three past papers and example answers, you've been to tutorials and you've got a good idea of how to answer the questions and you go to the exam, as in a lot of exams, especially me where you feel like you go into it quite blind.

Hanna et al.[56] found that their participants also wanted model answers but reflected that a comprehensive model answer could stifle independent learning and hamper the ability to apply knowledge. Haggis[62] posits that requests such as Gavin's, for example essays, are an attempt by students to "concretise the abstractions" of fundamental concepts such as "argument" and "evidence" that they find highly opaque. The challenge of this finding for those designing and delivering pharmacy education is to find a way to address the opaqueness of these abstractions without encouraging students to resort to mimicry.

Like Bonnard in The French Window, participants appeared to be using a variety of different strategies in their assessment practices both in terms of how they approached assessments and of alleviating stress. In comparing participants' strategies associated with assessment to Bonnard's The French Window, which has an interesting and unconventional construction of background and foreground and with the subject side-lined, the strategies described by participants have been highlighted and have brought to the foreground the complex meshwork surrounding their learning and the practices associated with assessment.

Red roofs at Le Cannet—The affective dimension

The fifth painting chosen was Red roofs at Le Cannet[63] to represent the affective dimension expressed about learning and more commonly about assessment. In this study, participants' description of assessment and their reflections on it was given in quite dramatic language at times evoking the affective dimension.

Participants expressed a number of emotional responses to assessment and to feedback; primarily negative emotions hence the choice of a painting with a foreboding air. Bonnard, as a colorist, generally painted with bright colors which are usually associated with positive emotions. Few of his paintings are dark and convey a sense of gloom as the sky over the Red roofs at Les Cannet does.

Kat and Jessica described frustration, usually in response to failure;

I wasn't expecting to fail as I was really confident with what I was doing, so I was more frustrated at myself because I know I can do it.

(Jessica)

This experience of disappointment at failing an assessment was commented on by a number of participants. For Ewan it generated annoyance with himself for not preparing as well as he felt he should have;

I was annoyed at myself as well for failing it because I knew that I probably hadn't done as much work for that.

He also expressed concern that he felt he was letting others down by failing;

I feel as if I've let people down in some respects. Sort of, Mum and Dad, who've, sort of, done so much to try and get me through and get me to uni and all that, and sort of, to have to go to them and say "I've failed."

Lisa described feeling disheartened when she found out she had not done as well as she expected but explained that it could still motivate her to do better next time;

the worst one is if you've not done well and you feel like you should have done well. That's disheartening, but … when you've not done well and you get feedback that erm … you've not done well, but you, you think like all that went really bad—it's still horrible to get like that final … thing there, but … it does motivate you.

Kat described a situation where she recognized she had invested a lot of time and emotional effort into an assignment and as a result was really disappointed when she received negative feedback;

that was for an essay so I was quite into that and when I got my feedback back it was, that was quite a, I took it quite personally. I was quite disappointed when I got it back and I got a poor mark and I thought oh I really went for that ....

Georgia also described her defensiveness and nervousness in response to feedback;

I should maybe erm be more neutral and just open, you know, about, you know, learning, so yeah I think it's just our human nature ... yeah, we are like defensive, you know, and it's erm just like they can send me down so but I would be nervous first when I receive it but I still want to see it, you know, because I know that it's going to help me.

Fritz et al.[64] identified that the "emotional and psychological investment in producing a piece of work has a much stronger effect on the student than the relatively passive receipt of subsequent feedback" and Kat's experience of emotional and psychological investment appears to echo this. Rust[58] argues that because of this emotional investment, subsequent repetition of the task is more likely to be carried out by replication of the previous attempt, including mistakes, despite these being highlighted in the feedback.

Other potent emotions expressed included shock at failing (Donna), panic during written exams (Victoria) and fear of failure. In response to being asked how she got through learning a subject she struggled with, Kat laughed and responded "would fear be an acceptable answer?" She explained that fear of failure was a motivator for her;

I want to pass, want to pass my exams, erm ... I don't .... ohhh ... I don't like to fail things, err ... and I don't like to feel stupid and that is a big motivator.

Crossman[37] identified very similar emotional responses from students in relation to assessment; disappointment, a sense of failure, anxiety, hurt, frustration, stress, loathing and hatred were all noted. As with this study, the expression of emotion when describing assessment was "frequent, potent and deeply embedded in the data" and similar to the overall emphasis in this study, all the emotions noted by Crossman were negative. Basson and Rothman[65] have explored positive emotion regulation strategies of pharmacy students and determined that students who flourished were more likely to use adaptive positive emotion regulation strategies. The findings of this study indicate that this is worthy of further exploration by pharmacy schools.

Pride was discussed by a number of participants in this study. Tracy et al.[66] have explored pride and differentiate between hubristic and authentic pride with the latter being "quiet satisfaction we take from our work, our relationships, our fitness, or even the cleanliness of our homes" and the former as "ego-driven pride" that leads to bragging and comparing ourselves to others. In this study, pride was expressed as a positive emotion, the only one expressed in this study. Lisa described the feeling of pride in doing well;

it's just a natural feeling if you've done well like—yes I've done well and that's great because I feel like I've deserved it.

Lisa also described not wanting to "lose face" in front of other people;

I think that's more of a ... a pride thing, than a lot of ... I like to know things myself because I don't feel ... that I can contribute like in group discussion a bit, if I don't know exactly what I'm on about.

Tracy et al.[66] assert that students who experience a lack of pride due to a poor result buckle down and work harder the next time. It seems the lack of this emotion regulates people's behavior to work harder, not the presence of it.

Similar to the emotional response evoked by Bonnard's dramatic sky in Red roofs over Le Cannet, assessment evoked a strong negative emotional response in these participants. Crossman's findings[37] and the findings from this study would indicate that "assessment is clearly not a neutral context, although educational professionalism has cultivated the myth that it is." Crossman[37] concludes that "Higher Education would do well to consider further how teaching and learning occurs in a particular human context in which individuals interact, conduct relationships and experience feelings about these relationships and pharmacy schools should be aware of these relationships and emotions in assessing and providing feedback to students."

A white interior—Assessment constrains free thinking

The sixth painting chosen was A White Interior[67] and this links to the theme that "assessment constrains free thinking" and to the difference between learning for assessment and learning for understanding.

Participants expressed views about taking control of their learning. Kat explained that learning for her own sake is a free process which assessment can constrain;

exams in my head are so tied with fear and trying to do things, cramming, you know trying to do things in that last week, I can't really disassociate exam time from positive learning experiences … when you're just learning for your own sake, when you just want to find things out, it's a very free process … but when you're trying to learn for an exam, you're forcing your brain to go down one route … and sometimes it's quite, quite difficult and that's why the rote learning has to come in.

Kat felt that the negative emotions surrounding assessment inhibited her from the learning experiences that she perceived as positive.

In relation to this free-thinking process, in the White Interior, it appears that Bonnard has not allowed convention to constrain his thinking; his construction of the painting challenges the conventions of perspective, alongside an element of mystery emerges with the floor metamorphosing into a body. Bonnard contrasts the use of the white, which is rarely used by colorists and the bright and dark colors of outside in achieving this effect. The challenge around assessment in pharmacy curricula design is to harness this free thinking and the enjoyment of learning described by Kat without allowing assessment, which in higher education is still required for "certification" or "qualification" purposes, to constrain these.

Similarly, Diane contrasted learning for herself and learning for assessment explaining that;

"learning for you [is] a lot more than just to get through an exam … it's more work but it's more enjoyable, you feel you get more out of it." She relates this enjoyable learning to a final year module which takes a problem-based learning approach; "there isn't that much teaching … a lot of it is up to you, and so, you really have to be organised from the start to know where you want to go … you have to kind of keep the, I suppose, the aims of what your trying to learn in view the whole time, it puts a lot of responsibility on you, but that's good … because you're always … taking control of your own learning and you're knowing where you want to go with it."

Echoing the experience of participants in this study, Entwistle and Entwistle,[68] in their series of studies exploring student understanding, found that students described the experience of understanding satisfying and complete. Their students also believed understanding to be irreversible and this links to Kat's experience of an eureka moment;

wow I get that now, that's brilliant … when you look back … it's really hard to think of them because once they're there they're as smooth as anything else so you can't pick them out individually because they're just part of your understanding.

Elderfield[69] explains how in The White Interior, as with many others of Bonnard's paintings, his construction of the painting challenges the eye to move rapidly backwards and forwards across the picture. The views expressed by participants in this study create a call for pharmacy educators to be mindful of moving their view backwards and forwards across the curriculum to ensure that it is designed in a way that ensures that students will demonstrate "performances of understanding."[70] When participants in this study felt part of the learning, were enjoying it and were in control of it, they felt that they understood. Biggs and Tang[70] argue that when students "really" understand concepts they act differently in contexts involving this concept and are capable of using it in unfamiliar or novel contexts, i.e., performances of understanding; a desired outcome for professional development in curricula such as pharmacy.

Reflections and conclusions

Using Bonnard's art in analysis has provided an additional way of extending the analysis of participant's assessment practices. Aligning with Bonnard's technique of foregrounding the unexpected or diverting attention away from the obvious has allowed illumination of these practices and previously unnoticed aspects of pharmacy students' learning practices.

In relation to Bonnard's Coffee,[35] it became clear that participants' conception of assessment as the summative examination was strong and consequently influenced their views of feedback. In Dining Room in the Country,[42] the nature of the assessment impacting on participants' learning practices was explored; MCQs tended to foster rote learning which participants perceived as negative. Participants recounted understanding the relevance of some of the topics previously studied; it would have been good if this had happened earlier at the time of studying these topics and this will be a challenge for ongoing curriculum design. Following on from this, perceived relevance to the future and the topics being assessed appeared to heavily influence participants' learning.

Feedback was explored using Nude in a Mirror.[35] Perceptions of lack of feedback and the feelings expressed on receiving feedback have had an influence on participants' learning. The idea of diffraction[58] as an alternative way of conceptualizing feedback was triggered by Bonnard's composition of the painting.

The French Window[59] enabled exploration of strategies used by students; curriculum design appears to have a significant influence on participants' learning with "load and dump" strategies reported. An overcrowded curriculum with no time for reflection or consolidation could be part of this. These issues were acknowledged by the course management team, under the leadership of the researcher, and were taken into account in curriculum redesign with reduction in both the numbers of modules and the assessment load across the course to attempt to allow students time to reflect, develop and learn for understanding.

There appears to be a significant emotional element to pharmacy students' learning often not acknowledged by literature or in teaching, learning and assessment practices and this was explored further using Red roofs at Le Cannet.[63] In comparing A White Interior[67] with assessment constraining free thinking, there appeared to be consequences of what participants described as "learning for themselves" and the creative processes that assessment appeared to inhibit. The challenge for pharmacy educators is to design learning activities and assessments that harness this "learning for themselves."

In keeping with the ethos of interpretivistic research, this study has not attempted to generalize findings but instead presents data about the way human beings (pharmacy students in one pharmacy school) progressively construct meanings about the world (their assessments and learning) in their lives.[71] Using art has added another dimension to help make sense of these data. There were a number of new insights gained from using this approach as well limitations. It could be argued that art creates an unnecessary distraction, and that the data could have been explored without Bonnard's paintings but like Tepper[20] the researchers would argue that arts-based inquiry fostered "deep, reflective learning and engagement" in this project. Some of the findings and analysis, for example diffraction, would not have emerged without the use of art. Limitations of the approach were that although some comparisons were nuanced and subtle and offered new insights, others were a little contrived, for example the discussion of emotions using Red roofs at Le Cannet.[63] Using art in research in this way appears not to have been used before (and certainly not in pharmacy education), and therefore, the process of achieving this was iterative and explorative. This means there was no previous work or structured methodology to guide the researcher, and therefore, the researcher's multiple positions (pharmacist, educator, artist, researcher) have had an influence on the findings. Subjectivity[33] as a positive attribute is an important conceptual underpinning of qualitative research unlike scientific or positivistic research where subjectivity is viewed as bias or a negative trait and these multiple "selves" (particularly the researchers art background) have enriched the study's findings.

Herman[5] asserts that "when an artist makes a penetrating observation, it often foreshadows a more formal one by a scientist and when science completes a convincing demonstration it can have the same aesthetic appeal as a work of art. One common denominator between the two spheres is the attempt to gain a deeper understanding of humanity's condition" and this study demonstrates the use of art in gaining a deeper understanding of the impact of assessment on pharmacy students' learning.

Combining art and science has enabled new insights into the data and may be a helpful technique to use in other types of pharmacy research. Other types of research that may benefit from the approach adopted in this study are where new insights into healthcare services, educational tools, assessments or curricula are desired. The approach adopted could potentially be adapted to using any form of art, including theater, poetry or music.

In conclusion, use of art in the innovative and unique way described in this chapter has enriched the analysis of data in this study, enabling the unnoticed to become visible and alternative interventions to be proposed. The richness provided by viewing the data through a fine art lens has enhanced the insight from the findings and this chapter offers a methodological approach which other researchers could consider to enhance their own findings.

Questions for further discussion

1. Which aspects of your practice would benefit from viewing through an alternative lens?
2. How might you use art (or other humanities) to enhance your understanding of human experience?
3. How might you adopt creative approaches to either collection or analysis of data?

Application exercise/scenario

Visit an Art Gallery and choose a piece of art that "speaks to you." Try and sit or stand for a while and look at it both from a distance and close up. Have a look at the curators' description and do some further research either via textbooks or online. Consider the following questions:

1. What struck you about this piece of art and caught your attention?
2. What message was the artist trying to project?
3. What insight can you gain from this piece of art or how does this piece of art challenge your thinking?
4. Can you apply any of this insight to my practice or to your learning?

Appendix: Assessment practices

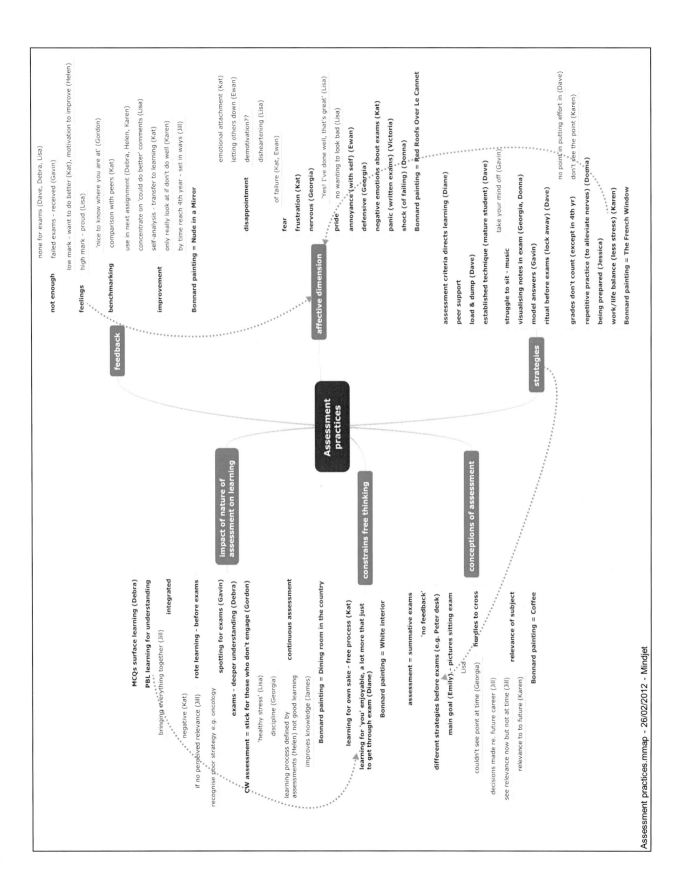

Assessment practices.mmap - 26/02/2012 - Mindjet

feedback

not enough
- none for exams (Dave, Debra, Lisa)
- failed exams - received (Gavin)
- low mark - want to do better (Kat), motivation to improve (Helen)

feelings
- high mark - proud (Lisa)
- 'nice to know where you are at' (Gordon)

benchmarking
- comparison with peers (Kat)
- use in next assignment (Debra, Helen, Karen)
- concentrate on 'could do better' comments (Lisa)

improvement
- self-analysis - transfer to learning (Kat)
- only really look at if don't do well (Karen)
- by time reach 4th year - set in ways (Jill)

Bonnard painting = Nude in a Mirror

affective dimension
- emotional attachment (Kat)
- letting others down (Ewan)
- demotivation??
- disheartening (Lisa)
- of failure (Kat, Ewan)

- disappointment
- frustration (Kat)
- fear
- nervous (Georgia)
- pride
- 'Yes! I've done well, that's great' (Lisa)
- annoyance (with self) (Ewan)
- no wanting to look bad (Lisa)
- defensive (Georgia)
- negative emotions about exams (Kat)
- panic (written exams) (Victoria)
- shock (of failing) (Donna)

Bonnard painting = Red Roofs Over Le Cannet

strategies
- assessment criteria directs learning (Diane)
- peer support
- load & dump (Dave)
- established technique (mature student) (Dave)
- take your mind off (Gavin)
- struggle to sit - music
- visualising notes in exam (Georgia, Donna)
- model answers (Gavin)
- ritual before exams (lock away) (Dave)
- grades don't count (except in 4th yr)
- no point in putting effort in (Dave)
- don't see the point (Karen)
- repetitive practice (to alleviate nerves) (Donna)
- being prepared (Jessica)
- work/life balance (less stress) (Karen)

Bonnard painting = The French Window

impact of nature of assessment on learning
- MCQs surface learning (Debra)
- PBL learning for understanding
- integrated
- bringing everything together (Jill)
- rote learning - before exams
- negative (Kat)
- spotting for exams (Gavin)
- exams - deeper understanding (Debra)
- if no perceived relevance (Jill)
- recognise poor strategy e.g. oncology
- CW assessment = stick for those who don't engage (Gordon)
- 'healthy stress' (Lisa)
- discipline (Georgia)
- continuous assessment
- learning process defined by assessments (Helen) not good learning
- improves knowledge (James)

Bonnard painting = Dining room in the country

constrains free thinking
- learning for own sake - free process (Kat)
- learning for 'you' enjoyable, a lot more that just to get through exam (Diane)

Bonnard painting = White interior

- assessment = summative exams
- 'no feedback'

conceptions of assessment
- different strategies before exams (e.g. Peter desk)
- main goal (Emily) - pictures sitting exam
- Lisa
- hurdles to cross
- couldn't see point at time (Georgia)
- relevance of subject
- decisions made re. future career (Jill)
- see relevance now but not at time (Jill)
- relevance to to future (Karen)

Bonnard painting = Coffee

Assessment practices

References

1. Clark TR, Gruber J, Sey M. Revisiting drug regimen review. Part II. Art or science? *Consult Pharm*. 2003;18:506–513.
2. Taylor J, Rocchi M. The art and science of counselling patients on minor ailments/OTC medicines. *Selfcare*. 2018;9.
3. Thomas P. Combining art and science in healthcare. *London J Prim Care (Abingdon)*. 2016;8:19–20.
4. Panda SC. Medicine: science or art? *Mens Sana Monogr*. 2006;4:127–138.
5. Herman J. Medicine: the science and the art. *Med Humanit*. 2001;27:42–46.
6. Saunders J. The practice of clinical medicine as an art and as a science. *Med Humanit*. 2000;26:18–22.
7. Francis G. Medicine: art or science? *Lancet*. 2020;395:24–25.
8. Anon. The 'art' and 'science' of medicine. *JAMA*. 1963;184:142–143.
9. Peplau HE. The art and science of nursing: similarities, differences, and relations. *Nurs Sci Q*. 1988;1:8–15.
10. Jasmine T. Art, science, or both? Keeping the care in nursing. *Nurs Clin North Am*. 2009;44:415–421.
11. Guba EG. *The Paradigm Dialog*. Newbury Park, CA: Sage; 1990.
12. Chu L. Research in development context: the lens through which researchers view the world. In: *Towards Data Science*; 2020. https://towardsdatascience.com/research-in-a-development-context-the-lens-through-which-researchers-view-the-world-838c9b03dcaf. Accessed 8 April 2021.
13. Fenwick T. Re-thinking the 'thing': sociomaterial approaches to understanding and researching learning in work. *J Work Learn*. 2010;22:104–116.
14. Edwards RM. *Opening the Door on Student Learning: Using Artefacts to Explore Pharmacy Students' Learning Practices* [[online] Doctor of Education Thesis]. University of Stirling; 2013. http://hdl.handle.net/1893/16412. Accessed 8 April 2021.
15. Bonnard P. *Bowl of Milk. Oil on Canvas*. London: Tate Gallery; 1919.
16. Watkins N. *Bonnard: Colour and Light*. London: Tate Gallery; 1998.
17. Minneapolis Institute of Art. *Dining Room in the Country by Pierre Bonnard*; 2009. https://collections.artsmia.org/art/1240/dining-room-in-the-country-pierre-bonnard. Accessed 28 November 2020.
18. Nickson G. *Bonnard: Drawing Color, Painting Light*; 2009. http://artcritical.com/2009/03/09/bonnard-drawing-color-painting-light/. Accessed 28 November 2020.
19. Fritz et al. 2000. Cited in Rust C. The impact of assessment on student learning: how can the research literature practically help to inform the development of departmental assessment strategies and learner-centred assessment practices? *Act Learn High Educ*. 2002;3:145–158.
20. Tepper SJ. Art as research: the unique value of the artistic lens. *GIA Read*. 2013;24(3). https://www.giarts.org/article/art-as-research-unique-value-artistic-lens. Accessed 8 April 2021.
21. General Pharmaceutical Council. *Future Pharmacists: Standards for the Initial Education and Training of Pharmacists*. London: GPhC; 2011.
22. Husband AK, Todd A, Fulton J. Integrating science and practice in pharmacy curricula. *Am J Pharm Educ*. 2014;78:63.
23. Langley CA, Aheer S. Do pharmacy graduates possess the necessary professional skills? *Pharm Educ*. 2010;10:114–118.
24. Van Winkle L, Fjortoft N, Hojat M. Impact of a workshop about aging on the empathy scores of pharmacy and medical students. *Am J Pharm Educ*. 2012;76:9.
25. Bell JH, Edwards RM, Hutchinson SL. Objective structured clinical examinations (OSCES) in pharmacy undergraduate education. *Pharm Educ*. 2002;2:154.
26. Edwards RM. The RGU OSCE Experience. In: *Workshop Presented at Academic Pharmacy Group Seminar on Student Assessment*. vol. 14. London: RPSGB; September 2005.
27. Bron J, Bovill C, Veugelers W. Curriculum negotiation: the relevance of Boomer's approach to the curriculum as a process, integrating student voice and developing democratic citizenship. *Curric Perspect*. 2016;36:15–27.
28. Usher R. A critique of the neglected epistemological assumptions of educational research. In: Scott D, Usher R, eds. *Understanding Educational Research*. 1st ed. London: Routledge; 1996:9–32.
29. Crotty M. *The Foundations of Social Research: Meaning and Perspective in the Research Process*. London: Sage Publications; 1998.
30. Edwards RM, I'Anson J. Using artefacts and qualitative methodology to explore pharmacy students' learning practices. *Am J Pharm Educ*. 2020;84:7082.
31. Tattersall C, Powell J, Stroud J, Pringle J. Mind mapping in qualitative research. *Nurs Times*. 2011;107:20–22.
32. Buzan T, Buzan B. *The Mind Map Book*. Millennium ed. London: BBC Books; 2000.
33. Peshkin A. In search of subjectivity—one's own. *Educ Res*. 1998;17:17–22.
34. Whitfield S, Elderfield J, eds. *Bonnard*. London: Tate Gallery; 1998.
35. Bonnard P. *Coffee. Oil on Canvas*. London: Tate Gallery; 1915.
36. Bonnard P. *Nude in a Mirror. Oil on Canvas*. Venice: Galleria Internazionaled'ArteModerna di Ca'Pesaro; 1931.
37. Crossman J. The role of relationships and emotions in student perceptions of learning and assessment. *High Educ Res Dev*. 2007;26:313.
38. Isaacs T. Educational assessment in England. *Assess Educ Princ Policy Pract*. 2010;17:315–334.
39. Black P, Wiliam D. *Assessment and Classroom Learning. Assessment in Education*. Abingdon, UK: Routledge; 1998.
40. Hattie J. *Visible Learning*. Abingdon, UK: Routledge; 2009.
41. Leung SF, Mok D, Wong D. The impact of assessment methods on the learning of nursing students. *Nurse Educ Today*. 2008;28:711–719.
42. Bonnard P. *Dining Room in the Country. Oil on Canvas*. Minneapolis: The Minneapolis Institute of Arts; 1913. The John R Van Derlip Fund, 54.15.
43. Law J. *After Method: Mess in Social Science Research*. Abingdon, Oxford: Routledge; 2004.
44. Hargreaves DJ. Student learning and assessment are inextricably linked. *Eur J Eng Educ*. 1997;22:401–409.

45. Barnett R. *A Will to Learn: Being a Student in an Age of Uncertainty.* Maidenhead: Open University Press; 2007.
46. Entwistle NJ, Entwistle A. Contrasting forms of understanding for degree examinations: the student experience and its implications. *High Educ.* 1991;22:205–227.
47. Entwistle NJ, Tait H. Approaches to learning, evaluations of teaching, and preferences for contrasting academic environments. *High Educ.* 1990;19:169–194.
48. Entwistle NJ, Peterson ER. Conceptions of learning and knowledge in higher education: relationships with study behaviour and influences of learning environments. *Int J Educ Res.* 2004;41:407–428.
49. Hounsell D, Hounsell J. Teaching-learning environments in contemporary mass higher education. In: *BJEP Monograph.* British Psychological Society; 2007:1–22. Student Learning and University Teaching, Series II;.
50. Boud D. Ensuring that assessment contributes to learning. In: *Procedings of the International Conference on Problem Based Learning in Higher Education.* Sweden: University of Linkoping; 1995:13–20.
51. Gibbs G. *Improving the Quality of Student Learning.* Bristol: TES; 1992.
52. Oxford English Dictionary (OED). *Continuous Assessment.* Oxford: OED.
53. Hernandez R. Does continuous assessment in higher education support student learning? *High Educ.* 2012;64:489–582.
54. Crisp BR. Is it worth the effort? How feedback influences students' subsequent submission of assessable work. *Assess Eval High Educ.* 2007;32:571.
55. Price M, Handley K, Millar J, O'Donovan B. Feedback: all that effort, but what is the effect? *Assess Eval High Educ.* 2010;35:277–289.
56. Hanna L, Hall M, Hennessey J. An exploration of feedback provision in a pharmacy degree programme from students' perspectives. *Pharm Educ.* 2012;12:10–13.
57. Brockbank A, McGill I. *Facilitating Reflective Learning in Higher Education.* Buckingham: Society for Research into Higher Education; 1998.
58. Haraway DJ. *The Haraway Reader.* New York: Routledge; 2004.
59. Bonnard P. *The French Window. Oil on canvas.* Private Collection; 1932.
60. Rust C. The impact of assessment on student learning: how can the research literature practically help to inform the development of departmental assessment strategies and learner-centred assessment practices? *Act Learn High Educ.* 2002;3:145–158.
61. Langley CA, Wilson KA, Jesson JK. Learning with other health professions in the United Kingdom MPharm degree: multidisciplinary and placement education. *Pharm Educ.* 2020;10:39–46.
62. Haggis T. Constructing images of ourselves? A critical investigation into 'Approaches to Learning' research in higher education. *Br Educ Res J.* 2003;29:89.
63. Bonnard P. *Red Roofs at Le Cannet. Oil on Canvas.* Private Collection; 1941.
64. Fritz CO, Morris PE, Bjork RA, Gelman R, Wickens TD. When further learning fails: stability and change following repeated presentation of text. *Br J Psychol.* 2000;91:493–511.
65. Basson MJ, Rothmann S. Flourishing: positive emotion regulation strategies of pharmacy students. *Int J Pharm Pract.* 2018;26:458–464.
66. Tracy JL, Cheng JT, Robins RW, Trzesniewski KH. Authentic and hubristic pride: the affective core of self-esteem and narcissism. *Self Identity.* 2009;8:196–213.
67. Bonnard P. *White Interior.* Oil on canvas, Grenoble: Musée de Grenoble; 1932.
68. Entwistle NJ, Entwistle A. Revision and the experience of understanding. In: Marton F, Hounsell D, Entwistle NJ, eds. *The Experience of Learning.* Edinburgh: Scottish Universities Press; 1997.
69. Elderfield J. Seeing Bonnard. In: Whitfield S, Elderfield J, eds. *Bonnard.* London: Tate Gallery; 1998:33–52.
70. Biggs JB, Tang C. *Teaching for Quality Learning at University: What the Student Does.* 3rd ed. Maidenhead: McGraw-Hill/Society for Research into Higher Education & Open University Press; 2007.
71. Scott D. *Reading Educational Research and Policy.* London: RoutledgeFalmer; 2000.

Chapter 17

Evaluating benefits and harms of deprescribing using routinely collected data*

Frank Moriarty[a], Wade Thompson[b], and Fiona Boland[c]

[a]School of Pharmacy and Biomolecular Sciences, RCSI University of Medicine and Health Sciences, Dublin, Ireland, [b]Women's College Hospital Research Institute, Toronto, ON, Canada, [c]Data Science Centre, RCSI University of Medicine and Health Sciences, Dublin, Ireland

Objectives

- Explain the advantages and disadvantages of analyzing routine data to assess benefits and harms of deprescribing.
- Determine the design aspects to be considered when emulating a target trial of deprescribing.
- Identify the types of bias that the active comparator new user design may mitigate against.
- Describe how a propensity score can be constructed and used to evaluate the effects of deprescribing.
- Appraise various analytical options that could be used to address deprescribing research questions.

Introduction

Deprescribing is defined as "the planned and supervised process of dose reduction or stopping of medication that might be causing harm, or no longer be of benefit." It aims to address inappropriate polypharmacy, a common problem among older persons.[1] Deprescribing should form part of prescribing practice, involving ongoing review of the need for a medication and its appropriateness when issuing repeat prescription for patients.[2] However, deprescribing can be challenging to implement in practice, compounded by various factors including the predominance of treatment guidelines which only recommend initiation or intensification of treatment without guidance on reducing or stopping medications.[3]

Indeed, lack of guidance and resources to support deprescribing is a common barrier cited by healthcare professionals along with fear of negative consequences after stopping a medication.[4,5] Both healthcare provider fear and lack of guidance may stem from the limited available evidence on the benefits and harms of deprescribing many medications commonly used among older persons.[5] This ultimately contributes to inertia and limits uptake of deprescribing in practice.[4,5] There are few randomized controlled trials (RCTs) evaluating the benefits and harms of deprescribing, with examples in certain therapeutic areas including hypertension, dementia and osteoporosis.[6,7] In addition to the usual challenges of conducting RCTs, those involving older adults and deprescribing present additional challenges including the time required for outcomes of interest to accrue, obtaining ethical approval, concern about lack of equipoise, and potential participants having difficulty completing consent or other trial processes.[8,9] Therefore, quantitative deprescribing research is often small, single-arm, short-term pilot studies, or observational studies describing outcomes among patients who had medication(s) deprescribed compared to those who continue taking the medication(s). These studies frequently focus on measures of prescribing appropriateness, and often lack information on clinical or patient-reported outcomes.[10] Like all observational research, there is potential that deprescribing (i.e., a medication being discontinued) may be influenced by measured or unmeasured confounders, and may be more likely to occur for patients with a poor prognosis or who have had a poor response to treatment or an adverse effect. These, among other factors, may confound the relationship between deprescribing and certain outcomes, both beneficial and adverse.

---

*This article was published in Research in Social and Administrative Pharmacy, vol 18, Moriarty F, Thompson W, Boland F, Methods for evaluating the benefit and harms of deprescribing in observational research using routinely collected data, pages 2269-2275, Copyright Elsevier 2022.

Contemporary Research Methods in Pharmacy and Health Services. https://doi.org/10.1016/B978-0-323-91888-6.00036-3
249

Advances in the field of pharmacoepidemiology and causal inference in recent years have yielded new approaches to assess benefits and harms of medications in observational research using routine datasets, such as electronic health record or claims data. These methods, including emulation of a target trial, active comparator new user designs, and use of the prior event rate ratio or propensity scores, can reduce confounding and produce results that more closely reflect those from RCTs.

Such methods have been described and applied in the context of prescribed treatments; however, there has been less consideration of how these may be used to evaluate benefits and harms of deprescribing in observational research. While the role of pharmacoepidemiology research in older adults has been discussed previously,[11] and emulation of a target trial has been proposed as a way to leverage existing data to generate evidence on deprescribing,[12] there appear to be no papers that have specifically discussed how pharmacoepidemiological approaches may apply to questions about deprescribing. This chapter provides a conceptual overview of select research approaches and considerations for applying these to research on deprescribing using large routinely collected datasets. This discussion is framed using two illustrative research questions relating to deprescribing benzodiazepines and low-dose acetylsalicylic acid (aspirin). These are commonly prescribed medications, identified as priority targets for deprescribing, and the rationale for these are described in Table 1. After the discussion of various approaches, the last section considers some of the key challenges in applying causal inference approaches to deprescribing research questions, and makes recommendations to help support improvements in the use of these approaches.

TABLE 1 Summary of the clinical questions and rationale for deprescribing in these cases.

Drug/class of interest	Clinical question	Rationale for using observational data to address this deprescribing question
Benzodiazepines	Among older adults treated with long-term benzodiazepines, does deprescribing reduce the risk of fractures compared to continuing benzodiazepines?	• Long-term benzodiazepine use is a prevalent and well recognized form of potentially inappropriate prescribing, and has been identified as a priority area for deprescribing[13,14] • Although benzodiazepines may be indicated for short-term prescription for anxiety and insomnia, they have been associated with increased risk of fractures among older persons,[15] and it is therefore of interest whether discontinuation of benzodiazepine reduces risk of these outcomes compared to those who continue • As fractures may be a relatively rare outcome, an observational study may be preferable to answer this question rather than (or before) conducting an RCT
Acetylsalicylic acid (aspirin)	Among adults aged 60 years and over without previous cardiovascular disease (i.e., for primary prevention) treated with low-dose acetylsalicylic acid (aspirin), does deprescribing provide a net benefit over 10 years compared to continuing aspirin?	• There is limited evidence on the effects deprescribing aspirin among people taking it for primary prevention. Cumulative evidence suggests prescribing for primary prevention provides little to no benefit in reducing risk of major adverse cardiovascular events, but increases risk of intracranial or major bleeds[16–18] • The US Preventive Services Task Force (2016) recommends that starting aspirin among adults aged 60 years and over should be an individual one, and should consider 10-year cardiovascular risk[19] • However, this evidence relates to initiation and the converse cannot be assumed to apply to deprescribing among patients who have been taking aspirin for primary prevention for years or decades[20] • An observational study among adults in Sweden who had been continuously taking aspirin for at least 12 months found a 28% higher rate of cardiovascular events among those who discontinued aspirin compared to those who continued[21] • The rationale for answering this question in an observational study is the long time frame over which outcomes are to be evaluated

Emulating a target trial

The aim of target trial emulation (the application of design principles from RCTs to the analysis of observational data) is to improve the quality of observational research when a comparator trial is not available, feasible or ethical. It requires defining all aspects of the target trial, including the eligibility criteria, treatment assignment, follow-up period and outcomes, as illustrated in Table 2.[22]

Using large administrative datasets can present challenges because the data were not collected for research purposes. The quality of the data must be checked as recording of required data may be inconsistent or vague. Furthermore, several different codes may be used to represent the same medication or condition. For example, if using the World Health Organization's (WHO) Anatomical Therapeutic Chemical (ATC) classification, or International Statistical Classification of Diseases and Related Health Problems (ICD) all relevant/potential codes must be identified. Before proceeding with the emulation of a target trial, high-quality validation studies are recommended, if not already completed, to assess the consistency and accuracy of the coding of variables of interest within the database.[22] Furthermore, in the case of deprescribing the feasibility of emulating a target trial depends on the rates of deprescribing and size of the database being used, to ensure sufficient numbers of individuals have the medication of interest deprescribed and to allow assessment of outcomes, so that analysis will be powered to detect a true effect if one is present.

Eligibility criteria

The elements of an ideal trial for the question at hand should be emulated as much as possible, including eligibility criteria. In a typical trial, participants would generally be asked about their medical history and medications to assess eligibility.

TABLE 2 Design aspects for hypothetical target trials for emulation to estimate the effects of benzodiazepine and low-dose aspirin deprescribing, and considerations for emulating such trials using observational data.

	Eligibility criteria	Treatment strategies	Assignment procedures	Outcomes
Benzodiazepine	Adults aged 75 years and over who have been prescribed a benzodiazepine for 5 years	(1) Continuing to take a benzodiazepine or (2) Benzodiazepine dose tapering and discontinuation	Participants will be randomly assigned to either strategy at baseline and will be aware of the strategy to which they have been assigned	A fracture diagnosed by X-ray or other imaging within 3 years of baseline
Aspirin	Adults aged 60 years and over who have been prescribed low-dose aspirin regularly for 3 years and who have no history of previous cardiovascular disease or events	(1) Continuing to take aspirin or (2) Stopping aspirin		A major adverse cardiovascular event (cardiovascular death, or nonfatal stroke or myocardial infarction), or a major hemorrhage diagnosed within 10 years of baseline
Considerations for target trial emulation	Definition of taking the medication may require use of a measure of adherence to establish regular use (e.g., a medication possession ratio of >80%). Assessment of cardiovascular disease history may be based on a comprehensive list of ICD disease and procedure codes indicative of cardiovascular disease	Definition of tapering as a treatment strategy may be less challenging as it still involves receipt of a prescription, compared to stopping which will be based on absence of a prescription. Stopping aspirin could be defined as the absence of a prescription by the end of coverage of the previous prescription	A grace period could be applied in the case of stopping aspirin to avoid misclassifying those with a gap in coverage as stopping	Definition of outcomes requires consideration of a range of relevant ICD condition and procedure codes indicative of outcome occurrence. In cases of deprescribing, individuals who had a medication deprescribed may be subject to greater monitoring leading to higher detection of outcomes

However, using routine data for emulation may require assumptions to be made based on the available data (e.g., prescriptions over a certain period of time, validity of ICD codes). In emulating a deprescribing trial, being currently prescribed the medication of interest, and using it as prescribed (i.e., adherent), will generally be part of the eligibility criteria. There are limitations in determining adherence using routinely collected data, for example, there may be delays in the recording of prescriptions, and individuals may refill their prescription early, or have a short gap in coverage due to hospitalization. Defining regular use could be based on number of prescriptions in a given time period, the proportion of days covered (PDC), or the medication possession ratio (MPR). MPR is the sum of the days' supply of a medication from the first to the last prescription in a particular time period, divided by the number of days in the time period. It is a relatively straightforward calculation, however, can lead to overestimation in individuals who refill their medications early and underestimation in those who have a short gap in coverage. Hence, a minimum acceptable cut-off for MPR (e.g., $\geq 80\%$) can be used to classify individuals as being currently prescribed the medication of interest. There may also be additional clinical considerations. For example, to identify individuals with aspirin treatment for primary prevention, it would be necessary to ensure they do not have cardiovascular disease (e.g., based on hospitalization and procedure data). Further consideration of selecting optimal eligibility criteria and treatment strategies is given in the active comparator new user section below.

Time zero

When individuals meet the eligibility criteria, they are assigned to a treatment strategy (e.g., the treatment or the comparator group). This is known as time zero of follow-up (i.e., time of randomization). Individuals are then followed from time zero until the end of follow-up. It is vital that meeting the eligibility criteria, time zero and treatment assignment coincide for successful trial emulation and can help minimize bias. Several scenarios where these do not coincide and can result in trial emulation failures are outlined elsewhere.[23]

Defining time zero can be a challenge. With observational data, it is generally best to emulate time zero by defining it as the time when individuals meet the eligibility criteria and initiate a treatment strategy. As described above, for deprescribing research it is important to ensure individuals are taking the medications of interest regularly at time zero in order to be eligible. In some trials, eligibility is determined by events that can only occur once. However, in the context of deprescribing research, an individual may meet the eligibility criteria at multiple time points. For example, a person may start and stop benzodiazepine treatment multiple times over the course of several years, or may continue for the full study period. In such instances one could choose one of the multiple eligibility times as time zero (e.g., the time of first eligibility or a random time) or include the majority or all eligible times (requires emulating multiple nested trials).

Including a grace period

Grace periods are used to reflect real life. For example, people may refill their prescription late, or individuals may have a short gap in coverage due to a hospitalization. Therefore, partly to avoid misclassifying people who continued a medication as having discontinued, a grace period to the end of a prescription might be attached. Over this grace period, a person is deemed to continue unless they do not redeem or receive another prescription during this time, in which case it can be assumed deprescribing occurred (e.g., on the last day of the grace period). It may also be useful to conduct sensitivity analyses varying the grace period to assess its impact on outcomes.

Allowing a grace-period raises some issues; if an individual experiences the outcome of interest within the grace period, which strategy of the target trial would the individual have been assigned to? One option is to randomly assign the individual to one of the strategies. However, another option is to use clones, i.e., create two exact copies of the individual and assign one to each of the treatment strategies.[22] The clones are then censored at the time their data deviated from the strategy to which they were assigned. If the individual experiences the outcome of interest within the grace period, then both clones experience it which prevents bias that could arise if the individual was randomly assigned to one strategy. However, such approaches can introduce challenges, for example if individuals (clones) are assigned to both strategies, an intention-to-treat analysis is not possible. To allow for intention-to-treat analysis individuals must be randomly assigned to one strategy.

Outcomes

Typically, observational data cannot be used to emulate a target trial with systematic and blind outcome ascertainment. Furthermore, prescribers are generally aware of their patient's medications, in particular when deprescribing, which could influence the prescriber to look for specific outcomes. For example, an increased incidence of adverse drug withdrawal events may be observed as prescribers are monitoring individual's deprescribing and are aware of potential effects. Careful consideration and selection of outcomes least prone to ascertainment bias is important. Ascertainment bias can occur when there is more intense surveillance for outcomes among individuals deprescribing than among individuals continuing on the medication.[24] Furthermore, some outcomes may be more at risk of confounding by indication. A change in prognosis or diagnosis of a life-limiting illness can frequently be a trigger for deprescribing, and therefore, associations with all-cause mortality can be biased if, for example, prescribers deprescribe low-dose aspirin, when a patient is approaching end of life.

Active comparator, new user design

The active comparator new user (ACNU) approach shares similarities to target trial emulation in resembling the intervention part of an RCT. Often, target trials' eligibility criteria and treatment strategies will reflect an ACNU design. The sample of individuals included in an ACNU study are those newly initiated on the medication of interest, or a suitable therapeutic alternative (the active comparator) and this cohort are then followed up and compared over time.[25] This approach aims to reduce a number of biases (see Table 3).

Options for comparison include nonusers, active comparators, or inactive comparators.[28] Comparing those who are deprescribed to those who continue taking the medication of interest will account for one form of confounding by indication, in that all participants have at one point been prescribed the treatment of interest, e.g., benzodiazepines for insomnia. However, there may be other factors relating to indication, e.g., severity or prognosis, which may still differ between groups. The impact of these differences may vary depending on the outcomes being considered, as discussed previously.

TABLE 3 Select biases of treatment comparisons in observational studies that can potentially be mitigating using the active comparator new user design.

Bias	Explanation	Impact
Confounding by indication	Where an indication leads to selective (de)prescribing of a treatment and is also related to the outcome	Confounding by indication can make exposure to the treatment appear harmful. This may be most pronounced when comparing individuals who are started on a treatment compared to nonusers, or in the case of deprescribing, those who are deprescribed due to frailty, for example, versus those who continue. This can be reduced by considering an active comparator
Healthy user bias	When evaluating preventive treatments, individuals who are healthy and engage in other healthy behaviors may be more likely to initiate or continue such treatments.[26] A preventive treatment may also be prescribed less frequently (or deprescribed more frequently) for individuals who are frail or with poor prognosis, and these individuals may have an increased baseline risk of poor outcomes	Both of these mechanisms can exaggerate the beneficial effects of a preventive treatment, or the harmful effects of deprescribing (depending on the outcome)
Healthy adherer bias	Those who adhere to preventive treatment are more likely to adhere to other healthy behaviors and are less likely to have experienced a deterioration in function	This is illustrated by a metaanalysis showing a mortality benefit associated with adherence to placebo among participants in RCTs[27]
Access to healthcare[28]	Those who are prescribed a treatment may have differential access to healthcare or uptake of healthcare services compared to those not prescribed any treatment	This could make treatment appear more beneficial if access to healthcare is associated with better outcomes, or less beneficial if those accessing healthcare are those with higher illness burden. Less use of healthcare will also relate to lower surveillance and detection of outcomes
Depletion of susceptibles	Patients who develop adverse effects or do not respond after starting a treatment are unlikely to remain on the treatment, and so prevalent users are those individuals who are more likely to tolerate and obtain benefits from the treatment[29]	For example, higher rates of venous thromboembolism are observed in the first year of use of hormone replacement therapy relative to subsequent years of use.[30] Regarding benefits, observational studies comparing prevalent users of statins for secondary prevention to nonusers showed exaggerated mortality reductions, whereas studies comparing new users to nonusers found a benefit more reflective of RCTs[31]

There may also be an "indication" for discontinuation or deprescribing, such as development of a new symptom suspected to be an adverse drug effect, a deterioration in function, or a fall that triggers medication review.

True active comparators (e.g., comparing outcomes in those prescribed one of two alternative antihypertensive drugs) likely have little applicability for deprescribing research. An exception may be examining individuals taking two similar potentially inappropriate medications to determine if deprescribing one has more impact compared to the other. An example may be patients on both benzodiazepine and nonbenzodiazepine (Z-drug) hypnotics, to compare deprescribing benzodiazepines or Z-drugs with regard to reinitiations and falls.

A further alternative may be to compare those who are deprescribed the medication of interest to those who continue the medication of interest but are deprescribed or discontinue another unrelated treatment. Some trials of deprescribing have randomized individuals in the intervention group to switch (immediately or gradually) to a placebo, to blind patients and their healthcare professional. Emulating such a trial using existing data sources is infeasible since placebos are not routinely used. However, using an active comparator that is inactive for the outcome of interest has been proposed as a means of emulating trials which use placebos.[32] Using this approach, like blinded placebo-controlled trials, patients in both groups would undergo similar procedures, but one group would be subject to a dummy or inactive intervention.[32] The comparator should be used in a similar context as the treatment of interest, for example, both being used for the long-term treatment of a chronic disease.[28] Consideration should be given to eligibility criteria and whether to restrict to individuals with indications for both treatments, or only those taking both treatments.[32] This warrants attention from researchers, as such choices can result in different causal effects being estimated, a topic expanded on by Huitfeldt et al.[32]

By comparing to patients who have a medication deprescribed that is inactive for the outcome of interest, this may account for some of the unmeasured factors that may affect both deprescribing of the medication of interest and general prognosis. It can also ensure individuals in the comparison group had similar access to healthcare and opportunity to receive the exposure of interest, e.g., they attended their doctor/clinic and received a prescription.[28] However, it may be challenging to identify a relevant comparator medication. A large sample may be required to identify sufficient numbers of patient who are deprescribed the medication of interest, and restricting the comparison group may further impact this. For example, considering the case of aspirin deprescribing and risk of cardiovascular events or major hemorrhage, those deprescribed aspirin could be compared to those who continue aspirin but are deprescribed their bisphosphonate for fracture prevention (assuming bisphosphonate use does not affect cardiovascular events or major hemorrhage, with the exception of gastro-intestinal bleeds or ulceration which are an adverse effect of bisphosphonates).

The new user aspect of the typical ACNU design (selecting new users of the treatment of interest or active comparator) means the groups are aligned at similar points in treatment (and potentially their disease course or prognosis), and accounting for beneficial/harmful effects associated with treatment duration. Compared to an alternative prevalent user design (i.e., including individuals who are prescribed the medication or comparator of interest regardless of their duration of treatment), new user designs address the issue of depletion of susceptibles (see Table 3).

For deprescribing research, considering newly deprescribed patients (i.e., new nonusers) is important, as those whose medication was deprescribed at some point in the past are likely to be those who have not experienced any adverse consequences of deprescribing (e.g., adverse drug withdrawal events or return of condition). Longer term use before deprescribing/discontinuation may also be an important consideration, as discontinuation in someone who recently started a medication may be due to an adverse drug effect or lack of benefit. Also, for certain drug classes such as benzodiazepines, any physiological tolerance may not have developed. While this may be relevant to answer questions about safety and effectiveness of deprescribing after a short period of use, a more common clinical focus is deprescribing among long-term users.

Prior event rate ratio

The prior event rate ratio (PERR) has been proposed as a measure which controls for unmeasured confounding in pharmacoepidemiological studies.[33] It uses the outcome rate in the period after exposure to a medication divided by the rate in a period before exposure. The PERR is the ratio of this rate ratio in the exposed group and the rate ratio in an unexposed or other comparator group, similar to difference-in-difference analysis used in economic studies. This can account for time-stable within individual factors which may differ between groups. However, it cannot control for any time-varying factors or other temporal changes after exposure that alter the ratio of the outcome between the exposed and unexposed groups independent of the effect of therapy. Furthermore, outcomes such as mortality, or any event that is also an exclusion criteria for the study cannot be analyzed.[33] Evidence from simulation studies indicates that in the presence of unmeasured confounding, the PERR can produce less biased estimates compared to conventional analytical methods,[34] and is often consistent with RCTs.[35–37] However, where prior events affect the likelihood of subsequent exposure (e.g., episodes of dyspepsia reducing the likelihood of diclofenac prescription), the PERR estimates are more biased than conventional estimates.[34]

In the context of deprescribing research, this may present a challenge where an adverse event or symptom among users of a medication may potentially influence the likelihood of deprescribing, and also be an outcome of interest following deprescribing. For instance, among benzodiazepine users, prior falls may be associated with deprescribing (i.e., where an older patient falling and being hospitalized may trigger a comprehensive geriatric assessment and medication review) and falls are also an important outcome of interest in evaluating the benefits and harms of deprescribing. Similarly, occurrence of dyspepsia or gastrointestinal ulceration can encourage deprescribing of aspirin, and these are also outcomes of interest that deprescribing may improve. The PERR may also be unsuitable for evaluating low-dose aspirin deprescribing and cardiovascular events as an outcome, because prior cardiovascular events would be an exclusion criteria if considering use for primary prevention. Surveillance bias may also apply, where there is greater monitoring and detection of events after deprescribing compared to before, unrelated to the effect of deprescribing. Therefore, the application of the PERR may be limited to specific cases where outcomes of interest will not influence the likelihood of the medication of interest being deprescribed or inclusion in the study.

Propensity score approaches

The propensity score is defined as "the probability of treatment assignment conditional on observed characteristics."[38] In the context of observational research in deprescribing, this is the probability of a medication being discontinued or continued. Propensity scores are of particular interest for observational research in deprescribing because in routine clinical practice, deprescribing is influenced by a complex interplay of characteristics such as life expectancy, comorbidities, concomitant medications, frailty, and patient preferences, among other factors.[39] Thus, the characteristics of a group of people whose medication has been deprescribed will likely be different from those who continued the medication. For an observational study evaluating the outcomes of deprescribing, this clearly has the potential to introduce confounding. Propensity score methods aim to balance the two groups based on measured covariates such that the distribution of known covariates is similar between those discontinuing a medication and those continuing.[40,41] Garrido et al. provide a comprehensive overview of propensity scores, including how to construct and implement them in observational research.[41] Propensity scores are typically created using a logistic regression model, where the treatment (i.e., deprescribing or continuation) is a dependent variable and potential confounders are explanatory variables.[41] After ensuring similar distribution of propensity scores between the two groups,[41] the created propensity score can then be used to compare the groups. This most commonly involves matching individuals who share similar propensity scores in the treatment (deprescribing) group with those in a comparison (continuation) group or using weighting techniques. These methods are described in detail elsewhere.[38,41,42] Overlap weighting has recently been proposed as a technique to emulate RCTs.[43] Overlap weighting is where the emphasis is put on the target population with the most overlap in observed characteristics (i.e., could appear with substantial probability in the treatment or comparison group) and individuals in the tails of the propensity score distribution are down-weighted. After ensuring covariate balance between groups,[44] the effect of treatment on outcomes is then estimated.

A critical step in creating propensity scores is selecting covariates, which will be factors that are potential confounders. This is particularly important in deprescribing studies, as there is a high potential for confounding given the complexity of older adults, who often have multiple comorbidities and take many medications. There are several practical and statistical considerations for selecting confounders.[41,45] Notably, identification of confounders should be carried out in close consultation with clinical experts with subject matter expertise, and based on previous literature, to ensure proper confounders are defined. A major consideration in constructing propensity scores is that they are based on *measured* confounders. One challenge with observational studies of deprescribing is that potentially relevant confounders such as patient preferences and goals, frailty, and function, can be difficult or impossible to capture in a valid and reliable way from data sources. Thus, there may still be potential for unmeasured confounding that might bias outcome measurement. While methods to capture frailty in routinely collected healthcare data have been proposed,[46,47] it is often unclear how well these methods capture the true clinical picture of frailty and the functional state of older persons.[48,49] Therefore, if using propensity scores, it is important researchers acknowledge such limitations where relevant. The E value, defined as the minimum strength an unmeasured confounder would need to have with the treatment and outcome to explain away any observed association, conditional on the measured covariates, can help evaluate the potential for unmeasured confounding.[50] This can help create transparency around how robust an observed association is to unmeasured confounding. Another point to consider is that individuals may change over the study period, for example people may start a new medication, stop one they were taking at baseline, or acquire a new disease during follow-up. Thus, depending on the duration of the study, it may be important to account for time-varying confounding.[51,52] One proposed approach to account for time-varying confounding is the use of g methods, which includes the parametric g formula, g estimation of structural nested models and marginal structural models.[51–53] Compared to standard regression approaches (e.g., linear, logistic, Cox regression) where the values of confounders are fixed, these methods allow for more flexible treatment pathways, and can thus incorporate situations where the value of a confounder changes over time (while also minimizing bias when time varying confounders are affected by previous exposure).[51–53]

Self-controlled designs

Self-controlled designs use each individual as their own control, so like the PERR, these designs control for measured and unmeasured confounders which are stable over time within each individual, but not time-varying confounding.[54] However, unlike the PERR, self-controlled designs are "case only," and include only individuals who have experienced the outcome of interest. Self-controlled approaches have been most often used to evaluate drug safety,[55] assessing the short-term effects of transient exposures on outcomes or events with sudden onset. Given the frequent focus on deprescribing among patients who have been taking a medication long term, the applicability of these designs may be limited to specific relevant situations, e.g., acute effects of discontinuing a medication.

The case-crossover design involves assessing exposure at the time of occurrence of the outcome, and at earlier reference time point(s).[56] Those with discrepant exposure are compared in the analysis, and individuals with consistent exposure are omitted, meaning this approach is inefficient/underpowered where exposure tends to be chronic with a low prevalence of crossover.[54] Estimates may be biased if there is an upward trend in exposure in the source population over time, which would lead to a higher chance of being exposed at the outcome time point compared to earlier time points. This can be mitigated by using variations of this design, such as the case-time-control design (which accounts for trends in a control group without the outcome), or alternative approaches such as the self-controlled case series.[54,57]

The self-controlled case series requires an intermittent exposure and acute outcome, and has been used extensively in evaluating vaccine safety.[58] Each individual's observation time is divided into "risk periods" during and for a defined time after exposure, and "control periods," where an individual is unexposed. The incidence rate of the outcome in "risk periods" is compared to that in "control periods" to evaluate the association of interest. All of an individual's observation time is evaluated, including that which is after the outcome occurrence, which mitigates the risk of bias due to trends in exposure over time.[54] However, like the PERR, occurrence of the outcome should not be associated with subsequent likelihood of exposure, and therefore, it is not suitable for evaluating established effects.

As these designs are only amenable to exposure effects that are transient, one potential application may be to evaluate short-term risk of an event, such as a physiological withdrawal reaction or condition exacerbation, shortly after discontinuation (e.g., risk of hospitalization for heart failure following discontinuation of loop diuretics). The point of discontinuation/deprescribing and shortly after could be used to define the "risk period(s)" in a self-controlled case series design. They could be considered to evaluate deprescribing in scenarios where exposure is intermittent (for example, considering patients whose benzodiazepine is stopped, and then restarted at a later date, and the risk of fracture). Applying such designs in this context could involve a reversal of the perspective of "risk" and "control" periods, so that the period following deprescribing would be considered as the risk period, compared to control periods where the medication was prescribed. However, the temporal relationship between periods of exposure and nonexposure is not explicitly included, and lack of exposure to the medication of interest is often not equivalent to deprescribing after a period of use. The focus on transient effects and intermittent exposure also increases the risk of misclassification bias occurring and affecting the results. Certainty that individuals have actually stopped their medication when classifying them in the deprescribing category may be particularly important in this context. Hence for many deprescribing situations where duration of use and cumulative exposure may be relevant to benefits and harms of deprescribing (for reasons like dependence and tolerance in the case of benzodiazepines), such self-controlled designs may have limited utility.

Instrumental variables

Instrumental variable (IV) analysis has been described elsewhere in detail[59]; however, this section provides a brief summary of this approach and principles relevant to deprescribing research questions. An IV is a factor that is available within an administrative data source, that is assumed to relate to a treatment of interest, but does not relate to the outcome of interest either directly or indirectly via unmeasured variables. IV analyses typically focus on a subsection of individuals where some measured factor (an IV) is strongly determinant of which treatment they receive, and thus can be similar to random/pseudorandom assignment of exposure to some patients.[60] An effective IV can be assumed to control for known and unknown individual characteristics that may affect outcomes. IV analysis has been used across medical interventions, including to evaluate medication effectiveness and safety. IVs used in this context include prescriber preference, regional variation, institution/facility prescribing patterns, or calendar time (e.g., before or after a policy change).[60,61] Some of these instrumental variables, if available, could potentially be applied to evaluate deprescribing. However, IV analysis has largely been used to address research questions comparing benefits and harms of alternative treatments, rather than a treatment versus no treatment. Hence, for a research question comparing continuation of a medication to deprescribing it, it may be challenging to identify a suitable IV that meets the necessary assumptions. Moreover, previous commentators have urged caution in the use of IV analysis in general, as its validity is contingent on several assumptions, some of which are untestable.[60] Furthermore, even when comparing relatively interchangeable treatment options, a suitable IV can be difficult to identify. Hence, it may be prudent to limit such analyses to specific situations where a fortuitous natural experiment can provide a plausible instrument.[62]

Acknowledging these reasons for potential limited applicability, examples of potential IVs to evaluate deprescribing can be considered. Taking the example where national guidelines were introduced in Denmark in 2008 restricting renewal of driving licenses for patients on long-term benzodiazepines,[63] current benzodiazepine users who attended an appointment with their physician before and after this guideline change could be compared. In this case, the timing of the patient's consultation (before or after the guidelines change) could be considered as an IV in evaluating the effects of benzodiazepine deprescribing. Alternatively, data from a facility where some prescribers have a strong preference for deprescribing aspirin among older adults taking it for primary prevention could be evaluated, using the prescriber preference as the IV. However, in both these cases, it is likely that the proposed IV may relate to relevant outcomes via mechanisms other than deprescribing alone, such as through increased surveillance and detection of adverse events.

Discussion

This chapter has discussed a number of methods used in pharmacoepidemiology and comparative effectiveness research, and considered how they may be applied to answer deprescribing research questions. This is not an exhaustive list of approaches, and other methods may also be relevant to specific deprescribing research questions.

A major challenge with applying these methods is defining deprescribing as a treatment strategy. In routinely collected data, it is challenging to differentiate purposeful stopping of medication (i.e., deprescribing, typically accompanied by comprehensive medication review, active follow-up and monitoring) from patients stopping on their own (i.e., nonpersistence). In cases of nonpersistence, a comparison with individuals who persist with their medication may be subject to healthy adherer bias, while in cases of genuine deprescribing, we may expect individuals whose medication has been deprescribed to be frailer than those who continue. Therefore, evidence of benefits/harms of medication cessation from one group may not be fully applicable to the other. Medication deprescribing or discontinuation is likely to be captured via a lack of further prescription or dispensing after a period of regular use, incorporating a grace period to avoid misclassifying delayed filling of prescriptions as deprescribing. However, the precise definition will vary depending on the database (e.g., electronic health record (EHR) versus claims data for prescribing/dispensing), how it captures prescription duration (i.e., explicitly or inferred based on quantity and dosing), and the medication and outcomes of interest. For instance, deprescribing of low-dose aspirin could be defined based on an abrupt absence of prescriptions, whereas for benzodiazepines, dose tapering over time with or without complete cessation would be expected. The introduction of an activity/billing code for deprescribing within EHR systems to indicate planned stopping or dose reduction of a medication would mitigate some of the challenges of defining deprescribing.

A further limitation of using routine data sources is that certain outcomes of interest may not be recorded in available datasets and therefore cannot be investigated in such studies. This is particularly true of patient-reported outcomes, limiting the ability to consider potential return of a condition or adverse drug withdrawal events following deprescribing of medications for symptomatic treatment. This is also relevant for factors such as patient preferences—for example, patients with life-limiting illness may prioritize symptom control (and avoidance of adverse effects) over long-term prevention, and thus analysis of the benefits and harms of deprescribing for this population using routine data may be limited. However, technological advances with EHRs mean that collection of patient-reported outcomes in routine care is increasingly possible, and more widespread integration of this may facilitate further deprescribing research.[64] However, in the absence of this, applying these comparative effectiveness research approach may require a pragmatic approach in considering which scenarios and research questions would observational research using routine data be most feasible and of value. For instance, focusing on outcomes captured routinely and most accurately in administrative/EHR data sources, or outcomes over the longer term due to the time it would take to conduct a prospective observational study or RCT to investigate.

Although there have been several methodological advances in pharmacoepidemiology and comparative effectiveness research in recent decades, and these approaches are readily applied to deprescribing research questions, it is still important to recognize the limitations of these approaches. Even with rich data for large numbers of individuals, allowing for optimal design and analysis choices to reduce confounding, the potential for unmeasured confounding still persists, and although challenging, RCTs of deprescribing are possible.[65] Therefore, at best, it would be prudent to consider such observational studies as exploratory and hypothesis generating, which may provide evidence to support evaluation of particular deprescribing research questions in RCTs.

Questions for further discussion

1. What are the key differences in evaluating deprescribing of a medication compared to prescribing of a medication within observational research?
2. Can observational research on benefits and harms of deprescribing be useful for clinical decision making, given the biases and limitations?
3. What are the fundamental enhancements to routinely collected data that would facilitate higher quality observational research to evaluate deprescribing?

Application exercise/scenario

Your research team is aiming to answer the following question using the target trial emulation approach: "Among women aged 65 years and older, residing in long-term care, who have been taking alendronate for 4 to 5 years, does deprescribing alendronate affect 2-year risk of hip fractures compared to continuing to take alendronate?" Describe (i) the design characteristics of a suitable target trial, (ii) how you would operationalize these in an idealized routine dataset, and (iii) anticipated challenges in doing this.

References

1. Wastesson JW, Morin L, Tan ECK, Johnell K. An update on the clinical consequences of polypharmacy in older adults: a narrative review. *Expert Opin Drug Saf.* 2018;17(12):1185–1196. https://doi.org/10.1080/14740338.2018.1546841.
2. De Vries TPGM, Henning RH, Hogerzeil HV, Fresle DA, Haaijer-Ruskamp FM, Van Gilst RM. *Guide to Good Prescribing—A Practical Manual.* Geneva, Switzerland: World Health Organisation; 1994. http://apps.who.int/medicinedocs/pdf/whozip23e/whozip23e.pdf. Accessed 31 May 2018.
3. Moriarty F, Pottie K, Dolovich L, McCarthy L, Rojas-Fernandez C, Farrell B. Deprescribing recommendations: an essential consideration for clinical guideline developers. *Res Soc Adm Pharm.* 2019;15(6):806–810. https://doi.org/10.1016/j.sapharm.2018.08.014.
4. Anderson K, Stowasser D, Freeman C, Scott I. Prescriber barriers and enablers to minimising potentially inappropriate medications in adults: a systematic review and thematic synthesis. *BMJ Open.* 2014;4:e006544. https://doi.org/10.1136/bmjopen-2014-006544.
5. Doherty AJ, Boland P, Reed J, et al. Barriers and facilitators to deprescribing in primary care: a systematic review. *BJGP Open.* 2020;4(3). https://doi.org/10.3399/bjgpopen20X101096.
6. Page AT, Clifford RM, Potter K, Schwartz D, Etherton-Beer CD. The feasibility and effect of deprescribing in older adults on mortality and health: a systematic review and meta-analysis. *Br J Clin Pharmacol.* 2016;82(3):583–623. https://doi.org/10.1111/bcp.12975.
7. Thio SL, Nam J, Van Driel ML, Dirven T, Blom JW. Effects of discontinuation of chronic medication in primary care: a systematic review of deprescribing trials. *Br J Gen Pract.* 2018;68(675):e663–e672. https://doi.org/10.3399/bjgp18X699041.
8. Clough AJ, Hilmer SN, Kouladjian-O'Donnell L, Naismith SL, Gnjidic D. Health professionals' and researchers' opinions on conducting clinical deprescribing trials. *Pharmacol Res Perspect.* 2019;7(3):476. https://doi.org/10.1002/prp2.476.
9. Provencher V, Ben MW, Tanguay-Garneau L, Bélanger K, Dagenais M. Challenges and strategies pertaining to recruitment and retention of frail elderly in research studies: a systematic review. *Arch Gerontol Geriatr.* 2014;59(1):18–24. https://doi.org/10.1016/j.archger.2014.03.006.
10. Aubert CE, Kerr EA, Maratt JK, Klamerus ML, Hofer TP. Outcome measures for interventions to reduce inappropriate chronic drugs: a narrative review. *J Am Geriatr Soc.* 2020;68(10):2390–2398. https://doi.org/10.1111/jgs.16697.
11. Laroche M-L, Sirois C, Reeve E, Gnjidic D, Morin L. Pharmacoepidemiology in older people: purposes and future directions. *Therapies.* 2019; 74(2):325–332. https://doi.org/10.1016/j.therap.2018.10.006.
12. Krishnaswami A, Steinman MA, Goyal P, et al. Deprescribing in older adults with cardiovascular disease. *J Am Coll Cardiol.* 2019;73(20): 2584–2595. https://doi.org/10.1016/j.jacc.2019.03.467.
13. Farrell B, Tsang C, Raman-Wilms L, Irving H, Conklin J, Pottie K. What are priorities for deprescribing for elderly patients? Capturing the voice of practitioners: a modified Delphi process. *PLoS One.* 2015;10(4):e0122246. https://doi.org/10.1371/journal.pone.0122246.
14. Pottie K, Thompson W, Davies S, et al. Deprescribing benzodiazepine receptor agonists: evidence-based clinical practice guideline. *Can Fam Physician.* 2018;64(5):339–351.
15. Donnelly K, Bracchi R, Hewitt J, Routledge PA, Carter B. Benzodiazepines, Z-drugs and the risk of hip fracture: a systematic review and meta-analysis. *PLoS One.* 2017;12(4):e0174730. https://doi.org/10.1371/journal.pone.0174730.

16. Zheng SL, Roddick AJ. Association of aspirin use for primary prevention with cardiovascular events and bleeding events. *JAMA*. 2019;321 (3):277. https://doi.org/10.1001/jama.2018.20578.

17. Moriarty F, Ebell MH. A comparison of contemporary versus older studies of aspirin for primary prevention. *Fam Pract*. 2020;37(3):290–296. https://doi.org/10.1093/FAMPRA/CMZ080.

18. McNeil JJ, Nelson MR, Woods RL, et al. Effect of aspirin on all-cause mortality in the healthy elderly. *N Engl J Med*. 2018;379(16): 1519–1528. https://doi.org/10.1056/nejmoa1803955.

19. Bibbins-Domingo K. U.S. Preventive Services Task Force. Aspirin use for the primary prevention of cardiovascular disease and colorectal cancer: U.S. Preventive Services Task Force recommendation statement. *Ann Intern Med*. 2016;164(12):836–845. https://doi.org/10.7326/M16-0577.

20. Truong C. Update on acetylsalicylic acid for primary prevention of cardiovascular disease. *Can Med Assoc J*. 2019;21(65):481–482. https://doi.org/10.1111/resp.12721.

21. Sundström J, Hedberg J, Thuresson M, Aarskog P, Johannesen KM, Oldgren J. Low-dose aspirin discontinuation and risk of cardiovascular events: a Swedish Nationwide, Population-Based Cohort Study. *Circulation*. 2017;136(13):1183–1192. https://doi.org/10.1161/CIRCULATIONAHA.117.028321.

22. Hernán MA, Robins JM. Using big data to emulate a target trial when a randomized trial is not available. *Am J Epidemiol*. 2016;183(8): 758–764. https://doi.org/10.1093/aje/kwv254.

23. Hernán MA, Sauer BC, Hernández-Díaz S, Platt R, Shrier I. Specifying a target trial prevents immortal time bias and other self-inflicted injuries in observational analyses. *J Clin Epidemiol*. 2016;79:70–75. https://doi.org/10.1016/j.jclinepi.2016.04.014.

24. Haut ER, Pronovost PJ. Surveillance bias in outcomes reporting. *JAMA*. 2011;305(23):2462–2463. https://doi.org/10.1001/jama.2011.822.

25. Lund JL, Richardson DB, Stürmer T. The active comparator, new user study design in pharmacoepidemiology: historical foundations and contemporary application. *Curr Epidemiol Rep*. 2015;2(4):221–228. https://doi.org/10.1007/s40471-015-0053-5.

26. Shrank WH, Patrick AR, Brookhart MA. Healthy user and related biases in observational studies of preventive interventions: a primer for physicians. *J Gen Intern Med*. 2011;26(5):546–550. https://doi.org/10.1007/s11606-010-1609-1.

27. Simpson SH, Eurich DT, Majumdar SR, et al. A meta-analysis of the association between adherence to drug therapy and mortality. *BMJ*. 2006; 333(7557):15. https://doi.org/10.1136/bmj.38875.675486.55.

28. D'Arcy M, Stürmer T, Lund JL. The importance and implications of comparator selection in pharmacoepidemiologic research. *Curr Epidemiol Rep*. 2018;5(3):272–283. https://doi.org/10.1007/s40471-018-0155-y.

29. Johnson ES, Bartman BA, Briesacher BA, et al. The incident user design in comparative effectiveness research. *Pharmacoepidemiol Drug Saf*. 2013;22(1):1–6. https://doi.org/10.1002/pds.3334.

30. Renoux C, Dell'Aniello S, Brenner B, Suissa S. Bias from depletion of susceptibles: the example of hormone replacement therapy and the risk of venous thromboembolism. *Pharmacoepidemiol Drug Saf*. 2017;26(5):554–560. https://doi.org/10.1002/pds.4197.

31. Danaei G, Tavakkoli M, Hernán MA. Bias in observational studies of prevalent users: lessons for comparative effectiveness research from a meta-analysis of statins. *Am J Epidemiol*. 2012;175(4):250–262. https://doi.org/10.1093/aje/kwr301.

32. Huitfeldt A, Hernan MA, Kalager M, Robins JM. Comparative effectiveness research using observational data: active comparators to emulate target trials with inactive comparators. *eGEMs*. 2016;4(1):20. https://doi.org/10.13063/2327-9214.1234.

33. Tannen R, Weiner M, Xie D. Replicated studies of two randomized trials of angiotensin-converting enzyme inhibitors: further empiric validation of the 'prior event rate ratio' to adjust for unmeasured confounding by indication. *Pharmacoepidemiol Drug Saf*. 2008;17:671–685. https://doi.org/10.1002/pds.

34. Uddin M, Groenwold R, van Staa T-P, et al. Performance of prior event rate ratio adjustment method in pharmacoepidemiology: a simulation study. *Pharmacoepidemiol Drug Saf*. 2015;24:468–477. https://doi.org/10.1002/pds.3724.

35. Tannen RL, Weiner MG, Xie D. Use of primary care electronic medical record database in drug efficacy research on cardiovascular outcomes: comparison of database and randomised controlled trial findings. *BMJ*. 2009;338(7691):395–399. https://doi.org/10.1136/bmj.b81.

36. Scott J, Jones T, Redaniel MT, May MT, Ben-Shlomo Y, Caskey F. Estimating the risk of acute kidney injury associated with use of diuretics and renin angiotensin aldosterone system inhibitors: a population based cohort study using the clinical practice research datalink. *BMC Nephrol*. 2019; 20(1). https://doi.org/10.1186/s12882-019-1633-2.

37. Rodgers LR, Dennis JM, Shields BM, et al. Prior event rate ratio adjustment produced estimates consistent with randomized trial: a diabetes case study. *J Clin Epidemiol*. 2020;122:78–86. https://doi.org/10.1016/j.jclinepi.2020.03.007.

38. Austin PC. An introduction to propensity score methods for reducing the effects of confounding in observational studies. *Multivar Behav Res*. 2011; 46(3):399–424. https://doi.org/10.1080/00273171.2011.568786.

39. van der Ploeg MA, Streit S, Achterberg WP, et al. Patient characteristics and general practitioners' advice to stop statins in oldest-old patients: a survey study across 30 countries. *J Gen Intern Med*. 2019;34(9):1751–1757. https://doi.org/10.1007/s11606-018-4795-x.

40. Austin PC. The use of propensity score methods with survival or time-to-event outcomes: reporting measures of effect similar to those used in randomized experiments. *Stat Med*. 2014;33(7):1242–1258. https://doi.org/10.1002/sim.5984.

41. Garrido MM, Kelley AS, Paris J, et al. Methods for constructing and assessing propensity scores. *Health Serv Res*. 2014;49(5):1701–1720. https://doi.org/10.1111/1475-6773.12182.

42. Austin PC, Stuart EA. Moving towards best practice when using inverse probability of treatment weighting (IPTW) using the propensity score to estimate causal treatment effects in observational studies. *Stat Med*. 2015;34(28):3661–3679. https://doi.org/10.1002/sim.6607.

43. Thomas LE, Li F, Pencina MJ. Overlap weighting. *JAMA*. 2020;323(23):2417. https://doi.org/10.1001/jama.2020.7819.

44. Austin PC. Balance diagnostics for comparing the distribution of baseline covariates between treatment groups in propensity-score matched samples. *Stat Med.* 2009;28(25):3083–3107. https://doi.org/10.1002/sim.3697.

45. Kim DH, Pieper CF, Ahmed A, Colón-Emeric CS. Use and interpretation of propensity scores in aging research: a guide for clinical researchers. *J Am Geriatr Soc.* 2016;64(10):2065–2073. https://doi.org/10.1111/jgs.14253.

46. Clegg A, Bates C, Young J, et al. Development and validation of an electronic frailty index using routine primary care electronic health record data. *Age Ageing.* 2016;45(3):353–360. https://doi.org/10.1093/ageing/afw039.

47. Gilbert T, Neuburger J, Kraindler J, et al. Development and validation of a hospital frailty risk score focusing on older people in acute care settings using electronic hospital records: an observational study. *Lancet.* 2018;391(10132):1775–1782. https://doi.org/10.1016/S0140-6736(18)30668-8.

48. O'Caoimh R, Cooney MT, Cooke J, O'Shea D. The challenges of using the hospital frailty risk score. *Lancet.* 2018;392(10165):2693. https://doi.org/10.1016/S0140-6736(18)32424-3.

49. Putot A, Hacquin A, Barben J, et al. Comment on: revascularization versus medical therapy in patients aged 80 years and older with acute myocardial infarction. *J Am Geriatr Soc.* 2021;69(1):274–275. https://doi.org/10.1111/jgs.16938.

50. Vander Weele TJ, Ding P. Sensitivity analysis in observational research: introducing the e-value. *Ann Intern Med.* 2017;167(4):268–274. https://doi.org/10.7326/M16-2607.

51. Mansournia MA, Etminan M, Danaei G, Kaufman JS, Collins G. Handling time varying confounding in observational research. *BMJ.* 2017;359:4587. https://doi.org/10.1136/bmj.j4587.

52. Pazzagli L, Linder M, Zhang M, et al. Methods for time-varying exposure related problems in pharmacoepidemiology: an overview. *Pharmacoepidemiol Drug Saf.* 2018;27(2):148–160. https://doi.org/10.1002/pds.4372.

53. Naimi AI, Cole SR, Kennedy EH. An introduction to g methods. *Int J Epidemiol.* 2017;46(2):756–762. https://doi.org/10.1093/ije/dyw323.

54. Hallas J, Pottegård A. Use of self-controlled designs in pharmacoepidemiology. *J Intern Med.* 2014;275(6):581–589. https://doi.org/10.1111/joim.12186.

55. Consiglio GP, Burden AM, Maclure M, McCarthy L, Cadarette SM. Case-crossover study design in pharmacoepidemiology: systematic review and recommendations. *Pharmacoepidemiol Drug Saf.* 2013;22(11):1146–1153. https://doi.org/10.1002/pds.3508.

56. Maclure M. The case-crossover design: a method for studying transient effects on the risk of acute events. *Am J Epidemiol.* 1991;133(2):144–153. https://doi.org/10.1093/oxfordjournals.aje.a115853.

57. Uddin MJ, Groenwold RHH, Ali MS, et al. Methods to control for unmeasured confounding in pharmacoepidemiology: an overview. *Int J Clin Pharm.* 2016;38(3):714–723. https://doi.org/10.1007/s11096-016-0299-0.

58. Weldeselassie YG, Whitaker HJ, Farrington CP. Use of the self-controlled case-series method in vaccine safety studies: review and recommendations for best practice. *Epidemiol Infect.* 2011;139(12):1805–1817. https://doi.org/10.1017/S0950268811001531.

59. Baiocchi M, Cheng J, Small DS. Instrumental variable methods for causal inference. *Stat Med.* 2014;33(13):2297–2340. https://doi.org/10.1002/sim.6128.

60. Ertefaie A, Small DS, Flory JH, Hennessy S. A tutorial on the use of instrumental variables in pharmacoepidemiology. *Pharmacoepidemiol Drug Saf.* 2017;26(4):357–367. https://doi.org/10.1002/pds.4158.

61. Chen Y, Briesacher BA. Use of instrumental variable in prescription drug research with observational data: a systematic review. *J Clin Epidemiol.* 2011;64(6):687–700. https://doi.org/10.1016/j.jclinepi.2010.09.006.

62. Garabedian LF, Chu P, Toh S, Zaslavsky AM, Soumerai SB. Potential bias of instrumental variable analyses for observational comparative effectiveness research. *Ann Intern Med.* 2014;161(2):131–138. https://doi.org/10.7326/M13-1887.

63. Eriksen SI, Bjerrum L. Reducing prescriptions of long-acting benzodiazepine drugs in Denmark: a descriptive analysis of nationwide prescriptions during a 10-year period. *Basic Clin Pharmacol Toxicol.* 2015;116(6):499–502. https://doi.org/10.1111/bcpt.12347.

64. Ahmed S, Ware P, Gardner W, et al. Montreal accord on patient-reported outcomes (PROs) use series—paper 8: patient-reported outcomes in electronic health records can inform clinical and policy decisions. *J Clin Epidemiol.* 2017;89:160–167. https://doi.org/10.1016/j.jclinepi.2017.04.011.

65. Bonnet F, Bénard A, Poulizac P, et al. Discontinuing statins or not in the elderly? Study protocol for a randomized controlled trial. *Trials.* 2020;21(1):342. https://doi.org/10.1186/s13063-020-04259-5.

Chapter 18

Understanding and addressing the observer effect in observation studies

Sofia Kälvemark Sporrong[a,b], Birgitte Grøstad Kalleberg[c], Liv Mathiesen[c], Yvonne Andersson[d], Stine Eidhammer Rognan[c,e], and Karin Svensberg[a]

[a]Department of Pharmacy, Uppsala University, Uppsala, Sweden, [b]Department of Pharmacy, Social and Clinical Pharmacy Research Group, University of Copenhagen, Copenhagen, Denmark, [c]Department of Pharmacy, University of Oslo, Oslo, Norway, [d]Hospital Pharmacies Enterprise, South Eastern Norway, Oslo, Norway, [e]Department of Pharmaceutical Services, Oslo Hospital Pharmacy, Oslo, Norway

Objectives

- Describe the observer effect in observation studies.
- Identify factors affecting the observer effect.
- Discuss measures that can be used to counteract the observer effect.
- Discuss how to investigate the observer effect in observation studies.

The observer effect

Observation studies shed light on people's actual behavior, rather than their self-report of such behavior. Such studies have been used in a range of real-world settings, including pharmacies and other health care settings. In pharmacies, observation studies have, for example, been used to explore patterns of work and encounters between staff and customers or prescribers.[1-3] In health care, observation studies have been used in many settings, for example, to explore interactions between patient and health care professional (HCP), or processes such as hospital discharge.[4-9]

Observational methods cover a range of practices: They can be unstructured and qualitative (recording what happens as it happens) and/or structured and quantitative (using some sort of coding scheme). The role of the observer can be everything from completely participant (going native), to only observing (nonparticipant). Observations can be overt (participants know they are being observed) or covert.[1,10-12] An advantage with observational studies, almost regardless of how they are performed, is the directness of the methods; what is being studied is what is happening in a real-life context. However, no method comes without challenges. For observational methods, these include that they are relatively time-consuming and often ethically troublesome.[11] One of the most frequently discussed disadvantages is the observer effect, which is the focus of this chapter. The observer effect was previously called the Hawthorne effect, but over the course of time, it has mutated to other labels such as the observer-expectancy effect or participant reactivity.[11,13] In this chapter, the label *observer effect* is used. The observer effect can be defined as "*any form of artifact or consequence of research participation on behavior*"[13] and implies that people tend to change their behavior if they know they are being observed.[13]

One psychological explanation of the observer effect is that if a participant is informed about or (sub)consciously has an idea of what behavior is studied, they might adapt to what they think is expected from them. Consequently, they may change their acting toward an "ideal" behavior compared to under normal circumstances, that is conformity and social desirability considerations are at play.[11-14] Hence, the observer effect can lead to erroneous conclusions being drawn from a study.

Studies explicitly exploring the observer effect in clinical health care practice include a study by Goodwin et al., which reported a small or no effect on physician encounters, except for patients with lower sociodemographic status.[15] However, they saw an initial effect the first day of observations, with encounters being on average 10% longer compared to the second day. Additionally, the majority of participants themselves reported no effect of the observer on the interaction (74% of patients; 55% of physicians).[15] Fernald et al. found no clinical difference on primary study outcomes when they explored the observer effect in a study on clinician management of skin and soft tissue infections in primary care.[16] A recent review of observation studies on hand hygiene concluded a variable and possibly transient observer effect. It varied between clinical specialty and across departments, and the magnitude ranged from −6.9% to 65.3%.[17]

Despite the focus which has been placed onto the observer effect, it is controversial; there are doubts about its actual existence, the mechanisms behind it, and the magnitude of the effect.[13,15,18,19] McCambridge et al. conducted a review of studies where the observer effect had been quantified (the majority of the included studies were conducted in the health care sector).[13] They concluded that results from the included studies were heterogeneous, and that "*there is no single Hawthorne effect. Consequences of research participation for behaviors being investigated have been found to exist/.../ although little can be securely known about the conditions under which they operate, their mechanisms of effects, or their magnitudes.*"[13]

The observer effect, including its magnitude, seems to depend on many known and unknown factors, including[12–15,20]

- The context, e.g., what kind of group is observed, their profession and/or sociodemographic characteristics.
- Study design, e.g., type of observation.
- The observers, including their personality, characteristics, and behavior.
- What is observed—what the participants are doing. This also includes the complexity of the observed behavior.
- Where observations take place.
- Observation intensity, e.g., timespan for observations and degree of observer presence.

Hence, the observer effect is difficult to quantify in a general sense, and particularly it is different to transfer results from a study setting to others. However, and connected to the factors that affect the observer effect, measures have been suggested to minimize it. Some of these are[11–13,15]

- Habituation, i.e., using longer observation periods, so that the observed get used to being observed.
- No, or limited, sharing of study hypothesis/aim, which reduces the risk of participants altering their behavior.
- Use of native observers, i.e., (type of) observers that are known in/to the context.
- Minimal interactions between observer and observed.
- Use of less obtrusive observation tools or clues of observers' presence.
- Awareness of field entry—that observers are aware of, e.g., how to behave, how to establish trust.

A need for new ways of understanding the observer effect has been suggested, for example, about whether, when, how, how much, and for whom research participation may affect behavior or other study outcomes, as research about this is scarce.[13,15] As stated above, it is difficult to generalize around the observer effect. Therefore, in order to understand its impact, it is important to monitor the observer effect in each specific study. This can be done in many ways, both quantitative (see e.g., McCambridge et al.[13] and Goodwin et al.[15]) but also in a qualitative way.

Exploring the observer effect in a specific study

In this chapter selected results from a follow-up study are presented and discussed (from the perspective of the observer effect).[21] The study investigated the observer effect in an observation study about medication communication.[22,23] By exploring research participation, from the perspectives of both the observed and the observers the aim was to increase the understanding of participants' experiences, including the observer effect. This also serves as an example of how the observer effect can be explored in a qualitative way.

Methods and context

In the original observation study, health care professionals (HCPs) and patients were observed, and hence these groups were interviewed in the follow-up study: HCPs in focus groups[11,24] and patients in individual interviews.[11] Additionally, the observers (two pharmacy students, and one pharmacist/researcher) were interviewed in a separate focus group. This third group was important to get "the other side," as the observers also reflected on the observer effect while observing.

More details on the methodology and results from the *observation study* can be found in the articles of Eidhammer et al.[22,23] However, some aspects of importance to understand the follow-up study are presented here. The observation study was conducted at a medical ward at a Norwegian hospital, during 4 months (September-December 2019). The aim was to "explore and understand the discharge process with a focus on medicines communication, from the patient perspective."[22]

The ward had clinical pharmacists working there on a regular basis, and staff were hence used to the pharmacist profession being around. The observers were identifiable, as they wore yellow t-shirts with the text "observer," but the observed knew that they were pharmacists or pharmacy students. They did not have any active role in the social setting and were only present in the patient's room during HCP encounters. Both written and oral information about the study, including study aim, was provided during several occasions. HCPs were provided this at information meetings before study start and when signing informed consent. Patients were informed in connection to their inclusion in the study. Additionally, a poster with information about the study hung on the wall at the ward during the full observation period.

In relation to the suggested measures to minimize the observer effect, observations were conducted for a long period of time (habituation); observers were clinical pharmacists or pharmacist students (native observers) and were instructed to limit interactions with the observed. However, the full study aim was shared (not limited), and the observers were fully visible to the observed, including notes-taking. There was no specific field entry strategy.

The *follow-up study* focused on the topic of being observed, to observe and the observer effect. Data were collected after observations had ended, when focus groups with the observed HCPs and observers were conducted by two persons who had no role in the observation study. HCPs who had participated (i.e., had given their written informed consent) in the observation study were eligible participants. Staff working at the ward recruited the HCP participants for the focus groups. A convenience sampling strategy was used,[11] but with the requirement that the three professions who had been mostly observed, should be represented (physicians, nurses, and nursing assistants). Additionally, the three observing pharmacist/students were invited to a separate focus group. Patients who had participated in the observation study were interviewed by the observers 1 to 2 weeks after the patient had been discharged from hospital. These interviews covered several topics related to the patients' hospital stay, but also included a question about being observed. All participants received information about the study beforehand and consented to take part. See Table 1 for information about the interviews and socio-demographic data for participants.

The data from the focus groups and interviews were analyzed and are presented together. The primary analysis was inductive[25] and resulted in five themes. For more details on how the follow-up study was conducted and analyzed see Svensberg et al.[21] For this chapter the results have been selected and reorganized.

In the quotations below, the following abbreviations are used; Assistant nurse (AN), Nurse (N), Observer (O), Patient (P), Senior consultant physicians (SCP) followed by a number for the specific participant and, if relevant, a focus group number.

Following up an observation study regarding the observer effect

In the following, the results from the follow-up study are presented and discussed in relation to the factors that are supposed to have an impact the observer effect, as well as actions suggested to counteract it (see above).

The context, and where observations take place: Overall experiences of being observed

The context in which observation takes place, and in addition where observations are conducted are two factors suggested to influence the observation effect. In this case, observations were conducted in the context of a hospital ward, involving HCPs and patients. Observations took place in the patient rooms, and only included encounters between HCPs and patients.

When discussing their overall experiences of being observed, the HCPs and patients described it as neutral, good, or, for some patients, the presence of the observers was experienced as very positive.

TABLE 1 Focus group and interview participants.[21]

HCP focus group

- Four focus groups with mixed professions; however, physicians were only present in one of them
- Lasted on average 23 min
- Participants were 3 senior consultant physicians, 9 nurses, 2 nursing assistants; age range 24–60, average 38; 3 male, 14 female; number of encounters participants had been observed (self-reported): one person one time, 4 persons 2–5 times, 3 persons 6–10 times and 5 persons over 10 times. One person had not been observed

Observer focus group: the 3 female observers. Lasted for 53 min

Patient interviews

- Ten patients were interviewed: 4 men and 6 women, ages 40–90 years. Their encounters with HCPs had been observed between 1 and 22 days

Both HCPs and patients said they were used to having people observing their encounters. HCPs stated that being observed by others, for example students, is part of their ordinary workday. Patients talked more about other HCPs (or students) observing: *P2:…when the doctors were present, there were often a couple of nurses, as well. They were just standing there and said nothing….* This also seemed to be true for other health care contexts: *P2: I did not think about it. When I go to the physicians, GP or other places, I'm so used to them asking "can he or she observe?"*

Generally, patients reported not being affected by the presence of the observers. They phrased this as *"I have not cared about that at all, I have pretended that you are not there"* (P1), or *"I knew that you should be there. This was not more disturbing, than anything else"* (P2).

However, a few HCP participants implicitly described the experiences as if they had a shadow after them or being bugged and judged.

When asked, the patients stated that they had not experienced any difference in HCPs' behavior during observations as compared to when not being observed:

Interviewer: Did you feel that there was any difference in how people talked, or something else that was different the day we were in the room? P3: No, I don't think so, at least it didn't feel that way.

As expressed by both HCPs and patients, it is commonplace that there are "observers," for example students, at a hospital ward, at least at the current one (which was a teaching hospital). Hence, having additional people present at an encounter was a familiar situation. Regarding the context and locations where observations took place, it seems as observations of HCPs and patients, conducted in the patients' rooms in the context of a hospital, create less observer effect than it would have in other settings. This is supported by Paradise et al., who concluded that HCPs have a high workload and have to focus on the patient and that HCPs in (teaching) hospitals always are observed.[18]

What is observed and sharing of study aim: How am I portrayed as a professional?

What is observed, for example what activity, has an impact on the observer effect, or to be more precise, what the observed think is observed. The latter will of course depend on what they get to know about the study. As stated previously, it was HCP-patient encounters that were observed in the observation study. This implies that behavior related to HCPs as professionals were part of the observations. The full aim of the study was shared with both HCPs and patients.

Some nurses and nursing assistants reflected on how they would be portrayed in the observations, and felt a need for changing and thinking about their behavior. One participant described a situation when she did not know how to respond to a patient. She did not like the thought of being described as unable to master the situation in the observer's notepad. The observers also described situations where they had experienced HCPs as nervous in relation to medication information and knowledge. The observers said they experienced this behavior also among senior consultant physicians, who did not report any of this in the focus group interview.

Although the study hypothesis was fully revealed to the observed both before and during the observation study, HCPs had a rather vague idea about it. For example, "discharge process" was not mentioned by the HCPs or the patients, although it was part of the study aim. HCPs several times and continuously seemed unsure, and for example described it as "*a research project having something to do with medications.*" There were different interpretations of what this "something" was, although medication information and communication often were mentioned.

The HCPs reported a potential effect on, and awareness of, their communication and information behavior regarding medication (use) in the presence of the observers, who they knew had expertise in pharmaceuticals. For example, some felt obliged to check that the medications they administered were accurate, if the information was correct or not, and they reflected on what and how much information they gave.

This illustrates a challenge with giving the right amount of information in the right way and at the right time, but also raises a question about how informed consent works in reality. In studies with longer time spans (using observations or other methods), it might be that participants should be reminded several times about what they have consented to make it possible for them to make an informed decision to participate or withdraw from the study later on in the process.

Regarding the observer effect it seems as full sharing of a study hypothesis/aim can turn into a limited sharing from the participant point of view. That the observed did not remember the discharge process part, can mean that they did not focus on, and hence not change their behavior in regard to discharge (apart from the medication communication that they did associate the observation study with).

The information part of informed consent is given high priority in many types of studies, but it could be that other factors are more important for what study participants think they are part of. In this case, the profession of the observers seemed to have an impact as pharmacists are associated with medications but not specifically with discharge.

The observers having a connection to pharmacy might have been more important to the focus on medications communication than the information about the study aim that HCPs received. That is, the presence of an observing pharmacist/ student per se raised the initial level of awareness of medication related behavior and communication at the ward as HCPs had a preunderstanding of what a pharmacist is and what they emphasize in their work. Consequently, for example a physician/medical student or nurse/nursing student would have had a different impact.

Medication communication is a complex behavior[26] with many components compared to, for example, hand hygiene,[17] which has been investigated in several studies. Even if especially the HCPs might have changed their behavior regarding information and communication on medications, the full "medication communication behavior" is difficult to change. For example, the quantity of medication communication can change without modifying the quality.

Observation intensity and habituation: Time as a factor

The intensity of observations is said to impact the observer effect.[14] In the observations study, observations were conducted for full (week-)days and several months. The long observation time could possibly lead to habituation, i.e., that the observer effect diminishes with time as the observed get used to being observed.

Both the observed and the observers referred to time as a critical factor regarding HCPs' behavior.

O3: I guess it's just that you get to be there for a long enough time, maybe. When we have been in the room a few times, they understand that it isn't that uncomfortable.

The first observation encounters were described as something different from ordinary practice, where HCPs, according to themselves, were more observant toward their own behavior on medication communication. However, these situations seemed to quickly become everyday life at the ward.

SCP3: No, maybe the very first time I heard it was medication information. Maybe I thought a little…, maybe I thought a little extra about it when I was with the patient. But other than that, I have not thought about it. I do not think I have behaved any differently. At least not thought about it.

SCP1: No, I gave medication information to a patient. I remember there was a pharmacist there. I think I would have done that anyway. /…/

N2: It has not made any difference. You got used to it very quickly too. /…/ But I would be if there are physicians in the room as well if I provide medication information. So you get used to it quickly.   (Focus group 1)

AN: I can be a little preoccupied with the girls. I'm kind of like that. Eventually I relaxed and was myself. /…/
Moderator: But if I understand you correctly, it was something that disappeared after a while, right?
N2: Yes, it kind of became more natural.
N3: Yes.

(Focus group 2)

The observers thought that rather than the presence of observers, stressing situations and lack of staff had an impact on HCPs' communication about medications.

The observers stated that in the beginning some HCPs had explained their behavior toward the patient immediately after the observed encounter.

O3: And I understand that certain physicians when leaving a room would say "now I said that because" and that they wanted to defend what they did, I understand that. But when you have done it a few times, maybe that effect disappears. But I think it's going to be there anyway, I think….

As seen above, there seems to have been an observer effect in the observation study, but both observers and the observed stated that it lessened with time, which suggests that *habituation* took place.[11,12]

The observer effect is usually thought to make people behave in a way that is more in line with what is socially desired. Hence, patients could have been exposed to better communication about medications as a consequence of the observations. As the observer effect diminishes with time, the pros and possible cons of the observations would not have lasted for long. Actually, both HCPs and patients considered the consequences for patients to have been small or nonexisting.

From the above, a hypothesis is that habituation takes less time in hospitals than in other settings, again since the context includes different groups of people (e.g., students) commonly observing HCP-patient encounters.

The (native) observers: Pharmacists and young women

The characteristics of observers can influence the observer effect, and use of native observers are suggested as a measure to counteract this effect. In the observation study, the observers were young, female, and pharmacists/students.

Many HCPs reported a feeling of safety, as they already "knew the observers," i.e., were familiar with clinical pharmacists at the ward. This can be illustrated by the fact that, outside observations, the observers were asked questions about medication use (see more under Study design below). The observers proffered a potential reason in that the HCPs were used to having clinical pharmacists in the interdisciplinary team, and hence forgot that they had an "observer role."

The observers thought that the fact that they were relatively young women and students reduced the intimidating effect on the HCPs compared to if they had, e.g., been an SCP.

HCPs described the observers overall as humble, nonobtrusive, and neutral. Also, that they seemed to "*understand the hospital culture*," and "*respected challenging situations*," for example, knew when to walk out of the room.

HCPs were used to clinical pharmacists working at the ward, which might have lessened the observer effect, i.e., even if the specific observers were mainly new, what they represented (pharmacists and students) was not. The characteristics of the observers has been described as important (e.g., profession, sex, age, ethnicity, and social class).[12,15,20] It has also been concluded from interview studies that the social status of the researcher has an impact (deference, social alignment) and that "…respondents' perceptions of the interviewer [their profession/social status] influenced the interview interactions."[20] Thus, in order to lessen the observer effect, it is important that observers are both native and nonthreatening to any hierarchy so as not to provoke performance anxiety among participants.[12]

Study design, nonobtrusive, and minimal interaction—Relations and observing the observers

The observation study was designed as an overt, but nonparticipant observation study. Therefore, the observed were aware of the observers, but the observers strived for not interacting in the observed encounters.[12] When observing, observers tried to place themselves somewhere in the room where they would not interfere with the HCP-patient encounter, hence a strategy to be nonobtrusive. This was also reported by HCPs who described observers as standing in the background, taking notes.

> N3: They kept very much to themselves in the background. Very quiet. Almost invisible.
> N2: I think they were very professional in the way they worked.
> N1: They have been very nice. Very sweet, all of them.
>
> (Focus group 3)

Also, patients reported that the observers were nonobtrusive, "*just standing in the background*" (P5), or

> I almost didn't see you [the observers] /…/ I think it was fine /…/ you didn't interfere with anything, you just were there
>
> (P6)

In the HCP focus groups there was much discussion about what the observers actually did, and it seemed clear that HCPs had been thinking about this. Much of their reflections were in regard to the time observers spent just waiting, which was seen as most of the time they spent at the ward—or as a patient said: "*you were in guard at the door!*" (P5).

> N3: But they sit mostly out in the corridor, don't they? I've seen them mostly there. Outside the room. /…/
> SCP2: I think they just waited, right?
> N3: I do not know, they are just sitting there.
>
> (Focus group 1)

There were discussions in the HCP focus groups about *what* the observers had observed and this was, according to the HCPs "everything," even though they earlier had agreed that the study was about medications.

Another aspect of the observers sitting in the ward corridor was, according to the HCPs, that people from outside the ward asked about who they were, mainly staff from other wards who happened to see them. The HCPs then reported just informing whoever asked that these were observers working on a research project. The fact that the observers wore yellow t-shirts, with "observer" written on them was seen as positive in several ways. First, that one could actually read what they were (the word observer in large print). Second, that the color differed from the HCPs mostly dressed in white, so that observers were not taken for HCPs; and third, that it was clear to all when the observers entered into a patient room.

> N1: Yes, because it's okay. Everyone is wondering what's going on. If it is a white coat, all patients and relatives come and ask for help. If it says "I'm just there", then everyone else knows it too.
> AN: Yes, fine to wear.

N2: And yellow color stands out. "Observer". Clearly what the role is. So there was not much doubt. I think they got to sit pretty much in peace.

(Focus group 3)

Minimal interaction between observers and observed is a strategy suggested to decrease the observer effect.[11] This was the practice of observers, and also what HCPs reported. HCPs stated that they had mainly not talked to the observers during the observations. Still, some said they had tried to ask medication-related questions but received a reply from observers that they were only there to observe and could not help.

N3: So I kind of tried to consult and hear if they [i.e. the observers] agreed with me. But I was told that "no, I don't want to answer". They were just supposed to observe without providing any more information. They expect me as a nurse to know what I am supposed to. I do not know. But if you ask them any questions, they said why they could not answer it.

(Focus group 3)

Some communication had, however, taken place outside observations. Some HCPs reported having asked the observers outside the patient's room in regard to both medical issues, as well as practical, or other advice. This was typically by saying which patient they were going to see (when there were several patients in one room) so that the observers should know if it was the patient being observed or not.

N2: And so when we were going into a triple room, I tried to communicate a little with them before we went in, so that they understood if it was "that patient" or someone else. Because it was a little difficult for them to understand whether they should join in or not, when there are three or two others in the room. So that was fine.

(Focus group 2)

This was confirmed by the observers, who reported that after a while they understood some of the HCPs without having to speak to them, especially regarding practical issues, such as if the observer should enter the room or not. The observers also verified that during the observations they were asked questions for example about if a medicine had a specific medical indication or not. Additionally, when not observing they were asked questions about medications, typically for a specific patient, and not necessarily those observed. The observers also got questions about the reasons for them being there.

HCPs also reported a feeling of awkwardness, wondering whether they should debrief or not with the observers after the observed encounter. They compared it to having training of students, to whom they always explain everything about their behavior, whereas the observers *"just stood there taking notes"* with no further interactions with the HCPs. The observers, on the other hand, felt being in somebody's way and disturbing the relations among HCPs and patients, especially when sensitive topics where discussed. According to both HCPs and observers, the HCPs and the observing pharmacists interacted nonverbally, such as with a smile of understanding if something humorous had occurred or with a nod if the HCPs wanted their confirmation in some medication related question. Several HCPs stated that a possibility to interact more may have made some situations less awkward. One pointed out that they recognized the observers' faces, but knew nothing about their names or them as persons, even though they had spent months at the ward.

According to the observers, they and the patients seldom spoke with one another during the observations. Still, the observers built relations with the patients outside and during the observing situations: by eye contact or small talk in the corridor. Patients were reported to use metaphors like *"my guardian"* to describe the observers' role during their hospital stays. One of the patients said she saw one of the observers *"almost as my daughter"* (P7).

Even though the observers were instructed not to interact with the observed, interactions seemingly took place. On the one hand, the observers seemed to have avoided answering medication-related questions, which seems to have made some HCPs feel somewhat insecure. On the other hand, all groups of participants talked about their "silent relationship" with some warmth. Practical nonverbal communication took place according to both observers and HCPs, hence relationships were built. At least some of the patients also built relationships with the observers. The length of observations per patient might have had an impact, but seeing that patients met so many HCPs during their stays (up to 50 were recorded in the observation study), for some patients the observers were the most familiar person to them during their hospital stay, and their presence per se created some feeling of security.

It is difficult to conclude on the impact of the minimal interaction strategy in this particular case as (HCPs') insecurity might lead to passivity. In any case, it is essential to have a common approach, when being several observers. The silent relationship, acknowledged by all parts (also patients) shows that rapport can be created without that many words, between observers and observed. The suggested minimal interaction strategy should be discussed in relation to specific observation studies. It is not possible to avoid relating to other human beings when spending so much time in the same (limited) space, so in cases where observers are physically "in the same room" the relevant question is not whether relations are built, but rather, what do these relations look like and how can they impact study results.

Field entry

There was no conscious strategy for field entry, i.e., how to enter into when observations take place. However, it seems as the *reciprocity model* of gaining entry was unconsciously used.[12] This model implies that there are reasons for the observed to cooperate, as there is something in it for them. In this case, the focus on developing work in a way that would benefit patients would be a mutual goal for all parts involved, including the observers. HCPs also mentioned that they did not associate the study with judging them as individual professionals. Instead, they felt that they and the observers (i.e., pharmacists) were part of the same interdisciplinary team working toward the same goal, wanting to improve patient care.

Patton writes that "While the observer must learn how to behave in the new setting, the participants [the observed] in that setting are deciding how to behave toward the observer."[12, p. 253] In this specific case, using native observers certainly helped, as they at least to some degree knew how behavior works in the context. Also behaving in a respectful way and the silent relationships established would have contributed to the observers being tolerated when entering the field.

The observed patients and HCPs also observed the observers: they speculated about what the observers were doing, what they observed, what they wrote. HCPs also tried to help them, and the patients expressed warm feelings toward them. The latter also related to observer characteristics (age and gender), like with the patient who called one of the observers "my daughter." To be noted is that the silent relationship between HCPs and observers was, among other things, used to protect patient integrity, which is an ethical challenge when conducting observations of vulnerable groups.

Following up your observation study

The reported research aimed to explore the observer effect through HCPs and patients' experiences of being observed in a hospital setting, and in addition, observers' experiences from an observation study. Some of the factors suggested to minimize the observer effect are habituation, no sharing of study hypothesis, use of native observers, minimal interactions, less obtrusive observation tools, and awareness of field entry.[11,12,14,15] In the observation study, several, but not all of these measures were taken into consideration. To that end, this chapter has attempted to show the experiences and reflections of observed and observers, and in addition to reflect on consequences of how the observation study was presented and conducted.

The follow up study (i.e., focus groups and interviews) has several limitations; these are further discussed in Svensberg et al.[21] However, to summarize the results, there seems to have been some initial observer effects, such as a temporary modification of HCPs medication communication behavior in the presence of observers who were pharmacist/students, i.e., native to the context. However, this diminished after the first observation encounters; hence, habituation took place. This rather quick habituation could partly be because patients and HCPs in the hospital context are used to having extra persons, for example students, present in their encounters. Being an inpatient in a hospital often means constant surveillance, if not by HCPs so by other patients in the same room. Additionally, HCPs work in an "open landscape" where they can see each other, and in addition often have other people watching them (students, patients, next of kin). The "unthreatening" appearance of the observers seems to have contributed to diminishing the observer effect in this specific context. In relation to the characteristics and social status, trained students might be suitable in order to decrease the observer effect.

Even though a minimal interaction strategy was used, observers and the observed still built rapport. Medication communication in hospital settings is a complex behavior. The complexity can per se make it difficult totally to change behavior, and hence contribute to diminish the observer effect.

As the observer effect depends on so many factors, it is difficult to generalize from or transfer results. Some aspects such as presence of student observers can probably be transferred to other contexts. However, when planning any observation study it is important to take into account the factors that are present in the specific study. How observers enter the field, how they behave, their knowledge about the context and culture, how the study is presented are all part of if the observed accept both the study and the observers. All of this is important for the success of the observations and hence the validity of the results. Furthermore, the researcher should reflect beforehand on the complexity of the behavior being studied in relation to the study aim, potential effect of revealing the study aim, appropriate dress codes, the study context and how accustomed the people under study are to natural "observers."

It is suggested that an important strategy to understand the impact of the observer effect poststudy is through explicitly interviewing the observed and the observers about their experiences, using someone not connected to the observation study. This could be done immediately after observations—to reduce recall bias—but also while/after analyzing data to further explore the presence, nature and impact of an observer effect in the specific study. This is as aspects important for data interpretation can be revealed.

Questions for further discussion

1. In this chapter, we have presented an example of the observer effect at a hospital ward. Discuss how you think this differs from the observer effect in other settings, for example a classroom or a pharmacy.
2. Discuss how you think you would react to being observed at your workplace or when studying (or any other activity you do). Elaborate around factors such as type of observation, observer characteristics, observation intensity and what would be observed.

Application exercise/scenario

Design a hypothetical observation study. Focus areas could for example be medication practices in a nursing home, what people do in the laboratory, or staff-customer interaction in the pharmacy. Describe an aim, a setting, who would observe, for how long, what would be observed and how. Especially elaborate on how you would try to counteract the observer effect.

After doing this, reflect on what strengths the study would possibly have, and what limitations, not least regarding the observer effect.

Acknowledgments

The authors want to thank Helene Berg Lie and Kajsa Bengtsson who conducted patient interviews, further Anne Mette Njaastad and Mina Dybdal, who helped with recruitment for the focus groups.

The follow-up study was partly funded by the Hospital Pharmacies Enterprise, South Eastern Norway. The funding body had no involvement in any parts of the study.

References

1. Da Costa FA. Covert and overt observations. In: Babar ZUD, ed. *Pharmacy Practice Research Methods.* Singapore: Springer Singapore; 2020.
2. Seiberth JM, Moritz K, Herrmann NS, Bertsche T, Schiek S. What influences the information exchange during self-medication consultations in community pharmacies? A non-participant observation study. *Res Soc Adm Pharm.* 2022. https://doi.org/10.1016/j.sapharm.2021.03.015 [in press].
3. Trausch N, Green JA. Direct observation of telephone communication between community pharmacies and prescribers in New Zealand. *Int J Clin Pharm.* 2018;40:1005–1009.
4. Flink M, Ekstedt M. Planning for the discharge, not for patient self-management at home—an observational and interview study of hospital discharge. *Int J Integr Care.* 2017;17(6):1.
5. Laugaland K, Aase K, Waring J. Hospital discharge of the elderly—an observational case study of functions, variability and performance-shaping factors. *BMC Health Serv Res.* 2014;14:365.
6. Ekdahl AW, Linderholm M, Hellström I, Andersson L, Friedrichsen M. 'Are decisions about discharge of elderly hospital patients mainly about freeing blocked beds?' A qualitative observational study. *BMJ Open.* 2012;2(6):e002027.
7. Dyrstad DN, Laugaland KA, Storm M. An observational study of older patients' participation in hospital admission and discharge—exploring patient and next of kin perspectives. *J Clin Nurs.* 2015;24(11–12):1693–1706.
8. Fylan B, Marques I, Ismail H, et al. Gaps, traps, bridges and props: a mixed-methods study of resilience in the medicines management system for patients with heart failure at hospital discharge. *BMJ Open.* 2019;9(2):e023440.
9. Pollack AH, Backonja U, Miller AD, et al. Closing the gap: supporting patients' transition to self-management after hospitalization. In: *Proceedings of the SIGCHI Conference on Human Factors in Computing Systems CHI Conference 2016*; 2016:5324–5336.
10. Bowling A. *Research Methods in Health—Investigating Health and Health Services.* 2nd ed. Milton Keynes, UK: Open University Press; 2002.
11. Robson C. *Real World Research: A Resource for Social Scientists and Practitioner-Researchers.* 4th ed. Blackwell Publishers; 2016.
12. Patton MQ. *Qualitative Research & Evaluation Methods.* 3rd ed. Thousand Oaks, CA: Sage Publications; 2002.
13. McCambridge J, Witton J, Elbourne DR. Systematic review of the Hawthorne effect: new concepts are needed to study research participation effects. *J Clin Epidemiol.* 2014;67:267–277. https://doi.org/10.1016/j.jclinepi.2013.08.015.
14. Chen LF, Vander Weg MW, Hofmann DA, Reisinger HS. The Hawthorne effect in infection prevention and epidemiology. *Infect Control Hosp Epidemiol.* 2015;36:1444–1450. https://doi.org/10.1017/ice.2015.216.
15. Goodwin MA, Stange KC, Zyzanski SJ, Crabtree BF, Borawski EA, Flocke SA. The Hawthorne effect in direct observation research with physicians and patients. *J Eval Clin Pract.* 2017;23:1322–1328. https://doi.org/10.1111/jep.12781.
16. Fernald DH, Coombs L, DeAlleaume L, West D, Parnes B. An assessment of the Hawthorne effect in practice-based research. *J Am Board Fam Med.* 2012;25:83–86. https://doi.org/10.3122/jabfm.2012.01.110019.

17. Purssell E, Drey N, Chudleigh J, Creedon S, Gould DJ. The Hawthorne effect on adherence to hand hygiene in patient care. *J Hosp Infect.* 2020;106:311–317.

18. Paradis E, Sutkin G. Beyond a good story: from Hawthorne effect to reactivity in health professions education research. *Med Educ.* 2017;51:31–39.

19. Levitt SD, List JA. Was there really a Hawthorne effect at the Hawthorne plant? An analysis of the original illumination experiments. *Am Econ J Appl Econ.* 2011;3:224–238.

20. Richards H, Emslie C. The 'doctor' or the 'girl from the University'? Considering the influence of professional roles on qualitative interviewing. *Fam Pract.* 2000;17:71–75.

21. Svensberg K, Kalleberg BG, Mathiesen L, Andersson Y, Eidhammer Rognan S, Kälvemark Sporrong S. The observer effect in a hospital setting—experiences from the observed and the observers. *Res Soc Adm Pharm.* 2021;17:2136–2144. https://doi.org/10.1016/j.sapharm.2021.07.011.

22. Eidhammer Rognan S, Kälvemark Sporrong S, Bengtsson K, et al. Discharge processes and medicines communication from the patient position. A qualitative study at an internal medicines ward in Norway. *Health Expect.* 2021;1–13. https://doi.org/10.1111/hex.13232.

23. Eidhammer Rognan S, Kälvemark Sporrong S, Bengtsson K, et al. Empowering the patient? Medicines communication during hospital discharge: a qualitative study at an internal medicines ward in Norway. *BMJ Open.* 2021;11:e044850.

24. Kitzinger J. Qualitative research: introducing focus groups. *BMJ.* 1995;311:299.

25. Malterud K. Systematic text condensation: a strategy for qualitative analysis. *Scand J Public Health.* 2012;40:795–805.

26. Manias E. Medication communication: a concept analysis. *J Adv Nurs.* 2010;66:933–943.

Chapter 19

An introduction to how realist research can inform pharmacy practice and policy

M.J. Twigg[a], K. Luetsch[b], I. Maidment[c], and D. Rowett[d]

[a]School of Pharmacy, University of East Anglia, Norwich, United Kingdom, [b]School of Pharmacy, The University of Queensland, St Lucia, QLD, Australia, [c]School of Life and Health Sciences, Aston University, Birmingham, United Kingdom, [d]Clinical & Health Sciences, University of South Australia, Adelaide, SA, Australia

Objectives

- Describe the reasons why a realist approach is useful for pharmacy practice research.
- Describe the key components of a realist logic of analysis: context, mechanisms, and outcomes.
- Reflect on the necessary steps and factors to formulate and answer your research question using realist logic.
- Apply some of the key concepts of realist approaches to a research question in your area of practice.

Outline

The purpose of this chapter is to give the reader an overview of realist approaches to evaluation and synthesis in pharmacy practice research. It will provide a brief introduction and signpost the reader to key articles that have been published in the last 20 years by leaders in the field. These articles have been chosen as accessible examples for someone new to this theory-driven, interpretive approach; they explain key concepts in realist research or illustrate examples of how these principles have been applied. Clinicians and academics interested in this area will find a wide range of resources to guide them and may start their realist journey by being involved in a realist research project, for example, being a member of a stakeholder advisory group.

Two case studies then further exemplify how realist approaches assist in developing a program theory of when and why pharmacy services may be effective and how recipients of health care services make choices.

Background

The design and introduction of pharmacy services and programs is increasingly framed by implementation science and its theory-based approaches.[1,2] Theories, models and frameworks informing the development of health care services are also utilized by pharmacy researchers and practitioners to facilitate the translation of best evidence into practice.[3,4] Even when theory-driven design and implementation processes lead to initial success, the long-term sustainability of programs is not guaranteed and may rely on balancing fidelity with adaptability.[5]

The majority of programs aimed at improving pharmacy practice, health care and health outcomes are complex interventions, considering the quantity and interlinkage of components within the experimental interventions, the difficulty and range of behaviors required by those delivering or participating in the intervention, the organizational levels they target and the range and variability of outcomes. Once programs are adopted more widely into practice the context of their implementation begins to vary, and a significant degree of flexibility or tailoring to context is inevitable.[6] The triple threat of complex pharmacy programs and their reliance on participants with varying motivations and capacities that play out in complex, adaptive systems, confounds our understanding of how and why their effectiveness in routine day-to-day practice can be achieved. This may be related to the evidence, which is selected in informing the design and implementation of programs. Experimental or quasiexperimental designs are necessary to establish effectiveness of interventions,[7] but will inevitably limit considerations of the complexity of most pharmacy practice programs and consequent service models. Effect size can tell us whether a program has achieved its intended or desired benefits, or caused inadvertent harm, in

Contemporary Research Methods in Pharmacy and Health Services. https://doi.org/10.1016/B978-0-323-91888-6.00041-7

271

the context and at the time it was delivered, but still leaves policy makers and health care funders guessing how similar programs or services will affect different populations in different contexts.[8]

Closing the loop between evidence-informed, theory-based implementation and evaluation calls for evidence syntheses and evaluation research which develop theory by analyzing and incorporating complexity rather than ignoring it, informing future program and implementation design. Implementation design and evaluations which pay attention to the multiple interacting influences that contribute to a particular outcome, increase the chances of recognizing and eliciting which parts of a program and its implementation are pivotal to its success, which external factors influence the way it works, who will benefit most from it and under which circumstances.[9] A focus on emergent causality will potentially answer many questions which experimental studies designed with a linear, cause-and-effect model in mind are unable to answer.[10]

Realist research offers particularly useful approaches to inform theory-driven evaluation and implementation. Realist syntheses of existing evidence and literature can guide the design and implementation of a program by developing models of causality and theories which explain why it may show effect, particularly when effect relies on social contingency, as in the case of healthcare programs.[11] Realist evaluations of programs then assist in testing or refining these program theories, establishing new ones and creating further causal links to observed outcomes.

The role of realism

Many authors have discussed the provenance of realism which contemporarily is applied in health care and social policy evaluation, and there are a number of readings, for a teaser,[12,13] overview,[14–16] or in-depth discussion.[11,17,18] For its discussion on how to conduct realist research and how it could advance knowledge, enrich pharmacy practice evaluations and policy design, this chapter draws on scientific realism in evaluation research as described and applied by Pawson and Tilley[11,19,20] in addition to two case studies of applied realist research. These two cases, based on our own research, are examples of a realist synthesis of existing literature and an evaluation related to medicines management.

Generative causation

A major distinction between realist and traditional (experimental and positivist) pharmacy practice research is in the definition and exploration of causation.[21] Within traditional experimental research paradigms, causation is taken as a direct relationship between the intervention and the outcome. Randomized controlled trials and systematic reviews/metaanalyses are constructed to "control" for certain variables in order to increase the likelihood of identifying "cause and effect." Randomized controlled trials (RCTs) compare "intervention on" with "intervention off" and may produce statistically accurate evidence of efficacy or effectiveness, but often leave the user none the wiser about where to target resources, how to adapt the tested intervention to different settings or maximize impact. However, scientific realism argues that this cause and effect is less linear, context-dependent, and acts through (often) multiple mechanisms that cannot be directly observed. By understanding how modifying the context allows or facilitates particular mechanisms to "fire" (activate) leads to a more nuanced understanding of how outcomes and outcome patterns are achieved, rather than just whether they *were* achieved. This moves the research from a *correlational* causation perspective to a *generative* causation perspective, which can prove to be more informative when trying to understand how an intervention works in any given setting and therefore how it can be adapted in other settings with different contexts. A realist approach to research can be thought of as applying realist logic to analysis rather than a specific set of methodologies or methods. Indeed, realist research is agnostic to methods—it is reflected in how relevant data are collected, analyzed, and interpreted.

Contexts, mechanisms and outcomes

Following the argument that realist research focuses on generative rather than correlational causation means that there are some key conventions surrounding data analysis, interpretation, and presentation. A realist logic of analysis focuses on the context in which an intervention or program is implemented, the mechanisms it activates in these specific contexts and the outcomes which are generated. These elements can be summarized in a contexts (C), mechanisms (M) and outcomes (O) heuristic to explain the contingency of outcomes on how mechanisms are activated in specific contexts. Other additions can be found in the literature to supplement these, including intervention (I), agency (Ag) and actor (Ac). However, these are not commonplace, and researchers need to think carefully about introducing additional variables into the causal pathway and how they influence the causal chain of events. A brief definition for C, M and O is below:

Contexts: this refers to the environment, culture, infrastructure, people, expertise, experience, relationships, behavior, and resources (to name a few) that exist in a particular setting where the intervention is implemented. Changes in these contexts result in the mechanism "firing" and so understanding context is a fundamental part of undertaking realist research.

Mechanisms: these are a central tenet of a realist approach to research and are essential to linking contexts with outcomes. They are often hidden and not always observable. They can be thought of as "firing" or "activating" in response to a particular context in order to produce an outcome or outcome pattern. A mechanism is said to exist at all times but only becomes detectable when it is activated in a particular context. Further reading on the definition of mechanisms and how they relate to mechanisms in other schools of research can be found here.[22–24]

Outcomes and outcome patterns: these are the resultant effects of context-dependent mechanisms "firing." They can be proximal or distal and often describe the intermediate outcomes along an intervention implementation chain, in other words, they do not need to solely relate to the primary outcome that would traditionally be reported in an RCT.

Once identified, these Cs, Ms., and Os need to be configured to properly achieve the goal of forming a theory of generative causation. While recognizing and reporting a list of Cs, Ms. and Oscan be useful, only their linkage through CMO configurations allows us to develop a theory of when or under which circumstance (C), an outcome will occur because a mechanism has been activated.[25–27] Examples of these can be found in the literature,[28,29] with Jagosh et al. outlining that often an outcome in one CMO configuration can, in turn, be a context in another.

Program theory and middle range theory

The CMO configurations (CMOcs) that are formed when contexts (C) are connected with outcomes (O) through mechanisms (M) are referred to as program theories (PT), and there is specific guidance relating to the level at which these can be "pitched." Firstly, the use of the term "program theory" can be confusing, as it can relate to different levels of theory. For example, one author may refer to an individual CMOc as a PT, whereas others may use PT to refer to a collection of CMOcs that have, themselves, been configured together to illustrate an overall theory of the intervention being examined (see case one below for an example of this approach). This latter approach of outlining the overall program aligns more closely with the concept of a logic model as it usually charts all components of the intervention and the interactivity between them. However, the difference is that a realist approach uses the configuration of C, M and O to express the theory of how the program works, why, how and in what circumstances.

An important thing to note is that at whatever level the PT is located they are ideally framed as a "middle range theory." There are many chapters and papers exploring the notion of a middle range theory, with some key ones cited here.[11,30] Middle range theory is one that is located in the middle range; it is not too abstract (by trying to account for everything in that field, e.g., theoretical domains framework, diffusion of innovation theory, theory of planned behavior, etc.) nor too specific (by focusing on one very specific context, setting, environment, person, etc.). By positioning these CMOcs in the middle range, the researcher develops theories that on the one hand allow generalization but can also be empirically tested. As a test of this, a reviewer of realist research has to be able to read the PT/CMOcs and think of it as a theory explaining the phenomena under investigation but also see how it can be tested in future work.

The use of substantive theory (e.g., theory of planned behavior, communities of practice) in realist syntheses and evaluation is also important and can be used to inform individual PTs, CMOcs, or overarching PTs. An example is shown in case study two below where Normalization Process Theory[31] has been used to assist Maidment et al. with their understanding of medication management in older people.[32,33] This is a clear example of where substantive theory, located at a higher level of abstraction than a middle range theory, can be helpful in guiding the interpretation of the data and helping to explain mechanisms or outcomes.

Development of program theories

The overall aim of realist research is to develop PTs (or series of them), and this can be achieved in a number of different ways. In both realist reviews and evaluation, this is usually prefaced with an initial PT that may be arrived at through a scoping review or stakeholder consultation. A realist review is often followed by a realist evaluation that will use the already developed PT to inform the data collection. The realist analysis of new data then will confirm/refute/refine the PT developed from existing literature. In contrast to traditional systematic reviews of experimental studies, realist reviews are deliberately iterative in their process and require a degree of forward and backward movement through the literature and data. As such, realist reviews, in particular, often appear less linear as the process of searching, extracting and analyzing merge into one as the PT evolves over the course of the study. Booth et al. have written extensively on this subject and their description of the iterative process of literature searching and review is described well elsewhere.[34,35]

Final presentation and critique

Throughout the process of realist research consideration must be given to the presentation of the data in the final report. A particularly helpful resource here are the RAMESES standards[36] which can be found at www.ramesesproject.org/. These standards are central to the development, conduct and reporting of realist research and provide guidance throughout a project.

Case studies

What follows are two case studies as examples of realist research from within pharmacy practice. These case studies are illustrative approaches to realist research; there are many others available, which have been cited in this chapter.

Case study 1

A realist synthesis of pharmacist-conducted medication reviews in primary care after leaving hospital: what works for whom, and why?

Overview

Luetsch et al. conducted a realist synthesis to establish for whom, under which circumstances, how and why a pharmacist-conducted medication review (MR) may be of benefit for people who return to primary care after a hospital admission.[37] Systematic reviews regularly attest to the heterogeneity between studied MR programs, interventions and the outcomes they achieve and a realist synthesis potentially explains some of the ambiguity. The aim was to add to the significant body of work in this area by examining what leads to observed outcomes (whether desired or undesired by program designers and implementers). Making sense of how an MR functions as a healthcare intervention in a given context, which mechanisms it activates to produce context-sensitive outcomes facilitates the identification of components or aspects which may be essential in achieving benefits for patients, healthcare professionals, and the system in which it is implemented. Identification of underlying, generative mechanisms which are triggered by particular aspects of an intervention or program, in this case an MR, in specific contexts, lies at the center of realist enquiry.[24]

Realist review of the literature

An initial program theory was developed, supported by a literature search, experience and discussions by the authors, and framed by the steps patients and healthcare professionals take in completing an MR. This initial theory centered on three questions that summarized the patient and professional journey when initiating or participating in the MR process: what makes it happen?, what happens? and what happens next?. This "scaffold" allowed the team to map their journeys and points of contact and interaction, eliciting how and why they chose to engage with invitations to participate in an MR, using guidance from realist training materials and literature then provided the structure for the extraction of comprehensive data supporting the refinement into a final program theory.[22]

One of the main differences to other reviews conducted in this area was the systematic retrieval of a broad range of documents.[17] These included trial protocols, which often make underlying assumptions of why an MR should have a positive effect explicit, conference abstracts of mainly qualitative studies, which provided stakeholder experiences and opinions, program evaluation reports, which yielded fine-grained detail supporting the inference of mechanisms, and PhD theses, granting insight into why interventions were not as successful as anticipated. This was in addition to studies customarily included in systematic reviews, which usually investigated existing service models or adaptations in the posthospital-discharge setting. These, however, often provided little detail regarding the exact nature of the intervention or program, how patients and healthcare professionals engaged with the MR and each other. The inclusion of other types of literature and policy documents allowed the research team to fill gaps and compare intention with actual implementation in the process of generating program theory.

Instead of appraising the quality of documents under consideration through application of standard criteria, their inclusion into the realist synthesis was predicated on their relevance to the development of theory, with relevance shifting during different developmental phases. Although even poorly designed studies can yield information which adds to or supports theory,[38] rigor in intervention or study design and implementation was assessed by examining whether methods used to generate data were appropriate to answer the research questions, were employed with reliability and consistency and could credibly generate reported findings. Additionally, the trustworthiness of selected data was considered by ascertaining whether they had been obtained empirically and through a cross-examination of outcomes of similar studies conducted on MR in general.[17] When documents seemed highly relevant but lacked depth of information, authors were contacted to obtain additional or missing detail to enable judgments of trustworthiness and rigor.

Development of program theory—Literature synthesis

Once data relating to contexts (C), intervention (I), outcomes (O), and potential mechanisms (M) were extracted, they were iteratively linked into CMO configurations (CMOcs). This process is central to realist logic, as it is not only the identification of relevant CMOcs but also their linkage and configuration which establishes generative causation and underpins program theory development as to what works for whom, under which circumstances and why. At this stage all researchers involved in the synthesis had to be prepared and familiar with the literature under investigation and realist philosophy of science to engage in the stimulating academic endeavor of discussing and arguing over how interventions influence context, contexts, mechanisms and outcomes link together, when and how a mechanism becomes context in a different CMOc, and which of the many CMOcs to finally abstract into program theory. This high level of engagement may differ from approaching research meetings where one person reports and others agree or tweak. At times realist expertise external to the discipline of pharmacy could have been of benefit, to arbitrate when it was difficult to come to an agreement, or challenge potential bias when the small research group created an echo chamber of similar voices.

The final program theory based on the synthesis of 66 documents points to components that would appear essential for the success of an MR performed by pharmacists for patients in the community after they have been discharged from the hospital. The realist synthesis allowed the identification of contextual and program mechanisms as causal factors which make a MR work. Based on the available documentation and literature, it describes the structures which ideally are put in place to maximize review benefits for people who left hospital but also their agency and choices within the MR process. Many outcome differences were accounted for through consideration of nuances in medication review program activities and implementation, but also differences in the contexts of their implementation.

Implications

The program theory, described here as a diagram of interlinked CMOcs (Fig. 1) could be applicable to most health systems in which pharmacists, patients, and physicians navigate the transition from hospital to community.

A number of key messages based on the program theory are of relevance to future MR program design, implementation and policy development (Box 1).

Case study 2: MEMORABLE[a]

Overview

MEMORABLE (MEdication Management in Older people: Realist Approaches Based on Literature and Evaluation) took a realist approach to synthesizing literature and the personal accounts of older people living in the community, their families (informal carers), and practitioners of their behaviors managing medicines, relationships with and support by others at multiple layers of health and social care.[32,33] An understanding of how older people and their carers manage complex medication regimens then provided the basis for a framework outlining medication management as a complex process and recommendations for interventions and improvements.

Stakeholder involvement

MEMORABLE was supported by working groups providing governance and management support, of which two were instrumental in taking a realist approach:

1. A multidisciplinary research team providing oversight and expertise, including older people, practitioners, academics with expertise in realist and information management methodologies and experience in patient and public involvement and engagement (PPIE).

a. MEMORABLE was funded by the HS&DR Programme (project number 15/137/ 01) and the full report is available in NIHR Journals Library. It presents independent research funded by the National Institute for Health Research (NIHR). The views and opinions expressed by authors in this publication are those of the authors and do not necessarily reflect those of the NHS, the NIHR, NETSCC, the HS&DR Programme, or the Department of Health and Social Care. The views and opinions expressed by the interviewees are those of the interviewees and do not necessarily reflect those of the authors, those of the NHS, the NIHR, NETSCC, the HS&DR Programme or the Department of Health and Social Care.

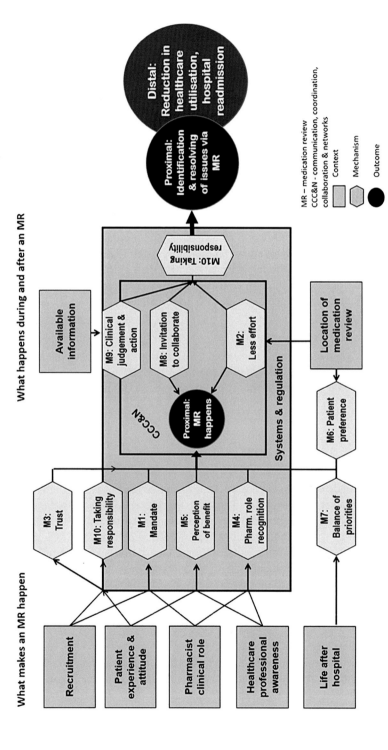

FIG. 1 Program theory of pharmacist-conducted medication reviews in primary care after leaving hospital. (*Reproduced with permission from Luetsch K, Rowett D, Twigg MJ. A realist synthesis of pharmacist-conducted medication reviews in primary care after leaving hospital: what works for whom and why?* BMJ Qual Saf 2021;30(5):418–430, copyright CC BY-NC, BMJ Publishing Group Ltd.)

BOX 1 Key messages for medication reviews after hospital discharge

- Ensure stakeholders have awareness of and perceive a benefit from the medication review.
- Accommodate patients' preferences, needs and capabilities in terms of timing and location.
- Coordinate the medication review process.
- Ensure pharmacists performing the medication review have access to relevant patient information.
- Encourage or enable pharmacists to establish collaboration with other healthcare professionals involved in the medication review and to take responsibility for outcomes.

---

2. A stakeholder group of practitioners, older people and their family (informal) carers. They provided advice and feedback to the research group on the veracity of emerging evidence, program theories and proposed interventions, ensuring recommendations were appropriate, practicable and potentially making a difference for everyone involved.

Both groups advised on the dissemination strategy, which was proactive from the start of the project and added to its credibility. This strategy involved creating a website, registering the study protocol on PROSPERO, and publishing the results in a peer-reviewed journal,[39] which enabled the principal investigator to utilize publicly available documents. This strategy also helped to establish credibility for MEMORABLE when discussing it with stakeholders and potential participants.

The realist research process

Developing the research protocol and early informal theorizing by stakeholders assisted in establishing an initial program theory about how medication management might work for older people. This guided an initial systematic search and review of literature. Potential explanatory factors were extracted and used to develop context, mechanism, and outcome configurations (CMOcs) related to the research questions. Searches were then extended iteratively, informed by initial findings and consequently established contexts and mechanisms, which, for example, included burden and shared decision making, and a subset of articles from the initial search containing causal accounts related to medication management was later included. Review of the literature led to refinement of CMOcs and mapping a tentative medication management process, supporting the development of a number of candidate program theories. Although several substantive theories of interest were considered at this stage, none could be sufficiently evidenced from the literature to support the complex process model which had been developed.

Realist evaluation

A realist evaluation exploring mechanisms and driving program theory development further was then added by conducting and analyzing 50 realist informed interviews with older people, family carers and practitioners. This added key strengths and innovation to MEMORABLE and encouraged stakeholders to directly articulate their "real world" challenges and capture the burden associated with medication management from their perspective. Realist interviews facilitate gleaning program theories in the early stages of development and later invite interviewees to comment on developing program theories, allowing researchers to refine and consolidate them.[40,41] These interviews substantially offset the limitations of the literature on the subject and allowed particular lines of inquiry to be followed up in more detail. However, they did increase the duration (and therefore cost of the project), due to the ethical approval processes and additional researcher time needed. Both data sources (literature synthesis and interviews) were then combined to establish theoretical understandings of medication management by older people.

Program theory development

Medication management, as an implementation process, was abstracted into a five-stage model (Table 1), breaking down the complexity of medication management processes.

These five stages were then categorized into overarching stages of medication management:

a. Individual stages (1, 3, and 4), where older people (sometimes with support from a family carer) balance routines, coping, and risks.

b. Interpersonal stages (2 and 5), where older people have contact with a practitioner, again sometimes with support from a family carer.

TABLE 1 Five stages of medication management.

Stage	Stage 1 Identifying the problem	Stage 2 Acquiring a diagnosis and/or medications	Stage 3 Starting, changing or stopping medications	Stage 4 Continuing to take medications	Stage 5 Reviewing/ reconciling medications
Who/ doing what	Older person identifies that something is wrong	Older person and practitioner agree on the problem and how to treat it. A prescription is issued and dispensed	Older person adjusts daily medication routine to include new medication and/or adjusts or omits current medication	Older person fits new routine into day-to-day life	Practitioner confirms safety and efficacy of medication Older person and practitioner agree appropriateness, adherence and fit with day-to-day life

Family (informal) carers can be involved at any stages

Having established the stages of medication management as complex interventions, Normalization Process Theory (NPT) was identified as an existing substantive theory to frame and explain processes and behaviors. NPT articulates how new activities are introduced and made both routine and are sustained through work by those involved.[31] Substantive theories can progress understanding when making sense of CMOcs and in this case NPT provided a lens and structure to understand the work required when managing medications at an individual, interpersonal and system level and was applied to each of the five stages.

The synthesis of a realist review of the literature and interview findings established that older people/family carers and practitioners may have different priorities in relation to medication management. Practitioners focused on process goals such as optimization, adherence, or deprescribing. Whereas quality of life, fitting medications into their day-to-day lives, and reducing the burden of medication management were important for older people.

Implications

A key finding of MEMORABLE was the relationship between workload associated with medication management and capacity (Table 2), how they fluctuated, and its impact in terms of burden on the older person. For example, workload increased with polypharmacy and capacity decreased with cognitive impairment; both were likely to increase overall burden, whereas burden decreased if the medication regimen was simplified.

Burden was often not obvious to practitioners. Older people developed and established routines in dealing with medications, when medications changed burden potentially increased, at least temporarily.

Two potential interventions were identified and proposed from MEMORABLE. First, because medication management burden is often hidden, it needs to be identified. Second, the provision of "individualized information" for older people and family carers, to enable them making sense of complex diagnoses and medications; and find ways to fit medication into their day-to-day lives, thus mitigating the substantial burden.

These findings informed key messages for practitioners to assess burden (Box 2).

TABLE 2 Relationship between workload, capacity and burden.

What capacity does the older person have? What is the workload?	Increasing/high capacity	Decreasing/low capacity
Increasing/high workload: may be high workload in general or may spike at times of change and uncertainty	Burden: coping	High burden: not coping—high workload and low capacity risk
Decreasing/low workload	No burden: coping	Burden: not coping—low capacity risk

---

BOX 2 Key messages for practice from MEMORABLE

When prescribers initiate a new medication or change a dose they should routinely address burden: "How are people coping with managing their medications?" "Will a change increase their medication management burden and how can we address it together so they can cope?"

Discussion

As illustrated by the case studies, realist research exhibits a degree of agnosticism with regards to the design and methods used to establish relevant contexts, mechanisms, and outcomes. Realism provides the underlying philosophy of science, with realist research questions informing the choice of methodological approach. This allows realist researchers to draw on a wide range of evidence and methods.[42] Many contributions to this book outline methods with relevance to realist research, by supporting the generation of trustworthy findings or ensuring rigor of intervention and study design.

The aim of most realist research, whether synthesis of existing evidence or evaluation of programs or behaviors, is to increase knowledge and certainty as to how and why interventions or programs work, while accepting that knowledge can only ever be partial and incomplete. As it is grounded in the acceptance and analysis of complexity the application of standardized formulae would pose the inherent danger of a technical or reductionist approach; dealing with complexity is complex in itself. Heterogeneity of programs, which is unavoidable even when they are implemented with exceptional consistency and fidelity, their desired and undesired outcomes, and the observations and varied findings of studies describing them reflect what actually happens in the real world. Attempts to standardize complex interventions, reducing their natural variation and controlling the context of their implementation may be necessary to establish initial effectiveness but will reach a limit, and at the same time limit the applicability, in the wider environment, of any findings derived from their observation and analysis. At the same time, realist logic can assist in the identification of essential ingredients in contexts and programs which facilitate the activation of mechanisms, which cause desired (or undesired) outcomes. For example, the realist synthesis of postdischarge MR identified mechanisms, which are ideally in place in various contexts and activated by the intervention, describing some of the essential ingredients of the MR process which are likely to lead to a beneficial outcome, e.g., a reduction in healthcare utilization. It also made clear that these have to be combined with sensitivity to context and responsiveness to emergence and rivalry. Valuing complexity, acknowledging uncertainty and variations of context mean recommendations for a standardized approach to MR are likely to be futile. Though the same ingredients may well be essential in many contexts, the exact recipe will be adjusted for local context and adaptations.

In its approach to data collection and analysis realist research integrates other theories that help to explain findings and underpin program theories. As MEMORABLE demonstrated, often substantive theories can help build the theory development in the specific real-world clinical environment under investigation, helping to explain what happens and why. The addition of a realist evaluation involving stakeholders aided the process of identifying the appropriate theory, which supported the generation of final program theory. Opening the treasure trove of existing social and scientific theories will allow pharmacy practice researchers to leave the confines of deterministic cause and effect models and empiricism behind, and gain new insights into how and why their programs work through a combination of theory-integrating and -driven evaluations and evidence syntheses.

Ultimately, pharmacy and healthcare programs are funded and implemented to improve the clinical outcomes in healthcare and thus create benefit for people in need of care. Realist research is now recognized as a strategy to inform the decision-making of funders and policy makers as to where to allocate resources, which services and programs to fund.[6,43] Pharmacy practice researchers have ample scope to support this process by first developing, then iteratively refining pharmacy practice program theories and generating new evidence through realist evaluations and syntheses. Making program theories applicable and translatable into practice includes providing clear messages about what seems the best way forward based on the most relevant evidence currently available and theory-driven knowledge development to increase their relevance to policy makers, funders, stakeholders and program participants. This links with an implementation science approach, with program theories identified through realist research informing the implementation of a new or modified pharmacy service or practice program and forming the basis for the next round of theory driven analysis or evaluation.

A downside to realist research in the traditional sense is the requirement for considerable content and methodological expertise, and the length of time it can take to develop program theory, particularly when it includes real world, lived experience. When decisions around program implementation have to be made within short timeframes, the scope of analysis and

---

BOX 3 Example of rapid realist review

Maidment and colleagues conducted a realist review on the role of community pharmacy in supporting the public health agenda in relation to Covid-19. Due to the urgency of the situation and narrow research question, a rapid realist review was conducted that took approximately 12 months from initial concept to publication. The team decided to primarily focus the review on the role of community pharmacy in the vaccination program in order to narrowly define the scope and limit the time required for the review.

Key challenges included the constantly published policy recommendations and academic publications. The team aimed to ameliorate this key challenge by strong stakeholder engagement and producing broad fundamental recommendations primarily designed for policy-makers.[45]

---

review may have to be narrowed. Instead of aiming at the development of theory that is transferable across many domains, reviews of evidence may have to focus on the "theory-driven identification of contextually relevant interventions that are likely to be associated with specific outcomes within a particular set of parameters."[44] Rapid realist reviews often work backwards from the desired outcome in the quest of identifying interventions and programs which will activate the mechanisms needed to achieve the outcome in a specific context of interest. Box 3 provides an example of a rapid realist review in relation to the pandemic of 2020.

While still applying the realist logic and constructs they may be able to provide answers to highly focused research questions in a time responsive manner, addressing more immediate needs in informing policy.

Conclusion

Based on the practical applications and experiences of employing realist logic to pharmacy relevant practice programs and patient behaviors a number of key recommendations were developed for those who may be considering starting with realist research in pharmacy practice including: embracing available realist research guidance, expertise, training materials and courses; involving a wide range of expertise, experience and program stakeholders at all stages of theory development; focusing on generative causation and developing a program theory to advance the conceptualization of outcomes; and drawing on existing theories to help make sense of data and CMOcs.

Generating a more nuanced understanding through realist research of how pharmacy services contribute to overall healthcare supports all stakeholders in the refinement and targeting of programs, successful adaptations to local contexts and resources, which, in turn, may lead to their greater effectiveness.

Resources and groups

Many resources and groups exist internationally to support the development and experience of realist researchers. There is an active community ready and willing to support colleagues looking to explore and use this approach to research. The best place for any researcher looking for further information is the RAMESES Project website: www.ramesesproject.org/. On this website you can sign up to a mailing list and become part of the realist community. This mailing list will also signpost to upcoming training events and groups running seminar series.

Questions for further discussion and application exercise/scenario

The following questions are designed to facilitate further discussion within your research group and can also be used as an application exercise for your students or research group.

1. Reflecting on your practice and research, is there a particular area where obvious explanatory mechanisms for why something is happening the way it does have not been explored and would be helpful to explore?
2. Thinking about your example above, what would constitute contexts or mechanisms which influence outcomes?
3. What would a realist research question look like for your example above?
4. What sources of data would help you answer your realist research question? How would these sources differ from a nonrealist research project?
5. Which methods of data collection would be appropriate to answer your realist research question?

References

1. Smith MA, Blanchard CM, Vuernick E. The intersection of implementation science and pharmacy practice transformation. *Ann Pharmacother.* 2020;54(1):75–81.

2. Weir NM, Newham R, Dunlop E, Bennie M. Factors influencing national implementation of innovations within community pharmacy: a systematic review applying the consolidated framework for implementation research. *Implement Sci.* 2019;14(1):1–16.

3. Bauer MS, Damschroder L, Hagedorn H, et al. An introduction to implementation science for the non-specialist. *BMC Psychol.* 2015;3(1):1–12.

4. Curran GM, Shoemaker SJ. Advancing pharmacy practice through implementation science. *Res Social Adm Pharm.* 2017;13(5):889–891. https://doi.org/10.1016/j.sapharm.2017.05.018. [Epub 2017 Jun 1; 28619650].

5. Crespo-Gonzalez C, Benrimoj SI, Scerri M, Garcia-Cardenas V. Sustainability of innovations in healthcare: a systematic review and conceptual framework for professional pharmacy services. *Res Soc Adm Pharm.* 2020;16:1331–1343.

6. Craig P, Dieppe P, Macintyre S, et al. Developing and evaluating complex interventions: the new Medical Research Council guidance. *BMJ.* 2008;337:a1655.

7. Krass I. Quasi experimental designs in pharmacist intervention research. *Int J Clin Pharm.* 2016;38(3):647–654.

8. Cartwright N, Hardie J. *Evidence-Based Policy: A Practical Guide to Doing It Better.* Oxford: Oxford University Press; 2012.

9. Greenhalgh T, Papoutsi C. Studying complexity in health services research: desperately seeking an overdue paradigm shift. *BMC Med.* 2018;16:95.

10. Westhorp G. Using complexity-consistent theory for evaluating complex systems. *Evaluation.* 2012;18(4):405–420.

11. Pawson R, Tilley N. *Realistic Evaluation.* London: Sage; 1997.

12. Wong G. Getting started with realist research. *Int J Qual Methods.* 2015;14(5):1–2.

13. Luetsch K, Twigg M, Rowett D, Wong G. In search for gold—the relevance of realist reviews and evaluations to pharmacy research and policy development. *Res Soc Adm Pharm.* 2020;16(6):836–839.

14. McEvoy P, Richards D. Critical realism: a way forward for evaluation research in nursing? *J Adv Nurs.* 2003;43(4):411–420.

15. Pawson R, Greenhalgh T, Harvey G, Walshe K. Realist review-a new method of systematic review designed for complex policy interventions. *J Health Serv Res Policy.* 2005;10(1_suppl):21–34.

16. Williams L, Rycroft-Malone J, Burton CR. Bringing critical realism to nursing practice: Roy Bhaskar's contribution. *Nurs Philos.* 2017;18(2):e12130.

17. Emmel N, Greenhalgh J, Manzano A, et al. *Doing Realist Research.* London: Sage; 2018.

18. Maxwell JA. *A Realist Approach for Qualitative Research.* London: Sage; 2012.

19. Pawson R. *Evidence-Based Policy: A Realist Perspective.* London: Sage; 2006.

20. Pawson R. *The Science of Evaluation: A Realist Manifesto.* London: Sage; 2013.

21. Greenhalgh T, Wong G, Jagosh J, et al. Protocol—the RAMESES II study: developing guidance and reporting standards for realist evaluation. *BMJ Open.* 2015;5(8):e008567.

22. Wong G, Westhorp G, Pawson R, Greenhalgh T. Realist synthesis. In: *RAMESES Training Materials.* London: The RAMESES Project Web Site; 2013. https://www.ramesesproject.org/media/Realist_reviews_training_materials.pdf.

23. Van Belle S, Wong G, Westhorp G, et al. Can "realist" randomised controlled trials be genuinely realist? *Trials.* 2016;17(1):313.

24. Dalkin SM, Greenhalgh J, Jones D, et al. What's in a mechanism? Development of a key concept in realist evaluation. *Implement Sci.* 2015;10(1):1–7.

25. Wong G, Greenhalgh T, Westhorp G, et al. RAMESES publication standards: realist syntheses. *BMC Med.* 2013;11(1):21.

26. Wong G, Westhorp G, Manzano A, et al. RAMESES II reporting standards for realist evaluations. *BMC Med.* 2016;14(1):96.

27. Van Belle S, Wong G, Westhorp G, et al. Can "realist" randomised controlled trials be genuinely realist? *Trials.* 2016;17(1):1–6.

28. Jagosh J, Bush PL, Salsberg J, et al. A realist evaluation of community-based participatory research: partnership synergy, trust building and related ripple effects. *BMC Public Health.* 2015;15(1):725.

29. De Brún A, McAuliffe E. Identifying the context, mechanisms and outcomes underlying collective leadership in teams: building a realist programme theory. *BMC Health Serv Res.* 2020;20(1):261.

30. Marchal B, Kegels G, Van Belle S. Theory and realist methods. In: *Doing Realist Research.* 1st ed. Los Angeles: Sage Publications; 2018:80–89.

31. May C, Finch T. Implementing, embedding, and integrating practices: an outline of normalization process theory. *Sociology.* 2009;43(3):535–554.

32. Maidment I, Lawson S, Wong G, et al. Towards an understanding of the burdens of medication management affecting older people: the MEMORABLE realist synthesis. *BMC Geriatr.* 2020;20:1–17.

33. Maidment ID, Lawson S, Wong G, et al. Medication management in older people: the MEMORABLE realist synthesis. *Health Serv Deliv Res.* 2020;8(26).

34. Booth A, Briscoe S, Wright JM. The "realist search": a systematic scoping review of current practice and reporting. *Res Synth Methods.* 2020;11(1):14–35.

35. Booth A, Wright J, Briscoe S. Scoping and searching to support realist approaches. In: *Doing Realist Research.* London: Sage; 2018:147–166.

36. Wong G, Westhorp G, Pawson R, Greenhalgh T. *RAMESES Standards*; 2013. https://www.ramesesproject.org/.

37. Luetsch K, Rowett D, Twigg MJ. A realist synthesis of pharmacist-conducted medication reviews in primary care after leaving hospital: what works for whom and why? *BMJ Qual Saf.* 2021;30(5):418–430.

38. Pawson R. Digging for nuggets: how 'bad' research can yield 'good' evidence. *Int J Soc Res Methodol.* 2006;9(2):127–142.

39. Maidment I, Booth A, Mullan J, et al. Developing a framework for a novel multi-disciplinary, multi-agency intervention(s), to improve medication management in community-dwelling older people on complex medication regimens (MEMORABLE)—a realist synthesis. *Syst Rev.* 2017;6(1):1–8.

40. Manzano A. The craft of interviewing in realist evaluation. *Evaluation.* 2016;22(3):342–360.

41. Pawson R. Theorizing the interview. *Br J Sociol.* 1996;47:295–314.

42. McEvoy P, Richards D. A critical realist rationale for using a combination of quantitative and qualitative methods. *J Res Nurs.* 2006;11(1):66–78.

43. Moore GF, Audrey S, Barker M, et al. Process evaluation of complex interventions: Medical Research Council guidance. *BMJ.* 2015;350:h1258.

44. Saul JE, Willis CD, Bitz J, Best A. A time-responsive tool for informing policy making: rapid realist review. *Implement Sci.* 2013;8(1):1–15.

45. Maidment I, Young E, MacPhee M, et al. A rapid realist review of the role of community pharmacy in the public health response to COVID-19. *BMJ Open.* 2021;e050043.

Chapter 20

Application of process philosophy with organization and management science in pharmacy and health services research

Phillip Woods

School of Pharmacy and Medical Sciences, Griffith University, Gold Coast Campus, QLD, Australia

Objectives

- Review how the gap between theory and its practice can be understood.
- Review an alternative perspective: "practical rationality," arising from a process philosophical viewpoint, that redefines how the lived experience of practice, and the theory about such practice, can relate more closely.
- Illuminate a "style of thinking" that must accompany a process philosophical way of thinking.
- Consider a range of theoretical perspectives and congruent methodologies that are appropriate for enacting research that is capable of narrowing the theory-practice gap.

Introduction

> *We say the acrobat on the high wire maintains her stability. However, she*
> *does so by continuously correcting her imbalances.*
>
> (Tsoukas and Chia,[1] p. 572, also citing Bateson[2])

In recent decades, a "journey of concern" for pharmacist practitioners around the world can be loosely described as: the continuous development of pharmacy practice toward meeting the evolving pharmaceutically related health care needs of societies.[3–6] Pharmacy practice research (PPR), increasingly enabled by social pharmacy research (SPR), has a critical role in helping to understand, inform, and preempt pharmacy practice so it can move to meet societal needs.[7–11] Pharmacy practice researchers use different research approaches to try to clarify the direction, activity, and effectiveness of different aspects of this journey. The overarching purpose of PPR is to develop diverse knowledge that will assist those on the journey.

For many years, PPR has been encouraged to follow the lead of the larger and growing domain of health services research that has been drawing methodologically and theoretically from other disciplines like economics, sociology, anthropology, and psychology.[12] This has broadened perspectives and analysis, as well as to produce different "qualities" of knowledge. However, the dominant approach in PPR over decades has been through quantitative research methodologies.[5,8,13] Quantitative methodologies have served, and will continue to serve PPR and SPR well. But complex social phenomena that underpin "the social practice" of pharmacy require the deployment of more diverse perspectives and methodologies that offer better ways to explore and understand human performance.[5,14]

Qualitative research approaches in PPR and SPR have been increasing and represent a solid research domain in medicine and healthcare.[14,15] Qualitative approaches offer contributions concerning the myriad influences of human attitudes, beliefs, experiences, and understanding, upon healthcare practice and social engagement.[14–16] But while qualitative research holds much promise for advancing answers to research questions that cannot be addressed solely by quantitative approaches, the rigor of much qualitative research has been criticized from a variety of perspectives.[15] Key criticisms center on a range of issues from poor integration of essential theory in research processes and outcomes to the related problem of

Contemporary Research Methods in Pharmacy and Health Services. https://doi.org/10.1016/B978-0-323-91888-6.00006-5

poor quality data analysis.[14-16] However, putting the imperfections of both qualitative and quantitative approaches aside, researchers can ponder something more pragmatic; that is, are PPR and SPR outcomes satisfactorily addressing the profession's most pressing needs?

It appears that the answer to this question is "no," at least in relation to the speed and depth of uptake of "professional pharmacy services." Internationally, the progression from PPR and SPR findings (the theory) to practical implementation (the practice), has been reported as disappointing.[17-21] As highlighted in the pharmacy literature: *"There is a well-described and on-going problem with the translation of existing knowledge to the delivery of health care"*[22] (p. 902). The more fundamental problem of a "gap" between what we know (the theory), and what practitioners do (the practice) is not limited to pharmacy practice or even health practices more generally. The problematic gap between theory and practice is also highlighted in organization and management science (OMS).[23]

OMS is concerned with very broad and interdisciplinary studies that seek to improve the understanding of both organization (structures) and organizing (actions) at scales that span from the actions of individuals to global scale concerns. Progress within the OMS domain is being made in developing perspectives and research methodologies that bridge the theory-practice gap in ways that complement the more dominant natural sciences approach in understanding work practice, and how to change it.

The purpose of this chapter is to entice the imagination of PPR researchers who are interested in considering paradigm perspectives that profoundly alter virtually all taken-for-granted assumptions about how "reality" is perceived, experienced, and then conceived. Such perspectives invite the comprehension of new and different qualities of knowledge that become available. Referring mainly to the literature of OMS, the chapter begins by describing how the theory-practice gap can be understood. Discussion will then move to consider a radically alternative perspective, arising from a philosophy of process, that redefines how to "see" the relationship between theory and practice. Such a perspective requires a "style of thinking" that must accompany a philosophy of process. Finally, consideration will be given to a range of theoretical perspectives and congruent methodologies that are appropriate for enacting research that is capable of narrowing the theory-practice gap, including two examples from pharmacy practice research.

Different thinking may enable development of research processes and outcomes that capture a logic of pharmacy practice that more closely reflects practitioners' experience of that practice. When the logic of pharmacy practice is more closely understood from the perspective of practitioners, new possibilities for meaningful intervention and change may arise. What follows is a discussion regarding how we might better understand the theory-practice gap.

How can the theory-practice "gap" be better explained and understood?

OMS scholars Sandberg and Tsoukas[23] assert that the theory-practice gap as reported in management research literature has hitherto located its causes through one of two pathways: either problems with how knowledge is communicated to practitioners (knowledge transfer), or problems caused by poor or insufficient collaboration between researchers and practitioners regarding practitioner problems (knowledge production). In PPR, the knowledge transfer problem is being increasingly acknowledged and treated through the expansion of dissemination and implementation sciences in pharmacy research.[22,24,25] A common approach for improving the implementation of theory into practice (including novel professional pharmacy services) is by theoretically fracturing an entire implementation process into abstracted but logical domains that permit a more manageable and stepwise implementation application. Examples are the Medical Research Council Framework,[26] adapted for pharmacy by Garcia-Cardenas et al.,[25] and the Consolidated Framework for Implementation Research,[27] asserted by some as the most widely cited and utilized implementation framework today.[24]

Research initiatives that accentuate increased collaboration between researchers and practitioners as a means of improving implementation of theory into practice (i.e., knowledge production) are less common in PPR. One recognized method is the application of the philosophy and practice of action research (AR). Pharmacy researchers Sørensen and Haugbølle[28] describe the key idea of AR as the researcher and practitioner working together to resolve practice problems that the practitioner is actually experiencing. In AR, the researcher and participant learn together and coproduce knowledge. The researcher ensures application of scientifically rational principles that include studying the problem systematically, leading the theoretical analysis and synthesis, and ensuring that adaptations or interventions are informed primarily by theoretical considerations. Practical considerations while important are secondary.

The dominant methods used for improving knowledge transfer and knowledge production, share a common foundation; specifically, that planned changes in practice are derived from and driven by "correct" scientifically rational theories. The theories in the form of generalizations arise from the identification of correlations as a basis for assigning causal relationships. Causal relationships if found (the theory) are then proffered to inform the enactment of practice. This is the highly valuable and time-tested natural sciences approach. But as already stated, this theoretical approach seems to deliver knowledge that has poor translation when it comes to practitioners enacting the theory in practice.

With these insights in mind, other OMS scholars[29–33] according to Sandberg and Tsoukas,[23] have suggested more *fundamental* considerations as to what causes the gap between theory and practice. They suggest that the gap is caused by mostly taken for granted assumptions that researchers make about (i) how practitioners actually experience their practice reality and (ii) what quality of knowledge is "practically rational" for them to enact.[23] It is suggested that theories produced by scientifically rational approaches do not actually capture "the logic of practice"[34] as experienced by practitioners while practicing.[35] The lived experience[36] of practitioners is qualitatively and experientially very different from the sterile theoretical abstractions that are offered to guide them. Such theories are removed from the highly specific and personally experienced social contexts and "ways-of-doing" that are already habituated and embedded at a particular time.[23] Put another way, practitioners may see the "wisdom" of new theoretical ideas, but implementation becomes much more challenging than the theory suggests.

Consider the example of learning to drive a motor vehicle. Most people when learning to drive a car for the first time, personally experience a theory-practice "gap." They struggle with the real-time practical application of correct driving implementation theory. Competent driving performance when achieved does not so much "exist" as an identifiable set of discrete steps that must be consciously placed in correct sequential order in a context of rules.[37] Rather, competent driving from the driver's perspective, like life itself, "continuously occurs" seamlessly as an integrated flow of processes, much of which is engaged beyond consciousness.[38,39] A great deal of practice and repetition is required to integrate (interpret) scientifically rational driving theory into competent driving practice. Different practitioners are more or less competent at accomplishing the necessary theory-to-practice interpretations of practice change on-the-run. This reveals something of how the theory-practice gap arises and is experienced.

Simply put, scientifically rational theories, while valuable, are not close to how we *actually live* (i.e., practice), making difficult the theory implementation into the flow of already existing real life. With this idea in mind, some PPR academics are calling for more holistic research approaches that better incorporate context, particularly the complex social contexts of pharmacy practice. For example, Maher et al. call for a "…reconsideration of the types of research designs that provide the types of knowledge that is contextual and particularistic"[40] (p. 644). To provide knowledge types that are personally contextual and particularistic implies having a prior understanding of the lifeworld of practitioners, *before* attempting to instruct them as to where we are sure they would better be.

Modern scholars[23,36,41] highlight that to better understand the lifeworld of practitioners from their own perspective, it should be considered that every practitioner is immersed in their own meaningful understanding of their identity in their own world; that they are entwined uniquely in their daily unfolding social contexts and mostly habituated actions; and that time is an experienced phenomenon, inseparably integrated with both emerging context and actions.[23] These aspects characterize the flowing logic of living and practice. To develop more useful and implementable explanatory pathways and theories for and about practice and practice change, approaches and methods that begin with understanding practice in a way that is more practically rational should be used. So, what is an alternative approach that affords the development of knowledge that is closer to the practitioners' experienced logic of practice?

How can pharmacy practice be understood in a more practically rational way?

As suggested earlier, scholars point toward reviewing and reconceptualizing the basic assumptions regarding how practitioners actually experience their practice reality, from day-to-day.[23] Then the promise is that researchers can conceive a different, more practically identifiable quality of knowledge that invites new possibilities for intervention and practice change.

OMS scholars Sandberg and Tsoukas explicate a radically alternative framework of "practical rationality" for approaching the understanding of practice life.[23] They suggest three ideas that contrast with the underlying assumptions of scientific rationality. First, practical rationality suggests that human reality is fundamentally constituted by *entwinement*, where: "…we are never separated but always already entwined with others and things…" (p. 343).

To illustrate the experienced meaning of this statement, think back to your last journey as a car driver to somewhere familiar. Unless you were a novice, it is most likely you did not consciously experience every individual transaction with necessary driving objects—the indicator lever, foot pedals, traffic light symbols, random passing movements of other cars and pedestrians, etc. While you may not have been unconscious to these transactional events, it is likely that your experience of transacting with them was more like a flowing holism. Or as the philosopher Bourdieu has put it, we act "…'on the spot,' 'in the twinkling of an eye,' 'in the heat of the moment,' that is, in conditions which exclude distance, perspective, detachment and reflection"[34] (p. 82). The exclusion of distance, perspective, detachment, and reflection reveals that we were closer to a state of entwinement with the world in our drive, than to a state of pressurized, linear, conscious deliberation with every issue. Entwinement, it is proposed, is our most basic (but not only) state[34,36] while driving, managing, practicing pharmacy, and living.

Second, and related to the idea of entwinement, is the aspect of *embodiment* in our lived experience.[23,36] Embodiment, while referring to our bodies, does not stay limited to that. The concept includes material things in relation to the body when a particular practice is being engaged. Citing the philosopher Merleau-Ponty,[42] Dall'Alba and Sandberg explain that the "lived-body is the means by which we are entwined with, and have access to our world…"[36] (p. 107). Going back to the experience of your last car driving journey, it is not difficult to acknowledge that the driving engagement incorporated a type of seamlessness between ourselves (the body) and the material car control objects, the car itself, as well as the technologies that underpin them—an experience of bodily unity with material things and their workings as we engage in driving. Correct and competent driving seems to arise from this entwined-embodied state, without the need to make countless deliberate and conscious decisions. Practical rationality in contrast to scientific rationality recognizes that human agency-in-action is fundamentally embodied within the world, in its entwined and dynamic engagement with the world.[23,34,41,43]

Third, where theory arises from scientific rationality, time and context are regarded as important, but time and context-as-experienced are absent in the rendering of theory.[23] When we reflect on life as it is actually lived, there are no stationary moments that allow the neat "insertion" of an implementation or adaptation step. Time and context are always moving, evolving, and changing. Time and context are inseparable from the already existing interconnected and unfolding processes that we recognize as living. Take, for example, the professional competency standards for pharmacists, which can be understood as "rational theories of competence" for pharmacy practice. An illustrative example of one such standard (a competency contingency theory) belongs to Domain 4 as maintained by the Australian Pharmaceutical Society: Leadership and management.[44] Standard 4.4 is titled "*Participate in organisational planning and review*" (p. 15). This competency standard provides five enabling competencies that are designed to assist practitioners adapt toward the achievement of this standard. These are to

1. Undertake strategic and/or operational planning.
2. Develop a business plan and monitor performance.
3. Establish suitable premises and infrastructure.
4. Undertake workforce planning.
5. Develop and maintain supporting systems and strategies (p. 15).

This package of scientifically rational theory is certainly helpful in defining "what" is required to achieve participation in *organizational planning and review*, but the theory is exclusive of time and context. While competency standards are not designed for the purpose of explaining "how," all five necessary competencies are reliant on timing and tempo in relation to the emergent context.

So *how* do we assume such scientifically rational adaptation steps are implemented by competent practitioners in real life? It seems that translation is expected to be accomplished by somehow interpreting the steps or statements into many meaningful (new) processes and the "stirring-in" of these processes into the already existing and moving processes of work life. Each new adaptation step factually represents a Trojan horse of processes that require "integration" into existing and flowing life, rather than an "implementation," perhaps like the insertion of a new jigsaw puzzle piece into an already stable picture. Until the practitioner engages in the labor of practically interpreting (translating) what are effectively "*generic propositional statements*"[23] (p. 342), the steps remain sterile and difficult "objects" to transform into a work life that is experienced as flowing entwined-embodiment through time. In contrast to scientifically rational theories, practical rationality is a perspective that understands that human action as experienced cannot be separated from time, or complex evolving circumstance.[23]

Developing a radically different and practically rational understanding of pharmacy practice invites us to understand practice holistically as "flowing-process" that captures (i) the meaningful totality in which practitioners are immersed within a lifeworld, (ii) the situational uniqueness of a moving context as it relates to practitioners and what they do, (iii) time-as-experienced by practitioners within their unfolding lifeworld, and therefore (iv) dynamic relationships, within resultant explanations.[23] For research approaches to examine practice this way means focusing on "the doing" of pharmacy practice—that is, to develop understandings of practice by taking a process approach. While qualitative methodology will be a dominant choice with such an approach, moving toward a practically rational understanding of human practice is more fundamental than choosing qualitative over quantitative.

To fully grasp the practically rational perspective, some have suggested that a fundamental mental movement is required even beyond the notion of "different theoretical perspective or social paradigm"[45] (p. 584). What is required is a fundamentally different "style of thinking."[45] Such a style of thinking requires us to go further in re-examining presuppositions regarding what reality-as-experienced is (ontology), the human relation to that reality, and the nature of knowledge (epistemology), that arises from such an understanding.[46] For social pharmacy researchers to think and research in a *practically* rational way, "prior *organization of mentalities* and modes of thought"[46] (p. 4) are required. To assist with this (re)organization, the next section begins by contrasting different ways of conceiving "process" and "processes," and ends with a summary to assist researchers in comprehending a process philosophical perspective.

How can (re)organizing mentalities be better understood?

There is more than one way to understand "process." The scientifically rational view mostly considers processes as mechanisms to explain practice outcomes, a perspective often referred to as the "variance"[47] or "substance view."[48] A practically rational view is to consider that practice *is* process: the "process view."[47,48]

The substance view

The most commonly understood notion is that processes *happen to* people/organizations (social entities).[49] Process happenings are assumed to occur with some form of sequential structure over a time period. Typically, studies that assume this view examine if there is a causal relationship between a measurable change in some aspect of an entity over time, as a consequence of process input (the variable).[50] An "entity" might be a practitioner or organization performance measure. A process input variable might be some category of training, tool usage, or different operational method. Fig. 1 demonstrates a generalized diagram of this common research approach for interrogating the effectiveness of process(es).

The main idea of this normalized understanding of process is that social entities were and remain relatively stable, as processes occur around them.[49] That is, processes are secondary phenomena in reality, in contrast to entities that are assumed as primary.[49] Change for an entity as caused by processes, is not assumed to alter the fundamental "substance" of the entity, although the entity may "contain" different constituents as a result of the processes (e.g., a practitioner may gain a skill attribute). Time is understood as an external constant.

Context is not directly included in the cause-effect findings. This sort of process understanding informs researchers *if* an intervening process has had an effect, but not exactly *how* that effect became constituted within the entity. That is, how the processes and the entity actually engage with each other to produce the change remains obscure. This perspective and research practice is founded upon what is termed a substance philosophy,[51] or substance ontology.[33] Research that assumes the substantive ontological approach for understanding how knowledge can bring about change is common.

A substance view example

An illustration is provided in a commentary by Hohmeier et al.,[52] who highlight existing methods from implementation science and a pharmacy case study. They suggest how implementation rates of new patient care services may be increased. Their analysis focused on methods of improving processes of "prioritization" of tasks within already over full and complex workloads. Within a case study participant group of third-year doctor of pharmacy students, the use of a prioritization matrix tool (henceforth "the tool"), to aid thinking in a more systematic way was explored. The tool's use was shown to be positively correlated with subjectively reported improvements in both rating and ranking various medication related

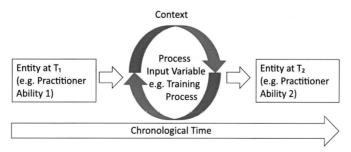

FIG. 1 Diagrammatic generalization of how process(es) are understood and researched when understood from the perspective of the substance view, or substance ontology.

problems, offered as challenges. The tool was thus shown to have positive potential as a prioritization skill improvement resource.

The valuable contribution of this commentary and its conclusions are not in question, but its philosophical approach is a demonstration of a "substance" view of reality, knowledge, and how process(es) act to change human performance. That is, if objectified knowledge (e.g., use of the tool, applied as the independent variable) is provided with training, then its embedded common sense will be engaged (somehow) by practitioners who will then act rationally to do things in a different way. That is, practitioners used to act in an old way, but with the tool and training they act in a new way. The "substance" of the practitioner has not fundamentally changed, as they now act in a new way. Practitioners simply possess a new skill (Fig. 1). While this is the most common perspective of how knowledge "insertion" leads to change, supported by rational behavior theories,[53] it is not the only the perspective.[46,54]

It is definitely advantageous to know about the potential effectiveness of this tool. As the authors point out, the tool is directed toward the "how-to-do" skills, rather than the "what-to-do" list. But the "how-to" revelation of the tool only goes so far. The findings do not actually reveal much about how, precisely, the tool was actually engaged by members of the participant group who operationalized its use in each case. For example, while the results from participants uncovered some new perspectives that were delivered by the tool, *how* materials, old beliefs as well as thinking and acting processes were altered/discarded in each consultation, through engaging with the tool, remain obscure. The authors lean on abstract phrases such as "paradigm shift" and "systematic thinking," to explain the changes in practitioner performance.

These phrases deliver some useful descriptive language as to "what" took place when the tool was used, but neither phrase explains "how" the tool (independent variable) acted upon practitioners (the entities) through their lived experiences. The "black boxes"[50] of "paradigm shift" and "systematic thinking" need to be opened up, so as to understand how the tool actually works to alter practice. To accomplish this opening-up, a different process-perspective of reality, knowing and emergent practice is likely needed.

The process view

A radically alternative understanding of "process" is afforded from a perspective of process philosophy, or an ontology of becoming.[33,45] An ontology of becoming reminds us that stable entities that simply make knowledge adjustments are in fact an illusion. From the process perspective, change *is* the primary and continuous phenomenon, where an "entity" (person or organization) is but a dynamic "eddy of comparative stability, in a sea of process,"[55] (p. 1) and thus not really an "entity" at all. Rather than the "person" or "organization" being the primary constitutor of processes, the reverse notion is prioritized. That is, interrelated emerging processes are regarded as the primary constitutor of both person and organization, and therefore their performance.[45]

With this view, practitioners, patients, universities, or pharmacies are not independent, relatively unchanging structures that bump about in a surprising world. Rather these "are collective social orders *brought about* through (continuous) human interactions"[33] (p. 282, italics added for emphasis). That is, both intentional and nonintentional (mainly social) processes, continuously (re)constitute both people and organizations through time. How people or organizations perform through time arises from the swirling nexus of processes that constitute them. Thus, people and organizations can be considered as secondary "effects" of processes that are considered as primary, even though people and organizations can influence the very processes that constitute them. Processes and people/organizations thus mutually constitute each other.[35] All of life then is rendered as a continuous unfolding transformative becoming.[33] If processes are considered as the primary phenomenon in the production of performance, then understanding emergent process patterns becomes the focus for scrutiny in particular contexts.

The task of process research is to be attentive to unfolding practice performance that can be explained "in terms of the repeated (process) patterns found in a certain series of interrelated events"[56] (p. 65, as cited by Langley and Tsoukas[49]). The research focus thus moves toward examining dynamic unfolding patterns of actions that reveal *how* performance arises. Theoretical process explanations speak in terms of patterns of action, practices, activities, and choice making,[57] revealing the "how" and "why" of performances and outcomes through time. When explanations speak in terms of *how practitioners (or patients) do what they do*, the explanations are likely to feel more familiar to the practitioner, that is, more "practically rational" from the perspective of the practitioner. Rather than time and context remaining external in explanatory findings, both become included when explanations arise in terms of dynamic patterned happenings. The key features of process explanations of practice are that they are holistic, dynamic, open ended, and context specific.

A process view example

There is a growing interest in process philosophical research approaches in the domain of public health policy.[54] While research to-date into public health problems and solutions has delivered much improvement, such as dropping smoking rates in many nations, progress is generally slow when it comes to people and their habits of living.[58] This stickiness of human habituation has motivated public health researchers to look for different ways to approach understanding how human living practices interrelate with the emergence of health problems. Rather than using scientifically rational psychological and individualistic behavior theories, there are increasing calls for use of paradigmatically different social theories to think through both the nature of public health issues and therefore new approaches to their potential solution.[54,58]

With reference to tobacco smoking, Blue et al.[58] suggest looking at smoking, not as associated with factors such as individual characteristics and social determinants of health, but as a dynamic practice. The practice of smok-*ing* (with emphasis on the verb) is viewed as a "doing" that is also constituted by several interwoven and inseparable aspects such as materials, various symbols, particular evolving contexts, repeated bodily actions, other social interactions, consuming foods and drinks, etc., that change over time. This process view of smok-*ing* expands its understanding toward a more encompassing notion of patterned practice that holds strong co-constituting allegiances with other patterned practices such as consuming certain drinks and socializing. Blue et al. suggest that practically understanding the nature of key practice bundles and how they interrelate and co-evolve over time, provides new "sites"[59] for intervention. For example, improvements may be available by diminishing unhealthy practices (e.g., sedentariness) by slowly introducing new healthier practices that are less conducive to smoking practice (e.g., exercise routines). Or the banning of smoking in restaurants and other eating locations has aided breaking the association between the practice of smoking and some eating and drinking practices.[58]

Diagrammatic representations of the process view

It would be convenient to be able to provide diagrammatic illustration of how this theoretical approach could be generally represented, as a contrast to the illustration of Fig. 1. However, process ontology means focusing on reality as it unfolds; that is, a segment of actual lived experience where people, their actions, the context and time are particular. An ontology of process does not permit conceptually dividing a generalized reality into relatively stable idealized boxes (e.g., structures and processes) that interact linearly, as per Fig. 1. Consequently, there is no generalized or standardized way to demonstrate a process or practice view of some aspect of life and work. Diagrammatic representations can only be particular to each research case. Often narrations best preserve the complexity of human interactions that include actions, time, specific contexts, emotions, motivations, and perceptions.[23,60]

However, creative illustrations of life-as-process are available in the literature. Sandberg and Tsoukas[23] cite a range of diagrammatic representations within the literature that capture the holistic, open-ended and context-specific nature of human processes, that include "bidirectional arrows, recursive patterns (and) circular interactions..."[23] (p. 352). Examples offered are diagrams by the organizational researcher Orlikowski[61] (p. 410) that utilize double-ended arrows and recursive patterning to illustrate how organizational structure and human agency interrelate. Orlikowski shows "how people, as they interact with a technology in their ongoing practices, enact structures which shape their emergent and situated use of that technology"[61] (p. 404). Diagrammatic recursive patterning is effectively used by management researchers Sandberg and Pinnington[62] (p. 1162) who propose a different way of understanding professional competence as (enacted) "ways of being." Also, the pharmacy practice researcher Woods[63] has utilized recursive patterning and circular arrows as diagrammatic devices to illustrate his reconceptualization of pharmacist "managerial capability" as an unfolding set of enacted but integrated relational processes (p. 244). (This study is discussed further in a later section.) Finally, Feldman[64] dedicates her edited chapter to explaining how to bypass the use of arrows connected to boxes by illustrating three alternative diagrammatic strategies, informed from theory. Feldman illustrates how actor-network theory,[65] action nets,[66] and narrative network analysis[67] can inform diagrammatic designs that preserve the particular dynamic, situated and relational nature of practice, without the use of arrows and boxes.

In summary, and as an aid to "organizing mentalities," Table 1 provides a summary of how researchers can imagine the world through the contrasting ontological perspectives of substance versus process.

Methodological considerations: How can "the doing" of practice be explored?

Process philosophy offers a spacious thinking orientation, rather than a doctrinal prescription.[49] From this viewpoint, it is possible to illuminate the patterns of actions and social relations that daily activity (practice) brings into being.[75] Appropriate methodologies are able to deliver dynamic explanations regarding research questions focusing on "the how" of

TABLE 1 The contrasting perspectives that arise from ontologies of substance versus process.

Research criteria	Perspective: ontology of substance	Perspective: ontology of process
The *primary* phenomenon of reality: What is real?	Entities, individual people and organizations, that variously respond to interventions and contextual circumstances	Patterns of emergent relational interactions, that are influenced by, and that coincidently influence unfolding context
What is the "normal state" of existence?	A resting state with occasional visitations of small to big change	Continuous change where all aspects of existence are moving and dynamic, where change only varies in apparent amplitude and/or scale
Change can be...	Categorized rationally and managed with rational counteractions, whose outcomes can be measured at discrete points in time	Understood as continuous unfolding movement along paths of observation,[68] where responses also unfold as endless participatory patterned actions, through time
Sociological studies deal with...	Results, effects or outcomes. Reporting obeys certain rules that determine "truth" of connections between causes that produce effects	Social process relations (including the context in which they emerge), that constitute and produce practices, effects, and outcomes. Reporting reassures "authenticity"[69,70] of social action and shows how actions produce effects
The fundamental unit of analysis is...	Stable "units" or entities (commonly nouns) such as individual people, structures, culture, gender, etc., that produce some aspect of stabilized *organizat-ion*	The dynamic relational processes (commonly verbs) that occur between individuals and groups (and their materials) in unfolding actions of *organiz-ing*[71–73]
Analytical thinking is concerned with...	"Things" that contribute to some aspect of *organizat-ion*	Patterned actions that reflect the logic of *organiz-ing*[74]

Based on the OMS contributions of Chia R. From modern to postmodern organizational analysis. *Organ Stud.* 1995;16(4):579–604; Nayak A, Chia R. Thinking becoming and emergence: process philosophy and organization studies. In: Lounsbury M, ed. *Philosophy and Organization Theory.* Emerald Group Publishing; 2011:281–309.

practice phenomena such as strategizing, leading, learning, supporting, implementing, managing, etc., that arise from everyday activity. There is broad scope for considering suitable methodologies that can illuminate patterned, dynamic, and unfolding phenomena over time. From a process perspective, collecting data is concerned with capturing evidence of interconnected life-processes-in-action, often focused on an aspect of some larger process of concern.

Broadly, data collection for exploring human performance seeks to capture (i) the meaningful and unfolding contextual totality in which people are entwined, and from which anticipations and choices arise; (ii) the situational uniqueness that is characteristic within the actions and relations that people engage; and (iii) time-as-experienced by people as they accomplish their performances.[23] Gathering data that encompasses "temporality, flow, activity and emergence"[49] can be approached through several broad theoretical perspectives that include symbolic interactionism,[76] actor-network theory,[65,77] and practice theory.[78,79] Methodologies that are consistent with process ontology include hermeneutic phenomenology,[80] phenomenography,[81] ethnography,[82] constructivist grounded theory,[63,83,84] and narrative approaches.[60] Suitable data collection methods that support these methodologies[23] include phenomenological lifeworld interviewing,[85] observing through shadowing,[86] and qualitative research diaries.[87]

Options for analyzing process data are similarly broad given the theoretical and methodological choices available, with intellectual groundings provided by OMS contributors such as Pettigrew,[88] Langley[89] and in a compilation by Langley and Tsoukas.[90] Indeed, the handbook edited by OMS scholars Langley and Tsoukas[90] provides an excellent starting point for pharmacy and health services research scholars who wish to expand their inquiries regarding to how to approach and conduct research informed by process philosophy.

The relevance of using the more practically rational process perspective, to complement scientifically rational theories, is that process theories can show how patterned unfolding processes and practices interrelate and come together *to produce* some aspect of human life or work. Such theories generally offer narrative descriptions that illuminate the fundamental mechanisms—that is, *what people actually do*—and potentially provide novel perspectives and possible sites for influencing change.

Methodological examples from pharmacy practice research

While pharmacy practice studies framed by process philosophy may be few, examples are two recent studies by Burrows[80] and Woods.[63] Burrows drew on hermeneutic phenomenology in her longitudinal study of how pharmacy practice was understood, enacted, and developed in a cohort of graduating pharmacy students. Differing individual ways of understanding the meaning of "pharmacy practice" were shown to be highly influential for how later learning processes were chosen and integrated into practice, thus influencing practice development trajectories through time. Embedded processes of understand-*ing* shape many other ongoing processes that constitute an individual's particular and unfolding expression of practice in pharmacy. Burrows' insight was that early educational intervention in broadening and deepening how pharmacy practice is understood may fundamentally influence future practicing performance and direction.[80]

Woods' study[63] utilized a constructivist mode of grounded theory[84] to explore how capable pharmacist managers competently managed their pharmacies during a period of turbulent business conditions. Rather than viewing managerial capability as caused by some collection of skills, attitudes, and abilities, Woods' reconceptualized the concept of "managerial capability" as an unfolding process, where managers engaged in a range of iterative (mostly) social processes that produce incremental knowledge-in-action, or "knowing-as-they-go." This "wayfinding" perspective[68] accentuates how managerial capability emerges as an effect of patterned social relations, involving relationships that unfold within an emergent and continuously changing social arena. Shifting focus to exploring the social relations that constitute managing-in-action provides a very different perspective for understanding how managerial capability "happens," and how it might be adjusted.

The Burrows and Woods studies utilize a process philosophical orientation to show a partial but novel view of the mechanisms that deliver respective emergent outcomes. While both studies are ultimately "about" people and their performances, analysis and synthesis of data focuses on the unfolding processes that constitute both people and performances over time. The ontological ordering of processes as fundamentally prior to people and performances is the hallmark of a process philosophical orientation. Findings are not reported as static snapshots of practices. Rather, they invoke an imagery of movement, that is, of practic-*ing*. Explaining practice phenomena by means of actions and "doings" is ontologically closer to practitioners' lived experience and are more "practically rational" than the dominant "scientifically rational" concepts of logical abstraction.[23] The gap between practice and how researchers theoretically report it narrows.

Conclusion

This chapter comments on the valuable works of others, published in constellations of books and journals over the past century, mainly in the domain of organization and management science. It discusses what are undeniably challenging ideas, concepts, and "ways of seeing." If this chapter has a particular value, it is mostly through its invitation to investigate a wider and more authoritative literature.

As elegantly expressed by the American Pragmatist philosopher William James: "The intellectual life of man consists almost wholly in his substitution of a conceptual order for the perceptual order, in which his experience originally comes"[91] (p. 33). A process philosophical orientation enables the reprioritization of the perceptual order that reflects life through how-it-is-lived and experienced. Process philosophy enables the development of practical and usually more complex understandings of human life that give a closer, more realistic and dynamic representation of how performances are accomplished.[23,35,89,92] Such understandings can narrow the gap between *what* we think a phenomenon is (the theory) and *how* it actually happens (the practice).[23] The promise is that pathways showing how practice improvements can be made, become visible. The emphasis on process analysis through time brings together context, emotion, meaning, action, directionality, and anticipatory decision-making. This is how we live. It provides the opportunity for research that may be able "to catch reality in flight"[93] (p. 270).

Questions for further discussion

1. Think about the "gap" between theory and practice: Why is it that a person who cannot ride a bike, can read the "How to ride a bike" instruction manual (the theory), and even memorize it, but still not be much more able to *actually* ride a bike (the practice) at the end of such study? What type of knowledge do they gain by reading/memorizing the manual? What type of knowledge is missing to create this competence gap? *How* (precisely) does this person gain the "missing knowledge" that would result in them conquering the bike riding feat? [Also, think of other common "practices": dancing, swimming, car driving, pharmaceutical dispensing, etc.]

2. Continuing from the questions above: If they did gain this missing bike riding knowledge (or is it "know-ing"?), how would they communicate this "knowing" to someone else? Could they write a better "how-to" manual? [Tip—Read:

Cook SN, Brown JS. Bridging epistemologies: the generative dance between organizational knowledge and organizational knowing. *Organ Sci.* 1999;10(4):382–390.]

3. The American Pragmatist philosopher William James is noted to have said: "The intellectual life of man consists almost wholly in his substitution of a conceptual order for the perceptual order, in which his experience originally comes"[91] (p. 33). Discuss what you think he meant in his comment regarding the intellectual substitution of the "conceptual order" over the "perceptual order" [in social research]. How and why would the reporting/narrating of a "perceptual order" of human life be closer to human lived experience? How is his comment relevant to the dominant research approaches concerning social pharmacy and pharmacy practice? What research approaches can be considered if researchers decided to capture more of the "perceptual order" of human life (viz. some aspect of social pharmacy or pharmacy practice)?

Application exercise/scenario

The common pharmacy activity of dispensing pharmaceutical prescriptions is a central practice for the pharmacy profession around the world. What is involved in this practice is highly explicated in documents ranging from competency standards, set by professional bodies, to atomistic procedural explanations (listed procedure steps) that individual organizations provide. There may even be research publications that articulate lists of "facilitators and barriers" to good dispensing practice. But all of this explanatory knowledge is of a certain type: rationalistically conceptualized explanations of abstract notions regarding "what is to happen to do dispensing," generally. What this type of explanation misses is "how it is actually performed and accomplished" (practically), through time, in a particular context (e.g., in a particular setting), on a particular day.

Using what has been learned from this chapter, describe how you might develop a research approach that results in an alternative "process philosophical explanation" of the phenomenon of pharmaceutical dispensing. Consider the following questions:

1. What aspects of the phenomenon of pharmaceutical dispensing will you focus upon to design your data collection?
2. What will be your primary "unit of analysis" for this study?
3. Describe how your analytical thinking will be directed in your research analysis and synthesis processes.
4. What forms of data collection might be suitable for accomplishing this study? Justify your choices.

[Tip: for the first 3 questions above, the notes contained in Table 1 in the chapter may be useful.]

References

1. Tsoukas H, Chia R. On organizational becoming: rethinking organizational change. *Organ Sci.* 2002;13(5):567–582.
2. Bateson G. *Mind and Nature: A Necessary Unity.* vol. 255. Bantam Books New York; 1979.
3. Thorlby R, Maybin J. *A High-Performing NHS? A Review of Progress 1997–2010.* The King's Fund; 2010.
4. Speedie MK, Anderson LJ. A consistent professional brand for pharmacy—the need and a path forward. *J Am Pharm Assoc.* 2017;57(2):256–260.
5. Scahill S. Placing "culture" at the center of social pharmacy practice and research. *Res Soc Adm Pharm.* 2013;9(1):1–3.
6. Mossialos E, Courtin E, Naci H, et al. From "retailers" to health care providers: transforming the role of community pharmacists in chronic disease management. *Health Policy.* 2015;119(5):628–639.
7. Roberts R, Kennington E. Pharmacy practice research has an impact on each and every pharmacist. *Pharm J.* 2010;284(7593):267–268.
8. Winit-Watjana W. Research philosophy in pharmacy practice: necessity and relevance. *Int J Pharm Pract.* 2016;24(6):428–436.
9. Sheridan J. What is social pharmacy? An Overview. *Jpn J Soc Phrm.* 2015;34(2):141–145.
10. Sorensen E, Mount J, Christensen S. The concept of social pharmacy. *The Chronic.* 2003;101:7.
11. Babar Z-U-D, Scahill S, Nagaria RA, Curley LE. The future of pharmacy practice research—perspectives of academics and practitioners from Australia, NZ, United Kingdom, Canada and USA. *Res Soc Adm Pharm.* 2018;14(12):1163–1171.
12. Bond C. The need for pharmacy practice research. *Int J Pharm Pract.* 2006;14(1):1–2.
13. Hadi MA, Closs SJ. Ensuring rigour and trustworthiness of qualitative research in clinical pharmacy. *Int J Clin Pharmacol.* 2016;38(3):641–646.
14. Guirguis LM, Witry MJ. Promoting meaningful qualitative research in social pharmacy: moving beyond reporting guidelines. *Int J Pharm Pract.* 2019;27(4):333–335.
15. Lau SR, Traulsen JM. Are we ready to accept the challenge? Addressing the shortcomings of contemporary qualitative health research. *Res Soc Adm Pharm.* 2017;13(2):332–338.
16. Bradbury-Jones C, Taylor J, Herber O. How theory is used and articulated in qualitative research: development of a new typology. *Soc Sci Med.* 2014;120(Supplement C):135–141.
17. Roberts AS, Benrimoj SI, Dunphy D, Palmer I. *Community Pharmacy: Strategic Change Management.* North Ryde, Sydney, Australia: McGraw-Hill Australia Pty Ltd; 2007.

18. Benrimoj SI, Feletto E, Wilson L. *Building Organisational Flexibility to Promote the Implementation of Primary Care Services in Community Pharmacy.* Canberra: Pharmacy Guild of Australia and the Department of Health and Aging; 2010. http://6cpa.com.au/wp-content/uploads/Building-Organisation-Flexibility-to-Promote-the-Implementation-of-Primary-Care-Service-in-Community-Pharmacy-Full-Final-report.pdf. Accessed 1/11/2020.

19. Desselle SP, Zgarrick DP, Alston GL, eds. *Pharmacy Management: Essentials for All Practice Settings.* 3rd ed. McGraw-Hill Companies; 2012.

20. Garcia-Cardenas V, Perez-Escamilla B, Fernandez-Llimos F, Benrimoj SI. The complexity of implementation factors in professional pharmacy services. *Res Soc Adm Pharm.* 2017;14(5):498–500.

21. Palinkas LA, Aarons GA, Horwitz S, Chamberlain P, Hurlburt M, Landsverk J. Mixed method designs in implementation research. *Admin Pol Ment Health.* 2011;38(1):44–53.

22. Seaton TL. Dissemination and implementation sciences in pharmacy: a call to action for professional organizations. *Res Soc Adm Pharm.* 2017;13(5):902–904.

23. Sandberg J, Tsoukas H. Grasping the logic of practice: theorizing through practical rationality. *Acad Manag Rev.* 2011;36(2):338–360.

24. Curran GM, Shoemaker SJ. Advancing pharmacy practice through implementation science. *Res Soc Adm Pharm.* 2017;13(5):889–891.

25. Garcia-Cardenas V, Fernandez-Llimos F, Rosing CV, et al. Pharmacy practice research—a call to action. *Res Soc Adm Pharm.* 2020;16(11):1602–1608.

26. Craig P, Dieppe P, Macintyre S, Michie S, Nazareth I, Petticrew M. Developing and evaluating complex interventions: the new Medical Research Council guidance. *BMJ.* 2008;337:979–983.

27. Damschroder LJ, Aron DC, Keith RE, Kirsh SR, Alexander JA, Lowery JC. Fostering implementation of health services research findings into practice: a consolidated framework for advancing implementation science. *Implement Sci.* 2009;4(1):1–15.

28. Sørensen EW, Haugbølle LS. Using an action research process in pharmacy practice research—a cooperative project between university and internship pharmacies. *Res Soc Adm Pharm.* 2008;4(4):384–401.

29. Chia R. Ontology: organization as "world-making". In: Westwood R, Clegg SR, eds. *Debating Organization: Point-Counterpoint in Organization Studies.* Oxford: Blackwell Publishers; 2003:98–113.

30. Mintzberg H. Developing theory about the development of theory. In: Floyd SW, Wooldridge B, eds. *Handbook of Middle Management Strategy Process Research.* Cheltenham, UK: Edward Elgar Publishing; 2017:177–196.

31. Clegg SR, Kornberger M, Rhodes C. Learning/becoming/organizing. *Organization.* 2005;12(2):147–167.

32. Weick KE. The generative properties of richness. *Acad Manag J.* 2007;50(1):14–19.

33. Nayak A, Chia R. Thinking becoming and emergence: process philosophy and organization studies. In: Lounsbury M, ed. *Philosophy and Organization Theory.* Bingley, UK: Emerald Group Publishing; 2011:281–309.

34. Bourdieu P. *The Logic of Practice; Translated by Richard Nice.* Cambridge: Polity Press; 1990.

35. Tsoukas H. Don't simplify, complexify: from disjunctive to conjunctive theorizing in organization and management studies. *J Manag Stud.* 2017;54(2):132–153.

36. Dall'Alba G, Sandberg J. Learning through and about practice: a lifeworld perspective. In: Billett S, ed. *Learning Through Practice: Models, Traditions, Orientations and Approaches.* Dordrecht: Springer; 2010:104–119.

37. Dall'alba G, Sandberg J. Unveiling professional development: a critical review of stage models. *Rev Educ Res.* 2006;76:383–412.

38. Sztompka P. *Society in Action: The Theory of Social Becoming.* University of Chicago Press; 1991.

39. Pettigrew AM. The character and significance of strategy process research. *Strateg Manag J.* 1992;13:5–16.

40. Maher JH, Lowe JB, Hughes R, Anderson C. Understanding community pharmacy intervention practice: lessons from intervention researchers. *Res Soc Adm Pharm.* 2014;10(4):633–646.

41. Sandberg J, Dall'Alba G. Returning to practice anew: a life-world perspective. *Organ Stud.* 2009;30(12):1349–1368.

42. Merleau-Ponty M. *Phenomenology of Perception.* London & New York: Routledge & Kegan Paul; 1945/1962 [C. Smith Translation].

43. Taylor C. Engaged agency and background in Heidegger. In: Guignon CB, ed. *The Cambridge Companion to Heidegger.* Cambridge [England]/New York, NY: Cambridge University Press; 1993:317.

44. Pharmaceutical Society of Australia. *National Competency Standards Framework for Pharmacists in Australia.* Canberra, ACT: Pharmaceutical Society of Australia; 2016. https://my.psa.org.au/s/article/2016-Competency-Framework. Accessed 24 October 2019.

45. Chia R. From modern to postmodern organizational analysis. *Organ Stud.* 1995;16(4):579–604.

46. Tsoukas H. Introduction: why philosophy matters to organization theory. In: Chia R, Tsoukas H, Chia R, eds. *Research in the Sociology of Organizations: Philosophy and Organization Theory.* Emerald Group; 2011:1–21.

47. Bansal P, Smith WK, Vaara E. New ways of seeing through qualitative research. *Acad Manag J.* 2018;61(4):1189–1195.

48. Weik E. In deep waters: process theory between Scylla and Charybdis. *Organization.* 2011;18(5):655–672.

49. Langley A, Tsoukas H. Introduction: process thinking, process theorizing and process researching. In: Langley A, Tsoukas H, eds. *The Sage Handbook of Process Organizational Studies.* Sage Publications; 2016:1–26.

50. Van de Ven A. Suggestions for studying strategy process: a research note. *Strateg Manag J.* 1992;13(Special Issue):169–188.

51. Rescher N. *Process Metaphysics: An Introduction to Process Philosophy.* Albany, NY: SUNY Press; 1996.

52. Hohmeier KC, Shelton C, Havrda D, Gatwood J. The need to prioritize "prioritization" in clinical pharmacy service practice and implementation. *Res Soc Adm Pharm.* 2020;16(12):1785–1788.

53. Shove E, Pantzar M, Watson M. Promoting transitions in practice. In: *The Dynamics of Social Practice: Everyday Life and How It Changes.* London, UK: Sage Publications; 2012:139–164.

54. Shove E, Pantzar M, Watson M. *The Dynamics of Social Practice: Everyday Life and How It Changes.* London, UK: Sage Publications; 2012.

55. Rescher N. Process philosophy. In: *Process Philosophical Deliberations.* Berlin/Boston, Germany: De Gruyter; 2006:1–26.

56. Farmer RL. *Beyond the Impasse: The Promise of a Process Hermeneutic.* vol. 13. Macon, GA: Mercer University Press; 1997.

57. Langley A, Tsoukas H. Introducing perspectives on process organization studies. In: Hernes T, Maitlis S, eds. *Process, Sensemaking, and Organizing.* vol. 1. Oxford, UK: Oxford University Press; 2010:1–27.

58. Blue S, Shove E, Carmona C, Kelly MP. Theories of practice and public health: understanding (un) healthy practices. *Crit Public Health.* 2016;26 (1):36–50.

59. Schatzki TR. *The Site of the Social: A Philosophical Account of the Constitution of Social Life and Change.* University Park, PA: Pennsylvania State University Press; 2002.

60. Rantakari A, Vaara E. Narratives and processuality. In: Langley A, Tsoukas H, eds. *The Sage Handbook of Process Organization Studies.* London, UK: Sage Publications; 2016:271–285.

61. Orlikowski WJ. Using technology and constituting structures: a practice lens for studying technology in organizations. *Organ Sci.* 2000;11(4):404–428.

62. Sandberg J, Pinnington A. Professional competence as ways of being: an existential ontological perspective. *J Manag Stud.* 2009;46(7):1138–1170.

63. Woods PS. *Pharmacists Managing Capably: A Grounded Exploration and Reconceptualisation of Managerial Capability* [Doctoral thesis]. Gold Coast, QLD: Griffith Business School, Griffith University, Queensland, Australia; 2018.

64. Feldman MS. Making process visible: alternatives to boxes and arrows. In: Langley A, Tsoukas H, eds. *The Sage Handbook of Process Organization Studies.* London, UK: Sage Publications; 2016:625–635.

65. Latour B. *Reassembling the Social: An Introduction to Actor-Network-Theory.* Oxford: Oxford University Press; 2005.

66. Czarniawska B. On time, space, and action nets. *Organization.* 2004;11(6):773–791.

67. Pentland BT, Feldman MS. Narrative networks: patterns of technology and organization. *Organ Sci.* 2007;18(5):781–795.

68. Ingold T. To journey along a way of life. In: Ingold T, ed. *The Perception of the Environment: Essays on Livelihood, Dwelling and Skill.* London, New York: Routledge, Taylor & Francis Group; 2000:219–242.

69. Lincoln YS, Guba EG. But is it rigorous? Trustworthiness and authenticity in naturalistic evaluation. *New Dir Progr Eval.* 1986;30:73–84.

70. Amin MEK, Nørgaard LS, Cavaco AM, et al. Establishing trustworthiness and authenticity in qualitative pharmacy research. *Res Soc Adm Pharm.* 2020;16(10):1472–1482.

71. Langley A, Tsoukas H. Introduction: process thinking, process theorizing and process researching. In: Langley A, Tsoukas H, eds. *The Sage Handbook of Process Organization Studies.* London, UK: Sage Publications; 2017:1–25.

72. Weick KE. *The Social Psychology of Organizing.* Reading, MA, USA: Addison-Wesley; 1979.

73. Weick KE, Sutcliffe KM, Obstfeld D. Organizing and the process of sensemaking. *Organ Sci.* 2005;16(4):409–421.

74. Jarzabkowski P, Lê J, Spee P. Taking a strong process approach to analyzing qualitative process data. In: Langley A, Tsoukas H, eds. *The Sage Handbook of Process Organization Studies.* London, UK: Sage Publications; 2016:237–251.

75. Feldman MS, Orlikowski WJ. Theorizing practice and practicing theory. *Organ Sci.* 2011;22(5):1240–1253.

76. Dionysiou DD, Tsoukas H. Understanding the (re)creation of routines from within: a symbolic interactionist perspective. *Acad Manag Rev.* 2013;38 (2):181–205.

77. Czarniawska B. Actor-network theory. In: Langley A, Tsoukas H, eds. *The Sage Handbook of Process Organization Studies.* London, UK: Sage Publications; 2016:160–173.

78. Sandberg J, Tsoukas H. Practice theory: what it is, its philosophical base, and what it offers organization studies. In: Mir R, Willmott H, Greenwood M, eds. *The Routledge Companion to Philosophy in Organization Studies.* New York, NY, USA: Routledge; 2016.

79. Nicolini D. *Practice Theory, Work, and Organization: An Introduction.* Oxford, UK: Oxford University Press; 2013.

80. Burrows J. *Becoming Pharmacists: Exploring Professional Development of Pharmacists Following Graduation* [Doctoral thesis]. Brisbane, QLD: School of Education, University of Queensland; 2019.

81. Sandberg J. Understanding human competence at work: an interpretive approach. *Acad Manag J.* 2000;43(1):9–25.

82. Van Hulst M, Ybema S, Yanow D. Ethnography and organizational processes. In: Langley A, Tsoukas H, eds. *The Sage Handbook of Process Organization Studies.* London, UK: Sage Publications; 2016:223–236.

83. Charmaz K. Grounded theory as an emergent method. In: Hesse-Biber SN, Leavy P, eds. *Handbook of Emergent Methods.* New York: The Guilford Press; 2008:155–170.

84. Charmaz K. The power of constructivist grounded theory for critical inquiry. *Qual Inq.* 2016;23(1):34–45.

85. Kvale S. *InterViews: An Introduction to Qualitative Research Interviewing.* Thousand Oaks, CA: Sage Publications; 1996.

86. McDonald S. Studying actions in context: a qualitative shadowing method for organizational research. *Qual Res.* 2005;5(4):455–473.

87. Symon G. Qualitative research diaries. In: Cassell C, Symon G, eds. *Essential Guide to Qualitative Methods in Organizational Research.* London, UK: Sage Publications; 2004:98–113.

88. Pettigrew A. What is processual analysis. *Scand J Manag.* 1997;13(4):337–348.

89. Langley A. Strategies for theorizing from process data. *Acad Manag Rev.* 1999;24(4):691–710.

90. Langley A, Tsoukas H, eds. *The Sage Handbook of Process Organization Studies.* London, UK: Sage Publications; 2016.

91. James W, Hare PH. *Some Problems of Philosophy.* vol. 7. Harvard University Press; 1911/1979.

92. MacKay B, Chia R, Nair AK. Strategy-in-practices: a process philosophical approach to understanding strategy emergence and organizational outcomes. *Hum Relat.* 2021;74(9):1337–1369.

93. Pettigrew AM. Longitudinal field research on change: theory and practice. *Organ Sci.* 1990;1:267–292.

Chapter 21

Design and application of the simulated patient method in pharmacy and health services research

Jack C. Collins[a], Wei Wen Chong[b], Abilio C. de Almeida Neto[c], Rebekah J. Moles[a], and Carl R. Schneider[a]

[a]*The University of Sydney School of Pharmacy, Faculty of Medicine and Health, The University of Sydney, Sydney, NSW, Australia,* [b]*Centre of Quality Management of Medicines, Faculty of Pharmacy, The National University of Malaysia, Kuala Lumpur, Malaysia,* [c]*Neto Psychological Consulting, Pyrmont, NSW, Australia*

Objectives

- Describe the simulated patient method and a brief history of its use.
- Compare and contrast observational methods used in pharmacy practice and health services research.
- Discuss relevant considerations required at the design, implementation, and evaluation phases of simulated patient studies.
- Describe applications of the simulated patient method, including mixed-methods, communication analysis, and audit and feedback.

Introduction

Background and overview

In health services research, numerous observational methods can be utilized to investigate and characterize practice and behavior.[1] The use of "simulated" or "standardized" patients has become increasingly popular as the technique of choice in observational research, as it allows researchers to witness the true-to-life response of healthcare practitioners to predetermined scenarios in a naturalistic setting.[2–4]

This chapter aims to provide readers an overview of the simulated patient method, a brief history of its use, where it is situated, as compared to other observational methods, and considerations for designing, implementing, and evaluating studies using this method. The approach is to provide an overview and "how to" guide for health services researchers, ranging from those who are new to the simulated patient method, to those who have experience in conducting simulated patient studies, and builds on a published methods paper by the authors.[5] Although the focus of this chapter is primarily pharmacy practice research, these concepts and considerations can be applied to other healthcare disciplines.

A simulated patient (SP) may be called a number of synonyms (Box 1). This individual is trained to go to a practice site and enact a predetermined scenario, while being indistinguishable from a genuine patient, to assess aspects of the care or service received or other aspects of the practice site, such as the environment.[4,6]

The SP method can be utilized in health services research for several purposes. First, it can be used simply as an audit of current practice to characterize how a particular aspect of care is provided (e.g., to determine how many practitioners provide appropriate care in response to a standardized scenario).[7–9] It can also be used to observe the effect of an intervention on practitioners' behavior (e.g., after providing training to practitioners on a specific aspect of care, SP observations can be used to determine if training is translated into behavior).[10,11] Finally, it can also be used as a component of an intervention in its own right, where following the SP visit, feedback is provided to the practitioner to facilitate behavior change.[12–14]

BOX 1: Synonyms for simulated patient[3,6]

Covert participant
Covert shopper
Disguised shopper
Mystery client
Mystery shopper
Pseudo customer
Pseudo patient
Pseudo patron
Shopper patient
Simulated client
Standardized actor
Standardized
patient
Surrogate client
Surrogate shopper
Test buyers
Undercover patient

Application and brief history of the simulated patient method

Customer observers ("mystery shoppers") have been used to audit service quality in retail and business settings, such as supermarkets and banks, for many years.[4] Similarly, healthcare may be considered a service-orientated industry where the patient is a consumer of the healthcare service, and, as such, the SP method has been used to examine care or service quality in the healthcare practitioner's naturalistic practice setting.[3,15]

Although SP studies have been conducted in nonhealth service industries since at least the 1940s,[16] SP studies in healthcare have their genesis in a study conducted in 1973 by Rosenhan, in which 8 SPs were instructed to go to mental hospitals and feign just one symptom of schizophrenia, hearing voices.[17] Seven of the 8 SPs were diagnosed with schizophrenia and admitted to hospital. In no case was their simulation detected by healthcare practitioners. At discharge, the 7 SPs received the diagnosis of "schizophrenia in remission."[17]

Rosenhan's study[17] induced anxiety, resentment among practitioners, and controversy concerning both the merit of his conclusions and the competence of the staff involved.[18,19] Such resentment is particularly prone to occur if the observation is very critical or undertaken without prior consent. SP research often results in critical reports of practitioner behavior. In a Dutch study, 4 SPs visited 39 general practitioners complaining of headaches, diarrhea, shoulder pain, and diabetes. General practitioners' performance was reported to have been "substandard."[20] This type of research, of course, is not unique to medicine. Pharmacists have also been criticized based on SP studies. For example, in a British study, SPs posed as parents requesting community pharmacist advice for the treatment of their child's diarrhea. It was reported that 70% of the pharmacists recommended inappropriate treatment.[21]

SP methods, however, do not have to be purely observational, punitive, and negative. Some more recent studies have evolved to focus on the implementation of skills in the practice of healthcare through performance feedback and coaching, as part of continuous professional development.[12,13,22–24]

Comparison with alternative methods

In addition to the use of SP methodology as described, other approaches to the measurement of actual healthcare practitioner behavior in the naturalistic environment include self-reported behavior, exit surveys, documentation abstraction, and nonparticipant observation (Table 1). Alternatively, other approaches may be applied to measure behavior outside the naturalistic setting, through such methods as observation in a simulated environment or measurement of behavior in response to clinical vignettes.[33,34] As a result of removal of the behavior of interest from its naturalistic setting into a simulated environment, such measures are surrogates of actual behavior, with wide variation in their alignment to actual behavior in the practice setting.[35,36]

While all methods of measurement of healthcare practitioner behavior in the naturalistic environment have their advantages and disadvantages, the SP method is well suited and frequently used for the measurement of the quality of practitioner behavior.[37] The key reasons are that the SP method can provide sound internal validity as the scenario or experimental conditions are consistent for the entire sample.[38] Second, the researchers can develop a scenario such that there is a clear understanding of what is considered an appropriate response or outcome.[39] Accordingly, one can calculate the prevalence

TABLE 1 Comparison of methods to measure practitioner behavior in the practice setting.

Method	Examples	Advantages	Limitations
Reported behavior (historical)	Survey,[25] interviews,[26] focus groups[11]	• Large sample possible • Low-cost • High participation rate • Able to measure behavioral intent • Can target practitioners and service recipients	• Overt only • Limited external validity • Recall bias • Response bias • Practitioner time burden
Reported behavior (contemporaneous)	Exit survey,[27,28] time and motion study[29]	• Efficient • Low-cost • High participation rate • Able to measure behavioral intent • Can target practitioners and service recipients	• Overt only • Limited external validity • Response bias • Practitioner time burden
Documentation abstraction	Written record audit[30]	• Large sample possible • Low-cost • High participation rate • Low practitioner time burden • Can be used for experimental study designs • Individual consent may not be required	• Only practitioners targeted • Unmeasured discrepancy between performance and documentation
Observation (nonparticipant)	"Fly on the wall"[28]	• Overt or covert • High external validity • Can target practitioners and service recipients • Low practitioner time burden	• Unable to control conditions • Limited internal validity • Covert observation subject to increased ethical considerations • Overt observation potentially subject to observer effect
Observation (participant)	Simulated patient[3]	• Overt or covert • Efficient • High internal validity • Fair external validity (covert) • Can control script/scenario/simulated patient • Can be used for experimental study designs	• Covert observation subject to increased ethical considerations • Only practitioners targeted • Practitioner time burden • Overt observation subject to Hawthorne effect
Clinical vignettes	Role-play,[31] think-aloud[32]	• High internal validity • Able to capture behavioral intent • Can control conditions • Can be used for experimental study designs	• Limited external validity • Overt only • Only practitioners targeted • Practitioner time burden • Potentially subject to observer effect

of appropriate responses across a population sample as a measure of quality of practice behavior. Additionally, the method focuses on the key behaviors to be tested, rather than on proxy measures such as file records of interventions that are made by the practitioner. Additional advantages of the SP technique are that it is covert, thereby eliminating the possibility of a Hawthorne effect, as the subject is unaware of the measurement and thus does not alter their behavior or become reactive.[3] The SP method is also efficient. Large samples can be conducted in a reasonable timeframe, and response rates are not an issue as with voluntary surveys and interviews.[40] Finally, the method is an acceptable method of research by practitioners when consent is provided in advance.[22,24] In contrast to the wide-spread acceptance of SP methods, there is emergent critique that the artificiality or "fakery" of the method, despite rigorous effort to mimic natural conditions, may create a construct in which the subject provides a biased response, thereby affecting external validity.[41] Although this critique raises points which may warrant further investigation and consideration, the SP method remains a popular choice for researchers investigating practice behavior, is widely accepted, and presents advantages over other methods in this sphere (Table 1). The SP method may well still be regarded as the best choice for investigating practice behavior when executed appropriately.

Selecting a research method—Is the SP method appropriate?

When contemplating the use of the SP method in health services research, it is first necessary to develop and refine the research question. The researcher should consider what is being asked and which method of observation is best suited to answer the research question (consider Table 1). The SP method is ideally placed to investigate "actual" behavior of practitioners covertly. Conversely, it is less suited to obtain outcomes of the service or care provided due to the lack of "real" patients to follow-up and this may be more suitably answered with an alternative method such as a follow-up interview with patients after receiving the service or care.

The SP method has primarily been used to assess the performance of practitioners in the primary care setting. This is likely a result of the challenge in simulation of physiological symptoms in secondary and tertiary settings such as hospital wards where advanced diagnostic tools are more readily available and presenting complaints are often more serious in nature. Examples of primary care settings include general medical practice,[20] community pharmacy,[3] online pharmacies,[42] opticians,[43] telephone triage,[44] and hospital emergency departments.[45] The method has been widely used to measure performance of healthcare services in both high-resource and low-resource settings.[46–49]

In isolation, the SP method does not directly capture behavioral intent, attitudes, beliefs, or knowledge, and mixed-methods or other research methods are better suited to address research questions with a focus in these areas. For example, if the research question is to examine the knowledge of practitioners in a specific therapeutic area, the SP method may not be suitable as it captures the actual behavior of practitioners rather than their knowledge (although, of course, knowledge may inform behavior). On the other hand, if the research question is to examine the communication skills of practitioners during consultations or how practitioners respond to certain clinical presentations in a naturalistic setting, or the effect of an educational intervention on practice, the SP method is suitable. Alternatively, a combination of methods (mixed-method) study may be appropriate, whereby certain outcomes of interest are investigated using the SPs (e.g., communication skills, what outcome occurs in response to a request) and other outcomes are measured by sampling the same population with an alternative method (e.g., a questionnaire to assess knowledge, interviews to ascertain further information about why certain events occurred during the encounter).[50,51]

Study design and application of the simulated patient method

Sampling

An important consideration at the study development stage is the sampling and unit of measurement for analysis. Each SP visit/interaction can be considered a data point. These data points can be clustered by practice sites, individual practitioners, or by SPs. A large-scale study which intends to audit behavior across many practice sites with a single visit to each site, may consider each visit to be the representative sample for that site.[40] Conversely, a design where a smaller number of sites are visited to measure the effect of an intervention could either treat the visits as representative of that practice site[12] or of individual practitioners.[52] This may be determined by whether the research team can confidently and ethically identify individual practitioners at each site and whether this is necessary for the research question. In addition to treating the practice site or individual practitioners as the unit of measurement, it is also possible to make comparisons between the SPs, if the study is intended to compare how different SPs are treated, as conducted in a study investigating implicit racial bias in pharmacists.[50] The target sample size will need to be determined by the research team, following standard statistical considerations and procedures, and based on existing evidence in the area of investigation and the design and objectives of the study. Researchers may wish to seek statistical advice when determining an appropriate sample, particularly for experimental designs. Sampling strategy may be influenced by the consent approach required for the study (see "Ethical considerations" section in this chapter) and whether the sample is intended to be generalizable. For example, if a consent waiver is obtained for an entire region, the research team could theoretically sample all pharmacies in that region. Conversely, the requirement for individual consent may require consideration of the logistics involved in this process when deciding the sample and may result in defaulting to a convenience sample. If the sample is intended to be generalizable, more robust and purposive consideration of the intended sample may be required as opposed to a convenience sample. Finally, it is necessary to decide if audio and/or video recordings of the interactions are necessary for analysis and integrity of the data, or if data collection will be solely based on recall of SPs. This is an important consideration as recall bias has been highlighted as a potential limitation of the SP method.[3]

Scenario and script development

Once the research question and/or topic of interest have been decided, it is necessary to consider the development of scenarios and scripts for the SPs. The scenarios and scripts should be written so as to address the research question(s) and maintain a level of authenticity to real-life scenarios. Scripts may be generated through a review of the literature,[53] by the research team, or a team of experts with consensus on the content of the script.[23,54] The level of detail included in the scripts given to SPs can vary from a basic outline of the scenario and responses to anticipated questions to more detailed prompts for the SP or an algorithm-based script where the responses from the SP vary based on the management of the request by the practitioner.[55,56] It is also necessary to consider if the scripts are written with specific SPs in mind or if there is a need for them to be adjusted for individual SPs based on their demographics. For example, if the SP is male and the request is for emergency contraception, the script would need to be adjusted to state that the request is for a female.[51] Scripts may have their content validity assessed by an external panel during the development stage.[57] Content validity can be established using standard methods.[58] An additional quality control measure may be to conduct a pilot study with a smaller number of visits to pilot and refine the scripts and the data collection process.[39] Intentional changes made to the script throughout the data collection period may alter the results obtained, and this should be considered during the analysis and interpretation phases. Unintentional changes or SPs going "off-script," may also have an effect on the findings and may be excluded from analysis.[12,59]

An important aspect of the script is who the SP will approach and how the initial request will be opened. For example, in the context of community pharmacy, the SP may approach the first staff member they encounter, wait to be approached by a staff member, or directly seek a specific staff member such as a pharmacist. Each of these approaches may depend on whether the focus of the research question is to audit any staff (first staff member encountered), service quality (wait to be approached by a staff member), or pharmacists (directly ask for the pharmacist).

Once speaking to a staff member, the SP may then request a product by name, assistance with symptoms, assistance with the management of a self-diagnosed condition, or information. Visual cues such as empty packaging or written notes may also be used.[60] Examples of request methods are shown in Table 2. The method of request may play an important role in the performance of the staff and the subsequent results obtained, as evidence shows that different request types are managed differently.[7,25] For example, direct product requests have been demonstrated to be managed poorly compared to symptom-based requests in SP studies conducted in community pharmacies.[7] Any prompts, such as declaring use of a particular medicine,[56] provided by SPs may also alter the way practitioners respond to the original query.

Once the request has been made, the SP should follow the script provided and complete the interaction with the practitioner, including following any questioning and counseling made by the practitioner. At the design stage, it is necessary to consider if the SP will purchase any products if this is relevant to the scenario, when they will terminate the simulated interaction, and how the SP will respond if the practitioner detects them.

TABLE 2 Examples of methods of requesting assistance in community pharmacy.

Direct product request	Condition-based request	Symptom-based request	Visual cues
"Can I get some triamcinolone paste?"	"Can I get something for a mouth ulcer?"	"Can I get something for a sore mouth?"	A prescription from a dentist for triamcinolone paste
"Can I get some ibuprofen tablets?"	"Can I get something for a migraine?"	"Can I get something for a headache?"	An empty blister of ibuprofen tablets presented by the SP[a]
"Can I get some clotrimazole cream?"	"Can I get something for thrush?"	"Can I get something for an itch?"	An image of clotrimazole cream on the SP's smart phone

[a]*Simulated patient.*
Modified from Collins JC. *Community Pharmacy Faciliation of Consumer Self-Care in Australia* [PhD Thesis]. Sydney: The University of Sydney; 2020.

Selection and training of simulated patients

SPs may consist of people from various backgrounds, including students, trained actors, researchers, individuals with previous SP experience, people with lived experience of the target condition, and laypeople.[2,3] The selection of who takes on the role of SPs is based on a number of considerations, including the research topic and questions, target population, suitability to the tasks based on requirements of the scenarios and scripts, and previous experience as SPs. For example, recent studies have purposively recruited SPs from diverse backgrounds to reflect the population in the area,[50,61] and to investigate implicit bias among healthcare providers.[50,61] These considerations ensure that the recruited SPs are congruent with the scenario and particulars, resulting in increased authenticity. Researchers may choose to select SPs based on their scripts/scenarios or vice versa. Further face validation of the recruited SPs can be achieved by showing images/videos of the SPs to members of the intended target sample (e.g., practicing pharmacists[50]). The number of SPs in a single study is an important consideration and is described in the "Validity and reliability" section of this chapter.

Regardless of the background of the SPs, adequate training prior to commencing visits is important to ensure standardization and consistency of the simulated scenarios, in addition to minimizing the risk of detection by participants. Duration and number of training sessions may vary depending on the complexity of scenarios and roles of SPs in the study. Table 3 summarizes the key considerations for the training of SPs.

During the training session(s), SPs should be briefed about important study-specific information, as well as be familiarized with the scenarios given and any data collection requirements such as the use of concealed recording devices. A considerable part of the training may involve role-playing, in which SPs will be trained to enact the scenarios and to respond to situations that may arise during the visits. SPs should also be instructed on the visit process, including how to approach participants (such as directly speaking to the first person encountered or waiting to be approached) and how to manage detection (e.g., immediately terminating the interaction). SPs who are responsible for recording observations following their visits should be trained on the appropriate use of data collection tools and/or equipment. In some studies, SPs are also trained in providing performance feedback to participants, such as highlighting areas where the practitioner did well and where they could improve.[12,24] Other aspects to be covered during the training session may include ethical considerations, including ensuring the anonymity of participants and data confidentiality. SPs should be afforded ample opportunity to ask questions and clarify any issues related to the study.

As part of the study, researchers should consider how to assess the effectiveness of the training and readiness of SPs to perform the tasks entrusted to them. As part of the evaluation process, SPs can be provided a guide for self-assessment or self-reflection of their performance. An evaluation session can be conducted during rehearsals to assess the performance of SPs in terms of authenticity and level of congruency to scenarios, and reliability of SPs in completing data collection forms accurately. Pilot visits can also be carried out to examine the fidelity and face validity of the SPs from audio records of interactions or identification of the detection rate.[40]

Outcome measures

The outcome of interest is typically the performance of healthcare practitioners in providing clinical care.[2,3,6] Outcome measures may vary and be driven primarily by the research objectives of the study. A common outcome measure from SP studies is the competencies or performance of healthcare practitioners in the management of case presentations for both minor and major illnesses.[3,6] These are usually evaluated through the appropriateness of clinical actions of the healthcare practitioner, or appropriateness of outcomes, in response to simulated scenarios.[2,3,6,45] Examples of these outcomes may include the appropriateness of dispensing and supply of pharmaceutical products (usually in compliance with legal requirements and practice guidelines, e.g., legal handling of nonprescription medicines[62]), referral to a medical practitioner,[63] communication skills,[23] counseling points covered,[39,51] and the accurate demonstrations of devices (such as inhaler technique).[39,64] Other outcome measures could include how practitioners respond to a specific item request or assessment of the environment of the practitioner.[45,65] Appropriate outcomes for the scenarios may be determined a priori by the researchers based on practice guidelines, professional standards, and protocols developed by national and pharmaceutical organizations.[51,66–68]

The quality of counseling by a practitioner is usually measured through two main elements; questioning and advice-giving.[2,3,6] The practitioner's ability to gather information from the patient is measured through the types or number of questions asked or both. Similarly, the extent and content of advice and information provided to the patient are also measured. To analyze these measurements, some researchers have used scoring systems developed from established questioning protocols[12] (e.g., the WHAT-STOP-GO protocol developed by the Pharmaceutical Society of Australia[69] for nonprescription medicine requests or the WWHAM protocol from the United Kingdom[70]). Others have used case-specific

TABLE 3 Considerations for training of simulated patients.

Training component	Purpose	Suggested elements
Purpose of study	General understanding about study and SP[a] methodology	General orientation and briefing about • Training aims and objectives • Study objectives and research questions • Role expectations of SPs • Ethical considerations and confidentiality issues • Relevant details or facts related to study
Simulation scenarios	Internal validity (accurate portrayal of case) Consistency between visits Authenticity of performance	Training for role portrayal that involves • Introduction to case scenarios • Instructions on delivery of scenarios using prompts (if applicable) and scripts • Practice and rehearsal through role-playing of scenarios • Evaluation of SP role performance
Visit procedure	Minimize risk of detection	Instructions and advice on visit process including on • Rules for identifying and approaching participants • How to manage detection • How to respond to emerging situations during visit • Other particulars relevant to study (e.g., behavior and dress code)
Data collection	Reliability and accuracy of observations and documentation	Training in use of • Data collection tools to record observations and findings • Equipment (if applicable, e.g., recording devices)
Provision of feedback (if applicable to study)	Accurate and effective feedback to participants	Training on providing constructive performance-based feedback to participants
Assessment of training effectiveness	Fidelity (accuracy of SP performance) Face validity Reliability in observations	SP performance evaluation (in role portrayal, data collection, provision of feedback) can be carried out • During rehearsal sessions • During pilot visits • As part of ongoing scheduled visits Provision of continual feedback to improve performance SP's self-reflection or self-assessment after training

[a]Simulated patient.

checklists, assessment rubrics or scoring tools developed based on previous literature or reviewed by an expert panel in the area.[23,53,54] Additionally, SPs have also been used to measure the costs of the provision of care.[71,72]

Communication analysis and mixed-methods

In addition to quantitative assessment of the care or service provided, other applications of the SP method and analytical approaches may be used to measure further aspects of interactions between SPs and practitioners. An important outcome measure in health services research is the communication skills and behaviors of healthcare practitioners.[23] For communication behaviors to be measured effectively, interactions between SPs and practitioners should ideally be recorded. One method that may be useful in analyzing the interactions is the Roter Interaction Analysis System (RIAS).[73,74] The RIAS is a widely used quantitative coding system in studies of medical communication, with demonstrated reliability and predictive validity.[73] This system assigns each "utterance" (the smallest unit of expression) to mutually exclusive and exhaustive categories. Summary measures that reflect patient-centeredness, such as verbal dominance and a ratio of socioemotional and psychosocial statements to statements that further the biomedical agenda, can be measured using RIAS.[60,75,76] However, a potential drawback with this system is that it may not always capture the depth and complexity of human interactions.[77] A combination of RIAS with qualitative methods (such as discourse or conversational analysis) may be useful to study the dynamic interplay of the communication process. Content analysis[78,79] has also been employed to assess the quality and content of pharmacist counseling[80] and written responses to online drug information queries from SPs.[42] In addition to verbal and written communication, some studies have investigated the nonverbal communication of practitioners (such as facial expression)[23,81] or the interaction of practitioners with the surrounding environment and equipment such as computers,[82] via video-recording of the interactions.

Qualitative methods may be implemented to measure and analyze additional outcomes in SP studies. A recent study explored the use of discourse analysis as a novel method to investigate implicit racial bias among pharmacists.[50] Researchers have also reported qualitative descriptions of the experiences and perceptions of SPs concerning their interaction with practitioners.[50,83] Mixed-method approaches with SP studies may also enable structured or semistructured interviews with practitioners following the visits to better understand aspects of the interactions, such as why they made a certain recommendation.[51] Additionally, studies that had an educational focus and incorporated performance feedback to participants also recorded qualitative interview responses of practitioners' perceptions regarding SP methods as a training tool.[22]

Simulated patient visits with feedback

Audit and feedback is a theoretically grounded method of intervention, which has been shown to improve practitioner behavior in healthcare settings.[84,85] When audit and feedback is employed in SP studies in an interventional design, an educator provides feedback to the practitioner after the SP visit has been completed. Either the SP is the educator themselves or reports immediately to an educator (a member of the research team), who waits outside, on how the interaction with the healthcare practitioner was conducted. This may include reviewing any recordings made during the interaction or scoring the interaction on a data collection sheet. The educator (or SP) then enters the healthcare setting to discuss the observations made during the interaction with the healthcare provider and staff and provides performance feedback and coaching.[86]

When SP methods are used for educational (interventional) purposes, the SP visit provides an accurate assessment of practice behavior and performance feedback and coaching are used as a basis for further skills acquisition.[13,86] Performance feedback relates to how well the healthcare provider performed and feedback and coaching addresses what the healthcare provider can do to improve their performance. An important part of the feedback and coaching process may include self-assessment by the practitioner using a standardized scoresheet. This process allows the practitioners to examine and verbalize self-identified deficiencies or strengths in their practice, including verbalizing changes in practice behavior are needed, which may induce behavior change with repeated audit and feedback.[12,13]

Allowing the healthcare providers to appraise their own performance and making their own decision to modify the target behavior, as opposed to being told by the educator how to conduct themselves, minimizes the effect of "psychological reactance"; a phenomenon where individuals react negatively to being told how to behave and defy these instructions.[87] Through directing the healthcare provider's cognition toward making an "autonomous" decision to improve practice behavior, the educator averts this instinctual resistance to behavior change in the form of compensatory oppositional behavior, the phenomenon of psychological reactance, and increasing the likelihood of long-lasting practice behavior change.[88] Informing the practitioners of the upcoming SP visits during the study period may also influence practice behavior.[22] Participants may always be on their "best behavior" in anticipation of the visit and may falsely suspect some regular consumers to be SPs, thereby elevating the standard of practice.[12]

Validity and reliability

Many aspects of the design of SP studies can affect both internal and external validity. An advantage of the SP method is that it can offer a high degree of internal validity. Fig. 1 highlights some components of SP study designs which may present as a trade-off between internal and external validity. For example, using a smaller number of scenarios or variations of

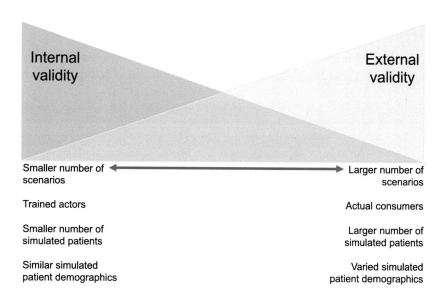

FIG. 1 Internal-external validity trade-off.[89]

Internal
validity

External
validity

Smaller number of
scenarios

Larger number of
scenarios

Trained actors

Actual consumers

Smaller number of
simulated patients

Larger number of
simulated patients

Similar simulated
patient demographics

Varied simulated
patient demographics

scenarios results in a high level of internal validity; however, this might come at the expense of being able to generalize findings across a range of different scenarios thereby constraining external validity. Similarly, the demographics and number of SPs may also influence the degree of internal and external validity. If it is imperative that the scenario is delivered consistently for each occasion, then a smaller number of trained actors with similar demographics would result in the greatest degree of internal validity as compared to using a larger number of actual consumers with demographic variation. These trade-offs must be considered during the design phase of the study and the most appropriate design selected based on the research question. For example, if it is sought to explore how practitioners respond to a variety of requests then this comes with a trade-off of internal validity.

The same principle applies to sampling. Multiple visits to a single practice site may provide a good indication of practice at that site but may be less indicative of what is occurring at other sites where a design with a smaller number of visits to multiple sites may be employed, thereby constraining external validity via reducing generalizability.

The reliability of documentation by SPs must be considered when analyzing and interpreting data. Strategies to improve the reliability of this data could include training in the use of the data collection sheets,[60] scoring from audio/visual recordings of the interactions,[63] and using a second SP who acts as a direct observer of the interaction between the SP and practitioner.[90] Recording of the interaction may be conducted with a concealed recording device, such as a smart phone, where permitted by local laws and ethical approval. Several studies in health services research have highlighted that SPs document interactions with practitioners with a good level of reliability when compared to audio recordings; however, deficiencies remain in documenting some aspects.[91–93]

Ethical considerations

As the SP method is primarily employed covertly, the informed consent of participants is an important ethical consideration during development of the study. King et al.[94] have articulated the options for provision of consent ranging from obtaining consent from every individual study participant, obtaining consent at the organizational level on behalf of employees, to obtaining consent at the system level such as consent being provided by a statutory authority or representative professional organization. Some researchers have requested and obtained ethical approval for a waiver of consent by appealing to the ethical principle of utility in performing the research.[94] Last, there are published studies in which the authors have justified conducting the research without formal ethical approval.[95]

As consent to participate in a SP study, particularly those with audio/visual recordings, may be required, this may result in the influence of the Hawthorne effect on the behavior by practitioners in SP studies. This risk may be mitigated by leaving a period of time between obtaining consent and conducting the SP visits, and by not informing practitioners of exactly when visits will occur and what the topics of interest are (subject to ethical approval). Although the potential influence of the Hawthorne effect may be considered detrimental to study designs which intend to audit usual practice or the effect of interventions, it may be useful in designs where SP visits are combined with feedback to modulate practice.

In these situations, practitioners may alter their behavior in anticipation of unannounced SP visits, which may itself lead to success of the intervention.[96]

A second ethical consideration when employing covert methodology is that a degree of deception is undertaken. At what point should disclosure be made and to whom should disclosure be made? As SP methods are employed to measure actual practice behavior, there is the opportunity to measure inappropriate practice.[62] The nature of the impropriety could range from suboptimal performance to illegal behavior. Researchers are required to consider in advance what behavior will be disclosed to a third party, for example, the reporting of illegal activity to an authority or the reporting of poor work performance to an organizational representative. Any such disclosure should be considered as part of the ethical approval process, and participants should also be aware of their level of identifiability in any dissemination of the research findings.[97]

Finally, researchers may wish to consider the burden of conducting the research on both the individual subjects and the healthcare system.[98] Depending on the consent model, participants may or may not be aware that the study is taking place. If participants are not aware, then resources may be diverted to the SP. The ethical justification and potential negative impacts of this should be considered during the study development stage. For example, a SP study conducted in a hospital emergency department may divert resources from patients who may need urgent medical care.

Reporting and dissemination

When it comes to reporting and dissemination of the completed study, standard reporting for observational (such as STROBE[99]) or interventional studies (such as TIDieR[100]) should be followed with some specific considerations applicable to the SP method. These considerations may include information on training of SPs and any modifications to or assessment of this training, ethical considerations (including approval to conduct the study), scenario descriptions including prompts/scripts, characteristics of SPs, detection rate of SPs by practitioners to determine fidelity, and the data collection process following a standard format such as CONSORT diagrams.[101] Finally, any missing or excluded visits/data should be discussed along with any reasons for exclusion.[102] A checklist designed specifically for SP studies in health services research implemented to audit practice (CRiSP) that complements existing checklists such as STROBE and CONSORT has been proposed to guide reporting of SP studies.[103] It may be necessary to consider if it is appropriate to disseminate the findings to practitioners that were included in the research or other interested parties such as professional bodies. Dissemination of any SP research should adhere to standard practices and principles, including anonymity of any participants where this is expected.

In summary, the SP method may be a suitable research tool to use in an observational study; however, there are many considerations that need to be taken into account at the outset of the study and throughout the implementation, evaluation, and reporting stages. Careful consideration should be given by the researchers at all stages of the study in order to ensure that the study is conducted ethically, purposefully and in a robust manner.

Questions for further discussion

1. What are the considerations and implications of the detection of SPs during an interaction?
2. What factors may influence the authenticity of SP interactions?
3. What are some advantages and disadvantages of the different methods for obtaining participant consent?
4. How might the experiences of SPs be used to inform data analysis and interpretation?

Application exercise/scenario

You are interested in evaluating how pharmacists and their pharmacy assistants provide information to parents of children suffering from coughs and colds. You have read the literature, which suggests that many parents use cough and cold medicines inappropriately, and you hypothesize that some on-site training may improve service provision. Design a simulated patient/caregiver study to evaluate practice and potentially change practice over time. Use the list of considerations in the Appendix to plan, implement, and evaluate your study.

Appendix

Summary of considerations for the design, implementation, and evaluation of simulated patient studies.

Phase	Component	Elements
Design	Planning	<ul><li>Determine topic(s) of interest</li><li>Develop and refine research questions</li><li>Determine purpose of SP[a] design<ul><li>Audit of current practice</li><li>Evaluation of intervention</li><li>As an intervention (with feedback and coaching)</li></ul></li><li>Determine outcomes of interest</li><li>Sampling considerations<ul><li>Unit of measurement (by practice site, individual practitioner)</li><li>Target sample size</li><li>Sampling strategy</li></ul></li><li>Equipment (audio/video recorder)</li><li>Data collection sheets (electronic or hard copy)</li><li>Logistics (site considerations including access to sites, timing of visits, paying for any products or services)</li><li>Ethical considerations (audio/video recording, obtaining ethical approval, consent from participating practitioners/sites, dissemination of results)</li><li>Budgetary considerations</li></ul>
	Scenario and script development	<ul><li>Develop scenarios based on research question(s) (number, topics, and variations)</li><li>Determine appropriate response or outcome (if applicable)</li><li>Develop data collection/scoresheets relevant to each scenario (electronic or hard copy)</li><li>Determine level of detail for scripts (prompts, responses to anticipated questions, room for ad-lib responses)</li><li>Establish content validity for scripts (literature review, expert panel feedback, pilot study)</li><li>Is script variation necessary between SPs?</li><li>Ensure scripts are authentic to real-life</li></ul>
	Selection of SPs	<ul><li>Consider demographics and number of SPs based on<ul><li>Research question(s)</li><li>Scenarios and scripts</li><li>Previous experience of SPs</li></ul></li></ul>
Implementation	Training of SPs	<ul><li>Duration and number of training sessions necessary</li><li>Location of training</li><li>Components of training</li><li>Training based on scenarios and roles of SPs e.g., do SPs also need to provide feedback?</li><li>Evaluation of training</li></ul>
	SP visits and data collection	<ul><li>Data collection during SP visits (written and audio/visual recordings)</li><li>Performance feedback and coaching</li><li>Data management (storage, access, cleaning)</li></ul>
Evaluation	Analysis	<ul><li>Units of measurement</li><li>Missing data and measurement error</li><li>Analytical methods (statistical and qualitative)</li><li>Relevant to outcome measures developed a priori</li><li>Data management (storage, access, cleaning)</li></ul>
	Reporting and dissemination	<ul><li>Follow reporting checklists where applicable</li><li>Ethical considerations (anonymity)</li><li>Dissemination to participants and interested bodies where relevant</li></ul>

[a]Simulated patient.

References

1. Caamaño F, Ruano A, Figueiras A, Gestal-Otero J. Data collection methods for analyzing the quality of the dispensing in pharmacies. *Pharm World Sci.* 2002;24:217–223.

2. Watson M, Norris P, Granas A. A systematic review of the use of simulated patients and pharmacy practice research. *Int J Pharm Pract.* 2006;14:83–93.

3. Björnsdottir I, Granas AG, Bradley A, Norris P. A systematic review of the use of simulated patient methodology in pharmacy practice research from 2006 to 2016. *Int J Pharm Pract.* 2020;28:13–25.

4. Wilson AM. The role of mystery shopping in the measurement of service performance. *Manag Serv Qual.* 1998;8:414–420.

5. Collins JC, Chong WW, de Almeida Neto AC, Moles RJ, Schneider CR. The simulated patient method: design and application in health services research. *Res Social Adm Pharm.* 2021;17(12):2108–2115.

6. Xu T, de Almeida Neto AC, Moles RJ. A systematic review of simulated-patient methods used in community pharmacy to assess the provision of non-prescription medicines. *Int J Pharm Pract.* 2012;20:307–319.

7. Horvat N, Koder M, Kos M. Using the simulated patient methodology to assess paracetamol-related counselling for headache. *PLoS One.* 2012;7: e52510.

8. Tsang MW, Resneck Jr JS. Even patients with changing moles face long dermatology appointment wait-times: a study of simulated patient calls to dermatologists. *J Am Academy Dermatol.* 2006;55:54–58.

9. Watson MC, Skelton JR, Bond CM, et al. Simulated patients in the community pharmacy setting. Using simulated patients to measure practice in the community pharmacy setting. *Pharm World Sci.* 2004;26:32–37.

10. Ratanajamit C, Chongsuvivatwong V, Geater AF. A randomized controlled educational intervention on emergency contraception among drugstore personnel in southern Thailand. *J Am Med Womens Assoc.* 2002;57:196–199.

11. Watkins K, Trevenen M, Murray K, Kendall PA, Schneider CR, Clifford R. Implementation of asthma guidelines to West Australian community pharmacies: an exploratory, quasi-experimental study. *BMJ Open.* 2016;6:e012369.

12. Collins JC, Schneider CR, Naughtin CL, Wilson F, De Almeida Neto AC, Moles RJ. Mystery shopping and coaching as a form of audit and feedback to improve community pharmacy management of non-prescription medicine requests: an intervention study. *BMJ Open.* 2017;7:e019462.

13. de Almeida Neto AC, Benrimoj SI, Kavanagh DJ, Boakes RA. Novel educational training program for community pharmacists. *Am J Pharm Educ.* 2000;64:302–307.

14. de Almeida Neto AC, Kelly F, Benrimoj SI. Shaping practice behaviour: novel training methodology. *Int J Pharm Pract.* 2001;9:203–210.

15. Rethans JJ, Gorter S, Bokken L, Morrison L. Unannounced standardised patients in real practice: a systematic literature review. *Med Educ.* 2007;41:537–549.

16. Xu L, He S. Analysis on the survey method of mystery shopping in hospitality management. In: Lee G, ed. *E-Commerce, E-Business and E-Service.* CRC Press; 2014:221–225.

17. Rosenhan DL. On being sane in insane places. *Science.* 1973;179:250–258.

18. Rabichow HG, Pharis ME. Rosenhan was wrong: the staff was lousy. *Clin Soc Work J.* 1974;2:271–278.

19. Wolitzky DL. Insane versus feigned insane: a reply to Dr. DL Rosenhan. *J Psychiatry Law.* 1973;1:463.

20. Rethans J-J, Sturmans F, Drop R, Van der Vleuten C. Assessment of the performance of general practitioners by the use of standardized (simulated) patients. *Brit J Gen Pract.* 1991;41:97–99.

21. Goodburn E, Mattosinho S, Mongi P, Waterston T. Management of childhood diarrhoea by pharmacists and parents: is Britain lagging behind the third world? *Brit Med J.* 1991;302:440–443.

22. Xu T, de Almeida Neto AC, Moles RJ. Simulated caregivers: their feasibility in educating pharmacy staff to manage children's ailments. *Int J Clin Pharmacol.* 2012;34:587–595.

23. Mesquita AR, Lyra Jr DP, Brito GC, Balisa-Rocha BJ, Aguiar PM, de Almeida Neto AC. Developing communication skills in pharmacy: a systematic review of the use of simulated patient methods. *Patient Educ Couns.* 2010;78:143–148.

24. Watson MC, Cleland JA, Bond CM. Simulated patient visits with immediate feedback to improve the supply of over-the-counter medicines: a feasibility study. *Fam Pract.* 2009;26:532–542.

25. Watson MC, Bond CM. The evidence-based supply of non-prescription medicines: barriers and beliefs. *Int J Pharm Pract.* 2004;12:65–72.

26. Jones LF, Owens R, Sallis A, et al. Qualitative study using interviews and focus groups to explore the current and potential for antimicrobial stewardship in community pharmacy informed by the theoretical domains framework. *BMJ Open.* 2018;8:e025101.

27. Collins JC, Schneider CR, El-Den S, Moles RJ. Self-care–seeking behaviors in the community pharmacy: a cross-sectional exit survey of Australian consumers. *J Am Pharm Assoc.* 2020;60:827–834.

28. Emmerton L. The 'third class' of medications: sales and purchasing behavior are associated with pharmacist only and pharmacy medicine classifications in Australia. *J Am Pharm Assoc.* 2009;49:31–37.

29. Cavaye D, Lehnbom EC, Laba T-L, El-Boustani E, Joshi R, Webster R. Considering pharmacy workflow in the context of Australian community pharmacy: a pilot time and motion study. *Res Social Adm Pharm.* 2018;14:1157–1162.

30. Williams M, Peterson GM, Tenni PC, et al. Drug-related problems detected in Australian community pharmacies: the PROMISe trial. *Ann Pharmacother.* 2011;45:1067–1076.

31. Akhtar S, Rutter P. Pharmacists thought processes in making a differential diagnosis using a gastro-intestinal case vignette. *Res Social Adm Pharm.* 2015;11:472–479.

32. Rutter P, Patel J. Decision making by community pharmacists when making an over-the-counter diagnosis in response to a dermatological presentation. *SelfCare.* 2013;4:125–133.

33. Lamé G, Dixon-Woods M. Using clinical simulation to study how to improve quality and safety in healthcare. *BMJ Simul Technol Enhanc Learn.* 2020;6:87–94.

34. Hd T, De Vries W, van het Loo M, et al. Guideline adherence rates and interprofessional variation in a vignette study of depression. *BMJ Qual Saf.* 2002;11:214–218.

35. Peabody J, Luck J, Glassman P, Dresselhaus T, Lee M. Should we use vignettes as a yardstick? A prospective trial comparing quality of care measurement by vignettes, chart abstraction, and standardized patients. *JAMA.* 2000;283:1715–1722.

36. Watson MC, Walker A, Grimshaw J, Bond CM. Why educational interventions are not always effective: a theory-based process evaluation of a randomised controlled trial to improve non-prescription medicine supply from community pharmacies. *Int J Pharm Pract.* 2006;14:249–254.

37. Weiner SJ, Schwartz A. Directly observed care: can unannounced standardized patients address a gap in performance measurement? *J Gen Intern Med.* 2014;29:1183–1187.

38. Schneider CR, Emery L, Brostek R, Clifford RM. Evaluation of the supply of antifungal medication for the treatment of vaginal thrush in the community pharmacy setting: a randomized controlled trial. *Pharm Pract.* 2013;11:132.

39. Schneider CR, Everett AW, Geelhoed E, Kendall PA, Clifford RM. Measuring the assessment and counseling provided with the supply of nonprescription asthma reliever medication: a simulated patient study. *Ann Pharmacother.* 2009;43:1512–1518.

40. Schneider CR, Everett AW, Geelhoed E, et al. Provision of primary care to patients with chronic cough in the community pharmacy setting. *Ann Pharmacother.* 2011;45:402–408.

41. Kingori P, Jones RD. Revelation or confirmation? *Med Anthropol Theory.* 2020;7:214–229.

42. Holmes ER, Desselle SP, Nath DM, Markuss JJ. Ask the pharmacist: an analysis of online drug information services. *Ann Pharmacother.* 2005;39:662–667.

43. Nie J, Zhang L, Gao J, et al. Using incognito standardised patients to evaluate quality of eye care in China. *Br J Ophthalmol.* 2021;105(3):311–316.

44. Montalto M, Dunt DR, Day SE, Kelaher MA. Testing the safety of after-hours telephone triage: patient simulations with validated scenarios. *Australas Emerg Nurs J.* 2010;13:7–16.

45. Xie Y, McNeil EB, Sriplung H, Fan Y, Zhao X, Chongsuvivatwong V. Assessment of adequacy of respiratory infection prevention in hospitals of Inner Mongolia, China: a cross-sectional study using unannounced standardized patients. *Postgrad Med.* 2020;132(7):643–649.

46. Madden JM, Quick JD, Ross-Degnan D, Kafle KK. Undercover careseekers: simulated clients in the study of health provider behavior in developing countries. *Soc Sci Med.* 1997;45:1465–1482.

47. Kwan A, Daniels B, Bergkvist S, Das V, Pai M, Das J. Use of standardised patients for healthcare quality research in low-and middle-income countries. *BMJ Glob Health.* 2019;4:e001669.

48. Brata C, Gudka S, Schneider CR, Clifford RM. A review of the provision of appropriate advice by pharmacy staff for self-medication in developing countries. *Res Social Adm Pharm.* 2015;11:136–153.

49. Brata C, Schneider CR, Marjadi B, Clifford RM. The provision of advice by pharmacy staff in eastern Indonesian community pharmacies. *Pharm Pract.* 2019;17(2):1452.

50. Collins JC, Mac Kenzie M, Schneider CR, Chaar BB, Moles RJ. A mixed-method simulated patient approach to explore implicit bias in health care: a feasibility study in community pharmacy. *Res Social Adm Pharm.* 2021;17:553–559.

51. Collins JC, Schneider CR, Moles RJ. Emergency contraception supply in Australian pharmacies after the introduction of ulipristal acetate: a mystery shopping mixed-methods study. *Contraception.* 2018;98:243–246.

52. Murphy AL, Gardner DM. A simulated patient evaluation of pharmacist's performance in a men's mental health program. *BMC Res Notes.* 2018;11:765.

53. Wazaify M, Elayeh E, Tubeileh R, Hammad EA. Assessing insomnia management in community pharmacy setting in Jordan: a simulated patient approach. *PLoS One.* 2019;14:e0226076.

54. Chong WW, Aslani P, Chen TF. Adherence to antidepressant medications: an evaluation of community pharmacists' counseling practices. *Patient Prefer Adherence.* 2013;7:813.

55. Mac Farlane B, Matthews A, Bergin J. Non-prescription treatment of NSAID induced GORD by Australian pharmacies: a national simulated patient study. *Int J Clin Pharmacol.* 2015;37:851–856.

56. MacFarlane BV, Bergin JK, Reeves P, Matthews A. Australian pharmacies prevent potential adverse reactions in patients taking warfarin requesting over-the-counter analgesia. *Int J Pharm Pract.* 2015;23:167–172.

57. Mirza N, Cinel J, Noyes H, et al. Simulated patient scenario development: a methodological review of validity and reliability reporting. *Nurs Educ Today.* 2020;85:104222.

58. Almanasreh E, Moles R, Chen TF. Evaluation of methods used for estimating content validity. *Res Social Adm Pharm.* 2019;15:214–221.

59. Watson M, Bond C, Grimshaw J, Mollison J, Ludbrook A, Walker A. Educational strategies to promote evidence-based community pharmacy practice: a cluster randomized controlled trial (RCT). *Fam Pract.* 2002;19:529–536.

60. Chong WW, Aslani P, Chen TF. Pharmacist–patient communication on use of antidepressants: a simulated patient study in community pharmacy. *Res Social Adm Pharm.* 2014;10:419–437.

61. Jumbe S, James WY, Madurasinghe V, et al. Evaluating NHS stop smoking service engagement in community pharmacies using simulated smokers: fidelity assessment of a theory-based intervention. *BMJ Open.* 2019;9:e026841.

62. Collins JC, Hillman JM, Schneider CR, Moles RJ. Supply of codeine combination analgesics from Australian pharmacies in the context of voluntary real-time recording and regulatory change: a simulated patient study. *Int J Drug Policy.* 2019;74:216–222.

63. Collins JC, Schneider CR, Faraj R, Wilson F, de Almeida Neto AC, Moles RJ. Management of common ailments requiring referral in the pharmacy: a mystery shopping intervention study. *Int J Clin Pharmacol.* 2017;39:697–703.

64. Khan TM, Azhar S. A study investigating the community pharmacist knowledge about the appropriate use of inhaler, eastern region AlAhsa, Saudi Arabia. *Saudi Pharm J.* 2013;21:153–157.

65. Collins JC, Schneider CR, Wilson F, de Almeida Neto AC, Moles RJ. Community pharmacy modifications to non-prescription medication requests: a simulated patient study. *Res Social Adm Pharm.* 2018;14:427–433.

66. Schneider CR, Gudka S, Fleischer L, Clifford RM. The use of a written assessment checklist for the provision of emergency contraception via community pharmacies: a simulated patient study. *Pharm Pract.* 2013;11:127.

67. Benrimoj SI, Gilbert A, Quintrell N, de Almeida Neto AC. Non-prescription medicines: a process for standards development and testing in community pharmacy. *Pharm World Sci.* 2007;29:386–394.

68. Benrimoj SI, Gilbert AL, De Almeida Neto AC, Kelly F. National implementation of standards of practice for non-prescription medicines in Australia. *Pharm World Sci.* 2009;31:230–237.

69. Pharmaceutical Society of Australia. *Standards for the Provision of Pharmacy Medicines and Pharmacist Only Medicines in Community Pharmacy.* Canberra: Pharmaceutical Society of Australia; 2006.

70. Sharpe S, Norris G, Ibbit M, Staton T, Riley J. Protocols: getting started. *Pharm J.* 1994;253:804–805.

71. McLeod PJ, Tamblyn RM, Gayton D, et al. Use of standardized patients to assess between-physician variations in resource utilization. *JAMA.* 1997;278:1164–1168.

72. Parwani V, Ulrich A, Rothenberg C, et al. National assessment of surprise coverage gaps provided to simulated patients seeking emergency care. *JAMA Netw Open.* 2020;3:e206868.

73. Roter D, Larson S. The Roter interaction analysis system (RIAS): utility and flexibility for analysis of medical interactions. *Patient Educ Couns.* 2002;46:243–251.

74. Roter DL, Stewart M, Putnam SM, Lipkin M, Stiles W, Inui TS. Communication patterns of primary care physicians. *JAMA.* 1997;277:350–356.

75. Cooper LA, Roter DL, Johnson RL, Ford DE, Steinwachs DM, Powe NR. Patient-centered communication, ratings of care, and concordance of patient and physician race. *Ann Intern Med.* 2003;139:907–915.

76. Helitzer DL, LaNoue M, Wilson B, de Hernandez BU, Warner T, Roter D. A randomized controlled trial of communication training with primary care providers to improve patient-centeredness and health risk communication. *Patient Educ Couns.* 2011;82:21–29.

77. Chou W-YS, Han P, Pilsner A, Coa K, Greenberg L. Interdisciplinary research on patient-provider communication: a cross-method comparison. *Commun Med.* 2011;8:29.

78. Krippendorff K. *Content Analysis: An Introduction to Its Methodology.* Sage Publications; 2018.

79. Holdford D. Content analysis methods for conducting research in social and administrative pharmacy. *Res Soc Admin Pharm.* 2008;4:173–181.

80. Olsson E, Ingman P, Ahmed B, Sporrong SK. Pharmacist–patient communication in Swedish community pharmacies. *Res Soc Admin Pharm.* 2014;10:149–155.

81. Liekens S, Vandael E, Roter D, et al. Impact of training on pharmacists' counseling of patients starting antidepressant therapy. *Patient Educ Couns.* 2014;94:110–115.

82. Montgomery AT, Lindblad ÅK, Eddby P, Söderlund E, Tully MP, Sporrong SK. Counselling behaviour and content in a pharmaceutical care service in Swedish community pharmacies. *Pharm World Sci.* 2010;32:455–463.

83. Queddeng K, Chaar B, Williams K. Emergency contraception in Australian community pharmacies: a simulated patient study. *Contraception.* 2011;83:176–182.

84. Ivers N, Jamtvedt G, Flottorp S, et al. Audit and feedback: effects on professional practice and healthcare outcomes. *Cochrane Database Syst Rev.* 2012;(6):CD000259.

85. Kluger AN, DeNisi A. The effects of feedback interventions on performance: a historical review, a meta-analysis, and a preliminary feedback intervention theory. *Psychol Bull.* 1996;119:254.

86. de Almeida Neto A. Changing pharmacy practice: the Australian experience. *Pharm J.* 2003;270:235–236.

87. Brehm JW. *A Theory of Psychological Reactance.* New York, NY: Academic Press; 1966.

88. de Almeida Neto AC. Understanding motivational interviewing: an evolutionary perspective. *Evol Psychol Sci.* 2017;3:379–389.

89. Collins JC. *Community Pharmacy Faciliation of Consumer Self-Care in Australia* [PhD Thesis]. Sydney: The University of Sydney; 2020.

90. Schneider CR. *Provision of Non-Prescription Medication by Community Pharmacists in Western Australia* [PhD Thesis]. Perth: The University of Western Australia; 2010.

91. Collins JC, Chan MY, Schneider CR, Yan LR, Moles RJ. Measurement of the reliability of pharmacy staff and simulated patient reports of non-prescription medicine requests in community pharmacies. *Res Social Adm Pharm.* 2021;17(6):1198–1203.

92. Werner JB, Benrimoj SI. Audio taping simulated patient encounters in community pharmacy to enhance the reliability of assessments. *Am J Pharm Educ.* 2008;72:136.

93. Luck J, Peabody JW. Using standardised patients to measure physicians' practice: validation study using audio recordings. *Br Med J.* 2002;325:679.

94. King JJ, Das J, Kwan A, et al. How to do (or not to do)... using the standardized patient method to measure clinical quality of care in LMIC health facilities. *Health Policy Plan.* 2019;34:625–634.

95. Granas AG, Haugli A, Horn AM. Smoking cessation advice provided in 53 Norwegian pharmacies. *Int J Pharm Pract.* 2004;12:179–184.

96. Cheo R, Ge G, Godager G, Liu R, Wang J, Wang Q. The effect of a mystery shopper scheme on prescribing behavior in primary care: results from a field experiment. *Health Econ Rev.* 2020;10:1–19.

97. Collins JC, Moles RJ, Penm J, Schneider CR. Ethical considerations for mystery shopper studies of pharmaceutical sales. *Bull World Health Organ.* 2020;98:375. 375A.

98. Steinman KJ. Commentary: key issues to consider for reviewing and designing simulated patient studies. *Int J Epidemiol.* 2014;43:903–905.

99. Vandenbroucke JP, Von Elm E, Altman DG, et al. Strengthening the reporting of observational studies in epidemiology (STROBE): explanation and elaboration. *PLoS Med.* 2007;4:e297.

100. Hoffmann TC, Glasziou PP, Boutron I, et al. Better reporting of interventions: template for intervention description and replication (TIDieR) checklist and guide. *Br Med J.* 2014;348:g1687.

101. Schulz KF, Altman DG, Moher D, Group C. CONSORT 2010 statement: updated guidelines for reporting parallel group randomised trials. *Trials.* 2010;11:32.

102. Narayan SW, Yu Ho K, Penm J, et al. Missing data reporting in clinical pharmacy research. *Am J Health Syst Pharm.* 2019;76:2048–2052.

103. Amaratunge S, Harrison M, Clifford R, Seubert L, Page A, Bond C. Developing a checklist for reporting research using simulated patient methodology (CRiSP): a consensus study. *Int J Pharm Pract.* 2021;29(3):218–227.

Section III

Qualitative, Hybrid, and Consensus-Gathering Approaches

Chapter 22

Moderation analysis with binary outcomes: Interactions on additive and multiplicative scales

John P. Bentley[a], Sujith Ramachandran[a], and Teresa M. Salgado[b]

[a]Department of Pharmacy Administration, University of Mississippi School of Pharmacy, University, MS, United States, [b]Department of Pharmacotherapy & Outcomes Science, Virginia Commonwealth University School of Pharmacy, Richmond, VA, United States

Objectives

- Identify research questions in pharmacy and health services research that require the use of moderation analysis with binary outcomes.
- Recognize statistical models that can be used to estimate effects when the outcome of interest is binary and describe basic concepts of moderation.
- Explain the meaning of interactions in the context of logistic regression.
- Summarize the challenges inherent in conducting moderation analysis when modeling binary outcomes.
- Interpret relevant statistical output including interpretations of interactions on additive and multiplicative scales.

Introduction

Clinical and social pharmacy researchers often have questions regarding contingencies of effects, seeking to examine under which conditions, or for which groups of individuals, an effect of interest exists or evaluating what variables might enhance, reduce, block, or reverse effects. For example, Paulus et al.[1] assessed whether alcohol use severity intensifies the relationship between pain and opioid misuse, and Basak et al.[2] examined whether the effect of perceived impact on relationship quality on hospital pharmacists' willingness to influence a physician's decision regarding an indication-based off-label medication order was different for different levels of the appropriateness of the medication order and the relative expert power of the pharmacist. Other examples, include Almeida et al.,[3] who explored differential relationships between adherence and glycemic control among groups defined by patients' family support, gender, and age, and Liddelow et al.,[4] who tested hypotheses concerning whether the intention-behavior relationship in terms of medication adherence was contingent on behavioral prepotency and self-regulation. Evidence of such contingencies can have implications for theory, practice, and policy. For example, resources can be allocated to groups most likely to benefit from interventions.

The evaluation of contingencies of effects is referred to as moderation analysis[5] and such questions are explored or tested by including interactions in statistical models. If the focal independent variable's (X) effect on some dependent variable (Y) depends on a third variable, termed a moderator (M), one can say that X's effect is moderated by or is conditional on M; furthermore, many would say that X and M interact in influencing Y.[5,6] Thus, a moderator effect is known as an interaction effect, and these terms are commonly used interchangeably. In the clinical trials literature, one may seek to evaluate whether a treatment effect varies across the levels of a baseline or demographic factor. This analysis is referred to as subgroup analysis, and statistical tests for interaction reflect a direct examination of whether the treatment effect on an outcome differs among different subgroups (i.e., an interaction between the treatment group and the baseline (or subgroup) variable).[7-9] Although there is some disagreement,[10-12] epidemiologists refer to this concept as effect-modification (or heterogeneity of effect), and moderators are called effect modifiers (and interaction and effect modification are typically used interchangeably). Greenland et al.[13] note that, in the absence of any bias, statistical interaction and effect modification are "logically equivalent," while VanderWeele and Knol[11] note that an interpretation of a finding as measure of effect

Contemporary Research Methods in Pharmacy and Health Services. https://doi.org/10.1016/B978-0-323-91888-6.00039-9

modification, causal interaction, or both "depends on what confounding factors have been controlled for." Knol and VanderWeele[14] outline the information needed to assess effect modification or interaction. Much like the conceptual and operational differences between associations and effects,[15,16] the distinction between effect modification and interaction is beyond the scope of this chapter, and the examples used throughout will assume no unmeasured confounding for simplicity of presentation of additional important concepts. The use of additional predictors to adjust for confounders is a straightforward extension and follows the principles of multivariable modeling.[17,18]

Much of the available literature for estimating and testing interaction effects is based on extensions of the linear model with continuous outcomes.[19,20] In this case (i.e., the linear moderation model), the regression coefficient for the interaction term (the product of the focal independent variable and the moderator variable as will be subsequently described) has an interpretation based on a departure from additivity (i.e., the effect of two variables together is different than the sum of the two individual effects). Binary (or dichotomous) outcome variables, such as prescription-medication misuse versus no misuse, medication adherence versus nonadherence, birth defect versus no birth defect, and future repatronization versus no future repatronization, are commonly encountered by clinical and social pharmacy researchers. A common statistical model used in epidemiologic and health care research for a binary dependent variable is logistic regression. When modeling interactions in a logistic regression model, the regression coefficient for the interaction term has an interpretation based on a departure from multiplicativity (i.e., the effect of two variables together is different than the product of the two individual effects). As will be discussed, there are alternative statistical models for binary outcomes, and some of these models lead to interpretations based on departures from additivity; furthermore, there are surrogate measures of interaction that can be calculated from logistic regression results (and other models) that are interpreted in terms of departures from additivity.

Interactions evaluated as departures from additivity versus departures from multiplicativity do not always agree, meaning one cannot always clearly identify the presence or absence of effect modification, as it may depend on whether one is focusing on interactions on an additive or multiplicative scale.[21] Although departure from multiplicativity may be meaningful in many contexts, from a public health perspective, interaction on the additive scale is often viewed as most informative.[9,11,13,14] This is analogous to potentially different public health implications between absolute effect measures (i.e., differences in occurrence measures) versus relative effect measures (i.e., ratios of occurrence measures).[16]

The purpose of this chapter is to describe a number of considerations when conducting moderation analysis with a binary outcome. It begins with a review of statistical models that can be used to estimate effects when the outcome of interest is binary, followed by a brief review of basic concepts associated with the linear moderation model. Two different examples will then be covered to illustrate how to estimate and interpret interactions in the context of logistic regression. Finally, the concepts of interaction as departures from additivity and multiplicativity will be explored with a focus on identifying which statistical models for binary outcomes lead to which measure of interaction along with a discussion of surrogate measures for estimating interaction on an additive scale.

Review of statistical models with binary outcomes

Generalized linear models (GLMs) are a family of models used for prediction of a variety of outcomes.[22] A GLM is commonly represented as Eq. (1) where a function of the expected value (or mean) of the outcome variable Y, depicted here as $f(E(Y))$, is expressed as a linear combination of a set of explanatory variables $X_1, X_2, X_3, ..., X_k$:

$$f(E(Y)) = \beta_0 + \beta_1 X_1 + \beta_2 X_2 + \beta_3 X_3 + ... + \beta_k X_k \tag{1}$$

In this equation, the β_is represent effects of the corresponding predictor variables. GLMs are regression models that can accommodate a variety of outcome variables based on a selected distribution of the dependent variable (called the random component) and a link function. The link function, $f(E(Y))$, specifies a function that relates the mean of the response variable on the left-hand side of Eq. (1) to the model (called the systematic component) on the right-hand side. In the simplest case, the ordinary linear regression model for a continuous response variable employs an identity link that directly models the mean of the outcome variable ($f(E(Y)) = E(Y)$) and assumes that the outcome follows a normal distribution. In the case of a binary response variable, there are several options. In a logistic regression model, one assumes a binomial random component and the link function is the logit function, which is the log of the odds of the outcome, as shown in Eq. (2), where p is the probability of the outcome.

$$f(E(Y)) = \log \left[\frac{p}{1-p} \right] \tag{2}$$

As a result of the use of this link function, the parameter estimates obtained from the logistic regression model do not represent the change in the expected outcome for a one-unit change in the predictor variable (as they would in linear regression) and must be interpreted with caution. Instead, the natural exponent of parameter estimates (e^{β_i}) from this model are commonly reported and can be interpreted as odds ratios (ORs), or the ratio of the odds of occurrence of the outcome for the different levels of the predictor variable. The procedure for estimation of ORs is shown elsewhere.[23] ORs have certain disadvantages. In the case of frequent outcome occurrence, ORs may overestimate the prevalence ratio or risk ratio (RR).[24] In addition, ORs are generally not as intuitive as RRs and are not considered preferable,[25,26] despite existing literature demonstrating the risks in misinterpretation associated with RR.[27]

In order to overcome the disadvantages of ORs, many researchers prefer alternative approaches to modeling binary response variables. The log-binomial model is an example of such an approach.[28] Like the logistic regression model, this model assumes a binomial distribution for the response variable, but the log-binomial model uses a log link function as shown in Eq. (3).

$$f(E(Y)) = \log(p) \tag{3}$$

Because of the log link, the natural exponent of parameter estimates from this model represents the ratio of probabilities or risks of the outcome—commonly referred to as a RR. RRs are often preferred to ORs because of their ease of interpretation. Another approach to this problem also uses a log link but employs the Poisson distribution as opposed to the binomial distribution, resulting in a model referred to as Poisson regression. For statistical inference, care should be taken to use a robust error variance estimator with this approach.[29] This model also yields RRs when coefficients are exponentiated.

Despite their ease of interpretation, these models have certain challenges. First, the log-binomial model, and sometimes the Poisson model, can result in estimation problems due to a lack of convergence. Second, the RR obtained from these models is not symmetric, i.e., the risk of success is not equal to the inverse of the risk of failure, which can potentially lead to confusion. The linear probability model overcomes this disadvantage by using an identity link function ($f(E(Y)) = E(Y) = p$) along with a binomial distribution (sometimes a normal distribution).[22,23,30] As a result of the identity link, this model directly predicts the mean of the outcome variable, which in the case of a binary outcome is simply the probability or risk. The advantage of the linear probability model is that the parameter estimates directly represent the difference in risk for each corresponding predictor without the need for exponentiation. This difference in risk of the outcome, referred to as risk difference (RD), is by far the easiest estimate to interpret and has the added advantage of being symmetric, unlike the RR.[23] However, it is important to bear in mind that no one measure of effect is superior to another and that interpretation of absolute and relative effect measures may lead to significantly different conclusions about the size of the effect depending on the size of the baseline risk. It is usually recommended that, whenever possible, researchers present both absolute and relative measures of effect to allow the reader to interpret the effect on their own.[31,32] Finally, one disadvantage of the linear probability model is that it can result in predicted probabilities outside the range of 0 to 1, leading to challenges in interpretation. The differences among these models, in terms of their link functions, distributions, and interpretations of their parameter estimates, are summarized in Table 1.[23,33] Other alternative models, such as the probit regression model or the Cox proportional hazard model, are also acceptable approaches for modeling categorical response variables.

Review of the linear moderation model

Moderation describes the influence of a variable M on the sign or strength of the relationship between two other variables, X and Y (Fig. 1). In other words, variable M interacts with X to determine their conjoint influence on Y. Moderators (M), as well as the variables (X) whose effects they moderate, can be categorical or continuous.[5,20]

TABLE 1 Some regression models used for modeling binary outcomes.

Model	Distribution	Link function	Measure of effect
Logistic	Binomial	Logit	Odds ratio
Log-binomial	Binomial	Log	Risk ratio
Poisson	Poisson	Log	Risk ratio
Linear probability	Binomial or normal	Identity	Risk difference

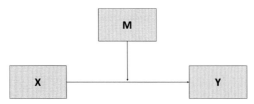

FIG. 1 Moderation model depicting the effect of variable M on the relationship between variables X and Y.

The linear moderation model, with a continuous outcome (Y), can be represented mathematically by the following equation:

$$Y = \beta_0 + f(M)X + \beta_2 M + e_Y \qquad (4)$$

where $f(M)$ is a linear function of M, $f(M) = \beta_1 + \beta_3 M$, which when substituted into Eq. (4) yields

$$Y = \beta_0 + (\beta_1 + \beta_3 M)X + \beta_2 M + e_Y \qquad (5)$$

Because the effect of X on Y is the most important effect being examined, X is also referred to as the *focal predictor*. The conditional effect of X on Y at different levels of M ($\theta_{X \to Y}$) is the linear function of M and is equal to $\beta_1 + \beta_3 M$ in Eq. (5). Thus, the conditional effect of X on Y is determined by β_3. If β_3 is equal to zero, the relationship between X and Y is linearly independent from M. The linear moderation model of the effect of X on Y by M is tested by inferring whether β_3 is different from zero.

Distributing X across the two terms in Eq. (5), results in the commonly presented simple linear moderation model, where the product term XM represents the interaction or moderating effect:

$$Y = \beta_0 + \beta_1 X + \beta_2 M + \beta_3 XM + e_Y \qquad (6)$$

Eq. (6) allows estimation of regression coefficients for X, M, and XM as predictors of Y in a linear regression model (typically using ordinary least squares). To infer whether the effect of X on Y is linearly moderated by M (i.e., whether these two variables interact), the p-value for the coefficient of XM or the confidence interval are used. Fig. 2 depicts the simple linear moderation model.[5,20]

For interpretation of the regression coefficients, consider Eq. (6). The interpretation of the regression coefficients β_1 and β_2 differs depending on whether or not XM is included as a predictor. When XM is included as a predictor, both β_1 and β_2 are *conditional effects*—β_1 represents the conditional effect of X on Y when M is equal to zero (if $M = 0$, then $\theta_{X \to Y} = \beta_1$) and β_2 represents the conditional effect of M on Y when X is equal to zero (if $X = 0$, then $\theta_{M \to Y} = \beta_2$). When XM is **not** included as a predictor (i.e., no moderation), β_1 and β_2 are *unconditional* or *partial effects*—β_1 represents the change in Y for a one-unit increase in X while holding M constant, and β_2 represents the change in Y for a one-unit increase in M, while holding X constant.

In the linear moderation model, β_3, the regression coefficient for the interaction term, indicates how the linear relationship between X and Y changes as M changes by one unit; as noted earlier, the effect of X on Y is a linear function of M. Stated differently, β_3 provides information regarding how much the difference in the expected value of Y between two cases that differ by one unit on X changes for a one-unit increase in M, leading to an interpretation of interaction as a difference between differences.[5,20] Thus, the effect of X (which is really a difference in expected value of Y for two cases that differ on X by one unit) is different as a function of another variable, in this case M. An alternative, but equivalent, way to interpret β_3 is that it denotes a deviation from the sum of the independent effects of the variables involved in the

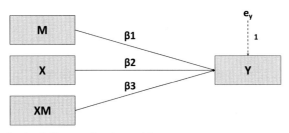

FIG. 2 Statistical diagram representing the simple linear moderation model.

interaction.[9,34] Because this deviation is from the sum of the independent effects of the other variables, the linear moderation regression model is said to evaluate an interaction on the additive scale.[9]

The interpretation of moderation can be further explored through plotting and probing the interaction. Additional details about this process and various extensions, such as the use of multiple moderators as well as multicategorical independent variables and moderators, can be found elsewhere.[19,20]

Interactions in logistic regression: Two examples

In general, two separate, yet related, research streams regarding modeling of interactions with a binary outcome can be observed. The first focuses on the interpretation of interactions in the context of logistic regression.[35,36] A second, broader literature is concerned with interpretations of interactions on additive and multiplicative scales with a focus on identifying which statistical models for binary outcomes lead to which measure of interaction as well as surrogate measures forestimating interaction on an additive scale.[9,11,13,14,37] This section will explore the former using two different examples that analyze simulated data based on the results of published research, while the next section will explore the latter using three different examples. All datasets are available at the following link: https://osf.io/pfysb/?view_only=cdbc99da247647a0976cb1f8f9c961d2.

Two binary predictors

Paulus et al.[1] examined the moderating role of alcohol use severity in the pain-opioid misuse relationship, hypothesizing that "those with more severe alcohol use would evidence a stronger positive relationship between pain and opioid misuse relative to those with less severe alcohol use." A conceptual model illustrating their hypothesis can be found in Fig. 3. Although the authors used continuous variables to represent the constructs and performed linear regression analysis to assess and probe for interaction, their study motivated the hypothetical summary data that appear in Table 2 (Example 1a), where both pain intensity and alcohol use severity are represented as binary variables (scored $0 =$ low and $1 =$ high) as is the dependent variable of whether or not the respondent misused opioids in the past 30 days (scored $0 =$ no and $1 =$ yes). Results of a logistic regression for the Example 1a data can be found in Table 3. A test of the interaction between pain intensity *(X)* and alcohol use severity *(M)* tests whether or not *X*'s effect on *Y* depends on *M* (i.e., does *M* moderate the $X \rightarrow Y$ relationship?). Such a test also assesses whether the two conditional effects of pain intensity at both levels of alcohol use severity are different. There is evidence of moderation in Table 3. The coefficient associated with the product term (pain

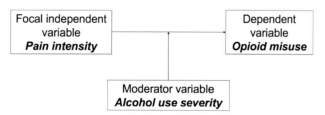

FIG. 3 Conceptual moderation model for Example 1a as motivated by Paulus et al.[1]

TABLE 2 Hypothetical probabilities and odds of opioid misuse as a function of pain intensity and alcohol use severity (Example 1a).

	Low alcohol use severity	High alcohol use severity
Probabilities		
Low pain intensity	$28/130 = 0.2154$	$15/65 = 0.2308$
High pain intensity	$49/195 = 0.2513$	$60/115 = 0.5217$
Odds		
Low pain intensity	$28/102 = 0.2745$	$15/50 = 0.3000$
High pain intensity	$49/146 = 0.3356$	$60/55 = 1.0909$

Note: Odds is the probability of an event occurring divided by the probability of the event not occurring or $\frac{R}{1-R}$.

TABLE 3 Logistic regression output for data from Example 1a (outcome = opioid misuse).

Predictor	Regression coefficient	Exponent of coefficient (odds ratio)	95% CI for odds ratio	p-Value
$\hat{\beta}_0$: Intercept	−1.2928	0.275	0.181, 0.417	<0.0001
$\hat{\beta}_1$: Pain intensity	0.2010	1.223	0.721, 2.075	0.456
$\hat{\beta}_2$: Alcohol use severity	0.0888	1.093	0.536, 2.229	0.807
$\hat{\beta}_3$: Pain intensity × Alcohol use severity	1.0900	2.974	1.254, 7.056	0.013

intensity × alcohol use severity), $\hat{\beta}_3$, is an estimate of the interaction, and the p-value (or the CI) provide support for a significant finding of moderation.

It is important to consider the meaning of the parameter estimates provided in Table 3. As with other applications of logistic regression, it is common to exponentiate coefficients to produce ORs (the coefficients are in the log-odds scale, which is not very intuitive). This has been done in Table 3, and CIs for these ORs are also provided. For the two lower-order terms (i.e., what some people refer to as "main effects"), these ORs are not unconditional main effects as defined in ANOVA terms, but rather conditional effects (or simple effects in ANOVA terms), and they are interpreted as:

- $e^{\hat{\beta}_1}$: The conditional OR for pain intensity when alcohol use severity $=0$ (i.e., is low): $0.3356/0.2745 = 1.223$.
- $e^{\hat{\beta}_2}$: The conditional OR for alcohol use severity when pain intensity $=0$ (i.e., is low): $0.3000/0.2745 = 1.093$.

The exponentiated coefficient for the product term, $\hat{\beta}_3$, is not an OR, but rather a ratio of two ORs, namely, the two conditional ORs reflecting the effects of one variable at each level of the other variable. In Example 1a, we will do this for the focal independent variable, pain intensity (the math also works if you switch the focal independent variable and the moderator):

- $e^{\hat{\beta}_3}$: Ratio of conditional ORs: $\frac{1.0909/0.3000}{0.3356/0.2745} = 2.974$

If the two conditional ORs are the same, then the ratio of the ORs will be 1. We can also describe $e^{\hat{\beta}_3}$ as the amount that the conditional OR for the outcome associated with one variable (the focal independent variable) is multiplied by for a one-unit increase (or state change if the independent variable is binary) of the other variable (or moderator). Thus, the OR for pain intensity for those with high levels of alcohol use severity is 2.974 times that for those with low levels. Researchers should report conditional ORs of interest along with CIs (see Jackson et al.[38] for an example). This is easily accomplished in the current situation by recoding the reference categories or, in more general situations, one can use the ODDSRATIO statement in SAS PROC LOGISTIC or Hayes' PROCESS macro (which is available for SPSS, SAS, and R).[20] For the data from Example 1a, the association of pain intensity with opioid misuse is stronger among those with high, but not low alcohol use (low alcohol use: OR = 1.223, 95% CI: 0.721–2.075, $p = 0.456$; high alcohol use: OR = 3.636, 95% CI: 1.836–7.201, $p = 0.0002$).

Two continuous predictors

It is possible for either or both of the focal independent and moderator variables to be continuous when modeling interactions in general and specifically with logistic regression. This next example (Example 1b) illustrates some considerations when assessing interactions between continuous variables in logistic regression. Liddelow et al.[4] evaluated whether the intention-behavior relationship in terms of medication adherence was moderated by a number of different variables, including one measure of the self-regulatory process, namely planning. They hypothesize that planning "will moderate the intention-behavior relationship, such that the association between intention and adherence will be weaker at low levels of" planning. This suggests that for individuals with high planning, intentions and behavior are more closely aligned. A conceptual model illustrating their hypothesis can be found in Fig. 4. Although the authors used continuous measures of the outcome, in our simulated example based on their work, the dependent variable is binary, whether or not the respondent exhibited medication adherent behavior (scored 0 = nonadherent and 1 = adherent). Similar to Liddelow et al.[4], intention is based on three items with a 1–7 response format (1 = strongly disagree and 7 = strongly agree) and averaged to form a single

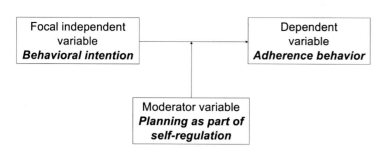

FIG. 4 Conceptual moderation model for Example 1b as motivated by Liddelow et al.[4]

TABLE 4 Logistic regression output for data from Example 1b (outcome = adherence behavior).

Predictor	Regression coefficient	Exponent of coefficient (odds ratio)	95% CI for odds ratio	p-Value
$\hat{\beta}_0$: Intercept	3.7513	42.575	9.37, 193.45	<0.0001
$\hat{\beta}_1$: Behavioral intention	−0.9356	0.392	0.272, 0.567	<0.0001
$\hat{\beta}_2$: Planning	−0.9045	0.405	0.253, 0.648	<0.0001
$\hat{\beta}_3$: Behavioral intention × Planning	0.2840	1.328	1.187, 1.487	<0.0001

score where higher scores indicate stronger intentions. Planning is represented by five items scored 1–5 (1 = strongly disagree and 5 = strongly agree) and averaged into a single variable with higher scores indicating a greater likelihood to plan. Results of a logistic regression for the Example 1b data can be found in Table 4.

The analytic approach taken is similar to that with binary independent variables with the exception that the independent variables are now interpreted in terms of one-unit increases rather than state changes. For example, the OR for intention when planning = 2 on a 5-point scale is 0.6924 (i.e., $e^{-0.9356+0.2840\times2}$) and 0.9198 ($e^{-0.9356+0.2840\times3}$) when planning = 3, which represents a one-unit increase in the moderator. The ratio of these two conditional ORs (0.9198/0.6924) is 1.328, which is $e^{\hat{\beta}_3}$. There is evidence of moderation in Table 4 (ratio of conditional ORs = 1.328, 95% CI: 1.187, 1.487, $p < 0.0001$). The ORs for the lower order terms still represent conditional effects (i.e., ORs conditioned on the other variable involved in the interaction being 0), but in the present case these coefficients are not meaningful as 0 is outside the range of possible values for either independent variable. This interpretational issue can be rectified by centering (see Hayes[20] for more information) or picking various values of the moderator to compute and evaluate conditional effects of the focal independent variable, what some refer to as probing the interaction using the pick-a-point approach or simple slopes analysis.[19,20] One straightforward approach is to pick low, medium, and high values of the moderator to examine these effects (one standard deviation below the sample mean, the mean, and one standard deviation above the mean; or the 16th, 50th, and 84th percentiles). Another approach to probe the interaction with a continuous moderator is the Johnson-Neyman technique, which locates value(s) of the moderator where the relationship between the focal independent variable and the outcome transitions between statistically significant and not significant.[39] All of these approaches can be automated using one of several publicly available macros, such as PROCESS.[20] In addition, plots of the moderated effects are often helpful, especially with continuous predictors. For Example 1b, three values of the moderator were selected: 1.6, 3, 4.6 (representing values at the 16th, 50th, and 84th percentiles). A plot of the findings can be found in Fig. 5. The results demonstrate that the intention-adherence behavior relationship was significant and negative at low planning, nonsignificant at mean levels, and significant and positive at high planning.

The scale of interaction: Additive and multiplicative interactions

Definitions and basic terminology

In moderation analysis, binary outcomes have led to an increased focus on the fact that measures of interaction and effect modification are scale-dependent; thus, it is possible to find different answers regarding interaction depending on whether

FIG. 5 Moderation of the association between intention and adherence behavior by planning. Note: Plot is on the probability scale.

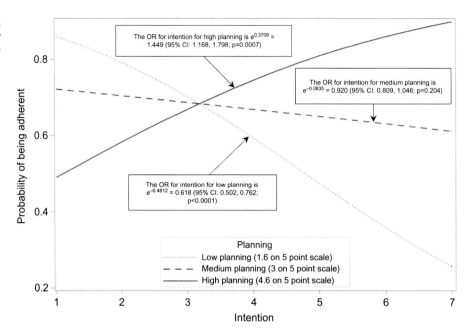

you are looking at the risk-difference scale (additive scale), the risk-ratio scale (multiplicative scale), or the odds-ratio scale (multiplicative scale). This could be extended to rates as well (i.e., rate-difference scale and rate-ratio scale), but rate and hazard models will not be covered in this chapter. Given this, researchers may need to consider both additive and multiplicative interaction.

In order to differentiate these concepts, consider a simple case where one has a binary outcome and two binary exposure (i.e., independent) variables, also called risk factors. There are four possible probabilities (i.e., risks) of the outcome associated with various combinations of the two exposures as outlined in Table 5. This 2×2 table also indicates terminology that will be used extensively in this section. For example, R_{11} represents the risk (or probability) of the outcome when one is exposed to both Factors 1 and 2, and R_{00} is the risk of the outcome when one is exposed to neither (i.e., both factors are absent).

As defined earlier, a departure from additivity (i.e., interaction on an additive scale) indicates that the effect of two variables together is different than the sum of the two individual effects. In other words, the difference between the combined effect and the sum of the two individual effects does not equal zero. This can be represented as:

$$(R_{11} - R_{00}) - [(R_{10} - R_{00}) + (R_{01} - R_{00})] = R_{11} - R_{10} - R_{01} + R_{00} \tag{7}$$

Eq. (7) is referred to as a measure of interaction on the additive scale[11] and is also known as the absolute excess risk due to interaction (AERI).[9] If this measure equals zero, that means no interaction on the additive scale, while a nonzero value suggests an additive interaction. An AERI >0 is sometimes called a positive or superadditive interaction (i.e., the combined effect is greater than the sum of the individual effects), and an AERI <0 is referred to as a negative or subadditive interaction (i.e., the combined effect is less than the sum of the individual effects).[9,11] Note that we can alternatively conceptualize AERI as the difference between differences as described earlier for the linear moderation model. In other words, the difference between two conditional RDs (simple effects in ANOVA terminology), the RD of Factor 2 at each level of Factor 1 (or vice versa):

TABLE 5 Assuming two binary exposure variables and a binary outcome variable, this 2×2 table represents the risks (or probabilities) of the outcome for the four combinations of the exposure variables.

	No exposure (Factor 2)	Exposure (Factor 2)
No exposure (Factor 1)	R_{00}	R_{01}
Exposure (Factor 1)	R_{10}	R_{11}

$$(R_{11} - R_{10}) - (R_{01} - R_{00}) = (R_{11} - R_{01}) - (R_{10} - R_{00}) = R_{11} - R_{10} - R_{01} + R_{00} \tag{8}$$

For this reason, an additive interaction when one has a binary outcome variable is also referred to as an interaction on the risk-difference scale or that one has risk-difference modification.[11,13]

Before describing interaction on the multiplicative scale, let us define the following RRs based on the components in Table 5:

$$RR_{11} = R_{11}/R_{00}$$

$$RR_{10} = R_{10}/R_{00}$$

$$RR_{01} = R_{01}/R_{00}$$

A departure from multiplicativity (i.e., interaction on a multiplicative scale) states that the effect of two variables together is different than the product of the two individual effects. In other words, the ratio of the combined effect to the product of the two individual effects does not equal one. This can be measured in one way as:

$$RR_{11}/(RR_{10} \times RR_{01}) \tag{9}$$

Eq. (9) is referred to as a measure of interaction on the multiplicative scale.[11] If this measure equals 1, that means no interaction on the multiplicative scale, while a value other than one suggests a multiplicative interaction. A value >1 indicates a positive multiplicative interaction and a value <1 is referred to as a negative multiplicative interaction. Note that we can alternatively conceptualize this measure as a ratio of RRs as was demonstrated in an earlier example using ORs from logistic regression rather than RRs. In other words, the ratio of two conditional RRs, the RR for Factor 2 at each level of Factor 1 (or vice versa):

$$(R_{11}/R_{10})/(R_{01}/R_{00}) = (R_{11}/R_{01})/(R_{10}/R_{00}) = RR_{11}/(RR_{10} \times RR_{01}) \tag{10}$$

For this reason, one form of multiplicative interaction when one has a binary outcome variable can be referred to as an interaction on the risk-ratio scale or that one has risk-ratio modification.[11,13] Such an interaction describes how much the conditional RR for the outcome associated with one exposure variable (the focal independent variable) is multiplied by for a one-unit increase (or state change if the independent variable is binary) of the other exposure variable (or moderator). Note that this derivation can be done with ORs rather than RRs, which would produce measures for interaction on the odds-ratio scale or odds-ratio modification. Odds-ratio modification, like risk-ratio modification, is also interaction on the multiplicative scale but with ORs as the measure of effect (association) rather than RRs.

To illustrate these concepts and calculations, Table 6 provides summary data from three studies. The first two, Examples 2a and 2b (panels 1 and 2) will be used here, while the data for Example 2c (panel 3) will be used later (as with the previous examples, raw datasets are available at: https://osf.io/pfysb/?view_only=cdbc99da247647a0976cb1f8f9c961d2). For Example 2a, there is risk-difference modification (i.e., interaction on the additive scale), as the AERI $= 0.036$ $\left(\frac{50}{1000} - \frac{10}{1000} - \frac{5}{1000} + \frac{1}{1000}\right)$, but no risk-ratio modification (i.e., interaction on the multiplicative scale), as the measure of interaction on the multiplicative scale in terms of RR equals 1 $\left(\frac{0.05/0.001}{(0.01/0.001) \times (0.005/0.001)} = 1\right)$. Note that the relative effects for mother's age and medication use are multiplicative: The RR for mother's age alone (i.e., 5) multiplied by the RR for medication use alone (i.e., 10) equals the RR for both factors together (i.e., 50) (i.e., there is no departure from multiplicativity). Likewise, the conditional RR of medication use at each of mother's age (and mother's age at each level of medication use) are homogeneous (i.e., the ratio of these conditional RRs is 1).

The measure of interaction on the odds-ratio scale in this example is also very close to 1 (i.e., 1.038). Example 2a reflects a situation of a rare outcome (generally considered to be a risk of outcome at all levels of the study variables of less than 0.1% or 10%). For relative effect measures (i.e., risk ratios, rate ratios, and odds ratios), no statistical interaction for one of these measures implies no statistical interaction for the others for rare outcomes.[13] This relationship does not generally hold when the outcome is common and the exposure variables both have effects. This is illustrated in Example 2b, where the outcome, future repatronization intent, is fairly likely. There is no clear indication of additive interaction (in the next section, we will show that a test for additive interaction in this example is not statistically significant). However, there is discrepancy when looking at two measures of multiplicative interaction: there is absolutely no interaction on the odds-ratio scale (i.e., the measure equals 1), but the measure of interaction on the risk-ratio scale is 0.875 and, as will be shortly demonstrated, is statistically significantly different from 1, providing evidence of negative multiplicative interaction.

TABLE 6 Summary data from three studies.

Panel 1. Hypothetical risk of child being born with a congenital heart defect as a function of medication use in early pregnancy and age of mother at birth—cases per 1000 (Example 2a)

	Mother's age < 35	Mother's age ≥ 35
Medication nonuser	$R_{00} = 1$	$R_{01} = 5$
Medication user	$R_{10} = 10$	$R_{11} = 50$

Data adapted from an example illustrated in Rothman[21]

Panel 2. Hypothetical odds and probability of future repatronization intent as a function of type of primary pharmacy and trust in pharmacy (Example 2b)

	Other type of pharmacy	Independent pharmacy
Low-to-moderate levels of trust	$R_{00} = 0.50$ $Odds_{00} = 1$	$R_{01} = 0.6667$ $Odds_{01} = 2$
High levels of trust	$R_{10} = 0.7143$ $Odds_{10} = 2.5$	$R_{11} = 0.8333$ $Odds_{11} = 5$

Data simulated for illustrative purposes
Note: Odds is the probability of an event occurring divided by the probability of the event not occurring or $\frac{R}{1-R}$

Panel 3. Cases (thrombotic stroke) and controls by exposure to oral contraceptives and hypertension status (Example 2c)

	No hypertension: Cases/controls	Borderline, moderate, or severe hypertension: Cases/controls
Oral contraceptive nonuser	26/165	54/129
Oral contraceptive user	17/25	38/23

Data from the Collaborative Group for the Study of Stroke in Young Women[40] and a similar example is illustrated in Rothman[21]

Statistical models of interaction

Although the tabulation approach to estimate interactions is useful conceptually and helps to visualize differences between additive and multiplicative interaction effects, in practice, researchers usually include a product term, or interaction term, for the two variables (i.e., the two exposures or the focal independent variable and the moderator variable) suspected to interact in a statistical model. Such models are utilized for several reasons: (1) simple tables are not possible if one or both of the variables are continuous, (2) multivariable adjustment for confounders is readily handled by statistical models, and (3) interactions among more than two variables can be more easily addressed in a statistical model.[9,37] Common statistical models for binary data were reviewed earlier. The linear probability model, logistic regression, and the log-binomial model can be applied to test for interaction between variables. Note that there are other potential models for binary outcomes and Cox regression can be used when one has time-to-event data (continuous) along with an indicator of event occurrence (binary). The interpretation of the regression coefficients, including for the interaction term, varies across these models.

Consider the case outlined earlier with a binary outcome and two binary exposure variables (Table 5). The exposures do not need to be binary, but this example is going to demonstrate how the parameter estimates from statistical models can be used to estimate interaction on the risk-difference, risk-ratio, and odds-ratio scales. Some possible statistical models and interpretations of model parameters can be found in Table 7. Using the specifications noted in the table, results of model estimation for the Example 2a data can be found in Table 8. Note the correspondence between the measures of interaction noted earlier and the results in Table 8:

- Additive: Interaction on the risk-difference scale (AERI) $= 0.036$ and $\hat{\beta}_3 = 0.036$ (95% CI: 0.029, 0.043; $p < 0.0001$).
- Multiplicative: Interaction on the risk-ratio scale $= 1$ and $e^{\hat{\beta}_3} = 1$ (95% CI: 0.645, 1.550; $p > 0.999$).
- Multiplicative: Interaction on the odds-ratio scale $= 1.038$ and $e^{\hat{\beta}_3} = 1.038$ (95% CI: 0.667, 1.616; $p = 0.869$).

TABLE 7 Select statistical models for evaluating interactions with a binary outcome.

Linear probability model (GLM distribution = binomial; GLM link = identity)

$R(Outcome = 1) = \beta_0 + \beta_1 exposure_1 + \beta_2 exposure_2 + \beta_3 (exposure_1 \times exposure_2)$

Interpretation of coefficients

- β_0: Risk or probability of the outcome when not exposed to either (R_{00})
- β_1: Conditional risk difference for the two levels of exposure$_1$ when unexposed to exposure$_2$ (i.e., exposure$_2$ = 0; $R_{10} - R_{00}$)
- β_2: Conditional risk difference for the two levels of exposure$_2$ when unexposed to exposure$_1$ (i.e., exposure$_1$ = 0; $R_{01} - R_{00}$)
- β_3: Measure of interaction on the additive scale or the AERI (i.e., $R_{11} - R_{10} - R_{01} + R_{00}$)

Log-binomial model (GLM distribution = binomial; GLM link = log)

$log\,[R(Outcome = 1)] = \beta_0 + \beta_1 exposure_1 + \beta_2 exposure_2 + \beta_3 (exposure_1 \times exposure_2)$

Interpretation of coefficients

- β_0: When exponentiated (e^{β_0}), risk or probability of the outcome when not exposed to either (R_{00})
- β_1: When exponentiated (e^{β_1}), conditional RR for the two levels of exposure$_1$ when unexposed to exposure$_2$ (i.e., exposure$_2$ = 0; R_{10}/R_{00})
- β_2: When exponentiated (e^{β_2}), conditional RR for the two levels of exposure$_2$ when unexposed to exposure$_1$ (i.e., exposure$_1$ = 0; R_{01}/R_{00})
- β_3: When exponentiated (e^{β_3}), one measure of interaction on the multiplicative scale, namely interaction on the risk-ratio scale (i.e., $RR_{11}/(RR_{10} \times RR_{01})$; also a ratio of two conditional RRs)

Logistic regression model (GLM distribution = binomial; GLM link = logit)

$logit\left[(R(Outcome = 1)] = log\left[\frac{R(Outcome=1)}{1-R(Outcome=1)}\right] = \beta_0 + \beta_1 exposure_1 + \beta_2 exposure_2 + \beta_3 \left(exposure_1 \times exposure_2\right)$

Interpretation of coefficients

- β_0: When exponentiated (e^{β_0}), odds of the outcome when not exposed to either (i.e., $R_{00}/(1 - R_{00})$)
- β_1: When exponentiated (e^{β_1}), conditional OR for the two levels of exposure$_1$ when unexposed to exposure$_2$ (i.e., exposure$_2$ = 0; $\frac{R_{10}/(1-R_{10})}{R_{00}/(1-R_{00})}$)
- β_2: When exponentiated (e^{β_2}), conditional OR for the two levels of exposure$_2$ when unexposed to exposure$_1$ (i.e., exposure$_1$ = 0; $\frac{R_{01}/(1-R_{01})}{R_{00}/(1-R_{00})}$)
- β_3: When exponentiated (e^{β_3}), one measure of interaction on the multiplicative scale, namely interaction on the odds-ratio scale (i.e., $OR_{11}/(OR_{10} \times OR_{01})$; also a ratio of two conditional ORs)

Notes: In this simplifying case, exposure$_1$ and exposure$_2$ both equal 0 when unexposed and 1 when exposed. *R* indicates risk (or probability) of the outcome and the outcome variable equals 1 when the event of interest occurs and 0 when the event does not occur. *AERI*, absolute excess risk due to interaction; *GLM*, generalized linear model; *OR*, odds ratio; *RR*, risk ratio.

The results for Example 2b (not included in the table):

- Additive: Interaction on the risk-difference scale (AERI) = -0.048 and $\hat{\beta}_3 = -0.048$ (95% CI: -0.119, 0.024; $p = 0.192$).
- Multiplicative: Interaction on the risk-ratio scale = 0.875 and $e^{\hat{\beta}_3} = 0.875$ (95% CI: 0.784, 0.976; $p = 0.017$).
- Multiplicative: Interaction on the odds-ratio scale = 1 and $e^{\hat{\beta}_3} = 1$ (95% CI: 0.694, 1.441; $p > 0.999$).

In the linear probability model, the regression coefficient for the product term estimates (or quantifies) departure from additivity, whereas in logistic regression and the log-binomial model (and other risk-ratio regression models as well as Cox regression) the regression coefficient for the product term estimates (or quantifies) departure from multiplicativity. Given these differences, it is possible for different regression models estimated from the same data to provide different answers with respect to questions of interactions. So, which model should one use and which type of interaction, additive or multiplicative, should be reported?

VanderWeele and Knol[11] note that measures of multiplicative interaction, typically based on the results of logistic regression, are most frequently reported primarily because standard software implementing this generally well-understood approach, logistic regression, will by default provide an estimate and CI of interaction on the multiplicative scale. Other practical reasons that the reporting of multiplicative interaction estimated in the context of logistic regression is more common include: (1) fewer problems with convergence in model estimation generally occur with logistic regression and (2) additional effort is required for obtaining measures of additive interaction with binary outcomes.[11] Furthermore, the inclusion of additional predictors for confounder adjustment is straightforward in the assessment of departure from multiplicativity, yet can create some issues for assessment of additive interaction depending on the measure used.[41] Even in the epidemiology and clinical trials literatures, where there is greater awareness of this issue, interactions on the additive scale are often not reported,[42] despite long-standing arguments that additive interaction has more public health

TABLE 8 Output for data from Example 2a (Table 6, Panel 1; Outcome = child being born with a congenital heart defect) from three statistical models: linear probability model, log-binomial regression model, and logistic regression model.

Panel 1. Linear probability model (distribution = binomial; link = identity)

Predictor	Regression coefficient	95% CI for regression coefficient	p-Value
$\hat{\beta}_0$: Intercept	0.001	0.0008, 0.0012	<0.0001
$\hat{\beta}_1$: Medication use	0.009	0.0076, 0.0104	<0.0001
$\hat{\beta}_2$: Mother's age	0.004	0.0024, 0.0056	<0.0001
$\hat{\beta}_3$: Medication use × Mother's age	0.036	0.0288, 0.0432	<0.0001

Panel 2. Log-binomial regression model (distribution = binomial; link = log)

Predictor	Regression coefficient	Exponent of coefficient (risk ratio)	95% CI for risk ratio	p-Value
$\hat{\beta}_0$: Intercept	−6.9078	0.001	0.0008, 0.0012	<0.0001
$\hat{\beta}_1$: Medication use	2.3026	10	7.717, 12.958	<0.0001
$\hat{\beta}_2$: Mother's age	1.6094	5	3.371, 7.416	<0.0001
$\hat{\beta}_3$: Medication use × Mother's age	<0.0001	1	0.645, 1.550	>0.9999

$RERI_{RR} = 36$ (95% CI: 25.417, 46.583; $p < 0.0001$) ($RERI_{RR}$, relative excess risk due to interaction based on risk ratios)

Panel 3. Logistic regression model (distribution = binomial; link = logit)

Predictor	Regression coefficient	Exponent of coefficient (odds ratio)	95% CI for odds ratio	p-Value
$\hat{\beta}_0$: Intercept	−6.9068	0.001	0.0008, 0.0012	<0.0001
$\hat{\beta}_1$: Medication use	2.3116	10.091	7.781, 13.087	<0.0001
$\hat{\beta}_2$: Mother's age	1.6134	5.020	3.380, 7.457	<0.0001
$\hat{\beta}_3$: Medication use × Mother's age	0.0372	1.038	0.667, 1.616	0.869

$RERI_{OR} = 38.468$ (95% CI: 26.992, 49.944; $p < 0.0001$) ($RERI_{OR}$, relative excess risk due to interaction based on odds ratios)

relevance.[9,11,13,14] As an example of why additive interaction is the more relevant public health measure, consider Example 2a. The conditional RD associated with medication use is 0.009 $\left(\frac{10}{1000} - \frac{1}{1000}\right)$ for mothers less than 35 years of age and 0.045 $\left(\frac{50}{1000} - \frac{5}{1000}\right)$ for mothers 35 years or older; these conditional RDs correspond to values of number need to harm (NNH) of 111 $\left(\frac{1}{0.009}\right)$ and 22 $\left(\frac{1}{0.045}\right)$, respectively. Such values suggest a clinically meaningful difference in risk of harm[43] associated with medication use for older mothers relative to younger mothers, a relationship that would have been completely missed if one examined solely multiplicative interaction. Additional arguments for using one scale instead of the other have been reviewed by VanderWeele and Knol,[11] but importantly, these authors recommend reporting interaction (and CIs) on both additive and multiplicative scales as both can be informative depending on the situation. Knol and Vanderweele[14] provide additional guidance and recommendations for reporting such analyses.

Other measures of interaction on the additive scale

In some situations, only RRs are reported or are available. In addition, in case-control study designs, without additional information, one cannot directly estimate risk differences or risk ratios (i.e., cannot use a linear probability model or log-binomial model to analyze such data). However, ORs can be estimated in case-control studies, which is a major reason why the logistic regression model is so widely used in epidemiology.[44] For rare outcomes, ORs closely approximate RRs. This also holds regardless of the rare outcome assumption for certain types of case-control designs.[45] So, how does one assess additive interaction when only RRs are available or one needs to use logistic regression (or another odds-based model), when these situations lead to interactions that have interpretations based on a departure from multiplicativity?

A number of measures of interaction have been proposed that operate as surrogates for the interaction parameter β_3 in the linear probability model, in essence providing an indication of the presence of additive interaction. These measures can be used in both cohort and case-control studies. Perhaps the most commonly reported is the relative excess risk due to interaction (RERI) (also called the interaction contrast ratio or ICR).[46] Although this measure can be used to assess the direction of additive interaction, it cannot be used to assess the magnitude as AERI can,[9] unless one knows R_{00}.[11] Although we cannot arrive at the additive interaction measure directly from RRs, consider dividing AERI (i.e., $R_{11} - R_{10} - R_{01} + R_{00}$) by R_{00} which produces the following:

$$\text{RERI} = (R_{11} - R_{10} - R_{01} + R_{00})/R_{00} = \text{RR}_{11} - \text{RR}_{10} - \text{RR}_{01} + 1 \tag{11}$$

Eq. (11) provides something like the measure of additive interaction but using RRs instead of risks. It is straightforward to see that if RERI $= 0$, there is no additive interaction; if RERI > 0, there is positive additive interaction; if RERI < 0, there is negative additive interaction. As described above, in certain situations ORs are close approximations of RRs and ORs can be used in Eq. (11). Thus, we can estimate RERI using the parameter estimates from logistic regression. A hazard ratio (HR) often approximates relative risk, so this method can be applied to Cox regression as well.[37] Based on the logistic regression model parameterized in Table 7:

$$\text{RERI} \approx \text{OR}_{11} - \text{OR}_{10} - \text{OR}_{01} + 1 = e^{(\beta_1 + \beta_2 + \beta_3)} - e^{(\beta_1)} - e^{(\beta_2)} + 1 \tag{12}$$

Formulas are available for calculation of standard errors (and thus p-values and CIs) for RERI[47]; bootstrapping can also be used.[48] Although approaches are generally not available in standard statistical software, Brankovic et al.[9] describe several sources that provide codes in SAS, R, and STATA for these calculations. In addition, spreadsheets that use standard output from statistical software to perform the calculations are available.[14] With sufficient sample sizes, various approaches should provide comparable CIs; with smaller sample sizes, bootstrapping may perform better in terms of accuracy of standard errors.[11]

Using the data in Example 2a and a publicly available spreadsheet tool,[14] the RERI calculated from the parameter estimates of the log-binomial model (Table 8) was 36 (95% CI: 25.417, 46.583; $p < 0.0001$) and from the logistic regression model it was 38.468 (95% CI: 26.992, 49.944; $p < 0.0001$), both indicating positive additive interaction consistent with the linear probability model even though there is no multiplicative interaction. Note that the absolute background risk in this example is 0.001 (i.e., R_{00}). With this knowledge, one can calculate AERI from RERI: $0.001 \times 36 = 0.036$ (3.6%).

As another example, consider the data in Table 6 panel 3 (Example 2c). These data come from a case-control study designed to assess whether the use of oral contraceptives and the presence of hypertension interact to increase the risk of thrombotic stroke.[40] A logistic regression model suggests a nonsignificant negative multiplicative interaction (measure of interaction on the odds-ratio scale: 0.915; 95% CI: 0.351, 2.386; $p = 0.855$), but the RERI calculated from the parameter estimates in the logistic regression model suggests that there is some indication of positive additive interaction (RERI $= 4.513$; 95% CI: -1.762, 10.788; $p = 0.159$).

These surrogate measures of interaction can be quite useful, but there are some special considerations, one of which has to do with the inclusion of additional predictors in the underlying statistical model to control for confounding. The adjustment for confounders by including additional predictors in a multivariable model is a straightforward extension in the assessment of interaction. However, the RERI and the attributable proportion (AP) due to interaction (another surrogate measure of additive interaction) may vary across levels of additional predictors included in a multivariable model (i.e., the value of these measures depends on the other predictors in the model) even though the parameter β_3 in the linear probability model indicating additive interaction does not.[9,11,41] To avoid this problem, Skrondal[41] recommends another surrogate measure, the synergy index (S), as the measure of choice since it is independent of confounder adjustment. A modified version of AP[49] also has this characteristic and should be considered for reporting.[9,11]

A second consideration is whether any of the exposures of interest are preventive factors rather than risk factors, as calculation of these surrogate measures can be problematic and lead to inconsistent findings when preventive factors are included in underlying statistical models. The simplest solution to this problem is to recode preventive factors into risk factors by assuming that an absence of the preventive factor is actually a risk factor.[21,50]

Finally, in the case of continuous exposure variables, sometimes the effects associated with something other than a one-unit change are of interest (e.g., 5-year difference in age or 10 mmHg change in blood pressure). Such assessments lead to a nonlinear transformation of the RERI and its CI. This issue, as well as the assessment of robustness of the RERI in such situations, is considered by Knol et al.[37] This cautionary note also applies to situations where the same amount of change (e.g., a one-unit change) occurs, but on different locations of the continuous scale. For example, the RERI measure of additive interaction for a change in a continuous exposure from 1 to 2 may not necessarily be the same as the RERI for a change in the continuous exposure from 4 to 5. Thus, the RERI can vary as a function of the levels of the exposures (i.e., independent variables) being compared.[11] As noted earlier, the interpretation of RERI provides information about the direction of additive interaction, not the magnitude. Researchers may need to investigate whether the sign of the RERI changes across various levels of the exposures (i.e., evaluate the robustness of the findings).

Conclusions

Exploration of contingencies of effects when modeling binary outcomes is common in social and clinical pharmacy research and the implications for such moderation effects can be significant for public health. However, the statistical models used to explore moderation are often not thoroughly evaluated. This chapter shows that the commonly accepted default of building an interaction term in a logistic regression model does not always provide the best solution to the research question. Researchers need to carefully evaluate whether their hypothesized moderation effects need to be evaluated on the additive or multiplicative scale and allow the theory to guide their choice of model selection and analysis. Where possible, interactions should be evaluated on both the additive and multiplicative scales, followed by thoughtful interpretation of the implications of their findings. While the concepts explored in this chapter are not particularly novel, they have not been widely adopted yet. Therefore, this chapter calls for a change in the status quo with respect to the exploration, interpretation, and usage of interactions in research.

Questions for further discussion

1. Describe some statistical models used for predicting binary outcomes. What are the advantages and disadvantages of each approach?
2. Provide an example of a moderation hypothesis from your area of research. The outcome variable should be binary, but the predictors can be either categorical or continuous. Please specify the form of the interaction as well [i.e., state whether the moderator (*M*) will increase or decrease the association between the focal independent variable (*X*) and the dependent variable (*Y*)]. Provide literature to support your hypothesis, if possible.
3. Which measure of effect would you prefer to report for a binary-outcome regression model? The odds ratio (OR) or the risk ratio (RR)? Why?
4. Describe an example where you believe evidence suggests that additive and multiplicative interactions may be different from each other (i.e., one is significant, but not the other). Cite your reasoning.
5. Imagine a recent publication demonstrates the interaction between two risk factors in the community that can increase individual risk of an adverse outcome. What are the public health implications of this study's findings if the interaction was additive but not multiplicative? Would these implications change if the interaction was also multiplicative? Explain.
6. What are some approaches to help improve reporting of AERI *and* RERI in published literature?

Application exercise/scenario

Part 1. Consider Examples 2a, 2b, and 2c described in this chapter. For each example, draw a conceptual moderation model similar to Figs. 3 and 4 that were provided for Examples 1a and 1b, respectively.

Part 2. Consider Examples 1a and 1b described in this chapter. Is there evidence of additive interaction for either example? Note that the datasets are available at: https://osf.io/pfysb/?view_only=cdbc99da247647a0976cb1f8f9c961d2. To answer the question, first calculate $RERI_{OR}$ from the logistic regression models for the two examples and then use one of the tools described in this chapter to estimate a 95% CI for $RERI_{OR}$. Then calculate $RERI_{RR}$ (and a 95% CI for $RERI_{RR}$) for the two examples after first estimating models that provide risk ratios (RRs) as a measure of effect. You should notice that the estimated $RERI_{OR}$ and $RERI_{RR}$ are somewhat different from one another in both Example 1 and Example 2. Why is that the case in these examples? Finally, for both examples provide estimates of the AERI from an appropriate generalized linear model. If you run into estimation (i.e., convergence) problems for any of these models, please refer to Spiegelman and Hertzmark[33] and Naimi and Whitcomb[23] (see reference list) for some guidance. Based on your analyses, provide a short summary of your findings for both examples.

References

1. Paulus DJ, Rogers AH, Bakhshaie J, Vowles KE, Zvolensky MJ. Pain severity and prescription opioid misuse among individuals with chronic pain: the moderating role of alcohol use severity. *Drug Alcohol Depend.* 2019;204:107456.
2. Basak R, Bentley JP, McCaffrey 3rd DJ, Bouldin AS, Banahan 3rd BF. The role of perceived impact on relationship quality in pharmacists' willingness to influence indication-based off-label prescribing decisions. *Soc Sci Med.* 2015;132:181–189.
3. Almeida AC, Leandro ME, Pereira MG. Adherence and glycemic control in adolescents with type 1 diabetes: the moderating role of age, gender, and family support. *J Clin Psychol Med Settings.* 2020;27(2):247–255.
4. Liddelow C, Mullan B, Boyes M. Understanding the predictors of medication adherence: applying temporal self-regulation theory. *Psychol Health.* 2021;36(5):529–548.
5. Rockwood NJ, Hayes AF. Mediation, moderation, and conditional process analysis: regression-based approaches for clinical research. In: Wright AGC, Hallquist MN, eds. *The Cambridge Handbook of Research Methods in Clinical Psychology.* New York, NY: Cambridge University Press; 2020:396–414.
6. Hayes AF, Rockwood NJ. Regression-based statistical mediation and moderation analysis in clinical research: observations, recommendations, and implementation. *Behav Res Ther.* 2017;98:39–57.
7. Assmann SF, Pocock SJ, Enos LE, Kasten LE. Subgroup analysis and other (mis)uses of baseline data in clinical trials. *Lancet.* 2000;355(9209):1064–1069.
8. Wang R, Lagakos SW, Ware JH, Hunter DJ, Drazen JM. Statistics in medicine—reporting of subgroup analyses in clinical trials. *N Engl J Med.* 2007;357(21):2189–2194.
9. Brankovic M, Kardys I, Steyerberg EW, et al. Understanding of interaction (subgroup) analysis in clinical trials. *Eur J Clin Investig.* 2019;49(8): e13145.
10. VanderWeele TJ. On the distinction between interaction and effect modification. *Epidemiology.* 2009;20(6):863–871.
11. Vander Weele T, Knol MJ. A tutorial on interaction. *Epidemiol Methods.* 2014;3:33–72.
12. Corraini P, Olsen M, Pedersen L, Dekkers OM, Vandenbroucke JP. Effect modification, interaction and mediation: an overview of theoretical insights for clinical investigators. *Clin Epidemiol.* 2017;9:331–338.
13. Greenland S, Lash TL, Rothman KJ. Concepts of interaction. In: Rothman KJ, Greenland S, Lash TL, eds. *Modern Epidemiology.* 3rd ed. Philadelphia, PA: Lippincott Williams & Wilkins; 2008:71–83.
14. Knol MJ, VanderWeele TJ. Recommendations for presenting analyses of effect modification and interaction. *Int J Epidemiol.* 2012;41(2):514–520.
15. Petitti DB. Associations are not effects. *Am J Epidemiol.* 1991;133(2):101–102.
16. Greenland S, Rothman KJ, Lash TL. Measures of effect and measures of association. In: Rothman KJ, Greenland S, Lash TL, eds. *Modern Epidemiology.* 3rd ed. Philadelphia, PA: Lippincott Williams & Wilkins; 2008:51–70.
17. Katz MH. Multivariable analysis: a primer for readers of medical research. *Ann Intern Med.* 2003;138(8):644–650.
18. Kleinbaum DG, Kupper LL, Nizam A, Rosenberg ES. *Applied Regression Analysis and Other Multivariable Methods.* 5th ed. Boston, MA: Cengage Learning; 2014.
19. Aiken LS, West SG. *Multiple Regression: Testing and Interpreting Interactions.* Thousand Oaks, CA: SAGE Publications; 1991.
20. Hayes AF. *Introduction to Mediation, Moderation, and Conditional Process Analysis: A Regression-Based Approach.* 2nd ed. New York, NY: The Guilford Press; 2018.
21. Rothman KJ. *Epidemiology: An Introduction.* 2nd ed. New York, NY: Oxford University Press; 2012.
22. Agresti A. *An Introduction to Categorical Data Analysis.* 2nd ed. Hoboken, NJ: John Wiley & Sons; 2007.
23. Naimi AI, Whitcomb BW. Estimating risk ratios and risk differences using regression. *Am J Epidemiol.* 2020;189(6):508–510.
24. Greenland S. Model-based estimation of relative risks and other epidemiologic measures in studies of common outcomes and in case-control studies. *Am J Epidemiol.* 2004;160(4):301–305.
25. Barros AJ, Hirakata VN. Alternatives for logistic regression in cross-sectional studies: an empirical comparison of models that directly estimate the prevalence ratio. *BMC Med Res Methodol.* 2003;3:21.
26. Deddens JA, Petersen MR. Approaches for estimating prevalence ratios. *Occup Environ Med.* 2008;65(7):481. 501–506.
27. Doi SA, Furuya-Kanamori L, Xu C, Lin L, Chivese T, Thalib L. Questionable utility of the relative risk in clinical research: a call for change to practice. *J Clin Epidemiol.* 2020;31171–31179. S0895-4356(20).
28. McNutt LA, Wu C, Xue X, Hafner JP. Estimating the relative risk in cohort studies and clinical trials of common outcomes. *Am J Epidemiol.* 2003;157 (10):940–943.
29. Zou G. A modified Poisson regression approach to prospective studies with binary data. *Am J Epidemiol.* 2004;159(7):702–706.
30. Cheung YB. A modified least-squares regression approach to the estimation of risk difference. *Am J Epidemiol.* 2007;166(11):1337–1344.
31. Moher D, Hopewell S, Schulz KF, et al. CONSORT 2010 explanation and elaboration: updated guidelines for reporting parallel group randomised trials. *Int J Surg.* 2012;10(1):28–55.
32. Vandenbroucke JP, von Elm E, Altman DG, et al. Strengthening the reporting of observational studies in epidemiology (STROBE): explanation and elaboration. *Int J Surg.* 2014;12(12):1500–1524.
33. Spiegelman D, Hertzmark E. Easy SAS calculations for risk or prevalence ratios and differences. *Am J Epidemiol.* 2005;162(3):199–200.
34. Szklo M, Nieto FJ. *Epidemiology: Beyond the Basics.* 4th ed. Burlington, MA: Jones & Bartlett Learning; 2019.
35. Jaccard J. *Interaction Effects in Logistic Regression.* Thousand Oaks, CA: Sage Publications; 2001.

36. Hayes AF, Matthes J. Computational procedures for probing interactions in OLS and logistic regression: SPSS and SAS implementations. *Behav Res Methods.* 2009;41(3):924–936.

37. Knol MJ, van der Tweel I, Grobbee DE, Numans ME, Geerlings MI. Estimating interaction on an additive scale between continuous determinants in a logistic regression model. *Int J Epidemiol.* 2007;36(5):1111–1118.

38. Jackson TH, Bentley JP, McCaffrey 3rd DJ, Pace P, Holmes E, West-Strum D. Store and prescription characteristics associated with primary medication nonadherence. *J Manag Care Spec Pharm.* 2014;20(8):824–832.

39. Bauer DJ, Curran PJ. Probing interactions in fixed and multilevel regression: inferential and graphical techniques. *Multivar Behav Res.* 2005;40 (3):373–400.

40. Collaborative Group for the Study of Stroke in Young Women. Oral contraceptives and stroke in young women. Associated risk factors. *JAMA.* 1975;231(7):718–722.

41. Skrondal A. Interaction as departure from additivity in case-control studies: a cautionary note. *Am J Epidemiol.* 2003;158(3):251–258.

42. Knol MJ, Egger M, Scott P, Geerlings MI, Vandenbroucke JP. When one depends on the other: reporting of interaction in case-control and cohort studies. *Epidemiology.* 2009;20(2):161–166.

43. Citrome L, Ketter TA. When does a difference make a difference? Interpretation of number needed to treat, number needed to harm, and likelihood to be helped or harmed. *Int J Clin Pract.* 2013;67(5):407–411.

44. Hosmer DW, Lemeshow S, Sturdivant RX. *Applied Logistic Regression.* 3rd ed. Hoboken, NJ: John Wiley & Sons; 2013.

45. Knol MJ, Vandenbroucke JP, Scott P, Egger M. What do case-control studies estimate? Survey of methods and assumptions in published case-control research. *Am J Epidemiol.* 2008;168(9):1073–1081.

46. Greenland S. Applications of stratified analysis methods. In: Rothman KJ, Greenland S, Lash TL, eds. *Modern Epidemiology.* 3rd ed. Philadelphia, PA: Lippincott Williams & Wilkins; 2008:283–302.

47. Hosmer DW, Lemeshow S. Confidence interval estimation of interaction. *Epidemiology.* 1992;3(5):452–456.

48. Assmann SF, Hosmer DW, Lemeshow S, Mundt KA. Confidence intervals for measures of interaction. *Epidemiology.* 1996;7(3):286–290.

49. VanderWeele TJ. Reconsidering the denominator of the attributable proportion for interaction. *Eur J Epidemiol.* 2013;28(10):779–784.

50. Knol MJ, VanderWeele TJ, Groenwold RH, Klungel OH, Rovers MM, Grobbee DE. Estimating measures of interaction on an additive scale for preventive exposures. *Eur J Epidemiol.* 2011;26(6):433–438.

Chapter 23

The use of ethnography in social pharmacy and health services research

Sofie Rosenlund Lau[a], Janine Marie Traulsen[b], Susanne Kaae[b], and Sofia Kälvemark Sporrong[b,c]

[a]Department of Public Health, University of Copenhagen, Copenhagen, Denmark, [b]Department of Pharmacy, Social and Clinical Pharmacy Research Group, University of Copenhagen, Copenhagen, Denmark, [c]Department of Pharmacy, Uppsala University, Uppsala, Sweden

Objectives

- Highlight ethnography's potential for pharmacy and health services research.
- Understand the epistemological basics of ethnographic research.
- Discuss when and why to use ethnography.
- Suggest how to embark on an ethnographic research project.

Introduction: Why ethnography?

Social pharmacy was once defined by Sørensen, Mount, and Christensen as a field concerned with "the social factors that influence medicine use, such as medicine- and health-related beliefs, attitudes, rules, relationships, and processes."[1] One central aim of social pharmacy is to understand the actions, behaviors, and motives of patients and relatives, healthcare professionals and policymakers, in their dealings with medications. It is by understanding what drives these actors in their relationships with medications and with each other, that social pharmacy can initiate solutions to optimize medication use. Ethnographic research is suitable for exactly that, with the overall aim to explore and interpret the cultural construction of a given social setting or phenomenon.[2,3]

Qualitative methods have increasingly gained recognition in social pharmacy and health services research[2,4] yet researchers in qualitative social pharmacy rarely spend much time studying what research participants *do* in their natural environments. By being present in the daily lives of patients, healthcare professionals, policymakers, and their social networks, ethnographers provide rich insight into "real world settings." More than other methods employed in health research, ethnography gives access to nuanced accounts of matters related to medication use and its underlying basis. With a focus on meaning-making, ethnography goes beyond description and, when informed by theory, offers interpretation. Therefore, this methodology can bring forward new understandings for medications' place in society and in individuals' lives.

This chapter provides insight into the nature of ethnography for social pharmacy and health services researchers and serves as an overall introduction to the principles of ethnography, including how to conduct an ethnographic research project and the possibilities and pitfalls of doing ethnography.

Ethnography at a glance

Contemporary ethnography developed in the early 20th century with its origins in American cultural anthropology and British social anthropology. The American roots are situated in the University of Chicago and developed at a time when Chicago was going through a period of immense social change resulting in poverty and social inequality. It was here that a group of social scientists developed a distinctive style of anthropology (known as The Chicago School) that is comparative and fieldwork based. These researchers sought to explore questions of social stratification, poverty, race, and ethnicity in the American urban setting, in ways that acknowledge the centrality of ordinary people's voices and their own viewpoints in social life. Social scientists, including Robert Park and Ernest Burgees, found the city to be a "natural laboratory" wherein life could be observed first-hand, thereby breaking with the more classic, abstract and theoretical practice of "arm-chair sociology" and moving toward a more direct, intimate study of daily living.[5]

The British roots can be traced back to one of the most influential anthropologists of the 20th century, Bronisław Malinowski. He is credited with transforming British social anthropology, concerned with historical origins and the writings of missionaries and travelers, into a discipline aimed at understanding the interconnections of social life through intense fieldwork. His 1922 publication: *Argonauts of the Western Pacific: An Account of Native Enterprise and Adventure in the Archipelagoes of Melanesian New Guinea*[6] is one of the first modern ethnographies and remains a key reference in contemporary ethnography. Malinowski spent 3 years participating in and systematically collecting data on the daily living of the local people in the Trobriand Islands. He was the first to systematically record and teach the basics of ethnographic fieldwork, pointing toward two main essentials: To learn about the culture or phenomenon being studied by spending time in the field, and, while doing this, "to grasp the native's point of view, his relations to life, to realize his vision of his world"[6] (p. 25).

Ethnography and pharmaceuticals—Some examples of former and contemporary research

So what is it that makes ethnography relevant for social pharmacy and health services research? Ethnography focuses primarily on the *social* aspects of the research object; that is, how a certain phenomenon unfolds among and between people. Since the mid-1980s, studies of pharmaceuticals have emerged in social science disciplines, including anthropology, sociology, science and technology studies (STS), and the history of medication.[7,8] van der Geest et al.[7] summarized it nicely:

> *Pharmaceuticals constitute a perfect opportunity for the study of the relation between symbols and political economy. On one hand, they are a part of the international flow of capital and commerce. On the other, they are symbols of hope and healing and of the promise of advanced technology. They are more thoroughly incorporated than blue jeans and popular music, and they are more desperately sought than Coca-Cola and videos. They allow individuals and peripheral communities to exercise more autonomy in health care but also create dependence on distant markets.*
>
> Ref. 7, p. 170.

The acceptance and widespread distribution of medications throughout the world makes ethnography a relevant research approach within at least three different settings: In the everyday life and social context of individual medication users, from an organizational perspective of state and industry, and in care practices.

From an everyday life perspective, many of the classic objects of interest in social pharmacy are inherently social. For instance, "pharmaceutical behaviors" such as nonadherence, experiences of effects, and side effects of medications, as well as information-seeking and shared decision-making, all include social practices and negotiations between and among users and healthcare professionals.

The research project described in Box 1 is an early example of the importance of studying local beliefs about pharmaceuticals in an attempt to understand their widespread use and improve safety. In a more recent ethnographic study aiming to understand the massive use of statins, Lau, Almarsdottir, and Oxlund show how, from the perspective of heart-healthy statin users, the medications provide an easy way to manage, not only the condition of elevated cholesterol as such, but *the risk* of future heart disease. The authors conclude that taking statins can be thought of as a "practice of anticipation," that is "a way to manage uncertain health futures and actively reorient possible future lives toward imagined safe and healthy trajectories."[10] Buying into the global construction of statins as safe and effective, some statin users become trapped

---

Box 1 The reinterpretation of western pharmaceuticals among the Mende of Sierra Leone, 1985

In a study from 1985, Bledsoe and Goubaud explored the use of western pharmaceuticals among members of a local Mende tribe in Sierra Leone.[9] To gain in-depth insight into local life, Bledsoe, an anthropologist, lived in a rural chiefdom and observed the extensive use of western pharmaceuticals among the local people. She decided to investigate local understandings of western medications and initiated observations and interviews with tribe members who took medications and the meanings they ascribed to them. She found that traditional beliefs about diseases and treatments were used as the explanatory framework for taking western pharmaceuticals. Also, that the efficacy of the medications where mainly assessed through qualities such as shape, color, taste, and consistency. While medications where often incorrectly administered, at times even in fatal doses, Bledsoe found that the reasons for using medications in these ways was rational once she understood the logic behind their actions. For instance, in traditional Mende medication, natural white chalk was used as a way to cool the skin when treating fever. Therefore, the Mende often chose white pills as a remedy for fever. Based on these findings, Bledsoe and Goubaud argued that, because of the globalization of western medications there is a need to take issues of safety seriously as the unregulated medication markets have consequences for public health.

between this pharmaceutical imaginary of statins as the way to keep future disease at bay and unpleasant experiences of statins in the present.[10]

On a structural level, the development, marketing, testing, and regulation of pharmaceuticals can likewise be investigated as social aspects of pharmaceuticals. A substantial part of medical anthropology has explored the *market-state nexus* of pharmaceuticals[11] as a way to point out the different roles of pharmaceuticals in international and national policy and local health institutions and as products in both formal and informal, legal, and illegal transactions.[8,11–14] For instance, Biehl has explored the ambiguous role of antiretroviral treatment in shaping Brazil's public health regime against AIDS, which fosters health for some while others are denied access or become stigmatized.[14]

Pharmaceuticals play a pivotal role in care settings as portable care technologies. A significant body of ethnographic literature explores the micropolitics of power in everyday care where health professionals are expected to make patients adhere to pharmaceuticals in specific ways and under specific circumstances and norms, which do not always fit well into other elements of everyday life.[15–17]

Finally, it is worth mentioning that today ethnography and ethnographers can be found studying the role of pharmaceuticals in people's lives in large pharmaceutical companies as well as through local pharmacies and in nursing homes. Healthcare research has learned not to lean too heavily on quantitative data when trying to understand patients' needs, wishes and expectations. Ethnographic "thick data" is proving valuable in capturing the patient insights from within the context of conversation communities. Ethnography can also be found today in collaboration with computer scientists employing a method known as Big-Thick Blending,[18] e.g., when observations derived from big data are blended with thick observations of the same social phenomenon. Other ethnographic studies have looked at social aspects of pharmaceuticals on different levels and from different perspectives (see more examples in Box 2).

Ethnographic epistemology

Engaging with ethnography involves engaging with a different way of understanding reality and of obtaining knowledge about reality. Especially when coming from a natural science-based research paradigm, it is important to be aware of some

---

Box 2 Suggestions for further reading, see also the chapter's reference list

Methodological papers and books:

Hammersley, M., Atkinson, P., 2007. Ethnography—Principles in Practice. Taylor & Francis.

Madden, R., 2010. Being Ethnographic. A guide to the theory and practice of ethnography. Sage Publications, London, Thousand Oaks, New Delhi, Singapore.

Reeves, S., Kuper, A., Hodges, B.D., 2008. Qualitative research methodologies: ethnography. BMJ 337, a1020. https://doi.org/10.1136/bmj.a1020.

Spradley, J.P., 1979. The Ethnographic Interview, in: The Ethnographic Interview. Holt, Rinehart and Winston, Inc., Florida, pp. 1–106. https://doi.org/10.1300/J004v08n02_05.

Emerson, Robert M., Rachel I. Fretz, and Linda L. Shaw., 2018. *Writing Ethnographic Fieldnotes*. 2. edition. Chicago: The University of Chicago Press.

Sismondo, Sergio, and Jeremy A. Greene. 2015. *The Pharmaceutical Studies Reader*. Chichester, England: Wiley Blackwell.

Sarah Pink. 2001. *Doing Ethnography: Images, Media and Representation in Research*. London: Sage.

Monographs and edited collections:

Mol, Annemarie, 2002. *The Body Multiple. Ontology in Medical Practice*. Duke University Press.

Petryna A, Lakoff, A. Kleinman A., 2006. *Global Pharmaceuticals: Ethics, Markets, Practices*. North Carolina: Duke University Press.

Jenkins, Janis H. 2009. *Pharmaceutical Self. The Global Shaping of Experience in an Age of Psychopharmacology*. Santa Fe. School for Advanced Research Press.

Mol, A., Moser, I., Pols, J. 2010. *Care in Practice. On tinkering in clinics, homes and farms*. Bielefeld. Transcript verlag.

Dumit, Joseph. 2012. *Drugs for Life. How Pharmaceutical Companies Define Our Health*. Duke University Press.

Ecks, Stefan. 2013. *Eating Drugs: Psychopharmaceutical Pluralism in India*. New York: NYU Press.

Whyte, Susan Reynolds. 2014. *Second Chances. Surviving AIDS in Uganda*. Durham and London. Duke University Press.

Kaufman, Sharon R. 2015. *Ordinary Medicine. Extraordinary Treatments, Longer Lives and Where to Draw the Line*. Durham and London. Duke University Press.

Adams, Vincenne. 2016. *Metrics. What counts in global health*. Duke University Press.

Wahlberg, Ayo. 2018. *Good Quality. The Routinization of Sperm Banking in China*. University of California Press.

fundamental features of ethnographic epistemology—that is, how the basic principles of ethnography dictate how and what can be known about the object of study. This opens a large discussion about the philosophy of science embedded in different research paradigms. This discussion is not within the scope of this chapter—we refer the reader therefore to the work of scholars such as Mason.[19] What is important here is to be aware that ethnography is anchored in a social constructivist research paradigm, which requires specific attention to the role of the researcher and to matters of reflexivity.

Constructivism

Ethnography is based on a research paradigm, which claims that there is no definite truth or reality waiting to be discovered (and therein measured or quantified). Reality as such does not exist as a neutral objective phenomenon that can be seen as a whole. Instead, reality (or realities in plural) is socially constructed at any given point in time by the ethnographer in conjunction with the research participants. This means that it is possible for another ethnographer to study the same topic in the same setting and produce different findings. This is because there are interpersonal differences between the researchers, the research participants, and the ever-changing context in which the research takes place. The aim of ethnography is therefore not to generalize about a certain phenomenon, but rather to describe in-depth the context which influences the shaping of the phenomenon and how this context gives rise to specific meanings in relation to the people (materiality, technologies, or knowledge) involved. For instance, to understand nonadherence to statins, it is not enough from an ethnographic viewpoint, to talk to statin users. It is also important to experience how the use of statins can change over time and in different settings and situations such as in the general practitioner's office in contrast to at home or while on holiday. Attitudes toward statin treatment, in this sense, is not a singular viewpoint but something that changes throughout the day, week or life, and which is deeply influenced by a large variety of interdependent factors on both a micro and macro level. Ethnography aims to describe these changing circumstances, which for instance shape the experiences of users.

The role of the researcher

Ethnography builds on a premise of intersubjectivity, which means a general awareness of and attentiveness to the fact that knowledge is constructed by humans who make choices about what they study, what they see and report, and how they interpret and write out their findings.[5,20] This also means that the researcher plays an active role in the making of ethnographic data. The quality aim is therefore not to avoid affecting the data, but rather to be explicit and transparent about this co-construction of knowledge. One way to reflect upon intersubjectivity is by actively locating the researcher in the empirical accounts, as is the case in the example in Box 5. Here, it is openly stated that the researcher was present during data collection, and that she was active in the data production by interacting with the study participants. Hence, transparency is of utmost importance in ethnographic research. This also means that as a researcher you need to look at your own background and experiences and reflect on how these influence your findings.

Reflexivity

Intersubjectivity is closely related to reflexivity. Being open and critical about the choices made throughout a research process and how they influence the findings is an important quality marker in ethnographic research. In other words, claims based on ethnographic research are conditional and partial, and must be taken seriously in the analysis and dissemination of ethnographic studies. In the ethnographic study on pharmaceuticals and eldercare (see Box 5), reflexivity could for example relate to what it means for the findings that the researcher followed the homecare workers into the homes of elderly people. What would be different if the researcher had recruited the elderly through their GPs, a senior center, or the local community? Further, what does it mean that the researcher is a young, female White? Would the findings have been different, if she was older, male or Black? Ethnographers take up such relevant questions of reflexivity and discuss them openly in the dissemination of their findings.

Doing ethnography

There are no simple guidelines or checklists for conducting an ethnographic study; there are however some basics on how to approach and practice ethnography. For example, it is important, if not essential, that the researcher emerges him/herself in the context of the fieldwork. This includes living in the field for a prolonged period, becoming familiar with the local

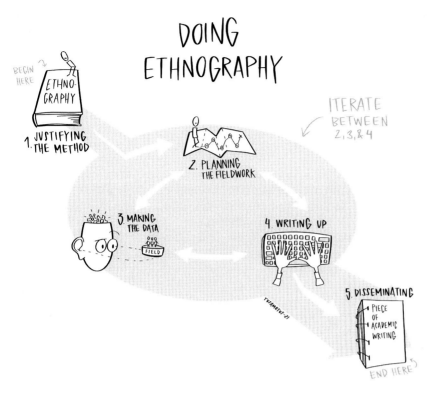

FIG. 1 Planning, making, writing ethnography. *Illustration by Kirstine Kolling,* Tusamotus

language and dialect, thereby becoming an active participant in the daily lives of participants. The researcher should also be aware of the "specific" ways of using methods for data creation. These include using everyday conversation as an interview technique and keeping a chronological record of observations in field notes. This means that the researcher should be aware of the importance of recording/ noting down unspoken and implicit information for use when analyzing and writing up the research.[21]

Fig. 1 suggests a framework for dividing an ethnographic project into 5 phases. First, one must justify the use of ethnography and make sure that the research approach fits with the research questions and objectives. Ethnography encompasses a specific way of thinking about reality and how to gain access to and knowledge about this reality. It also requires more time and resources when compared to other qualitative methods, including an open-mindedness on the part of the researcher (see "Is ethnography right for me?" section). However, once ethnography is found suitable for the research project, the process of doing ethnography consists of the following four phases: planning fieldwork, making data, writing up, and disseminating. These phases present a logical way of moving forward through an ethnographic project, thus are dependent on each other. Yet, they should not be understood as linear, but rather as an iterate process of moving to and from, in and out of the field. In the following, the phases are presented in more details.

Planning the fieldwork

Gathering ethnographic data is known as *doing fieldwork,* with the field referring to the specific sites or locations where the data collection takes place. Traditionally, ethnographers conducted fieldwork in unknown, often exotic places, and the field constituted a geographic site (e.g., a rural village on a tropical island). Today, however, the notion of the field is understood as more complex and multilayered.[20] In recent years, doing ethnography "at home" (places familiar to the researcher) and doing "multi-sited ethnography" (data collected from numerous social or geographic sites) has gained prominence.[20,22] Also, doing online ethnography has become popular (see Box 3).

When preparing an ethnographic research project, the field is actively constructed by the researcher(s), meaning that choices are made regarding the project's focus and how and where data can be obtained. Constructing a field helps to

---

Box 3 On-line ethnography

Currently, in an increasingly digitalized global world, online/virtual ethnography has become a widespread acceptable alternative to being physically present.[23,24] Developed in the 2000s, on-line ethnography analyzes how people interact in online communities and within the cultures created through computer-mediated social interaction. Data is gathered via blogs; Facebook groups; online diaries etc. Examples of this approach can be found in the literature on studies of on-line patient groups and associations, e.g., Kingod's work on Type-1 Diabetes.[25]

---

narrow in on the research objective and steer the project in a certain direction. If the research focuses on specific places, e.g., pharmacies or hospital wards, then it is obvious to center the fieldwork at these sites. If the research focuses on a broader or more widespread phenomenon, other conditions will guide the construction of the field. Fig. 2 provides a visual example of "a field" based on a study conducted by the first author which focused on pharmaceuticals and eldercare by "following the pharmaceuticals" in the lives of frail elderly. Frailty is a complex construct,[26] thus to make a practical demarcation, the project group decided to only include elderly over the age of 65 who received homecare including help with medication management. A homecare facility was chosen as the main *gate keeper*—meaning those who have access to the study participants. Gaining access to vulnerable elderly persons through homecare services turned out to be an effective sampling strategy as the homecare staff literally opened the doors to the homes of the elderly. These often homebound elderly would otherwise have been difficult to reach. Furthermore, homecare turned out to be an interesting site for obtaining knowledge about the role of pharmaceuticals and the tacit work required which helped retain pharmaceuticals as a pivotal element in keeping frail elderly in their homes.[27] Because GPs in Denmark prescribe the vast majority of all medications, general practice served as a secondary field site.

On sampling

Doing fieldwork means choosing specific cases to represent a larger cultural phenomenon. Cases can be understood as specific sites or people, projects, or technologies. The aim is to use the small number of cases for in-depth exploration of the researched phenomenon. As previously mentioned, ethnography has roots in social constructivist theory, where knowledge is partial and situated. From this perspective, obtaining a saturated or "representative" amount of data is

FIG. 2 An example of "a field" in an ethnographic project. *Illustration by Kirstine Kolling, Tusamotus*

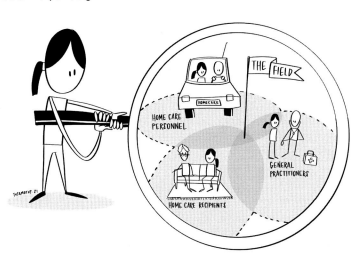

FOLLOWING THE PHARMACEUTICALS

meaningless and conflicts with the ontology that reality is fluid and ever changing. Instead, the ethnographic approach aims for richness and depth, and therefore it makes sense to stay longer with fewer participants, as opposed to spreading time out on several places and many different cases. Comparing contrasting cases (e.g., individuals, setting, or technologies) can be a great way to become aware of the differences across the same study object.

In the study on pharmaceuticals and eldercare, the researcher selected a sample of 10 elderly—a number which was possible for a single researcher to follow over approximately 1 year. The elderly were chosen with a reference to gender, age and health status as a way of getting access to different social contexts and experiences with medications. As explained in more detail below, the sample also included observations of homecare staff and interviews with GPs.

Making data

Ethnography is a multidimensional research methodology covering a range of (creative) qualitative methods, including but not limited to participant observation, interviews, focus groups, mapping, diaries, autobiographies, and a large variety of visual and audio methods. All fieldwork is unique and there is no standard recipe on how to conduct a fieldwork as such. During fieldwork, the researcher will often use a combination of observation, participation and talking to people (both formal and informal interviews).[20] Participant observation though, stands out as an essential part of doing ethnographic research, and therefore is the focus in this chapter. For other types of methods employed in ethnography, find inspiration in Box 2.

The following is an example of how the fieldwork was carried out in the project on pharmaceuticals and eldercare. The researcher initiated the fieldwork by following a public homecare service in a suburb of Copenhagen. During a period of 20 days, she followed different homecare workers on their daily rounds and "hung around" the homecare offices, including joining meetings of the different homecare teams. While "out driving" with the homecare staff, the fieldwork consisted of a mixture of participatory and nonparticipatory observations. Sometimes the researcher stood on the side, observing the practices and interactions between the homecare staff and the care receivers. Sometimes, she actively participated in care practices, for instance, by fetching equipment for the home care nurse, holding hands with the care receiver during care practices such as wound care or catheter change, or helping with simple tasks, e.g., cleaning a table or washing a face. These shifts between participatory and nonparticipatory observation is a typical way of making ethnographic data (see more in Refs. 20,28). Through the homecare staff, the researcher contacted 10 elderly persons interested in further participating in the study. She subsequently visited the elderly in their homes and carried out in-depth ethnographic interviews.[29] Most were visited twice (e.g., once with the homecare staff and once alone). Some were followed over several months. For example, one participant was interviewed twice at home, and followed for one entire day, followed to a diabetes clinic and a nursing clinic, and visited again at the end of the data collection period. Additionally, the researcher observed and interviewed 7 GPs, of which 5 were the personal GP of one or more of the elderly participants. A few times, the researcher observed GP home visits with elderly patients. When possible, and with permission from the participants, the researcher photographed the homes, thus creating a visual representation of the observations. Also, at one point the researcher invited an anthropologist who produced audio pieces from the homes of two of the elderly participants. This resulted in an in-depth sensorial representation of slices of everyday life (see Lau et al.[30]). Furthermore, the researcher collected written material during the fieldwork relevant for understanding the context of Danish eldercare, e.g., brochures on different diseases/health issues, announcement of services provided by the local community or policy papers related to both homecare management and general practice services. In total, the material collected for the present study consists of approximately 24 h audio recorded interviews, 200 pages of written observations, 150 photographs and 50 different documents collected between May 2019 and February 2020.

Writing ethnography

Ethnography comes from Greek and literally means "writing about people" (*Ethnos* means people, *graphe* means writing). A large part of doing ethnography goes into the production of ethnographic texts. Ethnography is thus both a practice or methodology and the textual product of that practice. The production of ethnographic texts is the art of bringing together the often-heterogeneous elements from the fieldwork. It is the writing together of fieldnotes, interview transcripts, and other documents or sensory materials (e.g., audio pieces or photographs). In the following, the process of writing ethnography is split into three stages: documenting (writing down), analyzing (writing out), and disseminating (writing up).[20]

Box 4 Template for structuring fieldnotes

Location:
Date, time:
   Observations:
   Try to stick to observable facts, reporting:
   Who
   What
   When
   Where
   What people do
   And what people say
Interpretations:
   What do my observations tell me in relation to the research question?
   What is the significance of what I have observed?
   Why did people act like this?
   How did the situation come to be like this?
Reflexivity:
   How was I perceived?
   How might I have influenced the data?
   How do I feel about what I have observed?
Next steps:
   Is there anything I would do differently next time?
   What leads might I follow up on?
   Have gaps been revealed?

Source: Skovdal and Cornish.[28]

Documenting—Writing down

The first stage is the process of documenting what is observed and experienced during fieldwork. Often, formal interviews are audio recorded; however, most other information is written down as *field notes*. A notebook will often accompany the researcher in the field for a continuous recording of observations and reflections. All kinds of observations, including what people said and did; the appearance of people and place; subtle experiences of sensations, smells, sounds, and feelings; and tentative analytical thoughts will be logged during or immediately after the observation has taken place. Writing up field-notes is a practice on its own. See Box 2 for suggestions on where to learn more about ethnography in practice. The production of field notes can be both open and dynamic or a relatively structured task. Skovdal and Cornish provide an example of a structured field note template in their methods book on Qualitative Research for Development[28] See Box 4.

It is advisable to spend time on writing field notes after each observation or at the end of each day in the field. All the details of specific experiences and further reflections are impossible to document in situ. Therefore, it is important to set aside ample time for the time-consuming process of writing down as many details as possible from the observations and related reflections. In the current project on pharmaceuticals and eldercare, the researcher always had a notebook with her. Notes could be written at the same time as observations during meetings of the homecare teams or during nonparticipatory observations. However, the researcher often participated actively in the care work, and therefore the documentation had to wait until back in the car or at the homecare office. Also, the researcher often found it inappropriate or awkward to write notes while observing the care work taken place as this took focus away from the often intimate moments between the elderly care recipients and the homecare staff. Finally, important knowledge often appears unexpectedly—"along the way"—in informal conversations for instance while having lunch in a GP clinic or while following a homecare worker to the car. It can be difficult to log these spontaneous conversations while they are happening. Therefore, most fieldnotes were produced after the observations took place often while commuting home or during a quiet time in the home care office.

Analyzing—Writing out

The next step, analyzing or "writing out" data is the process of ordering and transforming often incoherent field notes into coherent texts. This is the process of organizing messy notes so that the important parts can be securely stored and retrieved. In the study example, field notes from the notebook were rewritten into word documents, audio recordings were transcribed

---

Box 5 As a way to elaborate some central aspects of ethnographic research, an on-going ethnographic study conducted by the first author on pharmaceuticals and eldercare is used as an example throughout the following text. The study aims to explore the meanings and role of pharmaceuticals in old age as a way to inform and potentially strengthen pharmaceutical care in Danish eldercare. The project includes fieldwork in a public homecare facility and in the lives of 10 elderly individuals receiving homecare services. The project is funded by the Danish foundation Velux Fonden.

Betty, 79, is in bed when the care worker, Lisa, and I enter. She yawns loudly and complains about the early awakening. Lisa laughs affectionately and points out that it is almost 10 o'clock in the morning. "Well yes," Betty replies "But I'm a B, not a C person!" Lisa changes Betty's diaper and helps her to wash "below." She picks up a bowl with water so Betty can wash her face and upper body herself, but Betty refuses. "I need coffee. Coffee and cigarettes" she cries out loud. Betty searches on the crowded bedside table for the pack of cigarettes and lights one while coughing deeply and rattling. Lisa brings her a thermos with hot water for coffee and a bowl of oatmeal. Then she finds the box of medication pre-packaged by the pharmacy and tears off the small bag of morning pills. She checks the date and counts the number of pills before she pours them into a small glass, which she places in front of Betty. "Oh, I hate swallowing pills" Betty sighs and starts, one by one, fishing the pills out of the small glass and swallowing them loudly one at a time with a sip of coffee. Swallowing eight pills of different sizes takes time and Lisa waits patiently for all the pills to be taken. "Yes, I must make sure she swallows them" Lisa explains to me. "Why?" I ask. "It's part of the service here. They must be seen ingested, it is stated". Betty writhes a little, but otherwise remains silent. After breakfast, Betty has to go to the bathroom. This is done by Lisa guiding her into the wheelchair with the use of a sliding board and from there into the commode, which is in the room next to the living room. Betty's bathroom is too small for her to get in and out. While Betty is away, Lisa changes her bedding. She finds a pill in a hole in the mattress. Without saying anything, she shows me the pill and rolls her eyes. After Lisa leaves, I ask Betty why she's getting medication. "Yeah, I don't know. After all, it's the doctor when he comes. I just say yes!" she laughs and coughs before she continues: "And then they get so happy when you take those pills. I cannot tell you if I feel differently." Betty lights another cigarette and coughs again. "Yes, I can just as well enjoy the last thing I have in my life, right" she laughs referring to the cigarette. The tone becomes more serious "I do damn well as I please" She inhales, coughs and continues the sentence "… or whatever I can, right!" Betty leans back in bed with the smoke in her mouth as she zaps for something to watch on the TV. (Parts of this ethnographic piece is also presented in Lau.[32])

---

and documents were scanned, and finally everything was stored on a secured online drive. During this process, names were anonymized and personal data encrypted in a file only accessible to the researcher. Written consents were locked away.

This step is also about transforming the ordered data material into tentative analytical pieces. Box 5 is an example of the rewriting of field notes into a coherent text. When writing out data, ethnography includes three key elements: the production of thick descriptions, analytical generalization and social theory, which will be elaborated on briefly in the following (for further elaboration, see Lau et al.[31]).

Thick descriptions

Ethnographic research focuses on the context of the studied phenomenon. The purpose is to explore and describe the observed phenomenon in its specific spatial, temporal, and social context in order to say something about the phenomena in general. One way of accomplishing this is through the production of *thick descriptions*. According to Geertz,[33] making thick descriptions is the process of paying close attention to and documenting the contextual details of the observed event, and using these insights to extract the meanings, feelings, and worldviews that shape and inform social life (see also Oxford Reference).[34]

The example in Box 5 reveals how analysis is also an integral part of the process of transforming field notes to coherent text. By being present during the physical encounter between Betty and the homecare worker, various meanings of medication use became visible. For instance, Betty is assigned to what in homecare terminology is called "to be watched taken." This means that the homecare worker must ensure that Betty in fact swallows the medications. This precaution is in place because Betty's relatives and the homecare staff are not sure if Betty is compliant with taking her prescribed medications. However, through the observations it became obvious that Betty experienced the "watching" as coercive surveillance. If the homecare worker was not watching, Betty would occasionally skip a pill and hide it inside her mattress. This was her way of expressing autonomy. By avoiding a pill or two, Betty became empowered—proving that she was still an individual, self-reliant person. It was a way of caring for herself. This interpretation of the observation is supported by Betty's expression "*I do damn well as I please*," which reinforces her need for autonomy. However, when Lisa located the hidden pills, this reinforced her perception of Betty as a noncompliant patient, interpreted by the way Lisa rolls her eyes, thus implicitly stating, "Look, she is not compliant!" These observations thus provide rich insights into the local negotiations of medication use in eldercare. Further, it makes it possible to interpret these observations in relation to more general aspects of compliance and autonomy. Thick descriptions are thus not only about describing the nuances of what is being observed, but also about ascribing meanings to these observations by understanding what they mean from the perspective of the people under study.[33]

Analytical generalization

In ethnographic research, there is an ongoing circular flow between collecting data, analysis, and reading theory. This iterative process is often described as moving "in" and "out" of the field. In practice, the researcher will have some initial thoughts about what the findings will be; however, they might very well be completely different from what is actually observed during fieldwork. In the study from which the fieldnote excerpt was taken, the initial aim was to explore the reasons for the high levels of antidepressant use among the elderly. The aim was to understand the meanings of antidepressants from the perspectives of the elderly, their relatives, homecare staff, and GPs. However, after physically being present in the homes of the elderly, the researcher observed how, in daily life, the use of antidepressants disappeared among all other medications. As the fieldwork excerpt reveals, neither Betty nor her homecare worker seemed to notice which pill was the antidepressant or what the rest of the pills were for. Polypharmacy was present among all 10 research participants and this turned the focus of the study away from looking solely at antidepressants (and related topics such as depression, anxiety, and loneliness in old age) and toward understanding the meaning of multiple medication use in old age. Thus, the example highlights two critical aspects of ethnography: (1) Ethnography can make sure that research is relevant for real life. (2) Ethnographic analysis is not a fixed set of ideas; rather it is present from start to finish, as a continuous exercise in reflexivity.

The analysis is often driven by curiosity concerning a certain piece of the data: a wish to explore in more depth what is going on. In the example with Betty, it would be interesting to further unravel the relationship between autonomy and compliance. This would entail following up on Betty's ignorance toward her medications. Instead of taking her word about agreeing to whatever the GP prescribes, the aim would be to understand what this means from Betty's perspective. Has she given up trying to understand why she needs these medications? If so, why? Which surrounding factors contribute to this lack of engagement? For instance, what does it mean that the medications are hidden away and managed only by homecare workers?

In ethnography, the goal is not to generalize or construct patterns across the dataset, as is the case in quantitative research, but instead to provide depth and richness. Nevertheless, generalization occurs when one specific case or narrative is used to say something about a wider and more fundamental social phenomenon.[9] In the example above, Betty's experience of (and resistance to) being deprived of her autonomy can on a practice level, be used to make a generalization about the multiple understandings of noncompliance. On a broader level, her experience reveals a link between noncompliance and the ambivalence inherent in the values and norms in eldercare.

Use of theory

Ethnography is theory-informed, which means that engaging with ethnography also involves engaging with various theoretical works. Theory here can be understood on several levels, which is depicted here as a tree (see Fig. 3). The tree trunk is the philosophical underpinning of a given project and style of thought. The branches are the "grand" or substantial theories, which have been developed, adjusted, and discussed over a long period of time by many scholars. These theories differ fundamentally in extensiveness, credibility, and popularity, which can be thought of as the differences in lengths and thickness of the branches. The leaves are the concepts or ideas, usually developed by an individual or a few scholars and often applied in different combinations.

Reading articles, monographs, and other literature is the main way for getting familiar with (new) theory and is crucial in making ethnographic accounts theory based. In practice, this means searching the literature that is related to the research field one is working in, in order to gain insight and inspiration for the analysis.

The project on pharmaceuticals and eldercare is mainly inspired by social theories of care (which can be thought of as one thick branch leading to many other different theories and concepts). These theories provide a framework for understanding how care is constituted in everyday life from the perspectives of both care providers and care recipients, including the role pharmaceuticals play in the enactment of care.[8,35] For instance, the notion of the "logic of care" in contrast to the "logic of choice," brought forth by the Dutch philosopher and ethnographer Annemarie Mol, provides a theoretical basis for thinking about matters of adherence, autonomy, and patient choice in situations such as Bettys'.[16] According to Mol, the "logic of choice" dominates Western healthcare and highlights the notion that patients are individuals, capable of making free, rational choices in managing their disease. From the logic of choice perspective, care work resembles a linear process,

LEVELS OF THEORY

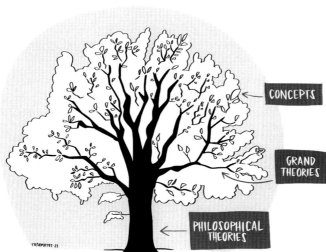

CONCEPTS

GRAND THEORIES

PHILOSOPHICAL THEORIES

FIG. 3 Different levels of theory: the tree trunk is the philosophical (ontology and epistemology), the branches the grand/substantial theories (developed and used over a long period of time by many scholars), and the leaves refer to single concepts/ideas (developed and used by an individual or only a few scholars). *Illustration by Kirstine Kolling, Tusamotus*

which is the case when Betty's homecare worker follows the guidelines for rational medication use. From the logic of care perspective, care work is flexible, an ever-changing phenomenon, attuned to what matters to the patient in the here and now, which might be different tomorrow. Hence, Mol argues for a less standardized, generalized approach to healthcare and instead centers healthcare on the local and specific needs of the individual patient. Following this approach, it would be relevant to ask what would happen if Betty were to be asked if something could be done to make medication use a more pleasant (rather than coercive) experience (see more in Lau[32]).

Applying theory makes it possible to make analytical generalizations: a bridge between the observations in several homes or clinics and a broader discussion of overarching issues related to eldercare. In general, various theoretical perspectives can be incorporated into ethnography, which means that researchers can find inspiration for their analysis in a variety of disciplines. What is critical here is not what kind of social theory is being used, but that it provides a plausible link between observing something and giving it meaning. For suggestions on where to look for theoretical inspiration, see Box 6.

Box 6 Where to look for theory?

It might be difficult for researchers in the pharmacy or health services research environment to become knowledgeable about social theory. One often hears questions like: where do you find your theoretical inspiration? The answer is—many places!
Places to look for theoretical inspiration:

- Become part of a social science research environment, at universities or virtually online.
  - Examples: Facebook groups for students or post graduates in anthropology, STS or sociology. Online research societies, e.g., MAAH (Medical Anthropology at Home), 4S (Society for Social Studies of Science).
  - Or online social research networks, e.g., ResearchGate and Twitter.
- Follow research blogs
  - For example—Somathosphere, a research blog that publishes news and short articles at the intersections of medical anthropology, science and technology studies, cultural psychiatry, psychology and bioethics.
- Subscribe to theory-driven research journals, e.g., Social Science and Medicine, Medical Anthropology, Sociology of Illness and Health, BioSocieties.
- Use Google and Google Scholar!! If interested in something specific, check out what Google suggests and find the original sources from there.

Note that becoming familiar with social science theories is not a straight-forward task for a scholar trained primarily in pharmacy or other natural science-based educations. Social theories are often similar to engaging with a new style of thought, new expressions and terminology, and new ways of presenting academic arguments. As with everything that is new, it takes time. The best way is to establish a reading group or network in order to read together and discuss what is read and learned.

Disseminating—Writing up

Dissemination or "writing up" ethnography is the process of creating and publishing coherent ethnographic arguments. According to Madden:

> *The act of ethnographic writing is a form of collating, reporting and interpreting at the same time; it is both systematic and artful, hence the anxiety many ethnographers have about the writing process. It is in the writing of ethnography that we finally realize what it is we want to say about our ethnographic experiences.*

Ref. 20, p. 153.

Ethnographic products can take on various formats and styles. To familiarize oneself and become comfortable with the ethnographic style, we recommend reading an assortment of ethnographic articles and monographs (see Box 2 for suggestions related to health and medicine).

Part of writing up is also the process of organizing data and ideas in a structured way so it can be read and understood by others. It is the process of matching the research question with the knowledge obtained during fieldwork and throughout the period of research. It builds on previous as well as new experiences and understandings. In the words of Madden: "… as ethnographers come to understand the overall picture of their ethnographic data […] they will sense they are making a movement from idea to explanation, from data to story, and in many cases from confusion to meaning"[20] (p. 148).

Finally, it is the process of making a coherent analytical argument—of combining the research context and what has been observed and experienced during fieldwork with relevant social theory in order to say something new and relevant about the cultural phenomenon under investigation. The study example used in this chapter is still in the writing-up process; however, it is already evident that the ethnographic contribution will focus on the role of pharmaceuticals in the *infrastructures of care*[27,36] (yet another "branch"—see Fig. 3). That is the arrangement of people, spaces, and technologies that, in this study, enable the welfare state to care for the elderly in Denmark. Previous research on medications' role in care infrastructures has focused mainly on the invisible work related to the use of chronic medications, primarily on how the procurement and practical arrangement of medications in peoples' homes are embedded features of daily living with chronic diseases. The continuous practices of communicating with healthcare professionals about prescription renewals, of going to the pharmacy and of organizing medications in the home, are all necessary elements for sustaining life with chronic illness. At the same time such practices are embedded in existing health care infrastructures (e.g., access to prescribed medications and reimbursement systems) but they are also in themselves *infrastructuring* ways of living with chronic diseases (e.g., having insulin-dependent diabetes takes a lot of planning). Thus, the practices are, at the same time, both enabling and prohibiting patients from living free, independent lives.[27] What this study wants to add is to show how these features of the infrastructures of pharmaceuticals slips under the radar in daily medication practices yet are fundamental for how care is provided and received—also in the context of public homecare for the frail elderly.

Ethics

Ethnographic research, as all research, requires that the people engaged in it are ethically responsible. Ethnographers gain access to private (and at times very intimate) moments in people's lives, and are responsible for ensuring the proper and respectful management of sensitive knowledge. An essential part of informed consent is being explicit about the researcher's role and where and how findings will be disseminated and potentially used. In the fieldwork on pharmaceuticals in eldercare, the researcher often found that the participants thought she was a nurse. Therefore, when encountering new persons, she made sure to present herself as a researcher conducting research on behalf of the university and repeated this fact when necessary. The terminology associated with doing research was unfamiliar and strange for many elderly participants. As such, the researcher spent time making certain that, as a minimum, the participants understood that she was interested in observing and understanding their everyday lives for the sake of improving eldercare in the future. It is the responsibility of the researcher to withdraw from situations where their presence is not fully accepted as well as to make sure that no one is directly or indirectly harmed by participating in the study. Overall, our experience is that the interrelatedness of ethnography, often makes participation a pleasant experience. Depending on the context of the study, most people are eager to share insights and experiences from their own life. Many other aspects of ethics are relevant when engaging with ethnography. During fieldwork, researchers can find themselves in situations, where deciding on what is the right thing to do can be difficult. This is especially true when engaging in fieldwork as a healthcare professional, you might be exposed to safety issues such as inappropriate uses or managements of medications. For information on ethics in ethnography, including how to withdraw from fieldwork, see for example Murphy and Dingwall.[37]

Is ethnography right for me—And how to go forward?

This final section sums up some of the main considerations prior to embarking on an ethnographic project and suggests ways to move forward.

Choosing an ethnographic approach can be linked to three overall considerations:

- Is ethnography suitable for gaining access to the knowledge I want?
- Does my understanding of reality, and how to make knowledge about reality, fit with ethnography?
- Do I have the resources necessary to conduct an ethnographic study?

Is ethnography suitable for getting access to the knowledge I want?

As described above, the main reason for engaging with ethnography is that the researchers want access to knowledge that is not visible alone through other methods such as interviews. In ethnography, the object of interest is observed in the course of everyday activities, and the researcher has the unique opportunity to understand these practices as they unfold in real life. Ethnography is usually applied when the object of study is a cultural phenomenon. Culture here, is not fixed, but is understood as the medium or context within which we live and engage in the complexities of everyday life.[38] See Box 7 for more examples on ethnographic projects on pharmaceuticals.

Therefore, if the knowledge you want can be accessed in-depth, and there is the opportunity to get close to and follow a few cases over a long period of time, then ethnography is a way to go.

Does my understanding of reality and how to make knowledge about reality fit with ethnography?

Second, referring to the above regarding ethnographic epistemology, one has to consider if the epistemological position of the researcher (how you think about reality and how to gain knowledge about reality) fits with the underlying philosophical principles of ethnography. As mentioned above, ethnography entails a specific way of thinking and doing research, which requires a specific mindset and role of the researcher. Doing fieldwork can be an intense and challenging task because it entails a personal investment on your part. According to Coffey: "Fieldwork is personal, emotional and identity *work*. The construction and production of self and identity occurs both during and after fieldwork. In writing, remembering and representing our fieldwork experiences we are involved in processes of self-presentation and identity construction"[42] (p. 1). For a researcher trained in, e.g., pharmacy or other health sciences and embarking on the first ethnographic project, it can be both quite a chocking and demanding task to let go of previous conceptions and experience the world in new ways and with new eyes.

As stated earlier, reflexivity is a main feature of ethnography, which means that in addition to the work of being a researcher, you also need to carefully follow your own development in the process of understanding. Hence, it is crucial to be aware that the world experienced by you as a researcher differs from the world experienced by the research participants. As a researcher it is a real challenge to try to, actively, see the world from the point-of-view of others, and actively reflect upon the differences between your own and the perceptions and experiences of others. The world that you enter as a

---

Box 7 Some other examples of ethnographic research projects on pharmaceuticals

- Going to the doctor with enhancement in mind—An ethnographic study of university students' use of prescription stimulants and their moral ambivalence.[39]
- Connecting Pills and People: An Ethnography of the Pharmaceutical Nexus in Odisha, India.[40]
- APOLLO-MM: An in-depth ethnographic case study of patients' and professionals' experiences and practices of polypharmacy.[41]

  In these examples the cultural phenomena under investigation are: use of prescription medications for non-prescription use (so called "study drugs") in Denmark and United States; the role of the pharmaceutical industry in therapeutic encounters in the capital of Odisha, India, and polypharmacy in older people in United Kingdom. For each project, the aim is to understand how these phenomena unfold among specific groups of people (here university students, doctors and patients, and elderly), by exploring in-depth the practices, experiences, negotiations and concerns that arise at the intersection of individual experiences, professionals at work and health care systems. Many other examples of ethnographic studies of pharmaceuticals are provided in Box 2, including research from non-western countries.

researcher can be very different from your own lived world, which can be difficult to understand and interpret, it can also challenge and change your own worldview. As a researcher you need courage to embark on this journey with an open mind.

Do I have the necessary resources to conduct an ethnographic study?

Finally, you have to consider if you have the resources needed to do an ethnographic study. Ethnography is a time-consuming endeavor. There is no consensus as to the time dimension for conducting ethnographic fieldwork.[38] However, typically fieldwork occurs over months, sometimes years and is often more time consuming than other methods. This is due to the data collection itself, but also to the management of the ethnographic data, and especially the writing of ethnographic analysis, which can be tedious. It is important to remember that ethnography is much more than a research method; it is a way of thinking about and approaching the world, including what kind of knowledge can be obtained about the world. This takes time and patience. Still, what this chapter hopefully has shown is that ethnography can illuminate some of the complexities of the social world and bring forward new ways of approaching matters highly relevant for social pharmacy and health services research.

Questions for further discussion

Discuss whether an ethnographic approach is suitable for the examples below. Then, discuss other suitable research approaches/methodologies:

1. Aims to obtain a deeper understanding of how pharmacy counseling affects patients' medicine taking behavior, and thereby possibly also their health status. This will be done by exploring the patients' responses to the counseling provided by pharmacy staff.
2. Aims to understand the experiences, perceptions, and suggestions of stakeholders who work with Direct to Health Professional Communication (DHPC) in European pharmaceutical companies taking into account the importance of the DHPC system and challenges identified at the sender (industry) level.
3. Aims to investigate the knowledge, attitudes and behaviors of patients and healthcare professionals in order to inform policymakers and other stakeholders of the specific reasons behind the current use of antibiotics.

Application exercises/scenarios

Designing an ethnographic study

Think of a culture or phenomenon you would like to study—and that can be researched through ethnography. Here are a few suggestions: what is the role of community pharmacies in society; how do medicine users educate themselves about medicines; what is the role of traditional medicines in patients' lives. You can look in the relevant parts of the chapter as you go.

Define the field

Reflect on sampling strategy, for example individuals and/or geographical, social or cultural factors.

How do you expect to make data (for example by participant observations, interviews) and for how long would you be in the field?

How would you document and make time for writing up field notes?

Reflexivity: what are your preconceptions and experiences with the culture/phenomenon? How would these differ from those of others within the field you would study? How may these differences impact your findings?

Observing and writing field notes

This exercise is best done together with at least one other person.

Find a place where you can train your observation skills and writing field notes. Make sure to choose a place where there are minimal risks for running into ethical issues—for example: a park, a city square, a shopping mall or a busy place at campus. Observe and take notes for approximately half an hour. For a suggestion on how to structure field notes see Box 4.

Afterwards: Consider how you will interpret your findings. If you were to transform these observations into an ethnographic research project, what could be the topic and research question?

Finally, try writing a short ethnographic text on behalf of your field notes. Get inspired by the example in Box 5.

References

1. Sørensen E, Mount JK, Christensen ST. The concept of social pharmacy. *Chronic Illn.* 2003;7:8–11.
2. Lau SR, Traulsen JM. Are we ready to accept the challenge? Addressing the shortcomings of contemporary qualitative health research. *Res Soc Adm Pharm.* 2017;13(2):332–338. https://doi.org/10.1016/j.sapharm.2016.02.014.
3. Bradbury-Jones C, Taylor J, Herber O. Use of theory in qualitative research: the degrees of visibility typology. *Soc Sci Med.* 2014;120:135–141. https://doi.org/10.1016/j.socscimed.2014.09.014.
4. Amin MEK, Nørgaard LS, Cavaco AM, et al. Establishing trustworthiness and authenticity in qualitative pharmacy research. *Res Soc Adm Pharm.* 2020;16(10):1472–1482. https://doi.org/10.1016/j.sapharm.2020.02.005.
5. O'Reilly K. Key concepts in ethnography. In: *Sage Key Concepts.* Sage Publications; 2009:29–33. https://doi.org/10.4135/9781446268308.
6. Malinowski B. *Argonauts of the Western Pacific.* London: Routledge and Kegan Paul; 1922.
7. van der Geest S, Whyte SR, Hardon A. The anthropology of pharmaceuticals: a biographical approach. *Annu Rev Anthropol.* 1996;25(1):153–178. https://doi.org/10.1146/annurev.anthro.25.1.153.
8. Hardon A, Sanabria E. Fluid drugs: revisiting the anthropology of pharmaceuticals. *Annu Rev Anthropol.* 2017;46(1). https://doi.org/10.1146/annurev-anthro-102116-041539.
9. Bledsoe CH, Goubaud MF. The reinterpretation of western pharmaceuticals among the Mente of Sierra Leone. *Soc Sci Med.* 1985;21(3):275–282.
10. Lau SR, Almarsdottir AB, Oxlund B. The pharmaceutical imaginary of heart disease: pleasant futures and problematic presents. In: Ballentyne PJ, Ryan K, eds. *Living Pharmaceutical Lives.* London, New York: Routledge; 2021:103–115.
11. Petryna A, Lakoff A, Kleinman A. *Global Pharmaceuticals. Ethics, Markets, Practices.* Durham and London: Duke University Press; 2006.
12. Dumit J. *Drugs for Life: How Pharmaceutical Companies Define Our Health.* London: Duke University Press; 2012.
13. van der Geest S. Anthropology and the pharmaceutical nexus. *Anthropol Q.* 2006;79(2). https://doi.org/10.1353/anq.2006.0020.
14. Biehl J. Pharmaceuticalization: AIDS treatment and global health politics. *Anthropol Q.* 2007;80(4):1083–1126.
15. Applbaum K. Getting to yes: corporate power and the creation of a psychopharmaceutical blockbuster. *Cult Med Psychiatry.* 2009;33(2). https://doi.org/10.1007/s11013-009-9129-3.
16. Mol A. *The Logic of Care: Health and the Problem of Patient Choice.* London, New York: Routledge; 2008.
17. Whyte SR. *Second Chances. Surviving AIDS in Uganda.* Durham and London: Duke University Press; 2014.
18. Bornakke T, Due BL. Big-thick blending: a method for mixing analytical insights from big and thick data sources. *Big Data Soc.* 2018;5(1):1–16.
19. Mason J. *Qualitative Researching.* 3rd ed. London, California, New Delhi, Singapore: Sage Publications; 2018.
20. Madden R. *Being Ethnographic. A Guide to the Theory and Practice of Ethnography.* London, Thousand Oaks, New Delhi, Singapore: Sage Publications; 2010.
21. Hobbs D, Wright R. *The SAGE Handbook of Fieldwork.* University of California Press/Sage Publications; 2006.
22. Marcus GE. Ethnography in/of the world system: the emergence of multi-sited ethnography. *Annu Rev Anthropol.* 1995;24(1):95–117. https://doi.org/10.1146/annurev.an.24.100195.000523.
23. Hine C. *Virtual Ethnography.* London: Sage Publications; 2000.
24. Kozinets RV. *What Is Netnography? SAGE Research Methods*; 2011. https://methods.sagepub.com/video/what-is-netnography.
25. Kingod N. The tinkering m-patient: co-constructing knowledge on how to live with type 1 diabetes through facebook searching and sharing and offline tinkering with self-care. *Health.* 2020;24(2). https://doi.org/10.1177/1363459318800140.
26. Grøn L. Old age and vulnerability between first, second and third person perspectives. Ethnographic explorations of aging in contemporary Denmark. *J Aging Stud.* 2016;39:21–30. https://doi.org/10.1016/j.jaging.2016.09.002.
27. Danholt P, Langstrup H. Medication as infrastructure: decentring self-care. *Cult Unbound J Curr Cult Res.* 2012;4(3):513–532. https://doi.org/10.3384/cu.2000.1525.124513.
28. Skovdal M, Cornish F. *Qualitative Research for Development.* Rugby, UK: Practical Action Publishing; 2015. https://doi.org/10.3362/9781780448534.
29. Spradley JP. The ethnographic interview. In: *The Ethnographic Interview.* Florida: Holt, Rinehart and Winston; 1979:1–106. https://doi.org/10.1300/J004v08n02_05.
30. Lau SR, Kristensen NH, Oxlund B. Taming and timing death during COVID-19: fragments of the quiet passing of an old man. *Anthropol Aging.* 2020;41(2):207–220. https://doi.org/10.5195/aa2020.319.
31. Lau SR, Kaae S, Kälvemark SS. Ethnography and its potential for studying the social in social pharmacy: an example of autonomy and pharmaceuticals in eldercare. *Res Social Adm Pharm.* 2022;18(1):2151–2156. https://doi.org/10.1016/j.sapharm.2021.04.003.
32. Lau SR. *Pharmacologic* and pharmaceutical care: an ethnographic study of the encounters between vulnerable elders, home care and medicines. *Tidsskrift for Forskning i Sygdom og Samfund.* 2021;18(35):73–94. https://doi.org/10.7146/tfss.v18i35.129994.
33. Geertz C. Thick description: toward an interpretive theory of cultures. In: *The Interpretation of Cultures.* New York: Basic Books; 1973.
34. Mark E, Ian F, Wendy O, Maria P. *A Dictionary of Social Research Methods.* Oxford University Press; 2016. https://www.oxfordreference.com/view/10.1093/acref/9780191816826.001.0001/acref-9780191816826-e-0410?rskey=Sl6mmp&result=412.
35. Whyte SR, van der Geest S, Hardon A. *Social Lives of Medicines.* Cambridge: Cambridge University Press; 2002.
36. Langstrup H. Chronic care infrastructures and the home. *Sociol Health Illn.* 2013;35(7):1008–1022. https://doi.org/10.1111/1467-9566.12013.
37. Murphy E, Dingwall R. The ethics of ethnography. In: *Handbook of Ethnography.* Sage Publications; 2001:339–351. https://doi.org/10.4135/9781848608337.n23.
38. Jeffrey B, Troman G. Time for ethnography. *Br Educ Res J.* 2004;30(4):535–548. https://doi.org/10.1080/0141192042000237220.

39. Petersen MA, Nørgaard LS, Traulsen JM. Going to the doctor with enhancement in mind—an ethnographic study of university students use of prescription stimulants and their moral ambivalence. *Drugs Educ Prev Policy*. 2015;22(3). https://doi.org/10.3109/09687637.2014.970517.

40. Seeberg J. Connecting pills and people: an ethnography of the pharmaceutical nexus in Odisha, India. *Med Anthropol Q*. 2012;26(2). https://doi.org/10.1111/j.1548-1387.2012.01200.x.

41. Swinglehurst D, Fudge N. Addressing the polypharmacy challenge in older people with multimorbidity (APOLLO-MM): study protocol for an in-depth ethnographic case study in primary care. *BMJ Open*. 2019;9(8). https://doi.org/10.1136/bmjopen-2019-031601.

42. Coffey A. *The Ethnographic Self Fieldwork and the Representation of Identity*. Cardiff, UK: Sage Publications; 1999.

Chapter 24

Video-reflexive ethnography applications in pharmacy and health services research

Faith R. Yong[a], Su-Yin Hor[b], and Beata V. Bajorek[a]

[a]*Discipline of Pharmacy, Graduate School of Health, University of Technology Sydney, Sydney, NSW, Australia,* [b]*Centre for Health Services Management, Faculty of Health, University of Technology Sydney, Sydney, NSW, Australia*

Objectives

- Describe possible uses of video-reflexive ethnography as a participatory action approach in pharmacy practice research.
- Define and apply the underlying principles of video-reflexive ethnography to a pharmacy setting.
- Justify the appropriateness of a video-reflexive ethnographic approach for a research objective.

Introduction

Participatory action research involves a large family of research approaches, characterized by their use of reflection and reflexivity, partnership with participants, and action (i.e., iterative cycles of reflection and action in changing practice).[1] By affirming individual experiences as knowledge which affects learning and practice,[2] research data are created through the interplay associated with researchers sharing their "power" with participants.[1,2]

Participatory action research is not new to pharmacy practice. Various participatory action research methods have been used in pharmacy studies, including participatory and social mapping, pictures/photovoice, spider-grams, ranking and scoring approaches, seasonal calendars, life histories, narratives and storytelling, problem trees, and human sculptures.[1] Such approaches have been utilized in the codesign and creation of pharmacy services,[3,4] in understanding how action research studies can change pharmacy work practices,[5] and in various hospital pharmacy quality improvement projects.[6,7] These methods are used for the exploration of subjective or social experiences, such as: power hierarchies, social relationships, personal satisfaction with services, and understanding physical or social conditions.[1]

In participatory research, the relationship between researcher and participants is key. Research teams must understand the study context well enough to both initiate and sustain engagement, in a way that is ethical and collaborative. The participatory research process itself can be multimodal and/or cyclical, requiring constant negotiation with participants and ongoing reflexivity from all parties involved.[1,2] This makes such research particularly suitable for disempowered and marginalized groups,[1,2] or constantly changing environments, such as the community pharmacy setting, due to the flexibility of the research process.[1,5] Participatory action research is also used for practice improvement, since changes often arise while research is in progress. Research outcomes, which are directly contributed by members of the target population, can also be transferrable to other settings.[1,2,5,8]

Video-reflexive ethnography (VRE) is a participatory methodology that has become increasingly popular in the last decade, and has been used to study and intervene in complex frontline healthcare practices.[9] VRE is a visual methodology which enables researchers and participants such as healthcare professionals or patients to collaborate in examining the "here and now" of healthcare. VRE uses video footage to undertake contextualized analysis, interpretation and amelioration of "mundane" everyday care practices. Thus in their everyday environment, the "taken-as-given" habits of practitioners (i.e., activities so routine that they become unremarkable or forgotten) can be seen in their complexity.[9]

Drawing on ethnographic and participatory research traditions, VRE researchers collaborate with study participants to record and select video footage of their everyday work practices. These videos are then replayed to participants in reflexive discussions facilitated by researchers. Viewing this footage makes "what is familiar strange,[10] enabling participants to approach their actions from a "third party" perspective on their actions within their context. Additionally, other ethnographic methods to understand the study context (e.g., researcher observation, documentary analysis) can be incorporated into the VRE process as required. The primary aim of VRE, on the whole, is to make the complexity of practitioners' care practices more visible and tangible to themselves and others, hence encouraging and inspiring new perspectives and insights into practice, and change.[9]

Below, the basic principles of VRE methodology are described in greater detail.

An overview of VRE study design considerations: The guiding principles of VRE

VRE, as a methodology, has developed its theoretical foundations from several fields: participatory action research, practice theory, educational philosophy, and science and technology studies.[9,11]

To understand how VRE differs from other participatory research methods, we describe its theoretical framework below, articulated in a set of four guiding principles: exnovation, reflexivity, collaboration, and care.[9]

Exnovation

VRE acknowledges that the creative enactment of everyday clinical practice often goes unnoticed, perhaps due to repetition (habit), or the distraction and pace of busy workplaces. Those using VRE seek to make visible this "local ecology of care," where the actions of a clinician can be seen as embedded in the workplace context. This process of *exnovation* is designed to make tangible the complexity of healthcare work, thus making visible the creativity, competence, and expertise of healthcare workers. In practice, this means that video-reflexive ethnographers are interested in how everyday practices unfold, creating (and making sense of) video footage of those practices in collaboration with front-line clinicians and patients.[9,11]

Reflexivity

As a common inclusion in pharmacy training and professional development plans,[12–14] pharmacists may be familiar with *reflection* as a personal activity for contemplating one's own actions, and an opportunity for learning.

Reflexivity, however, as described in VRE, also takes into account the context in which actions and behaviors happen, such that participants' actions and behaviors are framed within the impact of others' actions and behaviors, and vice versa.[11] In this way, reflexivity promotes critical awareness of individuals' conduct within layers of context, including their own backgrounds, the socio-political context of their workplaces, physical environment, their profession, and so on.[15] For researchers, their decisions (e.g., what should be recorded and played back, and how reflexive sessions are held and facilitated) are also determined through ongoing reflexivity. Reflexivity is expected from all parties involved (professionals, researchers and patients) and is necessary throughout all project stages.[16]

In practice, reflexive sessions involve researcher-facilitated viewings of recorded footage with participants. Participants may be those who are featured in the footage, colleagues, or others who are familiar with and/or have a stake in the practices shown. In viewing their footage, guided by researchers' questions, participants are invited to see their behavior, within its context, from different viewpoints, and to respond to the complexity of the local healthcare setting. This enables a critical review of healthcare practices by stakeholders, encouraging a reimagination of care: why do we work this way, is this appropriate, what else could be done, and what could be improved? Interestingly, researchers may find previous assumptions about their research question challenged at this stage. An example of researcher reflexivity is described later in this chapter.

Collaboration

In line with the principle of exnovation, which seeks to foreground and harness frontline actors' expertise and understanding of their own practices, VRE invites stakeholders (e.g., pharmacists, dispensary technicians, patients) to participate as coresearchers, working alongside researchers to create and analyze footage, and to reimagine and redesign work processes.

This collaboration is key, as stakeholders are active participants in the health care setting, with an experiential understanding of its inner workings. Since researchers work with stakeholders to decide what footage is significant and should be recorded, videos discussed in a reflexive session are inherently important to both the researchers and stakeholders. The researchers then take on the role of a curious facilitator to make sense of footage with participants.

This process allows them to create meaning from the recordings *together*, rather than separately, both at a distance from one another and the context at hand. The reflexive discussions arising from viewing the footage thus reflect researchers *and* stakeholders engaging in "sense-making" of the practices under scrutiny. Findings of a VRE study are therefore produced through both "insider" (i.e., stakeholders) and "outsider" (i.e., researcher) perspectives,[9,15] which may therefore be more readily translated into evidence-based, practical outcomes by combining theoretically-based researcher reflexivity, and experientially-based practitioner reflexivity.

Care

In this final principle, VRE researchers acknowledge that feelings of vulnerability are part of the VRE process: allowing one's behavior to be recorded and examined by oneself and important others, including colleagues and managers, can be stressful and confronting.[9] Video footage can be easily misused, for instance, for performance monitoring by management who may impose sanctions, further exacerbating the vulnerability of participants with low control or power (e.g., patients and healthcare workers lower in the medical hierarchy). Such outcomes would be contrary to the purposes of VRE: it is designed to support learning, rather than assign blame. This last principle of care, therefore, emphasizes the well-being of participants (and researchers) as a core tenet of this methodology. The collaborative and reflexive processes of VRE enable researchers to monitor and negotiate situations and participant relationships, for the purposes of ensuring that they are not adversely affected by research participation. Further understanding of the study context and participants can be helped by an initial observational stage, to aid in the process of caring for participants.[2,8,9] This is important because ensuring care for participants involves creating and maintaining their psychological safety, which enables open and frank discussion of recorded behaviors that are watched, edited and analyzed by others. This is done through respectful engagement, facilitation of open discussion, and an ongoing commitment to consent at every stage. For this reason, participants are regularly and continuously asked for their consent: to participate in the study, to be recorded, to have their footage kept and used, to have their footage shown to others, and so on. Much like the concept of a "just culture" in patient safety,[17] VRE aims to create a psychologically safe environment for clinicians to learn from observed footage and improve their care.

The researcher's role in VRE, then, is to protect participant wellbeing and ensure the research process is customized to allow full and honest participation. A synergistic effect should be occurring where ideally, clinicians are the experts leading the researcher through their everyday care practices. This process is, in turn, being facilitated and documented by the research team for further analysis and learning.

The potential for VRE applications in pharmacy practice research

Different approaches to community pharmacy research are necessary, given the complexity of pharmacists' behavior, attitudes and beliefs.[18–22] Unfortunately, the role of the community pharmacist is commonly misperceived by other healthcare professionals and the public alike, who may see them as little more than glorified medication shopkeepers.[23–27] These factors have perhaps resulted in a pharmacist workforce that can be wary of outsiders, including researchers,[28–30] since external parties do not seem to demonstrate understanding of pharmacists' everyday working challenges.

However, it has been said that pharmacists are more likely to engage in research where they have both a personal interest in the topic of research, and a belief that pharmacy practice research is beneficial, especially to their patients.[28–30] It could be the case, therefore, that participatory forms of research, like VRE, would be attractive to this population, particularly as this methodology requires engagement with front-line clinician knowledge, interests and the complexity of their work. Applying the participatory principle of "nothing about us without us"[31] into pharmacy practice, through research, could be transformational for the community sector.

As a novel participatory methodology in community pharmacy research, VRE does not just focus on the content of recorded footage alone. It may also involve reflexive discussions around: how the video footage was taken by researchers and/or participants (e.g., cinematographic choices, time of day chosen); facets of social/physical/interactional contexts that are not visible in footage (e.g., pharmacist glances/conversation to off-camera patients awaiting prescriptions); and the contextualization of everyday practices.[9,32,33] In other words, VRE acknowledges that the dynamics of interactional work and its context, wherein care is negotiated, given and received, can be both symbolic yet "invisible."[9,16,32] Through VRE, this "ecology of care" that practitioners work within, can therefore be explained by those steeped in its practices and environment, with its social, cultural, institutional and historical contexts. Within the VRE process, clinician care activities are acknowledged to be sensitive to the environment they are performed within. Thus, video footage is said to be "hologrammatic" and polysemic,[9] meaning participants often see "more" than is visible in the footage, allowing facilitators to probe for greater insights into the studied phenomena.

VRE has also been used as an intervention. Examples of previous VRE interventions in healthcare settings worldwide include improving: infection control in hospitals,[33,34] ICU clinical communication processes,[32] inpatient dementia care,[35] and shared decision-making in primary care,[36] involving both clinicians and patients. After successful completion of a VRE project, the methodology has been adopted in care settings as part of routine quality improvement, in a mode called "planned obsolescence" VRE.[9,37] Some examples include a neonatal intensive care unit in the Netherlands[9,38,39] which originally examined infant prognosis differences[40] and moral decision-making,[41] and a clinical handover initiative across several hospitals in Australia.[37,42] VRE presents an opportunity for clinicians to review and improve clinical performance without the threat of deregistration, insurance claims or litigation—improvement opportunities which can be rare for health professionals like pharmacists.[43–45] VRE has also been used in pharmacist populations as part of two multidisciplinary studies: Kaiser Permanente used VRE to improve transitional care in USA[46]; and a UK study protocol described using VRE to investigate polypharmacy review and interventions across 3 GP clinics and 4 community pharmacies.[47]

Although differing from VRE methodology, the use of video reflection itself in pharmacy practice education is well established, most commonly involving student reflection and improvement of their counseling practices.[48] In contrast, VRE has a broader focus on context and complexity, and a more comprehensive approach toward reflexivity.[49] Nonetheless, this suggests that pharmacists may be accustomed to video recording as an opportunity for reflection and learning.

Managing "distance": VRE in the pharmacy setting

Above, we described how VRE enables participants and researchers to examine and intervene in the complexity of everyday work practices. In doing so, this methodology may bridge the evidence-practice gap that characterizes much of health services research and policy-making.[50,51] In VRE, this is achieved by an interplay of closeness and distance: close engagement during research with practitioners and their actions embedded in their contexts; but also introducing "distance," through the researcher's (outsider) presence and perspective. Additionally, participants gain a kind of third-party perspective by watching their own footage. This "distance" serves to direct practitioners' attention and interest to formerly overlooked aspects of their practices, and to invite them to reimagine these practices. Thus evidence is both created and applied (e.g., in the improvement of everyday care processes),[32,49] by practitioners and researchers, close to the contexts of practice.

As a result of the COVID-19 pandemic, new challenges pertaining to distance have been introduced to research, e.g., physical distancing and travel restrictions for preventing community transmission.[52–55] To adjust to this new problem of distance, an adaptation of VRE in one pilot study is discussed, through reflexive engagement with the four guiding principles. As an example for readers, we describe this application in pharmacy practice research, and examine its potential, and challenges during a pandemic.

Use of VRE in an Australian community pharmacist research study: An adaptation for geographic restrictions and pandemic conditions

Cognitive pharmacy service (CPS) provision in community pharmacies requires further investigation, since pharmacists appear not to prioritize CPS routinely, despite demonstrating enthusiasm for them.[56–59] It appears that CPS provision may be of low priority for pharmacists, despite desiring to provide CPS.[56–59] This is especially important in the community pharmacy setting, where the pharmacy is run by one pharmacist (i.e., single-clinician pharmacies), since a prior study identified that these pharmacists experienced significant challenges in task prioritization.[60,61] This contrary pharmacist behavior of not prioritizing CPS (despite approving of it) is possibly explained as differing "front of stage" performance (i.e., how individuals may enact their professional role in front of a "significant audience" such as a client) and "backstage" behavior (e.g., covert eating behind the dispensary counter where patients cannot see, or how pharmacists prioritize tasks).[62,63] It could be that pharmacist CPS approval is a "front of stage" intention which cannot be enacted in practice, due to unaccounted-for processes that occur in the pharmacist backstage. VRE is a methodology which is designed to draw out the less visible practices of health professionals,[9] and could thus be used to examine backstage pharmacist behaviors. This "exnovating" process may assist in understanding how and why[11,35,40] CPS are not more commonly prioritized for delivery in the community pharmacy setting. The aim of this study was to explore the day-to-day (visible and less visible) work behavior of Australian community pharmacists, particularly their task prioritization considerations, and to pilot VRE feasibility and acceptability in the community pharmacy setting as a participatory research approach.

In the following sections of this chapter, using this study as an example, we provide a primer on how to conduct such a VRE study, following the guidelines set out in *Video-reflexive Ethnography in Health Research and Healthcare Improvement* by Iedema and colleagues.[9] Further details about this study are available in "Appendix" section.

Building a VRE research team

In order to engage with the pharmacist population, the research team assembled for this study consisted of a currently practicing community pharmacist completing her doctoral studies (FY), a professor who is a clinical and academic pharmacist and researcher (BB) and a health services researcher and social scientist (SH). This research team thus had expertise in pharmacy practice (FY and BB), extensive qualitative research experience (BB and SH) and advanced experience in VRE methodology (SH).

Study design and recruitment

Previous evidence suggests Australian pharmacists are more likely to participate in research if they have an interest in the topic, or have had previous research exposure.[28–30] In FY's experience, during informal discussions at conferences and in professional online forums, interest in this topic (i.e., work conditions limiting task prioritization of CPS provision) was repeatedly expressed by pharmacists and professional organizations. Ongoing work strain, which was associated by pharmacists with CPS provision,[60,61] concerned these potential participants, who stated a desire to provide CPS,[60,61] in line with research evidence.[64,65] As acknowledged in the VRE field, clinicians (such as pharmacists) may perceive participation in VRE research as "yet another thing they have to do."[9] At this stage, therefore, recruitment communication focused on the benefits of participating in the study, and the potential impact and uniqueness of this opportunity: to actively participate in the research, and "tell it as it is."[9]

In this study, pharmacists working in a single-clinician setting were chosen as the sample population: they would be more likely to have full autonomy over (1) their own practice, and (2) participation in the pilot study. It was still necessary to gain pharmacy owner consent, since the study would be performed in pharmacy premises during operating hours. The study did not preclude pharmacy owners from being present during study recording.

The recruitment strategy (through personal networks, closed pharmacist social media groups and through professional organizations) was informed by prior research experience, although limited by COVID-19 pandemic restrictions.

Ethical concerns

Due to the remote locations of some Australian community pharmacies and government-mandated physical distancing during the COVID-19 pandemic, a *participant-led* VRE approach was designed. Instead of researchers capturing video footage on site (as with traditional VRE approaches), participating pharmacists were asked to video-record their everyday work using their own devices. This approach limited the potential spread of COVID-19, and allowed participants to control what was used as study data). To avoid sensitive health information being recorded, a dummy audio plug was provided to disable audio recording on devices.

Minimizing study impact on participants and their clients

To minimize the burden of work for participants recording their own practices, who also had to deal with the changes in work during the pandemic,[52,53,55,66,67] several measures were employed to provide "care" for the participants, and others in the pharmacy environments:

First, use of participants' own devices to record video was designed to cut down on study complexity and logistical difficulties. Considering the remoteness of some of the potential participants, phone and tablet devices owned by the participants were deemed sufficient for video recording, and fixed location filming was recommended[9] to participants. Furthermore, recognizing that it would be unrealistic to obtain written consent for potentially hundreds of pharmacy clients and staff, researchers recommended that devices should be positioned to only capture the participating pharmacist, where possible.

Second, the research team created and provided template study posters and notices for pharmacy staff and clients, which included a QR code link to a video wherein a researcher explained the study. The study posters and notices were designed to be easily customized and printed on-site, and thereby displayed and made available around the pharmacy and in staff working areas. Thus, third parties would be informed and given the choice to view and delete any recordings they were in, even if the pharmacy staff and participant were too busy to provide study notices personally.

Third, to protect the privacy of third parties such as pharmacy clients and staff, submitted video footage of nonparticipant faces was later de-identified by FY, using videoediting software. Original videos were subsequently deleted. Participants were also asked to delete their own copies of footage involving third parties. These were important elements to consider since a VRE approach requires trust from participants and those who depend on them.[9] These additional steps were also taken to decrease participant research "work" to avoid recording staff/customers in their videos.

Fourth, as recommended for participatory research approaches (such as VRE) where participant collaboration is key,[1,9,16,20] multiple informal discussions with each participant were held before, during and after recording to establish rapport. This time was also used to reinforce the available researcher support for participants. In keeping with the principle of exnovation, a researcher (FY) consulted with participants to select routine practices for recording. Specific care was taken to consider what participant-researcher collaboration signified in this VRE study: although support and guidelines for video recording were provided, participants were asked to consider what *they* felt was important about pharmacist work, to choose what to record/submit, and to describe these clips in their own words during reflexive sessions.

Fifth, detailed written guidelines around participant recording were provided to participants as they were not likely to be experts in video recording, and to limit uncertainty they might experience about the technical process. This included: (1) diagrams to assist participants' understanding of what should be captured in videos, (2) step-by-step instructions on setting up the pharmacy for study participation, and (3) instructions about video upload to a confidential shared folder, with screenshots. These guidelines were typically provided after participants had returned their signed consent forms online, and provided a starting point for discussion with researchers about logistical issues. An adhesive wall device mount was also provided to participants who requested one.

Sixth, for secure data management, the REDcap survey platform[68,69] was used to record online consent, and to collect participant data (including nonidentifying demographic and workload information). Similarly, participant video recordings were uploaded to secure online shared folders. Participants were asked to limit the number and duration of recordings to prevent excessively long video upload times, and to minimize inconvenience to participants.[9]

Seventh, participant-submitted video footage was then reviewed for use by a researcher, based on participants' given justifications and the study objectives. If videos were too lengthy, the video footage was edited or played at double time during the reflexive session, so that the review of video footage would not take longer than half an hour. This was done to allow time for participants to comment at length, and for researchers to ask questions in the planned hour-long reflexive sessions. Some considerations for editing included extended periods when the participant was not in the camera frame, or when third parties crossed the screen and blocked the camera view. However, wherever possible, videos were not edited down for length, since it was possible that participants had unstated reasons for submitting footage. These processes were also intended to decrease participant and researcher fatigue in reflexive sessions, since participants generally scheduled these sessions after their workday. If agreed to by both researcher and participants, reflexive sessions were extended past an hour, or reconvened.

Caring for participants

A number of further measures were implemented to provide care for participants, considering their long working hours and multiple responsibilities.

First, FY periodically checked in with participants prior to, and during, the recording phase (around once/twice per week or fortnight) to offer assistance and receive progress updates. While this reinforced the researcher support available to participants, researchers were mindful not to contact participants too frequently (since this could be perceived as pressure that might cause participant stress).

Second, two strategies were adopted in case there were long delays between recording videos and reflexive sessions, being cognizant of limited participant availability and long working hours. (A) Reflexive sessions were scheduled as soon as possible, after participants were satisfied with their video recordings. (B) A template to capture information about each recorded clip was provided for participants (text fields included: file names, brief descriptions, and comments for researchers). These measures contributed to aiding participant recall, researcher understanding, and, where required, the selection of clips for reflexive sessions.

Third, it was decided that FY, as a current practicing community pharmacist, would conduct the reflexive sessions to assist in drawing out implied and assumed practitioner knowledge. Thus, during the online session, it was hoped that the participant would be able to focus on introducing work processes deemed important to task prioritization in the limited session time, without necessarily requiring detailed, in-depth explanations of the multiple, interwoven pharmacist work processes that are often multitasked.[21,22,57,70–79] This was also to mitigate potential "face threats" for participant psychological safety.[80,81] In order to decrease uncertainty and make clear researcher and participant roles, participants were asked to introduce the videos for their contextualized insights in the session, while the researcher facilitated the session (which included requesting participant insights on the clips viewed). An active listening approach was used by the researcher, as the facilitator, to elicit and confirm participant views. The "playing" and "pausing" of the video footage was not necessarily assumed to be the researcher's role, and was also negotiated with participants prior to each reflexive session. When the researcher was in control of the video during the session, videos were often paused to allow participants to complete their comments.

Coanalyzing VRE data and reflexivity

During VRE reflexive sessions, submitted videos underwent "coanalysis" by both participants and researchers, while watching and commenting on the video observations,[9] as described above. For this reason, all reflexive sessions were audio and video recorded, then transcribed. As mentioned above, VRE researcher and participant roles may be usefully negotiated before reflexive sessions, since these roles are often blurred in participatory action research,[1,2] including VRE.[9,37] Similarly, the participant-led adaptation led to shifting power relations between the researcher and participants. For instance, during video recording, researchers mainly provided assistance, while participants had the active role and agency of presenting themselves through their own selected video footage.[82] This power balance shifted during our one-on-one reflexive discussions, since the researcher actively hosted the session's structure and content as the facilitator. Other reflexive considerations included: relational/interpersonal reflexivity (i.e., how researchers navigated their relationships and interactions with participants); and collective reflexivity (i.e., how the research process and design affected study findings, outcomes and influenced learning).[9]

Reflexive sessions are considered part of the VRE data collection *and* data analysis processes.[9] Therefore, content analysis of the transcripts was used to further understand and interrogate nuances in the discussions. To do this, session audio was transcribed and verified by FY, and additionally made available to respective participants for verification. Each member of the research team was then involved in content analysis of transcripts. Content analysis followed a critical realist process where transcripts were read independently three times in quick succession by each researcher, and content themes were extracted during researcher reflection/reflexivity.[83] The themes were compared by the research team (including major and minor themes), until consensus was reached. Final results were sent to participants for checking.

This study obtained ethics approval from the UTS Human Research Ethics Committee (UTS HREC 20-5032).

Results

Overall, through video recording their practices and reviewing them with researchers, pharmacists were able to explain the complexities of their visible and nonobservable work on a procedural and personal level. As an example of participants for a VRE study, Table 1 is included in this book chapter: the study participants have differing characteristics, hail from different locations in Australia, and work in differing pharmacy types.

Results from this study are presented below in relation to the four guiding VRE principles, and the feasibility and acceptability of this participant-led approach to VRE in the community pharmacy setting are also discussed.

VRE principle 1: Exnovation

Participants' footage displayed their visible day-to-day work activities in their workplaces. Their comments "exnovated" the detailed systems, work processes, and tasks which were, for the most part, visibly situated in the dispensary. Their tasks and processes were described as requiring complete accuracy, for quality assurance of services. Specific colored prescription baskets, expressions, gestures or physical locations were used as symbolic codes for themselves, their staff and clientele (e.g., to indicate pharmacist availability or signal the progress of specific tasks in the overall workflow).

However, "less visible" work practices were more frequently mentioned in the reflexive sessions. Pharmacists primarily chose to describe administrative work and "checklist" tasks that related to compulsory operating guidelines and quality standard adherence, rather than clinically-focused processes.

For instance, task prioritization, or the immediate reorganization of their workflow, was spoken of often (i.e., when new and/or competing work demands presented). Situational awareness allowed pharmacists to respond rapidly by reprioritizing tasks, thus altering their immediate workflow (comprising physical, digital, and mental workspaces) accordingly. One pharmacist remarked that this prioritization process was an important and essential pharmacist competency.

CPS provision was either deferred to a set appointment time, or when more than one pharmacist or a dispensary technician was available to manage the separate CPS and dispensary workflows. These were spoken of as incompatible and competing workflows that were not usually multitasked, for fear of making errors. Quality assurance appeared to be a major consideration in not delivering CPS when working as a "sole" pharmacist:

> *If I feel I can't do a service properly, I would rather not do it [...] I might suggest to them that they come in during the week [when three pharmacists are available during one shift] (P3)*

Another challenge of the invisible work described was that the different systems/processes involved did not interact nor integrate with each other, with each requiring multiple and varying human interchanges. The pharmacists, as the middlemen, spoke at length about the hidden challenges of navigating between all these systems (which were implied to all be necessary to achieve good patient clinical outcomes). Since the pharmacy was an accessible retail environment, pharmacists did not have complete control over an unpredictable workload. Participants spoke of a type of powerlessness, feeling trapped between providing good patient care, patient demands, legislation, their own personal needs, and prescribers.

TABLE 1 Study participant details: an example from a pilot VRE study in the community pharmacy setting.

	Job status, gender, age, qualification[a]	Year of Australian registration, Number of pharmacy jobs, weekly hours in this pharmacy	Pharmacy prescriptions per day, # pharmacists/dispense technicians/pharmacy assistants in usual 9–5 week day shift	Pharmacy services (weekly^, monthly*, daily ~ estimate of S2/S3 inquiries personally handled)	State[b]	Pharmacy location (PhARIa, MMM, IRSD)[c]
Participant 1 (P1)	Owner, M, 30–34, BPharm	2013, 1 pharmacy job, 44 h	100–200, 1/0/3	^ 20–50 DAAs, * 1–5 Medschecks, * 0 HMRs/ RMMRs, * 6–10 facilities, ^ 0 vaccinations, ~ 11–20 inquiries	VIC	3 (inner regional Australia), 5 (rural/ remote), 1 (most disadvantaged)
Participant 2 (P2)	Owner, M, 40–44, MPharm	2009, 1 pharmacy job, 46.5 h	<100, 1/0/1 (+ 1 pharmacy student/ intern supervised in a year)	^ 20–50 DAAs, * 1–5 Medschecks, * 1–5 HMRs/ RMMRs, * 1–5 facilities, ^ 0 vaccinations, ~ 11–20 inquiries	TAS	5 (outer regional Australia), 5 (rural/ remote), 1 (most disadvantaged)
Participant 3 (P3)	Pharmacist in charge (part-time), F, 45–49, BPharm	2015, 2 pharmacy jobs, 10 h	201–400, 3/0/5 (+ 3 pharmacy students/ interns supervised in a year)	^ 51–100 DAAs, * 11–15 Medschecks, * 1–5 HMRs/ RMMRs, * 0 facilities, ^ peak of 201–300 vaccinations weekly in 2020, ~ 6–10 inquiries	QLD	1 (major city of Australia), 1 (metropolitan area), 1 (not rural), 3 (middling disadvantage)
Participant 4 (P4)	Pharmacist in charge (part-time), M, 30–34, BPharm	2011, 2 pharmacy jobs, 9 h	<100, 1/1/1	^ <20 DAAs, * 11–15 Medschecks, * 0 HMRs/ RMMRs, * 1–5 facilities, ^ peak of 1–50 vaccinations weekly in 2020, ~ 21–30 inquiries	NSW	1 (major city of Australia), 1 (metropolitan area), 1 (most disadvantaged)

[a]BPharm, Bachelor of Pharmacy (school entry degree); MPharm, Master of Pharmacy (graduate entry degree program).

[b]States of Australia: NSW, New South Wales; QLD, Queensland; TAS, Tasmania; VIC, Victoria.

[c]PhARIA, Pharmacy Area Remoteness Index of Australia, which into account the remoteness of the pharmacy location (professionally and geographically) in Australia, which determines federally-funded rural pharmacy allowances. MMM, Modified Monash Model, which categorizes locations according to remoteness and population sizes in Australia with respect to medical services, according to the five year Australian Census. IRSD, the Index of Relative Socio-economic Disadvantage which summarizes the relative economic and social conditions which disadvantage household and people in an area (i.e., income, qualifications and low-skilled occupations).

VRE principles 2, 3 & 4 (reflexivity, care and collaboration): Feasibility and acceptability

As is the norm with VRE studies, the ethics application took time to prepare and process due to patient privacy and third party consent considerations. Generally, pharmacist acceptability of this study was not high during the COVID-19 pandemic. Overall, it appeared that participants were more likely to participate if they had previous experience of research participation, prior interaction with the research team, or were from very remote or disadvantaged areas. Although trying to engage pharmacists in research has been reportedly difficult, it may be even harder to recruit them to a VRE study, particularly where the relationship between researcher and participant can be difficult to foster from a distance. It is, with some irony, that we note that we were asking pharmacists to do additional "work" for a study seeking to understand their workload issues, particularly in the context where workloads had increased in response to the impact of COVID-19 (as explained by our participants). In other words, the more usual VRE process (i.e., where a researcher works with participants on-site to record and conduct the study according to protocol) in nonpandemic scenarios may be more feasible and acceptable in the community pharmacy setting. The lengthy and involved nature of VRE methodology suggests that fewer steps in the research process for pharmacists are preferable, and could improve acceptability.

Regarding the use of VRE in the pharmacy setting, the following study findings are offered to illustrate addressing reflexivity, and to report the types of practical issues that may arise.

Logistical issues

During this pilot study, participants reported trialing video recording and problem-solving a range of pragmatic and logistic issues on their own. It seemed that participants preferred to personally handle these (or at least, try to) as if they had been delegated these research tasks, despite researcher assurances of their availability to provide support. For example, one participant downplayed their numerous attempts at video-recording over two weeks, finally reporting some "trouble." FY suggested that a pharmacy staff member could act as the participant's "research assistant" to record video clips, directed by the participant, solving the participant's practical issue of having to both record *and* provide quality care. This type of difficulty in completing research tasks was corroborated by another participant, who remarked, *"The issue with trying to capture footage for this particular project is that you can't predict when you have a bad day! And when you're having a bad day, you can't think, 'Oh I need to capture this,' because you're too busy focused on doing what you need to do."* In other words, work overload meant research participation would be the least of their concerns, and it is quite likely that participants in this pilot study did not submit footage of their busiest days. However, recording difficulties tended to be explained much later in the study process, during the reflexive sessions.

Also, requiring participants to record for the study meant that they were in charge of enforcing the study protocol in pharmacies. For example, researchers relied on participants to post study notices in pharmacy premises while recording, and to inform their staff and patients about the study. P2 and P4 spoke of receiving favorable reactions from staff and patients. However, video footage from P1 showed a pharmacy staff member gesturing at the camera in question, and as a result, this clip was not used in their reflexive session. This suggests that study protocols should be administered by researchers, or a proxy "research assistant" (e.g., pharmacy assistant who assists to record video, puts up study notices, communicates with researcher on behalf of the pharmacist etc.) whenever possible.

Technical issues

Although anticipated to be an issue, large video file sizes were only an issue for one participant who had trouble uploading to the shared research folder. To our knowledge, this step in uploading videos delayed the reflexive sessions of two participants by a day each, perhaps due to technological difficulties and poor internet speeds during the pandemic.

One unanticipated issue was that some participants used phones without an audio input port. This meant that the requirement to not record audio could not be followed, since it was not possible to eliminate the audio input manually. To address this, audio tracks were later deleted manually during third party de-identification by the researcher, and/or muted manually by the researcher while conducting reflexive sessions. It is possible that participants may have been relying on audio cues to remember why they had taken the video, since those using the "set recording" approach (as explained below) commented on not remembering why parts of the footage had been submitted.

Cinematography approaches

Two different approaches to video recording were used by the participants: placing the recording device in a set location overseeing the pharmacist's work (P1, P3), and use of a third party to follow the pharmacist in their work (P2, P4). This resulted in slight differences in the video recordings submitted and dynamics of the subsequent reflexive sessions.

The "set location" recordings looked visually similar to a CCTV recording. These recordings tended to be started by the participant, and left running for a period of time, during which they reported forgetting about the recordings. The clips had to be edited afterwards for length (by participant and/or researcher). In general, longer video files were submitted by these participants, which had an average duration of 6.5 min for 12 videos. During reflexive sessions, this meant there were longer periods of time when both participant and researcher were observing (rather than discussing) the video, and the videos for P3 had to be viewed in double speed to keep the session at a manageable duration. However, this approach also seemed to elicit more self-commentary about the participants' actions:

I'm working on two of 'em [baskets of prescriptions]! It is bizarre, like – because I think I try not to ever be working on two patients or things at a time (P3)

This included guessing their possible off-screen actions:

That's me running off, maybe looking for something? Maybe it's not in stock. Maybe I can't find it. (P1)

On the other hand, the use of a third party for video recording resulted in shorter video clips (average duration of 1 min for 10 videos) with a specific topic per video, where the participant actively explained their work in the short clips. Participants and staff also appeared more conscious of the recording device with this approach. There were fewer associated observational and reflexive remarks by participants. However, this approach seemed easier for participants to manage, since filming could be essentially delegated to a staff member.

Discussion: Using VRE in the community pharmacy setting

In this section, we discuss some of the practical and methodological findings that arose from the pilot study, with a view to informing how other researchers might wish to apply this methodology to the community pharmacy setting.

Firstly, a practical note—as with any time-poor health participants, one important consideration in conducting research with community pharmacists is the need to streamline the formal VRE process for this population. For example, we consider these steps as improvements to our study process:

- The data collection points that are required to be actioned by participating pharmacists themselves were limited. At minimum, the study would require an initial recruitment discussion with the participant, consultation on what would be appropriate to video, and their participation in reflexive sessions. After discussion with participants, researchers could lead the logistical work of the video recording in the pharmacy, which would then only require the participating pharmacist's input and approval.
- If the research team themselves cannot physically be present, this could be achieved by working with a proxy "research assistant" who is nominated by the participant (e.g., a dispensary technician, pharmacy assistant or pharmacy student) to complete research tasks on-site. The research team could then collect other ethnographic information required by attending the pharmacy themselves, and conducting interviews, perhaps with the assistance of the nominated research assistant.
- Finally, viewing pharmacies as a unit could be valuable to the research process, as pharmacists often work in teams by necessity, even when working as sole clinicians. Inclusion of other pharmacy team members may have additional benefits: (1) having other points of contact in the pharmacy (particularly when the study participant cannot be reached, due to workload), (2) other perspectives can be collected, and (3) they can work with other study participants on-site to solve logistical research issues as they arise.

Next, depending on the aims of the research, video-reflexive ethnography studies may need to follow the same requirements for informational power as other qualitative studies.[84] Although the sample size for our pilot study was small, with only four sites, it was sufficient for its primary purposes,[85] which were to explore a complex phenomenon and pilot a new methodology. In relation to representativeness, this study involved critical-case sampling[85]: single-clinician pharmacies represent the most basic community pharmacy work conditions in Australia and, thus, has implications across the sector.

With regard to the benefits of using VRE as a research methodology, we suggest that pharmacists may welcome it as a form of cultural brokerage.[86] Throughout the COVID-19 pandemic, despite being labeled as "essential workers" for their important roles in medication access, health promotion and education,[53] pharmacists reported feeling underrecognized.[52] Such sentiment presents an opportunity for greater research engagement within the profession, since the use of VRE as a participatory approach allows participants to directly contribute their lived experiences and perspectives, which may otherwise be inaccessible to "outsiders" (i.e., researchers), and enables them to "represent" the profession and its important role meaningfully. Through VRE, participants are able to provide detailed commentary about their work, in their specific context, explaining how and why they perform tasks in a particular way.

Interestingly, using their video footage, pharmacists in our study seemed to *preferentially* speak about their "unseen" care practices; knowledge of these invisible work processes may be instrumental in understanding pharmacist overload, reluctance to prioritize CPS, or engagement in research. This demonstrates the appropriateness of using VRE in this healthcare setting to "exnovate" pharmacist practice, where invisible work was described as a prominent feature. "Holo-grammatically," in viewing the videos, pharmacists were also able to recall specific details about the specific physical, digital, and mental workspaces they had been using, and describe the difficulties they faced through their practice in the COVID-19 pandemic. Reviewing their own work practices as third party observers through the video can also create opportunities for pharmacists and pharmacy staff to see how they work "at a distance," thus orienting and priming them to different perspectives, and opportunities for learning and improving practice.[87]

While validation of study findings with participants is encouraged in qualitative pharmacy research, the lack of front-line clinician involvement in other research processes (e.g., in analysis and formulating research questions) could limit the value, impact and translation of research findings into practice. Active engagement of front-line pharmacists in the research process (e.g., the formulation of research questions, data collection/extraction/analysis/interpretation) could increase pharmacy practice research translation into practice. This participatory approach may be empowering for pharmacists who may feel their professionalism is unseen, and their concerns about occupational health norms unheard. As described earlier, community pharmacists can be suspicious of outsiders like researchers. VRE as cultural brokerage, and communication of it, therefore, could possibly increase pharmacist research engagement.

Moving on to ethical issues, we emphasize the importance of trust between researchers and participants, particularly when considering the aforementioned reasons for low research engagement. In this study, relationship and trust-building required sustained engagement over a period of time for the VRE approach to be accepted as trustworthy. For instance, our participants seemed to implicitly trust that the research team would ensure privacy for their staff and clients captured on video. The importance of this step in building relationships between researchers and participants cannot be understated.

On a related topic, just as pharmacists have been documented to be tailoring their social interactions to others[88] (e.g., for those with language and health literacy barriers, or COVID vaccine hesitancy), pharmacist participants may also tailor their interactions with the researcher. Therefore, an active listening approach, which was used by the researcher in the study described, is crucial. Community pharmacists seemed to be acutely sensitive to the verbal and nonverbal communication of researchers and their perceived interest, and may have doubted the significance of their contributions; one participant asked, "Is there anything you need me to be talking about, rather than what I've been talking about?" VRE is a collaborative sense-making process,[9] so frequent verbal affirmation and engagement throughout the reflexive sessions can empower active participant collaboration in this setting.

As recommended for VRE in other healthcare settings,[9] backup methods for video-recording storage and transmission should be considered. It should be noted that the cinematographic framing of video in VRE can influence how subjects are viewed in a filmed clip.[89] Therefore, when a researcher negotiates and films healthcare practices, reflexivity regarding the cinematographic framing is expected. This chapter is an overview, introducing and advocating for the use of VRE to the pharmacy practice discipline, and interested researchers are strongly encouraged to read cited references, particularly the 2019 publication by Iedema and colleagues.[9]

Finally, we offer here a brief reflection on the participant-led model of VRE. Although a potential hurdle to recruitment, our participant-led VRE approach was novel, and aligned with the participatory principles of VRE. By limiting the researchers' input into video recording, participants took the lead in foregrounding their work practices, using their lived-in understanding of work contexts. For improved recruitment and acceptability, future use of VRE in similar work-related research could include: researcher-led video recordings negotiated with pharmacies (instead of solely con-sisting of participant-led recordings), and/or use of CCTV footage with assistance of the research team to ensure research proceeded ethically. This would remove the burden of administering VRE processes from pharmacists, avoid inadvertent protocol contravention by participants, and improve recruitment and efficiency in the VRE research process. Participants could then give input into (1) research aims and design, (2) when/where recording would be necessary (without having to think about the "how"), and (3) participate in reflexive sessions mostly with the "third-party" observational perspective (which may be preferable for eliciting reflexivity).

In a nonpandemic setting, having a research team filming on site, and a possible interventional VRE study design for increasing service quality or improving safety culture, could be attractive to community pharmacies. A remote participant-led approach with engaged parties, on the other hand, could be further refined by posting study notices about CCTV recordings between certain times, which are then reviewed and extracted with researcher assistance.

Implications

VRE is a promising alternative to in-person ethnography and other observational methods used in community pharmacy practice research, examining care and work practices as they are from moment to moment.[9] Participants are able to describe an invisible, complex web of systems within their care practices. They give detailed and contextualized insights into the "backstage" of their task prioritization thought processes, including their perceptions of how professional identity relate to their work. As a participatory action research approach, VRE holds some promise: it can be administered remotely (to some extent) and can be used to facilitate site-specific improvements in community pharmacy practice. Due to the time and active participation required, recruitment in the community pharmacy setting may require compensation for participants' time.

Limitations

Application of VRE methodology can be complex and time-consuming. The design and ethics application process may be lengthy, particularly if ethics committees are not familiar with such participatory action approaches. Further, the study process itself requires ongoing reflexivity and cooperation between participants and researchers. It may not be suitable nor practical for addressing all research questions, particularly since it requires acknowledging multiple perspectives and the complexity in everyday care practices. VRE methodology can be cognitively taxing, and thus, resource-intensive.

Future work

For community pharmacy and other pharmacist practice settings, VRE is a novel methodology. Its applications are therefore numerous: for example, in studying the communication between pharmacists and other health professionals, pharmacists and patients, and handover processes between pharmacists in the same pharmacies; in facilitating the quality improvement of dispensary processes and in CPS provision; in the implementation of CPS; in the examination of the dyads between pharmacy assistants, pharmacists, their clients, doctors and allied health professionals; and much more.

Conclusions

As an established methodology, VRE can engage with the complexity and contradictions in human behavior, which may be highly transformative in future pharmacy practice research. VRE can be effective in pharmacy settings as both an exploratory research approach and as an intervention. A key characteristic of VRE is the flexibility afforded to researchers in conducting research in return for ongoing reflexivity about methodological principles. For researchers, a thorough understanding of the theoretical underpinnings of VRE is therefore important to ensure its appropriate use.[9,18]

VRE presents an exciting opportunity for pharmacy practice researchers to answer complex research questions, such as the contrary behaviors of front-line clinicians who profess approval of cognitive pharmacy services but do not always provide them. It could also be an effective way to explore issues in the pharmacist workforce as it undergoes role transition.[90] Furthermore, it gives voice to front-line community pharmacists and other parties in the pharmacy practice settings. This engagement, in turn, may encourage research participation and future scholarship.

Questions for further discussion

1. Reflexivity is key to the VRE process, for both researchers and participants. Do you feel able, as a researcher, to be reflexive in your own research, and to articulate this reflexivity in communicating about your research? How could reflexivity improve the way research is conducted and reported in the pharmacy setting?
2. VRE tends to challenge the assumptions of researchers and participants, since it invites both researchers and participants to articulate and reflect on these assumptions in the process. This process of challenging one's own and others' assumptions needs to be done with sensitivity and care. What are some ways that researchers can create psychological safety for participants (and themselves) during reflexive sessions?
3. Given the site-specific nature of VRE studies and interventions, how can VRE researchers most effectively describe and translate the significance and impact of their work? Can this be built into VRE study design?

Application exercise/scenario

While working with community pharmacists to codesign the provision of a new diabetes screening service such as FIN-DRISC,[91] you become aware that pharmacy staff report difficulties in recruiting participants to the service. It is not clear whether this is due to the pharmacy clients and target population, the pharmacy staff, surrounding health professionals, the pharmacy leadership or something else entirely. Describe how VRE methodology could be applied to this situation to identify and address these issues.

Appendix

A. Online survey
B. Participant recording guidelines
C. Sample study information notice for pharmacy
D. Reflexive session questions

A. Online survey

	Personal details	
1.	**What age are you?**	**Under 25 years** **25–29, 30–34, 35–39, 40–44, 45–49,** **50–54, 55–59, 60–64, 65–69, 70–74,** **75–79,** **80 years old and over**
2.	What gender do you identify as?	Male Female Prefer not to say Self-described
	Pharmacy career	
3.	In which year did you first register as a pharmacist in Australia?	
4.	What pharmacy education degrees or certifications do you hold? *(tick boxes)*	☐ Bachelor of Pharmacy ☐ Masters of Pharmacy ☐ Graduate Certificate ☐ Diploma ☐ Advanced Diploma ☐ PhD ☐ AACP ☐ Other (please specify)
5.	How many jobs do you currently hold, including the pharmacy you will record yourself in?	*Number validation*
6.	For the pharmacy I'm recording myself in, my job description is: *(drop down list)* *Pharmacist Manager = responsible to owner for all store duties* *Pharmacist in Charge = in charge of regular day to day running of store*	Owner Pharmacist Manager Pharmacist in Charge Staff pharmacist Consultant Pharmacist Locum Other (please specify)
7.	How many weekly hours do you work in this pharmacy, on average?	*Number validation*
	About this Community Pharmacy	
8.	Postcode of workplace	*Postal code (Australia) validation*

Continued

—cont'd

About this Community Pharmacy ....

9.	During an average 9–5 shift on a week day, how many pharmacists work in this pharmacy (including yourself)?	*Number validation range: 1–10*
10.	How many dispensary technicians?	*Number validation range: 0–15*
	How many pharmacy assistants?	*Number validation range: 0–10*
11.	Average daily prescriptions dispensed	<100 100–200 201–400 >400
12.	Weekly DAAs provided	<20 20–50 51–100 101–150 151–200 >200
13.	Monthly Clinical Interventions delivered	*Number validation range: minimum 0*
14.	Number of Opioid Replacement Therapy clients	*Number validation range: minimum 0*
15.	Number of Staged Supply clients	*Number validation range: minimum 0*
16.	Monthly Medschecks provided (including Diabetes and Pain Medschecks) *Monthly claimable Medschecks in a month is 20.*	0 1–5 6–10 11–15 16–20
17.	Monthly HMR/RMMR workload *Maximum monthly HMRs/RMMRs currently claimable is 30.*	0 1–5 6–10 11–15 16–20 21–30
18.	Monthly number of nursing homes/aged care/disability/private hospitals serviced	0 1–5 6–10 More than 10
19.	In 2020, peak number of vaccinations provided in a week	0 51–100 201–300 401–500 1–50 101–200 301–400 More than 500
20.	Weekly screening services workload (cholesterol, diabetes, sleep apnea)	0 11–20 31–40 More than 50 1–10 21–30 41–50

—cont'd

About this Community Pharmacy ....

21.	Weekly blood pressure check workload	0 1–10 11–50 51–100 More than 100
22.	Daily estimate of S2/S3 inquiries handled personally	0 1–5 6–10 11–20 21–30 More than 30
23.	Yearly number of students/interns directly precepted or supervised	0 1 2 3 More than 3
24.	Monthly average number of educational seminars given (internally or externally)	0 1 2 3 4 5 More than 5
25.	Weekly average of case conferences (face to face or >15 min phone call with other health professionals)	0 1–5 6–10 11–20 More than 20
26.	Weekly average hospital discharge reconciliation workload	0 1–5 6–10 11–20 More than 20
27.	Weekly average number of extemporaneously compounding items	0 1–5 6–10 11–50 51–100 More than 100
28.	Weekly average of Away from Work certificates issued	0 1–5 6–10 11–20 More than 20
	Average daily number of patients who receive deliveries	*Number validation: minimum 0*
29.	Do you provide any other services not mentioned here?	Yes (please specify) No
30.	(Branching logic): Name of service/s:	
31.	(Branching logic): Quantity in a week:	

It is often said that pharmacists wear many hats. The following section has several descriptions of the hats that pharmacists can wear. During the upcoming reflexive sessions, we're interested in how you navigate these in your job, and want to use your answers to guide part of our discussion. Please answer as honestly as you can.

Please indicate below how much you agree or disagree that these descriptions reflect how you see yourself as a pharmacist. *(Strongly disagree, disagree, neutral, agree, strongly disagree)*

1. **Responsible generalist:**

    As a community pharmacist, I am the responsible "jack-of-all-trades" generalist in the store who does "everything."

2. **Accessible healthcare professional:**

    Community pharmacists such as me are accessible health care providers, ready to respond to whatever comes in the door.

3. **Medication expert:**

    As the pharmacist, I play a key role in the health care system by giving advice about the safe and effective use of medicines.

4. **Community asset:**

    As the pharmacist, I am a trusted healthcare resource that is deeply embedded in my community.

5. **Helper:**

    I became a pharmacist to help people with their health, taking on a caring, proactive role.

6. **Health promoter:**

    I support people in improving their health and preventing complications through health education, promotion and screening, particularly when they can't access other forms of care.

7. **Retailer:**

    As a pharmacist, I am a retailer. I dispense medications and supply other over-the-counter products, including vitamins and gifts.

8. **Protector**:

    In accordance with the law and pharmacist duty of care, I safeguard the use of, and access to, medications.

9. **Change agent**:

    Being a pharmacist, I adapt to the changing needs of patients and the healthcare system, transitioning my professional scope of practice where required.

10. *Organizational role—branching logic*

    Employee pharmacist:

    I am an employee pharmacist, fulfilling my professional duties by carefully balancing my employer's expectations and my duty of care to patients.

    Pharmacist proprietor:

    As the owner of my pharmacy, I ensure the business is financially viable in order to serve the community, and to provide an income for my staff and myself.

11. **Other**: If you believe there's another role you play as a pharmacist in your work, please label and describe it here. *(Free text response)*

Please rank how you feel these labels describe your day-to-day activities, where 12 is the most descriptive of your daily pharmacist work, and 1 is the least descriptive. (1–12)

12. Responsible generalist
13. Accessible health professional
14. Medication expert
15. Community asset
16. Helper
17. Health promoter
18. Retailer
19. Protector
20. Change agent
21. Employee pharmacist
22. Pharmacist proprietor
23. Other (self-description)
24. Feel free to comment on your ranking below. *(Free text response)*

B. Recording guidelines for pharmacists

Participant video recording guidelines
Over a period of two weeks, we would like you to:

- Record and submit a **minimum of 2** video recordings (i.e., ≥2 recordings over a period of 2 weeks). These recordings will serve as representative footage of your typical, everyday work as a pharmacist.
- Each video should be **no longer than 10 min** (i.e., maximum 10 min long), so that they can be easily uploaded to the secure UTS Onedrive folder. Clips of such length may take up to half an hour to upload, depending on your internet connection.
- If necessary, you can submit several shorter clips of your work to show or highlight different aspects of your work. However, if you submit a lot of footage to discuss in the follow-up 60 min reflexive session, we may ask you to choose only one or two recordings to discuss. Alternately, we can organize an additional reflexive session if you wish to review and discuss more footage.

Setup for the study
A. Displaying study signage
1. Print out pharmacy staff and customer information notices in the "Third party information notices":
   a. Pharmacy staff information notices are in the first three pages
      i. Print the information for each of your pharmacy staff to read on their shift. You can also send it as an email if practical.
      ii. Please discuss the practical implications with your staff: they will need to be able to explain to your customers what the study is about, and explain that customers can opt-out of the footage too.
      iii. Keep note of which staff do NOT want to be in the footage.
      iv. You will have to stop recording and turn off the equipment when they may be captured in the recording.
   b. Customer information notices are on pages 4 and 5.
      i. Print the information notices, and place them at points of contact with your customers: e.g., on the dispensary counter and consultation tables, before the study recording begins and during the study recording period
2. Please input the date period you'll be recording your work into the poster templates at the end of the "Third party information notices" document.
   a. Poster for informing pharmacy staff is on page 6
   b. Poster for informing pharmacy customers on page 7
3. Print the posters.
4. Display pharmacy customer posters at the points of interaction between the pharmacist and patient, beginning the week before recording, and for the two weeks you record within.
      Places you could display these posters include:
   a. Dispensary counters
   b. Waiting areas
   c. Consultation tables
   d. Counseling room/s
5. Display pharmacy staff posters in places where they will see it easily, e.g., the tea/lunch room area, behind dispensary counters for their reference.
6. Please keep note for *your own* reference which customers and staff opt-out of recording, as you will need to turn off the recording equipment during times they are in the pharmacy. (The research team does not need to know who opts out.)

B. Recording video guidelines
1. Choose the phone or tablet device you will record on. Ideally, this should be a device you do not use in your everyday pharmacist work. Alternatively, you could use a personally-owned video camera and tripod/mount. If security camera footage already records these areas, you can also use this footage—if possible, ensure that pharmacy customers, prescription information and the computer screen are not visible in this footage though.
2. If you use a phone or tablet device to record in your workplace, we will post you an adhesive phone/device wall mount and audio plug for ease of recording.
3. Using the front-view/selfie camera on your device, identify a location in your pharmacy to place your camera/device. This location should capture a clear view of the space/area in which you mostly work, such as the dispensary, front counter and/or counseling area.

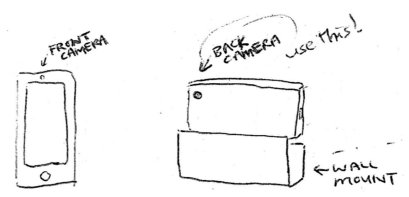

*Use **front** camera only to identify a location. When recording, the **back** camera is preferred.*

a. Ideally, the camera/device should be affixed (using the wall mount provided) to a wall, pillar or similar stable surface.

b. The device should be placed at a height which is one arms-length above your head, to capture an over-head view.

c. If at all possible, please choose a location where the device **cannot** capture customers/clients in the video recording. If possible, try to ensure prescription information and the computer screen are not visible.

4. You should have received a phone wall mount from the research team. This mount uses 3 M tape adhesive. Please follow the instructions to secure the wall mount in a horizontal orientation at the selected recording location.

5. **Take a test recording** using the *back-view camera* of your device in the selected location to ensure it captures what you want it to.

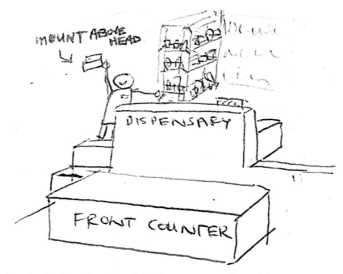

Mount device at arms-length above head, with a clear view of the places you normally work in.

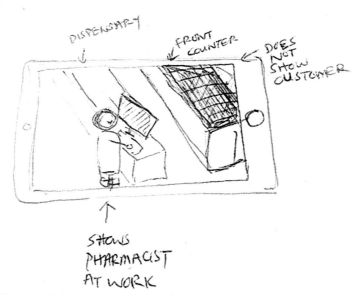

This is an example of what the footage might look like. If you can't avoid capturing your patients in the footage, you will need to be prepared to stop recording, to show the recording to the patient, and/or delete the footage upon customer request.

Recording tips

1. The back-view camera on your device is preferred since it has a higher resolution. However, if you have technical difficulties, the front-view camera can be used instead.
2. Since audio recording is not desired, to protect the privacy of your colleagues, patients and customers, please plug the audio plug we have provided to you into the audio jack (if your device has one).
3. Keep in mind that the length of video you can record will depend on your device's video capabilities and storage space. You may need to free up space on your device so you can record all that you may want to.
   How much space do I have on my device to record?
   To find out how much video recording time is on your device, you can follow this process:
   a. Record exactly one minute or 60 s of footage on your device. You can record anything as long as it's not in the dark and something is moving in the video.
   b. After recording the video, go to the Photo gallery or File Manager and check the file size of the video (e.g., 145 MB) by looking at the file "info." Record this down.
   c. Check how much free space is left on your device in Settings, then Storage. This number is usually given in GB. Convert this number to MB by multiplying by 1000.
   d. Divide the free space on your device by file size of the 60-s recording. This number will be the maximum number of minutes which you can take on your device.
4. You may find it easier to allow the device to continue recording at times when you expect certain pharmacist activities to take place. We suggest identifying these times beforehand so you can simply begin the recording at a specified time. You can separate these clips later into ten minute lengths later if necessary. Choose the videos you think are important to discuss in relation to normal pharmacist work, and decisions you have to make in prioritizing different tasks.
5. You can submit video recordings at any time to your assigned OneDrive folder. After doing this, you can delete the recording from your device to free up space. If you are doing this to make space for another recording, make sure you also delete the file from the "Deleted" folder in your Photo gallery or File Manager.

During recording period

1. You or the pharmacy staff will need to explain the study to customers during the study period. Here is an easy way for you to say it:

"I'm taking part in a research study to explain pharmacist work. As part of that, I'm recording short clips of myself working. No audio is being recorded. But if you're worried about being in the video, you're welcome to see the footage to confirm you're not in it. You also have the option to not run that risk: I can turn off the video recording equipment while you're here. I and the researchers will make sure none of your prescription information can be seen on the video. But let me know what's comfortable for you."

2. Make sure you place the posters and information notices where you normally interact with customers and around the pharmacy, particularly when you're recording.
3. Keep note of which pharmacy staff and customers do not want to be recorded.
4. Turn off video recording and equipment when these people may appear in the footage

Submitting/uploading the video recordings

We will assign to you a secure, unique OneDrive folder, shared only with the researcher Faith Yong, for submission of your video files. The link for this folder will be sent to your email once you complete the study consent form.

To upload to the folder:

1. Open the email invitation to the shared folder.
2. Click on the blue "Open" button.
3. This will trigger an email passcode to be sent to you. Enter this passcode within the next fifteen minutes.
4. Click on the three dots on the screen to click on the "Upload" button as below, and choose "File." You should be able to select your Photo gallery or navigate to your photos and videos and upload relevant files after this. Note that it can take up to half an hour to upload the video files, so don't close your device's internet browser window until it is finished uploading. You can leave it running in the background if you need it for other things, or even record more videos, but the OneDrive browser window should not be closed.

Please note that if you delete recordings from the shared folder, we will not have access to those recordings.

After uploading video files

1. For privacy and ethical reasons, please delete any videos that show pharmacy staff and customers in it from your device, cloud storage and Deleted folders. This is in keeping with the study information we have provided to your staff and customers.
2. We recommend that you provide a brief description to us of what happened in the video, in case you forget by the time we have the reflexive session.

To submit a brief description of the video files you send us, you can either (1) update the "Brief description" document in your OneDrive folder, or (2) email Faith at faith.yong@uts.edu.au, answering these questions:

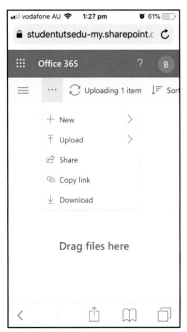 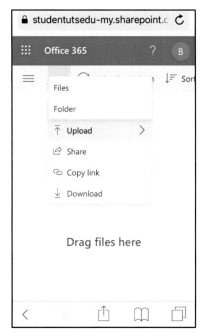

Screenshots which show you how to upload your videos to the research folder.

a. What happens in this recording?
b. Any other comments to the researchers?

If you have any questions or technical issues, you can contact Faith at faith.yong@uts.edu.au.

C. Sample information notice for pharmacy

UTS HREC 20-5032: EXPLORING COMMUNITY PHARMACIST WORK IN CONTEXT

WE ARE RECORDING
VIDEO IN-STORE*

[insert date range] 2020

NO AUDIO IS BEING RECORDED.

This is part of a research
study into pharmacist work.

*There is no change to your usual pharmacy services. We will not be recording video all day, and are not intending to capture the general public in these video recordings.
You can scan this QR code for an explanatory video →

Please tell our staff if:

- you want more information
- you don't want to be in the video**

**The staff will let the participating pharmacist know if you don't want to be in the video, so they can turn off the recording equipment while you're there.

D. Reflexive session questions

Welcome the participant.

Thanks for agreeing to be part of this research. We really appreciate your willingness to participate. As you know, we are conducting this study to explore pharmacist work in the community setting and how you make decisions around prioritizing different tasks. This session is expected to take about an hour.

In this session, we see you as a collaborator so we will be watching the footage, discussing and analyzing it together. If, at the end of this session, we find there's more to talk about, we can make another time to go over more footage or continue where we left off.

This session will be recorded so that nothing is missed in what you have to say. However, what is said in this session stays here. In the transcripts, we will anonymize any details that could identify you, the pharmacy, the staff or any customers/clients to protect everyone's privacy. If there are any times when you feel uncomfortable or need to leave the interview, please let me know so we can stop recording.

I. Watching the videos together

1. I've got your written summary of what happened in this video. As we watch this video, feel free to comment on what you want us to note specifically.

II. Guiding questions

2. What roles do you think you play as a pharmacist in the pharmacy?

3. We talked about (the activities in the recordings) earlier. Which roles would you assign the different activities to?

4. Tell me about your thought process. When there are conflicting priorities in your work, how do you decide what needs to be done first?

   If an example is needed and there is none in the videos supplied:

   For example, if there are ten prescriptions to check plus a new medication to explain, two flu vaccinations to give, a toddler with yellow crusty eyes, the wholesaler invoice is due and it's the first day for a new intern who has never worked in a pharmacy before.

5. I've got your answers from the online survey about different pharmacist descriptions. Could you tell me more about (descriptions of interest)?

6. One of our theories is that pharmacists' own definitions of their role could be a large factor in the way they handle conflicting work. What do you think?

7. If you had to choose three words to describe yourself as a person, what would they be?

   a. Why did you choose/not choose to describe yourself as a pharmacist?

References

1. Bradley H. Participatory action research in pharmacy practice. In: *Pharmacy Practice Research Methods.* Springer; 2015:91–105.
2. Baum F. Participatory action research. *J Epidemiol Community Health.* 2006;60:854–857.
3. Elliott RA, Lee CY, Beanland C, et al. Development of a clinical pharmacy model within an Australian home nursing service using co-creation and participatory action research: the visiting pharmacist (ViP) study. *BMJ Open.* 2017;7, e018722.
4. Dineen-Griffin S, Benrimoj SI, Williams KA, Garcia-Cardenas V. Co-design and feasibility of a pharmacist-led minor ailment service. *BMC Health Serv Res.* 2021;21:80.
5. Nørgaard LS, Sørensen EW. Action research methodology in clinical pharmacy: how to involve and change. *Int J Clin Pharmacol.* 2016;38:739–745.
6. van Buul LW, Sikkens JJ, van Agtmael MA, Kramer MH, van der Steen JT, Hertogh CM. Participatory action research in antimicrobial stewardship: a novel approach to improving antimicrobial prescribing in hospitals and long-term care facilities. *J Antimicrob Chemother.* 2014;69:1734–1741.
7. Loewenson R, Flores W, Shukla A, et al. Raising the profile of participatory action research at the 2010 global symposium on health systems research. *MEDICC Rev.* 2011;13:35–38.
8. Sørensen EW, Haugbølle LS. Using an action research process in pharmacy practice research—a cooperative project between university and internship pharmacies. *Res Social Adm Pharm.* 2008;4:384–401.
9. Iedema R, Carroll K, Collier A, Hor S, Mesman J, Wyer M. *Video-Reflexive Ethnography in Health Research and Healthcare Improvement: Theory and Application.* Florida, USA: CRC Press, Taylor & Francis Group, LLC; 2019.
10. Mannay D. *Visual, Narrative and Creative Research Methods: Application, Reflection and Ethics*; 2015.
11. Iedema R, Mesman J, Carroll K. *Visualising Health Care Practice Improvement: Innovation from Within*; 2013.
12. Fragkos KC. Reflective practice in healthcare education: an umbrella review. *Educ Sci.* 2016;6:27.
13. Austin Z, Marini A, Desroches B. Use of a learning portfolio for continuous professional development: a study of pharmacists in Ontario (Canada). *Pharm Educ.* 2005;5.
14. Micallef R, Kayyali R. A systematic review of models used and preferences for continuing education and continuing professional development of pharmacists. *Pharmacy.* 2019;7:154.
15. McHugh SK, Lawton R, Hara JK, Sheard L. Does team reflexivity impact teamwork and communication in interprofessional hospital-based healthcare teams? A systematic review and narrative synthesis. *BMJ Qual Saf.* 2020;29:672.
16. Collier A, Wyer M. Researching reflexively with patients and families: two studies using video-reflexive Ethnography to collaborate with patients and families in patient safety research. *Qual Health Res.* 2015;26:979–993.
17. Norden-Hagg A, Sexton JB, Kalvemark-Sporrong S, Ring L, Kettis-Lindblad A. Assessing safety culture in pharmacies: the psychometric validation of the safety attitudes questionnaire (SAQ) in a national sample of community pharmacies in Sweden. *BMC Clin Pharmacol.* 2010;10:8.
18. Hadi MA, José CS. Ensuring rigour and trustworthiness of qualitative research in clinical pharmacy. *Int J Clin Pharmacol.* 2016;38:641–646.
19. Winit-Watjana W. Research philosophy in pharmacy practice: necessity and relevance. *Int J Pharm Pract.* 2016;24:428–436.
20. Denzin NK, Lincoln YS. *The SAGE Handbook of Qualitative Research.* Thousand Oaks: Sage; 2011.
21. Yong FR. Instruments measuring community pharmacist role stress and strain measures: a systematic review. *Res Social Adm Pharm.* 2020.

22. Yong FR, Garcia-Cardenas V, Williams KA, Benrimoj SI. Factors affecting community pharmacist work: a scoping review and thematic synthesis using role theory. *Res Social Adm Pharm*. 2020;16:123–141.

23. Rieck A, Pettigrew S. How physician and community pharmacist perceptions of the community pharmacist role in Australian primary care influence the quality of collaborative chronic disease management. *Qual Prim Care*. 2013;21:105–111.

24. Schommer JC, Gaither CA. A segmentation analysis for pharmacists' and patients' views of pharmacists' roles. *Res Social Adm Pharm*. 2014;10:508–528.

25. van Eikenhorst L, Salema NE, Anderson C. A systematic review in select countries of the role of the pharmacist in consultations and sales of non-prescription medicines in community pharmacy. *Res Social Adm Pharm*. 2017;13:17–38.

26. Gidman W, Cowley J. A qualitative exploration of opinions on the community pharmacists' role amongst the general public in Scotland. *Int J Pharm Pract*. 2013;21:288–296.

27. Khan MU, Khan AN, Ahmed FR, et al. Patients' opinion of pharmacists and their roles in health care system in Pakistan. *J Young Pharm*. 2013;5:90–94.

28. Kuipers E, Wensing M, De Smet PAGM, Teichert M. Barriers and facilitators for community pharmacists' participation in pharmacy practice research: a survey. *Int J Pharm Pract*. 2019;27:399–402.

29. Awaisu A, Alsalimy N. Pharmacists' involvement in and attitudes toward pharmacy practice research: a systematic review of the literature. *Res Social Adm Pharm*. 2015;11:725–748.

30. Saini B, Brillant M, Filipovska J, et al. In: Saini B, ed. *Recruitment and Retention of Community Pharmacists in Pharmacy Practice Research*. Sydney, Australia: Faculty of Pharmacy, University of Sydney; 2005.

31. Bridges D. 'Nothing about us without us': The ethics of outsider research. In: *Philosophy in Educational Research*. Cham: Springer; 2017:341–361.

32. Carroll K, Iedema R, Kerridge R. Reshaping ICU Ward round practices using video-reflexive Ethnography. *Qual Health Res*. 2008;18:380–390.

33. Iedema R, Hor S, Wyer M, et al. An innovative approach to strengthening health professionals' infection control and limiting hospital-acquired infection: video-reflexive ethnography. *BMJ Innovations*. 2015;1:1–6.

34. Gilbert GL, Hor S, Wyer M, Sadsad R, Badcock C-A, Iedema R. Sustained fall in inpatient MRSA prevalence after a video-reflexive ethnography project; an observational study. *Infect DisHealth*. 2020;25:140–150.

35. Hung L, Phinney A, Chaudhury H, Rodney P. Using video-reflexive ethnography to engage hospital staff to improve dementia care. *Glob Qual Nurs Res*. 2018;5:1–10.

36. Mcleod HM. *Respect and Shared Decision Making in the Clinical Encounter, a Video-Reflexive Ethnography*. Dissertation, Minnesota, USA: Health Services Research, Policy and Administration, University of Minnesota; 2017.

37. Carroll K, Mesman J. Multiple researcher roles in video-reflexive ethnography. *Qual Health Res*. 2018;28:1145–1156.

38. Mesman J. *Boundary-Spanning Engagements on a Neonatal Ward: a Collaborative Entanglement Between Clinicians and Researchers*. Ashgate Publishing Ltd; 2015:171–194.

39. Pedersen KZ, Mesman J. A transactional approach to patient safety: understanding safe care as a collaborative accomplishment. *J Interprof Care*. 2021;1–11.

40. Mesman J. The origins of prognostic differences: a topography of experience and expectation in a neonatal intensive care unit. *Qual Sociol*. 2005;28:49–66.

41. Coeckelbergh M, Mesman J. With Hope and imagination: imaginative moral decision-making in neonatal intensive care units. *Ethical Theory Moral Pract*. 2007;10:3–21.

42. Iedema R, Merrick E. *HELiCS as a Tool for Ongoing Observation, Monitoring and Evaluation of Clinical Handover—Public Report on Pilot Study*. Sydney Centre for Health Communications UTS; 2009.

43. Lee YC, Wu HH, Hsieh WL, Weng SJ, Hsieh LP, Huang CH. Applying importance-performance analysis to patient safety culture. *Int J Health Care Qual Assur*. 2015;28:826–840.

44. Nordén-Hägg A, Kälvemark-Sporrong S, Lindblad AK. Exploring the relationship between safety culture and reported dispensing errors in a large sample of Swedish community pharmacies. *BMC Pharmacol Toxicol*. 2012;13.

45. Johnson SJ, O'Connor EM, Jacobs S, Hassell K, Ashcroft DM. The relationships among work stress, strain and self-reported errors in UK community pharmacy. *Res Social Adm Pharm*. 2014;10:885–895.

46. Neuwirth EB, Bellows J, Jackson AH, Price PM. How Kaiser Permanente uses video Ethnography of patients for quality improvement, such as in shaping better care transitions. *Health Aff*. 2012;31:1244–1250.

47. Swinglehurst D, Fudge N. Addressing the polypharmacy challenge in older people with multimorbidity (APOLLO-MM): study protocol for an in-depth ethnographic case study in primary care. *BMJ Open*. 2019;9, e031601.

48. Jin HK, Choi JH, Kang JE, Rhie SJ. The effect of communication skills training on patient-pharmacist communication in pharmacy education: a meta-analysis. *Adv Health Sci Educ*. 2018;23:633–652.

49. Iedema R. Creating safety by strengthening clinicians' capacity for reflexivity. *BMJ Qual Saf*. 2011;20:i83–i86.

50. Dopson S, Locock L, Gabbay J, Ferlie E, Fitzgerald L. Evidence-based medicine and the implementation gap. *Health*. 2003;7:311–330.

51. Lau R, Stevenson F, Ong BN, et al. Achieving change in primary care—causes of the evidence to practice gap: systematic reviews of reviews. *Implement Sci*. 2016;11:40.

52. Elbeddini A, Prabaharan T, Almasalkhi S, Tran C. Pharmacists and COVID-19. *J Pharm Policy Practice*. 2020;13.

53. Johnston K, O'Reilly CL, Cooper G, Mitchell I. The burden of COVID-19 on pharmacists. *J Am Pharm Assoc*. 2021;61:e61–e64.

54. Medina MS, Melchert RB, Stowe CD. Fulfilling the tripartite Mission during a pandemic. *Am J Pharm Educ*. 2020;84:ajpe8156.

55. Sousa Pinto G, Hung M, Okoya F, Uzman N. FIP's response to the COVID-19 pandemic: global pharmacy rises to the challenge. *Res Social Adm Pharm*. 2021;17:1929–1933.

56. Bond CM, Blenkinsopp A, Inch J, Celino G, Gray NJ. The effect of the new community pharmacy contract on the community pharmacy workforce. In: *Medicines & People: Turning Knowledge into Know-How.* The Pharmacy Practice Research Trust; 2008.

57. Gidman W. Increasing community pharmacy workloads in England: causes and consequences. *Int J Clin Pharmacol.* 2011;33:512–520.

58. Gidman WK, Hassell K, Day J, Payne K. The impact of increasing workloads and role expansion on female community pharmacists in the United Kingdom. *Res Social Adm Pharm.* 2007;3:285–302.

59. Luetsch K. Attitudes and attributes of pharmacists in relation to practice change—a scoping review and discussion. *Res Social Adm Pharm.* 2017;13:440–455.e411.

60. Yong F, Hor S, Bajorek B. Considerations of Australian community pharmacists in the provision and implementation of cognitive pharmacy services: a qualitative study. *BMC Health Serv Res.* 2021;21:906.

61. Yong F, Hor S, Bajorek B. *Australian Community Pharmacy Service Provision Factors, Stresses and Strains: A Qualitative Study.* unpublished; 2021.

62. Hardy ME, Conway ME. *Role Theory: Perspectives for Health Professionals.* Appleton & Lange; 1988.

63. Goffman E. *The Presentation of Self in Everyday Life.* London: Penguin; 1959.

64. Emmerton LM, Smith L, Lemay KS, et al. Experiences of community pharmacists involved in the delivery of a specialist asthma service in Australia. *BMC Health Serv Res.* 2012;12:164.

65. Roberts AS, Benrimoj SI, Chen TF, Williams KA, Hopp TR, Aslani P. Understanding practice change in community pharmacy: a qualitative study in Australia. *Res Social Adm Pharm.* 2005;1:546–564.

66. Koster ES, Philbert D, Bouvy ML. Impact of the COVID-19 epidemic on the provision of pharmaceutical care in community pharmacies. *Res Social Adm Pharm.* 2021;17:2002–2004.

67. Johnston K, O'Reilly CL, Scholz B, Georgousopoulou EN, Mitchell I. Burnout and the challenges facing pharmacists during COVID-19: results of a national survey. *Int J Clin Pharmacol.* 2021.

68. Harris PA, Taylor R, Minor BL, et al. The REDCap consortium: building an international community of software platform partners. *J Biomed Inform.* 2019;95, 103208.

69. Harris PA, Taylor R, Thielke R, Payne J, Gonzalez N, Conde JG. Research electronic data capture (REDCap)—a metadata-driven methodology and workflow process for providing translational research informatics support. *J Biomed Inform.* 2009;42:377–381.

70. Family HE, Weiss M, Sutton J. The effects of mental workload on community pharmacists' ability to detect dispensing errors. *Pharm Res UK.* 2013;1–121.

71. Lea VM, Corlett SA, Rodgers RM. Describing interruptions, multi-tasking and task-switching in community pharmacy: a qualitative study in England. *Int J Clin Pharmacol.* 2015;37:1086–1094.

72. Chui MA, Look KA, Mott DA. The association of subjective workload dimensions on quality of care and pharmacist quality of work life. *Res Social Adm Pharm.* 2014;10:328–340.

73. Gaither CA, Kahaleh AA, Doucette WR, Mott DA, Pederson CA, Schommer JC. A modified model of pharmacists' job stress: the role of organizational, extra-role, and individual factors on work-related outcomes. *Res Social Adm Pharm.* 2008;4:231–243.

74. Chui MA, Mott DA. Community pharmacists' subjective workload and perceived task performance: a human factors approach. *J Am Pharm Assoc.* 2012;52:e153–e160.

75. Schommer JC, Pedersen CA, Doucette WR, Gaither CA, Mott DA. Community pharmacists' work activities in the United States during 2000. *J Am Pharm Assoc (Wash).* 1996;2002(42):399–406.

76. Benrimoj SI, Frommer MS. Community pharmacy in Australia. *Aust Health Rev.* 2004;28:238–246.

77. Grasha AF, Schell K. Psychosocial factors, workload, and human error in a simulated pharmacy dispensing task. *Percept Mot Skills.* 2001;92:53–71.

78. Hassell K, Seston EM, Schafheutle EI, Wagner A, Eden M. Workload in community pharmacies in the UK and its impact on patient safety and pharmacists' well-being: a review of the evidence. *Health Soc Care Community.* 2011;19:561–575.

79. Chui MA, Mott DA, Maxwell L. A qualitative assessment of a community pharmacy cognitive pharmaceutical services program, using a work system approach. *Res Social Adm Pharm.* 2012;8:206–216.

80. Murad MS, Spiers JA, Guirguis LM. Expressing and negotiating face in community pharmacist-patient interactions. *Res Social Adm Pharm.* 2017;13:1110–1126.

81. Smith ME. *Fostering Psychological Safety through Facework: The Importance of the Effective Delivery of Performance Feedback.* The University of Texas at Austin; 2006.

82. Whiting R, Symon G, Roby H, Chamakiotis P. Who's behind the Lens? *Organ Res Methods.* 2018;21:316–340.

83. Leung DY, Chung BPM. Content analysis: Using critical realism to extend its utility. In: Liamputtong P, ed. *Handbook of Research Methods in Health Social Sciences.* Singapore: Springer Singapore; 2019:827–841.

84. Vasileiou K, Barnett J, Thorpe S, Young T. Characterising and justifying sample size sufficiency in interview-based studies: systematic analysis of qualitative health research over a 15-year period. *BMC Med Res Methodol.* 2018;18.

85. Suri H. Purposeful sampling in qualitative research synthesis. *Qual Res J.* 2011;11:63–75.

86. Pink S. *Doing Visual Ethnography.* 2nd ed. London: SAGE Publications, Ltd; 2007.

87. Iedema R. Video-reflexive ethnography as potentiation technology: what about investigative quality? *Qual Res Psychol.* 2021;18:387–405.

88. Duckett K. Community, autonomy and bespoke services: independent community pharmacy practice in hyperdiverse, London communities. *Res Social Adm Pharm.* 2015;11:531–544.

89. Luff P, Heath C. Some 'technical challenges' of video analysis: social actions, objects, material realities and the problems of perspective. *Qual Res.* 2012;12:255–279.

90. Latour B. Why has critique run out of steam? From matters of fact to matters of concern. *Crit Inq.* 2004;30:225–248.

91. Zhang Y, Hu G, Zhang L, Mayo R, Chen L. A novel testing model for opportunistic screening of pre-diabetes and diabetes among U.S. adults. *PLoS One.* 2015;10, e0120382.

Chapter 25

Reflexivity practice during ethnographic informed fieldwork

Sadaf Faisal[a] and Colleen McMillan[b]

[a]University of Waterloo School of Pharmacy, Kitchener, ON, Canada, [b]School of Social Work, Renison University College, University of Waterloo, Waterloo, ON, Canada

Objectives

- Define reflexivity and how it relates to the role of a pharmacist when conducting research.
- Understand the complexities related to the role of pharmacist-researcher.
- Explain how the concepts of positionality and intersectionality impact the pharmacist researcher during data collection.

Introduction

Ethnography is a qualitative research method originating from social anthropology and involves "learning about people from people" by immersing oneself into another's natural environment or culture.[1,2] The main focus of ethnography is to gain insight into social relations and the meanings related to the rituals, habits, and behavior of people through mindful observation. Various data collection methods can be utilized in ethnographic studies, such as, participant observations, field notes, in-depth interviews, and focus groups.[2] Additionally, an in-depth analysis is also required to interpret people's actions and behaviors in a substantial manner.[1] The main emphasis of an ethnographic study is to understand and learn about a culture or community through the lived experiences of the people by observing them, before drawing conclusions about their attitudes and behaviors.[2] Culture is a "set of guidelines which individuals inherit as members of a particular society."[3] The cultural aspects of the research in ethnography can be associated with things such as language, ethnicity, cuisine, customs.[4]

Numerous ethnographic studies have been conducted in nursing and healthcare.[4] The ethnographic research method was first utilized by Becker et al. in 1961 when he studied the lived experience of students in medical school in "*Boys in White*" by utilizing participant observations and interviews to collect data during their study.[5] After that numerous researchers used ethnography to understand the health care culture using various participant groups and study settings. For example, Goffman studied "the social world of the hospital inmate" in his study called "*Asylums*" based on year-long fieldwork at a psychiatric hospital with a nonspecified methodology.[6] Similarly, Glaser and Strauss conducted extensive fieldwork involving a combination of observations and interviews at six hospitals in their study titled "*Awareness of Dying.*"[7] During this study, researchers observed the dying process by observing patients and healthcare providers and reported how different stakeholders have different views and attitudes toward the dying process, which can impact patients' end-of-life care experiences.

There are three key principles of ethnographic research particularly related to the healthcare field: (1) investigating culture, (2) nature of knowledge, and (3) the role of the researcher.[4] When investigating a culture in the healthcare field, the culture-based approach can involve a particular disease condition such as heart disease, diabetes, and/or cancer, or a specific healthcare related behavior as a common characteristic of a group of people.[2,3] The second key principle of healthcare-related research is the nature of knowledge which demonstrates that "there is not one single objective truth or reality," the knowledge is co-created during the interactions, and can be interpreted in various ways depending on the situational context.[4] The role of the researcher is the third key principle and highlights that in ethnographic fieldwork, a researcher "does not arrive empty minded in the field" and therefore can never investigate a culture without incorporating their own knowledge of the world.[4] These influences can impact several aspects of research, ranging from the selection of

Contemporary Research Methods in Pharmacy and Health Services. https://doi.org/10.1016/B978-0-323-91888-6.00030-2

methodological approach to writing up the study findings for publication.[8] In addition to the researcher's personal beliefs, experiences, and knowledge that can have a deep impact on the research, their social location in the society and the socio-cultural circumstances of the study can also deeply influence the research.[9] By using the ethnographic approach, one can not only understand the lived experiences of patients suffering from particular illnesses, but can also illustrate and discover the complexities, attitudes, and behaviors of that shared culture and its impact on patients' illness in a detailed and thorough manner.[8] Since the ethnographic research method involves "hands-on, on the scene learning" this approach requires a high degree of self-awareness and self-reflection on the part of the researcher. Therefore, an important aspect of ethnographic research is reflexivity: a process of self-reference or self-explanation that involves examining one's personal reactions and the impact of the social location to situations that occur while working in the field.[10]

The concept of reflexivity is defined as "the process of examining oneself as a researcher and the research relationship."[11] It involves examining one's "conceptual baggage," meaning one's assumptions, bias, and beliefs around how knowledge is constructed and who is considered a knowledge holder. While a guiding principle of ethnographic research is to be intentional about practicing reflexivity, the complexity of human relationships eclipses even the most experienced interviewer leading to blind spots, which is not a bad thing. One of the joys of ethnography is giving yourself permission to experience emotions that seep unnoticed into the research/participant relationship. This is especially true when working toward establishing trust, a prerequisite for entry into recessed content held by the person you are interviewing. By incorporating the practice of reflexivity in ethnography, the researcher can recognize, address, and describe these possible influences on their findings. This acknowledgment of the researcher's influence using reflexivity practices is particularly important for ethnographic studies due to the close relationship fostered between the researcher and the culture they are studying.[9] The reciprocal nature of ethnography means that you may become aware of the information stored within yourself, which subconsciously informs how you conduct interviews as part of your data collection. Allowing such information to freely surface allows a researcher to become more attuned as a research instrument.[12] Reflecting upon why such emotions or feelings are surfacing is critical to developing authenticity and trust within the participant relationship.

Importance and challenges with rapport building

The negotiation of power

When doing qualitative interviewing one must quickly create an environment likely to building rapport in a very short period of time with a stranger, while retrieving personal information related to a research topic. A study by Willis and Todorov found that first impressions of an unfamiliar individual are composed within seconds, suggesting that the researcher has little control over the subconscious processes of the participant.[13] However, there are many areas the researcher can control toward fostering a positive, albeit quick, rapport. One such area is identifying the presence of power within the relationship between the researcher and participant, also referred to as the "researcher and the researched."[14] Perceptions of power held by the participant toward the researcher may be present and become entwined during the time rapport is trying to be established. While omnipresent, this dynamic may be amplified if the researcher is perceived as holding higher social status, more knowledge or other characteristics that make them appear as more privileged. Perceptions of power attached to the researcher are referred to as "expert power" and more common to certain professions including those within the scientific paradigm such as pharmacy.[15] The task of the researcher is to identify this dynamic in the moment and implement a strategy in which to flatten the power hierarchy as soon as possible. Failure to do so by the researcher will rupture rapport and result in an interview marked by posturing in an attempt to negotiate the power imbalance. Such posturing is often experienced as very nuanced as demonstrated by the following case.

Case example

The participant was happy to see the researchers. When we [researchers] walked into his [participant] apartment, he was drinking coffee out of a mug with a logo of a prestigious Ivy League school so I [one of the researchers] asked him where he went to school. He told me he received it as a gift from one of his grandchildren. He told us that he is a retired principal and that's how he met his wife who used to be a teacher in his school. This participant mentioned how other residents at the retirement home think of him as "some kind of tech wizard" as he uses Siri and is very familiar with iPhone etc. He told us that he bought an Apple computer MacBook this morning and attended the session at the Apple store about how to set up the computer. He was very interested in my [one of the researchers]'s life and asked a lot of questions about my life back home including education and journey as an immigrant. He also emphasized that two of his grandsons were doing their PhD [name of same university as the mug] and that he is familiar with the programme. He asked me [researcher] if she will invite him for her graduation and then added he knew only a few people could be invited.

Researcher memo note

As a researcher, I felt a bit surprised and awkward as he was very interested in my life story rather than the research project that he was participating in. His interest was more about why I am doing a PhD if I am a pharmacist, what would I do after my PhD, how this would change my social location in life. I entered a space of mixed and somewhat contradictory feelings. On one hand, he told me that he understood how much hard work is required to complete this degree after watching his grandchildren. Hearing that encouragement from someone made me feel good about my PhD journey right now. On the other hand, I asked myself why he chose to drink his coffee in this particular mug this morning? Why is it important for me to know where his grandchildren are attending school or that he just purchased an expensive laptop? Did the sharing of how others perceive him as a "tech wizard" meant to create a bond with me, intimidate me, or impress me? Were these attempts a way to build rapport or establish a "level playing ground?" I was holding all of these thoughts before the interview even started. The one feeling that clearly resonated was that of shifting power, whether that was my "conceptual baggage" or the participant's.

Negotiations of power are always present in the researcher-participant relationship, with varying degrees of visibility. The artifacts of power in this case, made explicit in the first few minutes of engagement, had to be identified, labeled, and navigated in the moment to allow the interview to continue in a manner that was comfortable and respectful to the participant. To maintain research professionalism, the researcher had to adopt a stance that would allow space for the participant to establish expertise and commonality of knowledge, his previous career in education, being university educated and skill level with technology, prior to moving forward with the interview.

Inner dialog

This case also highlights what is referred to as the unspoken inner or self-dialog, a form of reflexivity simultaneously occurring while attempting to build rapport with the participant.[14] Inner dialog or self-talk is described as;

The active listening intrinsic to in-depth interviewing "requires the researcher to look beyond the surface of the conversation for implicit analytic questions, alternative frames, and the content of categories created and used by the informant."[16] That is, "attention to meaning is far more complex than simply asking open-ended questions and allowing participants to speak extemporaneously. It requires a heightened sense of self-awareness about the researcher's personal understandings, beliefs, prejudices, and world view. Researchers bring to the research encounter considerable social, historical, and cultural baggage."[17]

The ability of the researcher to process *in the moment* content, manage interpersonal dynamics, practice presence, and formulate a plan on how to proceed with the interview is a complex process and can be experienced as emotionally draining. The importance of writing field notes after these types of encounters is paramount in order to identify and unpack the different discourses that occurred during the interview. Field notes also support the researcher to dissect the components of the exchange gaining valuable insights into their contributions.[18]

Case example

During the second home visit, the researcher took a few photographs of the participant's hands. On the next visit, when the researcher showed the participant those photographs, the first thing that she [participant] said was "Oh I never noticed that my hands look so old." She kept starring at those photographs and her hands back and forth for at least 5 minutes.

Field note written post interaction

This happened before too. The last time I was at one of other participants home and I showed her the photographs of her hands, the first thing she uttered from her mouth was "oh I am old… these are not my hands… are they really???" She [participant] was 81 years old, and I was thinking at that moment "if not like this how should your hands look like". But I kept myself quiet. I had the same reaction from another female participant today, who is in her late 80's. I kept thinking in my head while looking at her that if it would be a male participant, would I be getting the same response? Or is it just we females think about our aging process by comparing it with our physical beauty. I am not sure. Maybe I should pay attention to this specific scenario when I visit male participants and see how they react when they see their hand photographs.

Inner or self-dialog can present as both a possibility and limitation to the pharmacist-researcher. Of the three types of reflexivity identified by Rainford, inner self-dialog belongs to the category of autonomous reflexivity, defined as "a process that takes place within [our] own heads, relying solely on [our] own past experiences and knowledge to make sense of current internal conversations."[19] In other words, autonomous reflexivity is conversation a researcher has internally, while conducting an interview, that serves to make sense or answer questions in response to what the participant is saying. Such internal conversations can be very effective toward tailoring questions or probes to capture deeper material from the participant. For example, if a patient states, "I really dislike taking medication because of what happened with my pharmacist a couple of years ago," the researcher would likely engage in an internal dialog around such items as; "what happened, did a mistake occur, was the patient harmed, who was the pharmacist, do I know them, if I do know them what should I say, what does this mean for my study?" Such questions can be used to develop an interview probe that may reveal deeper emotions or experiences related to the research question and in this way be helpful. However, a lack of self-awareness or interviewing inexperience can just as easy flood the researcher with too much information resulting in internal noise with the researcher appearing distracted or overwhelmed. One way to avoid the latter is to practice a technique referred to as "holding and releasing."[12] This technique allows the researcher to decide what information is needed, hence holding, and what information needs to be released or externalized, allowing the researcher to be emotionally present and available to the participant.

Navigating professional versus personal boundaries

Boundaries are the framework within which the research-based relationship occurs and refers to the line between the private and personal life of the pharmacist and participant. Boundaries are a foundational concept in the Code of Ethics reflected in The Regulated Health Professions Act.[20] Supported by this legislation it could be assumed that, except for behaviors of a sexual nature or obvious conflicts of interest, the issue of boundaries when doing research is clear and simply requires following a set of guiding practice principles augmented by the legislation. This is not the case. In practice-informed research, boundaries are experienced at times as conflictual, porous, and fluctuating and in fact pose more commonly than anticipated. Pharmacists assume a dual set of responsibilities when they embark upon research, that unless an intentional effort is made to be mindful to be reflexive, research activities in the field can touch upon two important ethical concepts, nonmaleficence, and beneficence. The principle of nonmaleficence requires "an intention to avoid needless harm or injury that can arise through acts of commission or omission."[20] The beneficence principle refers to "actions that promote the well-being of others," in this case, the patient.[20] Although these two principles are more commonly seen in practice literature, they also transfer over to research, specifically in qualitative research where the establishment of a relationship based upon trust is critical. The following memo note demonstrates how close the relationship between personal and professional boundaries can become during fieldwork.

Field note

During the home visit, we [researchers] found a few expired medications in her [participant] plastic containers. As a pharmacist, ethically it is my [one of the researchers] obligation to make sure that safe use of medications is being practiced at the patient's home. But I did not want to say it out loud as I was present in her home as a researcher and I did not want to make her feel that there is some safety concern. I politely advised her to take her expired meds to the pharmacy so they can dispose them off for her. Participant also inquired about one of the OTC products she was using, she wanted to know if something better is available for her to purchase. At that point, I struggled a bit as to how to respond. I was there as a researcher not as a pharmacist, but she was also aware that I am a practicing pharmacist and she wanted an answer from me. I also did not want to advise her on a product as I felt I may be over-stepping if she has a pharmacist who she sees regularly.

Pharmacists who engage in ethnographic research, and particularly involving sensitive topics, need to be able to conduct ongoing assessments of the impact of the research on both the participants and themselves. For example, data collection gained through one-to-one interviews or focus groups requires the researcher to deliberately create a safe, affective environment for the participants to share their story or narrative, which often includes intimate details. While accessing this personal information is considered to be a privilege within the context of qualitative interviewing, it can pose a unique challenge to pharmacists who have been trained in the scientific paradigm, which reifies objectivity or at the very least, neutrality. Should the pharmacist-researcher experience any degree of dissonance between earlier education training and ethnographic informed interviewing, however nuanced this tension may be, the participant will notice and the premise of trust within the research relationship is jeopardized. Campbell refers to this task as "researching the researcher, a much-needed new [and critical] area of investigation" (p. 9).[21] While qualitative researchers have historically been acquainted with this benchmark of interviewing trustworthiness, researchers from the sciences including pharmacists, are gaining a new appreciation toward the subjectivity of the research process and for methodological approaches such as ethnography. Part of the reason for this new appreciation relates to the shift occurring within health research, from the recognition that relying only on quantitative measures loses valuable data due to the standardization of the data collection tools. Stories of lived experiences related to health issues by participants have attained greater significance from funding sources and policymakers.[22] Such stories, widely considered to be rich sources of understanding a health-related condition or topic, are lost when only quantitative measures are used and valuable information fails to reach clinical decision-making processes, potentially impacting patient care. Gaining confidence in shifting from a positivist (quantitative) to a postpositivist (qualitative) takes time and practice, specifically when adopting in-depth interviewing where professional boundaries become blurred in the quest to establish trust and authenticity.

Fluidity of being an outsider and insider

Researchers are considered to be an outsider if they are not the member of a certain culture, yet they engage in observing and describing that culture or the phenomenon under investigation.[1,4] Alternatively, researchers who are members of the community or culture being studied are considered insiders.[23] Moreover, the position of a researcher as an outsider or insider also depends on how much prior knowledge the researcher has about the culture they are studying instead of how they are situated in the community.[24,25]

Both approaches offer a rich and detailed collection of data and require the researcher to reflect on their own perspective and beliefs in order to provide legitimacy to their findings. This outsider/insider identity can be associated with the researcher's age, gender, profession or race. Participants may consider a researcher as an insider if they belong to the same gender, race, or age group. Similarly, if the researcher has a professional background similar to their area of research, they may be considered as an insider to some extent. The three key advantages of being an insider researcher identified by Bonner and Tolhurst are a deeper understanding of the culture or group of people, quick rapport building, and ability to immerse in the culture without any alteration.[26] These attributes help a researcher to identify and apply the best ways to approach the participants and create a good working environment more quickly. However, along with these advantages, being an insider can also cause some issues related to loss of objectivity due to familiarity, gain access to sensitive information creating ethical issues or biases due to previous knowledge.[27,28]

Unluer discussed his experiences as to how being an insider not only provided him access to data but also provided him the opportunity to gather detailed and trustworthy data.[29] Since his participants knew him, they never refused to participate in the study, showed him respect and shared their views in a detailed manner. On the contrary, he may have overlooked some of the routine behaviors or made assumptions without seeking any clarification. Berger shared her reasoning for considering herself as an insider with her immigrant participants due to the familiarity of challenges she faced as an immigrant. Her gender as a woman also helped her recruit women participants. Moreover, her awareness of their language and sensitivity to ask questions allowed her to gather the information that may have been missed by a nonimmigrant male researcher.[30]

A researcher usually chooses their area of research based on their personal experiences or professional experiences, which automatically grants them the position of an outsider due to their previous knowledge even before they enter into the fieldwork. They may not belong to the same age, gender, or race as the participant that they are studying, and this may make them an "outsider." Practicing pharmacists may face challenges associated with the dichotomy of being an insider and outsider depending on their area of practice and research interest while conducting ethnographic informed fieldwork. For example, if a pharmacist is practicing in a setting where most of their patients belong to the geriatric population and they decided to pursue research related to medication related issues in older adults, they may consider themselves as an "insider" of the group, as they would be already aware of a lot of medication-related challenges that this particular patient population is facing. Similarly, if a person is involved in the care of an older adult at their personal level, they would also be considered an "insider" due to their familiarity with the norms and social situations associated with the care of an older adult. This familiarity can help researchers' better access to the participants and also help them build rapport quickly. It has been argued that you must be an insider to understand the perspective of the participants or to gain their trust so they can share their experiences with great details. However, at the same time, if you are a part of that group, you may miss some important details as they will become nonsignificant for you as compared to someone who is seeing the participant's world from an outsider's eyes. If a pharmacist-researcher is already familiar with their participants due to their prior interaction, it makes the participants comfortable to share intimate details which they may not share with the researchers that they are not acquainted with. On the other hand, if the pharmacist does not belong to the culture based on their ethnicity, age group, or race, they may be considered as an "outsider." Pharmacist-researchers may assume the role of an insider-outsider while conducting ethnographic-informed research. However, this transition can be challenging and can impact the way information is being collected and knowledge is being generated. It is highly imperative to address the position of a pharmacist-researcher as an outsider-insider in healthcare-related fieldwork. The self-awareness of this fluidity between roles and its impact on the research process should be carefully considered. The practice of reflexivity can help a pharmacist-researcher to identify their position of being an outsider-insider and how that can impact their own assumptions in the field and can influence the data collection and interpretation of the results.

Positionality and intersectionality

Positionality is defined as the "position of the researcher in relation to social and political context of the study."[31] The social position of the researcher and the participant automatically introduces the concept of status and power into the interview, informing the ways the participant perceives the researcher or vice versa during their interactions.[32] Intersectionality is defined as "the study of the ways that race, gender, disability, sexuality, class, age, and other social categories are mutually shaped and interrelated."[33] While slightly different in definition, the two concepts share the similarity of understanding how different identities held by the researcher are performed and then perceived by the participant. Like the dynamic of power, the concepts of positionality and intersectionality are subtle yet present in some interviews, particularly so when cultural differences exist between the researcher and the participant.

Social position—Dual identities as pharmacist and researcher

Many pharmacist-researchers face the challenge of how to manage the dual identities of a pharmacist and a researcher when doing fieldwork. While this challenge is not new, it does acquire an additional layer of complexity when doing ethnographic research. Arber, who was a nurse by profession, reported her experience of managing the dual identities of a researcher and practitioner when she was conducting an ethnographic study in a hospice setting. She reported the process of choosing between the role of a researcher and nurse quite a challenge during her fieldwork.[34] Similar experiences were those of Hiller and Vears, two trained healthcare professionals who shared similar experiences and discussed how the researchers exhibited a dual role in the field and how the patient participants expected feedback regarding a clinical situation during study encounters, simply because of their awareness of the researchers' status as healthcare professionals.[35]

More specific to the pharmacy profession, researchers can encounter numerous situations where participants expect them to address a medication-related question, such as clinical advice about their treatment efficacy or managing side effects of their medications, due to the awareness of their professional role as a pharmacist. Pharmacists are one of the most trusted and accessible professionals in North America.[36,37] While this distinction is certainly valued, it can present as a challenge in some cases when doing fieldwork as participants see them as a pharmacist, rather than a researcher. As such, it is not unusual to be asked for advice about their medications-related issues. The dilemma of a pharmacist-researcher at that point is the struggle with how to respond in a way that protects the professional relationship while staying in a role as a researcher, as shown in the following example;

> She [the participant] seemed very proud to be in a research study and said that she was important and that these researchers were interested in learning more about her. There was an empty pill bottle on the container, the patient mentioned that she kept it over there to remind herself that she has to go to the pharmacy for a refill. While talking to the researchers, the patient inquired about one supplement she was not sure if she should take it or not.

At this juncture, the concept of positionality becomes less clear and has to be navigated carefully, especially when one is doing ethnographic research studying complex health behavior such as medication management.

The ability to establish participant trust while maintaining boundaries in the field when doing ethnographic work is critical and informs deep and genuine data collection. The need to reach stories that perhaps have not been shared before requires implicit respect, trust, and the ability to receive questions and hear experiences without judgment. The public position as a pharmacist can very well aid in a sort of *fiduciary trust* described as the trust that the person will act in others interest before their own,[38] perhaps assuming that since pharmacists already had their best interests as a healthcare professional, this would continue in their role as a researcher. This awareness can make participants more open and make them comfortable in granting entry to the researcher into their homes without condition.

Holding this trust, however, can also be experienced as tenuous. Participants may expect a certain level of advice giving, especially if the participant has known the researcher as a pharmacist in another context. In cases where a participant had a preexisting relationship with the pharmacist-researcher, while it can lessen the amount of time required to create an environment of trust, it can also comfortably default back to the preexisting relationship that was characterized by advice giving. To address this perplexity, pharmacist-researchers can make it clear to their participants that they are there as a researcher, not as a pharmacist and it would be best to speak with their pharmacist.

Intersectionality: Gender, age, culture, and race

A researcher's social position based on their gender or race can also influence their interaction with their participants. For example, Abdulrehman shared his experience of different approaches he had adopted with his male and female participants during fieldwork as being a male, his interaction with female participants was not something that was a norm for that culture.[39] Similarly, Purwaningrum and Shtaltovna explain the experience of two female researchers conducting research in Asia and how being females preclude them from certain interactions with their male participants.[40] While these domains of social location are influential when doing ethnographic research, it is the intersectionality, or the intersection of race, class, age, education, and gender that also shapes what occurs within an interview. The method of ethnography is highly compatible as interviews and fieldwork make explicit the complexities of individual identities and social dynamics.[41] An example will highlight how even preinterview conversation can contain multiple inferences to the researcher's race, education, gender, and culture, all sites of social location that have no relationship to the focus of the ethnographic study on medication adherence.

Case example

> She [participant] asked me [researcher] about my accent in a very polite way. She said, "I can hear an accent, so where are you from?". When I [researcher] told her [participant] my country of origin, she mentioned that she has some "very nice friends from there [country]." She then mentioned how her friends have done so well here [country name] and how I [researcher] will be fine here too. She continued her conversation about if I am already a pharmacist, why am I doing a PhD, is it because I will earn more money?

As illustrated, the questions posed to the pharmacist-researcher were external to the research question, but with the participant shifting the focus to the researcher's "inside world," the onus rested upon the researcher to manage at the moment to avoid a relational rupture in the interview, while concurrently processing how such questions impacted her.

Discussion

Reflexivity practice is a critical tool that can support a pharmacist-researcher to develop self-awareness about their own implicit assumptions, bias, beliefs, and attitudes during ethnographic informed fieldwork. Moreover, it can help identify various challenges related to dual identity and multiple social positions that a pharmacist-researcher may face during their study encounters. The social positions of a pharmacist can greatly assist or become impediments when accessing the inner world of participants during the trust building stage. Being aware of inner dialog, dual identities, the presence of power, and how different personal and professional identities intersect and inform the data collection represents reflexivity strategies but more importantly acknowledges the "self" as a research instrument.

A pharmacist-researcher should practice reflexivity throughout their fieldwork. Reflexivity enriches data collection by being mindful of the multiple complexities and junctures ethnographic research assumes. Adopting a reflexive stance offers deeper, more meaningful data and in the process urges the pharmacist researcher to extend themselves into fieldwork terrain that is not typically taught in academia, may be initially uncomfortable, but ultimately produces knowledge that is mutually grounded within the experiences of the participant and researcher.

Questions for further discussion

1. How do you navigate the power issues that emerge between the researcher and participant while preserving trust and rapport?
2. How much time do you allow for extra conversation during an interview that is unrelated to the research topic?
3. How do you leave a situation without breaking the rapport and feeling your participants rejected? Or when it is evident the participant is trying to extend your time?

Application exercise/scenario

You are a female pharmacist, from a migrant family, and born in an overseas country. Your ethnic background is a minority group in the country where you are living. You continue to practice as a pharmacist while being part of a research group which is conducting qualitative research related to medication usage. During the study project, you visit older adult participants in their homes, to conduct one-on-one semistructured interviews. You represent a different cultural group than most of the participants you visit, in terms of race and socio-demographic background. During one of the visits, a male participant queries you on the costs of his medications. He tells you that "it is well known" that pharmacists can provide samples of medicines. He strongly insinuates that you should provide him with free samples as a way of acknowledging his participation in your study. He adds "that as an immigrant you can understand how limited money can be, and the limited support from the government." He ends the conversation by asking if your parents still live in "your home country" and how drug reimbursement works there. You say nothing but feel overwhelmed with the myriad dynamics that just occurred in this brief transaction.

(a) How do you navigate this case where you concurrently recognize the importance of maintaining rapport while deciding to address, or not address, the assumptions and questions directed to you by the participant?

(b) What power issues are embedded in this case? Identify and describe how you would address?

References

1. Jones J, Smith J. Ethnography: challenges and opportunities. *Evid Based Nurs.* 2017;20(4):98–100. https://doi.org/10.1136/eb-2017-102786.
2. Goodson L, Vassar M. An overview of ethnography in healthcare and medical education research. *J Educ Eval Health Prof.* 2011;8:4. https://doi.org/10.3352/jeehp.2011.8.4.
3. Hodgson I. Ethnography and health care: focus on nursing. *Forum Qual Soc Res.* 2000;1(1):2–7. https://doi.org/10.17169/fqs-1.1.1117.
4. Draper J. Ethnography: principles, practice and potential. *Nurs Stand.* 2015;29(36):36–41. https://doi.org/10.7748/ns.29.36.36.e8937.
5. Becker H, Geer B, Hughes E. *Boys in White: Student Culture in Medical School.* Chicago, IL: Chicago University Press; 1961.
6. Gambino M. Erving Goffman's asylums and institutional culture in the mid-twentieth-century United States. *Harv Rev Psychiatry.* 2013;21(1):52–57.
7. Andrews T, Nathaniel A. Awareness of dying revisited. *J Nurs Care Qual.* 2009;24(3):189–193.
8. Bloor M. The ethnography of health and medicine. In: Atkinson P, Coffery A, Delamont S, Lofland J, Lofland L, eds. *Handbook of Ethnography.* London: Sage Publication; 2001:177–187.
9. Davies CA. *A Guide to Researching Selves and Others.* 2nd ed. London: Routledge; 2002.
10. Finlay L. Negotiating the swamp: the opportunity and challenge of reflexivity in research practice. *Qual Res.* 2002;2(2):209–230. http://pdfs.semanticscholar.org/fcda/f5e6e0fd76e54e5ce2f4f8686669f7067c14.pdf.
11. Hsiung P-C. Teaching reflexivity in qualitative interviewing. *Teach Sociol.* 2008;36(3):211–226. https://doi.org/10.1177/0092055X0803600302.
12. McMillan C. Navigating emotions while establishing trust and rapport in autoethnography. In: Kleinknecht S, van den Scott LK, Sanders C, eds. *The Craft of Qualitative Research.* Toronto, ON: Canadian Scholars; 2012.
13. Willis J, Todorov A. First impressions: making up your mind after a 100-Ms exposure to a face. *Psychol Sci.* 2006;17(7):592–598. https://doi.org/10.1111/j.1467-9280.2006.01750.x.
14. Arendell T. Reflections on the researcher-researched relationship: a woman interviewing men. *Qual Sociol.* 1997;20:341–368. https://doi.org/10.1023/A:1024727316052.
15. Jhangiani R, Hammond T. *Principles of Social Psychology.* 1st ed. BC Campus. Open Educational Resources, Hewlett Foundation: Victoria, BC; 2014. Retrieved from https://opentextbc.ca/socialpsychology/.
16. Sankar A, Gubrium J. Introduction. In: Gubrium J, Sankar A, eds. *Qualitative Methods in Aging Research.* Newbury Park, CA: Sage Publications; 1994:vii–xvii.
17. Harding S. *Feminism and Methodology.* Bloomington, IN: Indiana University Press; 1987.
18. Phillippi J, Lauderdale J. A guide to field notes for qualitative research: context and conversation. *Qual Health Res.* 2018;28(3):381–388. https://doi.org/10.1177/1049732317697102.
19. Jon R. Making internal conversations public: reflexivity of the connected doctoral researcher and its transmission beyond the walls of the academy. *J Appl Soc Theor.* 2016;1.1. Retrieved 23 Apr. 2021 [Online].
20. Ministry of Health. *The Regulated Health Professions Act;* 2021. https://www.health.gov.on.ca/en/pro/programs/hhrsd/about/rhpa.aspx. Accessed April 21.
21. Campbell R. *Emotionally Involved: The Impact of Researching Rape.* 1st ed. New York, NY: Routledge; 2002.
22. McMillan C, Lee J, Hillier LM, et al. The value in mental health screening for individuals with spinal cord injury: what patients tell us. *Arch Rehabil Res Clin Transl.* 2019;2:100032. https://doi.org/10.1016/j.arrct.2019.100032.
23. Chacko E. Positionality and praxis: fieldwork experiences in rural India. *Singap J Trop Geogr.* 2004;25(1):51–63.
24. Griffith AI. Insider/outsider: epistemological privilege and mothering work. *Hum Stud.* 1998;21:361–376.
25. Merton RK. Insiders and outsiders: a chapter in the sociology of knowledge. *Am J Sociol.* 1972;78:9–47.
26. Bonner A, Tolhurst G. Insider-outsider perspectives of participant observation. *Nurs Res.* 2002;9(4):7–19. https://doi.org/10.7748/nr2002.07.9.4.7.c6194. 12149898.
27. Delyser D. Do you really live here? Thoughts on insider research. *Geogr Rev.* 2001;9(1–2):441–453.
28. Hewitt-Taylor J. Inside knowledge: issues in insider research. *Nurs Stand.* 2002;16(46):33–35. https://doi.org/10.7748/ns.16.46.33.s5. 12219545.
29. Unluer S. Being an insider researcher while conducting case study research. *Qual Rep.* 2012;17:1–14. https://doi.org/10.46743/2160-3715/2012.1752.
30. Berger R. Now I see it, now I don't: researcher's position and reflexivity in qualitative research. *Qual Res.* 2015;15:219–234. https://doi.org/10.1177/1468794112468475.

31. Coghlan D, Brydon-Miller M. *The SAGE Encyclopedia of Action Research*. London, UK: Sage Publication; 2014. https://doi.org/10.4135/9781446294406.

32. Knight W, Deng Y. Neither here n/or there: culture, location, positionality, and art education. *Vis Arts Res*. 2016;42:105–111.

33. Rice C, Harrison E, Friedman M. Doing justice to intersectionality in research. *Cult Stud Crit Methodol*. 2009;19:409–420. https://doi.org/10.1177/1532708619829779.

34. Arber A. Reflexivity: a challenge for the researcher as practitioner? *J Res Nurs*. 2006;11(2):147–157. https://doi.org/10.1177/1744987106056956.

35. Hiller AJ, Vears DF. Reflexivity and the clinician-researcher: managing participant misconceptions. *Qual Res J*. 2016;16:13–25. https://doi.org/10.1108/QRJ-11-2014-0065.

36. Canadian Pharmacist Association; 2012. https://www.pharmacists.ca/news-events/news/more-and-more-canadians-say-pharmacists-play-essential-role-in-canada-s-health-care-system/. Accessed April 22, 2021.

37. Crossley K. Public. In: *Pharmacy Career Winters*. vol. 13; 2019. https://www.pharmacytimes.com/view/public-perceives-pharmacists-as-some-of-the-most-trusted-professionals. Accessed April 26, 2021.

38. Ontario College of Pharmacists. *Code of Ethics*; 2015. https://www.ocpinfo.com/library/council/download/CodeofEthics2015.pdf. Accessed 22 July 2020.

39. Abdulrehman MS. Reflections on native ethnography by a nurse researcher. *J Transcult Nurs*. 2017;28:152–158. https://doi.org/10.1177/1043659615620658.

40. Purwaningrum F, Shtaltovna A. Reflections on fieldwork: a comparative study of positionality in ethnographic research across Asia. *Int Sociol Assoc*. 2017;7:1–13.

41. Narvaez RF, Meyer IH, Kertzner RM, Ouellette SC, Gordon AR. A qualitative approach to the intersection of sexual, ethnic, and gender identities. *Identity (Mahwah, N J)*. 2009;9:63–86. https://doi.org/10.1080/15283480802579375.

Chapter 26

Utilizing a cognitive engineering approach to conduct a hierarchical task analysis to understand complex patient decision making

Ashley O. Morris[a], Aaron M. Gilson[b], and Michelle A. Chui[a,b]

[a]*Social and Administrative Sciences Division, University of Wisconsin-Madison School of Pharmacy, Madison, WI, United States,* [b]*Sonderegger Research Center, University of Wisconsin-Madison School of Pharmacy, Madison, WI, United States*

Objectives

- Demonstrate that hierarchical task analysis (HTA) is a valid and reliable method for understanding complex decision-making.
- Show that an appropriately applied HTA method to carefully collected data can be used to describe *how* decisions are made and what knowledge informs them.
- Describe how HTA output provides rich detail about goals and subgoals that underlie complex cognitive processes.
- Demonstrate how HTA can be applied to pharmacy to understand and describe complicated tasks performed by patients, caregivers, and pharmacy staff.

Introduction: Hierarchical task analysis

Origins of task analysis

The term "cognitive task analysis" (CTA) first appeared in research in the early 1900s, following a century-long exploration of cognitive analysis in industrial workplace settings.[1] Primarily developed to express a need to help novices become more like experts, interest in understanding and measuring human cognition was building internationally among researchers from many fields, including ergonomics, psychotechnics, cognitive and/or industrial psychology, cognitive and human factors engineering (e.g., human-computer interaction), and systems engineering (e.g., human efficiency in work environments). The study of **psychotechnics** (the practical application of psychological techniques to alter human behavior),[2] from European psychology, included the earliest task analysis and job analysis methods, which showed significant value for diverse industry manufacturing jobs while saving resources like time and effort. At the same time, American behavioral psychologists were engaging in early forms of behavioral task analysis, such as time and motion studies[3] and training development,[4] the benefits of which were also generalizable to the industry setting.[1,5] CTA remained in human factors psychology and instructional design into the 1990s when an explosion of references to the method appeared in a number of fields, prominently in naturalistic decision-making, cognitive systems engineering, and in aviation,[6] military,[7] medical reasoning, and computer systems domains.[1] To date, a broad spectrum of CTA methods has been developed, captured, and disseminated in research.[8]

What is cognitive task analysis?

CTA is grounded in **constructivism**, an epistemological framework that resists the idea that knowledge can be completely formalized and classified because knowledge is constructed, rather than acquired, and is context- and individual-specific.[9] Constructivist methods instead focus on how the learner interacts and processes information and uses that information to guide the development of an intervention or generate change. Therefore, the context in which experts make decisions is highly valuable and informative. Based on a theory of human performance,[10] CTA is used to analyze qualitative data associated with **action research** (e.g., observations, open-ended survey questions, interviews with subject matter experts, walkthroughs, user trials, and documentation reviews), which focuses on iteratively developed transformative change by taking action (e.g., an intervention) and doing research (e.g., assessing that intervention). The goal of action research is knowledge elicitation or analysis, to measure the impact of the intervention or to illustrate the role of the intervention in the decision-making process.[11] Such an approach is beneficial for capturing unobserved knowledge, cognitive processes, and goal structures that underlie human behavior.[11]

Definitions

The term **cognitive** describes the mental processes and decisions that experts use to achieve a goal and/or solve a complex problem, where **experts** are individuals who have been exposed to new knowledge that is acquired and its use is practiced, to the point where it gradually becomes automated and nonconscious. **Automated knowledge** helps overcome limits on the amount of conscious information we can hold in "working memory" and free our minds to handle novel problems.[4] Yet it also causes experts to be unable to completely and accurately recall the decision knowledge and analytical skills that are an essential component of their expertise—even though they can solve complex problems using the knowledge they cannot describe.[4,9,11,12] This means that experts are largely unaware of how they decide and analyze their problems in a specialty area and are usually unable to verbalize what they do not realize that they know.

While focusing on the tasks that people are required to perform, CTA is a tool to help **novices**, beginner colleagues who are still learning the necessary declarative and procedural knowledge required as an expert, become more like experts by (1) eliciting the automated, nonconscious knowledge experts use to solve complex problems and perform demanding tasks and (2) applying findings. In other words, CTA helps us understand experts' underlying goal generation and decision-making, and the information processing that is required of the human operator to complete tasks. This analysis method can be used to inform the design of decision support in a system and developing tools to support human performance.

Examples of CTA applied to healthcare settings

CTA has been widely applied in healthcare and significant work has been done to guide researchers and healthcare practitioners toward realizing the importance of understanding cognitive task demands. CTA-based studies in healthcare began as early as 1995, and have addressed such diverse topics as necrotizing enterocolitis,[13] diabetes self-management,[14] influence of electronic health records on patient-doctor communications,[15] end-of-life decisions,[16] postanesthesia patient care handoff,[17] patient prioritization,[18] functional endoscopic sinus surgery,[19] and patient self-care decision-making.[20] The methodology is not only beneficial as a tool for eliciting the underlying cognitive decision-making of healthcare providers, but its output provides a particularly useful representation of the decision-making process in a way that can guide future research and inform the development of interventions in complex healthcare environments. In fact, a meta-analysis of CTA studies[21] identified that this method contributes between 12% and 43% more information for documenting performance-relevant processes than non-CTA approaches. Few studies have developed a CTA for patients,[14,22] while many have been conducted to improve training. A focus of other studies has been to assess the impact of an intervention or resource in a healthcare setting.[15,23]

What is hierarchical task analysis?

Hierarchical task analysis (HTA) is a practical, strong step-by-step methodology within the cognitive task analysis family of methods that capture the nonconscious knowledge that experts use to solve complex problems and perform demanding tasks. Compared to other CTA methods that can be employed to understand decision-making, HTA is commonly used to develop task knowledge structures of expert systems and capture operation sequences (e.g., goals, timelines, interactions).[11]

Using the HTA method, high-level **goals** are decomposed into a hierarchy of **subgoals**.[14] At each level of subgoals, a **plan**, which explains how a goal should be accomplished, directs the sequence and possible variance of **tasks** as statements of the conditions necessary to achieve the goal.[24,25]

Principles of hierarchical task analysis

According to Annett and colleagues,[26] the principles of HTA, in technical terms, are as follows:

1. "At the highest level we choose to consider a task as consisting of an operation and the operation is defined in terms of its goal. The goal implies the objective of the system in some real terms of production units, quality or other criteria.
2. The operation can be broken down into sub-operations each defined by a sub-goal again measured in real terms by its contribution to overall system output or goal, and therefore measurable in terms of performance standards and criteria.
3. The important relationship between operations and sub-operations is really one of inclusion; it is a hierarchical relationship. Although tasks are often proceduralised, that is the sub-goals have to be attained in a sequence, this is by no means always the case" (p. 4).[26]

Therefore, the three principles of HTA state that (1) HTA defines an operation in terms of its goals, which imply the objective of the system (e.g., to complete the highest-level task), (2) HTA goals and subgoals must be measurable, and (3) the relationship between goals and their subgoals must be hierarchical in nature. Furthermore, HTA output captures in aggregate all observed decision-making processes that inform the completion of a complex task. Accordingly, it should be noted that a single process can be carried out differently by each person, so variability within sub-goal completion is expected.

There are also some established requirements for interpreting the quality of a CTA (and, by extension, HTA) in published work. A "good" CTA is one that is valid, reliable, generalizable, appropriate in scope, complete, and useful.[27] Table 1 describes the expectations for each of these measurable characteristics.

When should you use hierarchical task analysis?

HTA requires more technical skill by the data analyst, compared to less technical CTA methods, but its output is more useful when seeking to develop an in-depth understanding of the high-level decision-making goals and subgoals necessary to achieve those goals. Both CTA and HTA methods can be used to understand tasks that require decision-making, problem-solving, memory, attention, and judgment,[29] but only HTA can be used to identify the goals that lead to certain decision outcomes. Only when this is identified can interventions target latent decision-informed behaviors that lead to adverse outcomes (e.g., unsafe OTC use). The HTA method was originally utilized to determine operation and training specifications, and remains a popular method for training.[5] HTA also has been used for a variety of research topics that require the representation of system subgoal hierarchies, including error prediction, workload assessment, and interface design.[30] As the breadth of the examples throughout this chapter will demonstrate, there are many additional opportunities to apply CTA and HTA in the healthcare setting.

Examples of HTA in healthcare

The case study included at the end of this chapter is one example of how HTA can be used to conduct pharmacy research: here, to investigate older adult OTC selection in the community pharmacy. Using HTA to investigate medication errors is not unprecedented. One study employed an HTA approach to investigate healthcare professionals' medication administration errors in the hospital setting, concluding that errors can occur at any of the five main stages: prescribing, documenting, dispensing or preparing, administering, and monitoring.[31] HTA results revealed that nurses, who are the health practitioners involved in the last link of the medication administration chain, carry the burden of medication errors that occur earlier in the administration process. Another study, by Colligan et al.,[32] found that quality and safety concerns identified by practitioners improved when they were looking at a hierarchical diagram rather than a process map flow diagram (the prevailing process mapping approach in healthcare). A particular advantage of HTA was the identification of additional clinical safety concerns when reading the hierarchical diagram that they had not otherwise observed through the alternative diagrammatic process.

What are the advantages and disadvantages of hierarchical task analysis?

Advantages of HTA

It is clear that HTA shares many of the same principal benefits of CTA (the task analysis approach that is most comparable), such as understanding unobserved knowledge, cognitive processes, and goal structures of expert user behavior, the ability to conceptualize automated decision-making processes and action steps, applicability within a naturalistic setting, and

TABLE 1 Six factors comprising cognitive task analysis quality.[28]

Trait	Description	Case study HTA evaluation[a]
Valid	• *Construct validity*: appropriate choice of methodology, reliance on domain practitioners as a source of information (either as the focus of analysis, or as members of the analysis team), observation of work practices and inspection of tools and artifacts in the work domain itself • *Face validity*: whether the relationship between the goals of the analysis and the analysis methods is apparent	• *Construct validity*: demonstrated by using HTA as the appropriate methodological approach for the goals of this research, recruiting participants that were older adults themselves, and collecting data in their natural work environment, which was studied closely in pilot work while developing the Senior Section intervention[13,22] • *Face validity*: the goals of this analysis (evaluating the Senior Section) and the analysis method (analyzing older adults as experts who need to use the Senior Section) align, so there is good face validity
Reliable	• Redundancy—did the analyst interview enough people, see enough tasks performed, watch activities under enough conditions that he or she started hearing and seeing the same things repeated, without novel information coming to light?	• This HTA is *reliable*: the analysis stopped only once data saturation was achieved and two coders participated in the analysis
Generalizable	• Did the analyst explicitly describe the systems aspects to which the analytic results generalize, and support that argument by making links from the participants and settings in which the analysis took place, to those of interest?	• This HTA is *generalizable* to older adults that live in this region and shop for OTC medications in a community pharmacy chain. Future work is needed to apply this HTA to other groups of older adults to ensure this output is generalizable to all older adults
Scope	• Is scope of the analysis appropriate for the design goals?	• The *scope* is appropriate: the HTA covered the entire decision-making process from experiencing symptoms to selecting an OTC to treat the medication. We are able to generalize the scope of the HTA diagram to the entire shopping experience surrounding the Senior Section
Complete	• It is usually impossible to guarantee completeness of coverage—not every variable, function, task, component, decision, etc. is going to be identified or addressed • Consider the constraints and challenges inherent in the work domain, and the knowledge, skills, and strategies that expert practitioners bring to bear on those problems	• This HTA output is *complete*: variety of goals and subgoals have been identified, recognizing that some goals may have been missed because we did not recruit participants that consider alternative decision processes (e.g., demographically different participants than that of this study)
Useful	• Did the analysis result in information that is useful for the design of a new decision aid or training program? • Does this analysis support knowledge elicitation from and participation of subject matter experts in the analysis process?	This HTA is *useful*: used to evaluate the impact of the Senior Section intervention on older adult OTC medication decision-making and can be applied prospectively to future iterations of the Senior Section and its implementation in pharmacy store chains

[a]See "A case study: Understanding how *older adults select over-the-counter medications from their community pharmacy using hierarchical task analysis*" section.

gaining valid insights from small sample sizes. HTA has the advantage of deriving valid conclusions from interviews and/or observational data collected from a small sample size of 3–15 expert participants.[16,17,20] As a result, HTA's rich data analysis approach generates output that is a particularly useful representation of the decision-making process, and does so in a way that can guide research and inform intervention development in complex healthcare environments.[16,17,33]

In addition to the aforementioned results from Colligan et al.,[32] which demonstrated HTA's clear benefit over other task analysis methods, other studies have noted further advantages. Hignett and colleagues described several additional advantages for using this method in healthcare—importantly, that HTA is preferred when discussing safety problems with

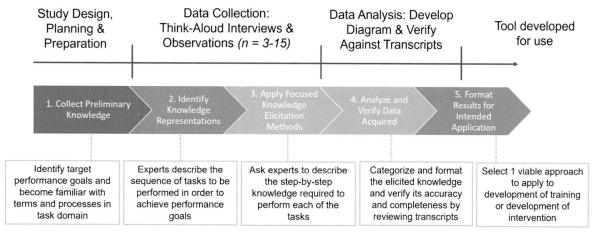

FIG. 1   CTA implementation follows the following 5 steps.[21]

colleagues because the environmental layout remains the same despite the process being carried out differently (unidentified variation in physical activities may still achieve the same cognitive goals).[26,34] This allows for differences in professional autonomy of practitioners with a shared focus on the goal to achieve, rather than the precise method used.

Disadvantages of HTA

Both HTA and CTA are characterized by being time and resource intensive, especially for the substantial resources required to develop the analysis output (e.g., an HTA diagram). However, the specificity and utility of the generated outputs far outweigh the costs associated with constructing it.[35] Furthermore, HTA provides procedural knowledge that is more human-centered, as it focuses on what the human operator will need to do when, how, and with what priority information. This makes HTA output less independent of the context of use,[36] but is valuable in the insights that its output provides.

A framework for conducting hierarchical task analysis

To be most effective, HTA must be considered throughout the lifecycle of the study. Fig. 1 describes the HTA process, according to Tofel-Grehl and Feldon.[21]

Stage 1: Collect preliminary knowledge

In the first stage, collect preliminary knowledge to identify target performance goals and review general knowledge about the task domain. Use this time to become familiar with the terms and processes that the experts use. Educating oneself on the unique language and terminology used by a group of experts can be challenging and time-intensive, so leave ample time for this activity by beginning exploration of terms and processes before and during the design, planning, and preparation phases of the study. Information learned in this stage will inform all phases of your study.

Stage 2: Identify knowledge representations

An expert's representation of knowledge provides valuable insight about the variety of tasks that surround the task under investigation and provides rich context for their decision-making. In this stage, experts describe the sequence of tasks to be performed for achieving their performance goals, which lays the foundation for the next stage of investigating the task of interest. Data for Stages 2 and 3 are typically collected simultaneously, during the data collection phase of the study.

Stage 3: Apply focused knowledge elicitation methods

For the task of interest, apply focused knowledge elicitation methods to capture the unobserved knowledge, cognitive processes, and goal structures that underlie human behavior. Ask experts to describe the step-by-step knowledge required to perform each subgoal of the task. Typical data collection methods include interviews, observations, focus groups, open-ended survey questions, walkthroughs, user trials, and documentation reviews.

Stage 4: Analyze and Verify data acquired

In this stage, categorize the knowledge elicited in the previous stage, verify the accuracy and completeness of the knowledge, determine the appropriate format to represent this knowledge, and validate all findings with experts. The example exercise provided at the end of this chapter offers an example for how one might analyze the data within the HTA framework. Findings can be validated by asking expert users to review the HTA output, or by applying the HTA to a new sample of experts that also complete this task. Keep in mind that sometimes experts are difficult to identify and recruit in the study and as stakeholders in the project, so asking expert users to reflect on the diagram is usually sufficient.

Stage 5: Format results for intended application

In this final stage, format study results for its intended application. Select one viable approach to apply to development of training or an intervention. For example, perhaps a particular subgoal proves to be challenging for novices to achieve. Upon further investigation, it may become clear that novices are missing clear declarative knowledge that informs the cognitive processes displayed by experts. Training could be developed to provide this declarative knowledge to the novice group.

A case study: Understanding *how* older adults select over-the-counter medications from their community pharmacy using hierarchical task analysis

Background

Over-the-counter (OTC) medications are nonprescription drug products that are considered safe and effective for use by the general public without healthcare professional oversight.[37,38] OTCs are widely available for purchase directly by consumers online and in any of the 750,000 mass-merchandize stores and 54,000 community pharmacies across the United States.[39] In 2019, OTC retail sales totaled US $32.2 billion,[40] with top sales in analgesics ($889 M), sleeping aids ($57 M), and upper respiratory medicines ($1207 M).[41] Unfortunately, widespread access combined with unmonitored use can cause consumers to overestimate the perceived safety of these products, which may increase the likelihood of unsafe use, a mistake that is both prevalent and costly.[42]

Painting the picture: Describing older adults' use of OTC medications

Older adults (aged 65 and over) account for 13% of the US population, but consume 30% of OTC medications.[43] What is unsettling about the prevalence of older adult OTC use is that certain OTC medications are associated with such geriatric outcomes as falls, worsened adherence, and increased frequency of adverse drug events (ADEs).[43] In fact, there is insurmountable evidence that older adults' OTC use often results in harm. For example, older adult use of nonsteroidal anti-inflammatory drugs to manage pain leads to 80,000 preventable ADEs each year,[42] and acetaminophen-related toxicities account for up to 50% of all acute liver failures annually.[44]

Indeed, older adults' self-medication behaviors carry risks and have critical safety implications. Instead of informing their provider,[28,45] older adults turn to the OTC medication aisles to manage sleeplessness, for which they take a variety of pain, allergy, and/or sleep products.[45,46] Their behavior illustrates an unawareness about underlying medical conditions that can disrupt sleep, and a lack of knowledge about safe OTC options to treat such symptoms, compounding ADE risk.[42] Cough, cold, and allergy medications (e.g., diphenhydramine and dextromethorphan) can cause dizziness, lethargy, and nausea, all of which can increase fall risk.[47] In addition, diphenhydramine can cause cognitive dysfunction, sleep disruptions, hepatic renal insufficiency and other anticholinergic side effects.[47] For these reasons, diphenhydramine and doxylamine are contraindicated for older adult use compared to other OTC treatment options, a fact supported by the Centers for Medicare and Medicaid Services.[42]

Older adults' decision-making for OTC selection and use

Older adults' safe OTC medication use can be particularly difficult to achieve because of age-related physiologic complexity, comorbidities developed over time, and a more robust medication list and regimen they are expected to follow. Not only do these factors contribute to more complex decision-making for older adults, but cognitive impairment can also become an issue. Given that most older adults are unfamiliar with the need to determine if OTC medications interact with their other medications or how to appropriately dose an OTC medication, a lack of provider awareness about their patients'

OTC use may further permit the duplication of therapies and dangerous overdosing.[42,48] Such factors demonstrate a critical reason for examining and intervening in OTC medication selection behaviors.

No study yet has taken a system-level approach to understanding the demands placed on older adults as they complete OTC selection tasks. Evidence suggests that an important aspect of selection behavior is understanding how older adults assess and make decisions about selecting an OTC medication. Task demand completion (e.g., identifying a product and following its instructions) relies on the interaction between the user, the task, and the package in the context of the community pharmacy environment.[49,50] Decision-making is influenced by individual patient-level factors, features of the medication product, and the context in which decisions are made.[37,51,52] In the retail pharmacy, older adults tend to seek OTC information to make decisions by reading drug labels and package inserts, asking a pharmacist or their doctor for help, looking online, and gathering information from family and friends.[53] This case study examines older adults' naturalistic decision-making in a community pharmacy setting, so that system-level interventions can be developed to effectively support older adults as they make tough OTC medication choices.

Research is beginning to explore the patient-level factors that inform decision-making that occurs in the pharmacy aisle. A variety of attempts have been made to improve older adult OTC safety, which can be categorized into three approaches:

- *Technological interventions.* One example of an effective technological intervention is an interactive game that educates older adults about OTC use, which has improved OTC safety, even for people with low health literacy.[54] In another example, an OTC consumer decision-making tool offers a variety of decision support mechanisms related to the sharing of knowledge and the usability of the technology.[55] However, although helpful in certain contexts, technological interventions have been criticized because they cannot systematically assess an older adult's mental model while shopping for an OTC and are not generalizable to the "real world" experience.
- *Educational interventions.* Another avenue of research has focused on healthcare provider interventions to alter older adult decision-making in a way that guides safer medication choices. One systematic review found that an extensive number of studies support the same conclusion: pharmacists are ideally placed to educate patients about self-medication practices and recommend medical advice when needed.[43] In addition, all community pharmacists should be expected to handle counseling for OTC medications in addition to educating patients on their prescription medications.[56]
- *Product redesign.* Some marketing and package design work has been implemented in response to the evidence that demonstrates that a person must perceive a message as a "warning," not only to comprehend the information but also to be able to encode the safety signal and take appropriate precautionary actions (e.g., not taking the medication). This work includes changes in formatting, font size, information order and language, and external tag placement.[49,57] Very little work has been done, however, to determine how to encourage older adults to read the label while in the pharmacy aisle.

The first system-level intervention: The Senior Section

The intervention in this case study represents a systematic effort to decrease older adults' selection/use of high-risk OTC medications. Participatory design[9] and human factors engineering[58] frameworks guided the redesign of community pharmacies' typical structural layout of their OTC aisles (called the Senior Section™), which promotes safe OTC use by facilitating pharmacy staff communication.[50] The Senior Section is shown in Fig. 2 and is comprised of the following features:

- A dedicated section of well-lit shelving stocked with a curated list of OTC medications that are safer for older adults.[59]
- Proximity and sight line to the prescription department to promote patient/pharmacy staff interactions about OTC medications.
- Tools to support older adults while they shop (e.g., lighted magnifying glass).
- Strategically placed signage to aid in selection of lower-risk OTCs for the treatment categories of allergy, cough/cold, sleep, or pain.[50]
- Shelving height to facilitate Senior Section use by older adults with visual or physical impairments.

The Senior Section is the first and only physical redesign intervention to demonstrate effectiveness in reducing OTC medication misuse in older adults without increasing pharmacist workload.[52,59] More detail about the design and development of the Senior Section can be found elsewhere.[42,52]

Although the Senior Section was designed principally to reduce OTC misuse, the data collection methods used (see below) were considered appropriate to assess patient decision-making when evaluating and selecting an OTC medication.

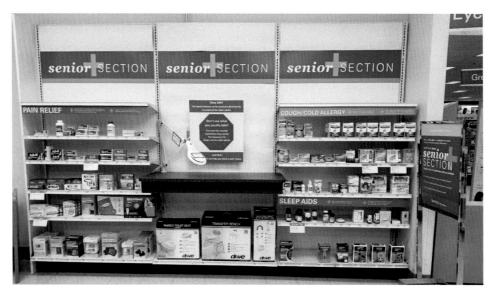

FIG. 2 The Senior Section intervention implemented in the Shopko Project.

Rationale for using hierarchical task analysis to understand older adult OTC selection decision-making

HTA tells us how older adults make decisions, how different amounts of prior knowledge influence decision processes, and how older adults categorize OTC products. As a result, a study which seeks to improve older adult medication safety by reducing errors during the OTC selection process aligns with the goals of HTA. Expert users can be described here as older adults who have had continuous, deliberate practice in solving problems in a domain, such as deciding which OTC medication(s) to select from their community pharmacy, such that their knowledge is automated and largely nonconscious. This approach makes it possible to draw out the automated decision-making processes and action steps older adults use while problem solving related to OTC medication selection. This enriched understanding of their decision-making may inform future intervention designs. For example, elements of the environment that facilitate safe OTC medication decision-making can be replicated in the intervention design, and instances where older adults fail to safely select OTC medication can be addressed during intervention development. In the pharmacy setting, decision-making comprises how consumers (e.g., older adults) make decisions, how prior knowledge influences decision processes, and how they categorize OTC products. Given the dozens of OTC medications on the market to treat particular symptoms, all with different attributes of values (risks, warnings, dosages, or ingredients) that present tradeoffs,[60] it is critical to understand how older adults navigate these intricacies when choosing to use an OTC medication. By applying HTA to consumers in the pharmacy setting, a systems-based approach is used to ascertain the usability, usefulness, and understandability of the community pharmacy OTC product aisles (work environment) and other system factors (technologies and tools, pharmacists) as the human operator (older adult) works to complete tasks.[15,55]

Not only is HTA applicable to older adults, OTC medications, and community pharmacies, this method of task analysis is particularly appropriate for this study because of the level of detail that can be interpreted, and its usefulness in the early stages of intervention development and iterative design.[35] For this study, HTA was used to understand older adult decision-making while they searched for and selected an OTC medication in a retail pharmacy setting, to manage or treat the symptoms of a minor illness not severe enough to see a doctor. The study objectives were to (1) characterize the cognitive decision-making process that older adults undergo when seeking to self-medicate with OTC medications in their familiar community pharmacy, and (2) demonstrate how HTA, a method of cognitive task analysis, can be used as a tool to evaluate the impact of a pharmacy intervention on their decision-making.

Methods

Study design and setting

A pre/postimplementation approach, using a think-aloud interview process, was conducted with older adults within a community pharmacy setting as they completed a hypothetical scenario to treat either pain, sleep, or cough/cold/

allergy symptoms. An HTA-based coding scheme was applied to the interviews to conceptualize older adult decision-making regarding OTC selection and use before and after Senior Section implementation. These methods were designed to conceptualize an understanding about the impact of a pharmacy intervention on OTC medication selection decision-making.

Three pharmacies in a Midwestern state were selected from within a single pharmacy chain to pilot the Senior Section. Each pharmacy was deliberately selected with the same physical layout and to represent communities with demographically similar patient populations, and were agreed upon by the study researchers and the pharmacy chain's corporate management.[61]

Data collection

Older adults participated in the study at the store location that was familiar to them, consistent with requirements of CTA, as described in Table 1.[5] Participants were equipped with an audio recording device and asked to choose a hypothetical symptom profile with which they were most familiar: pain, sleep, or cough/cold/allergy (see Table 2). These scenarios were developed to represent the typical scenarios that different types of older adult shoppers face when shopping for an OTC medication. Older adults were allowed to select whichever scenario was most relevant to them, because research shows that patients provide the most useful information about their decision-making when they can refer to a concrete, memorable episode (e.g., treating a cold in the past few months).[22]

Interviews began at the front of the store (during preimplementation), and then the older adult participant guided the researcher through the store to the pharmacy section where they were asked to think aloud while they shopped for an OTC medication to treat their chosen symptom profile. Conversely, at postimplementation, the researcher started each interview in front of the Senior Section, denoting the only change in data collection resulting from the Senior Section. The researcher observed the work and asked probing questions of the older adults while they interacted with the existing pharmacy system environment, which is a common task data collection technique for a think-aloud interview process.[35] The think-aloud session was completed once the participant selected an OTC medication in the aisle and indicated that this was the product that they would use to treat the chosen symptom profile.

Video recordings were used to collect data about the

(1) Physical tasks completed during the decision-making process, which may align with the cognitive tasks elicited during the think-aloud interview.
(2) Certain patient characteristics that may be of interest, such as gait and mobility (e.g., limp, use of a walker) and vision (e.g., glasses).
(3) *Interaction* between the participant and the products in their environment (e.g., with medication boxes, searching for correct one, pointing to things on the shelf, how quickly medication was selected).

The think-aloud process was identical for pre- and postimplementation, including the same probing questions guided by the SEIPS 2.0 model to target each component of the work system and how they influenced OTC medication selection and use, to elucidate factors important to older adults (see Supplementary Material in the online version at https://doi.org/10.1016/B978-0-323-91888-6.00027-2).[9,42] Think-aloud interviews took approximately 20 min to complete, although interview duration was highly variable across participants (range: 5–50 min).

TABLE 2 Study scenarios for three categories of symptoms.

Category	Scenario
Pain	*You are having soreness and muscle aches. You have not taken any medication to help with these aches yet. And it's not bad enough to call your doctor. So you're here at the pharmacy to look for a medication that can help you feel better. Show me how you would go about choosing a medication to help you feel better*
Sleep	*You are having some difficulty falling asleep or staying asleep. You have not taken any medication to help with this sleep problem yet. And it's not bad enough to call your doctor. So you're here at the pharmacy to look for a medication that can help you sleep better. Show me how you would go about choosing a medication to help you sleep better*
Cough/cold/allergy	*You are having symptoms related to a cold or allergies, like a runny nose, stuffy nose, cough, or congestion. You have not taken any medication for your symptoms yet. And it's not bad enough to call your doctor. So you're here at the pharmacy to look for a medication that can help you feel better. Show me how you would go about choosing a medication to help you feel better*

Data analysis of interview transcripts

CTA follows basic qualitative coding data analysis methods. Data analysis was conducted in two stages. In Stage 1, the video data for each older adult were inductively analyzed to become familiar with the tasks performed to select an OTC medication. Nonverbal behaviors, interactions with OTC products in the aisle (e.g., touching products, reading product labels, searching for specific products), and mobility were noted. This inductive review substantiated that these data were appropriate for a CTA, so the data were subjected to a second review to develop and test initial CTA pilot codes. During codebook development, it was apparent that HTA was a suitable analytical method. As a result, HTA was used in Stage 2 of analysis.

In Stage 2, the codebook was further refined and finalized using the transcripts to identify independent HTA goals, with a second coder assisting with this process. The stop-rule that determines the level of task decomposition for this CTA was determined by the extent of detail provided in the think-aloud interviews. The final codebook, a listed representation of the HTA, is shown in Table 3.

In total, 8 goals and 15 subgoals were identified as codes for this process. Goals 1 and 2 were predefined due to the structure of the study, while all other goals were deduced from study data, primarily identified by the video data analysis and then confirmed using a sample of interview transcripts for validity and completeness of the HTA. Video data were also analyzed in Stage 2 if the coder considered the interview transcript to be ambiguous, to provide more context and further corroborate the HTA codes. For example, some physical tasks that were not verbalized in the transcript were later confirmed by reviewing the video recordings. Data analysis was continued until data saturation was reached,[35] and resulting in a postimplementation sample size sufficiently powered for a CTA.[16,17,20]

Using the finalized codebook, a sample of transcripts were coded that were purposefully selected to reflect think-aloud processes interrupted only by interviewer probes for more detailed information (the reason for which is described in "Discussion" section). Two reviewers independently analyzed and coded the transcripts to identify explicit statements related to independent HTA goals. The reviewers met in-person to discuss each transcript and to identify and resolve coding discrepancies.

Results

Final HTA configuration

In this HTA, the overall goal of the task is Task 0: Treat OTC Symptoms with OTC. Eight goals (Table 3, left column) were identified, which comprised the tasks necessary to reach the overall goal. Goals 1–4 did not consist of subtasks, while goals 5, 6, and 7 had 10, 3, and 2, respectively. Goal descriptions are in Table 3. During the think-aloud process, participants verbalized what they were considering when making selection decisions (see examples in Table 3, right column).

An aggregated representation of the 12 participants included in the HTA is shown in Fig. 3. The sequence of goals (i.e., goals 1–8) was determined by averaging the order in which each goal appeared in all 12 transcripts. For example, goal 1 was the first goal to appear across all transcripts.

It should be noted that the symptom scenarios were always the same and included the same goal—to "treat the issue"—which provided structure for comparing the intervention effect between pre- and postimplementation participants throughout the decision-making process.

Prepost analysis

The average number of assessment factors considered preintervention was 6.33 factors. At postimplementation, participants considered only 3.14 factors on average. Table 4 shows the proportion of participants who considered each factor.

During the preimplementation phase, the most frequent factors considered were cost and quantity (78%), followed by regimen, past experiences, and generic vs brand name (all 67%). Alternatively, at postimplementation, past experiences were by far the single most frequent factor (at 71%), with the next-most-frequent factor being appropriateness of OTC medication for symptoms (57%). Although medication quantity and cost showed the highest occurrence at preimplementation, they were among the least deliberated at postimplementation (along with form and inactive ingredients, all at 14%).

Discussion

This HTA study, the first to investigate the holistic decision-making process surrounding OTC medication selection in the older adult's natural shopping environment, demonstrated that older adult decision-making is far more complex than just picking OTC medication off a pharmacy shelf. In the aggregated view of the older adult OTC medication model that the

TABLE 3 Final Codebook with goals, subgoals, plans (if applicable), term descriptions, and examples.

Goal	Subgoals	Plan	Final codes	
			Task description	Example participant quotes
0. Treat symptoms with OTC		Plan 0: 1–2, then 3–4 in any order, then 5–6 in any order, then 7, then 8	This is the highest-level goal that must be determined for the ensuing cognitive tasks to take place (not coded)	*Overarching goal aligns with the scenario provided to them in the study (see Table 2)*
1. Identify category of symptoms[a]			Given the nature of this study, participants identify the category of symptoms by assessing which category of sleep, pain, cough, cold, or allergy, they most frequently experience/identify with the most	*Interviewer: "So between sleep, pain, cough, colds, or allergy, what resonates more with you?" Participant: "Well, the allergies, asthma, that's my problem"*—Participant
2. Experience symptoms[a]			Given the nature of this study, "experience symptoms" is simulated by the interviewer, when they provide the scenario to the participant	*The participant is given the symptoms they are experiencing in the scenario (see Table 2)*
3. Locate OTC symptom category			This goal represents the cognitive effort to determine where a symptom-specific OTC category might be located	"I'm looking for signs. Well, I would think it would be here with health and beauty. Well, I don't see where their, even where their aspirin would be here, first aid. Okay. Well, we must be getting closer. Okay. Here's vitamins, health, wellness, pain relief, cough, flu, allergy, and ear care. All right. Well, we must be in the right area here. Let's see what they've got here"—Participant
4. Identify first OTC			This goal represents participant's cognitive identification of the first OTC option that they may or may not select to manage their symptoms (can be verbal or physical)	"I've tried this [doxylamine product], and I take maybe one every four months or something, so I don't use a lot"—Participant
5. Assess		Plan 5: 5.1–5.10 in any order	Participants assess the selected OTC using a variety of factors to determine whether an OTC should be selected and taken to treat their symptoms	—
	5.1 Assess quantity		The number of dosage units in the package	"Well, I'm getting 250 caplets for $17.99. I would probably look at it and get my calculator phone out and see which is the better deal. If I'm getting them here, I'm getting 100 caplets. They're both 650 mg. I'm getting 250. But then I also look and say, okay, I'm only taking one a day, so maybe I'm better off going the 100 caplets that take me 100 days versus 250 days, because I don't know on pain relievers if they lose their potency or not"—Participant
	5.2 Assess cost		The cost of the package	
	5.3 Assess form of medication		The form of the OTC medication could be liquid, tablet, caplet, soft-gel, dissolvable, etc.	"I want the dissolvable... I hate taking pills, and it works faster than the non-dissolvable, and that's what I wanted was to use it to get to sleep"—Participant "I usually go for the generic brand that is comparable to it, and then I like the, just the capsules... I have difficulty, a lot of difficulty swallowing, and so the smaller, the easier to go down, the better"—Participant

Continued

TABLE 3 Final Codebook with goals, subgoals, plans (if applicable), term descriptions, and examples—cont'd

Goal	Subgoals	Plan	Task description	Example participant quotes
			Final codes	
	5.4 Assess safety		The perception of medication risk	"The only other thing about ibuprofen, it's, it does have some effects on bleeding and blood pressure, sodium retention, and increases your risk for heart disease if you take it regularly, so I don't take it a lot"—Participant
	5.5 Assess strength		The amount of active ingredient per dosage unit	"And I'm only going to take one, so I can do extra strength with one"—Participant
	5.6 Assess regimen		The dosage, frequency, pattern of use, etc.	"Well, if 250 days, and I'm only taking one a day, there's some people that probably take maybe more than that a day. I'm only taking one a day, and as far as the regular arthritis, I'm not even usually taking one a day of the regular arthritis. The nighttime one, I am. The regular arthritis, I'm, like I said, maybe a couple a week"—Participant
	5.7 Assess past experiences		The participant's historical experience taking the selected medication	"[Camphor and menthol product], that reminds me of being a little kid and having rub on my chest, which I never was sure it worked. But it smelled good, so. I guess, no, probably I wouldn't take any of these"—Participant "But I know what to take from my past experiences"—Participant
	5.8 Assess appropriateness of OTC for symptoms		Relating the purpose of the selected OTC to the symptoms experienced	"I take [a pseudoephedrine hydrochloride product] for sinus and headache"—Participant "I tend to focus on this, you know, cold and flu [an acetaminophen, dextromethorphan, and doxylamine product] or there's chest congestion. There's a severe versus what looks like the mild for the [guaifenesin product]"—Participant
	5.9 Assess generic vs name brand		A comparison of generic and name brand products	"[This store] has a pain relief which has the same acetaminophen that [another acetaminophen product] has. So if this were, for example, on sale or if the [acetaminophen and diphenhydramine hydrochloride product] wasn't available, I'd know it's the same ingredient. It's basically the same thing under different packaging"—Participant
	5.10 Assess ingredients 5.10.1 Assess active ingredients 5.10.2 Assess inactive ingredients		Assess ingredients to best treat symptoms experienced Active = active ingredients Inactive = dyes, other formulation ingredients, emoluments	"Okay. So I have no idea what cetirizine is. It's an antihistamine. This one looks like it'd be pretty good for stopping, again, it's got corn starch in it, which is okay"—Participant

6. Consider alternative		Plan 6: 6.1, then 6.2–6.3 in any order	Considers an alternative OTC option	*After a first product is identified and assessed, any additional product identified and assessed is considered to be an alternative*
	6.1 Identify alternative OTC		Cognitively identifies an alternative OTC option that may be used to treat symptoms	
	6.2 Evaluate OTC	Plan 6.2: 5.1–5.10 in any order	Assess the selected OTC using a variety of factors to determine whether an OTC should be selected and taken to treat their symptoms	"I think the [pseudoephedrine hydrochloride product] is more of a decongestion, as whereas, the [loratadine product] is more of the antihistamine action, the anti-allergy action. And I've already taken both with knowledge of my doctor and pharmacist. But I have found I'm not taking the [pseudoephedrine hydrochloride product] particularly"—Participant
	6.3 Evaluate relative to other picked OTC(s)	Plan 6.3: 5.1–5.10 in any order	Assess the selected OTC in relation to another selected OTC using a variety of factors to determine whether an OTC should be selected and taken to treat their symptoms	—
7. Select treatment			Participant chooses a product	
	7.1 Select primary treatment		Participant chooses an OTC product(s)	"I would walk over here, and I would take [a loratadine product]. And I would probably take, in my case, a small one (Picks up a small box of [a loratadine product])"—Participant
	7.2 Select secondary treatment	Plan 7.2: 3, then 4, then 5–6 in any order	Participant chooses another product in relation to the primary treatment selected	"I would probably pick this one right here [loratadine product]… And if my nose is real stuffy, I will get these breathe strips"—Participant
	7.2.1 Decide that concurrent (OTC or non-OTC) product is needed		Participant may determine secondary treatment is necessary	
8. Treat			Marks the end of the think-aloud interview	"I would go with… the store brand, and I'd go with the 3 milligrams for $7.00"—Participant

aThese tasks/goals are predefined due to the structure of the study. All other tasks/goals were deduced from study interviews.

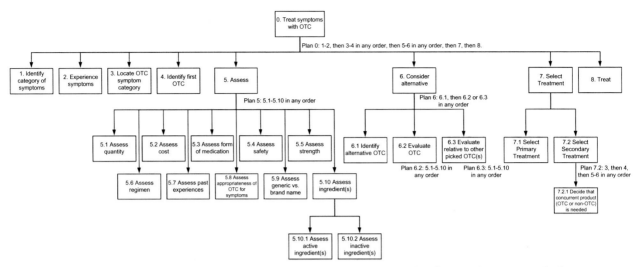

FIG. 3 The hierarchical task analysis representation of older adult decision-making in the selection of an over-the-counter medication.

TABLE 4 The extent that participants considered each assessment factor.

Factor	PRE $n = 9$ n (%)	POST $n = 3$ n (%)
Quantity	7 (78)	1 (33)
Cost	7 (78)	1 (33)
Form	5 (56)	0 (0)
Safety	4 (44)	1 (33)
Strength	4 (44)	1 (33)
Regimen	6 (67)	2 (67)
Past experiences	6 (67)	1 (33)
Appropriateness of OTC for symptoms	5 (56)	2 (67)
Generic vs brand name	6 (67)	0 (0)
Ingredients	5 (56)	0 (0)
Active ingredients	2 (22)	0 (0)
Inactive ingredients	0 (0)	0 (0)

HTA produced, system and individual-level factors that inform decision processes were identified and compared to prior profiles about shopping behavior. First, this HTA diagram, particularly the assessment factors regarding quantity (5.1), cost (5.2), form (5.3), strength (5.5), and generic versus brand name (5.9), aligns with the older adult decision-making processes described by Paliwal[62]:

- *Treatment decision-making*—deciding to take an OTC medication by themselves or deciding to seek a recommendation from a healthcare provider or family/friend.
- *Purchase decision-making*—obtaining information from the OTC medication label or from a pharmacist, comparing prices and deals among various options (and between generic or brand name), and making a final selection decision, typically choosing the product that has maximum and fast relief, at a lower cost, and in an easy to swallow dosage form.[62]

Second, these findings compliment other research indicating that the medication label and the community pharmacist are underutilized information sources.[57] Table 1 demonstrates how the HTA developed for this study complied with the six criteria for measuring the quality of CTA/HTA results: validity (construct and face), reliability, generalizability, scope, completeness, and usefulness.

Utility of HTA

For this study, an HTA was developed as a tool to evaluate the Senior Section's impact pre- and postimplementation. As shown in Table 4, prepost analysis of individual HTA subgoals demonstrated that the Senior Section altered the weight of each subgoal in their decision-making mental model. That is, factors that were most frequently considered during postimplementation were more aligned with medication safety concerns (e.g., appropriateness of OTC for symptoms), while factors considered important at preimplementation related more to superficial aspects of the OTC product (e.g., cost, quantity). This data analysis approach, which is novel for the pharmacy setting, allowed us to identify nuanced differences in older adult decision-making as they shop for OTC medications in the Senior Section.

HTA, as well as other CTA methods, have been used in other disciplines as a best practice method to understand expert decision-making, but this is the first study to apply HTA methodology to the community pharmacy space.[42] As such, this study contributes to a growing body of literature surrounding patient ergonomics.[22,63] HTA was particularly appropriate for this study because of the level of detail that can be interpreted, and its usefulness in the early stages of intervention development and iterative design.[35] This HTA can inform research to improve older adult OTC medication safety when shopping in a community pharmacy setting—conceptualizing systems-focused interventions that alter the salience of critical decision-making subgoals (e.g., safety-related assessment factors). Each subgoal presents an opportunity (e.g., a safe decision) and a threat (e.g., an unsafe decision or error). There is the potential to improve safety by simply addressing a single subgoal using a systems approach to the intervention development and implementation strategy. Safety-related subgoals should be targeted, including the importance of medication ingredients, strength, safety, appropriateness, and regimen.

Reviewing the video data confirmed that a pharmacist can be involved at many points along an older adult's decision-making process but may only be initiated when the older adult engages with the pharmacist. When pharmacists have the opportunity to engage with older adults about safe OTC medication selection, these HTA findings may help guide more patient-centric shared decision-making. These results can inform pharmacists' considerations about what is important to the older adult's mental model for selecting an OTC product. Such information can effectively supplement pharmacists' reliance on the Beers Criteria[59] to help older adults avoid harmful medication use. Given that determinations about older adults' safe OTC medication selection/use are often more complex than reflected by recommendations from a clinical guideline, HTA-informed decision profiles can provide pharmacists critical insights into safety issues that older adults may not be considering. For example, the pharmacist could make recommendations about such factors as safety, reduced strength, or appropriateness of OTC medication for symptoms, rather than having the older adult rely on such things as cost, form or quantity or not considering characteristics of the product that could result in potential harm.

Conclusion

Several advantages support using HTA for this research in the pharmacy environment. First, HTA elicits more detail than other task analysis methods, while maintaining clearly defined boundaries for the start and stopping points of the decision process. This method is particularly useful for defining healthcare providers' decision-making while completing complex care tasks. In addition, HTA is appropriate for providing rich information about the cognitive processes that guide patient behavior and interaction with healthcare systems. In this chapter's case study, this HTA approach was designed to clearly start at the time that the older adult first decided to treat their symptoms and stop when they decide which medication they intend to select to treat their symptoms. Second, HTA is relatively flexible in representing important goals that do not necessarily correspond to physical tasks at specific times, as it represents ongoing potential goals and subgoals that could be triggered at any time (e.g., asking a pharmacist for help).[34] The HTA developed in the case example was an aggregate representation of the older adult shoppers in the study, which allowed for us to develop a more complete representation of decision-making processes that may take place while any older adult shops for an OTC medication. However, the HTA process can be easily generalized to other patient age groups or those with different treatment needs. Third, HTA outputs make excellent tools for designing an intervention, or evaluating an intervention to improve its design.[56] For example, the

HTA diagram of older adult OTC selection can serve as a tool for future work in this space, as the Senior Section continues to be implemented in pharmacies. Importantly, the diagrammatic output can inform different intervention evaluations within a variety of healthcare systems.

Questions for further discussion

1. What are other healthcare applications that can benefit from the use of HTA as a tool to support quality improvement or other intervention-based change such as the older adult OTC medication selection model described in the extended example included in this chapter's case study?
2. What is the feasibility and limitations of applying HTA to address an issue relevant to your healthcare setting?
3. How might HTA be used to make healthcare-based research more patient-centered, aligning with the idea of patient ergonomics?

Application exercise/scenario

Take a moment to reflect on the tasks that you perform in your job. Identify one task you perform that requires more complicated decisions to be made, perhaps dependent on knowledge you've learned on the job or as you were trained to complete this task. Once you have identified this task, answer the following:

- In 3–4 words, describe this task. This is your highest-level *goal*, Goal 0. [to complete this task].
- Next, decompose Goal 0 into your next level of goals by describing Goal 0 in 3–5 steps, known as *goals*. Each goal should be described concisely, in a few words. As this is a process, label each goal from 1 to 5 in the order that they occur (*note*: remember that nonlinear processes can be represented in the plan, which you will add later).
- After you have completed a representation of Goals 0–5, you will want to add detail to each goal (Goals 1–5, as Goal 0 has already been described by Goals 1–5). Starting with the first goal and doing this for each goal thereafter, identify the *subgoals* required to achieve the main goal. Continue to identify subgoals until the overarching goal can no longer be broken down further (when the lowest-level goal describes an action or task that must be completed in order to achieve the cognitive goal).
- After you have roughly deconstructed your goals into appropriate subgoals that describe the complex decision-making that occurs in order to complete goal 0, you are ready to describe your plan. Your plan tells the viewer (of the HTA representation) the order in which you complete each cognitive goal and can be followed to help the viewer understand instances where certain goals may not be required in order to complete the overarching task. Each goal can have its own plan, and plans can refer to a single goal/subgoal or can span all goals in the HTA representation.

Now that you have completed a rough example of an HTA, reflect on this example. What stands out to you about the goals you identified? Is there any way that the completion of these goals could lead to unsafe or adverse outcomes?

If you would like to go a step further, you may choose to ask a colleague to create their own HTA representation of the same task. Note that this may require you to train your colleague on HTA as a data analysis and data representation method. After your colleague completes their HTA, compare the two HTA representations that you each developed. What is the same about the goals, subgoals, or actions you complete to achieve the overall task (Goal 0)? What is different? Are your plans similar or different? How could this diagram be used to inform training in your department?

References

1. Militello LG, Hoffman RR. The forgotten history of cognitive task analysis. *Proc Hum Factors Ergon Soc Ann Meet*. 2008;52(4):383–387. https://doi.org/10.1177/154193120805200439. 2008-09-01.
2. House R. *Definition of Psychotechnics*. https://www.dictionary.com/browse/psychotechnics.
3. Groover M. *Work Systems: Pearson New International Edition PDF eBook: The Methods, Measurement & Management of Work*. Pearson Higher Ed; 2013.
4. Clark RE, Estes F. Cognitive task analysis for training. *Int J Educ Res*. 1996;25(5):403–417.
5. Stanton NA. Hierarchical task analysis: developments, applications, and extensions. *Appl Ergon*. 2006;37(1):55–79.
6. Seamster T, Redding R. *Applied Cognitive Task Analysis in Aviation*. 1st ed. Routledge; 1997.
7. Kittinger R, Kittinger L, Avina GE. *Job Analysis and Cognitive Task Analysis in National Security Environments*. Springer; 2016:341–347.
8. Hoffman RR, Militello LG. *Perspectives on Cognitive Task Analysis: Historical Origins and Modern Communities of Practice*. Psychology Press; 2008.
9. Spinuzzi C. The methodology of participatory design. *Tech Commun*. 2005;52(2):163–174.

10. Salmon P, Jenkins D, Stanton N, Walker G. Hierarchical task analysis vs. cognitive work analysis: comparison of theory, methodology and contribution to system design. *Theor Issues Ergon Sci.* 2010;11(6):504–531.

11. Yates KA. *Towards a Taxonomy of Cognitive Task Analysis Methods: A Search for Cognition and Task Analysis Interactions.* University of Southern California; 2007.

12. Yates KA, Clark RE. Cognitive task analysis. In: *International Guide to Student Achievement.* vol. 1. New York: Routledge; 2012:1.1.

13. Militello LA. *Cognitive Task Analysis of Nicu Nurses' Patient Assessment Skills.* Los Angeles, CA: SAGE Publications Sage CA; 1995:733–737.

14. Lippa KD, Klein HA, Shalin VL. Everyday expertise: cognitive demands in diabetes self-management. *Hum Factors.* 2008;50(1):112–120.

15. Shachak A, Hadas-Dayagi M, Ziv A, Reis S. Primary care physicians' use of an electronic medical record system: a cognitive task analysis. *J Gen Intern Med.* 2009;24(3):341–348.

16. Dionne-Odom JN, Willis DG, Bakitas M, Crandall B, Grace PJ. Conceptualizing surrogate decision making at end of life in the intensive care unit using cognitive task analysis. *Nurs Outlook.* 2015;63(3):331–340.

17. Cole KM. *The Use of Cognitive Task Analysis for the Postanesthesia Patient Care Handoff in the Intensive Care Unit.* University of Southern California; 2015.

18. Chan T, Mercuri M, Van Dewark K, Sherbino J, Linberry M. How emergency physicians think: a cognitive task analysis of task and patient prioritization in a multi-patient environment. *West J Emerg Med Integr Emerg Care Popul Health.* 2016;17(4.1).

19. Corbett M, O'Connor P, Byrne D, Thornton M, Keogh I. Identifying and reducing risks in functional endoscopic sinus surgery through a hierarchical task analysis. *Laryngoscope Investig Otolaryngol.* 2019;4(1):5–12.

20. Holden RJ, Daley CN, Mickelson RS, et al. Patient decision-making personas: an application of a patient-centered cognitive task analysis (P-CTA). *Appl Ergon.* 2020;87:103107.

21. Tofel-Grehl C, Feldon DF. Cognitive task analysis-based training: a meta-analysis of studies. *J Cogn Eng Decis Mak.* 2013;7(3):293–304.

22. Holden RJ, Cornet VP, Valdez RS. Patient ergonomics: 10-year mapping review of patient-centered human factors. *Appl Ergon.* 2020;82:102972.

23. Stanton NA, Salmon PM, Walker GH, Baber C, Jenkins DP. *Human Factors Methods: A Practical Guide for Engineering and Design.* CRC Press; 2017.

24. Hornsby P. *Hierarchical Task Analysis.* UX Matters; 2010.

25. Shepherd A. *Hierarchical Task Analysis.* CRC Press; 2003.

26. Annett J, Duncan K, Stammers R, Grey M. Task analysis. In: *Department of Employment Training Information Paper 6.* London: HMSO; 1971.

27. Roth EM, O'Hara J, Bisantz A, et al. Discussion panel: how to recognize a "good" cognitive task analysis? *Proc Hum Factors Ergon Soc Ann Meet.* 2014;58(1):320–324. https://doi.org/10.1177/1541931214581066. 2014/09/01.

28. Sleath B, Rubin RH, Campbell W, Gwyther L, Clark T. Physician–patient communication about over-the-counter medications. *Soc Sci Med.* 2001;53 (3):357–369.

29. Usability.Gov. *Task Analysis;* 2021. Accessed June 24 https://www.usability.gov/how-to-and-tools/methods/task-analysis.html.

30. Annett J, Stanton NA. *Task Analysis.* CRC Press; 2000.

31. Lane R, Stanton NA, Harrison D. Applying hierarchical task analysis to medication administration errors. *Appl Ergon.* 2006;37(5):669–679.

32. Colligan L, Anderson JE, Potts HW, Berman J. Does the process map influence the outcome of quality improvement work? A comparison of a sequential flow diagram and a hierarchical task analysis diagram. *BMC Health Serv Res.* 2010;10(1):1–9.

33. Larson DL. *Using Cognitive Task Analysis to Capture Palliative Care Physicians' Expertise in In-Patient Shared Decision Making.* University of Southern California; 2015.

34. Hignett S, Banerjee J, Pickup L, et al. Comparing apples with apples: hierarchical task analysis as a simple systems framework to improve patient safety. In: *Presented at 2019 Healthcare Ergonomics and Patient Safety International Conference (HEPS 2019),* 3–5 July, Lisbon, Portugal; 2019.

35. Astiasuinzarra BT. *Compliation of Task Analysis Methods: Practical Approach of Hierarchical Task Analysis, Cognitive Work Analyses and Goals, Operations, Methods and Selection Rules.* Digitala Vetenskapliga Arkivet; 2011.

36. Miller CA, Vicente KJ. Comparison of display requirements generated via hierarchical task and abstraction-decomposition space analysis techniques. *Int J Cogn Ergon.* 2001;5(3):335–355.

37. Albert SM, Bix L, Bridgeman MM, et al. Promoting safe and effective use of OTC medications: CHPA-GSA National Summit. *Gerontologist.* 2014;54(6):909–918.

38. Buckley Jr JB. Food, drug and cosmetic law. *NYUL Rev.* 1953;28:301.

39. Association CHP. *Statistics on OTC Use.* CHPA.org; 2020. Accessed November 18, 2020 https://www.chpa.org/marketstats.aspx.

40. Association CHP. *OTC Use Statistics—OTC Medicines Retail Sales.* CHPA; 2020. Accessed November 18, 2020 https://www.chpa.org/OTCRetailSales.aspx.

41. Association CHP. *OTC Use Statistics—OTC Sales by Volume.* CHPA; 2020. Accessed November 18, 2020 https://www.chpa.org/OTCRetailSales. aspx.

42. Chui MA, Stone JA, Holden RJ. Improving over-the-counter medication safety for older adults: a study protocol for a demonstration and dissemination study. *Res Social Adm Pharm.* 2017;13(5):930–937. https://doi.org/10.1016/j.sapharm.2016.11.006.

43. Wagle KC, Skopelja EN, Campbell NL. Caregiver-based interventions to optimize medication safety in vulnerable elderly adults: a systematic evidence-based review. *J Am Geriatr Soc.* 2018;66(11):2128–2135.

44. Larson AM, Polson J, Fontana RJ, et al. Acetaminophen-induced acute liver failure: results of a United States multicenter, prospective study. *Hepatology.* 2005;42(6):1364–1372.

45. Gooneratne NS, Tavaria A, Patel N, et al. Perceived effectiveness of diverse sleep treatments in older adults. *J Am Geriatr Soc.* 2011;59(2):297–303.

46. Abraham O, Schleiden L, Albert SM. Over-the-counter medications containing diphenhydramine and doxylamine used by older adults to improve sleep. *Int J Clin Pharm.* 2017;39(4):808–817.

47. Glaser J, Rolita L. Educating the older adult in over-the-counter medication use. *Geriatr Aging.* 2009;12:103–109.

48. Shah S, Morris AO, Stone JA, Chui MA. *Older Adult Shopping Persona Types and Its Impact on Over-the-Counter Medication Misuse.* Los Angeles, CA: SAGE Publications Sage CA; 2020:124–128.

49. de la Fuente J, Bix L. A tool for designing and evaluating packaging for healthcare products. *J Patient Compliance.* 2011;1:48–52.

50. Reddy A, Lester CA, Stone JA, Holden RJ, Phelan CH, Chui MA. Applying participatory design to a pharmacy system intervention. *Res Social Admin Pharm.* 2019;15(11):1358–1367.

51. Ruiz ME. Risks of self-medication practices. *Curr Drug Saf.* 2010;5(4):315–323.

52. Stone JA, Phelan CH, Holden RJ, Jacobson N, Chui MA. A pilot study of decision factors influencing over-the-counter medication selection and use by older adults. *Res Social Admin Pharm.* 2020;16(8):1117–1120.

53. Shah S, Gilson AM, Jacobson N, Reddy A, Stone JA, Chui MA. Understanding the factors influencing older adults' decision-making about their use of over-the-counter medications—a scenario-based approach. *Pharmacy.* 2020;8(3):175.

54. Whittaker CF, Tom SE, Bivens A, Klein-Schwartz W. Evaluation of an educational intervention on knowledge and awareness of medication safety in older adults with low health literacy. *Am J Health Educ.* 2017;48(2):100–107.

55. Martin-Hammond AM, Abegaz T, Gilbert JE. Designing an over-the-counter consumer decision-making tool for older adults. *J Biomed Inform.* 2015;57:113–123.

56. Perrot S, Cittée J, Louis P, et al. Self-medication in pain management: the state of the art of pharmacists' role for optimal over-the-counter analgesic use. *Eur J Pain.* 2019;23(10):1747–1762.

57. Klein HA, Isaacson JJ. Making medication instructions usable. *Ergon Des.* 2003;11(2):7–12.

58. Holden RJ, Carayon P, Gurses AP, et al. SEIPS 2.0: a human factors framework for studying and improving the work of healthcare professionals and patients. *Ergonomics.* 2013;56(11):1669–1686.

59. Fick D, Semla T, Beizer J. American Geriatrics Society 2015 beers criteria update expert panel. American Geriatrics Society 2015 updated beers criteria for potentially inappropriate medication use in older adults. *J Am Geriatr Soc.* 2015;63(11):2227–2246.

60. Martin AM, Jones JN, Gilbert JE. A spoonful of sugar: understanding the over-the-counter medication needs and practices of older adults. *IEEE.* 2013;93–96.

61. Stats S. *Population Information and Statistics From Every City, State, and County in the US.* Retrieved on June, 22; 2016:2016.

62. Paliwal Y. *Understanding Over-the-Counter Medication Use and Decision-Making Among Community-Dwelling US Older Adults: A Mixed-Methods Approach.* Virginia Commonwealth University Scholars Compass; 2017.

63. Holden RJ, Valdez RS. *Town Hall on Human Factors and Ergonomics for Patient Work.* Los Angeles, CA: Sage Publications Sage CA; 2019: 725–728.

Chapter 27

Rapid turn-around qualitative analysis applications in pharmacy and health services research

Chelsea Phillips Renfro and Kenneth C. Hohmeier
University of Tennessee Health Science Center College of Pharmacy, Memphis, TN, United States

Objectives

- Describe how RAP can be used in pragmatic healthcare research studies.
- Illustrate the application of RAP to a qualitative research study in the healthcare setting.

Introduction

Research analytics and methodology is an essential part of determining outcomes in any project or trial. Methodologies are often categorized as quantitative or qualitative. Quantitative results are classified as a numerical value while qualitative results provide an open-ended, subjective component to results collected.[1,2] Additionally, mixed-methods approaches where quantitative and qualitative data analyses are combined are becoming popular in research conducted in the healthcare setting.[3] Qualitative research in the healthcare setting has seen a lag in adoption due to skepticism regarding the rigor, as many researchers are used to using quantitative research methodologies to produce an outcome, or due to validity and reliability evidence.[4] However, adoption of qualitative research methodologies has increased as many researchers have recognized the value of understanding participant viewpoints on actions, events, and relationships.[4] While the most common examples of qualitative methods are conducting focus groups and interviews, other examples include asking open-ended questions on survey instruments, field observations, or content analysis on newspaper articles.[5]

There are several different types of in-depth, traditional qualitative research approaches that can be used when working with qualitative data such as content analysis, thematic analysis, grounded theory, or phenomenology.[1] However, the foundation of all qualitative analysis is coding and categorizing the data to identify significant patterns.[5] While coding or categorizing data is one of the most important steps in the qualitative data analysis process, it is also one of the most time-consuming and cognitively demanding aspects of the process. The use of software to assist with qualitative analyses can help with coding and categorizing data; however, the software does not create the categories, code transcripts, identify patterns or draw meaning from identified patterns, which can be very time consuming.[6] For time-dependent research, this creates the larger problem of analyzing data rigorously and also within the allotted time frame.[7]

Rapid assessment procedures

Rapid assessment procedures (RAP) were developed by the World Health Organization for the need to quickly, accurately, and economically evaluate the quality of health care services.[7] This type of qualitative analysis provides the innovation needed to solve the problem of needing to analyze qualitative data rigorously within a short time frame. It is important to note that rapid should not be interpreted as rushed, but as an approach that emphasizes both rigor and analytical efficiency. While RAP has gone under many different names such as rapid qualitative assessment and rapid turn-around qualitative research, the process is the same.[7] RAP is an evidence-based methodology defined as "team-based qualitative inquiry using triangulation, iterative data analysis and additional data collection to quickly develop a preliminary understanding of a situation from the insider's perspective."[7] This analytical method, when compared to in-depth, traditional qualitative methodology, is a relatively underutilized method of decreasing turnaround time for results and outcomes to

Contemporary Research Methods in Pharmacy and Health Services. https://doi.org/10.1016/B978-0-323-91888-6.00022-3

become implemented and effect change. An example of this would be public health situations such as the COVID-19 pandemic where newly implemented programs need to be quickly assessed. By using RAP, researchers can have the opportunity to make changes in real time as results are provided in a shorter timeframe when compared to traditional qualitative methods, potentially creating even better outcomes.[8,9]

Considerations when designing a study using rapid assessment procedures

Designing a study using RAP to analyze qualitative data has common core features around methods and process that can be considered when designing the study. While it is not necessary to combine RAP with quantitative approaches, it can be used as part of a mixed-methods approach. For example, data gathered from semistructured interviews or focus groups can be combined with survey data or existing data sets. Another feature of RAP is that it is often used in projects which have a quick timeline from start to finish, which can last from a couple of weeks to a few months. In some instances, and to further improve qualitative data interpretation, it might be beneficial for the population of interest (e.g., representatives of population and institutions) to be involved in the research and evaluation process to allow for feedback in the design process. Another feature to be considered when designing RAP is a team approach to the research process. This includes planning, data collection, interpretation of findings, and presentation of results. This feature can be seen as a limitation to RAP as it can cause an increased workload and logistical burden on the research team due to the quick timeline.

Rapid assessment procedures methodology

RAP is performed in an iterative cycle of data collection and analysis.[10] Instead of waiting until all data are collected to perform the analysis, data are analyzed while they are being collected. Preliminary results then guide collection of additional data. While this iterative approach allows for data to be analyzed while being collected, it should be noted that traditional qualitative methods for developing and conducting focus groups or interviews would be used. To perform an iterative cycle of data collection and analysis, one analytic context that can be used is the Sort and Sift, Think and Shift approach which requires researchers to "dive in" by reading, reviewing, recognizing, and recording their observations during data analysis. "Stepping back" allows you to reflect, re-strategize, and re-orient after "diving in" analysis.[11] Use of the Sort and Sift, Think and Shift approach has been described below in an example of how RAP can be used in the pharmacy practice setting.

When approaching RAP, it is important to create an inventory of data contents. To do this, a systematic approach should be applied to move data collected into a templated summary.[12] The process to create this summary contains five main steps; however, it is important to note that this process can be tailored (e.g., summary template and matrix can be set up differently based on research team preferences and needs) to meet the research team's needs and the goals of the project. In the first step, a neutral domain name that corresponds with each interview question should be created (Table 1). Given that the interview questions have already been developed prior to collecting the data, neutral domains follow the intended concept of the research question. For instance, if a question asked a respondent to "Describe the planning process that occurred prior to implementation?" then a possible corresponding neutral domain may be "Preimplementation." Note that if the interview question was directly informed by theory, then the original theoretical domain may be used as the neutral domain. During the second step, the neutral domain can then be used to develop a summary template for use by the research team (Fig. 1). A summary template should include only the most relevant details about the interview or focus group, allowing for an at-a-

TABLE 1 Example of neutral domain development.

Sample interview question	Domain
Describe the planning process that occurred prior to implementation?	Preimplementation
To what extent might the implementation take a backseat to other high-priority initiatives going on now?	Implementation
How do you feel about the program (e.g., TennCare MTM) pilot being used in your setting?	Sustainment
To what extent is there a strong need for the program (e.g., TennCare MTM) Pilot?	Scalability

Transcript Summary		
Prepared by:	Initials	
Site:	#	
Respondent role	Community Pharmacist	
Neutral Domain #1	- Subdomain #1 - Subdomain #2 - Subdomain #3	*Supporting quote*
Neutral Domain #2	- Subdomain #1 - Subdomain #2	*Supporting quote*
...		

FIG. 1 Example summary template with neutral domains.

glance interpretation of the data by the entire research team (and not just by those who have specialized training in qualitative research methodology). Commonly included details include who prepared the summary, the study site identifier, subject or respondent role, neutral domain and subdomains, and supporting quotes. Subdomains may be sentences, sentence fragments, or a few words—although one should strive for the most concise descriptors possible to aid in quick interpretation (i.e., "Vaccines top priority" preferred over "Community pharmacists perceived vaccines as a higher priority than MTM and other clinical services").

A section should be included at the end for any other observations (e.g., a participant's tone during the interview) that do not fit into the neutral domains, as well as important quotations. Third, the summary template should be pilot tested with members of the research team to determine if the domains are intuitive, missing, or incorrectly labeled. All researchers who will be using the template should practice creating a summary using the same transcript/data to assess for consistency among researchers. For the fourth step, the transcripts/data should be divided across the team after establishing consistency across researchers. It is important to note that when creating summaries, researchers should make sure they are brief (max of 2 pages), thorough, organized, useful, and readable. The final step is transferring the summary into a matrix to streamline the process of noting similarities, differences, and trends.[13] The matrix format should be set up based on the purpose of analysis (e.g., by role, by site). Table 2 shows an example of how a matrix could be organized. The matrix allows you to quickly identify content in any domain, assess gaps in data, and develop memos or summaries based by domain, sites, or respondents. After finishing RAP, it is important to go back to the data and "dive in" by asking questions to identify any potential stories beyond the identified codes. Then "step back" and reflect on connections identified.[11,12]

In-depth qualitative analysis compared to rapid assessment procedures

Due to the quick timeline for analysis, some researchers struggle maintaining trustworthiness of RAP as compared to an in-depth, qualitative analysis.[7] One study by Gale et al. assessed the consistency of the findings from RAP as compared to an in-depth analysis for the evaluation of an opioid prescribing academic detailing program in the Veterans Health

TABLE 2 TennCare MTM Pilot case-based example of neutral domain development.

Sample interview question	Domain
How well does the TennCare MTM Pilot fit with existing work processes and practices in your setting?	Compatibility
To what extent might the implementation take a backseat to other high-priority initiatives going on now?	Relative priority
How do you feel about the TennCare MTM Pilot being used in your setting?	Beliefs
To what extent is there a strong need for the TennCare MTM Pilot?	Tension for change

Administration.[14] Consistency was defined as the similarity between findings as well as similarity between resources needed. The same research team used RAP to analyze the data followed by an in-depth analysis which included drafting a codebook, revising the codebook twice based on team consensus, and coding transcripts. In regard to consistency of findings, both RAP and in-depth analysis revealed similar themes in implementation of the academic detailing program. Comparing the resource intensity of RAP to the in-depth analysis showed that the in-depth analysis took approximately 10 weeks longer to analyze than RAP. Normally, this process might take longer as the research team was already familiar with the framework being used from conducing RAP prior to the in-depth analysis.

Application of rapid assessment procedures in the healthcare setting

Several studies implemented in the healthcare setting have used RAP methods to quickly move results to make changes. One study by Solomon et al. assessed HIV prevention programs within a community mental health center.[15] Rapid assessment procedures were used to analyze data collected from interviews and focus groups. Through use of RAP, areas for improvement in the program were able to be identified such as the failure between case managers to maximize their relationship with the patients to explain the importance of sexually transmitted infection and HIV education to a high-risk population. Determining this need over a few weeks versus a year-long study provides an opportunity to protect patients now as compared to them needing to receive potentially preventable treatment in the future.

In another study by Moloney et al., RAP was used to develop case studies and derive lessons learned from providing clinical interventions at the beginning of the COVID-19 pandemic.[16] As the world faces an unprecedented outbreak, this study implemented rapid analytics to progress clinical treatment at a quicker pace. Early findings from the use of RAP found that primary and secondary prevention strategies for COVID-19 could be incorporated into current treatment for patients who were at greatest risk for COVID-19 exposure. COVID-19 has brought the need for rapid qualitative analysis to the forefront of scientific research and Moloney et al. showed how healthcare within the United States and abroad can capitalize on it.

Application of rapid assessment procedures in pharmacy practice

Intervention overview

To support and improve primary care transformation through inclusion of medication therapy management (MTM), Tennessee's state Medicaid program (TennCare) implemented the TennCare MTM Pilot Program.[17] This program focused on implementing a patient-centered approach to MTM by integrating this pilot into an overarching TennCare Primary Care Transformation initiative which includes patient-centered medical homes (PCMH). The Primary Care Transformation initiative was designed to improve primary care through proactive management and coordination of a patient's healthcare experience. Nested within this initiative, the MTM pilot focused on four areas: (1) patient attribution through risk stratification, (2) reporting and documentation using a shared care coordination platform, (3) value-based reimbursement, and (4) evaluation of MTM-specific quality metrics. MTM services included medication therapy evaluation and monitoring, patient and prescriber education, care plan development, and a comprehensive medication review. The payment model for this program was established on a per month case rate based on targeted disease state or risk category.

Participants

Participants included the implementation team (e.g., pharmacists, physicians, nurses, support personnel, and administrators), implementation facilitators (e.g., University researchers, TennCare personnel), and managed care organizations (i.e., medical insurance companies contracted with TennCare to administer the Medicaid program to TennCare beneficiaries) in the state of Tennessee. The PCMH served as the center of the MTM pilot as it was intended to be the central location for the patient's entire medical and prescription record. Pharmacists practiced either within the PCMH or as a pharmacist at an external but nearby community pharmacy. Of note, the program spanned over 500 miles across three distinct regions of the state (east, middle, and west) and covered rural, urban, and suburban areas. In addition, three separate managed care organizations (MCOs) administered benefits for TennCare members. Key informants were recruited for the study via three separate emails sent over 4 weeks from implementation facilitators (TennCare and University of Tennessee Health Science Center College of Pharmacy researchers) to all participants within the program.

Methodology

The study aimed to explore the adoption, feasibility, acceptability and appropriateness of an implementation strategy to support the MTM pilot program in Tennessee. RAP was used to analyze qualitative data and provide real-time feedback on the MTM pilot program's implementation to TennCare in order for programmatic changes to be made. One member of the research team conducted nine in-depth, key informant interviews with nine participants as part of an early implementation assessment. The Consolidated Framework for Implementation Research (CFIR) provides 37 constructs organized into domains associated with effective implementation. Constructs underpinning the inner setting, characteristics of individuals, and process were used to develop a semistructured interview guide.[18] Interviews were audiotaped and transcribed. Field notes made during the interviews were added to the transcriptions.

To conduct RAP, researchers first created a neutral domain that corresponded with each interview question (Table 2). Next, the research team created a summary template to be used during data analysis (Fig. 2). The summary template was piloted with one transcript to allow for the research team to assess the usability, make any necessary changes, and develop consistency among the researchers conducting the analysis. Then, the transcripts were divided among the research team to develop summaries. A matrix (Table 2) was used to visualize data across participants and CFIR constructs. After completion of the analysis, the research team stepped back to reflect and re-strategize on the findings (Table 3). Formal RAP reports were delivered to TennCare personnel quarterly, with informal updates presented monthly during standing meetings (Table 4).

Implications from using rapid assessment procedures

The program officially started in July 2018. Interviews were conducted over the first quarter of 2019 to explore implementation processes, characteristics of individuals implementing the program, MTM pilot characteristics, and the inner setting or the PCMH or pharmacy. This data was compared against quantitative data including program reach and adoption as defined by rate of MTM claims billed per month and quantity of National Council for Prescription Drug Programs (NCPDP) numbers (i.e., discrete providers) billing per month.

RAP was used to provide real-time updates to the program (Table 3). For the purposes of formal interim and annual reports, as well as data dissemination via peer-reviewed manuscripts, traditional qualitative data analysis was used per the sponsor organization's request. This approach gave the project sponsor critical feedback as often as monthly and in real time, while still having the option to report to the legislature and Centers for Medicare and Medicaid Services results undergoing traditional qualitative research analysis. Neutral domains were drafted based on the Consolidated Framework for Implementation Research,[18] but was then further customized in collaboration with TennCare to match their internal

TABLE 3 TennCare MTM Pilot example matrix.

	Demographics	Relative priority	Tension for change
	Role, years in role, time at organization	Interviewee perception of importance of implementation within pharmacy	Degree to which individuals at pharmacy/PCMH perceives status quo needs to be changed
Interview 1	Ambulatory care pharmacist; role time: 1.5 years; organization time: 2 years	− Vaccines top priority − MTM growth area, high importance	− Competition leads to desire for differentiation from competitors
Interview 2	Community pharmacist; role time: 10 years; organization time: 3 years	− MTM high priority − Included in metrics for the pharmacy team	− Pharmacist experience with poorly managed program beneficiaries and sees pilot program as an opportunity to be change agent
Interview 3	Community pharmacist; role time: 2 years; organization time: 2 years	− Large emphasis placed on medication sync and vaccines over MTM	− Organization's 1 top management team recent turnover leading to fear of new initiatives and protection of status quo

FIG. 2 TennCare MTM Pilot example summary template with neutral domains.

Transcript Summary			
Prepared by:	KH		
Site:	10		
Respondent role	Community Pharmacist		
Relative Priority	- Vaccines top priority - MTM growth area, high importance	"…immunizations are still on the top of [the team's] mind, but yeah, we are making these MTMs happen because they are important for the pharmacy and the profession."	
Tension for Change	- Competition leads to desire for differentiation from competitors	"Look, we're a small independent pharmacy. We don't have the big name or advertising. The pilot gives us a way to partner with patient's physicians and expand our service offerings."	
…			

language and to further facilitate communication. Meetings within the research team refined the summary template over several meetings in early and mid-2019 to match data being collected. Data were transferred to a matrix to better visualize the data across multiple neutral domains and interviewees. The matrix tool was customized based on feedback within the University of Tennessee Health Science Center (UTHSC) research team and TennCare. From start to finish, the length of time to use RAP for this program was 4 months.

After an initial spike in participation through the end of 2018 and early 2019, a decline in both reach and adoption of the program was noted through summer of 2019. Monthly meetings between TennCare and UTHSC researchers allowed researchers to refine their analysis approach to meet real-time questions asked by TennCare personnel during those critical first two quarters of 2019. Four key programmatic changes were identified based on this rapid assessment, presented to TennCare, and changes were implemented during the fourth quarter of 2019 through the third quarter of 2020. These changes included: pharmacist reimbursement rate increases after a nationwide review of pharmacist MTM fee schedules, re-sequencing of care coordination tool training during credentialing process to increase the speed of program enrollment, duplicate documentation workaround using existing software limitations, and an eligibility expansion. Importantly, these barriers and the corresponding supporting data were not only used by the implementation facilitation team to make more informed decisions, but as concrete data from which key decision makers within the Tennessee Government could then approve those changes. Although several of these barriers and suggested changes were noted anecdotally by stakeholders within the project (e.g., conference calls with pharmacists, emails between implementation facilitators), it was the formal qualitative inquiry and use of RAP which provided both the adequate level of rigor and speed of analysis to allow for programmatic improvements to take place.

Future use of RAP

RAP offers a new tool in the arsenal of qualitative researchers, but there remain some unanswered questions and areas for future research. RAP may offer considerable reductions in time for analysis, but may also increase overall time spent in write-up of results.[19] The degree to which time may be saved in data analysis varies greatly and may be a function of both the techniques applied and the researchers themselves.[19,20] This should be of no surprise as data analysis is still heavily dependent upon manual coding procedures—meaning that even if researchers have more efficient procedures to code it does not guarantee that those researchers will spend less time on coding.

TABLE 4 Sample rapid assessment procedure timeline from Medicaid medication therapy management pilot project.

	Mar-19	Apr-19	May-19	Jun-19	Jul-19	Aug-19	Sep-19	Oct-19	Nov-19	Dec-19	Jan-20	Feb-20	Mar-20	Apr-20	May-20	Jun-20	July-20
Implementation stage	Early implementation										Middle implementation						
Qualitative data collection	X	X	X	X										X	X	X	X
Oral RAP briefings	X	X	X	X	X	X	X	X	X	X	X	X	X	X	X	X	X
Quarterly reports on overall evaluation status using RAP	X			X			X			X			X			X	
Formal interim report[a]					X			X			X			X			
Formal annual report[a]															X		

[a]Use of traditional qualitative data analysis methodology.

In our experience, a mutual understanding of the urgency for quick and rigorous data is key. The researchers and program sponsors which formed the project team were aware of the need for quick turnaround of data for program improvement and monitoring. This facilitated urgency in data interpretation while still relying on established RAP methods to ensure analytical integrity. It is our belief, that this mutually understood urgency within the team allowed for efficient data analysis and reporting, whereas RAP used for program assessment that is less obviously timebound or where urgency is not established may lead to increased analysis time.

Despite wide variations in time savings through the use of RAP, there is strong evidence to support consistent overlap in results between RAP and traditional qualitative research methods, such as thematic analysis.[19–21] Even at this early stage in the development, use, and study of RAP methods, there appear to be some general consensus around its application and usefulness. For instance, in health emergencies in the United States and abroad where there is both an urgent need for results and a rapidly evolving situation being studied (e.g., COVID-19, Ebola).[20] As was reported in the present paper, RAP is also useful for certain programmatic assessment—especially during early implementation periods when there is a need to quickly and fluidly understand implementation context from the field. Regardless of the reason to apply RAP, to make the most of this methodology it would seem that a mutually understood sense of urgency on the part of the research team performing the analysis is a critical factor for its successful application.

Conclusion

The benefit of using RAP is the potential to see changes made in real time that can affect patient healthcare immediately. Possible benefits in the profession of pharmacy could be seen in many areas, including disease prevention programming, medication therapy management and even guideline changes for the current global pandemic. Use of RAP provides key stakeholders and decision makers the ability to generate solutions to problems faster than before without compromising rigor, a method needed now in this rapidly changing healthcare environment. The progression of healthcare and clinical management is moving at an unprecedented rate, and RAP allows researchers to stay ahead by providing quicker results for better outcomes.

Questions for further discussion

1. In what type of project is RAP a preferred methodology over traditional in-depth qualitative analysis?
2. Beyond collecting interview and focus group data, what other types of data can be collected and assessed to aid in RAP?
3. What is meant by "dive in" and "step back" in RAP? How does this aid in the interpretation of data?
4. What is one advantage of RAP over in-depth qualitative analysis? What is one disadvantage?

Application exercise/scenario

You are interested in evaluating the effect of a naloxone-recommendation intervention in a regional community pharmacy chain. Although the intervention was designed based on a thorough review of the literature, its use outside of a few academic-affiliated pharmacies is limited. Moreover, you have already received substantial resistance from community pharmacy leadership who have been assigned to your research team as points of contact to aid in study implementation. These leaders believe the intervention is important, but may be unfeasible with other competing priorities for the pharmacy staff and within the existing pharmacy workflow. In addition to collecting clinical outcomes, you will be collecting barriers and facilitators to the implementation of the naloxone-recommendation intervention through in-depth semistructured interviews to inform future scaling of the intervention. What features of the study lend itself to an RAP approach? What data that is being collected could be used in RAP? What additional data should be collected to better interpret RAP findings?

References

1. Rosenthal M. Qualitative research methods: why, when, and how to conduct interviews and focus groups in pharmacy research. *Curr Pharm Teach Learn.* 2016;8:509–516.
2. Miles B, Huberman A, Saldana J. *Qualitative Data Analysis.* 3rd ed. Thousand Oaks, CA: Sage Publications; 2014.
3. Creswell JW, Plano Clark VL. *Designing and Conducting Mixed Methods Research.* Thousand Oaks, CA: Sage Publications; 2014.
4. Castleberry A, Nolen A. Thematic analysis of qualitative research data: is it as easy as it sounds? *Curr Pharm Teach Learn.* 2018;10:807–815.
5. Patton MQ. *Qualitative Research and Evaluation Methods.* 3rd ed. Thousand Oaks: Sage Publications; 2002.
6. Roberts K, Wilson R. ICT and the research process: issues around the compatibility of technology with qualitative data analysis. *Forum Qual Soc Res.* 2002;3, 58.

7. Beebe J. *Rapid Assessment Process: An Introduction.* 1st ed. Walnut Creek, CA: AltaMira Press; 2001.

8. Vindrola-Padros C, Chisnall G, Cooper S, et al. Carrying out rapid qualitative research during a pandemic: emerging lessons from COVID-19. *Qual Health Res.* 2020. 1049732320951526.

9. Holdsworth LM, Safaeinili N, Winget M, et al. Adapting rapid assessment procedures for implementation research using a team-based approach to analysis: a case example of patient quality and safety interventions in the ICU. *Implement Sci.* 2020;15. https://doi.org/10.1186/s13012-020-0972-5, 12.

10. McNall M, Foster-Fishman PG. Methods of rapid evaluation, assessment, and appraisal. *Am J Eval.* 2007;28:151–168.

11. Maietta RC, Mihas P. Sort & sift, think and shift: let the data be your guide. In: *Presentation at Research Talk Fall Seminar Series in Chapel Hill, NC*; 2017.

12. Hamilton A, Maietta R. Rapid turn-around qualitative research. In: *Presentation at 14th Annual Qualitative Research Summer Intensive in Chapel Hill, NC*; 2017.

13. Averill JB. Matrix analysis as a complementary analytic strategy in qualitative inquiry. *Qual Health Res.* 2002;12(6):855–866.

14. Gale RC, Wu J, Erhardt T, et al. Comparison of rapid vs in-depth qualitative analytic methods from a process evaluation of academic detailing in the Veterans Health Administration. *Implement Sci.* 2019;14(1):1–2.

15. Solomon PL, Tennille JA, Lipsitt D, Plumb E, Metzger D, Blank MB. Rapid assessment of existing HIV prevention programming in a community mental health center. *J Prev Interv Community.* 2007;33(1–2):137–151. https://doi.org/10.1300/J005v33n01_11.

16. Moloney K, Scheuer H, Engstrom A, et al. Experiences and insights from the early US COVID-19 epicenter: a rapid assessment procedure informed clinical ethnography case series. *Psychiatry.* 2020;83(2):115–127.

17. Woeppel J, Clark R, Underwood L, et al. The Tennessee medication therapy management program: a hybrid type 2 effectiveness-implementation trial study protocol. *Res Soc Adm Pharm.* 2020;16(3):315–320. https://doi.org/10.1016/j.sapharm.2019.05.018.

18. Damschroder LJ, Aron DC, Keith RE, Kirsh SR, Alexander JA, Lowery JC. Fostering implementation of health services research findings into practice: a consolidated framework for advancing implementation science. *Implement Sci.* 2009;4(1):1–5.

19. Taylor B, Henshall C, Kenyon S, Litchfield I, Greenfield S. Can rapid approaches to qualitative analysis deliver timely, valid findings to clinical leaders? A mixed methods study comparing rapid and thematic analysis. *BMJ Open.* 2018;8(10):e019993.

20. Vindrola-Padros C, Vindrola-Padros B. Quick and dirty? A systematic review of the use of rapid ethnographies in healthcare organisation and delivery. *BMJ Qual Saf.* 2018;27:321–330.

21. Johnson GA, Vindrola-Padros C. Rapid qualitative research methods during complex health emergencies: a systematic review of the literature. *Soc Sci Med.* 2017;189:63–75.

Chapter 28

Best practices in mixed methods for pharmacy and health services research

Deepika Rao and Olayinka O. Shiyanbola

Social and Administrative Sciences, School of Pharmacy, University of Wisconsin-Madison, Madison, WI, United States

Objectives

- Classify various mixed methods study designs and their applications.
- Identify and select appropriate integration strategies for mixed methods studies.
- Understand and describe types of legitimation, and address threats to legitimation in mixed methods research.
- Use new tools and techniques in designing, conducting, and writing mixed methods studies.
- Develop and report mixed methods research that meets quality criteria/recommendations.

Introduction to mixed methods

With an increasing focus on interdisciplinary teams in practice and research, mixed methods approaches to investigate complex health issues and systems have gained popularity in the health science fields. Pharmacy-related research is no exception. However, there is large variation in the rigorousness and depth of designing, conducting, and reporting mixed methods research.[1,2] This chapter will provide a brief introduction to mixed methods, describe the types of mixed methods study designs, discuss prior mixed methods research and their limitations, and make recommendations for future research including the use of novel tools in reporting mixed methods findings.

Although the definitions of mixed methods have evolved as the field developed, the most recent comprehensive definition by the 2018 National Institute of Health (NIH) report[3] states that mixed methods research focuses on questions that require contextual and multilevel perspectives. It employs rigorous quantitative and qualitative methods and involves multiple sources of data. Importantly, mixed methods research systematically integrates different types of data to strengthen findings and counterbalance weaknesses in individual methods of data collection. Mixed methods studies also offer opportunities to develop or integrate theory/frameworks into the study design during conceptualization, allowing for the design of data collection instruments and guiding the data analysis and interpretation.[4] The theory or framework usually serves as a common link between the different quantitative and qualitative approaches.[4-6] For example, Rao et al. conducted a mixed methods study to evaluate medication adherence changes in African Americans/Blacks with type 2 diabetes and explore the effect of psychosocial and interpersonal factors on these changes.[5] They used the Integrated Theory of Health Behavior Change for study conceptualization and to develop the quantitative questionnaires and interview guides. The theoretical constructs also linked the quantitative factors and qualitative themes together.[5]

"Multimethod" studies refer to various combinations of methods (two or more quantitative, two or more qualitative, two or more quantitative and qualitative methods). Mixed methods can be considered a subset of multimethods, not only requiring a combination of quantitative and qualitative techniques but also integration of the approaches at several points in the study process, including at the study design level, data collection, analysis, interpretation, and report of findings.[7] It is important to distinguish mixed methods research from multimethod studies which may include quantitative and qualitative approaches but do not systematically link the two approaches. Altogether, the focus on context of the research problem, theoretical basis of the study design, rigorous quantitative and qualitative data collection and analysis, and the deliberate integration of both types of data results in a more comprehensive understanding of the problem and possible solutions in mixed methods studies.

Contemporary Research Methods in Pharmacy and Health Services. https://doi.org/10.1016/B978-0-323-91888-6.00033-8

Methodological limitations in social pharmacy research and corresponding solutions

Despite the increasing popularity of mixed methods approaches in social and administrative pharmacy,[8–10] there are gaps in the techniques utilized in planning, conducting and reporting these studies. These limitations can be categorized into 3 areas: (1) lack of a specific mixed methods study design, (2) absence of systematic integration of quantitative and qualitative approaches and results, and (3) issues of credibility and validity in the mixed methods study. Failure to address these limitations in research can cause improper and insufficient use of mixed methods approaches and may ultimately lead to a lack of credibility in the findings. The three limitations and ways to address them are discussed below in detail.

Lack of specific mixed methods study designs

Many mixed methods studies found in the pharmacy literature state that a mixed methods approach has been utilized without clearly describing the exact study design that has been used or providing rationale for its use.[11] Each design comes with its own specific characteristics and related applications as described in Table 1. Without choosing a design for a study

TABLE 1 Study designs and their applications.

Study design	Phases	Application	Example studies[a]
Basic (core) designs			
Concurrent/ congruent	Qualitative and quantitative phases are conducted simultaneously and merged together	To gather complete data from multiple perspectives/analyze different aspects of the same research problem	Pharmacist perspectives on inappropriate antibiotic dispensing[12] Collaborative working relationships between pharmacists and physicians[13]
Explanatory sequential	Quantitative phase followed by qualitative phase	Used when quantitative findings need more explanation/context	Effect of psychosocial and interpersonal factors on medication adherence[5,14]
Exploratory sequential	Qualitative followed by quantitative phase	For the development of an instrument or intervention	Pharmacist prescribing activity in Scotland[15] Development of a measure of moral distress in UK pharmacists[16]
Advanced (complex) designs			
Intervention	Qualitative phase before/during/ after intervention (quantitative)	To embed qualitative phase within intervention Before: To recruit participants/ modify intervention During: To understand participant experiences After: To explain findings/ implementation outcomes	Antibiotic-prescribing educational intervention with the qualitative phase exploring acceptability[17] Effectiveness of a pharmacist-led pain management intervention with the qualitative phase focused on patient satisfaction in England[18]
Multistage	Multiple qualitative and quantitative phases	Used in program evaluation, intervention sustainment and dissemination	Implement and evaluate a pharmacy-based cardiovascular disease screening program[19] Evaluation of a pharmacist delivered electronic decision support system[20]
Case study	Converge qualitative and qualitative data from cases or compare quantitative case(s) with separate qualitative case(s)	For comparison of case studies	Comparing community pharmacies' performance on quality measures[21]
Community-based participatory/ social justice	Any basic design is threaded with a participatory/social justice lens	For a health equity/community engaged research project	Design a medication safety intervention using stakeholder input[22]

[a]*Examples are for illustrative purposes only.*

based on the research question, researchers may use designs that are inappropriate or suboptimal. Also, if the exact design is not described in a grant proposal or manuscript, it leaves reviewers and readers with multiple questions about the specific procedures involved. Finally, using a specific and appropriate study design along with a strong rationale for its use in proposals and manuscripts increases the trust and reliability of study findings.

Mixed methods designs and applications in social pharmacy

There are various mixed methods study designs that can be used in pharmacy depending on the research question and gap to be addressed. The three basic designs are "concurrent" (simultaneous quantitative and qualitative phases), explanatory sequential (quantitative followed by qualitative), and "exploratory sequential" (qualitative followed by quantitative). Researchers can use a concurrent design when more complete and corroborated results from multiple perspectives are needed. Examples include the use of a concurrent design to understand pharmacist perspectives on inappropriate antibiotic dispensing[12] or to explore collaborative working relationships between pharmacists and physicians.[13] Also, there are studies that have used explanatory sequential designs to study psychosocial and interpersonal factors affecting medication adherence.[5,14] Rao et al. used patient perceptions of these factors to explain the quantitative changes in medication adherence.[5] If instruments or interventions are to be designed in an area with limited prior research, an exploratory sequential design can be used. This design has been used to describe pharmacist prescribing activity in Scotland[15] and to develop instruments such as a measure of moral distress in UK pharmacists.[16]

Advanced mixed method designs are complex combinations or applications of the basic designs.[23] The "intervention design" can be used to enhance recruitment in experimental research, capture participants' experiences during a trial, or explain the outcomes of a clinical trial.[23] To our knowledge, advanced mixed method designs are less common in social and administrative pharmacy research. An intervention design for an antibiotic-prescribing educational intervention with the qualitative phase that explores acceptability has been reported.[17] Another mixed method intervention study in England evaluated the effectiveness of pharmacist-led pain management with the qualitative phase focused on patient satisfaction.[18] For the implementation and evaluation of programs, multiple qualitative and quantitative phases may be needed and an advanced mixed methods design called a "multistage study design" can be used.[24] For example, a multistage mixed method evaluation was used to implement and evaluate a pharmacy-based cardiovascular disease screening program[19] and a pharmacist delivered electronic decision support system.[20] Other advanced mixed methods include case studies, social justice, and community-based participatory designs. Comparing case studies using mixed method approaches is possible with a "case study design."[25] For example, a study compared cases of community pharmacies' performance on quality measures.[21] If conducting community-engaged work, a "social justice design" is a basic mixed methods design with a health equity based lens threaded throughout the study.[26] In these studies, qualitative data is usually collected to form or maintain partnerships or trust within underserved communities, identify priority issues in the community, design tailored programs, get feedback from stakeholders, or disseminate findings while quantitative data typically involves needs assessment surveys or outcomes such as program effectiveness.[27] Community-based participatory mixed methods designs seem to have limited use in pharmacy research but a protocol for a medication safety intervention developed using participatory approaches has been reported.[22] A summary of study designs with their phases, applications and exemplar studies is provided in Table 1.

Solution: Choosing appropriate study designs

It is extremely important to choose the mixed methods study design based on the research question. This will ensure that an appropriate and optimal study design is selected. One way to do this is to begin with the overall purpose of the study and the research gap to be addressed. Then, researchers can take an inventory of existing literature, potential sources of data available, and the potential application of mixed methods (see Table 1). Once the appropriate design is chosen, it is important to formulate separate specific aims for the quantitative, qualitative and mixed phases as well as a rationale describing why the study design is appropriate.

Absence of systematic integration of quantitative and qualitative phases

Systematic integration of both qualitative and quantitative phases , especially at one or more points throughout the study, is the cornerstone of any good-quality mixed methods study. Unfortunately, most studies in health sciences lack this integral aspect in their mixed methods research.[2,11,28,29] This leads to several problems, primarily the loss of critical advantages of mixed methods studies including the dependability of the research and quality of insights gained from a mixed methods approach. Integrating quantitative and qualitative findings allows researchers to conduct a third analysis of the data (mixed level) which provides more information than the individual phases alone, even if they are conducted in the same study. Integration is not achieved if quantitative and qualitative data are analyzed separately and then reported together within a manuscript; instead findings from both phases must be systematically mixed together.[30] For example, when using a concurrent design, after the analysis of the quantitative and qualitative phases, it is necessary to bring the phases together to systematically compare the findings. Researchers can then report the findings of this third analysis. Lack of integration in exploratory sequential designs leads to the development of instruments or interventions that are supposedly built on the qualitative phase, but the integration approach is not reported. Showing how each item in an instrument or each feature of an intervention is directly linked to themes or quotes from the initial qualitative phase will lead to clarity in the development of robust instruments/interventions.

Integration in mixed methods

There are three main points of integration that occur in any mixed methods study.[31] The first is at the design stage as described above. The second is at the methods level and the third is at the interpretation or reporting level (Fig. 1). There are four approaches to integration at the methods level in mixed research, as described below.

Merging

Merging is used commonly in mixed methods designs when data from both phases is brought together for mixed level analysis. This approach is used in concurrent designs to make comparisons, evaluate the complementarity between phases or even explore any divergence between findings. For example, Kaufmann et al. determined risk factors for drug-related problems by merging (called "triangulation" in the study) expert ratings and qualitative discussions.[32] This approach can also be used in sequential designs when both phases are completed. In an explanatory sequential study, researchers can use merging to understand qualitative thematic variations among groups differentiated on the basis of the previous quantitative results. In exploratory sequential studies, researchers can assess complementarity between their initial qualitative themes and quantitative scores on the developed instrument or intervention features. To make it easier to seamlessly merge the two databases, researchers can plan ahead and form "bridges" using theory or conceptual frameworks that help create links between the two. For example, in the medication adherence study, Rao et al. created interview guides that were parallel to their quantitative questionnaires based on theoretical constructs.[5]

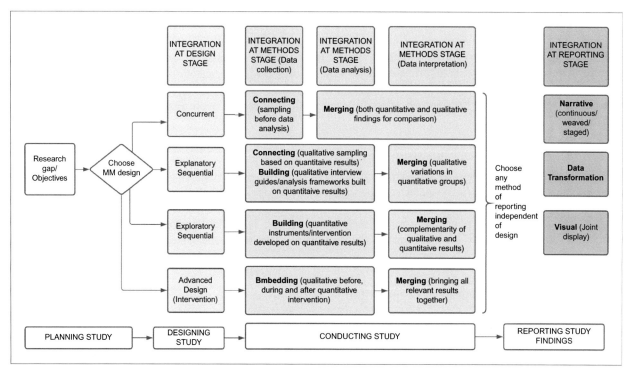

FIG. 1   Integration in mixed method studies.

Connecting

Connecting approach to integration is commonly used in explanatory sequential designs, where the qualitative data links to the quantitative data through the sampling frame. The participants in the qualitative phase are selected purposefully based on their responses to the initial quantitative measurements. Although not explicitly stated as connecting, in a study of prescribing errors, interviews were conducted with only those prescribers who made errors that were identified in the preceding quantitative phase.[33] Connecting can also be used in concurrent designs if the participants from the qualitative phase are selected from the quantitative phase before conducting quantitative analysis. This way, the two phases are connected through sampling, but the data collection and analysis of the two phases are still occurring almost simultaneously.

Building

A building approach to integration is used when results from one phase informs the data collection of the second phase. It is most commonly used in exploratory sequential designs where instruments or interventions are built on initial qualitative findings. For example, using themes or quotes to develop survey items or intervention features.[34] In explanatory sequential designs, qualitative interview guides can be built using initial quantitative scores, such as creating different versions of interview questions for participants based on their quantitative scores. A building approach cannot be used in concurrent designs as the data analysis of both phases must occur simultaneously.

Embedding

Finally, embedding integration occurs when one phase is linked to the other at multiple points throughout the study. Most commonly seen in intervention designs, where the intervention is the quantitative phase that links to multiple qualitative phases. The initial qualitative phase may be used to develop the intervention and inform the intervention sample using the building approach, while a qualitative phase during the intervention uses the merging approach to understand participant experiences. A follow-up qualitative phase using the connecting approach can purposefully sample participants who showed treatment effects to contextualize the intervention findings. Thus, the quantitative and qualitative phases are linked at multiple points during data collection and analysis. Although published separately, Hadi et al. used qualitative interviews during an intervention to explore participant experiences and evaluate patient satisfaction at the end of the intervention.[18,35]

Solution: Using appropriate integration strategies

As discussed above, certain integration strategies are applicable to specific designs. Researchers may also use more than one strategy within the same study if needed. In the explanatory sequential study on medication adherence, Rao et al. used the connecting approach during qualitative sampling and merging at the final interpretation stage.[5] Regardless of the specific strategies used, it is important to specify and describe how they were applied in the manuscript. In addition to the strategies at design and methods level described above, integration also occurs at the interpreting and reporting level through various ways including narrative or data transformation.[31] Narrative integration uses a written approach which can either be contiguous (results of quantitative, qualitative, and mixed phases reported one after the other), weaved (quantitative and qualitative results alternated by theme/theoretical construct) or staged (each phase reported in different publications). Data transformation involves transforming one data type into another (usually qualitative into quantitative) and integrating it together. More recently, visual approaches are being used for reporting integration, named "joint displays"[31] (details in section below).

Issues of credibility and validity in mixed methods research

Issues of credibility and validity in mixed methods studies stem from two main sources; the individual quantitative or qualitative phases and the mixed methods study overall. This chapter will mainly focus on the validity and credibility of the overall mixed methods study. It is important to note that quantitative and qualitative researchers approach validity and credibility issues very differently, primarily because of the differences in paradigms.[7] Postpositivist theories usually form the basis of quantitative research which relies on a "single truth,"[36] while constructivist theories used in qualitative research support the "multiple truths" idea.[37] Regardless, it is important to maintain high reliability and validity (if quantitative) or trust and credibility (if qualitative) in individual phases by following the set standards for the separate qualitative and quantitative strands, and completing the appropriate tests/procedures.

Legitimation of mixed method studies

Due to the differences in quantitative and qualitative terminologies, validity or credibility in mixed methods research is referred to as "legitimation."[38] Legitimation is described as the quality of the mixed methods study, including the quality of its individual phases, integration, conclusions and interpretations made.[38] The concept of legitimation is based on the Quantitative and Qualitative Legitimation Models,[38,39] both of which describe the threats to validity and credibility, respectively, that can occur at various stages of the study. This was adapted for mixed methods studies where threats to validity or credibility can be made worse due to the additive nature of mixed methods studies.[38]

There are 11 types of legitimation,[40] with "multiple validities" legitimation (validity of individual strands) being the most basic as compared to more advanced legitimation types described below. An advantage of mixed methods is the potential to overcome weaknesses of one phase with the strengths of the other. If this is not realized and specified in the research, the "weakness minimization" legitimation is not achieved. "Sample integration" legitimation is another important type to be considered with common threats to this legitimation occurring when researchers use unequal sample sizes in concurrent designs or the qualitative sample is not a subset of the initial quantitative phase in an explanatory design.[38,40] Some studies may also use a small sample in the quantitative phase of the exploratory design, similar to the initial qualitative phase, which undermines sample integration legitimation. "Sequential" legitimation is a type that considers the extent to which the later phase is appropriately built on the earlier phase. Explanatory designs where qualitative findings do not explain quantitative results or exploratory designs where the quantitative strand is not directly built on the qualitative findings are threats to sequential legitimation.[40] Finally, "integration" legitimation is also commonly threatened when quantitative and qualitative results are kept separate or the two phases do not address the same research topic. Other types of legitimation include commensurability, paradigm, emic-etic, multiple stakeholder, conversion, and pragmatic legitimation.[40]

Solution: Addressing threats to legitimation

Researchers must address issues of credibility and validity in mixed method studies and discuss their approach in manuscripts. Firstly, there should be focused attention to the validity of individual phases to ensure that threats to multiple validities legitimation are minimized. Threats to integration legitimation can be reduced if systematic procedures for integration as described above are followed. Researchers also must specify how strengths or weaknesses of one phase are augmented or minimized respectively by the other phase in their study. Using correct sampling procedures as directed by the study design and providing rationale for any deviations from the specified procedures are ways to ensure sample integration legitimation. Sequential legitimation can be addressed by choosing the appropriate qualitative sample and developing interview questions based on the initial quantitative results in the explanatory sequential designs, as well as explicitly stating how quantitative measures were developed based on qualitative findings in exploratory designs. Other types of legitimation[38,40] must also be addressed in the methods or limitation sections if applicable to the study. All 11 types of legitimation, their descriptions and ways to address potential threats to these legitimation types are summarized in Table 2.

Tools and techniques in mixed methods research

In addition to addressing the three common methodological gaps in mixed studies, researchers can use some tools and techniques to plan, conduct, and report mixed methods research effectively. We describe three useful tools.

Procedural diagrams

A procedural diagram is a drawing or figure that visually represents the study design, quantitative and qualitative data collection and analysis procedures, points of integration, and interpreting procedures in a mixed methods study.[41] Considering the complex nature of mixed methods studies and the multiple moving parts, visually communicating the entire study in one place becomes essential.[30] These diagrams are especially useful in research proposals, for dissertation presentations, grant applications, and journal manuscripts. They are also useful in planning studies with large multidisciplinary teams and communicating procedures efficiently when restrictions on length, words, and space apply. It is recommended to keep the diagram as simple as possible at the beginning and then start adding study content/methodological components to fit within a page. Some general guidelines include using squares/rectangles for individual phases, circles for the integration phase, using → for indicating flow, and using colors to show differentiation. These diagrams also consist of procedures (data collection/analysis/integration approach) and the resulting products.[42] Additionally, researchers can add aims, timeline, conceptual framework constructs, etc. if needed. Diagrams must have a descriptive title of the study and can show the priority

TABLE 2 Legitimation types with descriptions and ways to address threats to legitimation.[38–40]

Legitimation type	Brief description	Ways to address threats to legitimation
Multiple validities	Validity of quantitative and credibility of qualitative phase	Address potential threats to validity or credibility when designing the study
Weakness minimization	Weaknesses of one phase being compensated by strengths of other	Specify how weaknesses of one phase is minimized by the other phase
Sample integration	Appropriate sampling technique for both phases and integration of samples	Concurrent: Avoid unequal sample sizes or provide rationale for differences Explanatory: Qualitative sample must be a subset of quantitative sample Exploratory: Quantitative sample should not be the same size as qualitative sample
Sequential	Later phase appropriately built on earlier phase	Explanatory: Qualitative interview guides designed based on quantitative results Exploratory: Specify how the quantitative phase was directly built on qualitative findings
Integration	Successful integration of phases at study design, methods, interpretation, and reporting	Use appropriate integration strategies at design (Table 1), methods and reporting (described above) level (also see "Joint display" section)
Commensurability	Metainferences represent both the quantitative and qualitative lenses	Specify the cognitive switch from one lens to the other in manuscript Integration results should be presented with a mixed lens.
Paradigm	Successful integration of different quantitative and qualitative paradigms/philosophies	Specify the paradigm or philosophy used in the study
Emic-etic	Insider (participant) and outsider (observers/researchers) perspectives depicted	Balance both perspectives when reporting findings/provide rationale for imbalance
Multiple stakeholder	Addressing all stakeholder interests (especially in community-based research)	Include all stakeholder perspectives during planning, conducting, and disseminating study information
Pragmatic	Meeting research goals and providing actionable results	Specify how goals were met and state actionable suggestions

of the phase by using uppercase notations to describe the phase (QUAN/QUAL). We have created an example sketch of a procedural diagram that highlights these key elements (Fig. 2).

Although procedural diagrams have rarely been used in pharmacy-specific research, they are common in mixed methods publications within the social and administrative health sciences field.[43,44] It is important to note that diagrams may change as the study progresses, especially in complex designs. For example, Shiyanbola et al. initially planned a pharmacist-led health literacy intervention mixed methods study with the qualitative phase capturing patient perceptions postintervention, i.e., the core design used was explanatory sequential.[45] However, after pharmacist and expert input, they included a qualitative component during the intervention by audio-recording some of the pharmacist-led sessions, i.e., concurrent design. Below is the newly developed procedural diagram (Fig. 3).

Implementation matrix

In contrast to procedural diagrams that provide the big picture details of the study (bird's eye view), implementation matrices have more specific information regarding study procedures (forest-level view).[41] They can be included in proposal/manuscripts to communicate procedures visually rather than only in text (ground-level view).[41] Although some information may be repeated in the diagram and matrix, it is often useful to present multiple visuals of similar information to optimize communication to reviewers. Implementation matrices are tables that illustrate the overall mixed methods study

FIG. 2 Example sketch of a procedural diagram with the three key elements (procedures, products, merged data) highlighted.[41]

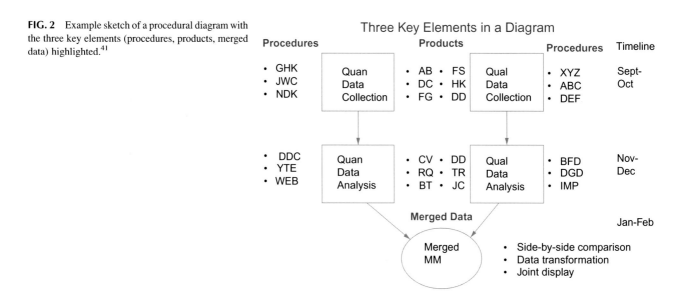

FIG. 3 Procedural diagram of an intervention mixed methods design to improve medication adherence among adults with diabetes using a health literacy/psychosocial support intervention.

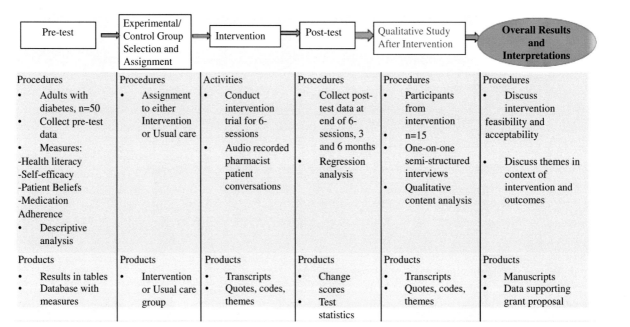

with the individual phases, corresponding aims, theoretical framework constructs, data collection and analysis procedures, outcomes or products, points of integration as columns, and each row detailing one phase of the study.[41] These matrices are especially useful in complex or advanced study designs. Apart from publications, implementation matrices can be useful in writing proposals, planning projects, communicating plans to reviewers, and conducting the study with teams. For example, we have included the implementation matrix we used for planning the medication adherence mixed methods study but did not publish (Table 3).[5] If it is included in publications/proposals, readers can easily digest information on all aspects of the study because it is presented in one location rather than at multiple places throughout the written text. It also increases the readers' confidence regarding the legitimation of the study procedures and scope of study.

TABLE 3 Implementation matrix of an explanatory sequential study of medication adherence in African Americans/ Blacks with type 2 diabetes.[5]

Study phase	Study aims	Data collection procedures	Data analysis procedures	Outcomes	Point of integration
Quantitative	To evaluate changes in medication adherence, key psychosocial, and interpersonal factors	• Convenience sample of $n=287$ English-speaking men and women ≥ 20 years old with type 2 diabetes who self-identify as Black/African American • Baseline and follow-up (6 months) mailed survey • Measures included: Belief about Medicines Questionnaire scale, Adherence Reasons-5 item scale, Self-efficacy for Adherence to Medication, Patient Perceived Involvement in Care scale, Medical Outcome Study Social Support scale, Health literacy screener, Patient Health Questionnaire	• SPSS software • Descriptive statistical analysis, mean differences (t-tests and ANOVA) bivariate correlations	• Adherence change score • Psychosocial and interpersonal factors score	Psychosocial and interpersonal factors chosen using the Integrated Theory of Behavior Change Model (ITHBC)
Qualitative	To explore patient perceptions of key psychosocial, and interpersonal factors	• Purposive sampling of 10 participants based on quantitative data • 60-min semistructured face-to-face interviews • Transcription of interview audio-recordings	Deductive and inductive content analysis	• Themes and quotes of patient perceptions of adherence changes	Participants who had a change in adherence scores included in sample [Connecting]
Mixed	To determine barriers and facilitators of type 2 diabetes medication adherence among African Americans/Blacks	• Match ITHBC constructs with quantitative scores and qualitative themes	• Back and forth analysis • Metainferences	• Joint display of barriers and facilitators of medication adherence	• Mean differences in construct scores and corresponding themes and quotes [Merging]

FIG. 4 Joint display of IPQ-R & culturally adapted (CA) IPQ-R items with sample quotes, themes and quantitative scores in an exploratory sequential study among African Americans with diabetes.[47]

IPQ-R Domains and Survey Items	Theme from Qualitative Focus Group and Sample Phrase Codes	Corresponding Adapted CA IPQ-R Items	Item Scores Mean (SD)	Average Item-Item Correlation
EMOTIONAL REPRESENTATION: My diabetes does not worry me Having this diabetes makes me feel anxious My diabetes makes me feel afraid	**FEAR OF DIABETES DIAGNOSIS AND DIABETES COMPLICATIONS** *"My daughter expect to get it now... she's so scared of getting it... I think diabetes scare you at first ... like if you see somebody with their limbs off, they ain't got no foot. It was usually diabetes that did that... or I'm blind, because I had diabetes. I don't want to be like that."* *"Right now, my father ...they cutting on his feet... I'm going to be in that situation one day... looking at my dad right now, getting ready to look like he's going to lose his legs... it scared the shit out of me... it scared me to death."*	I am worried about my children/grandchildren getting diabetes The experiences of my family and friends has led me to fear diabetes complications I am scared of having complications from my diabetes	2.5 (1.2) (61.9% agreed) 2.9 (1.3) (43.5% agreed) 2.4 (1.2) (64.5% agreed)	0.41 (All correlations were significant at 0.01 level)

Joint display

Joint displays are defined as, "a method to integrate data by bringing the data together through a visual means to draw out new insights beyond what is gained from separate quantitative and qualitative results."[31] Joint displays can be used for both planning a mixed methods study and for mixed analysis/interpretation. Using a joint display in the planning stage allows researchers to identify bridges between quantitative and qualitative phases such as matching survey items with interview questions based on common theoretical constructs. This makes the process of mixed analysis easier and can also be published as part of protocol papers. Joint displays for interpreting data can be used to make comparisons between quantitative and qualitative findings, explain initial quantitative results using subsequent qualitative findings, and examine whether qualitative findings are generalized by the subsequent quantitative results. The metainferences drawn after integration can then be included in the display for easy, visual communication and as an alternative to narrative methods of integration described above. Guetterman et al. have discussed the use of joint displays for mixed methods integration in health sciences in depth with description about various types of joint displays.[46] Side-by-side joint displays are most commonly used and can be used to depict the integration approach clearly. For example, Shiyanbola et al. used the building approach in an exploratory sequential design to culturally adapt and test a standardized questionnaire based on initial focus group data in African American populations.[47] Instead of simply stating that the questionnaire was developed based on initial qualitative data, they created a joint display of the original items, themes and quotes from focus groups, adapted items, and quantitative scores that showed congruence between qualitative and quantitative findings. Presented below is an example of a joint display of three such culturally adapted items (Fig. 4).

Publishing and reviewing mixed method studies

Mixed methods research offers authors the opportunity to present their findings in various manuscript formats and multiple publications. Common types of papers resulting from one mixed methods project include conceptual or protocol papers, quantitative-data only, qualitative-data only, empirical mixed methods results, and methodological papers.[41] However, it is important to note if using the staged approach to reporting findings, each paper must be complete on its own, with reported findings thoroughly answering the research question. This is possible if each phase has a separate research question and an overall mixed methods aim. For example, in an exploratory sequential design, qualitative themes may provide novel cultural context about a study population while also being used to develop a questionnaire. As the two objectives are different, findings can be reported separately. In general, it is always helpful to develop a publication plan before completing the study. This approach allows for the publishing of findings from earlier phases before the entire mixed methods study is completed and lets team members divide the publication writing responsibilities based on their expertise. A publication plan can include the article types, lead author(s), target journals, and intended audience. This approach works well for mixed methods research teams that are comprised of several team members with varying methodological skill sets and expertise.

Apart from the considerations that researchers must include in their studies and manuscripts, there are several tools and guidelines for reviewers to assess the quality of a mixed methods study.[28,48,49] Researchers may also use these tools to evaluate the quality and risk of bias of mixed methods studies included in scoping or systematic reviews. The Mixed Method Appraisal Tool (MMAT)[50] was specifically developed for this purpose and describes criteria for assessing quality of different types of mixed methods studies including randomized clinical trials, observational studies, and individual qualitative and quantitative phases. Similar to using Preferred Reporting of Systematic Reviews and Meta-Analyses guidelines and Consolidated Criteria for Reporting Qualitative research for systematic reviews and qualitative studies, respectively, journals must either include criteria such as the Good Reporting of a Mixed Methods Study (GRAMMS)[2] or MMAT[50] for mixed method studies as a requirement for publication or have general recommendations for authors.[28,48] Researchers in social and administrative pharmacy must stay abreast of new methodological innovations by reading journals such as the Journal of Mixed Methods Research, International Journal of Multiple Research Approaches, and Research in Social and Administrative Pharmacy if mixed methods criteria are required to be met for publication. Also, good quality writing of mixed methods studies is not limited to manuscripts only. Research proposals and grant applications for mixed methods research must also follow recommendations. The NIH Best Practices Report establishes review criteria that reviewers are recommended to use for grant proposal applications that use mixed methods approaches.[3] Recommendations for each section of the grant application, along with strategies for meeting the criteria and appropriate NIH scoring using the rating scale are included.

Recommendations for mixed methods research in social pharmacy

Based on the discussion of limitations in published studies and their potential solutions (including new tools), we have provided a checklist of considerations that can be used to conduct and report mixed methods studies in pharmacy (Table 4). The seven steps of mixed methods data analysis[41] have been used to develop some considerations included in the table (denoted Steps 1–7). In addition to the reporting recommendations included in the table, researchers may consider using other recommendations such as the GRAMMS or other published guidelines as appropriate.[2,51,52] Lastly, recommendations and guidelines may change as the field of mixed methods develops. Organizations such as the Mixed Methods International Research Association,[53] mixed methods programs at various universities and more notably the NIH Mixed Methods Research Training Program for the Health Sciences, offer various workshops, certificates, webinars, and trainings that can help social pharmacy researchers gain mixed methods skills and stay up to date with novel developments.

Conclusion

Altogether, mixed methods approaches present a significant number of advantages to research studies in pharmacy and can have varied applications. However, to optimally gain the advantages of mixed methods, researchers must avoid the three common methodological gaps of study design, integration, and legitimation. This chapter presented a detailed discussion on identifying and using the appropriate study design, systematically integrating findings from different datasets, and addressing threats to legitimation. Some important tools and techniques in the field, especially for writing mixed methods studies and proposals have been discussed. Finally, a checklist of recommendations for researchers to use at every stage of a mixed methods study has been included. There is a critical need for the development of mixed methods approaches in social pharmacy, which can only occur if researchers are well-trained in their use and continue to conduct rigorous mixed methods research.

Questions for further discussion

1. What topics or areas of social pharmacy research could mixed methods approaches be suitable for? What are the advantages of using mixed methods to answer research questions in these areas?
2. What are some common limitations in mixed methods publications? How would you identify these issues?
3. Compare and contrast the different tools and techniques useful in mixed methods. How would you use these tools in your own research?

Application exercise/scenario

Imagine you are designing a mixed methods study. Use your research area or choose one of the following research topics:

(a) Hypertension medication management.
(b) Pharmacist roles in HIV prevention and treatment.
(c) Pharmacist integration in interdisciplinary hospice care.

To develop your study proposal, answer the following questions:

1. What is your study titled? Describe the research context or problem to be addressed and develop your research question(s).
2. Choose an appropriate mixed methods study design and provide a rationale for your choice.
3. Select the appropriate integration strategies and evaluate the potential threats to legitimation.
4. Identify a conceptual or theoretical framework for your study proposal.
5. Organize your potential quantitative and qualitative data sources and sampling strategies in a table or figure.
6. Sketch a procedural diagram or implementation matrix for your study.

TABLE 4 Checklist of considerations for each stage of a mixed methods research project.[2,41,51,52]

Project stage	Considerations
Planning	✓ Identify the research gap and assess appropriateness for a mixed methods study ✓ Conduct a thorough literature review to search for similar studies, especially using mixed methods approaches ✓ Ascertain the overall purpose and research questions of the mixed methods study ✓ Evaluate available resources, data sources, and feasibility of conducting mixed methods studies ✓ Choose an appropriate study design (see Table 1) and provide a rationale for using it ✓ Write specific aims for each phase using appropriate terms for mixed methods aims (e.g., merge/explain/explore/integrate) ✓ Choose an appropriate theoretical or conceptual framework and consider any limitations of using it ✓ Develop specific plans for data collection and analysis, including mixed methods integration strategies to be used (consider creating a procedural diagram/implementation matrix) ✓ Plan for minimizing any threats to legitimation (see Table 2) ✓ Create timeline for each phase including sufficient time for mixed methods integration and interpretation ✓ Develop a publication plan for the project that includes journal options and content of each planned publication (e.g., quantitative, qualitative, mixed, methodological/protocol or literature review)
Conducting and analyzing	✓ Seek ethical approval (special considerations may apply for community-engaged research) ✓ Follow planned sampling and data collection procedures for each individual phase rigorously using the seven steps as stated below ✓ Step 1: Complete a data inventory at the end of data collection to identify any gaps ✓ Step 2: Frame analysis based on the research questions and conceptual framework ✓ Step 3: Conduct a preliminary analysis ✓ Step 4: Systematically integrate findings by matching quantitative and qualitative results and summarize results (consider using joint displays for mixed analysis) ✓ Step 5: Check for gaps, inconsistencies, and conflicting findings
Interpreting	✓ Step 6: Organize quantitative, qualitative, and mixed findings for reporting (choose integration strategy for reporting) ✓ Address any gaps or conflicting findings by rechecking study procedures, collecting more data, theorizing reasons behind conflicts, etc. ✓ Step 7: Make inferences for each research question and metainference for overall mixed methods results ✓ Consider the study limitations including threats to legitimation
Reporting	✓ Title: State the specific mixed methods design or allude to using a mixed methods approach ✓ Abstract: Mention mixed methods design and purpose of each phase along with integration approach ✓ Introduction: State the objectives for individual phases and the overall mixed methods purpose ✓ Study design: Describe the theoretical framework, specific mixed design used with justification and appropriate terminology (provide explanations as necessary or include procedural diagram) ✓ Data collection and analysis: Describe sampling procedures, data collection, and analysis of each phase, along with description of method-level integration strategies used (consider adding an implementation matrix especially if using an advanced design) ✓ Results: Clearly describe quantitative, qualitative and mixed methods results using narrative text or joint displays ✓ Discussion: Discuss findings from each phase (including implications of integration) along with any limitations including threats to legitimation ✓ Conclusion: Summarize overall study findings and provide implications including actionable strategies

References

1. Brown K, Elliott S, Leatherdale S, Robertson-Wilson J. Searching for rigour in the reporting of mixed methods population health research: a methodological review. *Health Educ Res.* 2015;30(6):811–839.
2. O'Cathain A, Murphy E, Nicholl J. The quality of mixed methods studies in health services research. *J Health Serv Res Policy.* 2008;13(2):92–98.
3. NIH. *Best Practices for Mixed Methods Research in the Health Sciences.* Bethesda: National Institutes of Health.: Office of Behavioral and Social Sciences; 2018.
4. Evans BC, Coon DW, Ume E. Use of theoretical frameworks as a pragmatic guide for mixed methods studies: a methodological necessity? *J Mixed Methods Res.* 2011;5(4):276–292.
5. Rao D, Maurer M, Meyer J, Zhang J, Shiyanbola OO. Medication adherence changes in Blacks with diabetes: a mixed methods study. *Am J Health Behav.* 2020;44(2):257–270.
6. Patton DE, Ryan C, Hughes CM. Enhancing community pharmacists' provision of medication adherence support to older adults: a mixed methods study using the theoretical domains framework. *Res Soc Adm Pharm.* 2021;17(2):406–418.
7. Johnson RB, Onwuegbuzie AJ, Turner LA. Toward a definition of mixed methods research. *J Mixed Methods Res.* 2007;1(2):112–133.
8. Hadi MA, Closs SJ. Applications of mixed-methods methodology in clinical pharmacy research. *Int J Clin Pharm.* 2016;38(3):635–640.
9. McLaughlin JE, Bush AA, Zeeman JM. Mixed methods: expanding research methodologies in pharmacy education. *Curr Pharm Teach Learn.* 2016; 8(5):715–721.
10. Ryan C, Cadogan C, Hughes C. Importance of mixed methods research in pharmacy practice. In: *Pharmacy Practice Research Methods.* Springer; 2020:137–154.
11. Hadi MA, Alldred DP, Closs SJ, Briggs M. Mixed-methods research in pharmacy practice: recommendations for quality reporting (part 2). *Int J Pharm Pract.* 2014;22(1):96–100.
12. Barker AK, Brown K, Ahsan M, Sengupta S, Safdar N. What drives inappropriate antibiotic dispensing? A mixed-methods study of pharmacy employee perspectives in Haryana, India. *BMJ Open.* 2017;7(3):e013190.
13. Snyder ME, Zillich AJ, Primack BA, et al. Exploring successful community pharmacist-physician collaborative working relationships using mixed methods. *Res Soc Adm Pharm.* 2010;6(4):307–323.
14. Johnson VR, Jacobson KL, Gazmararian JA, Blake SC. Does social support help limited-literacy patients with medication adherence?: a mixed methods study of patients in the pharmacy intervention for limited literacy (PILL) study. *Patient Educ Couns.* 2010;79(1):14–24.
15. Fisher J, Kinnear M, Reid F, Souter C, Stewart D. What supports hospital pharmacist prescribing in Scotland?—a mixed methods, exploratory sequential study. *Res Soc Adm Pharm.* 2018;14(5):488–497.
16. Astbury JL, Gallagher CT. Development and validation of a questionnaire to measure moral distress in community pharmacists. *Int J Clin Pharm.* 2017;39(1):156–164.
17. Lim R, Courtenay M, Deslandes R, et al. Theory-based electronic learning intervention to support appropriate antibiotic prescribing by nurse and pharmacist independent prescribers: an acceptability and feasibility experimental study using mixed methods. *BMJ Open.* 2020;10(6):e036181.
18. Hadi MA, Alldred DP, Briggs M, Marczewski K, Closs SJ. Effectiveness of a community based nurse-pharmacist managed pain clinic: a mixed-methods study. *Int J Nurs Stud.* 2016;53:219–227.
19. McNamara KP, Krass I, Peterson GM, et al. Implementing screening interventions in community pharmacy to promote interprofessional coordination of primary care—a mixed methods evaluation. *Res Soc Adm Pharm.* 2020;16(2):160–167.
20. Sawan M, O'Donnell LK, Reeve E, et al. The utility of a computerised clinical decision support system intervention in home medicines review: a mixed-methods process evaluation. *Res Soc Adm Pharm.* 2021;17(4):715–722. https://doi.org/10.1016/j.sapharm.2020.06.010 [Epub 2020 Jun 10; PMID: 32788083].
21. Adeoye-Olatunde OA, Lake LM, Strohmier CA, et al. Positive deviants for medication therapy management: a mixed-methods comparative case study of community pharmacy practices. *Res Soc Adm Pharm.* 2021;17(8):1407–1419. https://doi.org/10.1016/j.sapharm.2020.10.006 [Epub 2020 Oct 28; PMID: 33214124; PMCID: PMC8079557].
22. Chui MA, Stone JA, Holden RJ. Improving over-the-counter medication safety for older adults: a study protocol for a demonstration and dissemination study. *Res Soc Adm Pharm.* 2017;13(5):930–937.
23. Creswell JW, Clark VLP. *Designing and Conducting Mixed Methods Research.* 3rd ed. Sage Publications; 2017.
24. Mertens DM. *Mixed Methods Design in Evaluation.* vol. 1. Sage Publications; 2017.
25. Guetterman TC, Fetters MD. Two methodological approaches to the integration of mixed methods and case study designs: a systematic review. *Am Behav Sci.* 2018;62(7):900–918.
26. Ivankova NV. *Mixed Methods Applications in Action Research.* Sage; 2014.
27. DeJonckheere M, Lindquist-Grantz R, Toraman S, Haddad K, Vaughn LM. Intersection of mixed methods and community-based participatory research: a methodological review. *J Mixed Methods Res.* 2019;13(4):481–502.
28. Fàbregues S, Molina-Azorín JF. Addressing quality in mixed methods research: a review and recommendations for a future agenda. *Qual Quant.* 2017;51(6):2847–2863.
29. Wisdom JP, Cavaleri MA, Onwuegbuzie AJ, Green CA. Methodological reporting in qualitative, quantitative, and mixed methods health services research articles. *Health Serv Res.* 2012;47(2):721–745.
30. Clark VLP. Meaningful integration within mixed methods studies: identifying why, what, when, and how. *Contemp Educ Psychol.* 2019;57:106–111.
31. Fetters MD, Curry LA, Creswell JW. Achieving integration in mixed methods designs—principles and practices. *Health Serv Res.* 2013;48 (6pt2):2134–2156.

32. Kaufmann CP, Stämpfli D, Hersberger KE, Lampert ML. Determination of risk factors for drug-related problems: a multidisciplinary triangulation process. *BMJ Open.* 2015;5(3):e006376.

33. Ryan C, Ross S, Davey P, et al. Prevalence and causes of prescribing errors: the prescribing outcomes for trainee doctors engaged in clinical training (PROTECT) study. *PLoS One.* 2014;9(1):e79802.

34. Haggerty JL, Roberge D, Freeman GK, Beaulieu C, Bréton M. Validation of a generic measure of continuity of care: when patients encounter several clinicians. *Ann Fam Med.* 2012;10(5):443–451.

35. Hadi MA, Alldred DP, Closs SJ, Marczewski K, Briggs M. A mixed-methods evaluation of a nurse-pharmacist–managed pain clinic: design, rationale and limitations. *Can Pharm J.* 2013;146(4):197–201.

36. Ryan AB. Post-positivist approaches to research. In: *Researching and Writing Your Thesis: A Guide for Postgraduate Students.* MACE: Maynooth Adult and Community Education; 2006:12–26.

37. Schwandt TA. Constructivist, interpretivist approaches to human inquiry. In: *Handbook of Qualitative Research.* vol. 1. SAGE Publishing; 1994:118–137.

38. Onwuegbuzie AJ, Johnson RB. The validity issue in mixed research. *Res Sch.* 2006;13(1):48–63.

39. Onwuegbuzie AJ, Leech NL. Validity and qualitative research: an oxymoron? *Qual Quant.* 2007;41(2):233–249.

40. Johnson RB, Christensen L. *Educational Research: Quantitative, Qualitative, and Mixed Approaches.* SAGE Publications, Incorporated; 2019.

41. Fetters MD. *The Mixed Methods Research Workbook: Activities for Designing, Implementing, and Publishing Projects.* vol. 7. SAGE Publications, Incorporated; 2019.

42. Design SE, Delivery D. From theory to practice. *Field Methods.* 2010;18(3):1–20.

43. Berman EA. An exploratory sequential mixed methods approach to understanding researchers' data management practices at UVM: integrated findings to develop research data services. *J eSci Librariansh.* 2017;6:e1104.

44. Naughton F, Hopewell S, Lathia N, et al. A context-sensing mobile phone app (Q sense) for smoking cessation: a mixed-methods study. *JMIR Mhealth Uhealth.* 2016;4(3):e106.

45. Shiyanbola OO, Pigarelli DLW, Unni EJ, Smith PD, Maurer MA, Huang Y-M. Design and rationale of a mixed methods randomized control trial: ADdressing health literacy, bEliefs, adheRence and self-efficacy (ADHERE) program to improve diabetes outcomes. *Contemp Clin Trials Commun.* 2019;14:100326.

46. Guetterman TC, Fetters MD, Creswell JW. Integrating quantitative and qualitative results in health science mixed methods research through joint displays. *Ann Fam Med.* 2015;13(6):554–561.

47. Shiyanbola O, Rao D, Bolt D, Ward E, Brown C. APhA2020 abstracts of contributed papers: 22-an exploratory sequential mixed methods study to adapt the illness perception questionnaire for use with African Americans towards improving diabetes medication adherence. In: *Paper Presented at: Journal of the American Pharmacists Association*; 2020.

48. Guetterman T, Salamoura A. Enhancing test validation through rigorous mixed methods components. In: *Studies in Language Testing: Second Language Assessment and Mixed Methods Research.* Cambridge, UK: Cambridge University Press; 2016:153–176.

49. Heyvaert M, Hannes K, Maes B, Onghena P. Critical appraisal of mixed methods studies. *J Mixed Methods Res.* 2013;7(4):302–327.

50. Hong QN, Fàbregues S, Bartlett G, et al. The mixed methods appraisal tool (MMAT) version 2018 for information professionals and researchers. *Educ Inf.* 2018;34(4):285–291.

51. Schifferdecker KE, Reed VA. Using mixed methods research in medical education: basic guidelines for researchers. *Med Educ.* 2009;43(7):637–644.

52. Fetters MD, Molina-Azorin JF. A checklist of mixed methods elements in a submission for advancing the methodology of mixed methods research. *J Mixed Methods Res.* 2019;13(4):414–423.

53. Fischer B, Jones W, Tyndall M, Kurdyak P. Correlations between opioid mortality increases related to illicit/synthetic opioids and reductions of medical opioid dispensing-exploratory analyses from Canada. *BMC Public Health.* 2020;20(1):1–7.

Chapter 29

Using textual data in qualitative pharmacy and health services research

Laura Lindsey and Adam Pattison Rathbone

School of Pharmacy, Faculty of Medical Sciences, Newcastle University, Newcastle upon Tyne, United Kingdom

Objectives

- Describe types of textual data available to pharmacy and health service researchers beyond traditional interview and focus group transcripts.
- Discuss the benefits and challenges of using this data in relation to understanding social pharmacy and pharmacy practice.
- Describe ways to collect and analyze textual data in pharmacy research.
- Provide examples of how textual data can be used in pharmacy and health service research, and reflect lessons learned for researchers new to using this method.

Introduction

Qualitative research in social pharmacy

Qualitative research is a well-established branch of scientific enquiry.[1,2] It has long been the mainstay of historical, anthropological, psychological and sociological disciplines, and is now a recognized form of health research.[3,4] Qualitative approaches typically focus on rich data, capturing experiences, feelings, and emotions, to understand complex phenomenon.[2,5] Despite the inequality in prestige between qualitative and quantitative health research, qualitative approaches have gained traction with researchers in medical, nursing and pharmaceutical research.[6] Qualitative research has been used to examine patients' experiences of medication adherence contributing to practice and clinical guideline development, peer-reviewed publications and text-books on evidence-based medicine.[7–9] Healthcare professionals, policy makers and practitioners are using these findings to improve health outcomes, well-being and the experience of medication use globally.[10]

Transferring from quantitative research methods, which typically report validity based on large, representative sample sizes, to qualitative methods which often uses smaller samples of data, can be jarring.[11] Engaging with the philosophy, that research using smaller samples, uses rich and detailed data is valid and contributes to broader understanding of phenomenon, may be a crucial first step toward embracing interdisciplinary research methods for pharmacy researchers. Undertaking qualitative research does not necessarily require mastering specialist techniques or knowledge, however being interested in the meaning of things and an ability to reflect critically will help.[12] Qualitative research is a continuum, reaching from pragmatic approaches to theoretically driven philosophies. Fig. 1 portrays different layers and phrases commonly associated with qualitative research, demonstrating the fluidity across the layers and the ways these aspects of qualitative research are combined.

Types of textual data

Commonly used textual data in other disciplines can include data relating to experiences, such as narratives[13] or diaries, both unsolicited[14] and solicited.[15,16] Other textual data, that are not primarily created for research purposes but for communication or record keeping, are also used. Examples include blogs,[17] advertising,[18] medical records,[19,20] incident reports,[21] meeting transcripts,[22] and parliamentary proceedings,[23] textual data are commonly analyzed quantitatively, drawing inferences from frequencies,[24] for example a study in the United States looking at health messages in media found an increase in reporting over a 20 year period. In addition to frequency, topic and source media were also examined and

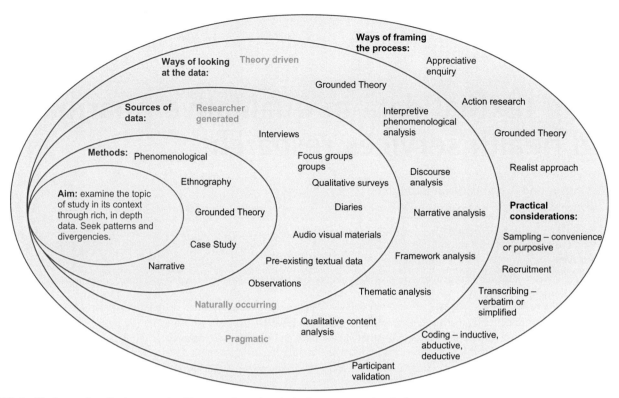

FIG. 1   The layers of qualitative research with commonly used methods, data sources and analysis.

provided new insights.[25] However, textual data can also be analyzed qualitatively, examining relationships between people, capturing perspectives and providing insights into complex social phenomenon. More commonly, interviews and focus groups, which can also be used to produce textual data once the audio recording of the encounter is transcribed into text, are used to examine these areas. However, existing forms of data such as those mentioned above can also be used to examine relationships, perspectives, and experiences.[16]

Using records as textual data

Records are powerful; they make things visible and traceable and act as mediators giving structure to social interaction.[26] Using textual data for research gives researchers two avenues, using them as a source for studying a specific subject or focusing on the nature of the documents themselves.[27] Analyzing records provides greater understanding of the process and meaning of social activities.[28] Qualitative research explores social elements of life through understanding character and process.[28] Official records, either public or private, are considered as a valuable data source by historians and social researchers.[27,29] There is a growing need for transparency across society, making records easier to access.[30,31] This data could be a valuable way of exploring elements of organizational life and practices in pharmacy, which may be harder to assess using interview or focus group methods of data collection. However, there has been a perceived lack of importance in this data source in social pharmacy research, beyond quantifying trends. This chapter describes the benefits and challenges of using existing textual data, how to gain access to this data and different approaches that can be adopted to analyze the data. The chapter also provides three exemplar cases[11,32,33] drawing on existing textual data to understand relational, organization and social phenomenon relevant to pharmacy and health services research.

Benefits and challenges of using existing textual data

Using large textual data sets broadens the horizons of pharmacy and health services research. Rather than limiting data collection methods to interviews and focus group, textual analysis of existing data opens new opportunities for understanding complex social and administrative pharmacy phenomenon that has implications for practice. Within pharmacy, different preexisting data sets may be available (see Table 1).

TABLE 1 Examples of sector specific sources of existing data suitable for qualitative social pharmacy research.

Setting or sector	Potential insights to be gained	Examples of proposed source of data
Community pharmacy	• Factors relating to practice • Power dynamics between people and organizations • Relationships between pharmacies and pharmacists	• "Near miss" incidents • Pharmacy Payment data (such as PharmOutcomes in United Kingdom) • Local Practice Committee meeting minutes • Local Professional Network meeting minutes • Support groups on social media
Hospital pharmacy	• Relationships between practice and guidelines • Presence of patient views in guidelines • Role of senior pharmacy managers • Senior pharmacy decision making • Pharmacy workforce and practice • Perceptions of side effects	• Treatment pathways • Clinical procedures and policy documents • Local Prescribing Formulary documents • Executive Board meeting minutes • Senior Pharmacy Managers meeting minutes • Support groups on social media • Patient or professional reports of adverse drug reactions
Regulatory authorities and industry	• Access to medications and pharmacy services • Perceptions of side effects	• Product submissions • Pharmacy premises registration documents • Pharmaceutical needs assessments • Patient or professional reports of adverse drug reactions
Commissioning and public health	• Relationships between commissioners and contractors • Commissioning decision making • Relationship between public and commissioners	• Formulary Committee meeting minutes • Communications to pharmacy contractors • Public Health messaging campaigns
Internet pharmacy	• Health and medicines information literacy • Relationship between pharmacy and the public	• Healthcare professional website interface • Patient website interface • Advertisement content • Image analysis • Video analysis • Social media content analysis

Complement quantitative findings

Utilizing the qualitative elements of data can improve and complement existing quantitative research findings, as can be seen with the Datix case study where medication error records were analyzed qualitatively, presented later in the chapter.[33] This interpretation of the data can improve our understanding as they represent first-hand, written accounts from the people directly involved in the phenomenon of interest. Another one of the case studies, the WhatsApp study,[34] demonstrates how qualitative analysis provide rich and detailed context to quantified data relating to incidents, episodes or experiences. Analyzing these immediate and often raw records of events can facilitate understanding of what it was like for people to experience a phenomenon and why what happened, happened.

First-hand accounts

Official documents are not necessarily impartial or autonomous.[27] Yet, there is an element of impersonality as the data creator who observed the event and recorded it, is not present when the researcher collects or analyzes the data. This element of impersonality can be advantageous, as it provides a narrative that would be likely to emerge differently from first-hand account in interviews or focus groups. Distortion exists in any account of social interaction[26] caused by the observer's choice of what to record and what to leave out. This provides unfiltered access to experiences of relationships and tensions between the person recording the data and their audience. Interpretations about what the person creating the data wanted to convey can provide insights into conceptions of power, autonomy and control experienced by an individual.

As shown in the WhatsApp case study later in the chapter, it is possible to explore relationships and hierarchy in a way that would have been more challenging if directly talking with the participants.[34]

Organizational considerations

Textual data in documents can characterize organizational communication through their form and material qualities.[35] Records typically include information about who did (or should do) what, when and where. Like a detective, qualitative researchers can use this data to paint a picture of different relationships between key characters in the records, from executives and managers, to individual pharmacists and support staff as was done in the case study utilizing meeting minutes.[32] Engaging with this data can identify gaps between individuals, professional groups and across hierarchies or professional boundaries. These inferences can support organizations to develop processes or procedures, as will be seen in the Datix case study where the health care providers reviewed the existing processes against the findings, or reflect organization cultures that could support workforce development, recruitment and retainment.

Longitudinal perspective

Qualitative analysis of textual data can also provide historical snapshots relating to a specific time and place. Many of the large data sets created by healthcare providers are purposefully date and time stamped, enabling qualitative researchers to map events and experiences over time. Analysis of policy documents might track the changing roles of pharmacy professional and support workers, as well as the consequent erosion of other roles. This can provide interesting and insightful findings, adding temporal context that can enable research to be placed within very specific periods of time. This also enables patterns to be identified over time, at different points in the day, week, month, or year or it allows comparison before and after a timepoint, as was the case in reviewing the medication-related error records before and after the introduction of ePMA in the Datix case study below. This data represents a lived history of a setting that can explain what and why something is happening now, by examining what happened before.

Data collection and storage

A practical advantage of using large data sets is that the data already exists. This can expedite data collection, avoiding laborious hours of coordinating and conducting interviews and focus groups, transcription and validation. In addition to saving time, it reduces human and financial costs as was the case with each of the case studies. Resources could be reallocated to support further research or dissemination activities. Although not always the case, large data sets may already be stored using standardized systems, such as electronic software or manual filing systems, which can improve the quality of data storage once it is transferred to researchers.

Although the impact of using large textual data sets in qualitative research is mostly positive, there are also disadvantages and draw backs researchers should be cognizant of before using this method.

Change in the context of the language

When using existing sources of data, the process of the creation of the text, the context in which it was created, and its role within the intended target audience, need to be considered.[28] In order to ascertain the authenticity and accuracy of the data, considering the role of and the reason for its creation is imperative before inferences and conclusions are made.[36] The textual data used in each case study, that will be presented, had a specific purpose it was originally created for. Researchers need to be aware of the original purpose of their data, whether it was to record an error or request for help, and how the intended audience were expected to perceive it.[27] Thus when analyzing existing textual data, it should be examined in the context of authenticity, representativeness, credibility and meaning.[27] The examination of the dynamics between the production, consumption and context of the data adds to the process of interpretation and analysis.[26] Accepting the content of a record or document without considering why and how it was produced is potentially misleading.

When considering the context, the ethics of the person behind the textual data the record represent should not be forgotten. Unlike researcher generated data that is gained with informed consent and the explicit permission of the participant[37,38] and data management plans in place for any future research use of the data,[39] working with preexisting textual data that was originally created for nonresearch purpose raises ethical questions. Even though the records are anonymous, legislation such as the General Data Protection Regulations in the European Union may prevent data being used for purposes other than that which it was collected for.[40] Guidelines are available which describe good conduct of reporting studies utilizing observational medical records[41]; however, limited work in social and clinical pharmacy has explored the theoretical ethical positions within this domain. A detailed, comprehensive and nuanced discussion is required to reconcile ethical challenges presented by using this data where consent cannot or has not been obtained from those generating the data.[42] Social and clinical pharmacists who engage with this method are best placed to contribute to this discussion and further work is needed to develop frameworks to navigate this complex issue.

Lack of participant checking or validation

Another drawback of analyzing large written data set is that participant checking, an established method of validation in qualitative studies, may not be possible. In participant checking, the researchers present findings to participants to ensure the inferences and understanding developed reflect the participants' experiences.[43,44] Not being able to go back to the original record makers can mean that the researchers' interpretations may have weaker perceived validity.[45] Without access to participants, researchers are unable to probe further into their interpretations of meanings, understandings and feelings that may only be briefly recounted in the data. The process of interpretation and analysis is solely dependent on the researcher's interaction and involvement with the text.[28] With the cases presented later, both the WhatsApp and Datix study benefitted from ongoing dialog with the data providing organization which offered a form of participant validation.

The role of the researcher can be harder without direct access to participants, as data may be incomplete or become fragmented over time. The data relies on the record maker to articulate their experiences in a way that provides sufficient information for qualitative researchers to gain understanding, while also being brief enough to provide quantifiable data for clinical utility. This data cannot always be easily found, clarified or replaced—particularly if systems of recording have changed or if staff have moved on. As with lack of agreement arising in the participant validation process[46] and the detail of reporting that brings validity to qualitative studies with researcher generated data,[45] researchers using existing data must report, openly and honestly, the completeness and quality of the data set to bring strength and validity to their findings. Additionally, researchers may engage with other methods to enhance trustworthiness, such as external audit and close reading technique.[47,48]

Collecting existing textual data

The data collection process itself, or rather the data recording process, has already been completed by others who have submitted, contributed, or prepared records in the data set. To utilize the data, it needs to be identified, accessed and extracted by the researcher. The ease of acquiring the data is affected by the ownership of the data, whether it is publicly available or requires permission to use.

Just as collecting new data requires good relationships between researchers, participants, stakeholders, and sometimes gate keepers, gaining access to existing data also requires building networks. When these data are not publicly available, access needs to be gained. Potential tools that might aid the process include offering honorary contracts or clinical roles to representatives of the data holding organization. Alternatively providing educational sessions, helping with service evaluations or quality improvement projects may also facilitate relationship-building. These exchanges should be considered mutuality beneficial and the researcher needs to highlight the benefits that the organization may receive from granting access to the data.

Creating trust and transparency through dialog will also help. A process for approval, authorship and acknowledgement, and agreeing on a dissemination strategy, can help facilitate access to textual data. Discussing and agreeing where data are kept, who has access and what training is required to access the data, can build trust between organizations and researchers. Drawing on an organization's objectives and areas of interest as well as building key relationships can expedite access to existing data sets. For example, opening up project proposals to clinical teams, inviting clinical colleagues to join existing research project panels or supervisory teams, and setting regular meetings to "feedback" on progress can help build rapport and trust.

Some data are also accessible publicly or via public powers. For example, in the United Kingdom, the Freedom of Information (FOI) Act[49] enables citizens to request access to data relating to specific events from public organizations, such as hospitals, healthcare trusts, universities, and public bodies including local authorities and Government departments.[50] The data holder has a legal obligation to respond to the request within 20 days, either providing the data or explaining why the data cannot be released, for example due to national security, propriety or the data does not exist. Similar acts around right to access information are in place in over 100 countries worldwide, with European countries providing the strongest access to information for third parties compared to other regions.[30,51] It is predicted that by 2025, 80% of all countries will have freedom of information legislation in place.[51]

Gaining access to data

Accessing large data sets can be challenging. These data sets, held by health systems or organizations, are often sensitive, relating to critical clinical incidents and near misses, or containing patient or professional identifiable data. Equally policy or procedural documents may have limited access to protect the integrity of an organizational brand. Data owners may be unwilling to allow access to data by researchers, as they fear how it may be used or interpreted and what the consequences for their organization or individuals may be. This is similar to collecting data, using focus groups, interviews or surveys, where organizations may be reluctant to allow research to take place.

Some data may be protected by legislation, where sensitive information must be withheld from the public. Although FOI requests can enable access to large data sets that include qualitative data, this has the potential to sour relationships between organizations and researchers. Limited studies have utilized data accessible via FOI for health research purposes.[52] Care should be taken when using this approach, ensuring long-term relationships are not sacrificed to meet short-term research goals. Time and resource are required for recruitment and data collection using interviews and focus groups, similarly, depending on the access requirements to the data, time and resource may be required to gain access to existing data sets.

Although there are challenges to gaining access to data, once data have been obtained, the next stage of the research will focuses on analysis. In the section below, this chapter describes two methods of analysis, content analysis and thematic analysis, and discusses how they can be used in health services research that uses textual data.

Data analysis

Once data has been collected or accessed, data analysis can take place. Most qualitative analytical methods that can be used for written transcripts of interview or focus group data are also applicable for large textual data sets. For example, content analysis or thematic analysis, used commonly in qualitative pharmacy research, is transferable to large data sets to identify key findings. A starting point of analysis is coding.

Considerations on coding

Coding is the starting point for most methods of qualitative analysis. This process can take three forms; inductive, deductive or abductive.[53,54] Deductive coding enables researchers to establish concepts, categories or units of interest that may be derived from existing literature or theory before looking at the data—in essence, a decision has to be made about which concepts to look for during coding. Inductive coding provides an alternative approach, enabling researchers to identify any data that is relevant to their research question and identifying categories, units and concepts of interests during coding— here coding is open to anything that can be seen *in* the data.[55] Abductive coding sits in between inductive and deductive, acknowledging that researchers will have some awareness of existing literature, theory and understanding of the phenomenon to which the data relates, but that researchers are looking to find *new* insights in the data, so will be open to finding new concepts in the data.[53] Inductive, deductive, and abductive coding represent how data are coded. This underpins the analytical thinking used to drive content or thematic analysis. In the next section, how to do both content and thematic analysis are discussed.

How to do content analysis

Content analysis of large, mostly written, data sets aims to identify what was said, by whom and when. This form of analysis can provide insights into experiences of the participants that created the written accounts by seeing patterns in language and sentence structure as well as revealing details about the object of the written record.[56] Examining the timing of events can provide inferences as to the external environment and contexts of when the record was made. Furthermore, focusing on content relating to people can identify factors, hierarchies, and relationships between individuals, groups and organizations.[57,58] Content analysis can identify meaning in the data,[59] for example how often someone speaks and has their contribution recorded in meeting minutes may indicate the relative importance of that person compared to other people in the meeting to the minute taker.

Content analysis can be conducted using a manual or computational approach or a combination of these.[60] A manual approach may highlight sections of data in different colors to observe patterns, use paper tabs to keep track of content within the data, or electronic software, such as NVivo, to help with the process to extract data and codify or store it. Manually working with large data sets requires a team effort. Alternatively, computational approaches utilizing algorithms can be used to automate some or all aspects of coding, which can reduce the need for human workforce.[61] However, there is an argument that especially with complex phenomena, combining computational and manual approaches is beneficial.[62]

Defining how the units and categories for analysis will be identified and then developing rules for coding is the starting point for analysis once the data source has been identified.[56,59] Once the units and categories have been agreed upon, the data would be analyzed, looking for content related to the specific information, such as communications relating to medication errors. A single researcher can work their way through the data set to identify and summarize the content according to the decided parameters. This can then be verified or cross checked by others if working in a team.[63] Alternatively, the team can distribute the identified data between themselves, which can speed up data analysis. Cross checking can still take place, as one member of the team verifies the work of another or through a whole team discussion.[56] A key part of this method is that the team agrees what the parameters or definitions of the phenomenon of interest are (e.g., medication errors) so a consistent approach is used by all researchers and the logic behind the decisions is visible to all.[54]

How to do thematic analysis

Thematic analysis is akin to content analysis; however, rather than capturing discrete categories of data, data are interpreted by the researcher, synthesized into themes that capture the nuance and meaning behind the data.[12] Thematic analysis uses a method of familiarization with the data (which can take some time with large data sets) followed by coding.[64] Coding uses words that mean something to the researcher to capture the essence or meaning of the data. Codes are compared with one another and where codes are similar, can be merged to form clusters. Coding and clustering continue so that ultimately, the underpinning meaning of the clusters are identified and can also be merged to form themes. Themes describe the experience of the participants that created the records, rather than the records themselves.[65] Themes should provide insights into what the experience is like and can include findings that relate to the absence of data (for example where coding identified information is missing) as well as relating to data that is in the data set.[64] Again, coding can be underpinned by a deductive, inductive or abductive approach.

Thematic analysis can be conducted manually or electronically.[66] Manual coding, similarly to content analysis, can use highlighters, tabs or index cards to keep track of codes, clusters and themes. Alternatively, software, such as NVivo, can be used to monitor code creation and compare codes, clusters and themes across the data set. A common method of summarizing thematic analysis is the "one sheet of paper method"[67] where the topic of interest (e.g., medication safety) is written in the middle of the page and the themes that have been identified are sequentially added to the page (like a mind map) until all of the themes (and data) that relate to the topic are included.

Examples of work

In this section, we describe examples of work using preexisting textual data to generate qualitative findings. Each subsection is a case study where qualitative methods were used to analyze textual data, our experiences as researchers during the study and the outcomes from the findings.

Using meeting minutes to identify how to promote discussion of clinical information

Board minutes from healthcare providers were analyzed to identify the nature of the content of discussion and assess the clinical content discussed.[32] These minutes were publicly available records of National Health Service (NHS) trust board meetings, recorded by secretaries and signed off by the board. The study examined the boardroom culture longitudinally (for 24 healthcare providers over 12-month period) and cross-sectionally (a stratified random sample of 60 providers at one time point). Meeting minutes were downloaded from trust websites, coding framework was developed based on a subsample. This framework was used to categorize the minute items as NHS agenda; organizational, financial, clinical, staff, and general issues; and positive comments or complaints. Of the content, 14.3% was clinical. Qualitative content analysis[59] identified behaviors encouraging clinical conversation, such as using fewer acronyms and encouraging dialog from nonexecutive directors and members of the general public. Common across providers with high clinical content was the CEO taking a lead in ensuring clinical issues were linked to all developments discussed; transparency and openness in allowing questioning by nonexecutive directors and regularly reviewing guidance on best practice. As well as synthesizing the findings across providers, three case studies were created, based on the longitudinal minutes to give more in depth view of the discussions taking place.

Attendance in person to collect this data through observation would have been time consuming and costly. Textual analysis provided insightful findings without the onerousness of physical data collection. Deciding on the coding framework to ensure reliability of coding was one of the challenges as in any qualitative project.[68] To improve reliability, a subsection of the data was individually coded by three researchers and then compared to identify and agree on codes. Being able to retrospectively analyze data longitudinally provides insights into what happened and relationships over time which may not be apparent in shorter studies.

Using incident reports to examine the impact of electronic prescribing on medication-related errors

There is textual data that is routinely collected for evaluating service provision and monitoring patient safety. An example is the Datix reports from the electronic incident recording system used in the United Kingdom in over 80% of the National Health Service.[69,70] Datix incident reporting forms are filled following incidents or near misses involving patients or staff, ideally within 24 h. This allows systematic reporting and investigating of incidents. Usually when these data are researched, the focus is on quantitative representation such as frequency and rate.[70–72] If qualitative methods are used, this is to explore the perceptions of the users of the system[73] rather than the content of the reports. Working with a local secondary-care healthcare provider, qualitative analysis of medication-related Datix entries before and after the introduction of an electronic prescribing and medicines administration (ePMA) system was conducted. The project utilized thematic analysis where the data are coded in small chunks and clustered into categories out of which themes that summarize data are formed.[64]

A total of 2236 anonymized reports were entered into NVivo, software that is used to organize and analyze qualitative data. Their length varied from two words to 2999 (mean 106 words). Inductive coding, where labels given to the data come from the data itself rather than existing theoretical thinking,[74] resulted in 1132 initial codes. Five themes were identified from these codes: prescribing process, administration errors, discharge process, context of errors and medication. The prescribing process picked up on factors associated with prescribing medication, which ultimately resulted in administration error. The theme "administration error" focused on types of errors that were made during the administration of medication. Potential errors which occurred when patients were transferred or discharged from hospital were grouped under the theme of "discharge process." The "context of errors" focused on factors not linked to a specific stage of the medication process but the context in which they happened. The theme, "medication," identified six types of medication that were involved in the majority of the errors.

Had the reports been purely analyzed quantitatively, the findings would have shown an overall reduction in medicine-related incidents since the introduction of the ePMA. What may not have been discovered is that human-related errors existed before, and persisted after, the introduction of the system. The findings also indicated that errors had changed in nature. For the healthcare provider involved, the qualitative analysis was valuable. They have since implemented changes to address human errors that had not been identified from their statistical analysis. The focus has been on improving training to empower users, such as tailored e-learning based on the person's role and access within the system as well as creating task-based competency assessment instead of knowledge based. Creation of quick lists or protocols with preset doses was also implemented to reduce the risk of prescription errors.

Furthermore, the qualitative analysis highlighted a contradiction to existing literature by showing that errors were, not only reduced in number, but also changed in nature. Many studies have suggested that duplicate administration was introduced or increased after electronic prescribing was implemented.[75–77] Yet the qualitative analysis showed that it had existed before ePMA, attributed to incorrect documentation of the administration or patient's self-administration, and errors due to a mixed economy in the transition period. The analysis of the reports was time consuming, taking 8 weeks of coding. Using software for coding was helpful to identify patterns and compare between time points in the data.

Using communication records on WhatsApp to explore relationships between junior and senior pharmacists delivering emergency services

An alternative to routinely and formally collected materials is using data that is collated informally in electronic communication records, such as messages on WhatsApp. In this project,[34] an extract of a collaborative WhatsApp group for a district hospital pharmacy department emergency service was content analyzed. To understand the context of the communication patterns and behavior qualitative content analysis was combined with quantification of certain terms to explore their usage.[59] The WhatsApp group included pharmacists and pharmacy technicians. It aimed to support junior pharmacists providing out-of-hours on-call emergency services, both clinical advice and information on sourcing medications in short supply. The extract included 1580 individual messages and over 300 communication events (periods of rapid messaging about a particular issue). Of the messages, 26% related to handover as junior pharmacists tried to identify who was on-call or was going to be on-call; 26% were procedural queries such as how to supply medications; 24% disseminated information to the whole staff, and 18% related to sourcing necessary equipment. Only 5% related directly to clinical queries. The messages were also analyzed according to staff seniority, 9% were from senior pharmacists, 39% from advanced pharmacists, 22% from specialist pharmacists, and 26% from junior pharmacist. Despite the group being set up to support junior pharmacists, the advanced pharmacists communicated the most. Their messages indicated a collective responsibility to correct the incorrect information being shared on the group by more junior members.

Analysis also identified messages were sent between 15:00 and 21:00 h, even by pharmacists not on-call; indicating members of staff were continuing to work outside of their usual working hours. Nonwork-related message content (e.g., jokes and photographs of social events) indicated the encroachment of work activities after hours led to a struggle to protect their work-life balance. Some members never sent a message on the group while others appeared to take "holidays" from messaging to protect their work-life balance.

A strength of using textual data in this study was that the interactions between senior, advanced, specialist and junior pharmacists were laid bare. Inferences could be made regarding the timing and phrasing of messages that were aiming to teach or to scold colleagues. A challenge in this study was formatting the data extract to maintain anonymity for group members and confidentiality of the issues discussed as it contained personal phone numbers, names, ward and hospital names as well as patient initials. Using textual analysis combining qualitative and quantitative elements enabled findings to present a coherent and rounded understanding of what it is like be part of a WhatsApp group. Presenting textual data in quantifiable ways is akin to information on participants demographics and study context, giving the reader a better understanding of the study and its rigor.[78]

Reflections from the examples of work

For both authors, the lack of participant validation was a challenge when working on the studies in question. Interaction and involvement with participants is central when working with researcher generated qualitative data such as interviews. Researcher generated qualitative data enables a dialog but in the case studies, there was no opportunity to ask from the minute taker how the meeting was, the junior pharmacist needing help out of hours if they felt supported or the nurse what their reflection on the reported medication error was. However, we feel that what is lost in the depth is gained in the breadth of data, this was especially noticeable with the analysis of Datix reports. Having textual data from prolonged period of time enabled patterns to be established. And because there was ongoing dialog with the health service provider whose records they were, it did not feel like the data were in isolation giving an element of interaction. In the analysis of board minutes, there was no interaction with the health care providers whose minutes were being analyzed, and this made the analysis process feel very detached and indifferent.

Conclusion

This chapter presents the case for using existing, routinely collected data in pharmacy and health services research. As an example, three case studies that drew on existing textual data available to pharmacy practice researchers were presented. Accessing existing data broadens the sources available for analysis in pharmacy and health services research. Engaging with textual data offers a wider temporal range of data subjects, rather than only subjects we can access here and now. Utilizing existing data from across geographies, jurisdictions, provinces and spaces can provide regional insights into human relationships with pharmaceutical products and practice. Disciplines like sociology, psychology, history or anthropology, possess a wealth of experience of using innovative methods to capture human experiences and inform our understandings of individuals, groups and societies in which we live. Adopting a wider range of data collection methods may provide new understanding and insights into social and clinical pharmacy practice.

Questions for further discussion

1. Other than interview and focus group data, what are other examples of textual data that can be used in social pharmacy and health services research?
2. What are the benefits and challenges of using textual data in social pharmacy and health services research?
3. How can textual data be analyzed in social pharmacy and health services research?
4. What are the differences and similarities between content and thematic analysis?
5. What approaches can be adopted to underpin the processes of analysis and how do these differ?

Application exercise/scenario

Find an online source of publicly available data, such as discussion forum, social media platform (that does not require login), a newspaper or an archive. Select keywords relevant to your area of interest (for example, if interested in medication errors, keywords could include medication errors and patient safety) and type them into the search function within your chosen platform. Extract a selection of the data that you have found into a word document and try coding it. How easy was it to search for the data? How relevant was the data that was identified in the search? What were the challenges in the process of downloading the data? How did you find the process of coding the data? What benefits could you perceive from working with data like this?

References

1. Malterud K. Qualitative research: standards, challenges, and guidelines. *Lancet (London, England)*. 2001;358:483–488.
2. Braun V, Clarke V. Novel insights into patients' life-worlds: the value of qualitative research. *Lancet Psychiatry*. 2019;6:720–721.
3. Kelly M. The role of theory in qualitative health research. *Fam Pract*. 2009;27:285–290.
4. Yardley L. Dilemmas in qualitative health research. *Psychol Health*. 2000;15:215–228.
5. Virdun C, Luckett T, Lorenz K, Davidson PM, Phillips J. Hospital patients' perspectives on what is essential to enable optimal palliative care: a qualitative study. *Palliat Med*. 2020;34:1402–1415.
6. Shuval K, Harker K, Roudsari B, et al. Is qualitative research second class science? A quantitative longitudinal examination of qualitative research in medical journals. *PLoS One*. 2011;6:e16937.
7. Kvarnström K, Airaksinen M, Liira H. Barriers and facilitators to medication adherence: a qualitative study with general practitioners. *BMJ Open*. 2018;8:e015332.
8. Jaam M, Hadi MA, Kheir N, et al. A qualitative exploration of barriers to medication adherence among patients with uncontrolled diabetes in Qatar: integrating perspectives of patients and health care providers. *Patient Prefer Adherence*. 2018;12:2205–2216.
9. NICE. *Medicines Adherence: Involving Patients in Decisions About Prescribed Medicines and Supporting Adherence*. London: National Institute for Health and Care excellence; 2009.
10. McHorney CA. The contribution of qualitative research to medication adherence. In: Olson K, Young R, Schultz I, eds. *Handbook of Qualitative Health Research for Evidence-Based Practice*. vol. 4. New York: Springer; 2016:473–494.
11. Rathbone AP, Jamie K. Transferring from clinical pharmacy practice to qualitative research: questioning identity, epistemology and ethical frameworks. *Sociol Res Online*. 2016;21:1–9.
12. Braun V, Clarke V. *Successful Qualitative Research: A Practical Guide for Beginners*. London: Sage; 2013.
13. Bruce A, Beuthin R, Sheilds L, Molzahn A, Schick-Makaroff K. Narrative research evolving: evolving through narrative research. *Int J Qual Methods*. 2016;15. 1609406916659292.
14. Jones RK. The unsolicited diary as a qualitative research tool for advanced research capacity in the field of health and illness. *Qual Health Res*. 2000;10:555–567.
15. Jacelon CS, Imperio K. Participant diaries as a source of data in research with older adults. *Qual Health Res*. 2005;15:991–997.
16. Ritchie J. The applications of qualitative methods to social research. In: Ritchie J, Lewis J, eds. *Qualitative Research Practice*. London: Sage; 2003.
17. Wilson E, Kenny A, Dickson-Swift V. Using blogs as a qualitative health research tool: a scoping review. *Int J Qual Methods*. 2015;14. 1609406915618049.
18. Roberts M, Pettigrew S. A thematic content analysis of children's food advertising. *Int J Advert*. 2007;26:357–367.
19. Merlin JS, Turan JM, Herbey I, et al. Aberrant drug-related behaviors: a qualitative analysis of medical record documentation in patients referred to an HIV/chronic pain clinic. *Pain Med*. 2014;15:1724–1733.
20. Leveille SG, Walker J, Ralston JD, Ross SE, Elmore JG, Delbanco T. Evaluating the impact of patients' online access to doctors' visit notes: designing and executing the OpenNotes project. *BMC Med Inform Decis Mak*. 2012;12:32.
21. Arnetz JE, Hamblin L, Essenmacher L, Upfal MJ, Ager J, Luborsky M. Understanding patient-to-worker violence in hospitals: a qualitative analysis of documented incident reports. *J Adv Nurs*. 2015;71:338–348.
22. Einstein KL, Palmer M, Glick DM. Who participates in local government? Evidence from meeting minutes. *Perspect Polit*. 2018;17:28–46.
23. Mackieson P, Shlonsky A, Connolly M. Increasing rigor and reducing bias in qualitative research: a document analysis of parliamentary debates using applied thematic analysis. *Qual Soc Work*. 2019;18:965–980.
24. Rourke L, Anderson T. Validity in quantitative content analysis. *Educ Technol Res Dev*. 2004;52:5.
25. Manganello J, Blake N. A study of quantitative content analysis of health messages in U.S. media from 1985 to 2005. *Health Commun*. 2010;25:387–396.
26. Prior L. *Using Documents in Social Research*. London: Sage; 2003.
27. Scott J. *A Matter of Record*. Cambridge: Polity Press; 1990.
28. Altheide DL, Schneider CJ. *Qualitative Media Analysis*. London: Sage; 2012.
29. Schwartz JM, Cook T. Archives, records, and power: the making of modern memory. *Arch Sci*. 2002;2:1–19.
30. Shepherd E. Freedom of information, right to access information, open data: who is at the table? *Round Table*. 2015;104:715–726.

31. Halstuk ME, Chamberlin BF. The freedom of information act 1966–2006: a retrospective on the rise of privacy protection over the public interest in knowing what the government's up to. *Commun Law Policy*. 2006;11:511–564.

32. Watkins M, Jones R, Lindsey L, Sheaff R. The clinical content of NHS trust board meetings: an initial exploration. *J Nurs Manag*. 2008;16:707–715.

33. Hogg H, Rathbone AP, Lindsey L. *Does ePMA Reduce Medicines Administration Errors? A Qualitative Thematic Analysis of Datix Reports*. Newcastle: Newcastle University; 2020:49.

34. Rathbone AP, Norris R, Parker P, et al. Exploring the use of WhatsApp in out-of-hours pharmacy services: a multi-site qualitative study. *Res Soc Adm Pharm*. 2020;16:503–510.

35. Riles A. *Documents Artifacts of Modern Knowledge*. Ann Arbor: University of Michigan Press; 2006.

36. Drew P. When documents speak: documents, language and interaction. In: Drew P, Raymond G, Weinberg D, eds. *Talk and Interaction in Social Research Methods*. London: Sage; 2006.

37. Hardicre J. Valid informed consent in research: an introduction. *Br J Nurs*. 2014;23:564–567.

38. World Medical A. World Medical Association declaration of Helsinki. Ethical principles for medical research involving human subjects. *Bull World Health Organ*. 2001;79:373–374.

39. Antonio MG, Schick-Makaroff K, Doiron JM, Sheilds L, White L, Molzahn A. Qualitative data management and analysis within a data repository. *West J Nurs Res*. 2019;42:640–648.

40. Mondschein CF, Monda C. The EU's general data protection regulation (GDPR) in a research context. In: Kubben P, Dumontier M, Dekker A, eds. *Fundamentals of Clinical Data Science*. Cham: Springer International Publishing; 2019:55–71.

41. Benchimol EI, Smeeth L, Guttmann A, et al. The reporting of studies conducted using observational routinely-collected health data (RECORD) statement. *PLoS Med*. 2015;12:e1001885.

42. Metcalf J, Crawford K. Where are human subjects in big data research? The emerging ethics divide. *Big Data Soc*. 2016;3. 2053951716650211.

43. Doyle S. Member checking with older women: a framework for negotiating meaning. *Health Care Women Int*. 2007;28:888–908.

44. Birt L, Scott S, Cavers D, Campbell C, Walter F. Member checking: a tool to enhance trustworthiness or merely a nod to validation? *Qual Health Res*. 2016;26:1802–1811.

45. Morse JM, Barrett M, Mayan M, Olson K, Spiers J. Verification strategies for establishing reliability and validity in qualitative research. *Int J Qual Methods*. 2002;1:13–22.

46. Caretta MA, Pérez MA. When participants do not agree: member checking and challenges to epistemic authority in participatory research. *Field Methods*. 2019;31:359–374.

47. Given LM. *The SAGE Encyclopedia of Qualitative Research Methods*. Thousand Oaks: Sage; 2008.

48. Allen M. *The SAGE Encyclopedia of Communication Research Methods*. Thousand Oaks: Sage; 2017.

49. HM Government. In: Government H, ed. *Freedom of Information Act 2000*. vol. 2000. London: The Stationery Office Limited; 2000. c.36.

50. Clifton-Sprigg J, James J, Vujić S. Freedom of information (FOI) as a data collection tool for social scientists. *PLoS One*. 2020;15. e0228392.

51. Relly JE. Freedom of information laws and global diffusion: testing Rogers's model. *J Mass Commun Q*. 2012;89:431–457.

52. Fowler AJ, Agha RA, Camm CF, Littlejohns P. The UK Freedom of Information Act (2000) in healthcare research: a systematic review. *BMJ Open*. 2013;3:e002967.

53. Jamie K, Rathbone AP. Using theory and reflexivity to preserve methodological rigour of data collection in qualitative research. *Res Methods Med Health Sci*. 2021. Epub ahead of print.

54. Graneheim UH, Lindgren B-M, Lundman B. Methodological challenges in qualitative content analysis: a discussion paper. *Nurse Educ Today*. 2017;56:29–34.

55. Kyngäs H. Inductive content analysis. In: *The Application of Content Analysis in Nursing Science Research*. Springer; 2020:13–21.

56. Bengtsson M. How to plan and perform a qualitative study using content analysis. *NursingPlus Open*. 2016;2:8–14.

57. Ceci F, Iubatti D. Personal relationships and innovation diffusion in SME networks: a content analysis approach. *Res Policy*. 2012;41:565–579.

58. Vaismoradi M, Turunen H, Bondas T. Content analysis and thematic analysis: implications for conducting a qualitative descriptive study. *Nurs Health Sci*. 2013;15:398–405.

59. Hsieh H-F, Shannon SE. Three approaches to qualitative content analysis. *Qual Health Res*. 2005;15:1277–1288.

60. Lewis SC, Zamith R, Hermida A. Content analysis in an era of big data: a hybrid approach to computational and manual methods. *J Broadcast Electron Media*. 2013;57:34–52.

61. Fu K-W, Liang H, Saroha N, Tse ZTH, Ip P, Fung IC-H. How people react to Zika virus outbreaks on twitter? A computational content analysis. *Am J Infect Control*. 2016;44:1700–1702.

62. Zamith R, Lewis SC. Content analysis and the algorithmic coder: what computational social science means for traditional modes of media analysis. *Ann Am Acad Pol Soc Sci*. 2015;659:307–318.

63. Schilling J. On the pragmatics of qualitative assessment: designing the process for content analysis. *Eur J Psychol Assess*. 2006;22:28–37.

64. Braun V, Clarke V. Using thematic analysis in psychology. *Qual Res Psychol*. 2006;3:77–101.

65. Vaismoradi M, Jones J, Turunen H, Snelgrove S. Theme development in qualitative content analysis and thematic analysis. *J Nurs Educ Pract*. 2016;6 (5):100–110.

66. Basit T. Manual or electronic? The role of coding in qualitative data analysis. *Educ Res*. 2003;45:143–154.

67. Ziebland S, McPherson A. Making sense of qualitative data analysis: an introduction with illustrations from DIPEx (personal experiences of health and illness). *Med Educ*. 2006;40:405–414.

68. Campbell JL, Quincy C, Osserman J, Pedersen OK. Coding in-depth semistructured interviews: problems of unitization and intercoder reliability and agreement. *Sociol Methods Res*. 2013;42:294–320.

69. Capstick B. *Datix*. London: RLDatix; 1986.

70. Leary A, Cook R, Jones S, et al. Using knowledge discovery through data mining to gain intelligence from routinely collected incident reporting in an acute English hospital. *Int J Health Care Qual Assur.* 2020;33:221–234.

71. Alrwisan A, Ross J, Williams D. Medication incidents reported to an online incident reporting system. *Eur J Clin Pharmacol.* 2011;67:527–532.

72. Mushcab H, Bunting D, Yami S, Abandi A, Hunt C. An evaluation of Datix implementation for incident reporting at Johns Hopkins Aramco healthcare. *J Patient Saf Risk Manag.* 2020;25:67–74.

73. Atwal A, Phillip M, Moorley C. Senior nurses' perceptions of junior nurses' incident reporting: a qualitative study. *J Nurs Manag.* 2020;28:1215–1222.

74. Skjott Linneberg M, Korsgaard S. Coding qualitative data: a synthesis guiding the novice. *Qual Res J.* 2019;19:259–270.

75. Hernandez F, Majoul E, Montes-Palacios C, et al. An observational study of the impact of a computerized physician order entry system on the rate of medication errors in an orthopaedic surgery unit. *PLoS One.* 2015;10:e0134101.

76. Joy A, Davis J, Cardona J. Effect of computerized provider order entry on rate of medication errors in a community hospital setting. *Hosp Pharm.* 2012;47:693–699.

77. Wetterneck TB, Walker JM, Blosky MA, et al. Factors contributing to an increase in duplicate medication order errors after CPOE implementation. *J Am Med Inform Assoc.* 2011;18:774–782.

78. Morse JM. *"What's Your Favorite Color?" Reporting Irrelevant Demographics in Qualitative Research.* Los Angeles, CA: Sage Publications Sage CA; 2008.

Chapter 30

Online focus group methodology: Recruitment, facilitation, and reimbursement

Matthew Halliday[a], Deanna Mill[a], Jacinta Johnson[b,c], and Kenneth Lee[a]

[a]*Division of Pharmacy, School of Allied Health, The University of Western Australia, Crawley, WA, Australia,* [b]*Division of Pharmacy, UniSA Clinical & Health Sciences, University of South Australia, Adelaide, SA, Australia,* [c]*SA Pharmacy, SA Health, Adelaide, SA, Australia*

Objectives

- Identify instances where online focus groups could be more appropriate than traditional focus groups.
- Recruit your own geographically diverse sample of participants using digital platforms.
- Facilitate online focus groups.
- Reimburse participants using online gift vouchers.

Introduction

The focus group

Focus groups have been a method for collecting qualitative data since first officiated by Merton et al.[1] in 1946. Facilitation of focus groups has not varied greatly over the greater part of a century, and they are widely used in health research and commercial marketing.[2] Compared to other qualitative data collection methods such as semistructured individual interviews, focus groups facilitate broad discussion among multiple participants to capture both deeper insight and differing ideas on a particular subject.[3,4] Focus groups have the advantage of facilitating idea elaboration among participants, helping elicit or debate ideas that may be missed by other methods.[3,5] This creates a unique environment for researchers to uncover new, creative ideas which can be employed to guide policy and practice as it relates to everyday life.[1–5]

Focus group discussions are extensively used in qualitative and mixed method studies relating to pharmacy practice as they provide rich insight into the experiences and perceptions of pharmacists, patients and their families or carers.[6] These explorations can delve into how particular policies or practices are experienced and provide feedback on how, and importantly why, participants have formed their experiences.[3] Studies employing focus groups traditionally involve a facilitator, a field note taker, and multiple participants meeting at a predetermined physical location chosen by the research team.[1,2,4]

Barriers to the traditional focus group method

Barriers commonly experienced with face-to-face facilitation include participant drop out/nonattendance, catering and venue hire costs, and difficulty targeting geographically diverse audiences.[4,7] Focus groups requiring physical attendance become impractical if recruiting participants from geographically-diverse locations.[4,7] Various studies reinforce the need for overrecruitment due to dropout rates as high as 50%, theorized to be due to inconvenience, personal traits such as shyness, and locational difficulties, especially with ill patients or traveling workers.[8–10] Another consideration is that hosting physical focus groups can be greatly time consuming for a number of reasons, including time spent searching for a suitable location, ushering of participants to the location, preparation time and financial costs for resource hand-outs, catering, and technology costs.[11,12] Dropout rates and costs are compounded by physical distance, as greater distances demand greater effort and hence inconvenience for the participant. As such, focus groups are often limited to having local participants and facilitators, impacting on their ability to capture broader perspectives.[4,13]

Contemporary approaches to the focus group method

Work has been conducted to address the shortfalls of face-to-face focus group discussions by naturally shifting qualitative research away from physical face-to-face facilitation. Marketing companies have trialed telephonic focus groups since the 1990s, and more recently in 2010, with asynchronous internet messaging boards with varying success.[7] Stewart and Shamdasani[7] remark on the potential advantages of synchronous real-time online focus groups over previous online and even physical methods. Tuttas[10] trialed four online platforms and then hosted four online focus groups with traveling nurses; this study covered the challenges and advantages of online focus groups, such as technical difficulties, platform appropriateness, and user friendliness.[10] Archibald et al.[14] further delved into addressing these challenges by using the unique features of the Zoom© videoconferencing platform as an interviewing medium[14,15]; in this case, the researchers used Zoom© due to the perceived advantages of it being intuitive, user friendly, containing inbuilt security as participants do not need to use personal emails to sign in as is required for other platforms,[7] and has recording capabilities to aid interview transcription.[14] However, it would stand to reason that any platform that allows simultaneous video conferencing with appropriate security and recording features could be used for this purpose.

An advantage that perhaps had not been previously considered by these researchers is the ability for online platforms to enable research to continue when physical distancing is required. The global SARS-CoV-2 (COVID-19) pandemic necessitates physical distancing (in many countries) to protect individuals from the spread of the virus. Physical distancing further strengthens the rationale for conducting focus group research online, as physical facilitation becomes unethical due to participant endangerment. While several studies have devoted phases of their research to utilizing online environments,[7,10,14] few studies have comprehensively described a completely online process for focus group recruitment and data collection.

The remainder of this chapter will provide an overview of how the focus group method can be adapted to be entirely online, with reference to one of our works[16] as the primary example, as well as brief references to other pharmacy-related research,[17-19] which have reportedly used online platforms for focus group facilitation.

Methods

Differences in approaches

Both traditional and online focus groups comprise of the same five stages: recruitment, confirmation and consent, preparation, facilitation, and reimbursement.[4,12] Fig. 1 briefly illustrates how each of these stages may look in both traditional and online settings.

Stage 1: Participant recruitment and advertising

Traditional recruitment strategies focus on using paper-based and/or in-person forms of advertising.[2-4] This approach can be readily adapted to an online setting such as by using digital advertising (e.g., digital flyers) on social media platforms, and email. The benefits of an online approach include no-to-low advertising cost, the ability to reach broad audiences, and the ability for more targeted advertising for the desired population.[14,16] Further, the performance of certain online advertisements can be tracked through analytics provided by certain social media platforms (e.g., how many times a Tweet has been viewed). These analytics can be useful to assess how much exposure the advertisements have received and their impact, which can then be used to refine and improve further recruitment strategies. For example, analytics may reveal certain times and days where more people view the advertisement; this will allow adjustment of the time/day for future advertisements to raise awareness of the study.

Of course, recruitment is population-dependent.[1,2,4,12] Thus, the recruitment strategy must reflect what would be most appropriate for the target population. For example, Twitter could be used if the researchers know that their target population use it and that they have an understanding of how they communicate on it (e.g., for pharmacists, #Pharmacists can be added to the recruitment tweet). Further, online strategies will only work if the target population have access to the internet. As such, it may be more favorable to use an all-online method for certain subgroups, such as younger participants in countries/regions with high internet penetration and usage.[14,16]

The online advertisement modality used depends on the platform it is being presented which comes with its own considerations as described in Table 1.

Traditional focus groups

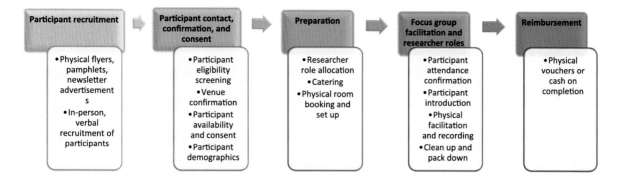

Online focus groups

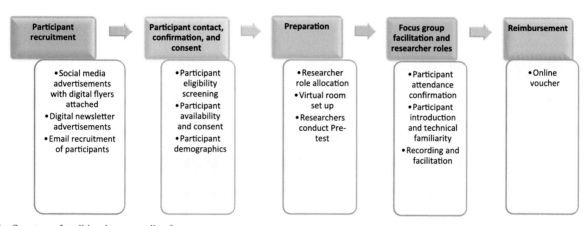

FIG. 1 Structure of traditional versus online focus groups.

TABLE 1 Online advertisement modality, considerations, and examples.

Modality	Considerations	Example from Halliday et al.[16]
Email	Consider whether to email potential participants directly or email others that could assist with recruitment (dependent on sampling strategy)	Pharmacists and pharmacist employers who were personally known to the research team, and professional bodies (advertised to members in newsletters) that represent and or train pharmacists, were contacted via email
Social media	Consider the platform(s) the target participants use or are likely to use For example, for Twitter, consider character limit and using visuals. Consider using relevant hashtags and tagging people or organizations that may be in contact with target participants	The research team tweeted advertisements from their personal accounts, created posts from their personal LinkedIn page, and created posts on member-only pharmacist-based Facebook pages
Online mass media	Consider which media outlets (pharmacy-specific or general) the target participants frequent	The research team contacted professional pharmacy bodies and societies to create media releases/newsletters

In the case of our study,[16] the target population were Australian community pharmacists, specialty practice pharmacists, hospital pharmacists, pharmacy assistants, and pharmacy technicians. Speciality practice pharmacists were classified as those practising in roles outside the traditional community and hospital pharmacist roles, such as those working in general practice, regulation, governance, or pharmaceutical industry. Participants were recruited either through multichannel online advertisements or from expressions of interest provided at the conclusion of a previous online survey study. Recruitment emails were sent directly to eligible populations from the research teams' professional networks, or indirectly via representatives of pharmacy organizations or pharmacy employers (Online snowballing). Pharmacy organizations and employers included large pharmacy banner groups, pharmacy wholesalers, academic organizations, pharmacy media (Australian Journal of Pharmacy) and professional bodies and societies (e.g., The Pharmaceutical Society of Australia, The Society of Hospital Pharmacists of Australia). These groups shared the study information with their employees, audiences and members via social media, direct email, e-newsletters, in-house presentations, and online articles. Social media platforms were also extensively used to aid recruitment; recruitment notices were posted on pharmacist-specific Facebook groups and the research teams' personal Twitter feeds and LinkedIn pages. See Fig. 2 for some examples of the advertisements used in this study.

Similarly, Popattia et al.[17] used a variety of online channels to recruit pharmacists in their qualitative study, which sought to evaluate the acceptability and feasibility of a new ethical framework for the sale of complementary medicines in Australian community pharmacies. Specifically, professional organizations and professional groups advertised the study via social media, and a number of pharmacy banner groups advertised the study through internal email distribution lists. Additionally, to ensure representation by pharmacists in regional and rural pharmacies, Popattia et al.[17] contacted 20 regional and rural pharmacies directly.

Once the advertising strategy has been decided, it is important to consider what to include in the advertisement. The way the information should be presented will vary according to the platform being used and its limitations. In general, we suggest that online advertisements should include a short summary that provides the study aim, study details, and

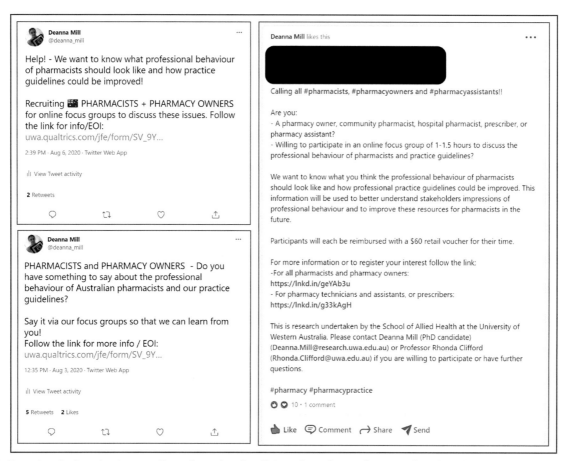

FIG. 2 Examples of online advertisements. *From: Screenshots from Twitter of actual tweets from an author of this chapter.*

participation requirements with a web link to the full participant information, contact details of the researchers, and an expression of interest (EOI) form that potential participants can complete online. The advertisements should be approved by a relevant human research ethics committee/institutional review board. Where possible, the advertisements should contain either a QR code or a direct URL link to the EOI for convenience for the participants. For example, the EOI form used in the online facilitation study[16] was generated and managed using the Qualtrics® platform.[20] However, any sufficient data collection website can be employed.

EOI forms should contain the full human research ethics committee approved participant information and any additional study information (e.g., logistics of meeting times or platform requirements). Within the EOI, it is important to ask for any details relevant to screening and selection according to the study participant inclusion/exclusion criteria (e.g., age, occupation, internet access) and participant contact details. It may be useful for scheduling purposes to ask participants' availability within or outside work hours, and to ensure adequate support for the individual in participating request an indication of familiarity with the videoconferencing software that will be used.

Stage 2: Participant contact, confirmation, and consent

At the conclusion of the EOI process, we recommend screening the EOI forms against the study's eligibility criteria. Both traditional and online focus groups need to have a mechanism to screen participants for eligibility; this will be dependent on the study's sampling strategy (e.g., maximum variation, convenience).[8] Eligible participants can be subsequently contacted and focus groups organized. The advantage of an online method in this aspect is that an online EOI can be linked with a questionnaire/online form. This questionnaire can automatically screen and exclude ineligible participants through their responses to the EOI form, reducing time spent on manual screening.[16] Online platforms also have the options of analytics, which can visualize participant data, identifying gaps or oversampling.

Confirming attendance to a focus group and consenting should be conducted once the participant is deemed eligible. As with face-to-face groups, this may be via email exchange between the researchers and participants or phone call. We suggest using multiple strategies such as sending a calendar invite, sending an email with the details, and following up nonresponders. Traditionally, confirming consent to participate would be done via a physical consent form, which is posted to participants to be signed or brought to the focus group session and completed prior to the discussion starting.[1,2] Online consent forms can be used and provided in the same manner as the EOIs (e.g., a link to an electronic form). Of note, it is important that data storage of digital information and ethical implications for this process are considered by the researchers and documented in their ethics approval as with the use of physical forms and storage (see "Ethical considerations" section for further considerations).

In our study,[16] potential participants who were deemed eligible were contacted by a member of the research team directly. This member emailed potential participants to ascertain their availabilities for the scheduled focus group discussions. If the participant confirmed availability for a focus group session, they were then emailed the study information again and asked to provide informed consent via an electronic consent form on the Qualtrics®[20] platform. The online consent form provided the study's participant information and a statement of consent with a section for an electronic signature. The form also requested demographic information and contact information required for participant reimbursement. All participant data and demographics were extracted from Qualtrics® and stored in a password protected Excel® spreadsheet, accessible only to the research team. This functioned as a running record for the study.

Familiarity with a study's chosen videoconferencing platform will vary among the participants, so additional information hand-outs such as "How to use" or "Tricks and tips" guides are important for smooth online group discussion facilitation and participant retention. For example, if participants do not know how to mute there will be background disruption to the group (ruining the quality of discussion and recording), or if they do not know how to join there will be higher dropout rates. The choice of platform is important and is population dependant. For example, some organizations may use Microsoft Teams© for their routine staff meetings, so employees may feel most comfortable using Microsoft Teams© as their platform for an internal focus group. In the context of pharmacy-related research, Cisco WebEx© and Zoom© have been used.[16–19] For example, Schellhase et al.[18] used Cisco WebEx© to facilitate focus group discussions with pharmacy students from the University of North Carolina at Chapel Hill, Purdue University, and the University of Colorado about their global health learning following completion of international advanced pharmacy practice experiences. Similarly, McEwen-Smith et al.[19] used Cisco WebEx© to facilitate focus group discussions with 4th year Master of Pharmacy students and students enrolled in the Overseas Pharmacist Assessment Programme across Schools of Pharmacy in the United Kingdom.

We[16] developed a "How to use Zoom©" self-help guide which was circulated with the attendance confirmation link to aid participants in using Zoom©. The guide covered setting up a Zoom© account and/or activating a link, trialing a test meeting to develop familiarity with the platform, and configuring device audio and video functions to ensure ease of use for the focus group. It was requested that participants change their Zoom© screen name to their preferred name, and to become familiar with the mute/unmute and chat functions. The researchers' contact details were listed to provide access to additional support. A version of this guide can be viewed in Fig. 3.

Stage 3: Online focus group facilitation and researcher roles

Pretesting

Once the focus groups have been arranged, researchers should take care to pretest and then pilot their discussion guides for their focus groups. This is an essential step for both online and face-to-face focus groups. The pretest involves the research team and several members of the targeted population who are not participating in the actual focus group sessions to meet and run through the questions of the discussion guide. During this process, researchers can "pause" the meeting to discuss if the questions made sense or are appropriate to the participants (e.g., phrasing, relevance, too open or closed), and what

Using Zoom
A Beginner's Guide

Due to this period of social distancing and self -isolation, our focus groups are being run through Zoom. Zoom is a computer program which facilitates online video calls with multiple participants. To use Zoom you will need an internet connection and a device with a camera and microphone. This may be a laptop, a smartphone, or a tablet.

Step 1. Visit https://zoom.us/ and set up an account, if you do not have one already. Click sign up and enter your email.

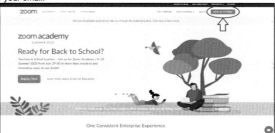

Step 2. You will receive an email with a link in it from Zoom. Click '**activate account**". You will be prompted to enter your name, and to choose a password. Make sure to check your spam folder if you do not receive it. This is what the email will look like:

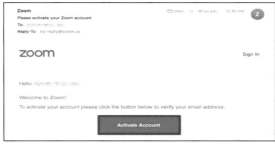

Step 3. In the next screen Zoom will offer to invite your colleagues to join. There is no need to do this, so click 'skip this step' in the bottom right-hand corner.

Step 4. From there you have the option to start a test meeting. Try it out to get a feel for how the program looks. At the edge of the screen, you have options to mute yourself, turn your camera on and off, or leave the call. To use these options on a computer, hover your mouse over each one and click.
These options will only be visible when you move your mouse over them, or tap for phones/iPads, and will disappear when you have the mouse elsewhere or tap again.

FIG. 3 Zoom guide. *From: Screenshots from Twitter of actual tweets from an author of this chapter.*

(continued)

Before starting the first meeting you will have to download the Zoom program to your computer. Zoom provides good step-by-step instructions for this.

Below: *The Zoom meeting window. This will look different on smartphones and tablets. You may be prompted to grant the app permissions, which it needs to work properly.*

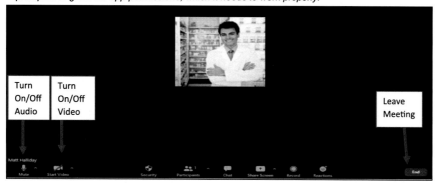

Step 5. To join a meeting that you have been invited to simply click the link that the host has sent you. Ensure your audio is enabled and your video is disabled at the bottom of the screen.

Note: Zoom will display the image of whoever is currently speaking. This means it is best to avoid having more than one person speaking at a time, as it can become confusing as the video switches back and forth.

Zoom Tips and tricks
Changing your name during a meeting!
You may wish to change your name during the meeting. To do this, click on 'Participants' at the bottom of your screen in the calling bar. Hover the mouse pointer above your name until you see the option to select 'More'. Once you see it, click on it, and select Rename. Enter your desired name in the text field and click on 'Ok' to confirm your selection.

Using the chat function during a meeting
If you wish to send a written message to everyone in the meeting, click on the 'Chat' icon at the bottom of your screen in the calling bar. The chat bar should appear to the right of the window. You can type a message into the chat box or click on the drop down next to 'To:' if you want to send a message to a specific person.

We are here for you.
For information online on getting Zoom setup please visit the Zoom help page which contains excellent tutorial videos: https://bit.ly/33LqDPz

If you are having difficulty getting Zoom set up, please reach out to our research team below

(Insert your contact details here)

FIG. 3 , CONT'D

responses and feedback the participants can provide to the facilitating team. While traditionally done in person, online pretests also assess the online platform appropriateness, flagging significant technical issues that may arise.

For example, in our study[16] the facilitation and discussion guide of the focus group were pretested on two occasions with two groups of Master of Pharmacy students (total participants $n = 8$). The pretests uncovered several impracticalities and solutions, such as not relying on the hand-raising feature in Zoom© as an indication a participant wants to speak and encouraging verbal input instead and limiting use of the chat function to technical support only. Both hand-raising and chat functions were difficult for the facilitator to monitor simultaneously while conducting the group discussions. Utilizing the share screen function to share presentation slides with the facilitator's questions and examples was found to be beneficial in keeping discussions on track. Furthermore, adding an additional role of a technical support team member also appeared essential to not overwhelm the facilitator with the technical aspects of the meeting, particularly if participants encountered technical issues during discussions. The researchers were also able to trial a number of recording options including those available on the platform and secondary back up recorders.

Pilot testing

After the pretest adjustments are implemented, a pilot test should be conducted with members of the targeted population. This is a full-dress rehearsal of the focus group and aims to demonstrate the flow, timing, and content of the formal focus groups. In physical focus groups, this provides the opportunity to find and setup an appropriate venue, plan seating arrangements, catering, and accessibility. Hosting the focus group online bypasses these considerations but does require researchers to become familiar with the technical aspects and basic troubleshooting for the chosen platform. Slides and other presentation materials are also likely to be used during the sessions, so any issues with these materials could be identified and resolved by the pilot session.

Facilitation

There are three phases to preparing and running online focus groups on the day that they are scheduled. These are comparable to the phases for face-to face focus groups. Researcher preparation and action before, during, and after each session is explained below[16]:

1. Before each focus group session (on the day)

    A member of the research team should confirm participant attendance of the scheduled focus group session (e.g., via e-mail or phone). This confirmation step should include a reminder to complete the consent form prior to the session start time. If participants remain uncertain on how to use the Zoom© platform, the contacting researcher should provide further instruction. We recommend the research team to be present 30 min before the allocated start time to open the Zoom© room and troubleshoot any technical issues including difficulty logging on, stable audio/visual connection, and calibrating microphones.

2. During each focus group session

    Participants should be instructed to join the Zoom© room 15 min before the allocated start time to ensure researchers can provide technical assistance if required. This also allows researchers to remind participants to complete their consent form if they had not already done so. When participants attend using their allocated Zoom© link, they should be redirected into a virtual waiting room and only allowed into the Zoom© room after researchers confirm that the participants have completed the consent forms. If a participant has not completed their consent form, a link can be sent privately via the chat function to allow immediate completion before the session commences.

    Participants should then be asked to join from a private area where they cannot be overheard and should be asked to agree to keep other participants' identities and the discussion confidential. Participants should then be informed that the session is recorded and to keep their audio and video on and if possible, throughout the discussion; this facilitates a natural flow of conversation, mitigates the occurrence of participants talking over one another, aids the facilitator and field note taker to capture both verbal and nonverbal communication and to aid the transcribers afterward. If the connection quality is poor, however, muting or turning off the video can help mitigate any disruptions and increase the quality and clarity of their audio input. Participants should be asked by the facilitator to state their name before speaking to aid in transcription, and also be reminded via the chat function by a second researcher during the session.

3. After each focus group session

    On conclusion of the Zoom© session, the technical support team member can close the Zoom© meeting. This triggers the program to produce an .mp4 recording, which then saves in a password-protected folder for transcription and analysis. Researchers can then discuss and debrief on the discussion and record their immediate thoughts about the content and facilitation of the discussion.

Researcher roles

Both face-to-face and online focus group discussions are conducted with two unique researcher roles, the facilitator, and a researcher to take field notes.[3,4,10] However, for the online focus group, a third role is required, which is the role of technical support.[16] The roles and responsibilities between traditional and online focus groups are described, compared, and contrasted in Table 2.

Stage 4: Reimbursement

At the conclusion of the focus group, it is common practice to provide participants with a gift voucher/card as a form of reasonable recompense for participants' time and participation. For online focus groups, an online retail voucher system is preferred as it allows more flexibility and ease for the researchers to store and record purchases and participant receipts compared to mailing physical vouchers. Furthermore, many online voucher systems allow the participant to choose from a

TABLE 2 Comparison of researcher roles between traditional and online focus groups.

Researcher roles	Traditional (face-to-face) focus group	Online focus group
Facilitator	• Is responsible for hosting and moderating discussion; asking structured questions from the discussion guide and ensuring adequate individual participation • Ensures the discussion stays on topic and that there is equitable time shared among the participants	• Responsibilities as for hosting and moderating face-to-face focus group meetings • Monitors all participants' videos simultaneously and pays attention to also engage participants without their videos enabled • This role requires a researcher with experience in conducting traditional focus groups and with familiarity in the online platform used
Facilitator support	• Is responsible for recording key interactions, non-verbal expressions, and quotes. This is to add additional context to the recordings as well as highlight key discussions points raised by the participants • Assists facilitator by raising talking points, assisting them to clarify points and ensuring that all participants are included in the discussion	• Responsibilities as for face-to-face focus group meetings but may use the chat feature of the online platform to privately send notes or talking points to the facilitator throughout the meeting, without disrupting the flow of the conversation
Technical support	Not essential	• Is responsible for providing technical assistance to participants during the session and recording the session • Needs to log in as an administrator or host within the online platform's room. For example, using Zoom© the technical support accepts consented individuals into the session via a virtual waiting room, records the session, and moves participants with technical difficulties into private "break out rooms," an inbuilt function of Zoom© • These break out rooms are used by the support researcher to test and trial a participant's audio or connection without disrupting the rest of the group in the discussion • Phone numbers of participants are also held by this researcher allowing them to contact participants if they drop out from the session unexpectedly • Is responsible for recording the session either using the videoconferencing platform and/or on an external recording device to ensure back-up if one recording fails

range of retailers, whereas physical cards are often limited to a range of retailers (e.g., supermarkets, department stores, and small goods stores). Online vouchers can be sent directly and instantaneously to participants' nominated email addresses and/or mobile phone numbers.

For example, in our study,[16] an online voucher system called Prezzee®[21] was used. Prezzee® allowed the researchers to choose their dollar value for the voucher and participants to exchange that for an online voucher of their choice to one of over 160 Australian retailers. One researcher emailed the voucher generated by Prezzee® to each participant within 48 h of the focus group discussion being complete, electronically saved receipts and recorded purchases in an Excel® spreadsheet.

Additional observations and important considerations of online facilitation

The following section includes some reflections and lessons-learned from the authors of this chapter.

Research observations

Based on our work,[16] there were several advantages that we observed

- Increased convenience for the participants and facilitators as they conducted the sessions within their own residences/ workplaces. This can be advantageous for multistate sessions as facilitators and participants can participate while in different States/Provinces/Territories and even time zones.
- The research team reported that discussion transcripts and data did not appear to vary from the quality usually provided by face-to-face focus groups.
- Facilitators reported that they observed less instances where participants talked over each other, compared to face-to-face groups they had previously facilitated. Fewer distractions during facilitation led to a smoother session.

Technical observations

Participants will vary in their observed technical expertise and familiarity with the video conferencing platform; however, all should manage to actively participate in the discussions. It is expected that participants will use a personal computer with web cameras or use mobile devices. The technical support role will need to be competent to work with technical difficulties with both systems and confident in contacting participants proactively via phone call if needed to ensure continued facilitation and support. Depending on the population sampled, some participants may require the focus groups to be outside of working hours, which means they may participate from their own homes. The location in which participants "call in" from can present unique distractions during the sessions, in particular, the unintentional input of small children or pets. Furthermore, multiple people participating from multiple locations may introduce various background noises that could distort participant voices and the quality of the recoding; this can be mitigated by limiting the number of participants per focus group, as adopted by Popattia et al.,[17] who limited each focus group to 4 to 6 participants.

In our study,[16] the solution to these distractions for the rest of the group was to mute the participant until they wished to speak, via the participant's own self-mute button or by the facilitator/technical support researcher. If the participant was less familiar with using the platform, the technical support researcher controlled the participant's mute button, muting the participant as necessary and unmuting when the participant indicated the desire to speak visually or via the chat function. This intervention mitigated interruptions to data collection and maintained flow throughout the discussion.

Technical difficulties can and will likely occur during online discussions. One such difficulty is poor audio and visual input because of unstable internet connection. Depending on the video conferencing software used, this issue can potentially be mitigated by turning off video input but leaving on audio, increasing audio input to an acceptable level. Furthermore, the minimum internet connection requirements to adequately participate should be communicated to participants prior to the session. This along with a suggestion to test their connection and the videoconferencing software in the location from where they will call in may help to further minimize these disturbances. A caveat however to turning off video for participants is that researchers are unable to record field notes on body language for these participants and the facilitator must be more vigilant and seek to include and check in with the audio-only participants more. Another technical issue includes malfunctioning microphones on a participant's chosen device. This issue can potentially be resolved via switching devices, such as between the participant's personal phone and computer. The audio of the new device should be checked in a breakout room by the technical support researcher before the participant is introduced back into the focus group.

Ethical considerations

Compared to traditional focus groups, where the research team sets the venue, the flexibility of an online environment means that participants can participate in a focus group discussion from a location of their choice. While this flexibility could reduce a potential barrier for participation, this also means that there is a potential for discussions to be overheard by people external to the focus group. When planning online focus groups, it is thus important to consider ways to protect participant privacy and confidentiality. We recommend considering requesting that all participants use headphones to maintain confidentiality of discussions from other participants, and to ask participants to choose a location where others are unlikely to overhear their discussions, as a way to protect their own privacy.

Similarly, it is important to have a data management plan appropriate for secure storage of digital data. While digital data can certainly be stored on local devices (e.g., desktop) with password-protection/encryption, given that online focus groups require a videoconferencing platform, it is important to review the platform's privacy and security statements to ensure that external parties do not have access to the data throughout the focus group session. Any cloud-based data must have an acceptable level of security to prevent unauthorized access. We recommend cross-referencing your jurisdiction/ institution's ethical and security standard requirements against the privacy and security statements across all digital platforms used in the research; this may include, but is not limited to, the platform used to capture information in the EOI process, videoconferencing platforms, and online gift voucher platforms.

Potential advantages and limitations of online focus groups

Hosting focus groups online brings many potential advantages over traditional face-to-face facilitation. These advantages include the potential for broader geographical recruitment, lower dropout rates, simplified logistics and management, and lower running costs. These potential advantages and disadvantages are explored in the following subsections.

Geographical-diverse recruitment and participation

Lower dropout rates and higher demographic/geographic diversity have been reported using the all-online focus group facilitation method.[16] This may be due to increased convenience, as the participant decides on what location is most convenient for them, usually their homes. Making the setting as comfortable as possible mitigates many external factors such as stressful or distracting environments, as described by Tausch and Menold,[8] which can affect communication and discussion. In this study, participants were not compelled by work distractions or time pressures to return to work and therefore likely felt comfortable discussing their views from their homes or self-chosen environments.[8] This provides an advantage over physical facilitation in an unfamiliar location. This comes with a trade-off with the increase of occurrence of home distractions such as small children, but these can be mitigated by coaching participants to find a quite space and by muting participants to limit disruption.

Conducting all aspects of the focus group process online creates an opportunity to host focus groups with participants joining from across a number of countries or continents, leading to a greater insight of practice across these areas, increasing transferability of a study's findings. Another added advantage is that accessibility is not hampered by physical distancing restrictions, such as those required due to a pandemic, unhampering data collection.

Low dropout rates demonstrate how accessible this method is for participants and how advantageous online facilitation can be for the researcher. For example, in the Halliday et al.[16] study, dropout rate (17%) was lower than reported in traditional focus group studies (up to 50%),[4,8,9] and demonstrated that demographically and geographically diverse participation is easily achieved.

Logistics

Logistically, when conducting focus groups online, researchers do not have to spend extensive time traveling to and setting up physical rooms, collecting refreshments or cleaning up afterwards, which reduces the time commitment for conducting a focus group session compared with traditional sessions.[8,19] While there is certainly financial costs associated with conducting online focus groups, much of these costs have the potential to be included in the infrastructure costs of the research institution (e.g., cost of videoconferencing software license, software license for EOI questionnaire platform). Traditional expenses such as venue hire and catering are thus saved in an online context, and thus the overall running costs for the online method can be comparatively lower.

The implementation of focus groups online is easy as readily available software (such as Zoom©) are highly intuitive and user friendly for both researcher and participant, with technological issues usually being minor.[16] Data can be stored securely online, can be made easily accessible to a geographically distributed research team, can be reliably backed up, and does not take up physical storage space.

Limitations

Online methodology is limited in its applicability and transferability to some specific study populations. The online method assumes that the targeted population is reasonably technologically literate and has access to internet and a suitable device to use the online platform. There is potential that when using an online method for the entire recruitment and facilitation process, that a subset of the community may be unable to participate. Particularly, those who do not readily use technology, those without the financial means to purchase the required devices, or those who do not have access to these resources such as developing regions and remote locations with no or poor internet connection. Anecdotally, older populations who may be less familiar with video-conferencing technology may feel frustration with an online method and may prefer face-to-face to feel included. These issues may be mitigated by offering a combination of face-to-face and online groups and/or supplementing the data with individual interviews conducted via telephone or face-to-face if appropriate for the study design.

These issues should be considered in future research when designing inclusion criteria, especially if studying vulnerable populations.

Another limitation that may arise with online facilitation is the potential risk to participants' privacy, as the researcher does not control the environment from which the participants are participating. Some participants may feel uncomfortable sharing their experiences in fear of nonparticipants listening in, as they cannot necessarily visually confirm other participants are joining from a private environment. Physical facilitation does not have this issue as participants can clearly see everyone in the room, and can confirm no nonparticipants are able to hear the discussion. As such, facilitators should ask participants to confirm that they are in a private area and should stimulate via their consent forms that participants cannot share other participants' information, even passively through not maintaining privacy. Facilitators can then confirm this postsession via asking participants for feedback on any concerns regarding privacy and whether they felt they were adequately able to participate.

Summary

The strengths of the online focus group method are manifold and for technologically engaged and literate study populations this method represents a useful alternative to traditional face-to-face focus group facilitation. A recent case study utilizing the method demonstrated low dropout rates, the ability to recruit demographically and geographically diverse participants, and successful facilitation with minimal technological issues.[16] This completely online approach enables research to be completed uninterrupted in situations where physical focus group facilitation is untenable, such as a pandemic as described in the case study. Like all methods, this mode of facilitation does include some limitations, which need to be managed and will not completely replace the face-to-face focus group method for all situations. Future research will need to consider how this method could be applied in different study populations, and should formally evaluate how the method is received by those conducting and participating in online focus groups.

Questions for further discussion

1. What are some potential roadblocks that could influence successfully running focus groups online?
2. Would the online focus group method described in this chapter be feasible and advantageous for individual structured interviews? Explain your answer
3. Compare and contrast the advantages and disadvantages of traditional focus group facilitation with online focus group facilitation. How can the limitations be addressed?
4. What populations of participants could see online focus groups as a barrier, and how could this affect data collection?

Application exercise/scenario

You are the lead data collection facilitator for a qualitative research project, which aims to recruit a target population of 100 employees from a global aid organization. The goal of this study is to explore the barriers and facilitators aid workers face within the organization when engaging affected communities in need. The organization plans to use your data as the basis of several internal reforms and requires diverse input from all levels of the organization. The employees of the global aid organization are spread across various countries and time zones, and range in age, roles, and technical literacy. While also based in a central city, aid workers frequently travel to underdeveloped areas and work unpredictable hours. The research team have agreed that a qualitative study using focus group discussions is the most appropriate approach to address the research aims. You have been provided with a modest budget to conduct the focus group discussions.

Discuss whether a face-to-face or online focus group approach would be the most appropriate research design to address the research aim. Design an efficient participant recruitment and facilitation plan for your targeted population, with explanation of how to address the potential study limitations in recruitment, sampling and obtaining a diverse sample, as well as in conducting the focus groups.

References

1. Merton RK. *The Focused Interview: A Manual of Problems and Procedures.* 2nd ed. New York, NY: Free Press; 1956.
2. Carey MA, Asbury J-E. *Focus Group Research.* 1st ed. New York, NY: Routledge; 2016.
3. Huston SA, Hobson EH. Using focus groups to inform pharmacy research. *Res Soc Adm Pharm.* 2008;4(3):186–205. https://doi.org/10.1016/j.sapharm.2007.09.001.

4. Fern EF. Introduction and conceptual framework. In: *Advanced Focus Group Research*. Thousand Oaks, CA: Sage Publications; 2001.

5. Seubert LJ, Whitelaw K, Boeni F, Hattingh L, Watson MC, Clifford RM. Barriers and facilitators for information exchange during over-the-counter consultations in community pharmacy: a focus group study. *Pharmacy (Basel)*. 2017;5(4):65. https://doi.org/10.3390/pharmacy5040065.

6. Jones LF, Owens R, Sallis A, et al. Qualitative study using interviews and focus groups to explore the current and potential for antimicrobial stewardship in community pharmacy informed by the Theoretical Domains Framework. *BMJ Open*. 2018;8(12):e025101. https://doi.org/10.1136/bmjopen-2018-025101.

7. Stewart DW, Shamdasani P. Online focus groups. *J Advert*. 2017;46(1):48–60. https://doi.org/10.1080/00913367.2016.1252288.

8. Tausch AP, Menold N. Methodological aspects of focus groups in health research: results of qualitative interviews with focus group moderators. *Glob Qual Nurs Res*. 2016;3. https://doi.org/10.1177/2333393616630466.

9. Jackson P. Focus group interviews as a methodology. *Nurs Res*. 1998;6(1):72. https://doi.org/10.7748/nr.6.1.72.s7.

10. Tuttas CA. Lessons learned using web conference technology for online focus group interviews. *Qual Health Res*. 2014;25(1):122–133. https://doi.org/10.1177/1049732314549602.

11. Coenen M, Stamm TA, Stucki G, Cieza A. Individual interviews and focus groups in patients with rheumatoid arthritis: a comparison of two qualitative methods. *Qual Life Res*. 2012;21(2):359–370. https://doi.org/10.1007/s11136-011-9943-2.

12. Morgan D. *The Focus Group Guidebook*. Thousand Oaks, CA: Sage Publications; 1998.

13. Thornton C. A focus group inquiry into the perceptions of primary health care teams and the provision of health care for adults with a learning disability living in the community. *J Adv Nurs*. 1996;23(6):1168–1176. https://doi.org/10.1046/j.1365-2648.1996.13214.x.

14. Archibald MM, Ambagtsheer RC, Casey MG, Lawless M. Using Zoom videoconferencing for qualitative data collection: perceptions and experiences of researchers and participants. *Int J Qual Methods*. 2019;18. https://doi.org/10.1177/1609406919874596,1609406919874596.

15. *Zoom [Computer Software]*. 5.0.2 (24046.0510). San Jose, CA: Zoom Video Communications; 2020. Available from https://zoom.us/.

16. Halliday M, Mill D, Johnson J, Lee K. Let's talk virtual! Online focus group facilitation for the modern researcher. *Res Soc Adm Pharm*. 2021. https://doi.org/10.1016/j.sapharm.2021.02.003. Published online.

17. Popattia AS, Hattingh L, La Caze A. Improving pharmacy practice in relation to complementary medicines: a qualitative study evaluating the acceptability and feasibility of a new ethical framework in Australia. *BMC Med Ethics*. 2021;2(3). https://doi.org/10.1186/s12910-020-00570-7.

18. Schellhase EM, Miller ML, Malhotra JV, Dascanio SA, McLaughin JE, Steeb DR. Development of a global health learning progression (GHELP) model. *Pharmacy (Basel)*. 2021;9(1). https://doi.org/10.3390/pharmacy9010002.

19. McEwen-Smith L, Price MJ, Fleming G, et al. How do pharmacy students select their pre-registration training providers? A mixed methods evaluation of the national recruitment scheme in England and Wales. *Int J Pharm Pract*. 2020;28:370–379. https://doi.org/10.1111/ijpp.12609.

20. *Qualtrics [Computer Software]*. Versions: 03/2020 to 09/2020. Provo, UT: Qualtrics; 2020. Available at: https://www.qualtrics.com/au/core-xm/survey-software/.

21. *Prezzee [Computer Website]*. Surry Hills, NSW, Australia: Prezzee Pty; 2020:2020. Available at: https://www.prezzee.com.au/.

Chapter 31

Consensus development methods: Use in the production of national and international frameworks and tools in health systems and policy making

Naoko Arakawa

School of Pharmacy, University of Nottingham, Nottingham, United Kingdom

Objectives

- Describe an overview of the consensus development approach and methods commonly used in health system and policy fields.
- Discuss examples of the application of consensus development methods at national and international levels for creating frameworks or tools in health systems and policy making.
- Discuss the importance of transparent decision-making processes and social accountability during the development of national and international frameworks or tools.

Introduction

In this ever-changing world, key decisions have to be made in healthcare systems and about health policies often under uncertain conditions or without complete objective evidence.[1–3] It is not uncommon for key decisions in healthcare systems and about health policies to be made based on informal group decision making.[2] However, various drawbacks of such an approach have been identified, including some individuals dominating discussions and decision-making processes, pressures from powerful individuals and the power imbalance of individuals in the group, skewed decisions being made because of individuals with strong opinions, and complex issues forgotten due to an unstructured process.[2,4]

When decisions are made at national or international levels, the impact of such decisions becomes even more pronounced, often affecting more stakeholders and sometimes entire populations. Decision making in health systems and about health policies at national and international levels could affect national and global health, and lead to inequality in the health of populations. In order to achieve transparent and socially accountable decision making for optimizing national and global health and achieving equitable health access, a framework or tool is often a useful guidance to set out a plan, organize a process of policy development, and implement a health service (e.g., Rütten et al.[5] and Kaufman et al.[6]). In the process of developing a framework or tool with a collective group of experts and key stakeholders, consensus development methods (CDMs) can be applied.

Understanding the different approaches and utilizations of CDMs can support researchers to ensure rigor, validity, and transparency in the use of CDMs and decision making for developing national and international tools and frameworks in health. This chapter provides an overview of different types of CDMs, and discusses the challenges and considerations in using CDMs for developing tools, frameworks and policies in health systems both nationally and internationally.

What are consensus development methods?

CDMs use a quantitative approach for synthesizing qualitative data, aiming to achieve general agreement, convergence of opinions, or resolution of inconsistencies in scientific information around a particular topic.[2,7,8] A complex process is involved in this consensus-based decision making.[4] CDMs assist such complex processes by offering a systematic approach

Contemporary Research Methods in Pharmacy and Health Services. https://doi.org/10.1016/B978-0-323-91888-6.00018-1

to synthesizing information and expert views.[1,9] The methods are widely used in the field of health, social care and well-being,[10] including pharmacy practice,[7] and are regularly applied to the development of clinical guidelines.[4,11] CDMs are officially used by the World Health Organization for guideline development.[12] The usefulness of CDMs in systematizing the complex processes of decision making has been demonstrated in the development of health and pharmacy policy tools and frameworks.[13–16] The process allows for transparent and accountable decision making.

CDMs usually involve repetitive interactions with a group of participants to reach a general agreement in the group. There are different types of CDMs available. The methods commonly consist of the Nominal Group Technique (NGT), Delphi Technique (DT), Consensus Development Conference (CDC), and RAND/UCLA appropriateness method (RAM). These differ in terms of anonymity, the number of participants, the use of face-to-face meetings, and time frame.

Nominal group technique

The Nominal Group Technique (NGT) is a highly structured and controlled small group process involving face-to-face group interaction.[3,7] The NGT was originally developed in the 1960s by Delbecq and Van de Ven in psychological studies, management science studies, and social work studies.[17] The NGT has four main stages: silent generation, round robin, clarification and voting/ranking.[7]

Silent generation is the first stage of NGT, where participants individually and silently list ideas or issues related to the particular topic in a written format.[17] Round robin is the second stage, when participants in turn state a single idea to the group one at a time around the room, then the chair continues to record one item from participants in sequence, until all group members have no more ideas to state.[7,17] The third stage of the NGT involves clarification where group members clarify, elaborate, defend or dispute the ideas listed, using a face-to-face focus group meeting.[17] During ranking, the last stage, participants rank the preferences, agreement, or appropriateness depending on what the NGT's aims are; ranking uses a structured questionnaire including Likert scales.[2,7,17] If the predefined level of consensus is not achieved, then the third and fourth stages are repeated until consensus is achieved. McMillan et al.[7] propose that the first two stages (i.e., silent generation and round robin) can be replaced by literature reviews or exploratory surveys.

Throughout the stages, controlled interactions with small groups of participants take place, with normally 5 to 12 people, depending on the aims and topics of the study.[1,2] Cantrill et al.[3] suggested that if a larger number of participants are required (i.e., more than 9 or 10 people), the participants may require dividing into two or more parallel or sequential groups. Participants of the NGT are "experts" in the topic or issue being investigated. This has an impact on the validity, credibility, reliability and acceptability of the findings of the method.[18,19] Careful consideration should be given to group composition regardless of different types of CDMs, as different stakeholder groups tend to produce different ratings. A systematic review conducted by Hutchings and Raine[20] summarized the impact on the selection of specialities depending on the aim of the study. However, the review also indicated that within defined specialist or professional categories, selecting particular individuals has little impact on the rating.[20]

The main advantages of the NGT include the ability to obtain relatively quick outcomes,[7] generating a large number of ideas,[1] and greater "ownership" of the decisions and tools developed by participants,[2] which can affect how the decisions or tools are implemented after the study. On the other hand, some limitations include relatively small number of participants,[2] and the difficulty in setting up face-to-face meetings.[7]

Delphi technique

The Delphi Technique (DT) is an iterative survey technique for group decision making which can occur without face-to-face interactions.[3] The DT was introduced by the RAND Corporation in the United States in the 1950s, as a means to forecasting the effects of atomic warfare in the United States.[4] Since the DT was first introduced, the method has been used in academic research, including science, technology, health, business, communication, education and policy analysis.[1,9] The DT can be applied within the pharmacy practice field. McMillan et al.[7] showcased examples which include a scoping exercise of future practice and education, developing criteria, indicators and definitions, and the more widespread utilization for clinical guidelines development.

The DT process includes collecting opinions/views on a particular issue, rating the agreement with each item/statement, and rerating the agreement with updated items/statements.[9] All stages are carried out using an anonymous questionnaire. This means participants never meet or interact in the DT.[4] Originally, the questionnaires were required to be distributed by mail, but recently this has been replaced largely by email or online questionnaires.[7] The rerating stage can be repeated as often as needed depending on the degree of agreement reached from the second stage, or until a predetermined number of rounds are completed.[1] In the first stage of the DT, opinions or views from experts are usually collected by open-ended questions[7] and analyzed using content analysis.[3] The results of the first stage are summarized and converted into a list of statements/items in a questionnaire to be distributed in the second phase.[7] The degree of agreement is commonly measured by a Likert Scale,[7] often with written feedback especially when the participant does not agree with the item.[1] After reconsidering a group median for each item, participants rerate the updated items again by a Likert Scale.[7] Some studies have modified the DT process, particularly the first stage, by replacing it with a literature review or qualitative study to explore in-depth opinions.[3]

The DT allows for repetitive interactions with a large number of participants,[9] which can range from 4 to 3000,[18] and presents no geographical barriers for conducting the study since the technique can be conducted remotely.[2] This flexibility, the option to have a large number of participants, and the relatively low resources needed are significant advantages of the DT. Potential disadvantages may be found in the fact that the participants do not engage with others nor are they exposed to their opinions and disagreements. Participants therefore may not change their opinions often; and it is argued that the agreement or consensus achieved is lower in level than that in NGT.[2] These disadvantages can be mitigated by combining the DT with other CDMs to have direct engagement with other participants, or providing feedback from participants in the next round of a Delphi survey to offer aggregated opinions or disagreements on items.

Consensus development conference

The consensus development conference (CDC) approach is a thoroughly face-to-face, interactive method to develop consensus among panel members at a public forum. CDCs were developed by the National Institutes of Health (NIH) in the United States in 1977.[4] CDCs are commonly used to evaluate and disseminate health care technologies for clinical practice.[21]

The CDC involves a series of intensive face-to-face interactions with panel members (about 10 people). Its process is more flexible compared to the previous two methods, using iterative face-to-face meetings of experts. A group of panel members are provided with evidence on a particular issue by a small group of experts (i.e., research team of the study) who are not involved in the decision-making process.[22] The panel members will then ask questions to presenters who present evidence to the panel members. After clarifying all issues, the panel group members will deliberate on the issue, directed by their chairperson, to attempt to reach consensus.[4]

The main advantage of the CDC technique is to foster dialog, debate and discussion.[14,22] Furthermore, the CDC method embeds a dissemination process of guidelines by holding a form of press conference at the end of each round.[21] The NIH, the developer of the CDC method, invited media representatives to the CDCs in order to hold press conference at the end of each round of public discussion. However, a significant drawback of the CDC method includes the high cost of holding the public forum, which usually lasts for more than 2 days. Due to the form of the public forum of the CDC method, time of hearing the evidence from experts is often limited as the use of conference venue and time to hold such an event is limited depending on budget and time of participants. This would lead to presenters being unable to cover all evidence related to the issue.[22] This could become a disadvantage of the method, as panel members may not be able to ask all relevant questions to inform their opinions. This would result in a possibly skewed decision.

RAND/UCLA appropriateness method

The RAND/UCLA Appropriateness Method (RAM) is a hybrid method combining the elements of both NGT and DT,[20] which was developed by the RAND corporation and University of California Los Angeles (UCLA) School of Medicine in the 1980s for a health services utilization study, measuring the overuse and underuse of medical and surgical procedures.[23] The RAM is commonly used in clinical practice for developing guidelines.[24] However, the method is also used in policy and organizational interventions.[24]

The RAM commonly involves 7 to 15 experts in the process.[23] The RAM consists of 5 stages, including (1) literature review to create a list of indicators for an intervention, (2) an expert panel to rate the appropriateness of the indicators of the intervention, measuring the degree of agreement on a 9-point Likert scale using an anonymous questionnaire, (3) a facilitated face-to-face meeting of the expert panel, to discuss areas of disagreement, and edit wording and definitions of the items, (4) the same expert panel privately rerating the appropriateness of updated items on the same 9-point Likert scale in an anonymous questionnaire, and (5) the research team categorizing indicators as appropriate, inappropriate, or uncertain, based on the group median rating.[3,20] Basic data analysis to determine agreement and disagreement is similar to that conducted for NGT and DT. However, the RAM uses more sophisticated analysis using the concept of Interpercentile Range (IPR) and Interpercentile Range Adjusted for Symmetry (IPRAS).[23] IPR was developed by investigators at the *Unidad de Investigación en Servicios de Salud* in Spain while developing and assessing new definitions of disagreement in order to apply to any panel size of expert panel group. The IPRAS was further developed to mitigate a disadvantage of using IPR—that identifying an indication as disagreement required the ratings to be smaller than the median values (i.e., the median values far from 5 on the 1–9 scale). This is described more comprehensively by Fitch and her colleagues in their RAND/UCLA Appropriateness Method User's Manual.[23] Having been developed by the same corporation—the RAND corporation, IPRAS data analysis has also been adapted to DT.[25] The use of IPRAS data analysis minimizes the effect of a different size of expert panel by identifying the degree of disagreement and the asymmetry of the data distribution of individual items.[23] This also provides an in-depth analysis of "disagreement" in searching the appropriateness of items in a tool when a panel does not reach consensus.[23]

How have CDMs been used at national and international levels?

Although Hutchings and Raine[20] state the growth of the use of formal CDMs (mentioned in "What are consensus development methods?" section) in the health field, a literature review conducted by the author and her colleague found that often formal CDMs were not used to develop consensus when developing tools or frameworks in a health system and about health policies at national and international levels. The review identified that over 60% of studies did not apply formal CDMs, instead, they used a series of flexible face-to-face meetings to exchange opinions to reach consensus on the topic of the study. These face-to-face meetings enable direct interactions between group members. However, compared to the formal CDMs introduced above, the unstructured process used to reach consensus introduces some drawbacks as described in "Introduction" section of the chapter. For this chapter, we have referred to this flexible series of meetings aiming to reach consensus, as consensus meetings (CMs).

For example, Kumanyika et al.[26] created a Community Energy Balance (CEB) Framework, using a series of CMs to reach consensus internationally. The CEB Framework was developed to identify and evaluate related implications of the excess obesity risk in African and other ethnic minority populations in order to prevent obesity. Panel members for the CMs included 6 experts, comprising experts in nutrition, obesity prevention and treatment, physical activity, marketing, cultural anthropology, public health, and social psychology. The draft framework was developed at a 2-day brainstorming session, followed by iterative consultations within the panel members to make it adaptable internationally for 2 years. The exact consensus threshold was not mentioned in the paper, which questions the transparency and validity of the consensus achieved.

Another example of nonformal CDMs is the development of a national performance indicator framework for the Dutch health system.[27] The framework was created for the purpose of continuing engagement and measurement of diverse aspects of health systems in the Netherlands, including mechanism, budgets, population, the quality of care, safety issues, and consumer satisfaction. The report covers the first phase of the development, including the construction of the framework and the selection of different indicator areas of the model. The project applied CMs to engage with multiple stakeholders ($n = 38$). Exact frequency and delivery of the meetings were not stated. However, the report stated that CMs were conducted monthly with all panel members. Consensus threshold was not mentioned in the report, similar to the first example of CM provided above.

A frequently adapted variation to CDMs in developing framework or tools in a health system or about health policies is to combine different CDMs.[28] Out of the formal CDMs introduced above, DT is often used as a main or part of a combination of methods. This is understandable considering the national and international geographical challenge. CDMs rely on experts to systematically develop consensus on a topic being investigated. When the investigating topic targets a national or international audience, experts often come from different cities, regions, or even countries. Therefore, using questionnaires in the process of the DT is beneficial in such cases. In recent years, online questionnaires have been used instead of postal questionnaires, which add a benefit to combining DT function with other CDMs in the process of consensus development, considering less resources and time are required when using online questionnaires.

An example of combining CDMs is a study conducted by Boers et al.,[29] which reported a process of framework development covering areas of core measurement in clinical trials in Rheumatology globally. This study used a combination of DT and CM to approach different groups of experts in the process of consensus development. CM was applied with 18 experts at a conference using a structured discussion to develop a draft framework based on a literature review. Then the draft framework was distributed to a larger group of experts ($n = 2293$) using the DT process to reach some degree of agreement. The study did not indicate the consensus threshold; thus, no clear definition of agreement was provided.

Another example of combining CDMs is a national study from Iran, conducted by Fazaeli et al.[30] The study was conducted to design a preliminary framework for an information system for assessing health system responsiveness. The study combined CM and DT, but also conducted qualitative interviews with panel members. DT was used for validating the preliminary framework, through applying two rounds of questionnaires via email. The final stage of consensus development employed CM via face-to-face discussions with panel members in order to view the feedback, review and discuss opinions provided by panel members about the appropriateness of each category and components of the framework. A consensus threshold was employed for DT, with 75% agreement defined as consensus. A 50% to 75% agreement was used as the threshold for discussion.

Unique environments to develop national or international frameworks or tools in health systems or about health policies raise some challenges that we need to consider in the process of applying and executing each type of CDM. Such limitations include geographical spread or representation of experts, fair selections and commitment of busy experts and policy makers, and costs associated with holding any face-to-face meetings. Balancing these challenges with a need to use CDMs for developing frameworks and tools for health systems and policies, it is not surprising that consensus methods evolve to be more flexible, and sometimes a combination of different methods is used to compensate for weaknesses of some methods. However, this doesn't mean that methods can compromise the rigor, validity, and transparency of the methods and results in order to achieve sound and socially accountable decision making. Unfortunately a systematic review of the literature on the development of national or global frameworks or tools in health systems or about health policies revealed that many papers did not report the numbers of consensus panel members or consensus thresholds.[28] Reporting this information has an impact on the quality of the report and affect the rigor and value of decisions made. This indicates that there is a great need for better understanding of CDMs in health systems and services research and policy development.

Discussion

We have seen several variations of CDMs since development in the 1950s and 1960s, and the growth in the use of methods over the last half a century. CDMs have been adapted for use in the healthcare field, often for clinical guideline development or health technology assessment. This chapter focused on the use of a consensus development approach in health policy and health system improvement outside of clinical guideline development. A literature review by the author and her colleague[28] and examples of studies provided in the chapter have shown a wide range of modifications of CDMs, and many have not followed any existing CDMs. This includes a variety of combinations of CDMs and unstructured face-to-face meetings or replacing the idea generation stage with a literature review. This is not consistent with the use of CDMs in creating clinical guidelines where intensive reviews and guidelines for formal steps of CDMs have been developed.[11,31] Humphrey-Murto et al.[1] criticize the lack of standardization in definitions of consensus, use of methods, and reporting of these methods saying that they would result in less certainty in the level of rigor or in the value of decisions made for interpretation of the outcomes.

However, high-level consensus development in international settings often encounters challenges of geographical and time issues due to panel members being from different countries. Considering these challenges, it is understandable that some consensus development processes take place in academic conference settings and are combined with other methods to utilize opportunities for meetings at conferences. Other processes are conducted on online platforms which mitigate the disadvantages of geographical issues and saves time compared with travel to face-to-face meetings.

As an example, the author applied NGT for developing a national competency framework for foundation level pharmacists in Japan. Adopting the FIP Global Competency Framework, a modified version of NGT as proposed by McMillan et al.[7] was utilized to establish consensus on behavioral indicators for the framework. The first two stages (i.e., silent generation and round robin) were replaced by an exploratory survey provided to panel members, evaluating the level of agreement on a 9-point Likert scale and identifying any reasons for disagreement using open-ended questions. The third stage of clarification used a face-to-face meeting of panel members to discuss disagreed items and those that required modification. The last stage of ranking applied an online survey form to assess the levels of agreement which confirmed the consensus of the panel members by setting the threshold for the median of individual item to be greater or equal to 7 on a 9-point Likert scale. Considering the geographical challenges of panel members to develop a national level framework, pre-and postsurveys (i.e., an exploratory survey of first/second stage and ranking survey at third stage) were conducted using an online survey. This enabled flexibility of time and locations for panel members and they only had to attend one face to face meeting.

A lack of consensus criteria reporting in published articles was identified in the systematic review conducted by the author and her colleague.[28] Scott and Black[32] showed that differences in consensus definitions led to differences in the sensitivity of consensus that panels would reach. This was revealed in their study which compared consensuses reached by two expert panels (one panel had a mix of 6 different experts—gastroenterologists, general physician, surgeon, general practitioner and radiologist, and the other had 8 general surgeons) assessing the appropriateness of a total of 272 indications for cholecystectomy, using NGT. The study exhibited that exclusion of outliers (i.e., those ratings that lie furthest from the median) increased the likelihood of having agreement from around 40% to 60%. Furthermore, stricter definitions of "agreement" and "disagreement" employed, led to a larger proportion of "disagreement" rating rather than "partial agreement," increasing the proportion of disagreement from 2% to 26%. For achieving transparent and rigorous consensus decisions in health, reporting the consensus threshold and criteria are essential. This indicates the need for rigorous planning of the consensus development process at national and international levels, especially with reference to any decisions made with respect to health systems and policies which can affect national and global health. Researchers and policy makers need to be aware of the consensus development methods for better decision-making processes. Creating a guidance of CDMs to develop national/international frameworks or tools in health systems and policies would be useful.

Conclusion

This chapter briefly presented four formal CDMs commonly used for decision making in health system and policy development, and examples of their uses in the field. There is a need to ensure quality of reporting in studies using CDMs, specifically, the elements of the consensus development process (e.g., the number of panel members and consensus threshold) as these are not always reported in studies. For better utilization and application of the consensus development methods in health system and policy development to guide transparent and socially accountable decision making, some standardization of the methods and reporting would be warranted while allowing for the necessary pragmatic adaptations needed by researchers.

Questions for further discussion

1. How do you choose the most suitable CDM for your study to develop national or international frameworks or tools to be used in the health system or for developing policy?
2. What elements should be considered to sustain the rigor of the CDM in the process of framework/tool development at a national or international level?
3. How could you modify a CDM to adapt it to your setting, while retaining the rigor of the method?

Application exercise/scenario

There is a need to develop a set of quality indicators of hospital pharmacy services in your country. There are several frameworks to assess quality of hospital pharmacy services which have been developed in different countries. However, the available frameworks from different countries were developed for different hospital pharmacy services and settings. You need to adapt these existing frameworks to the needs of your country's hospital services. What CDM can you use? How can you modify the CDM you planned to use in order to apply it to your setting while retaining the rigor of the CDM? Who will be your panel members, and why?

Declarations
Ethics

No requirement of ethical clearance.

Declaration of interest

None.

Author contributions

NA: concept development, original draft writing and edit.

References

1. Humphrey-Murto S, Varpio L, Gonsalves C, Wood TJ. Using consensus group methods such as Delphi and Nominal Group in medical education research. *Med Teach.* 2017;39:14–19.
2. Black N. Consensus development methods. In: Pope C, Mays N, eds. *Qualitative Research in Health Care.* 3rd ed. Oxford: Blackwell Publishing; 2006 [chapter 12].

3. Cantrill JA, Sibbald B, Buetow S. The Delphi and nominal group techniques in health services research. *Int J Pharm Pract*. 1996;4:67–74.
4. Murphy MK, Black NA, Lamping DL, et al. Consensus development methods, and their use in clinical guideline development. *Health Technol Assess*. 1998;2:i–iv. 1–88.
5. Rütten A, Gelius P, Abu-Omar K. Policy development and implementation in health promotion—from theory to practice: the ADEPT model. *Health Promot Int*. 2010;26:322–329.
6. Kaufman D, Roberts WD, Merrill J, Lai T-Y, Bakken S. Applying an evaluation framework for health information system design, development, and implementation. *Nurs Res*. 2006;55:S37–S42.
7. McMillan SS, King M, Tully MP. How to use the nominal group and Delphi techniques. *Int J Clin Pharm*. 2016;38:655–662.
8. Tammela O. Applications of consensus methods in the improvement of care of paediatric patients: a step forward from a 'good guess'. *Acta Pediatr*. 2013;102:111–115.
9. Jones J, Hunter D. Qualitative research: consensus methods for medical and health services research. *BMJ*. 1995;311:376.
10. Guzys D, Dickson-Swift V, Kenny A, Threlkeld G. Gadamerian philosophical hermeneutics as a useful methodological framework for the Delphi technique. *Int J Qual Stud Health Well Being*. 2015;10:26291.
11. Black N, Murphy DM, Lamping D, et al. Consensus development methods: a review of best practice in creating clinical guidelines. *J Health Serv Res Policy*. 1999;4:236–248.
12. World Health Organization. *WHO Handbook for Guideline Development*. 2nd ed. Geneva: World Health Organization; 2014.
13. Martin CM, Kasperski J. Developing interdisciplinary maternity services policy in Canada. Evaluation of a consensus workshop. *J Eval Clin Pract*. 2010;16:238–245.
14. Halcomb E, Davidson P, Hardaker L. Using the consensus development conference method in healthcare research. *Nurs Res*. 2008;16:56–71.
15. Calltorp J. Consensus development conferences in Sweden: effects on health policy and administration. *Int J Technol Assess Health Care*. 1988;4:75–88.
16. Beech B. The Delphi approach: recent applications in health care. *Nurs Res*. 2001;8:38–48.
17. Van de Ven AH, Delbecq AL. The nominal group as a research instrument for exploratory health studies. *Am J Public Health*. 1972;62:337–342.
18. Campbell SM, Cantrill JA. Consensus methods in prescribing research. *J Clin Pharm Ther*. 2001;26:5–14.
19. Grimshaw J, Russell I. Achieving health gain through clinical guidelines. I: developing scientifically valid guidelines. *Qual Health Care*. 1993;2:243–248.
20. Hutchings A, Raine R. A systematic review of factors affecting the judgments produced by formal consensus development methods in health care. *J Health Serv Res Policy*. 2006;11:172–179.
21. Fink A, Kosecoff J, Chassin M, Brook RH. Consensus methods: characteristics and guidelines for use. *Am J Public Health*. 1984;74:979–983.
22. James D, Warren-Forward H. Research methods for formal consensus development. *Nurs Res*. 2015;22:35–40.
23. Fitch K, Bernstein SJ, Aguilar MD, et al. *The RAND/UCLA Appropriateness Method User's Manual*. Santa Monica, CA: RAND; 2001.
24. Campbell JL, Fletcher E, Abel G, et al. Policies and strategies to retain and support the return of experienced GPs in direct patient care: the ReGROUP mixed-methods study. *Hearth Serv Deliv Res*. 2019;7.
25. Deshpande AM, Shiffman RN, Nadkarni PM. Metadata-driven Delphi rating on the internet. *Comput Methods Prog Biomed*. 2005;77:49–56.
26. Kumanyika S, Taylor WC, Grier SA, et al. Community energy balance: a framework for contextualizing cultural influences on high risk of obesity in ethnic minority populations. *Prev Med*. 2012;55:371–381.
27. ten Asbroek AHA, Arah OA, Geelhoed J, Custers T, Delnoij DM, Klazinga NS. Developing a national performance indicator framework for the Dutch health system. *Int J Qual Health Care*. 2004;16:i65–i71.
28. Arakawa N, Bader L. Consensus development methods: considerations for national and global frameworks and policy development. *Res Soc Adm Pharm*. 2022;18:2222–2229.
29. Boers M, Idzerda L, Kirwan JR, et al. Toward a generalized framework of core measurement areas in clinical trials: a position paper for OMERACT 11. *J Rheumatol*. 2014;41:978.
30. Fazaeli S, Ahmadi M, Rashidian A, Sadoughi F. A framework of a health system responsiveness assessment information system for Iran. *Iran Red Crescent Med J*. 2014;16:e17820.
31. Schünemann HJ, Wiercioch W, Etxeandia I, et al. Guidelines 2.0: systematic development of a comprehensive checklist for a successful guideline enterprise. *Can Med Assoc J*. 2014;186:E123.
32. Scott EA, Black N. When does consensus exist in expert panels? *J Public Health Med*. 1991;13:35–39.

Chapter 32

An overview of the Delphi technique in social pharmacy and health services research*

Sarah Drumm[a,b], Catriona Bradley[a], and Frank Moriarty[b]

[a]Irish Institute of Pharmacy, RCSI University of Medicine and Health Sciences, Dublin, Ireland, [b]School of Pharmacy and Biomolecular Sciences, RCSI University of Medicine and Health Sciences, Dublin, Ireland

Objectives

- Identify situations where the Delphi technique is a suitable method to achieve consensus.
- Appraise options for the design of the Likert scale used within a Delphi.
- Consider choices for the panel, consensus definition, type of feedback, and number of rounds within a Delphi.
- Explain the advantages and disadvantages of using the Delphi technique, and how to mitigate against the disadvantages.

Introduction

Consensus or group judgment methods are used to obtain opinions from a group of people with expertise in a particular area, and can be used for predicting future patterns, determining priorities, generating ideas, and solving problems.[1,2] Such methods of achieving consensus on an issue or problem are most valuable where evidence is equivocal and thus judgment must be relied upon, for example, in defining potentially inappropriate prescribing or diagnostic criteria,[3,4] or professional competencies.[5] There are different methods for this process, one of which is the Delphi technique or Delphi method (hereafter referred to as the Delphi). The aim is to reach agreement or a convergence of opinion, and the structured process allows for the effective amalgamation of information.[6,7]

Linstone and Turoff characterize the Delphi as "a method for structuring a group communication process so that the process is effective in allowing a group of individuals, as a whole, to deal with a complex problem" (p. 3).[8] Although the Delphi was traditionally used as a tool for forecasting, it has now been embraced for uses beyond predictive purposes, becoming widely used as a tool to aid decision-making by gathering expert opinion.[9–12] The most recent published pharmacy-related study that used the Delphi for forecasting (specifically the impact of internet supply of medicines on pharmacy) dates from 2002.[13] Although the term "consensus" is regularly used in connection with the Delphi, Linstone and Turoff state that:

> … it has often been necessary to correct the mistaken impression that the aim of Delphi is consensus. Our 1975 book clearly states that Delphi is "a method for structuring a group communication process", not a method aimed to produce consensus. The number of rounds should be based on when stability in the responses is attained, not when consensus is achieved.[14]

This differs from the original concept for the Delphi which was that it was "devised in order to obtain the most reliable opinion consensus of a group of experts."[15]

The Delphi is an iterative process involving the completion of questionnaires over several rounds with respondents often indicating their agreement/disagreement against a statement, typically by using a Likert scale with changes made in later rounds based on the feedback received. These statements, items or other inputs are most often based on a review of the literature, a first round consisting of open-ended questions, or both. With the Delphi there is no necessity for participants

---

*This article was published in Research in Social and Administrative Pharmacy, vol 18, Drumm S, Bradley C, Moriarty F, 'More of an art than a science'? The development, design and mechanics of the Delphi Technique, pages 2230–2236, Copyright Elsevier 2022.

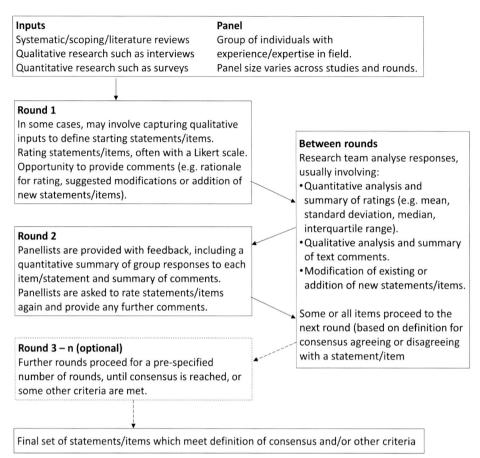

FIG. 1   Typical format and features of the Delphi.

to meet face-to-face.[2,16] Fig. 1 depicts the typical format and features of the Delphi.[8,17,18] Feedback on the results and comments submitted by respondents is usually circulated on an anonymous basis, allowing respondents to consider and potentially revise their stance, and rate the same statements again in the next round.[4,8,16,19,20] In many studies, the respondents are not known to each other which means that there is a double level of anonymity. Jones and Hunter point out that there are two types of agreement in a Delphi—the first is where respondents rate their agreement against the statement, and the second is the level to which they agree with one another.[21]

Data from a Delphi is interpreted using statistical analysis, the specifics of which are determined on a study-by-study basis.[8,16,22–24] As a Delphi deals with the content of the responses, and uses statistical analysis to determine levels of agreement, it can be regarded as both a qualitative and quantitative tool,[17,23] "deriving quantitative estimates through qualitative approaches."[21]

McMillan et al. note that "While consensus methods are commonly used in health services literature, few studies in pharmacy practice use these methods" (p. 655).[2] Examples of the use of a Delphi relevant to pharmacy education, research and practice, and design features of each, are outlined in Table 1.[25–32] The Delphi has wide applicability in pharmacy, and more broadly, health services research. The Delphi has been described as "more of an art than a science,"[8] and although evidence is equivocal on the optimal approach to the Delphi, a substantial literature exists to inform such design choices. This chapter provides an overview of design aspects/choices of the Delphi, the origins of the method, and advantages and disadvantages.

Mechanics of the Delphi

The panel

Typically, the panel chosen to complete a Delphi comprises those who have experience or expertise in a particular field—sometimes referred to as experts or specialists, or stakeholders who form a representative response group and who are affected by, or who work in the area.[8,33] Based on those selected, a certain level of knowledge about the field is presupposed

TABLE 1 Examples of recent studies (2016–20) relating to pharmacy/prescribing education, research, or practice that used the Delphi, and their key characteristics.

Study	Topic	Panel	Scale	Consensus	Rounds
Covvey and Ryan 2018[25]	Course objectives in a pharmacy curriculum	87 pharmacy educators in the United States who were engaged or interested in global health education	5-Point Likert scale from 1 (not at all important) to 5 (extremely important)	At least 85% of the panel selecting Extremely Important or Very Important	3
Drumm et al. 2020[26]	An accreditation framework for continuing education activities for pharmacists	Representatives of seven international accreditation organizations for pharmacist continuing education	5-Point Likert scale from 1 (Strongly Disagree) to 5 (Strongly Agree)	At least five of seven panelists selecting Agree or Strongly Agree	4 (with a face-to-face meeting before the final round)
Penm et al. 2019[27]	Definition of medication reconciliation, and essential components of medication reconciliation	24 international experts in the area (leadership in publications, education, professional interest, and participation in the area of medication reconciliation)	4-Point Likert scale from Strongly Disagree to Strongly Agree	At least 80% of the panel selecting Agree or Strongly Agree	3
Watson et al. 2019[28]	Pharmacists' roles in disasters	15 national and international experts on health aspects of disaster management, advancing practice of pharmacy, and knowledge of pharmacists' roles in disasters	5-Point Likert scale from 1 (Strongly Disagree) to 5 (Strongly Agree), switching to a 4-point scale after round 1 with the neutral mid-point option removed	At least 80% of the panel selecting Agree or Strongly Agree	3
Gibbins et al. 2017[29]	Strategies for managing nonprescription combination analgesics containing codeine misuse/dependence in a community pharmacy setting	40 experts within the fields of pharmacy and drug misuse and/or dependence in Australia	6-Point Likert scale from 1 (Strongly Disagree, or Very Ineffective) to 6 (Strongly Agree or Very Effective)	Median greater than the fourth point on the 6-point Likert scale, a maximum interquartile deviation (interquartile range/2) of 1, and ≥80% of panelists selecting agreement or effectiveness (highest 3 groups on the Likert scale)	3 (the first asking open-ended questions which formed the basis of items included in rounds 2 and 3)
Jebara et al. 2020[30]	A framework for the potential development and implementation of pharmacist prescribing in Qatar	33 health professionals (Director level) involved in prescribing, policymakers, leading administrators, senior educators and regulators, patient safety and quality assurance managers in Qatar	6-Point Likert scale from Strong Disagree to Strongly Agree	At least 70% of the panel selecting Agree or Strongly Agree and less than 15% selecting Disagree or Strongly Disagree	2

Continued

TABLE 1 Examples of recent studies (2016–20) relating to pharmacy/prescribing education, research, or practice that used the Delphi, and their key characteristics—cont'd

Study	Topic	Panel	Scale	Consensus	Rounds
Rankin et al. 2018[31]	Core outcomes for trials aiming to improve appropriateness of polypharmacy in older people in primary care	111 international healthcare experts and a public participant panel of 41 older people from Northern Ireland	9-Point Likert scale from 1 (limited importance) to 9 (critical importance)	At least 75% of the panel rating an outcome as critical (7–9)	3
Barry et al. 2016[32]	Indicators of prescribing appropriateness in children	18 GPs, pharmacists and pediatricians from the United Kingdom and Ireland	5-Point Likert scale from 1 (Strongly Disagree) to 5 (Strongly Agree)	At least 75% of the panel selecting Agree or Strongly Agree	2

A search of PubMed for papers including "Delphi" and either "pharmacy" or "prescribing" in their title/abstract over a 5-year period 2016–20 identified 196 papers. Examples were selected to reflect education-, research-, and practice-related studies.

and one would imagine that these would be the most appropriate respondents in a study. This may not always be the case however as Linstone and Turoff noted that "a specialist is not necessarily the best forecaster" as they can focus on the smaller details of something without being able to consider the bigger picture and that in a drive for homogeneity and conformity, there is a risk that the "tyranny of the majority" can overwhelm a respondent whose views may be in opposition to the group but who in fact may have superior insight (pp. 566–567).[8] Therefore, it is important to ensure the composition of the panel reflects the desirable balance of expertise; however, as Delphis are typically anonymous, the identity or credentials of respondents do not influence the group judgment. Examples from pharmacy and prescribing literature illustrate panels being selected based on their expertise in the research topic area, typically including relevant healthcare professionals working in research, educational and/or patient care roles (Table 1). However, patients are also an important stakeholder group that may be included in panels as experts by experience. For example, a Delphi to identify core outcomes for trials aiming to improve appropriateness of polypharmacy in older people in primary care included a large number of older adults on its panel.[31]

There is no defined agreement on what constitutes the optimum panel size, with examples ranging from 5 to more than 1000 respondents.[5,17,20] Loo noted that:

The careful selection of a relatively small panel according to a set of relevant criteria for the particular study (i.e., purposive selection) can yield valuable data for management or policy decision-making. Large, random samples are not the only option for such purposes (p. 767).[34]

The important consideration is that the correct expertise is represented on the panel, rather than just filling it for the sake of reaching an arbitrary number. A systematic review identified a majority of Delphis included ≤25 respondents,[20] while in the Delphi carried out by Dalkey and Helmer seven respondents were used.[15]

Likert scale

A Likert scale is commonly used in a Delphi as a tool to measure attitudes and opinions. It is a collection of Likert items, where the respondent is provided with a statement and they indicate on a scale their level of, for example, agreement or disagreement with it.[35–41] It is a quantitative instrument, and characteristics of a classic Likert scale include that it has several items arranged horizontally in an ordinal manner around a neutral middle moving from one end of a continuum to the other with the items approximately equidistant from each other.[35,36,42,43] The scale can be described as both ordinal and interval if it meets the following criteria: there are two or more categories, they can be ordered or ranked, e.g., from high to low, and the interval is equally spaced.[44] A nominal or categorical scale is similar to an ordinal scale, but the items are not ordered.

The language used in the statement must be coherent, avoiding double-barreled questions, leading questions and double negatives.[35,42,45] The items in the scale typically range from "strongly disagree" to "strongly agree" with the respondent selecting a corresponding number, e.g., strongly disagree = 1 and strongly agree = 5.[36,46] Scales can be arranged in the opposite order, with the agreement label at the lower scoring end. This is used particularly when negatively worded statements are used.[46] However, empirical evidence suggests using ascending or descending order does not impact on the validity of responses.[47]

Scale design choices include the number of points, whether there is a midpoint, and labeling of points. Scales often consist of 4–9 points. An odd number of points is more common, with the central point indicating that the respondent neither disagrees nor agrees. A smaller number of points may be unreliable when a respondent does not fit precisely into a category, e.g., "moderately agree," and they can therefore be inconsistent with their responses if surveyed on multiple occasions.[48,49] A greater number of items can allow respondents to select a response closer to their actual opinion, although including similarly-named items such as "moderately agree" and "slightly agree" may make it difficult for them to determine which accurately represents their opinion.

Inclusion of a central point allows for a neutral response for indecisive or ambivalent participants.[12,45,46,50] The "central tendency bias" describes how respondents prefer to avoid the extreme ends of a scale, preferring instead to remain in a more neutral central position (which is variously referred to as "neither agree nor disagree," or "undecided"), encouraging respondents to engage in satisficing.[24,42,45,51,52] Despite suggestions that omitting the mid-point is advantageous in pushing respondents into a more definitive position,[8] evidence suggests forcing a choice may evoke a negative response when they are truly ambivalent, and skew responses to the negative.[53] Published examples of Likert scales more generally,[53] and within Delphis in the pharmacy field (Table 1), have tended to use odd numbers of points which include a neutral central point.

Using labels only for the extreme ends of the scale can reduce the risk of central tendency bias, but this measure can introduce another bias where the respondents choose a label they understand rather than one without a label where they may be unclear on what the item is.[52] A 5-point scale reduces the risk of respondent uncertainty as with the extremes labeled, and the central point representing a neutral stance, there are just two points where the respondent is required to infer what the items are. A recent study evaluated how different types of Likert scales (3, 5, and 9 points) can impact the level of consensus in a Delphi study among patients to identify treatment goals, and identified no difference in reliability between the scales.[54] Overall, evidence is equivocal on the optimal scale design, as different approaches will typically reduce risk of some bias(es) at the expense of increased risk of others, and so the best choice is dependent on the context and purpose of the scale.[53] However, a proposed framework based on several experimental studies recommends that for opinion measurement a 5- or 7-point scale be used (the latter for respondents with high cognitive and verbal abilities and familiar with questionnaires), and fully labeled where responses are to be summarized directly using means and frequencies.[53]

Effect of feedback

The provision of feedback is another key component. It is often termed "controlled feedback" as it is the facilitator of the Delphi who determines what feedback will be given to respondents.[16,17,22,23,55,56] Feedback can take the form of a numerical summary of ratings, narrative comments including rationale for ratings, or both.[57] The effect of feedback can vary, as respondents have several options when selecting their response depending on where their original response fell in comparison to the group. The first option is to keep their original response which may or may not be within the range of the group's responses. The second is that having viewed the feedback, they disagree with the majority and choose a response at the other end of the scale. The third is that should their initial response be an outlier from the group, the feedback might convince them to choose a response that will move the group closer to achieving consensus.[58] Evidence suggests there is more movement among those whose responses were furthest from the mean after the first round, and with participants receiving feedback, scores move toward the mean.[4,59] Rowe et al. observed that the reason that the Delphi "works" is due to a combination of the iterative process, which allows respondents to reflect on their answers, and the effect of the feedback particularly where a rationale or further information is provided rather than just statistical data.[18]

Bolger and Wright propose that for a Delphi, process gain should be achieved through "virtuous opinion change" which they define as where the respondents whose scores are further from the "truth," which presumably refers to the majority opinion, need to change their scores more than those whose scores were closer to the truth, and that the direction that the scores move in needs to be toward that "truth."[60] The use of feedback would be instrumental in attaining this level of process gain.

How feedback is presented to the panel can have an impact on responses. Participants have reported being influenced similarly by statistical summaries of ratings and written comments from other panelists.[61] An experimental study of a Delphi focused on architecture has investigated the effect of feedback, where randomized panelists receive different forms of feedback (summary of ratings plus rationale, or rationale alone).[57] They found increased disagreement in the rationale alone group (along with a lower rate of drop-out); however, panelists expressed a preference to receive both summary ratings and rationale. Where panels include a mix of experts, feedback could be presented separately for each disciplinary or expert group. This was investigated in a randomized trial where healthcare managers and family physicians participating in a Delphi of primary care quality indicators received either feedback from only their own professional group or the full panel.[62] The results indicated polarized scores in the former group, whereas receipt of collective feedback moderated scores, reducing the difference between manager and physician ratings.

Consensus

Prior to beginning the Delphi, a decision must be made on what constitutes consensus, e.g., the point when a percentage of the votes fall within a prescribed range.[63] The specifics of this vary from study to study. Diamond et al. reviewed 100 Delphi studies published between 2000 and 2009 and found that the definition for consensus was only provided in 72 of the studies, 64 a priori. They believe that "failure to adequately define and use criteria for consensus challenges the notion that the results of a Delphi study reflect the consensus of the group of experts."[20]

There are several ways in which one can analyze data to determine whether consensus has been reached. These include evaluating interval scale statistics, include the mean, median or mode (measures of central tendency), or using standard deviation and interquartile range (measures of dispersion).[23,24,64] Where responses are skewed, the median should be used as outliers can have a disproportionate effect on the mean.[16,24] Nominal scale statistics, i.e., the percentage or frequency of responses,[40] can also be used as an alternative or a complement. For instance to interpret the data from Likert scales, Likert proposed using a table with percentages and sigma values (standard deviation) with the sigma deviation taken from the mean.[35] Using an average when analyzing the results of ordinal Likert scales can be problematic, as it does not account for variability nor provide answers to make actionable decisions, as it would be erroneous to interpret an average result as "Strongly Agree and a half."[51] To display the data, histograms, Likert charts, heat maps or scatterplots can be used.

A systematic review of Delphi studies identified the most common definition for consensus was percent agreement (25 of 100 studies), with 75% being the median threshold to define consensus (range 50%–97%),[20] with many examples in the pharmacy literature using similar (Table 1). It has been suggested that the consensus level should be determined by the importance of the topic, so for serious or life or death issues, 100% may be required whereas for something relating to establishing a preference, a simple majority (i.e., 51%) might be the appropriate level.[65] Several studies propose using the stability of responses over rounds as a more reliable alternative to using percentages, while others caution that stability of responses should not be confused with consensus.[17,24,55,58] The standard deviation and interquartile range as measures of the spread of responses can also be used, with low spread indicating respondents are largely in agreement.[16,19,23,24] Consensus can be defined as responses meeting several conditions, as a single measure may not capture consensus.[64] For example, a Delphi to achieve consensus on management strategies for misuse/dependence of nonprescription combination analgesics containing codeine used three parameters to define consensus, including the span of the interquartile range, the median, and ≥80% of respondents.[29]

Another consideration is that although consensus is the goal of a Delphi, dissensus can also be an interesting result as it identifies where there may be issues, or where more information is required for respondents to make an informed choice.[8] More recently some Delphis have been undertaken with the specific aim of dissensus rather than consensus, where the investigator looks to explore a range of opinions with the aim of achieving the greatest possible variance in order to expose a multiplicity of positions.[66,67]

Steinert proposed that a Delphi based on dissensus would result in a "stable bipolar distribution" rather than a "stable consensus" as seen in the typical Delphi (p. 293).[66] The proposed methodology is that participants are requested to provide insights that have not already been inputted to ensure maximum variation, and that the number of rounds is determined a priori. It is recommended by Steinert that this approach would be particularly suited to areas that are as yet unexplored. Van de Linde and Van der Duin carried out a Delphi to investigate social trends as an aid to predict trends in future radicalization.[67] The structure of the study consisted of two anonymous rounds followed by a face-to-face meeting at which the discussion focused on areas of dissensus, defined here as trends with a difference of at least two points. As this study was looking to explore new notions of future radicalization, using dissensus allowed a broad range of opinions to be considered rather than just achieving agreement, typically the aim of a classical Delphi. The outputs of the dissensus Delphi include both the points of difference and participants' opinions and views on these, hence Steinert's characterization of this as an exploratory research tool.[66]

Number of rounds

There is no set number of rounds for a Delphi but as Linstone and Turoff observed:

…in all early forecasting Delphis…a point of diminishing returns is reached after a few rounds. Most commonly, three rounds proved sufficient to attain stability in the responses; further rounds tended to show very little change and excessive repetition was unacceptable to participants (p. 223).[8]

The number of rounds for some Delphis can be linked to the determination of consensus, for example where rounds are held until consensus is achieved, or where the last rounds carried out show no significant difference.[4,16,24,68] The optimal number of rounds appears to be 2 or 3, with larger numbers inducing participant fatigue.[17,24,68] As mentioned, in some studies, the first round of the Delphi is an exploratory phase using a qualitative methodology, e.g., open-ended questions or interviews, before moving to a quantitative phase which solicits feedback on these items. Other Delphis begin directly with the quantitative survey element.[69]

Retention of respondents over successive rounds is important, and number of rounds and other design choices should be considered to minimize loss to follow up, such as the format of feedback.[57] Typically, a round in the Delphi is completed concurrently by all participants, before the results are summarized, and feedback provided when inviting the panel to complete the subsequent round. However, rounds can also be conducted in real time, so the responses of those who participate early in a round will be visible to those who respond later, and may influence their responses.[70] Overall, this may result in less time required, and thus may reduce drop-out.[70]

Origins of the Delphi

In July 1962 a memorandum was produced for the Research and Development, or Rand, Corporation, by Norman Dalkey and Olaf Helmer entitled *An Experimental Application of the Delphi Method to the Use of Experts*.[15] The report was a revised version of a classified report, *The Use of Experts for the Estimation of Bombing Requirements* (1951), with the aim of making the report suitable for a wider audience.[71] The original report remains classified so this abridged version is still used today.[72] The report described:

an experiment in the use of the so-called "DELPHI" [sic] method, which was devised in order to obtain the most reliable opinion consensus of a group of experts by subjecting them to a series of questionnaires in depth interspersed with controlled opinion feedback (p. v).[71]

The report described how an "experiment" which was described to participants as a study, had been carried out 10 years earlier with the aim or goal of obtaining expert opinion on the optimal locations in the USA for bombing, by asking experts to imagine themselves to be a Soviet strategic planner, and to consider the number of A-bombs required. The report detailed the process of the Delphi with questions centered on a problem, requiring the respondent to provide a rationale for their answers, in addition to considering what information they required to arrive at a more confident answer. Dalkey and Helmer believed that this "controlled interaction" avoided the pitfalls of more conventional forms of discussions such as round-tables, which could potentially inhibit independent thought and lead to hasty answers. The feedback element allowed the respondent to consider factors that they may have overlooked previously and correct any misconceptions they may have had.[71] The concept of using opinion, which can be controversial, was something that Dalkey expanded upon proposing that opinion falls between knowledge at one end of the information spectrum as it is verifiable and evidence-based, and speculation at the other end as it not generally based on evidence.[73]

The name Delphi does not appear after the first page of Dalkey and Helmer's report, and is capitalized when used. The capitalization suggests an acronym, although as the project was carried out for the US Air Force, that might reflect how air force projects are designated. The name Delphi refers to the oracle at Delphi in Greece where the Pythia, the high priestesses of the Temple of Apollo, acted as a medium for Apollo. The priestesses were, appropriately for studies involving pharmacy, potentially under the influence of ethylene drifting from the intersection of two fault lines on which the temple was built, and which produces an altered state of consciousness, similar to descriptions of the Pythia while in their mantic sessions.[74,75] They enigmatically translated the prophecies, or oracles, of Apollo for the pilgrims who sought assistance. Much has been written about how the rationale for choosing the name was due to the Oracle's skills at forecasting, interpretation and insight, although as noted by Marchais-Roubelat and Roubelat, Dalkey and Helmer, the originators of the Delphi, did not and have not explained the origin or rationale for the name.[9,17,21,76] The name appears to have been first used as a joke at Rand due to the idea of forecasting and Dalkey and Helmer were not very fond of it, particularly as it evoked the image of a priestess disseminating obscure information.[64,77] Dalkey noted that:

In some ways, it [the name] is unfortunate—it connotes something oracular, something smacking a little of the occult—whereas as a matter of fact, precisely the opposite is involved (p. 6).[72]

Cuhls describes the monastery at Delphi as "the largest database of the ancient world" as information was written down on metal and stone plates, accumulated, ordered and preserved there.[78] Many of the pronouncements of the Oracle could be described as being ambiguous, or even obscure, and required "careful investigation and reflection."[79] This obscure language could pose difficulties when interpreted by a mortal, with a famous example of this supplied by King Croesus of Lydia who in 560 BCE destroyed his own empire by going to war. He misinterpreted the words of the oracle which related that a great empire would fall if Croesus went to war, but did not specify whose empire this referred to.[76] Without wishing to labor the point too heavily, it is certainly true that results from any questionnaire must also be reflected upon and scrutinized to ensure the correct readings are derived from them.

The Oracle at Delphi was consulted for a number of purposes but one of the primary ones was related to politics and war, and this is appropriate given that the first use of the Delphi was with the objective of gaining expert opinion on the probability of an enemy attack during the cold war.[10,20] This fits with the way in which Rand envisaged its use in that although it was initially used for military projects, they proposed that it could be used for other purposes such as planning economies.[11]

Advantages and disadvantages

Advantages to using the Delphi include that it can be completed by respondents in different geographical locations in their own time which allows for reflection, and it is cost effective.[8,22] The structured method encourages participation from all group members while avoiding the issue of heterogeneity or of a dominant member or manipulation, as can sometimes be seen with focus groups.[2,8,16,23] Participants in Delphis have commented that it is inclusive, comprehensive, rigorous, systematic and efficient while giving them a personal stake in a project and allowing them to feel involved in the development of the research.[9,19,69]

The Delphi process attributes the same weight to all responses and follows a social constructivist approach, where "the contribution of each individual in the context to the creation of a reality is recognised."[22,80] Studies on questions that require expert judgment have demonstrated that when compared with traditional survey formats, the statistical aggregate produced by group decision processes such as a Delphi, where several individual judgments are assessed, is superior to the average of individual responses.[56,59] Greason notes further advantages to the Delphi as "Using a qualitative Delphi approach to explore ethics and policy in LTC [long-term care] resulted in deeper, more rich findings on ethics, an area seldom empirically, or qualitatively, explored" (p. 2) and as it:

> *iteratively aims to establish consensus on "ways forward" and produce tangible and applicable outcomes in underexplored areas, it involves up to stage three of the knowledge transition portion of Graham's Knowledge to Action-Ethics cycle, which "represents the process of knowledge creation and its translation into practice and policy" (p. 7).*[33]

The use of multiple rounds which allow participants the time and space to present their views, and reflect on their opinions of others as well as their own "sets a strong foundation for further knowledge translation and mobilization" (p. 9).[33]

The Delphi is not without its critics. Sackman reviewed a number of Delphi studies against the American Psychological Association "Standards for Educational and Psychological Tests and Manuals" (1966).[81] He commented that the "conventional Delphi is basically an unreliable and scientifically unvalidated technique in principle and probably in practice" (p. vi) noting approximately 200 potential drawbacks to the Delphi including sampling; the concept of the expert; group vs individual opinion; poor questionnaire design; whether the consensus is authentic; whether the questions, responses and results are meaningful; the presentation of descriptive results; the reliability and validity; whether a systematic review has been performed ahead of time; the dropout rate; the use of central tendency and the analysis and interpretation of findings. The Delphi's use of multiple rounds mean that the process can take longer to complete than other methods, but it also asks the respondents to spend longer participating than other methods do which can lead to attrition.[2,23,69] Some participants in Delphis missed the chance for face-to-face group interaction which can allow for lively debate and discussion.[4,19]

Helmer described Sackman's piece as a "singularly vituperative attack based almost exclusively on … misconception," and an issue of the journal *Technological Forecasting and Social Change* was subsequently dedicated to the Delphi.[82] Sackman declared that "The future is far too important for the human species to be left to fortune tellers using new versions of old crystal balls. It is time for the oracles to move out and for science to move in" (p. 73).[81] His claim that the Delphi neglects standard experimental guidelines for scientific methods can be contrasted with the opinion of Linstone and Turoff who note that "in its design and use Delphi is more of an art than a science" (p. 6).[8] A report by Helmer and Rescher (1958) entitled *On the Epistemology of the Inexact Sciences* describes how the social sciences were part of the inexact sciences whereas psychology, from whence Sackman derived his framework, can be viewed as one of the exact sciences perhaps indicating that methods for gathering opinions were not designed to be scientific, thereby obviating the necessity to adhere to the strictly scientific methods espoused by Sackman.[83]

In spite of Sackman's "vehement attack" (p. 146),[59] the process is still in use which perhaps indicates that with the correct preparation, many of the issues as described by Sackman can be mitigated. It is worth noting that the review carried out by Sackman took place just 10 years after the publication of the details of the Delphi process and the number, and potentially the quality, of the studies was significantly less than is available today.

The Nominal Group Technique, another consensus method, is one that "appears to be used more commonly with lay people than the Delphi Technique, although the reason why is not clear. Lay people may feel more comfortable participating in a face-to-face meeting, than in a relatively complex survey."[2] Additionally the use of the word "expert" when describing the panel of a Delphi could potentially be seen as exclusionary by some who may perceive it as referring to, for example qualified health professionals, rather than people with experience in the area under discussion which may include patients, patient advocates and other "lay" stakeholders. Pharmacy-related Delphi studies have included patients as part of their panel, and may be appropriate for many types of research objectives, e.g., identifying core outcomes for trials in a certain clinical area.[31] However, an advantage of the Delphi is its anonymity which may promote inclusion where there is a mixed panel of health professional and patient experts or other form of traditional hierarchy. While anonymity is hugely important in studies allowing participants to feedback candidly, it is particularly important in the health sciences for a number of reasons, including ensuring patient comfort in providing details on their experiences, and to guarantee that no potentially identifying patient information is included in the study.

Woudenberg cautioned that the consensus achieved in a Delphi was not based on genuine agreement but instead was due to the pressure to conform to the group.[59] However, this could be said of any group judgment method, and it is hoped with any study that respondents are able to make informed decisions based on their experience and expertise combined with taking the comments of their fellow respondents into consideration.

Conclusion

The nebulous beginnings of the Delphi and the fact that the original report is still classified lend a certain air of intrigue to its development. However in the intervening period, the method has been extensively used and refined, with some degree of variation in aspects of its design. This suggests it is widely applicable, and flexible for use for a variety of purposes. As Greason (2018) cautions, a Delphi should not be viewed as providing the solution to a question but rather a way forward as:

> adopting a qualitative Delphi method to explore ethics and policy in LTC brought the findings further than typical methods used in this area of research and resulted in agreed upon solutions and ways forward, there can still be significant challenges to connecting the findings to meaningful change.[33]

The Delphi's geographical neutrality and web-based format has advantages over methods that require face-to-face meetings. Certainly with the Covid-19 situation, techniques such as the Delphi offer a viable and pragmatic approach to attaining consensus.

As discussed in this chapter it is important that decisions on the design choices are made at the planning stage to ensure the reliability and validity of the Delphi. Whether or not the Delphis that are undertaken today remain true to that first conceived of by Dalkey and Helmer is another matter, but as it has evolved it has taken a shape that hopefully provides answers clearer than those of the original Oracle at Delphi.

Questions for further discussion

1. How can patients and the public be effectively involved and engaged as part of a Delphi?
2. What aspects of conducting a Delphi would benefit from further empirical investigation to provide evidence to inform design choices?
3. Are there modifications to the Delphi that could mitigate the disadvantages of this approach?

Application exercise/scenario

You are a researcher interested in how technology has influenced pharmacy practice since the onset of the COVID-19 pandemic. Describe how you would design a Delphi study to achieve consensus on research priorities in this topic area. In your answer, outline all aspects of the Delphi conduct, and provide rationale for your design choices.

References

1. Fitch K, Bernstein SJ, Burnand B, et al. *RAND/UCLA Appropriateness Method User's Manual*. RAND Corporation; 2001.
2. McMillan SS, King M, Tully MP. How to use the nominal group and Delphi techniques. *Int J Clin Pharmacol*. 2016;38(3):655–662. https://doi.org/10.1007/s11096-016-0257-x.
3. O'Mahony D, O'Sullivan D, Byrne S, O'Connor MN, Ryan C, Gallagher P. STOPP/START criteria for potentially inappropriate prescribing in older people: version 2. *Age Ageing*. 2015;44:213–218. https://doi.org/10.1093/ageing/afu145.
4. Graham B, Regehr G, Wright JG. Delphi as a method to establish consensus for diagnostic criteria. *J Clin Epidemiol*. 2003;56(12):1150–1156. https://doi.org/10.1016/S0895-4356(03)00211-7.
5. Janke KK, Kelley KA, Sweet BV, Kuba SE. A modified Delphi process to define competencies for assessment leads supporting a doctor of pharmacy program. *Am J Pharm Educ*. 2016;80(10). https://doi.org/10.5688/ajpe8010167.
6. Pope C, Mays N. Qualitative research: reaching the parts other methods cannot reach: an introduction to qualitative methods in health and health services research. *BMJ*. 1995. https://doi.org/10.1136/bmj.311.6996.42.
7. Di Zio S, Castillo Rosas JD, Lamelza L. Real time spatial Delphi: fast convergence of experts' opinions on the territory. *Technol Forecast Soc Chang*. 2017;115:143–154. https://doi.org/10.1016/j.techfore.2016.09.029.
8. Linstone HA, Turoff M. *The Delphi Method—Techniques and Applications*. Reading, MA: Addison Wesley; 1975.
9. Gupta UG, Clarke RE. Theory and applications of the Delphi technique: a bibliography (1975-1994). *Technol Forecast Soc Chang*. 1996;53(2):185–211. https://doi.org/10.1016/S0040-1625(96)00094-7.
10. Rowe G, Wright G. The Delphi technique as a forecasting tool: issues and analysis. *Int J Forecast*. 1999;15(4):353–375. https://doi.org/10.1016/S0169-2070(99)00018-7.
11. Landeta J. Current validity of the Delphi method in social sciences. *Technol Forecast Soc Chang*. 2006;73(5):467–482. https://doi.org/10.1016/j.techfore.2005.09.002.
12. Ecken P, Gnatzy T, von der Gracht HA. Desirability bias in foresight: consequences for decision quality based on Delphi results. *Technol Forecast Soc Chang*. 2011;78(9):1654–1670. https://doi.org/10.1016/j.techfore.2011.05.006.
13. Holmes ER, Tipton DJ, Desselle SP. The impact of the internet on community pharmacy practice: a comparison of a Delphi panel's forecast with emerging trends. *Health Mark Q*. 2002;20(2):3–29. https://doi.org/10.1300/J026v20n02_02.
14. Linstone HA, Turoff M. Delphi: a brief look backward and forward. *Technol Forecast Soc Chang*. 2011;78(9):1712–1719. https://doi.org/10.1016/j.techfore.2010.09.011.
15. Dalkey N, Helmer O. *An Experimental Application of the Delphi Method to the Use of Experts*. California: Rand Corporation; 1962. https://doi.org/10.1287/mnsc.9.3.458.
16. von der Gracht HA. Consensus measurement in Delphi studies. Review and implications for future quality assurance. *Technol Forecast Soc Chang*. 2012;79(8):1525–1536. https://doi.org/10.1016/j.techfore.2012.04.013.
17. Hasson F, Keeney S, McKenna H. Research guidelines for the Delphi survey technique. *J Adv Nurs*. 2000;32(4):1008–1015. https://doi.org/10.1046/j.1365-2648.2000.t01-1-01567.x.
18. Rowe G, Wright G, McColl A. Judgment change during Delphi-like procedures: the role of majority influence, expertise, and confidence. *Technol Forecast Soc Chang*. 2005;72(4):377–399. https://doi.org/10.1016/j.techfore.2004.03.004.
19. Hanafin S, Brooks A. *The Delphi Technique: A Methodology to Support the Development of a National Set of Child Well-Being Indicators*. National Children's Office: Dublin; 2004.
20. Diamond IR, Grant RC, Feldman BM, et al. Defining consensus: a systematic review recommends methodologic criteria for reporting of Delphi studies. *J Clin Epidemiol*. 2014;67(4):401–409. https://doi.org/10.1016/j.jclinepi.2013.12.002.
21. Jones J, Hunter D. Qualitative research: consensus methods for medical and health services research. *BMJ*. 1995;311(7001):376. https://doi.org/10.1136/bmj.311.7001.376.
22. Hanafin S. *Review of Literature on the Delphi Technique*. National Children's Office: Dublin; 2004.
23. Hsu CC, Sandford BA. The Delphi technique: making sense of consensus. *Pract Assess Res Eval*. 2007;12(10):1–8.
24. Trevelyan EG, Robinson N. Delphi methodology in health research: how to do it? *Eur J Integr Med*. 2015;7(4):423–428. https://doi.org/10.1016/j.eujim.2015.07.002.
25. Covvey JR, Ryan M. Use of a modified Delphi process to determine course objectives for a model global health course in a pharmacy curriculum. *Am J Pharm Educ*. 2018;82(8):6358. https://doi.org/10.5688/ajpe6358.
26. Drumm S, Moriarty F, Rouse MJ, Croke D, Bradley C. The development of an accreditation framework for continuing education activities for pharmacists. *Pharmacy*. 2020;8(2):75. https://doi.org/10.3390/pharmacy8020075.
27. Penm J, Vaillancourt R, Pouliot A. Defining and identifying concepts of medication reconciliation: an international pharmacy perspective. *Res Social Adm Pharm*. 2019;15(6):632–640. https://doi.org/10.1016/j.sapharm.2018.07.020.
28. Watson KE, Singleton JA, Tippett V, Nissen LM. Defining pharmacists' roles in disasters: a Delphi study. *PLoS One*. 2019;14(12). https://doi.org/10.1371/journal.pone.0227132.
29. Gibbins AK, Wood PJ, Spark MJ. Managing inappropriate use of non-prescription combination analgesics containing codeine: a modified Delphi study. *Res Social Adm Pharm*. 2017;13(2):369–377. https://doi.org/10.1016/j.sapharm.2016.02.015.
30. Jebara T, Cunningham S, MacLure K, et al. A modified-Delphi study of a framework to support the potential implementation of pharmacist prescribing. *Res Social Adm Pharm*. 2020;16(6):812–818. https://doi.org/10.1016/j.sapharm.2019.09.005.
31. Rankin A, Cadogan CA, Ryan C, Clyne B, Smith SM, Hughes CM. Core outcome set for trials aimed at improving the appropriateness of polypharmacy in older people in primary care. *J Am Geriatr Soc*. 2018;66(6):1206–1212. https://doi.org/10.1111/jgs.15245.

32. Barry E, O'Brien K, Moriarty F, et al. PIPc study: development of indicators of potentially inappropriate prescribing in children (PIPc) in primary care using a modified Delphi technique. *BMJ Open.* 2016;6(9). https://doi.org/10.1136/bmjopen-2016-012079.

33. Greason M. Connecting findings to meaningful change: the benefits of using qualitative Delphi in empirical ethics and policy research in long-term care. *Int J Qual Methods.* 2018;17(1). https://doi.org/10.1177/1609406918803271.

34. Loo R. The Delphi method: a powerful tool for strategic management. *Policing.* 2002;25(4):762–769. https://doi.org/10.1108/13639510210450677.

35. Likert R. A technique for the measurement of attitudes. *Arch Psychol.* 1932;140:44–53.

36. Uebersax J. Likert Scales: Dispelling the Confusion. 2006. http://john-uebersax.com/stat/likert.htm. (Accessed November 15, 2020).

37. Carifio J, Perla RJ. Ten common misunderstandings, misconceptions, persistent myths and urban legends about Likert scales and Likert response formats and their antidotes. *J Soc Sci.* 2007;3(3):106–116. https://doi.org/10.3844/jssp.2007.106.116.

38. Rattray J, Jones MC. Essential elements of questionnaire design and development. *J Clin Nurs.* 2007;16(2):234–243. https://doi.org/10.1111/j.1365-2702.2006.01573.x.

39. Johns R. SQB methods fact sheet 1: Likert items and scales. *Surv Res Netw.* 2010;1(March):1–11. https://www.ukdataservice.ac.uk/media/262829/discover_likertfactsheet.pdf.

40. Brown J. Likert items and scales of measurement? *Shiken JALT Test Eval SIG Newslett.* 2011;15:10–14. http://hosted.jalt.org/test/bro_34.htm.

41. Claveria O. A new metric of consensus for Likert-type scale questionnaires: an application to consumer expectations. *J Bank Financ Technol.* 2021. https://doi.org/10.1007/s42786-021-00026-5.

42. Krosnick J, Presser S. Question and questionnaire design. In: Marsden P, Wright J, eds. *Handbook of Survey Research.* 2nd ed. Bingley: Emerald Publishing; 2010:263–313.

43. Louangrath PI, Sutanapong C. Validity and reliability of survey scales. *Int J Res Methodol Soc Sci.* 2018;4(3):99–115.

44. Wu H, Leung SO. Can Likert scales be treated as interval scales?—a simulation study. *J Soc Serv Res.* 2017;43(4):527–532. https://doi.org/10.1080/01488376.2017.1329775.

45. Johns R. *Survey Question Bank: SQB Methods Fact Sheet 1: Likert Items and Scales*; 2010. https://www.sheffield.ac.uk/polopoly_fs/1.597637!/file/likertfactsheet.pdf. Published. Accessed November 15, 2020.

46. Warmbrod JR. Reporting and interpreting scores derived from Likert-type scales. *J Agric Educ.* 2014;55(5):30–47. https://doi.org/10.5032/jae.2014.05030.

47. Maeda H. Response option configuration of online administered Likert scales. *Int J Soc Res Methodol.* 2015;18(1):15–26. https://doi.org/10.1080/13645579.2014.885159.

48. Kuncel RB. Response processes and relative location of subject and item. *Educ Psychol Meas.* 1973;33(3):545–563. https://doi.org/10.1177/001316447303300302.

49. Kuncel RB. The subject-item interaction in itemmetric research. *Educ Psychol Meas.* 1977;37(3):665–678. https://doi.org/10.1177/001316447703700309.

50. Meshkat B, Cowman S, Gethin G, et al. Using an e-Delphi technique in achieving consensus across disciplines for developing best practice in day surgery in Ireland. *J Hosp Admin.* 2014;3(4):1. https://doi.org/10.5430/jha.v3n4p1.

51. Bishop PA, Herron RL. Use and misuse of the Likert item responses and other ordinal measures. *Int J Exerc Sci.* 2015;8(3):297–302.

52. Douven I. A Bayesian perspective on Likert scales and central tendency. *Psychon Bull Rev.* 2018;25(3):1203–1211. https://doi.org/10.3758/s13423-017-1344-2.

53. Weijters B, Cabooter E, Schillewaert N. The effect of rating scale format on response styles: the number of response categories and response category labels. *Int J Res Mark.* 2010;27(3):236–247. https://doi.org/10.1016/j.ijresmar.2010.02.004.

54. Lange T, Kopkow C, Lützner J, et al. Comparison of different rating scales for the use in Delphi studies: different scales lead to different consensus and show different test-retest reliability. *BMC Med Res Methodol.* 2020;20(1):1–11. https://doi.org/10.1186/s12874-020-0912-8.

55. Rowe G, Wright G, Bolger F. Delphi: a reevaluation of research and theory. *Technol Forecast Soc Chang.* 1991;39(3):235–251. https://doi.org/10.1016/0040-1625(91)90039-I.

56. Okoli C, Pawlowski SD. The Delphi method as a research tool: an example, design considerations and applications. *Inf Manage.* 2004;42(1):15–29. https://doi.org/10.1016/j.im.2003.11.002.

57. Meijering JV, Tobi H. The effect of controlled opinion feedback on Delphi features: mixed messages from a real-world Delphi experiment. *Technol Forecast Soc Chang.* 2016;103:166–173. https://doi.org/10.1016/j.techfore.2015.11.008.

58. Scheibe M, Skutsch M, Schofer J. Experiments in Delphi methodology. In: Linstone H, Turoff M, eds. *The Delphi Method: Techniques and Applications.* Reading, MA: Addison Wesley; 1975:262–287.

59. Woudenberg F. An evaluation of Delphi. *Technol Forecast Soc Chang.* 1991;40(2):131–150. https://doi.org/10.1016/0040-1625(91)90002-W.

60. Bolger F, Wright G. Improving the Delphi process: lessons from social psychological research. *Technol Forecast Soc Chang.* 2011;78(9):1500–1513. https://doi.org/10.1016/j.techfore.2011.07.007.

61. Turnbull AE, Dinglas VD, Friedman LA, et al. A survey of Delphi panelists after core outcome set development revealed positive feedback and methods to facilitate panel member participation. *J Clin Epidemiol.* 2018;102:99–106. https://doi.org/10.1016/j.jclinepi.2018.06.007.

62. Campbell SM, Hann M, Roland MO, Quayle JA, Shekelle PG. The effect of panel membership and feedback on ratings in a two-round delphi survey: results of a randomized controlled trial. *Med Care.* 1999;37(9):964–968. https://doi.org/10.1097/00005650-199909000-00012.

63. Miller L. Determining what could/should be: the Delphi technique and its application. *Proceedings of the 2006 Annual Meeting of the Mid-Western Educational Research Association. Columbus, Ohio*; 2006.

64. Giannarou L, Zervas E. Using Delphi technique to build consensus in practice. *Int J Bus Sci Appl Manag.* 2014;9(2):65–82.

65. Keeney S, Hasson F, McKenna H. Consulting the oracle: ten lessons from using the Delphi technique in nursing research. *J Adv Nurs.* 2006;53(2):205–212. https://doi.org/10.1111/j.1365-2648.2006.03716.x.

66. Steinert M. A dissensus based online Delphi approach: an explorative research tool. *Technol Forecast Soc Chang*. 2009;76(3):291–300. https://doi.org/10.1016/j.techfore.2008.10.006.

67. van de Linde E, van der Duin P. The Delphi method as early warning. Linking global societal trends to future radicalization and terrorism in the Netherlands. *Technol Forecast Soc Chang*. 2011;78(9):1557–1564. https://doi.org/10.1016/j.techfore.2011.07.014.

68. Boulkedid R, Abdoul H, Loustau M, Sibony O, Alberti C. Using and reporting the Delphi method for selecting healthcare quality indicators: a systematic review. *PLoS One*. 2011;6(6). https://doi.org/10.1371/journal.pone.0020476.

69. Fletcher AJ, Marchildon GP. Using the Delphi method for qualitative, participatory action research in health leadership. *Int J Qual Methods*. 2014;13(1):1–18. https://doi.org/10.1177/160940691401300101.

70. Gnatzy T, Warth J, von der Gracht H, Darkow IL. Validating an innovative real-time Delphi approach—a methodological comparison between real-time and conventional Delphi studies. *Technol Forecast Soc Chang*. 2011;78(9):1681–1694. https://doi.org/10.1016/j.techfore.2011.04.006.

71. Dalkey N, Helmer O. *The Use of Experts for the Estimation of Bombing Requirements: A Project Delphi Experiment*. Santa Monica: RAND Corporation; 1951. https://www.jstor.org/stable/2627117?seq=1.

72. Dayé C. How to train your oracle: the Delphi method and its turbulent youth in operations research and the policy sciences. *Soc Stud Sci*. 2018;48(6):846–868. https://doi.org/10.1177/0306312718798497.

73. Magnuson LA. *A Delphi study to understand relational bonds in supervision and their effect on rehabilitation counselor disclosure in the public rehabilitation program*. PhD dissertation, University of Iowa; 2012.

74. Spiller HA, Hale JR, De Boer JZ. The Delphic oracle: a multidisciplinary defense of the gaseous vent theory. *J Toxicol Clin Toxicol*. 2002;40(2):189–196. https://doi.org/10.1081/CLT-120004410.

75. de Boer JA. The Oracle at Delphi: The pythia and the pneuma, intoxicating gas finds, and hypotheses. In: Wexler P, ed. *History of Toxicology and Environmental Health: Toxicology in Antiquity*. vol. 1. Amsterdam: Academic Press; 2014:83–91.

76. Marchais-Roubelat A, Roubelat F. The Delphi method as a ritual: inquiring the Delphic Oracle. *Technol Forecast Soc Chang*. 2011;78(9):1491–1499. https://doi.org/10.1016/j.techfore.2011.04.012.

77. Turoff M, Hiltz S. Computer based Delphi processes. In: Adler M, Ziglio E, eds. *Gazing Into the Oracle: The Delphi Technique and Its Application to Social Policy and Public Health*. London: Kingsley; 1996:56–86.

78. Cuhls K, Blind K, Grupp H. *Innovations for Our Future; Delphi '98: New Foresight on Science and Technology*. Springer Science & Business Media; 2002.

79. Kindt J. Delphic oracle stories and the beginning of historiography: Herodotus' Croesus logos. *Class Philol*. 2006;101(1):34–51. https://doi.org/10.1086/505670.

80. Lincoln YS, Guba EG. *Naturalistic Inquiry*. London: Sage; 1985.

81. Sackman H. *Delphi Assessment: Expert Opinion, Forecasting and Group Process*. Vol. R-1283-PR. California: RAND Corporation; 1974.

82. O'Brien PW. The Delphi technique and educational planning. *Irish J Educ*. 1978;2:69–93. www.jstor.org/stable/30076717.

83. Helmer O, Rescher N. *On the Epistemology of the Inexact Sciences*. California: The RAND Corporation; 1958.

Chapter 33

Applying the Delphi technique in pharmacy and health services research

Myriam Jaam, Ahmed Awaisu, Alla El-Awaisi, Derek Stewart, and Maguy Saffouh El Hajj
Department of Clinical Pharmacy and Practice, College of Pharmacy, QU Health, Qatar University, Doha, Qatar

Objectives

- Provide an overview of the best practices related to the Delphi technique in pharmacy practice research.
- Highlight key methodological issues and areas of uncertainty pertaining to the Delphi technique in pharmacy practice research.
- Identify, critically appraise, and summarize strengths and limitations of pharmacy practice research studies utilizing the Delphi technique.
- Provide a guide for pharmacy practice researchers in using the Delphi technique.

Introduction

Consensus research methods are used in health services research to yield evidence derived through systematic means of measuring collective agreement and developing consensus from a group of subject matter experts.[1-5] While it is recognized that this evidence is of a lower level than that of metaanalyses of randomized controlled trials (RCTs), cohort studies, etc., these methods are justified in situations where there is a lack of scientific evidence and incomplete or contradictory evidence,[1,2,5,6] unanimity of opinion does not exist, and to enhance decision-making.[1,3-8] Consensus methods have particular merit in the development of statements of policies, guidelines, and performance indicators; hence, they are of relevance in the development, implementation, and evaluation of pharmacy services. There are many consensus methods reported in the literature, including, the Delphi technique, the nominal group technique, the RAND Corporation/ the University of California Los Angeles appropriateness method, the Glaser approach to consensus, and the consensus development conference.[9-11] Although several of these consensus methods are closely related and may serve the same purpose, there may be some primary differences in their design and utility. The Delphi technique is the most commonly reported and is a structured, isolated, indirect, multistage interaction method used to determine consensus through repetitive administration of anonymous questionnaires, usually across two or three rounds.[3,4,12] It intends to bring about opinions of different expects while preempting their social, political, and personal conflicts and regardless of their geographical locations.[13] Recent examples include studies of defining facilitators and barriers prior to system implementation,[14] defining professionals roles,[15] developing healthcare quality and key performance indicators to advance practices,[16-18] and setting standards for pharmacist prescribing.[19,20]

Despite its widespread utility, there is an acknowledged lack of standardized guidelines and criteria to support the Delphi technique study design, conduct, and reporting leading to inconsistent approaches and methodological difficulties.[3,4,8,21] There are also a number of key areas of considerable debate and conflicting opinions.[4,8] In this themed chapter, we provide the reader with a collation of best practices and highlight key methodological issues and areas of uncertainty pertaining to the Delphi technique, especially in pharmacy practice research. We identified, critically appraised, and summarized areas of strengths and weaknesses of recent studies utilizing the Delphi technique in pharmacy practice. However, this book chapter does not purport to be prescriptive or definitive guidelines for conducting Delphi methods but serves as a guide for pharmacy practice researchers in using the technique.

Contemporary Research Methods in Pharmacy and Health Services. https://doi.org/10.1016/B978-0-323-91888-6.00003-X

Key methodological considerations in using the Delphi technique

The Delphi technique was developed in the 1940s by the RAND Corporation as a means to forecast military events.[4,12] This was considered the "conventional Delphi" where a homogenous sample was used to bring about consensus. Later, the Delphi technique was used to create and modify policies and was referred to as "Policy Delphi." Unlike the conventional Delphi, policy Delphi aims at exploring conflicting opinions and raising an understanding of both consensus and disagreements about a particular topic, hence using a more heterogeneous sample.[22] Bloor and Wood (2006) defined the Delphi groups technique as, "a method for achieving consensual agreement among expert panelists, through repeated iterations (usually by email) of anonymized opinions and of proposed compromise statements from the group moderator."[23] It is a highly structured method of multiple rounds of questionnaires (mail or increasingly online), which ultimately aims to provide a consensus using the opinions and feedback of experts in a given field.[1–6,21,24] The basic principles and processes of the Delphi technique have remained fairly constant since its inception by the RAND Corporation, with the only real change being the use of email and online questionnaire administration and feedback of results. All in all, there are four key features of the Delphi technique as by Rowe and Wright "anonymity, iterations, controlled feedback and statistical aggregation of group responses."[13] The process of the Delphi technique steps are summarized below:

Problem definition

The first key consideration is to align the research problem (aim, objectives, questions) with the research method to ensure that a consensus approach is the most appropriate.[21] There should be a justification of the selection of the Delphi technique over other consensus approaches, with attention given to issues of researcher's abilities and skills, and availability of resources.

Selection of experts

The Delphi technique participants should be "experts in their field." McKenna (1994) defined expertise as "a panel of informed individuals[25]; hence there is a need to define selection criteria in relation to, for example, policy, practice, and research, and to consider the need for multidisciplinary representation, patient and public involvement, national versus international representation.[1,4,6,8,21,26–28] These considerations should be aligned with the research problem and the specific purpose of the consensus study. One key area of debate and uncertainty surrounds the number of experts to be recruited, with no gold standard method for estimating sample size. While published studies have reported expert sample sizes from 15 to several hundred according to reviews and methodological guidelines,[3,6,21,22,27,29] the range of expertise and participant representation are more important than the number. Typically, the sampling technique for the selection of the experts involves nonprobability sampling methods, particularly purposive or criterion sampling. Researchers should define the selection, sampling, and recruitment strategy as part of the study protocol and should avoid restricting experts to those within their own professional networks. Additionally, researchers should consider if they want to have a more homogenous sample or heterogeneous sample based on the study objective, keeping in mind a more heterogeneous sample may require a larger number of experts to yield sufficient results.[22] Another important factor to consider when selecting experts is one highlighted by Rowe and Wright whereby experts tend to hold to their opinions throughout the Delphi rounds as compared to the nonexperts who tend to change their opinion to match that of the group over subsequent rounds.[13] This phenomenon is termed "theory of error,"[13,22,30] which although not reported to be "problematic" but can be an interesting factor when analyzing the Delphi results. Moreover, a mix of experts can increase the reliability of findings.[22]

Statement development

The philosophical paradigms underpinning the Delphi technique are the subject of some debate. The statistical analysis of quantitative data generated from responses to a series of statements lends itself to a positivist or postpositivist stance and concepts of robustness (i.e., validity and reliability). The often need for a qualitative phase to aid statement development aligns more with interpretivism or social constructivism, and concepts of research rigor and trustworthiness (i.e., credibility, dependability, confirmability, and transferability). Others classify a mixed-methods or multimethod approach as being pragmatism.[5] Despite the philosophical stance taken, the development of a robust set of statements is clearly crucial to the Delphi technique, the meaning of "robust" is open to interpretation and should include consideration of the relevance of the content to the research problem. Further considerations surround generating a data collection tool that is likely to be internally valid, reliable, clear, and of an appropriate length. The terms "traditional Delphi" and "modified Delphi" frequently appear in the scientific literature, with the traditional approach having a phase of qualitative inquiry or unstructured questionnaire with the expert panel to aid statement development and the modified approach having statements largely developed through literature review. It could therefore be interpreted that these approaches could be polar opposites when, in fact, all Delphi studies should center on a systematic approach to statement development, irrespective of the descriptive term applied.

This systematic approach could include deriving statements from:

- Evidence syntheses (scoping reviews, systematic reviews, metaanalysis, metasynthesis)
- Published primary research (qualitative, quantitative, mixed methods) or primary research conducted with the expert panel
- Review of key documents (e.g., policy, guidance)

One further important consideration is the application of a theoretical framework or theoretical lens to statement development, which is likely to provide a more comprehensive reflection of all factors compared to a pragmatic approach. For example, in Delphi studies of implementation, the statements can be developed with reference to the Consolidated Framework for Implementation Research (CFIR).[31] CFIR is a synthesis of 18 published models, theories, and frameworks, described in five domains (Table 1).

Statements of implementation can be constructed around these five domains, with consideration of any evidence syntheses, primary research, and review of key documents. Attention also needs to be paid to the number of statements; one drawback of this systematic, comprehensive developmental approach is that it can produce a very large number of statements with negative consequences for later participation and response rates. It may be necessary to prioritize the statements by carefully reflecting on the research problem, or to conduct multiple studies.

Before moving to the Delphi technique data collection stage, it is wise to get feedback on the statements from trusted individuals with research and practice expertise in the area of research. It is, however, important to bear in mind that these individuals are not the Delphi expert panel hence they need to be given very clear instructions on what is expected in terms of reviewing for statement appropriateness, clarity, and number.

Once the Delphi technique is in progress, the experts can suggest including other statements and provide suggestions on statements that could be incorporated into further rounds with modifications. Care must, however, be taken to ensure that these statements are not reflecting the bias of the expert and it should be borne in mind that these additional statements have been developed through a systematic and comprehensive process.

Data collection and analysis

For data collection, a series of structured questionnaires are sequentially administered in rounds; typically there will be at least two rounds of questionnaire administration. Researchers should specify a priori whether there will be a set number of rounds or whether they will employ a "stopping guideline" based on expert responses. The questionnaires should be completed anonymously and the responses should be analyzed and summarized after each round and communicated to the experts. There is no interaction of the experts, with each unaware of who else is participating.

The Delphi statements are usually framed as Likert scale with the number of scale response categories varying across studies. While there is no agreement on the ideal number of response options, it is recognized that a small number may result in a lack of discriminatory power and a high number leading to unreliable results. It is not unusual for a high number of response options to be collapsed into a smaller number for the presentation of the study results. There is also a lack of

TABLE 1 CFIR domains and construct descriptions.[31]

Domain	Constructs
Intervention characteristics	Intervention source; evidence strength and quality; relative advantage; adaptability; trialability; complexity; design quality and packaging; cost
Outer setting	Patient needs and resources; cosmopolitanism; peer pressure; external policy and incentives
Inner setting	Structural characteristics; networks and communications; culture; implementation climate; readiness for implementation
Characteristics of individuals	Knowledge and beliefs about the intervention; self-efficacy; individual stage of change; individual identification with organization; other personal attributes
Planning	Planning; engaging; executing; reflecting and evaluating

agreement on the use of a scale-neutral midpoint or to have an even number of options forcing expert members to make a positive or negative judgment.

While these issues are important considerations for the researchers, the key consideration surrounds the definition and interpretation of consensus. In a systematic review of 100 Delphi studies, Diamond et al. concluded that "although consensus generally is felt to be of primary importance to the Delphi process, definitions of consensus vary widely and are poorly reported. Improved criteria for reporting of methods of Delphi studies are required."[32] The array of approaches to defining and measuring consensus is illustrated in Table 2. The "certain level of agreement" and the "measures of central tendency" are most frequently reported. There is, however, variation across studies in the cut-off levels set for consensus, with these often appearing arbitrary and having little justification.

Jünger et al. developed recommendations for "Guidance on Conducting and Reporting Delphi Studies (CREDES) in palliative care" based on the results of a systematic review.[34] One recommendation is that unless not reasonable due to the explorative nature of the study, an a priori criterion for consensus should be defined. This includes a clear and transparent guide for action on (a) how to proceed with certain items or topics in the next survey round, (b) the required threshold to terminate the Delphi process, and (c) procedures to be followed when consensus is (not) reached after one or more iterations.[32]

One further consideration related to the measurement of consensus surrounds data analysis. Following analysis of data from a Delphi round, it is likely (or hopeful) that consensus will be achieved for a number of statements. In many studies, these will be removed from further rounds which will focus on those statements not yet achieving consensus thus reducing the length of the questionnaire with potential impact on response rate. Others, however, recommend that statements achieving consensus be retained in a further round to allow exploration of stability of responses using appropriate inferential statistics.[35,36] According to *von der Gracht* stability is defined as "the consistency of responses between successive rounds."[33] Stability can be measured by statistically testing the difference in outcomes from two consecutive rounds and should be considered within the Delphi studies to provide more robust conclusions. It needs to be borne in mind that stability and consensus are not interchangeable terms as responses could be stable yet not be at a level for consensus and vice versa.

Controlled feedback is an important characteristic of the Delphi technique. Between each round of the Delphi, feedback should be solicited from experts, analyzed, and shared in subsequent rounds. Feedback can be summarized quantitatively reflecting on the group responses to Delphi items or qualitatively reflecting themes or opinions regarding specific items. Sometimes, arguments from individuals who are of opposed opinions to the group are also provided in subsequent rounds. Therefore, unlike in focus groups where opinions might be withheld due to social pressure, in the Delphi process, all feedbacks from all members are solicited and reflected upon especially when opinions are different from that of the group.[13,30]

TABLE 2 Approaches to defining and measuring consensus.

Methods	Description
Subjective criteria and descriptive statistics	
Stipulated number of rounds	The number of rounds of data collection is stated a priori
Subjective analysis	A judgment is made that another round would not significantly add to the results
Certain level of agreement	A consensus level of agreement is set, e.g., >80% of agreement for each statement. This may be extended to include consideration of disagreement, e.g., >80% and <10% disagreement
Measures of central tendency (e.g., median, interquartile range, mode)	A consensus level is set based on measures of central tendency
Average percent of majority opinions cut-off rate	Consensus is determined based on the total of the majority of agreements and disagreements as a percentage of total opinions expressed
Formal measures of agreement	Use of statistics such as Kappa, Cronbach's alpha, intraclass correlation
Coefficient of variation	Consensus is set based on a defined coefficient of variance
Postgroup consensus	Once the Delphi data collection is complete, agreement of consensus is sought from the expert members

Adapted from Diamond IR, Grant RC, Feldman BM, et al. Defining consensus: a systematic review recommends methodologic criteria for reporting of Delphi studies. *J Clin Epidemiol.* 2014;67(4):401–9; von der Gracht HA. Consensus measurement in Delphi studies. *Technol Forecast Soc Chang.* 2012;79(8):1525–36.

Study reporting and quality assessment

Many academic and scientific journals recommend that authors complete standardized reporting checklists as part of the submission process. While there is a myriad of checklists for many study designs (e.g., The Strengthening the Reporting of Observational Studies in Epidemiology [STROBE]) Statement[37] available on the EQUATOR (Enhancing the Quality and Transparency Of health Research) network website, the only Delphi checklist available is related to palliative care.[34] This checklist comprises four domains of the rationale for the choice of the Delphi technique; planning and design; study conduct; and reporting. Diamond et al. also proposed a four-domain Delphi technique quality assessment checklist comprising the following questions: were criteria for participants reproducible?; was the number of rounds to be performed stated?; were the criteria for dropping items clear? and; stopping criteria other than rounds specified?[32] Interestingly, little emphasis is placed on the processes of statement development and associated quality assurance measures.

Review of pharmacy practice Delphi technique studies

To understand how the Delphi technique is currently being utilized and reported in pharmacy practice research, a review was conducted by two researchers (MH and MJ) who have expertise in conducting a literature search and had several publications in peer-reviewed journals in the relevant field. The review was conducted of studies published from January 2015 to October 2020. The terms "pharmacy OR pharmacist" AND "Delphi" were searched as title and abstract terms in PubMed, with studies included if they used the Delphi method and reported pharmacy practice research. Studies reporting on pharmacy education and curricular development were excluded. No limits were applied to the search. Of the 122 hits identified, only 29 were judged to be potentially eligible and screened for full text. All 29 studies were included in the review, and relevant data were extracted independently by two researchers (MJ and MH) using a prepiloted data extraction tool.

Table 3 summarizes the characteristics, aims, designs, Delphi description, and quality of included studies.

Study characteristics

Most studies were conducted in European countries: United Kingdom[10,38,39] ($n=3$), Belgium[40] ($n=1$), Poland[41] ($n=1$), Spain[42] ($n=1$), Malta[43] ($n=1$), across Europe[44] ($n=1$), followed by United States[45–50] ($n=7$) and Middle Eastern countries[19,51–53] ($n=4$). Four studies were conducted at an international level,[15,54–56] two in Canada,[57,58] two in Brazil,[60, 61] one in Australia,[62] and one in Malaysia.[63] Studies were conducted across several pharmacy settings[15,19,38,43,44,49,54,62,63] ($n=9$), hospital only[40,42,47,55–58] ($n=7$), community pharmacy only[46,51,53,59,60] ($n=5$), critical care units[10,41,48] ($n=3$), three in primary or general care settings,[39,45,52] and one in ambulatory clinics.[61] The study setting was not defined in one study.[50]

Problem definition

All included studies aimed at using the Delphi method to achieve consensus among experts in the field. The studies aimed to study consensus over a range of areas including key performance/quality improvement indicators[41,42,49,52,53,61] ($n=6$), knowledge, roles, competencies[15,38,39,44,48,60,62] ($n=7$), performance tools and checklists[40,50,57,59] ($n=4$), medication errors and pharmacovigilance[10,51,58] ($n=3$), service optimization[19,43,47] ($n=3$), collaborative models of practice[45,63] ($n=2$), medication literacy or medication reconciliation[54,56] ($n=2$), payment models[46] ($n=1$), and identification of drug-related hospital admissions[55] ($n=1$).

Few articles have also described the expertise of the researchers conducting the Delphi process. For instance, Pouliot et al. highlighted that the researchers responsible for administering the survey and reviewing statements had over 30 years of expertise in the field along with two PharmD students.[54] This was similar to Penm et al.'s reporting where the research team had 30 years of experience in pharmacy reconciliation and included Ph.D. researchers.[56] On the other hand, Lima et al. indicated that the working group included university professors and Ph.D. students with expertise ranging from 5 to 25 years in pharmacy practice.[64] Three hospital pharmacists and a pharmacoeconomist conducted the Delphi process in Marine's work.[40] Hernandez described a scientific committee composed of five hospital pharmacists who delivered the Delphi process.[42] Smith et al. and Clay et al. described a research team composed of pharmacists with experience in pulmonary hypertension, and in the field of pharmacist-patient care interventions, respectively.[49,50] Conversely, Rault and Rocha did not describe the expertise of the researchers.[58,60]

TABLE 3 Characteristics and quality of included studies.

Author(s) Year of publication Country of data collection Setting	Stated study objectives	Experts	Number of experts Invited, agreed to participate, and completed all rounds	Item/statement Development	Number of rounds Mode	Consensus measure Description
Pouliot et al.[54] 2017 International Pharmacy (not specified)	To reach consensus on health literary related statements and a definition of medication literacy	Identified through literature review and responses to an international survey on medication literacy (self-identified or suggested) pharmacists, physicians, and academics	Invited: 50 Agreed: 28 Completed: 11	Literature search (PubMed, EBSCO, Google Scholar) identified 22 statements and open questions within a survey to pharmacists Identified 15 statements Total statements for round 1: 37; round 2: 62; round 3: 60; round 4: 1 definition. 1 definition was finalized	4 rounds Online (Research Electronic Data Capture)	A certain level of agreement • 10-point numerical scale (1 = no agreement, 10 = full agreement) • The consensus at >80% between agree and strongly agree
Lima et al.[61] 2018 Brazil Ambulatory care	This study aimed to develop and validate a KPI instrument for medication management services provided for outpatients	Identified through experts list and contained university professors and researchers in clinical pharmacy from various geographic regions	Invited: 16 Agreed: 11 Completed: 9	Systematic review[64] (PubMed/Medline, Scopus, Lilacs) and professional experience from the working group and other studies in clinical pharmacy areas. Total KPIs for round 1: 7; round 2: 8; instrument approved by experts with 6 KPIs	2 rounds Online (Google forms)	A certain level of agreement • Content validity index accepted at 0.78 or higher • 5-point Likert scale • Fleiss Kappa accepted at 0.70 or higher
Watson et al.[15] 2019 International Pharmacy (Not specified)	To acquire consensus from an expert panel of key opinion leaders within the field of disaster health on pharmacists' roles in disasters throughout the four disaster phases—prevention, preparedness, response, and recovery	National and international opinion leaders experts on health aspects of disaster management, advancing practice of pharmacy, and knowledge of pharmacists' roles in disasters.	Invited: 24 Agreed: 15 Completed: 15	Literature search and; interviews and surveys with international disaster health professionals. Total 46 roles for round 1; 43 roles in round 2; qualitative comments for round 3 43 items were accepted at the end	3 rounds Online (KeySurvey®)	A certain level of agreement • Round 1: consensus at 80% • Round 2: Confirm removing items using "yes" or "no" questions for items below 69% level; items between 70% and 79% presented again in a 4 point Likert scale

Study	Aim	Panel	Participants	Method/items	Rounds/mode	Consensus definition
Thevelin et al.[55] 2018 International Hospital	To develop a standardized chart review method to identify drug-related hospital admissions in older people caused by nonpreventable adverse drug reactions and preventable medication errors	Experts with academic or clinical expertise on the subject of drug-related morbidity in older patients	Invited: 29 Agreed: 15 Completed: 14	Literature search (PubMed). A total of 29 statements were identified for round 1; 15 statements were revised in round 2. 26 items were accepted at the end.	2 rounds Online (LimeSurvey)	Inter Quartile Range and median score • 5-point Likert scale • For each item, consensus measurement was based on the median Likert response and the inter-quartile range. • The following cut-off values of consensus were defined before data analysis: - a trigger should be retained if the median score on the 5-point Likert scale was ≥4 and the 25th percentile ≥4 (i.e., ≥75% of the experts considered the trigger as "relevant" or "absolutely relevant") - a trigger should be excluded if the median score was <3 and the 75th percentile <3 (i.e., ≥75% of the experts considered the trigger as "irrelevant" or "absolutely irrelevant") - no consensus for triggers that failed to meet either of the latter cut-off values."
Meredith et al.[59] 2019 USA Community Pharmacy	To use a modified Delphi method to develop standardized youth-friendly counseling tools that are sensitive to pharmacy workflow during pharmacist contraceptive prescribing.	A panel of experts across different disciplines, which included pediatric and adolescent gynecologists, adolescent medicine physicians, community and women's health pharmacists, and public health professionals.	Invited: NA Agreed: 9 Completed: NA	Researchers created a toolkit material based on published protocols from states with implemented programs. Experts commented on the tool. No item numbers were defined.	3 rounds Online (Qualtrics® platform)	Subjective analysis • The process was repeated until expert panel consensus was reached

Continued

TABLE 3 Characteristics and quality of included studies—cont'd

Author(s) Year of publication Country of data collection Setting	Stated study objectives	Experts	Number of experts Invited, agreed to participate, and completed all rounds	Item/statement Development	Number of rounds Mode	Consensus measure Description
Bourne et al.[10] 2018 UK Critical care units	(1) To evaluate the views of expert UK critical care pharmacists who participated on what combinations of resources they thought reduced medication errors and to classify the units by the level of combined resources available. (2) To investigate if there were significant differences in the pharmacist prescription intervention type, clinical impact, and rates according to unit resource classification using results from the previous study	Pharmacists members of the UK Critical Care Group "Expert Practice Development Group"	Invited: 18 Agreed: NA Completed: 13	Literature search with the addition of medication safety resources recommended in UK critical care practice. Total 15 items were identified for round 1; round 2: 13; round 3; 8 items. Consensus on top 5 combined medication error reduction resources was established	3 rounds Mode: Online (Delphi Decision Aid)	Measures of central tendency (mean, mode, median); and Certain level of agreement • Round 1: items <50% removed • Round 2: items with a median score of 4 or 5 were included in round 3 • 5 point Likert scale used
Al Juffali et al.[51] 2019 Saudi Arabia Community Pharmacy	This study aimed to adopt a theoretically- underpinned approach to derive consensus and prioritize medication safety problems in community pharmacy in Saudi Arabia	Three stakeholder groups: pharmacy users, professionals, and community pharmacists	Invited: 359 Agreed: 161 Completed: 102	Items derived from a qualitative study conducted by the authors[65]. A total of 119 items was generated; After piloting, the number of items was reduced to 84 items. Consensus achieved on 28 items.	3 rounds Online (SurveyMonkey and a paper questionnaire)	A certain level of agreement • 6-point Likert scale used • The consensus at >70%
Penm et al.[56] 2018 International Hospital	This study aimed to use feedback from an international cohort of healthcare professionals in the field of medication reconciliation to (1) develop a consensus definition of medication reconciliation and (2) define the essential components of medication reconciliation.	Experts were identified based on their leadership in publications, education, professional interest, and participation in the area of medication reconciliation	Invited: NA Agreed: 24 Completed: 17	Literature search (PubMed, EBSCO, Google scholar). 54 items were included in round 1; 60 in round 2; 28 in round 3. A total of 65 items had consensus. Round 4 was done to define medication reconciliation.	4 rounds Online (Research Electronic Data capture)	A certain level of agreement • >80% strong agreement • 70%–80% moderate to strong agreement were included in subsequent rounds

Study	Objective	Participants	Development	Rounds/Mode	Consensus definition
Jebara et al.[19] 2019 Qatar National level: Ministry of Public Health, healthcare settings, and healthcare institutions	To determine the levels of agreement among key stakeholders in Qatar regarding a framework for the potential development and implementation of pharmacist prescribing.	Leaders and directors representing medicine, nursing, pharmacy and pharmacy technicians, policy, quality, and patient safety, and academia.	Invited: 35 Agreed: 33 Completed: 30	Umbrella review of systematic reviews, systematic review of views on pharmacist prescribing,[70,71] recent qualitative interviews in Qatar, and pharmacist prescribing frameworks from other countries. A total of 47 statements were included in round 1; 15 in round 2. 38 items achieved consensus.	2 rounds Online (SurveyMonkey)	A certain level of agreement • >70% agreement
Knapp et al.[45] 2019 USA Clinics and community pharmacies	(1) To address workforce issues most likely to impact on pharmacists working in pharmacies with retail clinics; and (2) to develop recommendations that provide preliminary insights into the characteristics of an optimal model for successful collaborations in collocated facilities	Researchers with pharmacist workforce and pharmacy practice research experience	Invited: 8 Agreed: 8 Completed: 8	Developed by the research team from the literature on the topic. A total of 15 items were included in all "impact" rounds. A total of 12 items achieved consensus. Panelist provided initial recommendations for "optimization" round 1; 15 recommendations were provided in round 2 and 3; A total of 6 recommendations received consensus	3 rounds for "impact" 3 rounds for optimization Online (Qualtrics)	Measures of central tendency (mean, median, mode) • Round 1: 4 point numeric scale used; Consensus at ≥80% • Round 2: 3-point numeric scale was used • Round 3: ≥80% agreement
Marine et al.[40] 2018 Belgium Hospitals	To develop and validate a tool for a standardized comparison of clinical pharmacy practices that could be used in Belgian hospitals. The tool aims to measure Quality Indicators (QIs) and contextual factors relevant to the Belgian context.	Clinical pharmacists	**1st validation** 9 clinical pharmacists participated **2nd validation** 8 clinical pharmacists participated	A narrative literature review (PubMed, Google scholar) and focus groups. A total of 25 items were included in 1st validation; 13 items in the 2nd validation	3 rounds (2 rounds for 1st validation; 1 round for 2nd validation) Mode: NA	Measures of central tendency (mean, median, mode) • 5-point Likert scale was used • The consensus was a mean score ≥3.5. • kept the five highest-ranked items.
Krzyżaniak et al.[41] 2017 Poland NICU	(1) To identify a set of pharmacy-based key performance indicators in Donabedian's domains of process, structure, and outcome that can be used to benchmark the quality of pharmaceutical care provided to patients in Polish NICU settings. (2) To identify the minimum level of pharmacy services that should be consistently provided to NICU patients.	Key stakeholders involved in NICU care and were defined as hospital pharmacists, or pharmacists based in academia; leading medical doctors and nurses; people with hospital-based clinical pharmacy services experience; people with experience in NICU.	Invited: 29 Agreed: 16 Completed: 7	Based on two previous studies. A total of 30 pharmacist role items and 32 KPIs in rounds 1 and 2; Consensus was achieved for 28 pharmacist roles and 23 KPIs.	2 rounds Online (SurveyMonkey)	A certain level of agreement • 5-point Likert scale used • The consensus at ≥75%

Continued

TABLE 3 Characteristics and quality of included studies—cont'd

Author(s) Year of publication Country of data collection Setting	Stated study objectives	Experts	Number of experts Invited, agreed to participate, and completed all rounds	Item/statement Development	Number of rounds Mode	Consensus measure Description
Berenbrok et al.[46] 2020 USA Community pharmacies	To design a value-based payment model to incentivize pharmacists for increased administration of influenza, herpes zoster, pertussis-containing, and pneumococcal vaccines to adults at community pharmacies	Experts from community pharmacy practice, employer-sponsored health insurance, managed care, or value-based payment models, and academics.	Invited: 11 Agreed: 11 Completed: 9	Value-based model created by the project team. A total of 12 items in round 1 and round 2. Participants met in person after round 2 to build consensus on the model. Round 3 and 4 participants were asked to select between three goals	4 rounds Online (Qualtrics) and in-person meeting	Measures of central tendency (mean, median, mode) • 5-point Likert scale was used • No definition for consensus was provided
Maher et al.[62] 2020 Australia Clinical and regulatory pharmacy	To establish consensus on which competency items identified by the Association of Faculties of Pharmacy of Canada's Opioid Working Group are considered core competencies for Australian pharmacists in opioid supply and assess expert pharmacists' perceptions of how well these competencies are currently met by practicing pharmacists	Experts were registered pharmacists, and have content knowledge related to opioid supply above that of what is expected of a regular practicing pharmacist	Invited: 57 Agreed: 34 Completed: 27	Developed based on the Association of Faculties of Pharmacy of Canada Opioid Working Group's opioid set of competency statements; 37 items were included in round 1, 49 items for round 2. All items received consensus	2 rounds Online (Qualtrics)	A certain level of agreement • 6-point Likert scale used • The consensus at ≥75%
Gray et al.[38] 2016 UK Community pharmacies and dispensing doctor practices	To develop a set of characteristics of good pharmaceutical services that could be further refined into a quality improvement tool for use in CPs and dispensing DPs	Experts were pharmacists, dispensing GPs, dispensing staff at CPs and DPs, board members of CP and DP professional organizations, and laypersons.	Invited: 35 Agreed: 30 Completed: 22	A questionnaire administered by CPs and DPs results; and in-depth case studies of three CPs and four DPs informed the development of Delphi statements. A total of 23 items were included in rounds 1 and 2. All items were included and rated.	2 rounds Online or mailed paper copies	A certain level of agreement • 9-point numerical scale • Disagreement is defined as ≥30% of ratings in both the 1–3 and 7–9 tertiles

Study	Objective	Participants	Methods	Rounds/Mode	Consensus criteria
Awad et al.[57] 2017 Canada Hospital	Primary objective: To establish an urgency score to determine the priority of pharmacist consults at Chronic Viral Illness Service	Pharmacists working in an HIV outpatient hospital clinic in Canada	Invited: 20 Agreed: 16 Completed: 13	Scoring system based on a previously conducted study.[72] A total of 18 items were included in round 1; 20 items in rounds 2 and 3. All items were weighted using the Delphi.	3 rounds Online (LimeSurvey)	Coefficient of variation • 5-point continuous scale • The consensus was obtained with a CV<0.3 in the first and second round, • CV <0.5 in the third round
Hernández et al.[42] 2017 Spain Hospital	The objective of this study was to reach a consensus on the minimum set of data that would allow optimizing the pharmacotherapy follow-up of patients on biologic agents for chronic systemic inflammatory conditions, through a structured and standardized collection with an electronic tool in the hospital pharmacy	Hospital pharmacists with experience in the use of biologic agents. They were also promoters of research, education, and implementing new technologies in their work centers.	Invited: 30 Agreed: NA Completed: 21	Literature review. A total of 37 statements were included in both rounds. The consensus was achieved for all items.	2 rounds Online	A certain level of agreement • 5-point Likert scale • 75% level of agreement
Ignoffo et al.[47] 2016 USA Hospital	To estimate available BCOPs through 2020, to identify services BCOPs could provide to oncology patients, and to estimate their impact on the patient visit deficit/ to identify services that BCOPs could most reliably contribute to oncology patient care and to estimate how many patients visits BCOPs could provide.	Experts were academics and pharmacists with BCOP status and working pharmacists with residency	Invited: 15 Agreed: NA Completed: 13	Services were solicited from round 1 in Delphi and presented in round 2 with comments. A total of 13 services were finalized from round 3.	3 rounds Online (e-mail)	A certain level of agreement • 5-point Likert scale • 80% level of agreement
Atkinson et al.[44] 2017 International Pharmacists working in all settings	To produce a competence framework for PET in Europe	**Phase 1:** A panel consisting of the 13 consortial members All were academics with substantial experience in PET. **Phase 2:** A panel of community, hospital, industrial pharmacists and pharmacists working in other fields across Europe	Invited: NA Agreed: NA Completed: 410	Literature search. Individual round items NR. A total of 68 statements were finalized.	**Phase 1:** 3 rounds **Phase 2:** 2 rounds Online (SurveyMonkey)	Ordinal consensus: calculated as score= (frequency rank 3 + frequency rank 4) as % of total frequency • 4-point Likert scale used arbitrarily classified as: < 0.2 poor, 0.21– 0.4 fair, 0.41–0.6 moderate, 0.61–0.8 substantial, > 0.81 good

Continued

TABLE 3 Characteristics and quality of included studies—cont'd

Author(s) Year of publication Country of data collection Setting	Stated study objectives	Experts	Number of experts Invited, agreed to participate, and completed all rounds	Item/statement Development	Number of rounds Mode	Consensus measure Description
Pizzuto et al.[43] 2018 Malta Pharmacy (Not specified)	To investigate the perception of Maltese pharmacists to prescribe a selected number of antibiotics.	A heterogeneous group of five members was made up of three community pharmacists, one doctor, and one layperson.	Invited: 5 Agreed: 5 Completed: 5	A questionnaire was developed by the authors. A total of 36 questions were included in both rounds. 36 items were validated and included in the final version of the questionnaire.	2 rounds Mailed questionnaire	Consensus measure: NA • 5-point Likert scale 1 there is least agreement and 5 there is the highest agreement
Mubarak et al.[63] 2019 Malaysia Primary care clinics and community pharmacies	To seek consensus among different healthcare stakeholders for a "collaborative medication therapy management" model for chronic diseases in Malaysia which may involve CP and GPs in an active collaboration for the management of medicines and diseases.	A wide range of experts in practice and academia, including GPs, Family Medicine Specialists, clinical and community pharmacists, and nurses.	Invited: 38 Agreed: 34 Completed: 29	A systematic review (EBSCO, PubMed). A total of 132 statements in rounds 1 and 2. Consensus achieved on 119 statements.	2 rounds Online (QuestionPro)	A certain level of agreement; Kendall's coefficient of concordance; and measures of central tendency; ICC • Different Likert scales used • 85% level of agreement • Kendall's coefficient (less than 0.3, 0.3 to 0.5, 0.5 to 0.7, and 0.7 to 0.9 interpreted as weak, moderate, good, and strong agreement, respectively). • ICC (less than 0.3, 0.3 to 0.5, 0.5 to 0.7 and 0.7 to 0.9 indicate as weak, moderate, good and strong agreement, respectively)

Study	Objective	Panel	Participants	Items	Rounds/Mode	Consensus
Lat et al.[48] 2020 USA ICU	To delineate the activities of a critical care pharmacist and the scope of pharmacy services within the ICU	The task force included members representing a broad cross-section of critical care pharmacy practice (hospital, academia, administration, urban, rural, and clinical practice setting)	Invited: NA Agreed: NA Completed: 15	Literature search (PubMed) and review of the existing position paper on critical care pharmacy services. The number of items in each round NA. A total of 82 statements were finalized	3 rounds Mode: NA	A certain level of agreement and IQR • 9-point Likert scale • Consensus if 66% of members agreed
Smith et al.[49] 2019 USA Specialized clinics (pulmonary hypertension accredited centers for comprehensive care)	(1) To develop a consensus of best practice recommendations for the safe use of pulmonary hypertension pharmacotherapies by recruiting an expert panel of pharmacists and (2) To describe the pharmacist's role in the care of this patient population.	The panel consisted of the research coordinators and pharmacists with expertise in the management of pulmonary hypertension nominated by centers for pulmonary hypertension comprehensive care.	Invited: 16 Agreed: NA Completed: 13	Literature search (PubMed, and societal guidelines). A total of 24 recommendations included in round 1; 26 in round 2; 29 in round 3; and 26 in round 4. 26 recommendations were finalized.	4 rounds Online (SurveyMonkey) and group teleconferencing	Median score • 2-h teleconferencing with real-life modifications on items • 4- and 5-item Likert scale • panel consensus agreement (score of >3.75), equivocal (score of 2.5–3.75), or consensus disagreement (score of <2.5). • teleconferencing and dichotomous scale
Clay et al.50 2019 USA Not defined	To develop a pharmacist-patient care services intervention reporting checklist with interpretive guidance to be used in conjunction with existing primary reporting tools.	Round 1 and 2: Panels were researchers; expert pharmacists; current and former journal editors; academics, scientists, nonpharmacist clinicians, clinical trial specialists, students, and postdoctoral trainees Round 3: A new set of experts: a sample of established authors, peers of task force members, postdoctoral trainees, residency directors, pharmacy educators, current and former journal editors, and individuals with experience in conducting systematic reviews and metaanalyses	Round 1 and 2: Invited: NA Agreed: NA Completed: 16 Round 3: Invited: 179 Agreed: NA Completed: 30	A systematic review of systematic reviews and metaanalysis of pharmacy services. A total of 106 items were included in round 1. Round 2 involved testing the checklist. 9 items were included in round 3. A total of 9 items were finalized.	3 rounds Conference calls, checklist testing, and online (Qualtrics)	NA • Round 1: labeling items as 1(critical), 2 (optional), or 3 (unnecessary). • Round 3: denote if (1) the intention of the element was understandable and (2) an element should be included

Continued

TABLE 3 Characteristics and quality of included studies—cont'd

Author(s) Year of publication Country of data collection Setting	Stated study objectives	Experts	Number of experts Invited, agreed to participate, and completed all rounds	Item/statement Development	Number of rounds Mode	Consensus measure Description
Shawahna et al.[52] 2019 Palestine Primary care clinics	To develop and achieve consensus on KPIs of healthcare activities delivery by pharmacists to patients with epilepsy visiting epilepsy clinics as outpatients in primary care practice.	Experts in possession of academic qualifications or degrees qualifying for a healthcare profession; having a license to practice one of the healthcare fields directly involved in providing care to women with epilepsy (medicine, pharmacy, or nursing), and providing services to more than 5 women with epilepsy per month	Invited: 40 Agreed: 40 Completed: 40	Literature review (MEDLINE, EMBASE, COCHRANE, CINAHL, SCOPUS, and Google Scholar) 41 items were included in rounds 1; 12 items in rounds 2 and 3. A total of 8 KPIs achieved consensus.	3 rounds Mode: NA	A certain level of agreement; median and IQR • Round 1: 9 points Likert scale • 60% or more panelists needed to agree • Round 2 and 3: 9 point Likert scale • median 1–3 with IQR of 2 or less item was not important; 4–5 or IQR of more than 2, the item is equivocal and 7–9 with IQR of 2 or less item is important.
Shawahna et al.[53] 2017 Palestine Community Pharmacies	This study sought to develop a consensual core list of important knowledge items that community pharmacists should have on women's health issues in epilepsy	Panelists were licensed pharmacists with at least 10 years' experience in Palestine, with knowledge in women's issues in epilepsy, and interact with more than 5 women with epilepsy. The panel also included educators who taught courses related to epilepsy and women's health.	Invited: 30 Agreed: 30 Completed: 30	Interviews with experts and a review of the literature. 70 items were included in round 1; 17 items in round 2: A total of 68 items were finalized.	2 rounds Email	Median and IQR • 9-point Likert scale • The consensus at a median of 7–9 and IQR of 0–2,

Study	Objective	Panel	Sample	Methods	Rounds/Platform	Consensus definition
Rault et al.[58] 2019 Canada Hospital	The goal of this study was to develop good pharmacovigilance reporting practices	Directors of pharmacy of all Quebec hospitals	Invited: 30 Agreed: NA Completed: 25	Brainstorming sessions with three pharmacists and four pharmacy residents, literature review, and a survey of directors of hospital pharmacy. A total of 41 statements were included in round 1; round 2 NR; a total of 37 statements were finalized	2 rounds Online (SurveyMonkey)	Mean score • 9-point Likert scale • Average of ≥7 was considered as good statements • Average of <7 was modified in first round and eliminated in second round.
Karampatakis et al.[39] 2019 UK General Practice	The purpose of this study was to reach a broad consensus among experts on what general practice-based pharmacists' activities should be recorded on the general practice clinical computer systems	Pharmacists or pharmacy technicians working in general practice and involved in coding general practice-based pharmacists' activities either at a local or national level along with other national experts holding senior general practice-based pharmacists' roles and widely engaged on national committees.	Invited: 29 Agreed: NA Completed: 16	Two members of the research team screened the general practice computer system to identify codes, and focus groups were conducted.[73] A total of 81 codes were included in round 1; 59 in round 2; 34 in round 3. The final consensus was reached on 10 codes.	3 rounds Online (Bristol Online Survey)	A certain level of agreement • 5- and 6-point Likert scale and dichotomous scale • Levels of agreement: (51% in Round 1, 70% in Round 2, and 80% in Round 3
Rocha et al.[50] 2018 Brazil Community pharmacies	The objective of this study was to develop and validate the content of an instrument to support pharmaceutical counseling for dispensing prescribed medicines.	Pharmacists with professional expertise in drug dispensing public health units, chain community pharmacies; academics and researchers in the field of drug dispensing	Invited: 40 Agreed: 29 Completed: 23	A systematic review[74] and brainstorming meeting with experts. The number of items in each round NR. A total of 11 items were finalized.	2 rounds Online (Google Forms)	Content validity index (CVI) • 5-point Likert scale • CVI of 0.80 was used to indicate agreement among the experts

KPI, key performance indicator; USA, United States of America; NA, not available; UK, United Kingdom; NICU, neonatal intensive care unit; CPs, community pharmacists; DPs, dispensing pharmacists; DPs, dispensing doctors; BCOPS, Board Certified Oncology Pharmacists; PET, pharmacy education and training; GP, general practitioner; ICC, intra-class correlation coefficient; ICU, intensive care unit.

Selection of experts

Pouliot et al. identified experts through literature search and self-identification through a survey sent to an international pharmacy organization.[54] They aimed at selecting 30 experts based on the norm of having 18 to 20 experts and accounting for a potential decrease in responses in subsequent Delphi rounds. Fifty invitation letters were sent out after being selected by what they defined as an "expert in the field" based on their leadership in publications, professional interests, and education. This approach was similar to Penm et al. where an invitation letter was sent to an international pharmacy organization and self-identification was used[56]; however, the experts were selected only if they were involved in implementing or evaluating a medication reconciliation program or policy and were self-declared to be fluent in English. On the other hand, Lima et al. produced an expert list that included people with different levels of expertise and professions including professors and researchers in the field.[64] Sixteen experts were invited to participate and a competence questionnaire was also used to assess their competence. Watson et al. purposively identified and selected 24 experts from various organizations including pharmacy, military, governmental and nongovernmental organizations. Snowballing technique was also used to account for the inherent bias of investigator selection. Out of 24, 15 consented to participate.[15] Similarly, Maher et al. used purposive sampling after creating a list of potential experts with predefined criteria and also supplemented their list with snowballing technique.[62] However, Thevelin et al., Meredith et al., and Berenbrok et al. might have fallen into this inherent potential bias as experts were selected based on their expertise or contacts with the research team.[46,55,59] Bourne et al. defined their experts as those who were included in a previous study with no additional experts added to the team.[10] This might have limited representation of the field. Purposive sampling was employed by Al Juffaili et al. but focused on selecting pharmacists working in different settings such as community, clinic, and chain pharmacies or working in different areas in the country. Additionally, they sent an invite to all pharmacists who participated in a previous study as well.[51] An interesting approach was used by Jebara et al., where a list of all experts was defined based on different professions and expertise and then five different experts were randomly selected from each field[19] Knapp et al. described selecting experts from an objective perspective, but this was not further clarified.[45] Marine et al. purposively selected hospitals across Belgium with at least one clinical pharmacist. It is not clear how the researcher selected the clinical pharmacists thereafter.[40] Krzyżaniak et al. described using both purposive and criterion sampling approach with a clear description of the selection criteria.[41] Gray et al. described using purposive sampling to select experts across different relevant fields to represent views of all stakeholders.[38]

Statement development

Included studies conducted a systematic review or described literature search as a mean of identifying statements or items included in the Delphi process, hence the "modified Delphi" approach described earlier. Few studies described the search process and stated the number of databases included ($n = 9$)[40,48,49,52,54–56,61,63] which ranged between one and five databases. Nonetheless, six studies indicated a literature search with no further description.[10,42,44,53,58,60] Five studies supplemented their literature search with experts' interviews[19,53,58–60] ($n = 5$), and one study used focus groups[40] to refine their statements. Furthermore, five studies used prior research conducted by the authors to inform the statements,[19,41,46,51,57] while three studies used specific articles within the same field[41,59,62] ($n = 3$). One study solicited the statements directly from round 1 of the Delphi process,[47] and Gray et al.[38] used questionnaire results to pin out the statements.

Concerning the application or use of theory or framework in the Delphi process, Knapp et al. described using the Collaborative Theory to structure the survey used and to ensure capturing all relevant parameters related to their study.[45] Similarly, Jebara et al. used the earlier described Consolidated Framework for Implementation Research (CFIR) to capture all key elements related to the research.[19] Additionally, Al Juffaili used the Human Factors Framework to explore factors affecting patient safety and guide the development of relevant statements.[65]

With regards to reviewing the Delphi questionnaire, a total of ten studies described the review and the piloting process which was mainly conducted to ensure clarity and understanding. Al Juffali et al.,[51] and Karampatakis et al.[39] piloted the Delphi questionnaire on 15 experts and three experts, respectively. Krzyżaniak and Shawahna[53] briefly described that the questionnaire was piloted on a small number of experts for readability and comprehensiveness. On the other hand, Maher[62] piloted the questionnaire through interviews for clarification and understanding while in three studies, the questionnaire was reviewed by experts for face and content validity including wording, convenience, understanding, and design-related aspects. Shawahna et al. piloted their questionnaire on five newly graduating pharmacists for time, clarity, and ease of understanding,[52] while Rault et al. described that the questionnaire was pretested iteratively by the five experts to ensure maximum clarity and understanding for each statement.[58]

Data collection and analysis

The majority of included studies used online surveys for data collection ($n = 19$). Four studies used a combination of different data collection methods. For instance: Berenbrok et al. used an online survey and an in-person meeting.[46] Four studies did not clearly state their method of data collection. The majority of studies had three rounds of Delphi ($n = 12$), followed by two rounds ($n = 11$).

Defining Delphi rounds a priori or using preset stopping criteria is important to be documented as described earlier. Only eight articles described an a priori number of rounds,[39–41,43,44,49,56,63] nonetheless, all studies defined their consensus.

Most studies had a certain level of agreement as a consensus measure in their Delphi method ($n = 11$) and three studies reported measures of central tendency for consensus. Six studies had used more than one measure for consensus. For instance, Bourne et al. used measures of central tendency and a certain level of agreement for consensus,[10] and Shawahna et al. used a certain level of agreement for Delphi round 1 and median and interquartile range (IQR) for Delphi rounds 2 and 3.[52] Three, three, and four studies considered that consensus was achieved for statements with more than 70%, 75%, and 85% agreement, respectively. Stability was investigated in two articles only. For Watson, stability was achieved after three Delphi rounds; however, it was not examined statistically; the authors described that experts no longer continued to revise their ranking of items.[15] On the other hand, Mubarak et al. achieved stability after the second round and this was examined statistically.[63]

Reported limitations related to Delphi in included studies

The majority of studies reported limitations concerning their Delphi method. The most common limitations included: the use of virtual technology which may limit the richness of arguments versus face-to-face meetings or focus groups and restricts participation to those who have internet access. Furthermore, the inadequate response rate to Delphi surveys; the small number of panelists, the high number of dropouts between the first and the last Delphi rounds, selection bias, and the limited diversity of panelists or opinion leaders. Other limitations include the restricted number of Delphi rounds where additional rounds may have led to a definitive consensus of participants.

Important highlights from the review

Following a structured approach in selecting the expert panel is of great importance to have valid results and to reflect true consensus. Eight articles highlighted that the experts identified and selected by investigators might have added an inherent bias to their results. Therefore, it is suggested to follow the approach presented by Okoli[66] and applied by Mubarak et al.[63] in order to have a true reflection from experts in the field. Interestingly, three articles by Marine, Atkinson, and Pouliot reflected on the need to consider the native language of participants when selecting the panels or drafting the questionnaire items or statements for the Delphi. The authors indicated that the Delphi items might have been misunderstood because of language barriers, therefore, affecting the overall validity of the consensus process.[40,44,54] This might affect the validity of the overall consensus of the process.

Pouliot et al.[54] emphasized that the time gap between rounds might have contributed to the high dropout rates seen in their study. In fact, attrition bias was raised as a limitation in four studies.[41,49,54,55] It has to be noted that there is no solid recommendation in relation to the suitable time frame for Delphi studies. Okoli[66] reflected that attrition is not common with Delphi studies as compared to other study designs, yet this was not truly reflected in the Delphi studies conducted in the past 5 years. It is interesting to note that the approaches used by Mubarak et al.[63] aided in maintaining full participation.

Additionally, Okoli,[66] von der Gracht,[33] and Boulkedid[16] all reflect on the importance of maintaining the anonymity of panels throughout the Delphi process. In fact, anonymity is a major advantage of the Delphi method over other consensus methodologies. Nonetheless two studies[56,64] indicated that live meetings would have allowed for exploring disagreements within the expert panel. It is very important to maintain anonymity, "a fundamental Delphi characteristic,"[33] and use other modes such as structured qualitative feedback to reflect on disagreements.[33,66]

Almost all identified Delphi studies highlighted the lack of standardization due to lack of guidelines and reporting tools. Studies need to fully describe the Delphi method used to enhance credibility and transferability of results.[16] The majority of researchers relied on previous studies and methodology papers such as the ones presented by Boulkedid, von der Gracht, and Okoli to apply Delphi.[16,33,66] This highlights the urgent need to develop a comprehensive, reliable, and quality assessment tool.

It has been suggested that findings from consensus methods are explored and discussed further while considering the theoretical basis and context for the research.[67] Despite that theory can be applied to the various stages of research processes, it is advisable to consider it from the initial stages of planning to provide a framework for analysis and discussion as this will enhance the research rigor and robustness leading to findings that are of relevance and impact.[68] As an example, Jebara et al. used the Consolidated Framework for Implementation Research (CFIR) to guide the development of the statements in the Delphi method and provide comprehensive coverage of key factors needed for the implementation.[19]

An exemplary case study

A concrete research that illustrates a good utilization of the Delphi methodology is the one conducted by Mubarak et al. for the purpose of developing a model for pharmacy practice in Malaysia.[63] A "ranking-type" Delphi[66] was conducted to build consensus on all dimensions needed for a "collaborative medication therapy management" model for chronic diseases. The authors highlighted that using the Delphi method would overcome bias, hierarchy- and communication-related barriers in seeking physical consensus among competing stakeholders (defined as clinical pharmacists, general practitioners, and nurses).

A total of 38 experts were identified by adopting the five-step process demonstrated by Okoli et al.[66]: (1) preparing knowledge resource nomination worksheet; (2) populating the worksheet with names; (3) nominating additional experts; (4) ranking experts based on qualifications and; (5) inviting experts. Twenty-nine experts participated in both round 1 and round 2 of the study. An interesting approach adopted by Mubarak et al. was the use of three reminders, thank you note, providing an honorarium equivalent to US$24.30, and conducting face-to-face interviews between the rounds to eliminate attrition bias. Results demonstrated that these approaches indeed eliminated attrition.

With regards to the questionnaire items, a modified Delphi approach was used whereby the first-round items were obtained through extensive literature search resulting in 132 items classified into 11 themes. Six external reviewers were sought for face and content validity (through content validity index). The updated questionnaire was then uploaded to the "QuestionPro" web-based survey tool. The authors indicated that a web-based survey reduced time and resource utilization to obtain consensus.

In addition to the consensus measure, the researchers investigated the stability of responses before concluding the Delphi process. A certain level of agreement (i.e., $\geq 85\%$ indicates high consensus level, and $\leq 74\%$ indicates poor or no consensus), Kendall's coefficient of concordance, Intraclass Correlation Coefficient, Wilcoxon signed-rank test of stability, and measures of central tendencies were all utilized in this study. The second round was informed by the quantitative data and qualitative comments from the first round. The consensus was measured after confirming stability (which was accomplished after the 2nd round) and was achieved on 119 items out of 132 items. The authors presented a model as a figure and provided several recommendations for the Ministry of Health, community pharmacy leadership, general practitioners' leadership, and for the Ministry of Education.

Recommendations for researchers thinking about using Delphi in their research

Researchers need to demonstrate the methodological rigor for the Delphi technique that they use to enhance the credibility, reliability, and validity of their findings. This can be achieved by having a clear definition for the study objectives, justification for the used process along with a clear description and sufficient details of the scientific evidence provided to participants, the selection processes including the credentials of the panel of experts, the planned number of rounds and when to terminate the process, the initial questionnaire and the process of determination of items, the definition of group consensus, the reporting of findings and response rates, the type of feedback provided to the panel after each round, and assurance of maintaining anonymity.[5] Moreover, Landeta has shared his pearls on wisdom in effectively executing Delphi approach.[69] These include:

- The need for institutional support to facilitate the recruitment of the expert panel;
- The research team need to have expertise in running the Delphi method and the topic being discussed;
- The research team need to be able to select a good panel of experts who will effectively contribute to the topic under discussion and actively engage throughout the different steps of the process;
- The need to arrange an orientation session to the panel of experts from the outset of the process to provide further information about the topic being discussed, the various steps involved in the process, and answer any questions that may arise;
- Piloting the survey questions to ensure face and content validity;
- Encouraging qualitative feedback from a panel of experts;

- Thanking the panel of experts for their valuable participation and sharing with them the results through a personalized letter or a concluding session to present research findings.

Questions for further discussion

1. Is the Delphi technique the only research approach in studies determining consensus? If there are other approaches, what factors should be taken into account in selection? Are any approaches more suited to specific research aims and questions?
2. Considering that the Delphi technique will generate low-level evidence compared to methods such as randomized controlled trials, what approaches should be taken to enhance robustness and rigor?
3. Is a qualitative phase always a necessary step in conducting the Delphi technique? In what circumstances will it add value?
4. When and how should theories or theoretical frameworks be considered in conducting the Delphi technique? If being used, is one theory or framework more suitable than others?
5. Is there an optimal approach to determining consensus? If no, what factors should be considered in defining consensus and the measurement approach? How can validity and reliability be enhanced?

Application exercise/scenario

Select one of the included studies in Table 3 that is of interest to you and answer the following questions:

- Reflect on the five steps of the Delphi technique discussed in this chapter (problem definition, selection of experts, statement development, data collection and analysis, and reporting and quality assessment) and describe how these steps have been applied?
- What approach was used to define and measure consensus?
- How could have the Consolidated Framework for Implementation Research (CFIR) been applied?
- What challenges did the authors encounter?
- Make a list of learning points you would implement within your research?

Identify a topic of interest to you and describe how the Delphi technique could be of value to use?

References

1. Jones J, Hunter D. Qualitative research: consensus methods for medical and health services research. *BMJ*. 1995;311(7001):376.
2. Halcomb E, Davidson P, Hardaker L. Using the consensus development conference method in healthcare research. *Nurse Res*. 2008;16(1):56–71.
3. McMillan SS, King M, Tully MP. How to use the nominal group and Delphi techniques. *Int J Clin Pharmacol*. 2016;38(3):655–662.
4. Waggoner J, Carline JD, Durning SJ. Is there a consensus on consensus methodology? Descriptions and recommendations for future consensus research. *Acad Med*. 2016;91(5):663–668.
5. Humphrey-Murto S, Varpio L, Gonsalves C, et al. Using consensus group methods such as Delphi and nominal group in medical education research. *Med Teach*. 2017;39(1):14–19.
6. Humphrey-Murto S, Varpio L, Wood TJ, et al. The use of the Delphi and other consensus group methods in medical education research: a review. *Acad Med*. 2017;92(10):1491–1498.
7. Black N, Murphy M, Lamping D, et al. Consensus development methods: a review of best practice in creating clinical guidelines. *J Health Serv Res Policy*. 1999;4(4):236–248.
8. Brady SR. Utilizing and adapting the Delphi method for use in qualitative research. *Int J Qual Methods*. 2015;14(5), 1609406915621381.
9. Fitch K, Bernstein SJ, Aguilar MS, et al. *The Rand/UCLA Appropriateness Method User's Manual*. Santa Monica: Rand; 2001.
10. Bourne RS, Shulman R, Jennings JK. Reducing medication errors in critical care patients: pharmacist key resources and relationship with medicines optimisation. *Int J Pharm Pract*. 2018;26(6):534–540.
11. Fink A, Kosecoff J, Chassin M, et al. Consensus methods: characteristics and guidelines for use. *Am J Public Health*. 1984;74(9):979–983.
12. de Villiers MR, de Villiers PJ, Kent AP. The Delphi technique in health sciences education research. *Med Teach*. 2005;27(7):639–643.
13. Rowe G, Wright G. The Delphi technique as a forecasting tool: issues and analysis. *Int J Forecast*. 1999;15(4):353–375.
14. Hopf YM, Francis J, Helms PJ, et al. Linking NHS data for pediatric pharmacovigilance: results of a Delphi survey. *Res Social Adm Pharm*. 2016;12 (2):267–280.
15. Watson KE, Singleton JA, Tippett V, et al. Defining pharmacists' roles in disasters: a Delphi study. *PLoS One*. 2019;14(12), e0227132-e.
16. Boulkedid R, Abdoul H, Loustau M, et al. Using and reporting the Delphi method for selecting healthcare quality indicators: a systematic review. *PLoS One*. 2011;6(6), e20476.

17. Fernandes O, Gorman SK, Slavik RS, et al. Development of clinical pharmacy key performance indicators for hospital pharmacists using a modified Delphi approach. *Ann Pharmacother.* 2015;49(6):656–669.

18. Aljamal MS, Ashcroft D, Tully MP. Development of indicators to assess the quality of medicines reconciliation at hospital admission: an e-Delphi study. *Int J Pharm Pract.* 2016;24(3):209–216.

19. Jebara T, Cunningham S, MacLure K, et al. A modified-Delphi study of a framework to support the potential implementation of pharmacist prescribing. *Res Social Adm Pharm.* 2020;16(6):812–818.

20. Ryan K, Amir LH, Barnett C. Delphi study of pharmacology experts to derive international recommendations for medicine use in lactation. *Res Social Adm Pharm.* 2014;10(5), e15.

21. Hasson F, Keeney S, McKenna H. Research guidelines for the Delphi survey technique. *J Adv Nurs.* 2000;32(4):1008–1015.

22. Kezar A, Maxey D. The Delphi technique: an untapped approach of participatory research. *Int J Soc Res Methodol.* 2016;19(2):143–160.

23. Bloor M, Wood F. *Keywords in Qualitative Methods.* Thousand Oaks, Calif: SAGE Publications Ltd; 2006.

24. Campbell SM, Cantrill JA. Consensus methods in prescribing research. *J Clin Pharm Ther.* 2001;26(1):5–14.

25. Hugh M. The Delphi technique: a worthwhile research approach for nursing? *J Adv Nurs.* 1994;19:1221–1225.

26. Crisp J, Pelletier D, Duffield C, et al. The Delphi method? *Nurs Res.* 1997;46(2):116–118.

27. Powell C. The Delphi technique: myths and realities. *J Adv Nurs.* 2003;41(4):376–382.

28. Baker J, Lovell K, Harris N. How expert are the experts? An exploration of the concept of 'expert' within Delphi panel techniques. *Nurs Res.* 2006;14(1):59–70.

29. Akins RB, Tolson H, Cole BR. Stability of response characteristics of a Delphi panel: application of bootstrap data expansion. *BMC Med Res Methodol.* 2005;5, 37.

30. Rowe G, Wright G, Bolger F. Delphi: a reevaluation of research and theory. *Technol Forecast Soc Chang.* 1991;39(3):235–251.

31. Damschroder LJ, Aron DC, Keith RE, et al. Fostering implementation of health services research findings into practice: a consolidated framework for advancing implementation science. *Implement Sci.* 2009;4(1):50.

32. Diamond IR, Grant RC, Feldman BM, et al. Defining consensus: a systematic review recommends methodologic criteria for reporting of Delphi studies. *J Clin Epidemiol.* 2014;67(4):401–409.

33. von der Gracht HA. Consensus measurement in Delphi studies. *Technol Forecast Soc Chang.* 2012;79(8):1525–1536.

34. Jünger S, Payne SA, Brine J, et al. Guidance on conducting and REporting DElphi studies (CREDES) in palliative care: recommendations based on a methodological systematic review. *Palliat Med.* 2017;31(8):684–706.

35. Trevelyan EG, Robinson PN. Delphi methodology in health research: how to do it? *Eur J Integr Med.* 2015;7(4):423–428.

36. Holey EA, Feeley JL, Dixon J, et al. An exploration of the use of simple statistics to measure consensus and stability in Delphi studies. *BMC Med Res Methodol.* 2007;7(1):52.

37. von Elm EAD, Egger M, Pocock SJ, Gotzsche PC, Vandenbroucke JP. The strengthening the reporting of observational studies in epidemiology (STROBE) statement: guidelines for reporting observational studies. *Ann Intern Med.* 2007;147(8):573–577.

38. Grey E, Harris M, Rodham K, et al. Characteristics of good quality pharmaceutical services common to community pharmacies and dispensing general practices. *Int J Pharm Pract.* 2016;24(5):311–318.

39. Karampatakis GD, Ryan K, Patel N, et al. Capturing pharmacists' impact in general practice: an e-Delphi study to attempt to reach consensus amongst experts about what activities to record. *BMC Fam Pract.* 2019;20(1):126.

40. Cillis M, Spinewine A, Krug B, et al. Development of a tool for benchmarking of clinical pharmacy activities. *Int J Clin Pharmacol.* 2018;40(6):1462–1473.

41. Krzyżaniak N, Pawłowska I, Bajorek B. Quality pharmacy services and key performance indicators in Polish NICUs: a Delphi approach. *Int J Clin Pharmacol.* 2018;40(3):533–542.

42. Calleja Hernández M, Herrero Ambrosio A, Lamas Díaz MJ, et al. Pharmacotherapy follow-up of patients under treatment with biologic agents for chronic inflammatory systemic conditions: an agreement among hospital pharmacists for the standardized collection of a minimum set of data. *Farm Hosp.* 2017;41(n01):31–48.

43. Attard Pizzuto M, Camilleri L, Azzopardi LM, et al. Exploring views of pharmacists on antibacterial prescribing: a Maltese perspective. *Int J Pharm Pract.* 2019;27(3):256–263.

44. Atkinson J. The production of the PHAR-QA competence framework. *Pharmacy (Basel).* 2017;5(2):19.

45. Knapp KK, Olson AW, Schommer JC, et al. Retail clinics colocated with pharmacies: a Delphi study of pharmacist impacts and recommendations for optimization. *J Am Pharm Assoc.* 2020;60(2):311–318.

46. Berenbrok LA, Renner HM, Somma McGivney MA, et al. A conceptual value-based incentivization model of adult immunization for community pharmacists. *J Am Pharm Assoc.* 2020;60(6):835–842.

47. Ignoffo R, Knapp K, Barnett M, et al. Board-certified oncology pharmacists: their potential contribution to reducing a shortfall in oncology patient visits. *J Oncol Pract.* 2016;12(4):e359–e368.

48. Lat I, Paciullo C, Daley MJ, et al. Position paper on critical care pharmacy services: 2020 update. *Crit Care Med.* 2020;48(9):e813–e834.

49. Smith ZR, Rangarajan K, Barrow J, et al. Development of best practice recommendations for the safe use of pulmonary hypertension pharmacotherapies using a modified Delphi method. *Am J Health Syst Pharm.* 2019;76(3):153–165.

50. Clay PG, Burns AL, Isetts BJ, et al. PaCIR: a tool to enhance pharmacist patient care intervention reporting. *J Am Pharm Assoc.* 2019;59(5):615–623.

51. Al Juffali LA, Knapp P, Al-Aqeel S, et al. Medication safety problems priorities in community pharmacy in Saudi Arabia: a multi-stakeholder Delphi study using the human factors framework. *BMJ Open*. 2019;9(11), e032419.

52. Shawahna R. Development of key performance indicators to capture in measuring the impact of pharmacists in caring for patients with epilepsy in primary healthcare: a Delphi consensual study. *Epilepsy Behav*. 2019;98(Pt. A):129–138.

53. Shawahna R. Which information on women's issues in epilepsy does a community pharmacist need to know? A Delphi consensus study. *Epilepsy Behav*. 2017;77:79–89.

54. Pouliot A, Vaillancourt R, Stacey D, et al. Defining and identifying concepts of medication literacy: an international perspective. *Res Social Adm Pharm*. 2018;14(9):797–804.

55. Thevelin S, Spinewine A, Beuscart JB, et al. Development of a standardized chart review method to identify drug-related hospital admissions in older people. *Br J Clin Pharmacol*. 2018;84(11):2600–2614.

56. Penm J, Vaillancourt R, Pouliot A. Defining and identifying concepts of medication reconciliation: an international pharmacy perspective. *Res Social Adm Pharm*. 2019;15(6):632–640.

57. Awad C, Canneva A, Chiasson C-O, et al. PHIRST trial—pharmacist consults: prioritization of HIV-patients with a referral screening tool. *AIDS Care*. 2017;29(11):1463–1472.

58. Rault P, Mégroureche É, Labarre JS, et al. Determination of good pharmacovigilance reporting practices in Quebec hospital pharmacies using a modified Delphi method. *Pharmacoepidemiol Drug Saf*. 2019;28(7):985–992.

59. Meredith AH, Wilkinson TA, Campi JA, et al. Use of the Delphi method to enhance pharmacist contraceptive counseling materials. *J Pharm Pract*. 2019;34:678–684.

60. Rocha KSS, Cerqueira Santos S, Boaventura TC, et al. Development and content validation of an instrument to support pharmaceutical counselling for dispensing of prescribed medicines. *J Eval Clin Pract*. 2020;26(1):134–141.

61. Lima TM, Aguiar PM, Storpirtis S. Development and validation of key performance indicators for medication management services provided for outpatients. *Res Social Adm Pharm*. 2019;15(9):1080–1087.

62. Maher E, Nielsen S, Summers R, et al. Core competencies for Australian pharmacists when supplying prescribed opioids: a modified Delphi study. *Int J Clin Pharm*. 2020;43:430–438.

63. Mubarak N, Hatah E, Aris MAM, et al. Consensus among healthcare stakeholders on a collaborative medication therapy management model for chronic diseases in Malaysia; a Delphi study. *PLoS One*. 2019;14(5), e0216563-e.

64. Lima TM, Aguiar PM, Storpirtis S. Evaluation of quality indicator instruments for pharmaceutical care services: a systematic review and psychometric properties analysis. *Res Social Adm Pharm*. 2018;14(5):405–412.

65. Al Juffali L, Al-Aqeel S, Knapp P, et al. Using the human factors framework to understand the origins of medication safety problems in community pharmacy: a qualitative study. *Res Social Adm Pharm*. 2019;15(5):558–567.

66. Okoli C, Pawlowski SD. The Delphi method as a research tool: an example, design considerations and applications. *Inf Manage*. 2004;42(1):15–29.

67. Foth T, Efstathiou N, Vanderspank-Wright B, et al. The use of Delphi and nominal group technique in nursing education: a review. *Int J Nurs Stud*. 2016;60:112–120.

68. Stewart D, Klein S. The use of theory in research. *Int J Clin Pharmacol*. 2016;38(3):615–619.

69. Landeta J. Current validity of the Delphi method in social sciences. *Technol Forecast Soc Chang*. 2006;73(5):467–482.

70. Jebara T, Cunningham S, MacLure K, et al. Stakeholders' views and experiences of pharmacist prescribing: a systematic review. *Br J Clin Pharmacol*. 2018;84(9):1883–1905.

71. Stewart D, Jebara T, Cunningham S, et al. Future perspectives on nonmedical prescribing. *Ther Adv Drug Saf*. 2017;8(6):183–197.

72. Wong A, Gigure P, Robinson L, et al. Survey of healthcare professionals on the role of pharmacists in an outpatient HIV clinic setting. *Can J Infect Dis Med Microbiol*. 2015;26(Suppl B).

73. Karampatakis GD, Ryan K, Patel N, et al. How do pharmacists in English general practices identify their impact? An exploratory qualitative study of measurement problems. *BMC Health Serv Res*. 2019;19(1):34.

74. Boaventura TC. *Working Process of Pharmaceutical Dispensing: Systematis Reviews*. São Cristóvão: Federal University of Sergipe; 2016.

Section IV

Quantitative Approaches and Analytical Considerations

Chapter 34

Using prescription drug databases for comorbidity adjustment: A remedy for disaster or a prescription for improved model fit?

Mitchell J. Barnett[a,b], Vista Khosraviani[a], Shadi Doroudgar[a,c], and Eric J. Ip[a,c,d]

[a]*Clinical Sciences, Touro University-College of Pharmacy, Vallejo, CA, United States,* [b]*Iowa Board of Pharmacy, Iowa Department of Public Health, Des Moines, IA, United States,* [c]*Department of Medicine-Primary Care and Population Health, Stanford University, Stanford, CA, United States,* [d]*Internal Medicine, Kaiser Permanente Mountain View Medical Offices, Mountain View, CA, United States*

Objectives

- Define comorbidity or severity of illness and describe how it relates to health services research.
- List common approaches (techniques or methodologies) widely available to health service researchers for conducting comorbidity or severity adjustments using administrative or claims data.
- Describe potential advantages and disadvantages of using diagnostic claims data to create a comorbidity index and adjust for comorbidity or severity of illness.
- Describe potential advantages and disadvantages of using pharmacy claims data to create a comorbidity index and adjust for comorbidity or severity of illness.
- Be able to identify limitations of using claims data to adjust for patient differences in comorbidity or severity of illness.

In health services research, information on patient comorbidity is generally culled from three main or primary types of patient-level information when taken from administrative or claims data sources. These include inpatient diagnostic data, outpatient or ambulatory diagnostic data, and information from outpatient prescription drug files. Information collected from all three of these has been utilized, with varying degrees of success, to identify comorbid conditions in patients for purposes of severity or risk adjusting.

Broadly defined, comorbidity is any underlying patient condition or state that may affect the outcomes for the patient. Comorbidity has also been defined as the existence or occurrence of any additional disease during the clinical course of a patient who has an index disease under study.[1] A comorbidity index (CI) is a measure that, when conducting statistical analyses, will control for the potential influence of those illnesses on an outcome of interest. Comorbidity adjustment in health services research is vital in cases where randomization of treatments or comparison groups are not practical, ethical, or are simply too costly or time-intensive to undertake. Comorbidity adjustments, also called case-mix, or severity adjustments, may also be utilized in randomized control trials to reduce remaining bias; ensure that patient types have been evenly distributed among treatment arms, sites, institutions or providers; or to provide complementary information.

As noted by Iezzoni, researchers attempting to control or adjust for patient differences historically included only select patient attributes, such as age and gender, into their models.[2] Later attributes considered important by researchers included race, ethnicity, and socioeconomic factors, with measures attempting to gauge comorbidity or severity being relatively newer. It should be noted that controlling for severity and comorbidity is almost always done in conjunction with the more traditional measures, i.e., age, gender, and socioeconomic variables, rather than posing as proper substitutes. In other words, severity adjustments should be thought of only as an additional or adjunct measure to be considered to further refine models.

Severity adjustment measures may also serve a purpose beyond research. To give just one brief example, imagine a situation where provider report cards, listing aggregate patient outcomes, are distributed to clinic providers along with their leadership or management team. Furthermore, suppose that these report cards include benchmarking or reference points that show the clinic and the providers at the clinic to be performing poorly relative to their peers. However, what if the providers at the clinic in question are known for their expertise, and, therefore, the peers that make up the reference or comparison group routinely send their most difficult or challenging patients to the clinic for care? Shouldn't the clinic in question be given "credit" for electing or being selected to receive the more severe or onerous cases? As this simple example illustrates, adjustments when benchmarking are important, and comparisons of unadjusted outcomes, for research or other purposes, may lead to improper interpretation.[3]

Methods

The chapter first presents a history (timeline shown in Fig. 1) and narrative of the major diagnostic measures in use over the last four decades for comorbidity adjustments before focusing on comorbidity information gathered from outpatient prescription drug files or prescription file sources. The chapter next reviews the advantages and disadvantages (shown in Fig. 2) of utilizing prescription drug information relative to diagnostic information and summarizes published articles in which comparisons between prescription drug and diagnostic information are made. A review of English language studies found on PubMed, Medline, Embase or CINAHL published between January 1990 and December 2020. Prescription data for comorbidity adjustments was utilized as the search criteria for prescription drug articles. Initial search terms included "prescription and medication measures and indexes," "pharmacy," "pharmacy claims and pharmacy information systems," "risk adjustment and risk assessment," "severity of illness," "comorbidity," and comorbidity scores. In addition, references for the articles included were reviewed to identify any other remaining relevant published studies. Over 100 potential full text pharmacy or medication-based articles were screened for further review, from which 50 were retained. Excluded articles included those which did not incorporate a prescription or medication-based measure, did not report patient or policy outcomes, and were a commentary or letter or were duplicate publications.

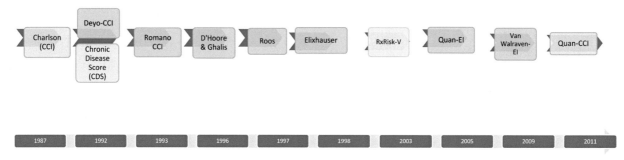

FIG. 1 Chronological development of free or shareware comorbidity measures.

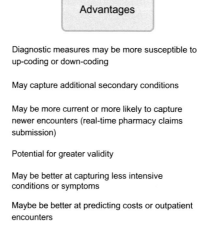

FIG. 2 Potential advantages and disadvantages of prescription measures (compared to diagnostic measures) for use with comorbidity adjustment.

Advantages	Disadvantages
Diagnostic measures may be more susceptible to up-coding or down-coding	May be worse at predicting mortality, inpatient encounters or utilization over relatively short time frames
May capture additional secondary conditions	May be suspectable to formulary restrictions or prior approval procedures
May be more current or more likely to capture newer encounters (real-time pharmacy claims submission)	May not be captured if patient is non adherent or obtaining medications outside of network/formal channels
Potential for greater validity	NDCs may not be universal and require updating
May be better at capturing less intensive conditions or symptoms	Some medications may have more than one indication which may not be appropriately captured
Maybe be better at predicting costs or outpatient encounters	More than half of the prescription-based models have yet to be validated externally
	Inferring a diagnosis from a prescription may result in error as a prescription may be used preventively or to confirm a diagnosis

Review of Charlson comorbidity index

Developed in 1987 by Mary Charlson et al., the Charlson Comorbidity Index (CCI) is arguably the first, the most utilized, and the most studied comorbidity measure. A contemporary search on PubMed finds over 10,500 citations for the original 1987 article. The original CCI was derived from 559 patients admitted for inpatient medical services at a New York hospital.[4] A chart review was conducted after discharge to collect information about the patient's comorbid conditions present at the time of admission and used to predict one-year mortality. A total of 19 comorbid categories were identified and subsequently assigned a score of 1 to 6 to create a weighted composite CCI. The CCI was validated on a second cohort of 685 women with breast cancer admitted to Yale University teaching hospital in the 1960s. The original CCI was found to be a good predictor of survival as measured by hazard ratios derived from a Cox proportional hazards regression. Since then, the CCI has been adapted for use with administrative data using ICD-9-CM codes and, subsequently ICD-10-CM codes, from inpatient or outpatient data and used to estimate an abundance of outcomes including: inpatient admissions, length of stay (LOS), hospital readmissions, outpatient visits, utilization, costs, and more subjective measures such as health-related quality of life (HRQoL). Different weights have often been utilized to predict different outcomes. Consistent findings regarding the CCI note that is a much better predictor of outcomes than age and gender alone.[5] Further, the CCI has generally been found to be a better predictor of mortality than readmissions. Although chart review usually uncovers additional diagnoses not captured in the CCI, some studies have found the CCI comparable to self-reported diagnoses when used for severity adjustment.[6] While obtaining comorbidity from chart review or patient history may outperform indices obtained from administrative data in some instances, they are much more time and resource-intensive, leaving a distinct advantage for administrative sources.

Adaptations in the CCI have been numerous, and several have resulted in gradual improvements in model fitting over the original CCI. More common adaptations include Deyo et al. (Deyo-CCI), Romano et al. (Romano-CCI), and Roos et al. (Roos-CCI). Deyo was one of the first modified CCIs (1992) and included 17 comorbid conditions.[7] The most current Deyo-CCI uses ICD-10-CM codes and has outperformed the original ICD-9-CM version with regards to hospital mortality.[8] While the Deyo variant of Charlson is the most commonly used, the Romano-CCI is likely superior to the Deyo-CCI, the original CCI, and other versions of the CCI (e.g., Quan-CCI, D'hoore-CCI, Roos-CCI, et al.).[9–11] The Romano-CCI (also referred to as the Dartmouth-Manitoba-CCI), adaptation includes broader definitions, encompassing more codes for peripheral vascular diseases, complicated diabetes, and malignancy.[10] Romano has also been an advocate of researchers deriving their empirical weights depending upon population and outcome. The term "empirical weights" in a study simply indicates that the authors did not change any categories or comorbidities, but derived new weights calibrated to their dataset as opposed to using the original published weights. It should be noted that many studies that used Romano in fact used empirical weights as recommended by Romano's paper. Therefore, the higher performance of Romano in predicting outcomes may partially reflect the impact of using empirical weights in general.[9] Most of the common CCI adaptions have been adapted for use with ICD-10-CM codes, in addition to earlier ICD-9-CM codes, thus allowing comparisons across times, regions and institutions. Finally, it has also been suggested that ICD-10-CM versions capture "more information" than their ICD-9-CM counterparts and may outperform existing ICD-9-CM coding algorithms.[12]

Review of Elixhauser comorbidity index

The original Elixhauser comorbidity index (EI) was developed by Anne Elixhauser et al. in 1998 and mapped 30 chronic conditions from ICD-9-CM codes (Elixhauser).[13] Output from the EI resulted in 30 categorical or indicator variables and was found to be a significant predictor of LOS and hospital charges. Subsequently, the EI was shown to have acceptable to excellent predictive ability of in-hospital mortality. Revisions of the EI included the removal of cardiac arrhythmias (29 categories) and the reconsideration of cardiac arrhythmias with the bifurcation of hypertension into uncomplicated and complicated (currently 31 categories). The revised EI has been shown to be a significant predictor of LOS and in-hospital charges, and it has generally been shown to have good to excellent predictive ability with regards to mortality. The EI was developed further; seminal work by Van Walraven et al. converted the 31 categories into a single weighted EI score (VW-EI). The VW-EI has been shown to have a similar predictive ability as the individual indicator variables.[10,14]

Charlson comorbidity index vs. Elixhauser comorbidity index

EI is generally accepted as similar or superior to the CCI in its prediction of prognoses.[15–17] In more direct comparisons to CCI, both show poor to excellent ability to predict depending on the outcome variable and the patient population. In a 2017 systematic review, Yurkovich reported nine studies in which the EI outperformed the CCI, four studies in which the CCI outperformed the EI, and four studies with no significant difference between the two.[10] When predicting mortality, C statistics have generally been used, where a predictive model with perfect discrimination has a C statistic of 1.0 and a model with no discrimination has a C statistic of 0.5, namely, a coin toss. C statistics have generally been found to range from 0.63 to 0.88 and 0.61 to 0.86 for the EI and CCI, respectively. The correlation between higher C statistics and better control for confounding has been demonstrated, where C statistics between 0.7 and 0.8 can be considered acceptable and between 0.8 and 0.9 excellent.[18,19] Recent literature has also shown an advantage of the EI over the CCI.[20–22] Although similar in semantics, a key distinction is that the EI was developed exclusively for use with administrative data, whereas the CCI was developed in another context (chart review) and later adapted for use with administrative data. Studies that also explored combining outpatient diagnoses with the original inpatient diagnoses found in the CCI and EI have generally found improvements in model fit.[9]

There is only partial overlap in the comorbidities that the CCI and EI cover, and many diseases are not covered by either. This has led to attempts to either combine the CCI and EI or expand them to use disease states notable to the patient population being studied. Combined measures include two studies that each reported a better ability to predict mortality when combining CCI and EI.[23,24] The combined comorbidity score (CCS), which includes only common CCI and EI conditions, has also been found to result in a better model fit.[25] Compared with baseline variables such as age and gender, comorbidity adjustment methods better predict long-term than short-term mortality, and the EI seems to be the better predictor for this outcome. For short-term mortality, recalibration with empirical weights seems more important than the choice of comorbidity measure.[9] The reader is reminded that while the CCI and EI were developed in patients with an inpatient event, adding outpatient diagnoses may moderately improve mortality prediction. In addition, any diagnostic-based measure is likely less useful than an algorithm which includes clinical data, such as the proprietary Acute Physiology Assessment and Chronic Health Evaluation, versions III or IV (APACHE-III or APACHE-IV). A summary of some of the common nonproprietary diagnostic-based measures, along with links to sites containing their computer code (i.e., macros), is shown in Table 1.

TABLE 1 List of commonly used "freeware" comorbidity measures.

Comorbidity measure	Link(s) to SAS software computer macros or coding information	ICD-9-CM, ICD-10-CM, AHFS, ATC or NDC based
Charlson (CCI)	http://mchp-appserv.cpe.umanitoba.ca/Upload/SAS/_CharlsonICD9CM.sas.txt	ICD-9 or ICD-10
Deyo CCI	http://mchp-appserv.cpe.umanitoba.ca/concept/Charlson%20Comorbidities%20-%20Coding%20Algorithms%20for%20ICD-9-CM%20and%20ICD-10.pdf https://github.com/kpwhri/CharlsonMacro	
Romano CCI	http://mchp-appserv.cpe.umanitoba.ca/viewConcept.php?conceptID=1098	ICD-9 or ICD-10
Roos	http://mchp-appserv.cpe.umanitoba.ca/concept/Archived_Charlson_Concept_Info.html	ICD-9
D'Hoore and Ghalis	http://mchp-appserv.cpe.umanitoba.ca/Upload/SAS/med_Charlson_3DigitCodes.sas.txt	ICD-9 or ICD-10
Quan	http://mchp-appserv.cpe.umanitoba.ca/Upload/SAS/ICD9_E_Charlson.sas.txt	ICD-9 or ICD-10
Elixhauser (EI)	https://www.hcup-us.ahrq.gov/toolssoftware/comorbidityicd10/comorbidity_icd10.jsp	ICD-9 or ICD-10
Van Walraven EI	https://rdrr.io/cran/icd/man/van_walraven.html http://mchp-appserv.cpe.umanitoba.ca/viewConcept.php?conceptID=1436	ICD-9 or ICD-10
Quan EI	http://mchp-appserv.cpe.umanitoba.ca/viewConcept.php?conceptID=1436#QUANSCODE	ICD-9 or ICD-10
CDS	https://sph.unc.edu/files/2013/12/CDS_Intro.doc	NDC
RxRisk-V	https://rdrr.io/github/eribul/classifyr/man/rxriskv.html (trying to find better links)	NDC

Review of pharmacy measures

The original chronic disease system (CDS) was the first widely recognized attempt to gauge comorbidities based on patient-level prescription data. The underlying notion was that patients with chronic conditions were more likely to use pharmacotherapy and the number of prescribed drugs was hypothesized to increase with the number of chronic conditions.[26] Developed in 1992 by von Korff et al., the CDS utilized a panel of experts to map 17 chronic diseases from prescription claims.[27] The 17 conditions were then weighted, and a composite score comprised of eight categories was created. Clark et al. updated the original CDS in 1995 to include 28 categories (Clark-CDS).[28] In both versions of the CDS, disease conditions were identified using associated prescription drugs used for such conditions, i.e., the use of antidiabetic agents corresponds to diabetes. A person filling a prescription for a drug included in the algorithm is considered to have the chronic condition associated with that drug. As a result, it has been noted that the Clark-CDS has high specificity, but only moderate sensitivity, causing it to sometimes underestimate the number of diseases associated with a patient.

Notable adaptions of the Clark-CDS include those by Malone et al. (CDI) in 1999 and Fishman et al. (RxRisk) in 2003.[29,30] These versions greatly expanded the number of chronic conditions, to 54 and 57 conditions, in the CDI and RxRisk, respectively, in addition to mapping new drugs into chronic conditions. More recent adaptions have included a revised RxRisk for use in VAMC patients (RxRisk-V) by Sloan et al. in 2003 and attempts to combine prescription and diagnostic measures such as the one by Corrao et al. (CMS) in 2017.[26,31] Further revisions have included adaptions for use in non–U.S.-based patient populations and for use in specific disease states (e.g., prostate cancer) and specific patient populations (e.g., Medicaid-RxRisk). A final prescription-based index is the medication-based disease burden index (MDBI), developed to deal with prior issues identified by Clark and Fishman.[32] However, current validation studies show the MDBI to be a weaker predictor than RxRisk-V.

Although the original CDS was used to predict one-year mortality, hospitalization and ambulatory visits, the various adaptions have been used to predict a variety of additional outcomes. These include, in addition to those previously mentioned, ambulatory costs, total costs, functional status and risk of infection. Predictive ability for the prescription measures has generally been found to range from $R^2 = 0.05$ to 0.15 for expenditures, $R^2 = 0.15$ to 0.40 for utilization with C statistics of 0.60 to 0.80 for mortality. The known prescription comorbidity measures are summarized in chronological order for the reader in Table 2.

General methodological concerns with using prescription-based measures for risk adjustment include: (1) only drugs prescribed specifically for treating certain chronic conditions can be used to assign subjects to these chronic conditions; (2) inferring a diagnosis from a prescription (e.g., chicken and egg paradox where a prescription is being used preventively or to confirm a diagnosis), (3) prescription dispensing data may not indicate patient use and often fails to capture adherence; and; (4) more than half of the prescription-based models have yet to be validated externally.[16,33,34] More specific concerns or problematic issues include drugs which may be available over-the-counter (OTC) and by prescription (either at the same or different doses), and drugs that are susceptible to wide variations in practice patterns rather than the severity of illness. Common examples of the latter include antibiotics and drugs for insomnia.[35] Medication indices may also require more frequent updating relative to diagnostic measures, as new medications come on the market or as new uses for existing medications become standard practice. Lastly, prescription data may lack information on drugs received from a friend or family member, procured from outside the country, or when supplies from previous prescription fills are utilized.

Advantages of prescription measures

Diagnostic measures may be subject to upcoding for a more favorable reimbursement, or down-coding if the provider is only interested in documenting the primary or presenting symptom. Research has suggested that salaried physicians record fewer diagnoses relative to their fee-for-service peers.[35] Diagnostic data may also miss secondary conditions, particularly when gathered from an acute inpatient event. Diagnostic measures may miss some conditions that prescription-based measures capture. For example, even though most providers now require regular, often yearly visits, scheduling delays may result. Such delays would mean that even 12-month queries would not capture all of a patient's diagnoses. Select diagnoses (e.g., quadriplegia) may be captured only once, or infrequently.[35] With such diagnoses, even a review of several years' worth of inpatient and outpatient diagnostic data may miss the diagnosis. Pharmacy data may be timelier and updated more frequently (often at the point of service in real time) than diagnosis data. Prescriptions may have greater validity, as there are legal requirements for pharmacies to report dispensations that do not exist for reporting of diagnoses.[29] Unlike diagnostic data, which involve some degree of uncertainty and discretion in the assignment of diagnosis codes, the National Drug Codes (NDCs) used in pharmacy data are linked to a specific product and a clinical course of action. Further, diagnostic indices were originally used to predict one-year mortality (CCI) or length of stay, hospital charges, and in-hospital

TABLE 2 Summary of 35 published articles concerning the use of prescription drug information for comorbidity or severity adjustment.

RF#	Title	Authors	Journal, Year	Findings	Comments
27	A chronic disease score from automated pharmacy data[a]	Von Korff M, Wagner EH, Saunders K	Journal of Clinical Epidemiology, 1992	$N = 122{,}911$ Time = 1985–1986 Region = Washington state Baseline model = age, gender and healthcare visits. Outcome(s) = One-year hospitalization and mortality, ambulatory visits. ORs ranged from 1.00 to 9.84. $R^2 = 0.18$ for ambulatory visits	Identified 17 chronic conditions, each scored 1 to 3. Composite scores were subsequently grouped into 8 categories. Model fits for mortality and hospitalization were not presented, although odds ratios increased for each increase in CDS category.
53	Replicating the chronic disease score (CDS) from automated pharmacy data	Johnson RE, Hornbrook MC, Nichols GA	Journal of Clinical Epidemiology, 1994	$N = 6324$ Time = 1990–1991 Region = Oregon and Washington state. Baseline model = age and gender Outcome(s) = Social, physical function (RAND-36) and depression. Following year healthcare visits and hospitalizations. R^2 for CDS ranged from 0.01–0.36. Less impressive for depressive measures	Validated CDS on subsequent sample population. Model fit (R^2) for following year healthcare visits and hospitalizations similar to previous Van Korff (CDS) models.
54	The use of prescription claims databases in pharmacoepidemiological research: the accuracy and comprehensiveness of the prescription claims database in Québec	Tamblyn R, Lavoie G, Petrella L, Monette J.	Journal of Clinical Epidemiology, 1994	$N = 65{,}349$ Time = 1990 Region = Quebec Baseline model = N/A Outcomes = Validating pharmacy claims. Concluded prescription claims represent accurate means of determining drugs dispensed to individuals.	May be limitations in using drug database for dosing information.

TABLE 2 Summary of 35 published articles concerning the use of prescription drug information for comorbidity or severity adjustment—cont'd

RF#	Title	Authors	Journal, Year	Findings	Comments
28	A chronic disease score with empirically derived weights	Clark D, Von Korff M, Saunders K, Baluch W, Simon G.	Medical Care, 1995	N = 254,994 Time = 1992–1993 Region = Washington state Baseline model = age and gender Outcome(s) = 6-month outpatient costs and PCP visits. Empirical weighting improved R^2 for 6-month outpatient costs from 0.16 to 0.23, and 6-month PCP visits from 0.04 to 0.13	Marked improvement over original CDS as measured by R^2 Utilized 28 categories vs. 17 CDS-Clark Developed to predict: total costs, ambulatory costs, and ambulatory visits
55	Development and estimation of a pediatric chronic disease score using automated pharmacy data	Fishman PA, Shay DK	Medical Care, 1999	N = 81,119 Time = 1992–1993 Region = Washington state Baseline model age and gender Outcome(s) = One-year total costs, ambulatory costs, primary care costs and PCP visits $R^2 = 0.06, 0.17, 0.01$ and 0.02 for one-year total costs, ambulatory costs, primary care cost and PCP visits, respectively.	Validated CDS in pediatric population (PCDS) 26 categories
56	Pharmacy costs groups: a risk-adjuster for capitation payments based on the use of prescribed drugs	Lamers LM	Medical Care, 1999	N = 55,907 Time = 1993–1995 Region = Holland Baseline model = age and gender and region and disability. Outcome(s) = 6-month total costs $R^2 = 0.10$	Pharmacy-based Cost Group (PCG) 23 chronic conditions. Can further group into 6 categories depending on number of chronic conditions. R^2 approximately twice the baseline model

Continued

TABLE 2 Summary of 35 published articles concerning the use of prescription drug information for comorbidity or severity adjustment—cont'd

RF#	Title	Authors	Journal, Year	Findings	Comments
29	Development of a chronic disease indicator (CDI) score using a Veterans Affairs Medical Center medication database[a]	Malone DC, Billups SJ, Valuck RJ, Carter BL.	*Journal of Clinical Epidemiology*, 1999	$N = 246$ Time = 1997 Region = Rocky Mountain Baseline model = N/A Outcome(s) = Correlation with chart review and CDS $R^2 = 0.43$ and 0.66 for chart review and CDS, respectively	54 chronic disease categories CDI identifies individual classes and all are weighted equally. CDS uses weights. Predicted chronic diseases, not outcomes.
57	Preoperative drug dispensing as predictor of surgical site infection	Kaye KS, Sands K, Donahue JG, Chan KA, P Fishman P, Platt R.	Emerging Infectious Diseases, 2001	$N = 563$ Time = 1992 and 1997 Region = Boston area hospitals Baseline model = age and gender and procedure duration Outcome(s) = 30-day postsurgery infection Higher OR 2.6 (95% CI = 1.5–4.7) for patients with high CDS	C statistic not presented.
35	The Medicaid Rx model pharmacy-based risk adjustment for public programs.	Gilmer T, Kronick R, Fishman P, Ganiats TG	*Medical Care*, 2001	$N = 362,370$ disabled, 401,557 adults and 1,094,385 children. Time = 1990–1999 Region = CA, CO, GA, TN Baseline model = CDPS Outcome(s) = 12-month total costs $R^2 = 0.06$ to 0.15 for prescription models. Diagnostic models were better at predicting expenditures for disabled, models performed similarly for TANF beneficiaries.	SSI and TANF patient population. Developed model (Medicaid Rx) to classify subset of NDCs into categories for risk assessment and risk-adjusted payment. Medicaid Rx excluded categories from CDS, but added acute conditions. 49 total categories. Diagnostic based CDPS uses 56 categories mapped into 18 major categories. Models combining diagnostic and prescription data were superior.

TABLE 2 Summary of 35 published articles concerning the use of prescription drug information for comorbidity or severity adjustment—cont'd

RF#	Title	Authors	Journal, Year	Findings	Comments
58	Chronic disease score as a predictor of hospitalization	Putnam KG, Buist DSM, Fishman P, Andrade SE, Boles M, Chase GA, Goodman MJ, Gurwitz JH, Platt R, Raebel MA, Chan KA	Epidemiology, 2002	$N = 29,247$ women Time = 1995 Region = Nationwide (8 HMOs) Baseline model = age and gender and CCI Outcome(s) = One-year hospitalization One-year total costs, outpatient costs and outpatient visits. C statistics = 0.68–0.71	Considered two versions of the CDS: CDS-Clark and CDS-Fishman. Clark CDS outperformed Fishman CDS. CDS > CCI
30	Risk adjustment using automated ambulatory pharmacy data	Fishman PA, Goodman MJ, Hornbrook MC, Meenan RT, Bachman DJ, O'Keeffe Rosetti MC.	Medical Care, 2003	$N = 1,536,867$ total sample $N = 106,245$ validation Time = 1995–1996 Region = Nationwide (8 HMOs) Baseline model = age and gender Outcome(s) = future total costs $R^2 = 0.09$	RxRisk revised CDS into 57 categories RxRisk also compared with propriety ACG and HCC models HCC > RxRisk > ACG R^2 (future total costs) of HCC = 0.15 and ACG = 0.09
31	Construction and characteristics of the RxRisk-V: a VA-adapted pharmacy-based case-mix instrument	Sloan KL, Sales AE, Liu CF, Fishman P, Nichol P, Suzuki NT, Sharp ND	Medical Care, 2003	$N = 126,075$ VAMC Time = 1998 Region = West Coast. Baseline models = age and gender Outcome(s) = Concurrent costs and one-year total costs $R^2 = 0.18$ and 0.10 for concurrent and one-year total costs, respectively.	RxRisk-V 45 categories. Linked drug names to NDC
50	Improved comorbidity adjustment for predicting mortality in Medicare populations	Schneeweiss S, Wang PS, Avorn J, Glynn RJ	Health Services Research, 2003	$N = 466,794$ Time = 1994 Region = NJ and PA states Baseline model = age and gender, CCI-Romano and EI Outcome(s) = one-year mortality C statistic = 0.70 (CDS-1)	30 categories (updated to map newer drugs) Avoid using pharmacy data over diagnostic data unless diagnostic data inferior. Simple sum of number of prescriptions may be a reasonable predictor. EI = Romano > CCI > CDS-1 > Age and gender for one-year mortality prediction

TABLE 2 Summary of 35 published articles concerning the use of prescription drug information for comorbidity or severity adjustment—cont'd

RF#	Title	Authors	Journal, Year	Findings	Comments
33	The Pharmacy-based Cost Group model: validating and adjusting the classification of medications for chronic conditions to the Dutch situation	Lamers LM, van Vliet R CJA	Health Policy, 2004	$N = 6,353,716$ Time = 1997–1999 Region = Holland Baseline models = age and gender and urbanization and disability Outcome(s) = 12-month total costs $R^2 = 0.09$	Used 22 categories from CDS Removed drugs treating acute conditions and drugs prescribed in less than half of relevant diagnoses.
59	Development and validation of a diabetes mellitus severity index: a risk-adjustment tool for predicting health care resource use and costs	Joish VN, Malone DC, Wendel C, Draugalis JR, Mohler MJ	Pharmacotherapy, 2005	$N = 734$ Time = 1998–2002 Region = Arizona state Baseline model = age and gender Outcome(s) = one-year total costs and ambulatory costs $R^2 = 0.06$ and 0.10 for total and ambulatory costs, respectively.	VAMC diabetic patients Adding diagnostic and clinical lab data, e.g., A1C, LDL, etc. via the diabetes severity index (DSI), markedly improved the models.
60	Utility of the chronic disease score and Charlson comorbidity index as comorbidity measures for use in epidemiologic studies of antibiotic-resistant organisms	McGregor JC, Kim PW, Perencevich EN, Bradham DD, Furuno JP, Kaye KS, Fink JC, Langenberg P, Roghmann MC, Harris AD	American Journal of Epidemiology, 2005	$N = 4112$ Time = 1998–2001 Region = Maryland State Baseline model = CCI Outcome(s) = MRSA and VRE infection during admission C statistics = 0.47–0.67	Tested CDS in predicting MRSA and VRE
61	Comorbidity risk-adjustment measures were developed and validated for studies of antibiotic-resistant infections	McGregor JC, Perencevich EN, Furuno JP, Langenberg P, Flannery K, Zhu J, Fink JC, Bradham DD, Harris AD	Journal of Clinical Epidemiology, 2006	$N = 57,785$ Time = 1998–2003 Region = Maryland state Baseline model = CDS Outcome(s) = MRSA and VRE infection during admission C statistics = 0.60–0.65	Modified CDS added 4 additional categories to CDS. Modified CDS, CDS-MRSA and CDS-VRE are better at predicting MRSA and VRE than CDS.
32	Development and validation of the medication-based disease burden index (MDBI)[a]	George J, Vuong T, Bailey MJ, Kong DCM, Marriott JL, Stewart K	Annals of Pharmacotherapy, 2006	$N = 317$ Time = N/A Region = Australia Baseline model = age, CCI and CDS Outcome(s) = Correlation with CCI and CDS. $R^2 = 0.10$ and $R^2 = 0.28$, respectively	MDBI 20 categories

TABLE 2 Summary of 35 published articles concerning the use of prescription drug information for comorbidity or severity adjustment—cont'd

RF#	Title	Authors	Journal, Year	Findings	Comments
46	Adapting the RxRisk-V for mortality prediction in outpatient populations	Johnson ML, El-Serag HB, Tran TT, Hartman C, Richardson P, Abraham NS	Medical Care, 2002	$N = 724,270$ Time = 2002 Region = Nationwide Baseline model = age and gender and race, CCI-Deyo Outcome(s) = one-year mortality C statistic = 0.78	NSAID and COX-2 VAMC patients Updated RxRisk-V by adding 26 categories RxRisk-V = 45 categories RxRisk-V2 = 71 categories RxRisk-V2 > RxRisk-V > CCI-Deyo > baseline demographics Individual RxRisk-V categories slightly better than composite measure
62	Development and validation of a medication intensity scale derived from computerized pharmacy data that predicts emergency hospital utilization for persistent asthma	Schatz M, Zeiger RS, Vollmer WM, Mosen D, Apter AJ, Stibolt TB, Leong A, Johnson MS, Mendoza G, Cook EF.	The American Journal of Managed Care, 2006	$N = 1079$, $N = 24,370$ Time = 2000–2003 Region = CA, WA and OR Baseline model = age and gender Outcome = one year asthma related ED or inpatient admission C statistics = 0.52–0.69	Persistent asthma patients in single HMO New asthma medication intensity score derived from asthma related pharmacy outpatient claims (e.g., oral-corticosteroid and beta-agonist inhalers).
38	Validity of medication-based comorbidity indices in the Australian elderly population	Vitry A, Wong SA, Roughead EA, Ramsay E, Barratt J	Australian and New Zealand Journal of Public Health, 2009	$N = 791$, $N = 213,191$ Time = 1992 Region = Australia Baseline model = age and gender, education and income. Outcome(s) = 6-month mortality HR = 1.08, 95% CI = 1.05–1.11 for RxRisk-V HR = 3.69, 95% CI = 2.26–6.02 for MDBI	Patients 65 and older Compared the MDBI (developed for use in Australian patient populations) and RxRisk-V. RxRisk-V has 45 categories MDBI has 20 categories. HR = 1.09, 95% CI = 1.09–1.09 ($N = 213,191$) For Australian patients, RxRisk-V preferable over MDBI Overall model fit statistics not presented
63	A medication-estimated health status measure for predicting primary care visits: the Long-Term Therapeutic Groups Index	Dhabali AA, Awang R.	Health Policy and Planning, 2010	$N = 30,466$ Time2004–2005 Region = Malaysia Baseline model = age and gender and race and income and marital status. Outcome(s) = primary care visits $R^2 = 0.34$ (increase of 0.19 from baseline)	Long-Term Therapeutic Group Index (LTTGI) Mapping somewhat unclear. Drugs were mapped into therapeutic classes deemed chronic (e.g., statins, diuretics, calcium channel blockers, etc.) then summed for a total LTTGI score.

Continued

TABLE 2 Summary of 35 published articles concerning the use of prescription drug information for comorbidity or severity adjustment—cont'd

RF#	Title	Authors	Journal, Year	Findings	Comments
64	Explaining primary healthcare pharmacy expenditure using classification of medications for chronic conditions	Vivas D, Natividad Guadalajaraa N, Barrachinaa I, Trillo J-L, Usób R, lena de-la-Pozaa E	Health Policy, 2011	N = 625,246 Time = 2008–2009 Region = Spain Baseline model = age and gender and payment Outcome(s) = one-year pharmacy expenditures $R^2 = 0.57$	Comorbidity measures captured from hospital encounters may help predict pharmaceutical expenditures. CDS-Spain = 18 categories mapped from ATC CDS = 25 categories
65	Identifying patients with chronic conditions using pharmacy data in Switzerland: an updated mapping approach to the classification of medications	Huber CA, Szucs TD, Rapold R, Reich O	BMC Public Health, 2013	N = 913,612 Time = 2011 Region = Switzerland Baseline model = age and gender and region Outcome(s) = N/A CDS-Swiss = 22 categories	CDS-Swiss = 22 categories mapped from ATC Estimated portion of population with a condition, not validated with an outcome. CDS-Swiss from ATC may be useful in identifying comorbidity
16	The predictability of claim-data-based comorbidity-adjusted models could be improved by using medication data	Bang JH, Hwang SH, Lee EJ, Kim Y.	BMC Medical Informatics and Decision Making, 2013	N = 247,712 Time = 2007–2008 Region: South Korea Baseline model = CCI, EI Outcome(s) = in-hospital mortality C statistics CCI = 0.63–0.88 ECCI = 0.64–0.88 EI = 0.70–0.92 EEI = 0.71–0.92 Majority of C statistics in enhanced models within 95% CI of original CCI and EI, (Exception EI AMI)	ECCI and EEI tried to improve predictability of models using CCI and EI indices by using medication data; prescription data used to infer omitted comorbidities. Missing comorbidities included 8 out of 17 Charlson comorbidities, and 14 out of 31 Elixhauser comorbidities. Predictabilities of comorbidity-adjusted diagnostic models improved, but likely only small improvements.
66	The prevalence and ingredient cost of chronic comorbidity in the Irish elderly population with medication treated type 2 diabetes: A retrospective cross-sectional study using a national pharmacy claims database	O'Shea M, Teeling M, Bennett K	BMC Health Services Research, 2013	N = 445,180 Time = 2010 Region = Ireland Baseline model = age and gender Outcome(s) = Identifying comorbidities using RxRisk-V Prevalence of 35 of 45 RxRisk-V conditions higher in T2DM patients relative to non-T2DM patients.	T2DM patients 65 and older Categorized nonconcordant (non-T2DM) and concordant (T2DM) conditions. Individuals with T2DM had nearly 3 × the number of comorbid conditions. Not really validating RxRisk-V, just showing how it can be used to classify patients for research.

TABLE 2 Summary of 35 published articles concerning the use of prescription drug information for comorbidity or severity adjustment—cont'd

RF#	Title	Authors	Journal, Year	Findings	Comments
10	A systematic review identifies valid comorbidity indices derived from administrative health data	Yurkovich M, Avina-Zubieta JA, Thomas J, Gorenchtein M, Lacaille D.	Journal of Clinical Epidemiology. 2015	N = Systematic review 76 articles, of which 13 were based on pharmacy data. Time = 1992–2009 Region = Developed world Baseline model = Varied Outcome(s) = Costs, visits, readmissions and mortality among others. C statistics = 0.53–0.71 (depending on outcome) R^2 = 0.01–0.36 (depending on outcome)	Two categories of comorbidity indices were identified: those based on diagnoses from hospitalization or outpatient data, and those based on medications, using prescription data. Ability of indices to predict ranged from poor to depending on the specific index, outcome, and study population. Diagnosis-based measures, particularly EI and CCI-Romano resulted in higher ability to predict mortality while prescription-based measures, particularly the RxRisk-V, did well at predicting utilization.
25	Ccmparative Performance of Diagnosis-based and Prescription-based Comorbidity Scores to Predict Health-related Quality of Life.	Mehta HB, Sura SD, Sharma M, Johnson ML, Riall TS.	Medical Care, 2016	N = 140,046 Time = 2005, 2007–2012 Region = Nationwide (MEPS) Baseline model = age and gender, CCI, EI, CDS, HRQoL-CI Outcome(s) = mental and physical HRQoL R^2 = 0.13–0.20 (mental HRQoL) R^2 = 0.20–0.44 (physical HRQoL)	HRQoL-CI = 44 categories Combining prescription-based scores improved prediction of HRQoL-CI HRQoL-CI+CDS > EI +CDS > CCI+CDS for mental HRQoL HRQoL-CI+CDS > EI+CDS = CCI+CDS for physical HRQoL Highly dependent on disease state.
26	Developing and validating a novel multisource comorbidity score from administrative data: a large population based cohort study from Ita y	Corrao G, Rea F, Mirko MD, Palma RD, Scondotto S, Fusco D, Lallo A, Maria L, Belotti B, Ferrante M, Addario SP, Merlino L, Mancia G, Carle F	BMJ Open, 2017	N = 3 × 500,000 Time = 2006–2008 Region = Italy Baseline model = age and gender Outcome(s) = 12-month mortality, C statistic = 0.78	Patients 50 and older MCS = 46 categories (18 diagnostic, 6 prescription and 22 from both) mapped into 5 categorical scores MCS > CCI = EI = CDS One year mortality, 5 year mortality, 1 and 5 year hospital admissions and 2 year hospital costs showed association with MCS

TABLE 2 Summary of 35 published articles concerning the use of prescription drug information for comorbidity or severity adjustment—cont'd

RF#	Title	Authors	Journal, Year	Findings	Comments
67	Assessing and predicting drug-induced anticholinergic risks: an integrated computational approach	Xu D, Anderson HD, Tao A, Hannah KL, Linnebur SA, Valuck RJ, Culbertson VL	Therapeutic Advances in Drug Safety, 2017	$N = 575,228$ Time = 2001–2013 Region = Nationwide (sample from 102 managed care programs) Baseline model = N/A Outcome(s) = Anticholinergic incidents $R^2 = 0.83$	Patients 65 and older Rx derived comorbidity measures may be used to fine tune or further refine clinical assessments (weak)
68	The impact of pharmacy-specific predictors on the performance of 30-day readmission risk prediction models	Kabue S, Liu V, Greene J, Kipnis P, Lawson B, Rinetti-Vargas G, Liu V, Escobar G	Medical Care, 2019	$N = 350,810$ Time: 2014–2015 Region: California sate Baseline model = age and gender, LOS, and site. Illness severity and comorbidity point score (LAPS2, COPS2) Outcome(s) = 30-day readmission C statistic = 0.71 Pharmacy score (RxDxCG)	Patients 18 and older Aggregate Pharmacy Score (APS) Comorbidity Burden Score (CBS) RxDxCGs = 21 categories mapped from Verisk software (proprietary). Potential value in adding prescription-based diagnostic cost groups (RxDxCG) Goal to develop comprehensive parsimonious model relatively easy to instantiate by clinicians unfamiliar with complex modeling techniques. Despite high C statistic, proprietary nature of measure likely limits its use
69	Development and validation of a medication regimen complexity scoring tool for critically ill patients	Gwynn ME, Poisson MO, Waller JL, Newsome AS	American Journal of Health Systems Pharmacy, 2019	$N = 130$ Time: 2016–2017 Region: Georgia sate Baseline model = age and gender. Outcome(s) = ICU LOS, inpatient mortality and patient acuity. $R^2 = 0.04$, N/A, 0.17	Adult MICU patients. A total of 39 medications (e.g., vancomycin) or regimens (e.g., mechanical ventilation) likely to be used in a MICU scored 1-3 ×. Measure significantly related to ICU LOS, mortality and patient acuity. Unclear if computerized or chart review.
51	Modified-Chronic Disease Score (M-CDS): Predicting the individual risk of death using drug prescriptions	Iommi M, Rosa S, Fusaroli M, Rucci P, Fantini MP, Poluzzi E.	PLoS One, 2020	$N = 492,273$ Time:2016–2018 Region: Bologna Italy Baseline model = age and gender Outcome(s): one-year mortality and one-year hospitalization. C statistics = 0.76–0.77	Patient 50 and older 18 chronic conditions mapped into 6 categories. Objective to update original CDS to include changes in drug therapy. New measure referred to as modified CDS (M-CDS). Includes drugs marketed up to March 2019.

TABLE 2 Summary of 35 published articles concerning the use of prescription drug information for comorbidity or severity adjustment—cont'd

RF#	Title	Authors	Journal, Year	Findings	Comments
				for mortality and 0.67–0.71 for hospitalization M-CDS > CCI. M-CDS = multisource comorbidity score (uses drug and diagnostic info) in predicting 1-year mortality.	Collapsed categories, e.g., Alzheimer's ≥dementia, and removed drugs prescribed for conditions different from original CDS target. Minimum number of prescription fills = 2. Exception of MS and PUD, one and three prescriptions, respectively. Somewhat unclear if combined or summed into a composite score or used individual indicators.
70	A novel superior medication-based chronic disease score predicted all-cause mortality in independent geriatric cohorts.	Quinzler R, Freitag MH, Wiese B, Beyer M, Brenner H, Dahlhaus A, Döring A, Freund T, Heier M, Knopf H, Luppa M, Prokein J, Riedel-Heller SG, Schäfer I, Scheidt-Nave C, Scherer M, Schöttker B, Szecsenyi J, Thürmann P, van den Bussche H, Gensichen J, Haefeli WE	Journal of Clinical Epidemiology, 2019	N = 3189 Time: 2008–2009 Region: Germany Baseline model = age and gender Outcome(s): one-year all-cause mortality. C statistic = 0.73 to 0.79 and 0.64 to 0.66 for medCDS vs. CDS.	Medication-based chronic disease score (medCDS) Geared to medications used in Germany and a German population Utilized ATC ATC mapped to 29 categories and 6 chronic conditions, plus age and gender medCDS > RxRisk > = CDS > age and gender Lacked full presentation of some results.
36	A pharmaceutical dispensing-based index of mortality risk from long-term conditions performed as well as hospital record-based indices.	Stanley J, Doughty RN, Sarfati D. A	Medical Care, 2020	N = 2,331,645, N = 1,000,166 Time: 2011–2012 Region: New Zealand Baseline model = age and gender, CCI Outcome(s): one-year mortality and one-year hospitalization. C statistics = 0.92 vs. 0.92 for mortality C statistics = 0.68 vs. 0.71 for hospitalization	ATC codes mapped to 19 P3 conditions Combining CCI and P3 had little improvement P3 = CCI for mortality P3 > = CCI for hospitalization P3 + CCI > = CCI or P3

OR, Odds Ratio; PCP, Primary Care Provider; CDS, Chronic Disease Score; CDI, Chronic Disease Indicator; CCI, Charlson Comorbidity Score; CDPS, Chronic Disease Score; ACG, Ambulatory Care Groups; HCC, Hierarchical Coexisting Conditions; T2DM, Type 2 Diabetes; EI, Elixhauser Comorbidity Index; CCI-R, Charlson Comorbidity Score-Romano; CDS-1, Chronic Disease Score (2003 update); MDB¹, Medication-Base Disease Burden Index; HR, Hazard Ratio; ATC, Anatomical Therapeutic Chemical Classification Index; 95% CI, 95% Confidence Interval; AMI, Acute Myocardial Infarction; MEPS, Medical Expenditure Panel Survey; HRQoL-CI, Health-Related Quality of Life-Comorbidity Index; ECCI, Enhanced Charlson Comorbidity Index; EEI, Enhanced Elixhauser Comorbidity Index; MCS, Multisource Comorbidity Score; MS, Multiple Sclerosis; PUD, Peptic Ulcer Disease; MCI, Medicines Comorbidity Index; MICU, Medical Intensive Care; medCDS, Medication-based chronic disease score; P3, Pharmaceutical Prescribing Profile.
ªValues originally reported as r have been converted to R² for easier comparison.

death (EI), so they may be less useful for outpatient measures or outcomes relative to prescription-based measures. Lastly, prescription measures may capture less intensive chronic conditions not requiring hospitalization.[36]

Disadvantages of prescription measures

Diagnostic measures may be better at predicting mortality and outcomes with relatively shorter timeframes. Certain, potentially important, comorbidity measures, such as alcohol dependency, appear to be captured more frequently in diagnostic measures than prescription measures. Conversely, seizure conditions are captured more frequently by prescription measures relative to diagnostic ones.[31] Pharmacy severity measures may require frequent updating and are perhaps more susceptible to variations among regions or plans. Pharmacy benefit managers (PBMs) also frequently have a single preferred brand among a class of drugs and some brand name drugs within a class have sought out indications over their competitors. Other research has suggested that selective under-prescribing, based on comorbidity and age, respectively, is possible and that the absence of prescriptions to treat a condition does not necessarily indicate a lack of disease.[37] For example, a Type 2 diabetes mellitus patient may lack an active prescription drug on file due to controlling their blood glucose solely through nondrug measures or may have very poor adherence and rarely obtain his or her prescription drug. There also may be hurdles in working with prescription data not containing NDCs. However, there are several widely available proprietary and nonproprietary measures to crosslink AHFS, VAMC, and ATC categories, or drug names with NDCs.

Pharmacy vs. diagnostic measures

The diagnosis-based Charlson, Elixhauser, and combined comorbidity scores were derived to predict one-year mortality, in-hospital mortality, length of stay, and hospital charges, while the prescription-based chronic disease score (CDS) and the Veterans Affairs pharmacy-based index (Rx-Risk-V) were derived to predict healthcare utilization, cost, and mortality.[25] Perhaps not surprisingly, diagnostic measures have appeared to be better at predicting outcomes or prognosis, in particular short-term mortality, relative to prescription-based measures. Conversely, prescription-based measures have appeared to be better at predicting utilization rates or costs relative to diagnostic-based measures.[38] Generally, medication-based indices demonstrate a better ability to predict health care utilization outcomes, including prescription medication use, total costs, disease burden, and hospitalizations.[6,10,39,40] In direct comparisons, the RxRisk-V has been shown to have better prediction than CDS and better than Deyo-CCI. Specifically, the RxRisk-V has been found to be a better choice than EI or CCI for hospital expenditures.[39] However, the EI demonstrated a better ability to predict physician visits than the RxRisk-V.[40] Other studies have found prescription measures, such as the RxRisk, to be similar to diagnosis indices with regards to predicting readmissions, and LOS and hospital costs. However, overarching implications or generalizations are made difficult by many studies being performed on patient populations outside of the United Sates, on limited disease states (patients undergoing bypass surgery or cancer patients), and studies being geared toward a single outcome, i.e., mortality or rehospitalization. In addition, time of event or outcome (i.e., 30-day vs. 24-month mortality) has repeatedly been shown to widely influence model fit. Lastly, incremental improvements in severity adjustment measures obtained from diagnosis information would appear to make diagnosis measures preferable to prescription drug measures. However, new drugs, specifically targeted to chronic diseases, appear to show marked improvements in severity algorithms predicted from prescription drug claims.

A total of 15 studies were found directly comparing diagnosis-based and medication-based measures. A summary of these studies is presented in Table 3. In the six studies predicting mortality, results showed diagnostic measures to be preferable in five studies.[41–45] While only one study reported greater ability of the RxRisk-V measure to predict mortality relative to the Deyo-CCI.[46] Either greater or similar ability of the diagnostic measures to predict, relative to prescription measures, were found for readmission and visits.[40,41,47] Finally, in comparing costs, two studies were found where prescription-based measures outperformed diagnostic-based measures while two studies found relatively similar abilities to pretended to be better predictors of cost.[39,41,48,49]

Combining diagnostic and prescription

The literature is inconclusive on the value of adding prescription-based comorbidity scores to diagnosis-based scores to improve outcomes.[25] Although some studies have found that prescription-based data can improve the prediction ability of diagnosis-based scores, it remains poorly explored and likely to result in only marginal improvements.[16,35,47] Other studies have found a simple sum of the number of prescriptions may be a better predictor than a RxRisk measure when attempting to combine diagnostic with prescription data.[50] Further, difficulties in combining prescription data, which

TABLE 3 Comparison of diagnostic-based severity adjustment measures vs. prescription-based severity adjustment measures.

	Title	Authors	Journal, Year	Findings	Comments
47	Can pharmacy data improve prediction of hospital outcomes? Comparisons with a diagnosis-based comorbidity measure	Parker JP, McCombs JS, Graddy EA	Medical Care, 2003	$N = 6721$ Time = 1993–1995 Region = California state Comparison models = Deyo-CCI vs. CDS Outcome(s) = 30-day readmission and LOS C statistic = 0.68 vs. 0.68 $R^2 = 0.26$ vs. 0.26	Small improvements when combined Deyo-CCI likely preferable
41	Common comorbidity scales were similar in their ability to predict health care costs and mortality	Perkins AJ, Kroenke K Unützer J, Wayne Katon W, Williams Jr. JW, Hope C, Callahan CM	Journal of Clinical Epidemiology, 2004	$N = 3496$ Time = 1999–2001 Region = Indiana state Comparison models = Deyo-CCI vs. ACG vs. CDS Outcome(s) = one-year mortality, ambulatory visits, log total costs C statistic = 0.78 vs. 0.74 vs. 0.63 $R^2 = 0.08$ vs. 0.15 vs. 0.09 $R^2 = 0.08$ vs. 0.13 vs. 0.10	ACG performed best Deyo-CCI ~= CDS for visits and costs Deyo-CCI > CDS for mortality
42	Consistency of performance ranking of comorbidity adjustment scores in Canadian and U.S. utilization data	Schneeweiss S, Wang PS, Avorn J, Maclure M, Levin R, Glynn RJ.	Journal of General Internal Medicine, 2004	$N = 607,955$ Time = 1995–1997 Region = British Columbia, NJ and PA states. Comparison models = Romano-CCI vs. Deyo-CCI vs. Clark-CDS Outcome(s) = one-year mortality C statistic = 0.75–0.77 vs. 0.75–0.77 vs. 0.68–0.72	Results across 4 regions were relatively consistent.
59	Utility of the chronic disease score and Charlson comorbidity index as comorbidity measures for use in epidemiologic studies of antibiotic-resistant organisms	McGregor JC, Kim PW, Perencevich EN, Bradham DD, Furuno JP, Kaye KS, Fink JC, Langenberg P, Roghmann MC, Harris AD	American Journal of Epidemiology, 2005	$N = 4112$ Time = 1998–2001 Region = Maryland State Comparison models = Deyo-CCI vs. CDS Outcome(s) = MRSA and VRE infection during admission C statistics = 0.66 vs. 0.63	

Continued

TABLE 3 Comparison of diagnostic-based severity adjustment measures vs. prescription-based severity adjustment measures—cont'd

	Title	Authors	Journal, Year	Findings	Comments
40	Comparison of three comorbidity measures for predicting health service use in patients with osteoarthritis	Dominick KL, Dudley TK, Coffman CJ, Bosworth HB	Arthritis & Rheumatism (Arthritis Care & Research), 2005	$N=306$ Time=1998–2000 Region=NC State Comparison models=EI vs. Deyo-CCI vs. RxRisk-V Outcome(s)= number of physician visits, number of prescription drugs, and hospitalization. EI>= RxRisk-V>Deyo-CCI	Older VAMC patients
39	A comparison of comorbidity measurements to predict healthcare expenditures	Farley JF, Harley CR, Devine JW	American Journal of Managed Care Pharmacy, 2006	$N=20,378$ Time=2001–2002 Region=N/A Comparison models=EI vs. Romano-CCI vs. RxRisk-V Outcome(s)=one-year total utilization $R^2=0.11$ vs. 0.11 vs. 0.14	Correlations among the measures ranged from 0.24 to 0.56
46	Adapting the RxRisk-V for mortality prediction in	Johnson ML, El-Serag HB, Tran TT, Hartman C, Richardson P, Abraham NS	Medical Care, 2006	N=724,270 NSAID and CHF patients Time=2002 Region=Nationwide Comparison models=Deyo-CCI- vs. RxRisk-V Outcome(s)=one-year mortality C statistics=0.77 vs. 0.78, 0.65 vs. 0.69, NSAID and CHF, respectively	VAMC patients
48	The estimation power of alternative comorbidity indices	Baser O, Palmer L, Stephenson J	Value Health, 2008	$N=47,743$ Time=2002–2003 Region=Nationwide Comparison models=CCI vs. CDS Outcome(s) = Expenditures $R^2=0.01$ vs. 0.01	Migraine patients using triptans Low correlation between measures
49	Performance of comorbidity, risk adjustment, and functional status measures in expenditure prediction for patients with diabetes	Maciejewski ML, Liu C-F, Fihn SD	Diabetes Care, 2009	$N=3092$ Time=1997–2000 Region=N/A Comparison models =Deyo-CCI vs. RxRisk-V Outcome(s)=total expenditures $R^2=0.03$ vs. 0.03	Similar results were found for inpatient and outpatient expenditures

TABLE 3 Comparison of diagnostic-based severity adjustment measures vs. prescription-based severity adjustment measures—cont'd

	Title	Authors	Journal, Year	Findings	Comments
6	Seniors' self-reported multimorbidity captured biopsychosocial factors not incorporated into two other data-based morbidity measures	Bayliss EA, Ellis JL, Steiner JF	Journal of Clinical Epidemiology, 2009	$N = 352$ Time = N/A Region = N/A Comparison models = Quan-CCI vs. CDS Outcome(s) = Disease burden $R^2 = 0.17$ vs. 0.31	
43	Charlson and RxRisk comorbidity indices were predictive of mortality in the Australian health care setting	Lu CY, Barrett J, Vitry A, Roughhead E	Journal of Clinical Epidemiology, 2011	$N = 94,714$ Time = 2005 Region = Australian VA Comparison models = Deyo-CCI vs. RxRisk Outcome(s) = One-year mortality C statistic = 0.77 vs. 0.73	Unweighted CCI and RxRisk performed less well.
71	Predicting Infections After Total Joint Arthroplasty Using a Prescription	Inacio MCS, Pratt NL, Roughead EE, Graves SE	The Journal of Arthroplasty, 2015	$N = 11,848$ Time = 2001–2012 Region = Australian VA Comparison models = VW-EI vs. CCI vs. RxRisk-V Outcome(s) = 90-day post THA surgery C statistic = 0.57 vs. 0.56 vs. 0.54	
44	Evaluation of three comorbidity measures to predict mortality in patients undergoing total joint arthroplasty	Inacio MCS, Pratt NL, Roughead EE, Graves SE	Osteoarthritis and Cartilage, 2016	$N = 30,820$ THA = 11,848, TKA = 18,972 Time = 2001–2012 Region = Australian VA Comparison models = VW-EI vs. CCI vs. RxRisk-V Outcome(s) = 90-day and one-year mortality C statistic = 0.77 vs. 0.76 vs. 0.72 (90 days) C statistic combined (64 comorbidities) = 0.84	Relative findings similar for one-year mortality
72	Development and validation of a Medicines Comorbidity Index	Narayan SW, Nishtala PS	European Journal of Clinical Pharmacology, 2017	$N = 161,461$, $N = 149,729$ Time = 2012 Region = New Zealand Comparison = CCI vs. modified CDS for	MCI = 20 comorbidities CCI > MCI for mortality; MCI > CCI for hospitalization

Continued

TABLE 3 Comparison of diagnostic-based severity adjustment measures vs. prescription-based severity adjustment measures—cont'd

	Title	Authors	Journal, Year	Findings	Comments
				New Zealand (MCI) Outcome(s) = one-year mortality and hospitalization C statistic = 0.64 vs. 0.62 for mortality; HR 0.92 vs. 1.08 for hospitalization.	
45	Use of a medication-based risk adjustment index to predict mortality among veterans dually-enrolled in VA and Medicare	Radomski TR, Zhaoa X, Hanlon JT, Joshua M. Thorpe JM, Thorpe CT, Naples JG, Sileanu FE, John P. Cashy JP, Hale JA, Mor MK, Hausmann LRM, Donohue JM, Suda KJ, Stroupeg KT, Good CB, Fine MJ, Gellad WF	Healthcare, 2019	N = 271,184 Time = 2013–2015 Region = Nationwide Comparison = VW-EI vs. Deyo-CCI vs. RxRisk-V Outcome(s) = one-year and three-year mortality C statistic = 0.80 vs. 0.79 vs. 0.77 (one-year)	Dual MC and VAMC eligible Relative findings similar for 3-year mortality

OR, Odds Ratio; *PCP*, Primary Care Provider; *CDS*, Chronic Disease Score; *CDI*, Chronic Disease Indicator; *CCI*, Charlson Comorbidity Score; *CDPS*, Chronic Illness and Disability Payment System; *ACG*, Ambulatory Care Groups; *HCC*, Hierarchical Coexisting Conditions; *T2DM*, Type 2 Diabetes; *EI*, Elixhauser Comorbidity Index; *CCI-R*, Charlson Comorbidity Score-Romano; *CDS-1*, Chronic Disease Score (2003 update); *MDBI*, Medication-Base Disease Burden Index; *HR*, Hazard Ratio; *ATC*, Anatomical Therapeutic Chemical Classification Index; *95% CI*, 95% Confidence Interval; *AMI*, Acute Myocardial Infarction; *MEPS*, Medical Expenditure Panel Survey; *HRQoL-CI*, Health-Related Quality of Life-Comorbidity Index; *ECCI*, Enhanced Charlson Comorbidity Index; *EEI*, Enhanced Elixhauser Comorbidity Index; *MCS*, Multisource Comorbidity Score; *MS*, Multiple Sclerosis; *PUD*, Peptic Ulcer Disease; *MCI*, Medicines Comorbidity Index; *MICU*, Medical Intensive Care; *medCDS*, Medication-based chronic disease score; *P3*, Pharmaceutical Prescribing Profile.

may be "owned" by PBMs and not the patient's medical insurer or payer, may be present. In particular, attempts to link patients across data sources may become especially difficult if they are missing a unique common identifier and merges or matches are attempted.

Future of prescription measures

Future measures may include dosing frequency and route of administration, which could be used to further refine prescription-based severity models. One prior and notable weakness of prescription drug measures was their incompleteness. Prior to Medicare Part D in 2006, the bulk of older patients had only limited and spotted outpatient prescription drug coverage. The notable exemption being VAMC patients, with select cohorts being eligible to receive prescription drugs without regards to age, under the nationwide VAMC program, prior to Part D. Perhaps not surprisingly, the most prominent prescription drug measure, the Chronic Disease Score (CDS), was developed and validated for use in VAMC patients. Medicare Part D, enacted in 2006, has greatly enhanced the completeness and robustness of outpatient prescription drug databases. While voluntary, the vast majority of Medicare patients opt into Part D coverage. Therefore, outpatient prescription information for patients whom the comorbidity measures are likely most useful, namely older patients, has become more readily available. Perhaps not surprisingly, prescription drug databases have received renewed interest by researchers, including investigators interested in using the information for comorbidity or severity adjustments.

Current recommendations

In recent years there has been an increasing use of administrative databases as data sources for conducting clinical and epidemiological studies.[50] Advantages of administrative databases include their immediacy, good reliability, wide geographical coverage and ability to contain long follow-up periods that would be logistically and financially difficult via survey methods.[51,52] Disadvantages of administrative databases include the lack of information on lifestyle, social and economic characteristics and the presence of bias related to their observational nature. Additionally, administrative data may have inadequate control variables, be difficult to access due to patient confidentiality issues, and require additional time to determine sufficient qualitative information.[52] Our current recommendations are to use diagnostic data based on both inpatient and outpatient encounters going back a minimum of 12 months, and to use the EI methodology to calculate a Van Walraven summary score (if sample size is relatively small or a concern) or individual indicator variables with empirical sample derived weights (if sample size is sufficiently large). The VW-EI also has an advantage in studies where mortality is the primary outcome of interest. In studies where utilization is the primary outcome, RxRisk or RxRisk-V may be preferred, although combining with a diagnosis measure may also be considered. Our recommendation of diagnostic over prescription measures is driven more by likely familiarity of readers and reviewers with diagnostic measures and not necessarily because of weaker performance of prescription-based comorbidity measures relative to diagnostic measures. If researchers are determined to use the CCI methodology, the Romano-CCI is preferable over the Deyo-CCI, despite the Deyo-CCI being more commonly used. If diagnostic data is unavailable for a large percentage of patients, the RxRisk-V can serve as a valid measure of severity adjustment, especially if the primary outcome measure is resource use or the goal of the researchers is to control for disease burden. The utility of combined diagnostic and prescription measures or scores is likely limited, as is the utility of costly proprietary measures (e.g., ACG) over readily "free" measures or algorithms such as the RxRisk-V or the EI.

Despite shortcomings, potential advantages of prescription drug databases over diagnostic data exist, and include: (1) relative quick turnaround time or timeliness; (2) validity (i.e., generally not subject to excessive over-coding); (3) ability to fluidly map new therapies into conditions; and (4) relative little provider variance in coding preferences. Potential disadvantages of using prescription drug databases for severity adjusting include: (1) the need for continual updating as new therapies and new NDCs come onto the market; and (2) the difficulty in construct mapping of dispensations to eventual patient use and actual diagnoses. Whereas in most instances, a diagnosis-based measure is preferable, in some instances a medication approach may be preferable. Consider tradeoffs between sensitivity and specificity. In general, diagnostic measures tend to be higher concerning sensitivity, but medication measures generally have higher specificity. Regardless of the measure for comorbidity employed, researchers are urged to always include other patient-level factors in their models, such as age, gender, ethnicity, and other socio-economic data and to keep in mind that either a diagnostic or prescription-based measure is simply a time-saving proxy for a thorough chart review.

Questions for further discussion

1. You are asked to review an article under consideration for publication in a health services journal utilizing Medicaid data. The author's data set covered an entire state for a five-year time period. The authors state there was no need to adjust for differences in patient comorbidity, as all the patients in their study (by definition) had Medicaid and they only studied adult male patients. Discuss some potential issues with their approach.
2. You are interested in studying an outcome within a large patient cohort that is likely impacted by the presence of comorbid conditions or differences according to severity of the patient's illnesses(es). In addition to age, gender, race and insurance type, name three widely used techniques or indices that you can use with administrative data to help control for these differences.
3. When would using diagnostic measures or prescription drug measures for severity or comorbidity adjustment likely make little if any difference?

Application exercise/scenario

You are interested in studying one-year all-cause mortality and 30-day readmission rates in a large cohort of HMO patients using claims data. You have inpatient admission and outpatient visit data for 30,000 HMO patients admitted for pneumonia over a two-year time period, but lack access to individual patient clinical information such as laboratory data. The presence of several comorbid conditions (e.g., CHF, T2DM, COPD et al) have been closely linked to outcomes in pneumonia patients. Your research funds are limited, so you do not have the available resources to purchase proprietary adjustment software and decide to use one of the previously validated freeware or shareware algorithms. What are two widely available algorithms for comorbidity adjusting using diagnostic data found in the most inpatient and outpatient files? In the middle of your two-year study period, the HMO switched from using ICD-9-CM to using ICD-10-CM codes. Does this impact your decision on which adjustment measure to use?

After the study is completed, you discover you can now obtain outpatient prescription drug data for your study cohort. What factors might you consider in deciding if repeating your study using prescription claims data to better adjust for comorbidity is worthwhile? (Hint, look at model fit such as C statistic or R^2 in your existing diagnostic adjusted models). In addition, how complete is the prescription data? Do many HMO enrolless utilize out of network pharmacies or frequently move or change health plans?

References

1. Mukherjee B, Ou HT, Wang F, Erickson SR. A new comorbidity index: the health-related quality of life comorbidity index. *J Clin Epidemiol.* 2011; 64(3):309–319. https://doi.org/10.1016/j.jclinepi.2010.01.025.

2. Iezzoni LI. The risks of risk adjustment. *JAMA.* 1997;278(19):1600–1607. https://doi.org/10.1001/jama.278.19.1600.

3. Liu J, Larson E, Hessels A, et al. Comparison of measures to predict mortality and length of stay in hospitalized patients. *Nurs Res.* 2019;68(3): 200–209. https://doi.org/10.1097/NNR.0000000000000350.

4. Charlson ME, Pompei P, Ales KL, MacKenzie CR. A new method of classifying prognostic comorbidity in longitudinal studies: development and validation. *J Chronic Dis.* 1987;40(5):373–383. https://doi.org/10.1016/0021-9681(87)90171-8.

5. Schneeweiss S, Maclure M. Use of comorbidity scores for control of confounding in studies using administrative databases. *Int J Epidemiol.* 2000; 29(5):891–898. https://doi.org/10.1093/ije/29.5.891.

6. Bayliss EA, Ellis JL, Steiner JF. Seniors' self-reported multimorbidity captured biopsychosocial factors not incorporated into two other data-based morbidity measures. *J Clin Epidemiol.* 2009;62(5):550–557.e1. https://doi.org/10.1016/j.jclinepi.2008.05.002.

7. Deyo RA, Cherkin DC, Ciol MA. Adapting a clinical comorbidity index for use with ICD-9-CM administrative databases. *J Clin Epidemiol.* 1992; 45(6):613–619. https://doi.org/10.1016/0895-4356(92)90133-8.

8. Sundararajan V, Henderson T, Perry C, Muggivan A, Quan H, Ghali WA. New ICD-10 version of the Charlson comorbidity index predicted in-hospital mortality. *J Clin Epidemiol.* 2004;57(12):1288–1294. https://doi.org/10.1016/j.jclinepi.2004.03.012.

9. Sharabiani MT, Aylin P, Bottle A. Systematic review of comorbidity indices for administrative data. *Med Care.* 2012;50(12):1109–1118. https://doi.org/10.1097/MLR.0b013e31825f64d0.

10. Yurkovich M, Avina-Zubieta JA, Thomas J, Gorenchtein M, Lacaille D. A systematic review identifies valid comorbidity indices derived from administrative health data. *J Clin Epidemiol.* 2015;68(1):3–14. https://doi.org/10.1016/j.jclinepi.2014.09.010.

11. Nuttall M, van der Meulen J, Emberton M. Charlson scores based on ICD-10 administrative data were valid in assessing comorbidity in patients undergoing urological cancer surgery. *J Clin Epidemiol.* 2006;59(3):265–273. https://doi.org/10.1016/j.jclinepi.2005.07.015.

12. Quan H, Sundararajan V, Halfon P, et al. Coding algorithms for defining comorbidities in ICD-9-CM and ICD-10 administrative data. *Med Care.* 2005;43(11):1130–1139. https://doi.org/10.1097/01.mlr.0000182534.19832.83.

13. Elixhauser A, Steiner C, Harris DR, Coffey RM. Comorbidity measures for use with administrative data. *Med Care.* 1998;36(1):8–27. https://doi.org/10.1097/00005650-199801000-00004. 9431328.

14. van Walraven C, Austin PC, Jennings A, Quan H, Forster AJ. A modification of the Elixhauser comorbidity measures into a point system for hospital death using administrative data. *Med Care.* 2009;47(6):626–633. https://doi.org/10.1097/MLR.0b013e31819432e5.

15. Southern DA, Quan H, Ghali WA. Comparison of the Elixhauser and Charlson/Deyo methods of comorbidity measurement in administrative data. *Med Care.* 2004;42(4):355–360. https://doi.org/10.1097/01.mlr.0000118861.56848.eeno.

16. Bang JH, Hwang SH, Lee EJ, Kim Y. The predictability of claim-data-based comorbidity-adjusted models could be improved by using medication data. *BMC Med Inform Decis Mak.* 2013;13:128. https://doi.org/10.1186/1472-6947-13-128.

17. Stukenborg GJ, Wagner DP, Connors Jr AF. Comparison of the performance of two comorbidity measures, with and without information from prior hospitalizations. *Med Care.* 2001;39(7):727–739. https://doi.org/10.1097/00005650-200107000-00009.

18. Schneeweiss S, Seeger JD, Maclure M, Wang PS, Avorn J, Glynn RJ. Performance of comorbidity scores to control for confounding in epidemiologic studies using claims data. *Am J Epidemiol.* 2001;154(9):854–864. https://doi.org/10.1093/aje/154.9.854.

19. Hosmer DW, Lemeshow S. *Applied Logistic Regression.* 2nd ed. New York, NY: John Wiley & Sons; 2000.

20. Simard M, Sirois C, Candas B. Response to precision on the scope on the combined comorbidity index published in: validation of the combined comorbidity index of Charlson and Elixhauser to predict 30-day mortality across ICD-9 and ICD-10. *Med Care.* 2018;56(9):812–813. https://doi.org/10.1097/MLR.0000000000000955.

21. Buhr RG, Jackson NJ, Kominski GF, Dubinett SM, Ong MK, Mangione CM. Comorbidity and thirty-day hospital readmission odds in chronic obstructive pulmonary disease: a comparison of the Charlson and Elixhauser comorbidity indices. *BMC Health Serv Res.* 2019;19(1):701. https://doi.org/10.1186/s12913-019-4549-4.

22. Maron SZ, Neifert SN, Ranson WA, et al. Elixhauser comorbidity measure is superior to Charlson comorbidity index in-predicting hospital complications following elective posterior cervical decompression and fusion. *World Neurosurg.* 2020;138:e26–e34. https://doi.org/10.1016/j.wneu.2020.01.141.

23. Austin PC, Stanbrook MB, Anderson GM, Newman A, Gershon AS. Comparative ability of comorbidity classification methods for administrative data to predict outcomes in patients with chronic obstructive pulmonary disease. *Ann Epidemiol.* 2012;22(12):881–887. https://doi.org/10.1016/j.annepidem.2012.09.011.

24. Gagne JJ, Glynn RJ, Avorn J, Levin R, Schneeweiss S. A combined comorbidity score predicted mortality in elderly patients better than existing scores. *J Clin Epidemiol.* 2011;64(7):749–759. https://doi.org/10.1016/j.jclinepi.2010.10.004.

25. Mehta HB, Mehta V, Girman CJ, Adhikari D, Johnson ML. Regression coefficient-based scoring system should be used to assign weights to the risk index. *J Clin Epidemiol.* 2016;79:22–28. https://doi.org/10.1016/j.jclinepi.2016.03.031.

26. Corrao G, Rea F, Di Martino M, et al. Developing and validating a novel multisource comorbidity score from administrative data: a large population-based cohort study from Italy. *BMJ Open.* 2017;7(12). https://doi.org/10.1136/bmjopen-2017-019503, e019503. 29282274.

27. Von Korff M, Wagner EH, Saunders K. A chronic disease score from automated pharmacy data. *J Clin Epidemiol.* 1992;45(2):197–203. https://doi.org/10.1016/0895-4356(92)90016-g.

28. Clark DO, Von Korff M, Saunders K, Baluch WM, Simon GE. A chronic disease score with empirically derived weights. *Med Care.* 1995;33(8):783–795. https://doi.org/10.1097/00005650-199508000-00004.

29. Malone DC, Billups SJ, Valuck RJ, Carter BL. Development of a chronic disease indicator score using a veterans affairs medical center medication database. IMPROVE Investigators. *J Clin Epidemiol.* 1999;52(6):551–557. https://doi.org/10.1016/s0895-4356(99)00029-3.

30. Fishman PA, Goodman MJ, Hornbrook MC, Meenan RT, Bachman DJ, O'Keeffe Rosetti MC. Risk adjustment using automated ambulatory pharmacy data: the RxRisk model. *Med Care.* 2003;41(1):84–99. https://doi.org/10.1097/00005650-200301000-00011.

31. Sloan KL, Sales AE, Liu CF, et al. Construction and characteristics of the RxRisk-V: a VA-adapted pharmacy-based case-mix instrument. *Med Care.* 2003;41(6):761–774. https://doi.org/10.1097/01.MLR.0000064641.84967.B7.

32. George J, Vuong T, Bailey MJ, Kong DC, Marriott JL, Stewart K. Development and validation of the medication-based disease burden index. *Ann Pharmacother.* 2006;40(4):645–650. https://doi.org/10.1345/aph.1G204.

33. Lamers LM, van Vliet RC. The pharmacy-based cost group model: validating and adjusting the classification of medications for chronic conditions to the Dutch situation. *Health Policy.* 2004;68(1):113–121. https://doi.org/10.1016/j.healthpol.2003.09.001.

34. Tugwell P, Knottnerus JA. Clinical prediction models are not being validated. *J Clin Epidemiol.* 2015;68(1):1–2. https://doi.org/10.1016/j.jclinepi.2014.11.020.

35. Gilmer T, Kronick R, Fishman P, Ganiats TG. The Medicaid Rx model: pharmacy-based risk adjustment for public programs. *Med Care.* 2001;39(11):1188–1202. https://doi.org/10.1097/00005650-200111000-00006.

36. Stanley J, Doughty RN, Sarfati D. A pharmaceutical dispensing-based index of mortality risk from long-term conditions performed as well as hospital record-based indices. *Med Care.* 2020;58(2):e9–e16. https://doi.org/10.1097/MLR.0000000000001217.

37. Redelmeier DA, Thiruchelvam D, Lustig AJ. Cross-linked survey analysis is an approach for separating cause and effect in survey research. *J Clin Epidemiol.* 2015;68(1):35–43. https://doi.org/10.1016/j.jclinepi.2014.09.008.

38. Vitry A, Wong SA, Roughead EE, Ramsay E, Barratt J. Validity of medication-based co-morbidity indices in the Australian elderly population. *Aust N Z J Public Health.* 2009;33(2):126–130. https://doi.org/10.1111/j.1753-6405.2009.00357.x.

39. Farley JF, Harley CR, Devine JW. A comparison of comorbidity measurements to predict healthcare expenditures. *Am J Manag Care.* 2006;12(2):110–119.

40. Dominick KL, Dudley TK, Coffman CJ, Bosworth HB. Comparison of three comorbidity measures for predicting health service use in patients with osteoarthritis. *Arthritis Rheum.* 2005;53(5):666–672. https://doi.org/10.1002/art.21440.

41. Perkins AJ, Kroenke K, Unützer J, et al. Common comorbidity scales were similar in their ability to predict health care costs and mortality. *J Clin Epidemiol.* 2004;57(10):1040–1048. https://doi.org/10.1016/j.jclinepi.2004.03.002.

42. Schneeweiss S, Wang PS, Avorn J, Maclure M, Levin R, Glynn RJ. Consistency of performance ranking of comorbidity adjustment scores in Canadian and U.S. utilization data. *J Gen Intern Med.* 2004;19(5 Pt 1):444–450. https://doi.org/10.1111/j.1525-1497.2004.30109.x.

43. Lu CY, Barratt J, Vitry A, Roughead E. Charlson and Rx-risk comorbidity indices were predictive of mortality in the Australian health care setting. *J Clin Epidemiol.* 2011;64(2):223–228. https://doi.org/10.1016/j.jclinepi.2010.02.015.

44. Inacio MCS, Pratt NL, Roughead EE, Graves SE. Evaluation of three co-morbidity measures to predict mortality in patients undergoing total joint arthroplasty. *Osteoarthr Cartil.* 2016;24(10):1718–1726. https://doi.org/10.1016/j.joca.2016.05.006.

45. Radomski TR, Zhao X, Hanlon JT, et al. Use of a medication-based risk adjustment index to predict mortality among veterans dually-enrolled in VA and Medicare. *Healthc (Amst).* 2019;7(4). https://doi.org/10.1016/j.hjdsi.2019.04.003.

46. Johnson ML, El-Serag HB, Tran TT, Hartman C, Richardson P, Abraham NS. Adapting the Rx-risk-V for mortality prediction in outpatient populations. *Med Care.* 2006;44(8):793–797. https://doi.org/10.1097/01.mlr.0000218804.41758.ef.

47. Parker JP, McCombs JS, Graddy EA. Can pharmacy data improve prediction of hospital outcomes? Comparisons with a diagnosis-based comorbidity measure. *Med Care.* 2003;41(3):407–419. https://doi.org/10.1097/01.MLR.0000053023.49899.3E.

48. Baser O, Palmer L, Stephenson J. The estimation power of alternative comorbidity indices. *Value Health.* 2008;11(5):946–955. https://doi.org/10.1111/j.1524-4733.2008.00343.x.

49. Maciejewski ML, Liu CF, Fihn SD. Performance of comorbidity, risk adjustment, and functional status measures in expenditure prediction for patients with diabetes. *Diabetes Care.* 2009;32(1):75–80. https://doi.org/10.2337/dc08-1099.

50. Schneeweiss S, Wang PS, Avorn J, Glynn RJ. Improved comorbidity adjustment for predicting mortality in Medicare populations. *Health Serv Res.* 2003;38(4):1103–1120. https://doi.org/10.1111/1475-6773.00165.

51. Iommi M, Rosa S, Fusaroli M, Rucci P, Fantini MP, Poluzzi E. Modified-Chronic Disease Score (M-CDS): predicting the individual risk of death using drug prescriptions. *PLoS One.* 2020;15(10). https://doi.org/10.1371/journal.pone.0240899, e0240899.

52. Timofte D, Pantea Stoian A, Razvan H. A review on the advantages and disadvantages of using administrative data in surgery outcome studies. *J Surg.* 2018;14(3):105–107. https://doi.org/10.7438/1584-9341-14-3-1.

53. Johnson RE, Hornbrook MC, Nichols GA. Replicating the chronic disease score (CDS) from automated pharmacy data. *J Clin Epidemiol.* 1994;47(10):1191–1199. https://doi.org/10.1016/0895-4356(94)90106-6.

54. Tamblyn R, Lavoie G, Petrella L, Monette J. The use of prescription claims databases in pharmacoepidemiological research: the accuracy and comprehensiveness of the prescription claims database in Québec. *J Clin Epidemiol.* 1995;48(8):999–1009. https://doi.org/10.1016/0895-4356(94)00234-h.

55. Fishman PA, Shay DK. Development and estimation of a pediatric chronic disease score using automated pharmacy data. *Med Care*. 1999;37(9): 874–883. https://doi.org/10.1097/00005650-199909000-00004.

56. Lamers LM. Pharmacy costs groups: a risk-adjuster for capitation payments based on the use of prescribed drugs. *Med Care*. 1999;37(8): 824–830. https://doi.org/10.1097/00005650-199908000-00012.

57. Kaye KS, Sands K, Donahue JG, Chan KA, Fishman P, Platt R. Preoperative drug dispensing as predictor of surgical site infection. *Emerg Infect Dis*. 2001;7(1):57–65. https://doi.org/10.3201/eid0701.010110.

58. Putnam KG, Buist DS, Fishman P, et al. Chronic disease score as a predictor of hospitalization. *Epidemiology*. 2002;13(3):340–346. https://doi.org/ 10.1097/00001648-200205000-00016.

59. Joish VN, Malone DC, Wendel C, Draugalis JR, Mohler MJ. Development and validation of a diabetes mellitus severity index: a risk-adjustment tool for predicting health care resource use and costs. *Pharmacotherapy*. 2005;25(5):676–684. https://doi.org/10.1592/phco.25.5.676.63594.

60. McGregor JC, Kim PW, Perencevich EN, et al. Utility of the chronic disease score and Charlson comorbidity index as comorbidity measures for use in epidemiologic studies of antibiotic-resistant organisms. *Am J Epidemiol*. 2005;161(5):483–493. https://doi.org/10.1093/aje/kwi068.

61. McGregor JC, Perencevich EN, Furuno JP, et al. Comorbidity risk-adjustment measures were developed and validated for studies of antibiotic-resistant infections. *J Clin Epidemiol*. 2006;59(12):1266–1273. https://doi.org/10.1016/j.jclinepi.2006.01.016.

62. Schatz M, Zeiger RS, Vollmer WM, et al. Development and validation of a medication intensity scale derived from computerized pharmacy data that predicts emergency hospital utilization for persistent asthma. *Am J Manag Care*. 2006;12(8):478–484.

63. Dhabali AA, Awang R. A medication-estimated health status measure for predicting primary care visits: the Long-Term Therapeutic Groups Index. *Health Policy Plan*. 2010;25(2):162–169. https://doi.org/10.1093/heapol/czp051.

64. Vivas D, Guadalajara N, Barrachina I, Trillo JL, Usó R, de-la- Poza E. Explaining primary healthcare pharmacy expenditure using classification of medications for chronic conditions. *Health Policy*. 2011;103(1):9–15. https://doi.org/10.1016/j.healthpol.2011.08.014.

65. Huber CA, Szucs TD, Rapold R, Reich O. Identifying patients with chronic conditions using pharmacy data in Switzerland: an updated mapping approach to the classification of medications. *BMC Public Health*. 2013;13:1030. https://doi.org/10.1186/1471-2458-13-1030.

66. O'Shea M, Teeling M, Bennett K. The prevalence and ingredient cost of chronic comorbidity in the Irish elderly population with medication treated type 2 diabetes: a retrospective cross-sectional study using a national pharmacy claims database. *BMC Health Serv Res*. 2013;13:23. https://doi.org/ 10.1186/1472-6963-13-23.

67. Xu D, Anderson HD, Tao A, et al. Assessing and predicting drug-induced anticholinergic risks: an integrated computational approach. *Ther Adv Drug Saf*. 2017;8(11):361–370. https://doi.org/10.1177/2042098617725267.

68. Kabue S, Greene J, Kipnis P, et al. The impact of pharmacy-specific predictors on the performance of 30-day readmission risk prediction models. *Med Care*. 2019;57(4):295–299. https://doi.org/10.1097/MLR.0000000000001075.

69. Gwynn ME, Poisson MO, Waller JL, Newsome AS. Development and validation of a medication regimen complexity scoring tool for critically ill patients. *Am J Health Syst Pharm*. 2019;76(Suppl 2):S34–S40. https://doi.org/10.1093/ajhp/zxy054. 31067298.

70. Quinzler R, Freitag MH, Wiese B, et al. A novel superior medication-based chronic disease score predicted all-cause mortality in independent geriatric cohorts. *J Clin Epidemiol*. 2019;105:112–124. https://doi.org/10.1016/j.jclinepi.2018.09.004.

71. Inacio MC, Pratt NL, Roughead EE, Graves SE. Predicting infections after total joint arthroplasty using a prescription based comorbidity measure. *J Arthroplasty*. 2015;30(10):1692–1698. https://doi.org/10.1016/j.arth.2015.05.004.

72. Narayan SW, Nishtala PS. Development and validation of a medicines comorbidity index for older people. *Eur J Clin Pharmacol*. 2017;73(12): 1665–1672. https://doi.org/10.1007/s00228-017-2333-0.

Chapter 35

Handling missing data in surveys—Concepts, approaches, and applications in pharmacy and health services research

Ardalan Mirzaei, Stephen R. Carter, Asad E. Patanwala, and Carl R. Schneider

The University of Sydney School of Pharmacy, Faculty of Medicine and Health, The University of Sydney, Sydney, NSW, Australia

Objectives

- Identify the different classifications for missing data such as Missing Completely at Random, Missing at Random, and Missing Not At Random.
- Plan for missing data during survey design and item development.
- Understand a range of methods to handle missing data including deletion, imputation, and likelihood methods.
- Evaluate optimal techniques to report missing data.

Introduction

There are two types of people: 1) Those who can extrapolate from missing data.

—A random T-Shirt I saw

What is missing data?

Missing data is when an observation has no value assigned to it. For any particular dataset, missing data is present in cases where, for any item, an input has not been entered or generated. In surveys, a respondents' response value is not available for it to be taken further for analysis.

There are multiple reasons why surveys can have missing data. For example, respondents may have skipped questions, data coding caused variables to be counted as null or missing, the Internet may have cut out during data gathering with electronic devices, a page of printed information may be missing, or a response item is deemed invalid.

Whether intended or unintended, classifications for missing data have been developed to describe the type of missingness. Classifying missing responses allows for decisions to be made on how to handle missing data and when reporting, how to inform readers of the considerations that were taken to mitigate or minimize missing values.

A recent review into missing data in pharmacy literature highlighted that a low proportion of studies reported on how missing data were handled.[1] A lack of reporting can lead to bias in the interpretation of findings and validity of the research. The aim of this chapter is to introduce the concept of missing data, how missing data is categorized, and introduce common techniques to account for and report on missing data.

Classification of missing data

Before a decision could be made about what to do with the missing data, the type of missingness needs to be classified. Considerations for the handling of missing data require both subjective interpretation and objective analysis. With missing

Contemporary Research Methods in Pharmacy and Health Services. https://doi.org/10.1016/B978-0-323-91888-6.00017-X

data, objective analysis uses statistical methods to observe and measure missing data, while subjective analysis uses the past experience and knowledge of the analyst to identify and handle the missing data. Missing data may be classified according to the degree of randomness with three categories described; Missing at Random (MAR), Missing Completely at Random (MCAR) or ignorable missingness, and Missing Not at Random (MNAR), also known as nonignorable missingness.[2,3]

Missing completely at random

MCAR is when a missing value is not related to any other value in the dataset.[4,5] Conceptually, data that are MCAR are not usually attributed to a question in the survey or other phenomenon, whether observable or unobservable. Assume for example, a question being asked relates to income and is represented by the letter X_1, while another question relates to occupation and is represented by the letter X_2. In MCAR, the reason for X_1 (income) having a missing response is not because of X_1 (income) or X_2 (occupation), i.e., neither the survey question nor another confounder is the reason for the missing value. When MCAR is suspected, Little's Test of Missingness can be used to determine whether the missing values meet the specification of MCAR.[6] A significant P-value result indicates that we reject the null hypothesis and assume that a pattern exists to the missing data (not MCAR). Little's Test of Missingness is available in most statistical software packages.

Missing at random

Data classified as MAR have missing data, and the degree of missingness is associated with one or more of the observed (measured) variables in the dataset. Certain groups may not respond to a question, as a result of an underlying or confounding reason. For instance, individuals with high paying jobs may not be inclined to answer questions that relate to finance. This is both theoretically and conceptually true, as research indicates that higher income earners are more likely nonresponders of income questions.[7] Using the example from MCAR above where X_1 is income and X_2 is occupation. The reasons why X_1 (income) may not be reported is based on X_2 (occupation), where those with higher paying occupations are less inclined to provide a response.[8] Thus, in the case of MAR, the reason for X_1 having a missing response is based on X_2, another variable.

Missing not at random

MNAR, or data that contains nonignorable missingness, are data that do not meet the criteria of either MCAR or MAR. Unlike MCAR and the use of an objective statistical test, subjective analysis is required to ascertain whether data are MNAR. In MAR, there may be a correlation between an observable phenomenon and why data are missing, but not a direct cause. Data that are MNAR, on the other hand, can be attributed to an unobservable factor that is directly affecting the reason that the data values are missing. This can be the question itself being the cause of the missing response, or underlying assumptions.[5] Using another example in a survey of overall health, assume X_1 is a depression related question and X_2 is gender. X_1 (depression) can have a missing response based on X_2 (gender) where men are less likely to talk about depression. This case would be MAR. On the other hand, if it is the level of depression (X_1) that is causing the person to provide a null response, then the missingness is MNAR. This is where the cause of the missingness is the phenomenon that is being evaluated by the item itself, which in this case is X_1.

To summarize the three categories, assume X_1 is the variable with missing responses and X_2 is another variable:

MCAR = Neither X_1 nor X_2, can explain the missingness. Mathematically from Little's Test, "No pattern exists."
MAR = Missingness of X_1 is based on X_2, where X_2 is another variable in the dataset.
MNAR = Missingness of X_1 is based on X_1 itself or another phenomenon that is rarely observed. It cannot be attributed to another observable dataset variable.

Planning for missing data

Ideally, consideration of how to avoid missing data should be part of the initial survey design, sampling strategy, as well as the data analysis plan. Estimation of the proportion of missing data may be inferred from literature as well as pilot studies. The estimated proportion of missing data obtained allows for improved survey sample size calculation.

If participants forget to answer a question or refuse to answer a question, then that information will not be collected. Missing by design is when the survey design increases the likelihood of missing values.[9,10] This can happen when a response was provided, but the response was converted to a missing value. In attempting to minimize missing data, some researchers have the misconception "If I force them to answer, then there won't be anything missing." Some surveys are used to gather the perceptions or opinions of participants. In order to form an opinion, you need to have awareness, such as experience.[11] Experiences are especially needed in order to gather participants' perceptions. Participants of a survey might have a broad understanding of a topic, but when you are measuring their perceptions, it might be useful to consider "do they have awareness." If the respondent does not have awareness or knowledge of the topic, or simply has a lack of engagement with the topic and is forced to answer, they may display a behavior known as straight-lining.[12] Straight-lining is when respondents answer identical or a similar response in order to finish a survey. Their provided answers are not useable as they do not represent a true response to the question asked, and affected responses should be coded as missing.

The number of questions and anticipated time required for survey completion can also influence the amount of data that is missing. This is due to "survey fatigue" or loss of interest by participants with longer surveys. The appropriate survey length can vary, based on circumstances such as whether participants are reimbursed for their time,[13] the health of participants, administration via the web,[14] or environmental factors. For instance, cross-cultural surveys are well known to experience missing data.[15,16] Although several studies have demonstrated survey length impacts on response rates, this effect is inconsistent and not demonstrated for all surveys.[17] The planning phase of the survey should balance the need for comprehensiveness, versus the risk of reduced participant response, which could result in missing data. A longer survey in some circumstances could lead to less usable information. An additional contributor to survey burden is administering the survey more than once. That said, although it is known that response rates decrease when potential participants anticipate the need to respond to a survey on multiple occasions,[18] it is not apparent that increased frequency of survey administration increases missing data for survey responses. Mitigation efforts for survey fatigue may be made by increasing "survey engagement" via reducing question complexity,[19] increasing salience,[18] and gamification.[20] In summary, survey fatigue is a factor that may contribute to missing data, with its impact subject to *context*. A two-step strategy to address survey fatigue is to first optimize survey engagement during the planning phase, and, secondly, it is valuable to pilot the proposed survey instrument in the population and setting of interest, thereby accounting for context, to identify whether survey fatigue is contributing to missing data. Finally, the proportion of missing data identified during piloting should inform refinement of the proposed sampling strategy and data analysis plan.

Standard form versus filtered form questions

What is to be done when a respondent does not respond to a question? Schuman and Presser suggest two forms of questions: standard or filtered. In a standard question, there is an alternative response option, such as "I don't know." We may ask the standard form question, "Diabetes has a genetic link. Do you agree or disagree," and wait for a response of either "Agree" or "Disagree." However, how is a response to be recorded if a respondent answers "I don't know?" This response is a volunteered "don't know" response.[21] Questions which assess an attitude, opinion or belief can be subject to the respondent "not knowing."[21] These responses can be seen when survey data is collected in situations where the respondent and the interviewer can converse.[21]

An alternate form of questioning is the filtered form of questioning. In this example, we may first ask the participants "Diabetes has a genetic link. Do you have an opinion about that?" To which if they respond "Yes" it can then be asked "Do you agree or disagree?" Schuman and Presser demonstrate that differences in responses can be gathered by using either standard form questions and filtered forms.[21] Therefore, if persons have no opinion about a topic, it is inappropriate to force them to respond to a question. It should be noted that filtered form and standard form questions provide different results.[21] In interview-based surveys, the interviewer has the ability to ask filtered form questions; however, this is difficult in self-administered paper-based surveys. An alternative is to use self-administered surveys with the option of branching or providing the option to respond "I don't know" or "No opinion."

Electronic surveys

Causes of MCAR can arise from participants skipping or forgetting to complete a question. This missingness commonly occurs in a paper-based survey or in electronic surveys when forced responses[a] before progression is not implemented.[2]

In electronic surveys, we can force each question to be answered before allowing participants to progress through the survey. In paper-based surveys or telephone surveys, they may choose to say, "I don't know" or provide no response. Forcing the participant to have an opinion about a topic where the person cannot form an opinion may lead to a biased

---

a. Forced responses in electronic surveys is a parameter which requires every question to be answered before the participant can progress onto the next part, or before saving the data. This forces a participant to select a response even if all the available responses are not consistent with their thinking. However, it has the advantage as it can create a safety check to ensure the questions are being answered and minimize your missing data.

or inaccurate data. Branching to ask filtered form questions in an electronic format is an ideal way to overcome this issue. However, if standard form questions are required for the survey, then consideration should be made to providing other option(s).

Deliberate nonresponse and missingness

In interviewer-led questionnaires, item nonresponses from participants can be encoded by the interviewer according to a predefined data dictionary.[22] However, in self-administered surveys, it is sometimes difficult to specify an appropriate nonresponse. Durand and Lambert suggest the use of a "don't know" option to allow for participants to have "less guessing, reductions in the threatening nature of items, and decreased embarrassment due to erroneous answers to knowledge-oriented items."[23] When providing participants with the option of "I don't know" or "Not applicable (NA)," it is recommended that these cases are coded as missing, since it is unclear in the cases of ordinal, interval or ratio type data, how such responses should be valued. An obvious error, for example, in a 7-point Likert-type response scale, would be to code "I don't know" as zero or eight. If that were done, those answering "I don't know" would be coded as having extreme responses. This would introduce bias in the data analysis.

A potentially problematic approach is to code an attitudinal-type item such as "I don't know" as a neutral or mid-point response. Encoding an "I don't know" response as a "neutral" may be inappropriate, as these responses have qualitatively two different interpretations. Imagine exploring the effect of the direct-to-consumer advertising (DTCA) on perceptions of a drug in different populations. For example, a survey item might be "TV drug advertisements make me nervous" and participants may be offered a 7-point Likert response scale ranging from "Strongly Disagree to Strongly Agree" with "Neutral" response at the midpoint, along with "I don't know." In any population, we may expect to see a range of responses, including having no affective response to DTCA, where participants select "Neutral." We may also expect that some participants may not be exposed to TV advertisements and have no concept of what DTCA looks like and these would be able to select "I don't know." Consider the situation where "I don't know" was not offered but "neutral" was. If the survey were administered in a jurisdiction where DTCA were prohibited, many would have to select "Neutral," as a large proportion would not have been exposed to the DTCA and would be unable to form an opinion based on their experience with DTCA. Following mathematical transformation and analysis, it could be misinterpreted that within that jurisdiction the population had overall neutral feelings with respect to DTCA. A more appropriate approach would be to report the level of missingness and speak to and interpret the data with that in mind. Consider the alternative situation above, where the survey is administered in a country where DTCA is NOT prohibited, a high level of missingness could indicate that the population surveyed has low "exposure" because, for example, high wealth households tend not to watch TV at the same rate as low wealth households. Missingness in that item might provide information about household wealth.

In summary, when a respondent selects "I don't know," it may be a deliberate choice. It is important to code these responses as missing, and it is advised that the proportion of respondents opting for the "I don't know" response be reported. Missingness for this reason provides valuable information about how well a topic is conceptualized within or "available to" a population. High levels of missingness of a particular item (compared with others in the survey) suggest MNAR, and this will influence the analytical approach.

Analyzing data with missing values

Data can be missing at two levels, either the variable (item) level or the case (individual) level.[24] The item level nonresponse is where the data for a particular item is missing for a very high proportion of participants. For example, most respondents may have answered the whole survey, except that many have missed all the items regarding income, particularly if administered in a cohort of high wealth individuals. A nonresponse on the case level is where information pertaining to a particular respondent is missing. For example, a respondent may have missed a sequence of questions but completed the remainder of the survey. The pattern of missingness at both item and case level can be taken into consideration when deciding on the analytical approach to missingness.

Analytical methods to handle missing data are commonly available in statistical software. It is up to the researcher to understand and use the missing information appropriately. The purpose of this chapter is not to restate the existing principles and methods used in missing data analysis, but to guide the initial consideration that need to be made when planning the analyses of data with missingness. Table 1 provides a summary of common approaches to handling missingness for data analysis. As statistical software has become more accessible, there has been a shift to using imputation and likelihood methods over traditional deletion methods when handling missing data.[25]

TABLE 1 Possible methods to handling missing data.

Category	Method
Deletion methods	Complete case analysis (CCA)/list-wise deletion
	Available case analysis (ACA)/pair-wise deletion
Single imputation	Mean imputation
	Last value/observation carried forward (LVCF/LOCF)
	Regression methods (RM)
	Hot-deck imputation
	Cold-deck imputation
Multiple imputation	Multiple imputation (MI)
Other	Markov-chain imputation
	Missing-indicator method
Likelihood methods	Expectation-maximization algorithm
	Full information maximum likelihood
Indicator methods	Indicator method imputation
	Pattern mixture models

Adapted from Bennett DA. How can I deal with missing data in my study? *Aust N Z J Public Health* 2001;25:464–469.

Deletion methods

The traditional approach to handling missing values is list-wise deletion, also known as Complete Case Analysis (CCA). CCA is when the entire case that contains any missing data is removed from analysis. This is different from "ignoring" missing data. That is, in ignoring missing data, we analyze each variable with the data available for that data. In CCA, it does not matter if all the other items are answered completely, when one of the items for your analysis has a missing value, the entire case is removed prior to any analysis which would include that item. CCA can be tricky depending on variable importance. For example, if key variables for a study are "age," "sex," and "drug" where we wish to predict "mortality." If a variable of lesser importance, such as "education," has missing data, do we delete the whole case because it is missing a response for "education." In this example, as "education" does not help with identifying "mortality," we would only focus on the complete cases for the 4 variables only. Although this is an easy method to apply, there is the possibility of introducing bias if the included individuals vary from those excluded.[26] To address bias, a weighted CCA[4] can be considered, with methods such as inverse probability weighting,[26,27] calibration[28] or propensity weighting for nonresponse.[29]

Inverse probability weighting (IPW) assumes the data is MAR and uses the other variables to estimate the value of the missing values.[30] Marron and Wahed use a simple example with a small dataset of 6 respondents to estimate the missing values which we will use here. Assume 2 respondents did not have the value of "age" reported. However, we have their "gender" and their "years in college," which is complete. Respondent 1 could be a female in their first year of college, which we will call characteristic 1, and Respondent 2 could be a female in the 3rd year of college, which we will call characteristic 2. IPW works by identifying other *females in their first year of college* and pairing them with Respondent 1. Similarly Respondent 2 could be paired with *females in their 3rd year of college*. Assuming we have small dataset where only 1 other person can be paired with each characteristic. Thus, when we come to calculate the mean age of the cohort, CCA would remove the missing values and then calculate the mean age of only 4 respondents. IPW on the other hand, takes the observed ages of the respondents paired with characteristics 1 and 2, and increases the weight they have in calculating the mean. As there is 1 missing and 1 observed for characteristic 1 and 2, the observed age is doubled, effectively, making it average the age of "6" people.[30]

An alternative option is pair-wise deletion or Available Case Analysis. Pair-wise deletion does not delete the whole case as is done with CCA, it performs calculations with all the variables that are not missing but omits that part of the calculation that includes missing cases.[31] This allows us to use more of the data. Pair-wise deletion or exclusion can also be referred to as available-case analysis or excluding cases analysis-by-analysis. For example, assume we have 3 variables (hours studied, classes missed, and final score), for which we wish to do a Pearson's Correlation. Each variable has different missing cases, pair-wise deletion will take into account variables as 3 groups. From Fig. 1, Group A will have variables 1 and 2 together (study hours and missed classes), Group B will have variables 2 and 3 together (missed classes and final score), and Group C will have variables 1 and 3 together (study hours and final score). Therefore, assuming each variable had 4 unique cases of missingness that means each group will have 8 unique cases of missingness. This contrasts with list-wise deletion (CCA) in Table 2, as all cases with a missing value are removed from analysis, meaning each group has 12 cases removed. Pair-wise deletion or exclusion can also be referred to as available-case analysis or excluding cases analysis-by-analysis. However, in the discipline of psychology, the American Psychological Association (APA) discourages using pair-wise and list-wise deletion because of the tendency to produce biased results and the superiority of imputation and likelihood methods.[32,33]

Imputation methods

Imputation is the process of replacing missing data with substituted values, *before* the analysis occurs. One method to impute the missing values for many categories of data is similar response pattern imputation in which missing values are replaced by the values which were observed in similar cases, based for example on gender or age.[34] An option for ordinal or categorical values is to "replace by mean" or "mean substitution" where the mean values of the responses for that item are substituted into the missing value field.

Hair et al. has presented a summary of single imputation methods such as case substitution, cold- or hot-deck imputation, and regression imputation.[35] Case-substitution replaces the missing values with observations from a different dataset that matches the current dataset. That is, if similar studies have cases which are like the study dataset, one could replace the missing values with the sample observations from another study.[36] This method has its limitations and requires the researcher to be well versed in the previous studies. In hot-deck imputation, data from respondents with matching covariates are used to replace the missing values. Cold-deck imputation works like hot-deck imputation, but the information is

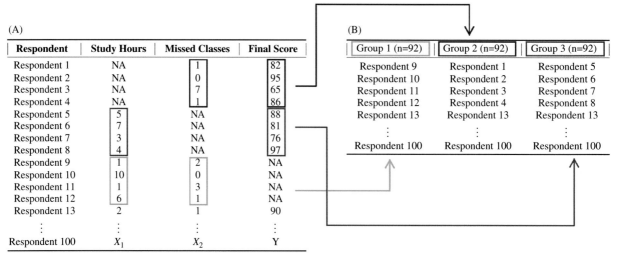

FIG. 1 Pair-wise deletion considering the complete cases for each pair group of variables.

TABLE 2 Comparison of pair-wise deletion and list-wise deletion for a Pearson's correlation of 100 respondents.

	Pair-wise deletion			List-wise deletion		
	Study hours	Missed classes	Final score	Study hours	Missed classes	Final score
Study hours	–	$r_1 (n=92)$	$r_1 (n=92)$	–	$r_1 (n=88)$	$r_1 (n=88)$
Missed classes	$r_1 (n=92)$	–	$r_3 (n=92)$	$r_1 (n=88)$	–	$r_3 (n=88)$
Final score	$r_2 (n=92)$	$r_3 (n=92)$	–	$r_2 (n=88)$	$r_3 (n=88)$	–

provided external or prior to analysis as opposed to the using the dataset. Regression imputation uses the available data in the dataset to build a regression model to predict the missing values. Regression methods may be better suited to analyses designed to predict outcome variables.[36,37]

Multiple imputation estimates a range of possible options for the missing value. The number of possible options is selected by the researcher. For example, the researcher may choose a number "M," and through multiple imputation methods, M possible values are provided to create M possible and complete datasets. These M datasets are then combined together to perform statistical analysis and generate a single summary finding.[37] It should be noted that multiple imputation draws results from a pooled estimate of a large number of random imputations, and therefore, the results obtained will be different, every time, as it is applied to a particular dataset. Multiple imputation is widely used and has, for instance, emerged as a leading approach for handing missing data in cross-cultural surveys because multiple imputation can account for error variance of imputed values.[15]

Likelihood methods

Likelihood methods may also be used when handling missing data without requiring the use of *prior* imputation.[38,39] With likelihood methods, values for variables that are missing are estimated *during* the analysis, and these values are used to replace the missing values. Algorithms are used to predict the most likely value of the missing variable—the value which minimizes the error of the model, based on all other observed parameters in the model. Expectation-Maximization (EM)[40] and Full Information Maximum likelihood (FIML)[24] are the most widely used of the likelihood methods. Compared with imputation methods, likelihood methods tend to be simpler to implement because the analyst does not have to make decisions about replacing data with imputed values, which requires considerable qualitative interpretation. Furthermore, since the results are always the same with the same dataset, the results are less prone to variability of interpretation and are more reproducible than imputation methods.[41] Likelihood estimation produces accurate standard errors for a range of analyses because the actual sample size is retained, unlike with multiple imputation.

Choice of method

The percentage of missing data at the item level, the case level, and complete survey dictates the different techniques used. It is difficult to have a rule of thumb for missing data. As Little and Rubin mention the "degree of bias and loss of precision depends not only on the fraction of complete cases and pattern of missing data, but also on the extent to which complete and incomplete cases differ, and on the parameters of interest."[4] It can, however, benefit researchers to use an initial framework approach handling missing data, until they have gained sufficient experience to justify choices based on theoretical and empirical foundations. As such, we have provided an example framework to approaching missing data in surveys. While there are some specialized analyses which requires specialized treatment (see below), a possible consideration is that if there is <5% missing data, then the technique of multiple imputation may not provide much benefit, and thus using a simpler single imputation approach may be appropriate.[32] However, if >10% of the data is missing, then there is more likely to be bias and as such multiple imputation techniques can be used.[37] Once there is >40% missing data, then imputation or likelihood methods can lead to results that are no more than hypothesis generating. Between 5% and 10% missingness is a gray area where the researcher should use a theoretical consideration of the phenomenon of interest, before deciding on which method to choose.

Once the type of missing data is ascertained, a decision needs to be made about how to deal with those missing observations. The three different levels of missingness that exist can help determine how to approach the handling of the data. If it can be determined and confirmed that the data is missing under MCAR, then imputations or deletions can be performed with minimal bias.[42] Thinking about the cause of why the data is missing, under MCAR, a respondent may not have answered the question, but this may be either an isolated case or mishandled error in collecting data. It does not reflect the nature of the question being asked. Assuming MCAR means that the missing data is a random sample of the complete data. The traditional approach is to perform a CCA. Removing the data in MCAR situations does not introduce bias; however, it does increase the standard error due to the reduced sample size.[24] The alternative approach would be to perform an imputation in order to estimate a response that the respondent may have answered, had they answered the question.

Data that are MAR can be imputed similarly to MCAR, but the procedures are more complex. As mentioned above, MAR data are categorized as MAR when other variables are related to the missing information. Therefore, in order to apply imputation techniques, ideally any variables which show observed correlation with missingness of a variable should be factored into the modeling process. While it would be tempting to include all the variables which correlated with the missing variable when creating an imputation model, the risk is that more variables increase the size of confidence intervals for the estimates and increase the chance that the imputation fails to provide any estimates at all. Enders suggests selecting variables for multiple imputation models when a variable has a correlation greater than $|0.4|$ with missing variable.[43] Tests of simulated datasets show that multiple imputation, EM and FIML methods work well with MAR data.[24]

Handling missing data that is MNAR is challenging yet appealing since many datasets will be MNAR. The concern is that parameter estimates using maximum likelihood and multiple imputation methods are generated while violating the assumptions underpinning them, resulting in bias. A relatively intuitive and simple method for understanding the impact of MNAR on multiple imputation estimates has been suggested by Rubin. He suggests conducting an ad-hoc sensitivity analysis of repeated analyses with a range of imputed values. In that method, the imputed values generated under the MAR assumption are multiplied by a constant to take into account that the imputed value may be biased (either too high or too low). Analyzing the imputed datasets helps understand how sensitive the parameter estimates are to the MAR violation. Other methods for handling MNAR in various situations are quite complex and include Heckman's selection model and a pattern mixture model. These methods are covered in a textbook by Enders.[43]

Fig. 2 shows the decision process and possible options that could be taken before running analysis. An example in handling missing data in surveys is provided in the Supplementary Materials in the online version at https://doi.org/10.1016/B978-0-323-91888-6.00017-X.

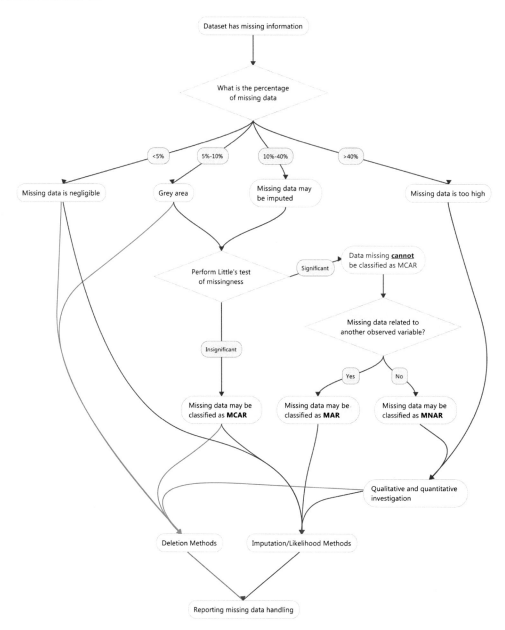

FIG. 2   Algorithm for handling missing data.

Missing data in special circumstances

Missing data in repeated measures

Of important mention is the missingness in trials and longitudinal studies. During the data gathering phase of these studies, loss of follow up can lead to missing entries. In clinical trials, patients may be withdrawn due to side effects or alternative treatments provided. At other times, patients drop out, with no indication of the cause, and this can also lead to missing values. Clinical trials papers and discussions on preventing and handling the missing values have been written at length.[44] Probably due to the nature of clinical trials and their purpose of providing demonstration of effect, the strategies to handle and prevent missingness and the influence of missing values are well considered. As part of integrating cohorts for epidemiological studies of metaanalysis, Rajula et al. suggest using deletion methods (CCA), single imputation methods, multiple imputation methods, or missing indicator methods.[45]

Missing data in factor analysis

The issue of missing data is well and truly manifest when techniques of factor analysis are used. Regardless of whether the intention is to simultaneously explore the number of dimensions and factor loadings using exploratory factor analysis (EFA), or whether hypotheses are tested to confirm factorial structure, where confirmatory factor analysis (CFA) is employed, or whether structural equation modeling (SEM) is used to test relationships between latent structures, missing data is a serious issue.

Exploratory factor analysis (EFA) is a technique used to identify the underlying structure of scale or questionnaire.[46] In EFA, a correlation matrix is created to observe patterns between variables, of which, the variables that have similar patterns (called factors) with a certain weight. These factor loadings are used to identify how are generalized to a wider population.

Within the discipline of social pharmacy research, EFA is conducted very frequently, and missingness is a big issue because it is often performed in exploratory studies, at the lower end of sample size recommendations. Sample size recommendations for factor analysis have traditionally used rules of thumb such as the either 10 cases to each item or minimum of 200 cases. However, it is now known that sample size requirements are highly sensitive to the size of factor loadings, number of items per factor and the size of the communalities, and these cannot be known in preliminary studies before the data is explored. When one considers, for example an EFA exploring the factorial structure of 20 items, there needs to be 20 out of 20 items without missingness or list-wise deletion would remove that case. In a simulation study, McNeish uses an example of a 3-factor model with 5 indicators for each factor, to show that with 5% missingness (for each item) a sample size of 240 is reduced to 180 and with 10% missingness the effective sample is reduced to 50 observations.[47] Even though maximum likelihood with list-wise deletion will lead to unbiased factor loadings when the data is MCAR, the representativeness of data is reduced drastically. There are a number of ways that EFA can utilize and incorporate information from cases, which would otherwise be missing if deletion methods were employed. McNeish therefore advises against deletion methods and recommends that a range of options for small datasets be considered including multiple imputation, EM and FIML. However, one of the problems of conducting FIML on small datasets with missingness is that the algorithms tend to fail to converge toward a replicable solution. McNeish showed that multiple imputation with predictive mean matching, prior to performing EFA, was the most superior method overall for accurately predicting the number of factors and factor loadings.[47] Following this, a novel and sophisticated method based on multiple imputation for conducting EFA in the presence of high level of missingness has been proposed by Nassiri et al.[48] Again, in simulations, the imputation method was compared with EM and FIML and was shown to provide the least biased estimates in the presence of higher levels of MCAR, MAR and even selected types of MNAR. Nassiri et al.'s method is available in an R package (https://ibiostat.be/online-resources/online-resources/expfactor).

The issue of missingness is important for CFA and SEM, where hypotheses regarding factorial structure and relationships between latent variables are tested. Here, the absence of bias in parameter estimation, along with accurate standard error size estimation is important to the validity of a range of statistical tests, including model fit. FIML has been shown to be superior to multiple imputation, for MCAR and MAR data, and affords a low chance of convergence failures.[49] FIML does require specialized software. It should be noted that likelihood methods rely on classical test theory and so assumes multivariate normality. Simply put, multivariate normality means that each of the variables, and certain mathematical combinations of the variables, in the analysis are normally distributed. This is not typical of 5-point Likert-type responses used in many surveys because these responses tend to yield data which is not normally distributed itself, and therefore, combinations of the variables are not multivariate normal. In order to manage excessive multivariate kurtosis, extensions of certain FIML programs use robust statistics. When there are departures from multivariate normality, robust statistics allow for reproducible parameter estimates to be generated with classical theory tests and are not overly affected by the presence of outliers. In regression analyses for example, the estimates of the standard errors of beta weights are less biased when robust statistics are used on multivariate nonnormal data. FIML with robust statistics are available in commercial products including SAS, STATA MPLUS (https://www.statmodel.com/), and EQS (http://www.mvsoft.com/eqs60.htm) and also in R.

Missing data as part of data integration

Data integration is the process of collecting various datasets and creating a combined dataset.[50] In linking datasets, item level information may be missing for some cases, or may not merge correctly. In building larger datasets by combining cross-sectional surveys, there is the possibility that items were not repeated in surveys, or their label coded names have changed. This creates an issue of missing items. Again, this results in missing data at both the item and case level, with missing data handling required to perform data analysis. An approach to handling missing data as part of record linkage has been explored by Fienberg and Manrique-Vallier.[51] In their paper, they describe Baker's work with breast cancer[52] and the use of the Expectation-Maximization (EM) algorithm. In the field of omics, multiple imputation[53] and Bayesian methods[54] have been used to handle the missing data.

Reporting on missing data

With multiple approaches available, it is important that the method/s of handling missingness are reported. Many fields require specifics in reporting on missing data, and this is left up to the researcher to determine. However, most readers would be interested in the responses to the following questions related to the missingness:

- What is the percentage of missing values?
- How did the missingness develop? Was it respondent allocated, administration related or other?
- How the missingness was classified (MCAR, MAR, MNAR)?
- Was item-level deletion performed and what were the criteria for deletion?
- Was a list-wise or pair-wise deletion performed?
- Was imputation performed? How?
- Was a likelihood method performed? Which method?
- What was the justification for the methods applied?

Missing data reporting should be presented in the results section. Tables reporting values can report the actual number (n) as well as those that are missing. An alternate approach is to report missingness and handling of missing data in the supplementary section for sake of conciseness.

As an example of reporting, the paper from Mirzaei et al. 2019 reports[55] missingness in a study conducting EFA as follows:

> *Therefore, a strategy was used to reduce the impact of missingness in this study. Items where more than 10% of the respondents answered "I don't know," were removed from the analysis. The rationale for this was that these items were likely to be poorly conceptualized by respondents and would not be a valid measure of service quality. As such, 7 items were excluded from the analysis with the entire "special services" subdimension requiring removal. Missing data were then handled using list-wise deletion.*

Summary

Missing data needs to be considered throughout the course of survey-based research, from planning through to reporting. This chapter has introduced multiple approaches for handling missing survey data and presented a guide for when these approaches should be used. It is essential to consider and report on missing data to accurately report the findings of a survey study.

Questions for further discussion

1. Which factors should be considered during the planning phase to minimize missing data?
2. What factors which may contribute to missingness will you evaluate during pilot testing?
3. What factors could influence the proportion of missingness for the choice of analysis method?
4. What assumptions are made when using imputation methods?

Application exercise/scenario

As an exercise, we are going to examine data that are in 3 forms of missingness. The datasets and respective code are available online. The original dataset is from the UCI Machine Learning Repository[56] and is of student performance at 2 secondary education Portuguese schools. The data has been simulated to contain missing data. The activities below are designed to not only have a researcher examine the missing data, but how analysis may differ when compared to the original data. The original analysis was performed in R; however, analyses and exploration of the data can be done using any statistical program.

There are four datasets; "Students_original.csv" which is the original dataset; "Students_MCAR.csv," which is the dataset with data missing completely at random; "Students_MAR.csv," which has data missing at random; and finally "Students_MNAR.csv," which has data missing not at random. The explanation of each column has been provided in a file called attributes. The objective is to do a regression to predict a student's *final grade (G3)*.

While attempting the regression, consider the following questions when preparing the data for performing an analysis.

Questions
1. Is there any missing data in this dataset?
2. What is the proportion of missing data per item and case? How much of the data is missing overall?
3. Can I visualize the missing information? Do the missing values show me any patterns?
4. What could be explanation for the missing data?
5. If I performed Little's test for Missing Completely at Random, what would be my result?
6. Are any variables correlated with each other?
7. What are the features I will use for analysis? If I perform a CCA, do I need to delete based on all the variables?
8. If I plan to use imputation methods, which method should I use? Could I use more than one method?
9. Finally, compare my analysis on the missing dataset to the original dataset. What was the difference?

References

1. Narayan SW, Yu Ho K, Penm J, et al. Missing data reporting in clinical pharmacy research. *Am J Health Syst Pharm.* 2019;76:2048–2052.
2. Allison PD. *Missing Data.* vol. 136. Thousand Oaks, CA, United States: Sage Publications; 2001.
3. Rubin DB. Inference and missing data. *Biometrika.* 1976;63:581–592.
4. Little RJ, Rubin DB. *Statistical Analysis With Missing Data.* John Wiley & Sons; 2002.
5. Vandenbroucke JP, von Elm E, Altman DG, et al. Strengthening the reporting of observational studies in epidemiology (STROBE): explanation and elaboration. *PLoS Med.* 2007;4:e297.
6. Little RJ. A test of missing completely at random for multivariate data with missing values. *J Am Stat Assoc.* 1988;83:1198–1202.
7. Turrell G. Income non-reporting: implications for health inequalities research. *J Clin Epidemiol.* 2000;54:207–214.
8. Aquilino WS. Telephone versus face-to-face interviewing for household drug use surveys. *Int J Addict.* 1991;27:71–91.
9. Little T, Rhemtulla M. Planned missing data designs for developmental researchers. *Child Dev Perspect.* 2013;7:199–204.
10. Pokropek A. Missing by design: planned missing-data designs in social science. *ASK Res Methods.* 2011;(20):81–105.
11. Rosenberg SW. Opinion formation, theory of. In: Wright JD, ed. *International Encyclopedia of the Social & Behavioral Sciences.* 2nd ed. Oxford: Elsevier; 2015:243–245.
12. Kim Y, Dykema J, Stevenson J, Black P, Moberg DP. Straightlining: overview of measurement, comparison of indicators, and effects in mail–web mixed-mode surveys. *Soc Sci Comput Rev.* 2019;37:214–233.
13. Dirmaier J, Harfst T, Koch U, Schulz H. Incentives increased return rates but did not influence partial nonresponse or treatment outcome in a randomized trial. *J Clin Epidemiol.* 2007;60:1263–1270.
14. Zhang C, Conrad F. Speeding in web surveys: the tendency to answer very fast and its association with straightlining. *Surv Res Methods.* 2014;8:127–135.
15. Dow MM, Eff EA. Multiple imputation of missing data in cross-cultural samples. *Cross-Cult Res.* 2009;43:206–229.
16. McGorry SY. Measurement in a cross-cultural environment: survey translation issues. *Qual Mark Res Int J.* 2000;3(2):74–81.
17. Rolstad S, Adler J, Rydén A. Response burden and questionnaire length: is shorter better? A review and meta-analysis. *Value Health.* 2011;14:1101–1108.
18. Porter SR, Whitcomb ME, Weitzer WH. Multiple surveys of students and survey fatigue. *New Dir Inst Res.* 2004;2004:63–73.
19. O'Reilly-Shah VN. Factors influencing healthcare provider respondent fatigue answering a globally administered in-app survey. *PeerJ.* 2017;5:e3785.
20. Keusch F, Zhang C. A review of issues in gamified surveys. *Soc Sci Comput Rev.* 2017;35:147–166.
21. Schuman H, Presser S. *Questions and Answers in Attitude Surveys: Experiments on Question Form, Wording, and Context.* Sage; 1981.
22. Laaksonen S. Missingness, its reasons and treatment. In: *Survey Methodology and Missing Data.* Springer; 2018:99–110.
23. Durand RM, Lambert ZV. Don't know responses in surveys: analyses and interpretational consequences. *J Bus Res.* 1988;16:169–188.
24. Dong Y, Peng C-YJ. Principled missing data methods for researchers. *Springerplus.* 2013;2:222.

25. Schafer JL, Graham JW. Missing data: our view of the state of the art. *Psychol Methods.* 2002;7:147–177.

26. Seaman SR, White IR. Review of inverse probability weighting for dealing with missing data. *Stat Methods Med Res.* 2011;22:278–295.

27. Seaman S, White I. Inverse probability weighting with missing predictors of treatment assignment or missingness. *Commun Stat Theory Methods.* 2014;43:3499–3515.

28. Lundström S, Särndal C-E. Calibration as a standard method for treatment of nonresponse. *J Off Stat.* 1999;15:305.

29. Roderick JAL. Survey nonresponse adjustments for estimates of means. *Int Stat Rev.* 1986;54:139–157.

30. Marron MM, Wahed AS. Teaching missing data methodology to undergraduates using a group-based project within a six-week summer program. *J Stat Educ.* 2016;24:8–15.

31. Lewis-Beck MS, Bryman A, Liao TF, eds. *Pairwise Deletion. The SAGE Encyclopedia of Social Science Research Methods.* SAGE Publications, Inc.; 2004.

32. Schafer JL. Multiple imputation: a primer. *Stat Methods Med Res.* 1999;8:3–15.

33. Wilkinson L. Statistical methods in psychology journals: guidelines and explanations. *Am Psychol.* 1999;54:594.

34. Jamshidian M, Mata M. 2—Advances in analysis of mean and covariance structure when data are incomplete. This research was supported in part by the National Science Foundation Grant DMS-0437258, In: Lee S-Y, ed. *Handbook of Latent Variable and Related Models*; 2007:21–44. https://www.sciencedirect.com/science/article/pii/B9780444520449500057#fn1. Amsterdam, North-Holland.

35. Hair JF, Tatham RL, Anderson RE, Black W. *Multivariate Data Analysis.* New Jersey: Pearson Prentice Hall; 2006.

36. Brown ML, Kros JF. The impact of missing data on data mining. In: *Data Mining: Opportunities and challenges.* IGI Global; 2003:174–198.

37. Bennett DA. How can I deal with missing data in my study? *Aust N Z J Public Health.* 2001;25:464–469.

38. Enders CK. A primer on maximum likelihood algorithms available for use with missing data. *Struct Equ Model Multidiscip J.* 2001;8:128–141.

39. Lee S-Y, Chiu Y-M. Analysis of multivariate polychoric correlation models with incomplete data. *Br J Math Stat Psychol.* 1990;43:145–154.

40. Dempster AP, Laird NM, Rubin DB. Maximum likelihood from incomplete data via the EM algorithm. *J R Stat Soc Ser B Stat Methodol.* 1977;39:1–38.

41. Schlomer GL, Bauman S, Card NA. Best practices for missing data management in counseling psychology. *J Couns Psychol.* 2010;57:1–10.

42. Donders AR, van der Heijden GJ, Stijnen T, Moons KG. Review: a gentle introduction to imputation of missing values. *J Clin Epidemiol.* 2006;59:1087–1091.

43. Enders CK. *Applied Missing Data Analysis.* New York, United States: Guilford Publications; 2010.

44. Laird NM. Missing data in longitudinal studies. *Stat Med.* 1988;7:305–315.

45. Rajula HSR, Odintsova V, Manchia M, Fanos V. Overview of federated facility to harmonize, analyze and management of missing data in cohorts. *Appl Sci.* 2019;9:4103.

46. El-Den S, Schneider C, Mirzaei A, Carter S. How to measure a latent construct: psychometric principles for the development and validation of measurement instruments. *Int J Pharm Pract.* 2020;28:326–336.

47. McNeish D. Exploratory factor analysis with small samples and missing data. *J Pers Assess.* 2017;99:637–652.

48. Nassiri V, Lovik A, Molenberghs G, Verbeke G. On using multiple imputation for exploratory factor analysis of incomplete data. Available at: *Behav Res Methods.* 2018. https://link.springer.com/article/10.3758/s13428-017-1000-9#citeas. [Accessed: 20 October 2020].

49. Enders CK, Bandalos DL. The relative performance of full information maximum likelihood estimation for missing data in structural equation models. *Struct Equ Model Multidiscip J.* 2001;8:430–457.

50. Doan A, Halevy A, Ives Z. 1—Introduction. In: Doan A, Halevy A, Ives Z, eds. *Principles of Data Integration.* Boston: Morgan Kaufmann; 2012:1–18.

51. Fienberg SE, Manrique-Vallier D. Integrated methodology for multiple systems estimation and record linkage using a missing data formulation. *Adv Stat Anal.* 2009;93:49–60.

52. Baker SG. A simple EM algorithm for capture-recapture data with categorical covariates. *Biometrics.* 1990;46:1193–1200.

53. Voillet V, Besse P, Liaubet L, San Cristobal M, González I. Handling missing rows in multi-omics data integration: multiple imputation in multiple factor analysis framework. *BMC Bioinf.* 2016;17:402.

54. Fang Z, Ma T, Tang G, et al. Bayesian integrative model for multi-omics data with missingness. *Bioinformatics.* 2018;34:3801–3808.

55. Mirzaei A, Carter SR, Chen JY, Rittsteuer C, Schneider CR. Development of a questionnaire to measure consumers' perceptions of service quality in community pharmacies. *Res Soc Adm Pharm.* 2019;15:346–357.

56. Dua D, Graff C. UCI Machine Learning Repository. 2019. http://archive.ics.uci.edu/ml. Irvine, CA: University of California, School of Information and Computer Science.

Chapter 36

Use of national databases and surveys to evaluate prescribing patterns and medication use

Rajender R. Aparasu and Sanika Rege

Department of Pharmaceutical Health Outcomes and Policy, College of Pharmacy, University of Houston, Texas Medical Center, Houston, TX, United States

Objectives

- Describe the NAMCS/NHAMCS, including survey content, sampling, data collection, and processing.
- Discuss the strengths and analytic considerations of the NAMCS/NHAMCS.
- Identify limitations and challenges of the NAMCS/NHAMCS.
- Provide a generalized approach for evaluating prescribing practices using the NAMCS/NHAMCS.

Introduction

Ambulatory care refers to the services provided by medical professionals in outpatient settings without the need for inpatient care.[1] These include the provision of health care at physician offices, hospital outpatient departments, urgent care, and ambulatory centers. Patients use ambulatory care services for multiple reasons, including treatment and curing of diseases, disease prevention, quality of life improvement, and disease knowledge.[2] Patients and payors prefer ambulatory care for cost and access considerations. However, the use and provision of ambulatory care can be optimal or suboptimal with respect to quality and cost. Therefore, understanding and evaluating ambulatory care utilization is important to inform patients, providers, payers, and policymakers. With increasing efforts to move health care delivery to ambulatory settings, there is a constant need to understand and evaluate ambulatory care practices.

The national health care surveys were designed by the National Center for Health Statistics (NCHS), the principal federal data collection agency under the Center for Disease Control and Prevention (CDC), to address the needs of policymakers, health care professionals, and researchers. The mission of the NCHS is "to provide statistical information that will guide actions and policies to improve the health of the American people."[3] They provide accurate and objective nationally representative data to serve the needs of policymakers and researchers. The national health care surveys that focus on ambulatory care include the National Ambulatory Medical Care Survey (NAMCS), the National Hospital Ambulatory Medical Care Survey (NHAMCS), the National Electronic Health Records Survey (NEHRS), and the National Survey of Ambulatory Surgery (NSAS). These provider-based nationally representative surveys aim to provide objective and reliable information regarding the provision and utilization of ambulatory care in the United States. These surveys involve unique sampling methods, data collection, and complex design features to provide generalizable national estimates of ambulatory care utilization.

The national surveys, especially the NAMCS and the NHAMCS, are valuable resources to pharmacy researchers because of their availability and generalizability. These cross-sectional surveys are often used to evaluate ambulatory care practices, especially prescribing practices. The surveys can address the nature, extent, and trends of prescribing practices in ambulatory settings. In addition, prescription drivers can be evaluated based on patient and provider factors. There are several methodological and practical considerations that make these national surveys useful to both novice and seasoned researchers. However, the data collection and design features should be carefully considered when analyzing the national survey data.[4] The purpose of this chapter is to provide an in-depth understanding of the NAMCS/NHAMCS, including

Contemporary Research Methods in Pharmacy and Health Services. https://doi.org/10.1016/B978-0-323-91888-6.00029-6

methodological considerations for evaluating prescribing practices in ambulatory care settings in the United States. This chapter starts with a detailed discussion of the NAMCS/NHAMCS, including survey content, sampling, data collection, and processing. This is followed by analyzing the strengths of these surveys and the analytic considerations of the NAMCS/NHAMCS. The limitations and challenges of the NAMCS/NHAMCS are also detailed to provide the context to undertake these studies. Finally, the generalized research approach is discussed by providing some examples and structural framework for evaluating prescribing practices using the NAMCS/NHAMCS.

Scope of the NAMCS and NHAMCS

The NAMCS is a national probability sample survey of visits to office-based physicians. The NCHS started the NAMCS in 1973, and it incorporated prescribing data in 1980.[5] It is conducted annually by the NCHS since 1989. The NAMCS is designed to provide objective and reliable information about the provision and utilization of medical care services provided at outpatient settings in the United States. Visit-level data are collected from nonfederal, office-based physicians who are mainly engaged in direct patient care. The NAMCS is limited to visits to office-based physicians not employed by the federal government and are classified as "office-based, patient care" by the American Medical Association (AMA) or the American Osteopathic Association (AOA); however, certain physician specialties such as anesthesiology, radiology, and pathology are excluded. In addition, the survey also includes providers at nonhospital private clinics and health maintenance organizations (HMOs). Due to the concerns that the NAMCS excluded office-based practices owned by hospitals, physicians classified as "hospital-employed" by the AMA were included in the sampling group starting in 2014.[6]

Beginning in 2006, the NAMCS added a sample of community health centers (CHCs), which included both physicians and nonphysician providers. In the period between 2006 and 2012, the CHC component did not include a nationally representative sample. However, the NAMCS included visits to CHC physicians with limited data from nonphysician clinicians such as physician assistants, nurse practitioners, and nurse-midwives. From 2012 onwards, the CHC component of the NAMCS data has been redesigned to include an independent national survey that allows computing the national estimates for CHCs.[7] Data from the CHC visits to physicians and nonphysician providers are available as separate public use files for the years 2012 and 2013, while the newer years are still in progress.[6]

The NHAMCS was developed to capture data in hospital ambulatory care settings such as emergency and outpatient departments in the United States.[8] The NHAMCS began in 1976, and annual data collection started in 1992.[8] The data for the NHAMCS are collected from emergency departments (EDs) and outpatient departments (OPDs) of noninstitutional general short-stay hospitals. The scope of the NHAMCS expanded to include hospital ambulatory surgery settings in 2009 and ambulatory surgical centers in 2010.[8] However, it excludes federal, military, and veteran facilities. The NHAMCS is especially important as hospital ambulatory visits represent a crucial component of the overall ambulatory care. In addition, the demographic and clinical characteristics of patients visiting hospital EDs or OPDs differ from patients in office-based settings.[9]

Outpatient clinics are considered within the scope of the NHAMCS if the physicians provided or supervised ambulatory medical care in the hospital. Other clinics providing ancillary services or those that do not require physician services or supervision are considered out of scope. Also, other settings such as freestanding clinics (physician practices located within hospitals but separate from OPDs) and ambulatory surgery centers/locations (in hospitals or independent) are also considered out of scope for the NHAMCS from 2008 onwards. The data for freestanding clinics are included in the NAMCS, while the data on ambulatory surgery centers/locations are captured as a separate NHAMCS component.[10] The OPD clinic definition excludes clinics that are rented out to physician groups, as they are included in the NAMCS. The OPD clinics providing chemotherapy, radiation, and physical therapy are also considered out of scope. Currently, the NHAMCS outpatient department and ambulatory surgery data are not available from 2012 to 2017 due to quality assurance issues, while emergency department data are available until 2017.[10] The OPD data were not collected due to budgetary issues in recent years. With regards to emergency care, EDs that were staffed 24 h a day or had an emergency service area were in scope for the NHAMCS. EDs or their services that are rented out in the hospital were also in-scope for the NHAMCS.

Sample design in the NAMCS and NHAMCS

NAMCS sampling

Both the NAMCS and the NHAMCS use a multistage probability sampling design with the physician and patient encounter as the final sampling unit.[6,10] The sampling procedure for the NAMCS involved three stages till 2011. The first-stage sample included the largest sampling unit referred to as the primary sampling unit (PSU) that contains a cluster of basic sampling units. This stage included 112 PSUs; each PSU refers to a geographic segment. Geographic segments can be further classified as counties/equivalents or towns and townships within the United States (including 50 states and the District of Columbia). The use of cluster sampling helps in obtaining a representative sample of geographically dispersed sampling units. Only a two-stage sampling procedure was used from 2012 onwards, and the PSUs were not utilized for the NAMCS. The first stage involved the selection of physicians, and the second stage involved the selection of visits within the practices.

The master files maintained by the AMA and the AOA are used to select probability samples of practicing physicians.[6] The master file maintained by the AMA contains up-to-date data on member and nonmember physicians in the United States, including those who graduated from foreign medical schools which meet requirements for the educational standards. The most recent data on physicians are collected from all physicians residing in the United States and all United States physicians living temporarily overseas using questionnaires. The AOA uses a similar procedure for maintaining its master file, which includes all persons who attend and graduate from osteopathic schools. The AOA also keeps its master file up-to-date by conducting surveys of persons in the file every 18 months.[11] The AMA and the AOA include over a million physicians, and about 3000 physicians are sampled for the NAMCS.

The first stage involved the stratified sampling of physician practices within the PSUs. Eligible physicians are stratified into 15 groups: general and family practice, osteopathy, internal medicine, pediatrics, general surgery, obstetrics and gynecology, orthopedic surgery, cardiovascular diseases, dermatology, urology, psychiatry, neurology, ophthalmology, otolaryngology, and a category including all other specialties, and may be sorted by census region, followed by metropolitan service area (MSA) status and practice type.[6] Within the specified strata and sorted region, metropolitan location, and practice type, about 60 physicians are randomly selected.

The second stage includes the selection of visits within the sampled physician practices and includes two steps. The first step involves randomly distributing the physician sample into 52 similar-sized samples and assigning each sample to one of the 52 weeks in the survey year. The second step involves the selection of a random sample of visits by the physician in the reporting week. Census Field Representatives mainly conduct visit sampling. This step has a variable sampling rate based on the interview carried out before the survey, with 100% sample considered for small practices to approximately 20% sample for very large practices. The recent data collection efforts include electronic health records data along with abstracted data.[6]

For the most recent NAMCS (2016), the sampling design did not factor specific states, which was done in previous years (2012–15) to allow state-based estimates. For the 2016 NAMCS, only a two-stage stratified sampling design was used (the first stage involved physician selection and the second stage involved visits selection).[2] The NAMCS oversamples certain populations. For instance, compared to primary care physicians, the NAMCS samples approximately twice the sample of physicians in smaller specialties such as dermatology.[12] This deliberate oversampling offers an advantage to evaluate patient care in smaller specialties better. Also, in 2006, the NAMCS oversampled CHCs, which led to improved reliability of estimates for CHC visits and capturing important findings regarding demographics of patients visiting these health centers.[13–15] There are over 14,000 CHCs, and about 100 CHCs are sampled for the NAMCS. The CHC sampling frame included the Federally Qualified Health Center (FQHC) with and without Section 330 funding and urban Indian Health Service outpatient clinics.

NHAMCS sampling

The sample design for the NHAMCS is similar to the NAMCS; it involves the use of a four-stage probability design and includes samples of PSUs, hospitals within these PSUs, clinics within hospital outpatient departments, and patient encounters within clinics/emergency service areas.[10] The PSU consists of a county, group of counties, or county-equivalents, towns, townships, minor civil divisions (specifically, some PSUs in New England), or a metropolitan statistical area (MSA). The hospital sampling frame and samples are updated if necessary, using hospital data from the IMS Health's Health Care Organizations (HCOS) database to remove out-of-scope hospitals and add new ones. Hospitals eligible for the NHAMCS are those with an average length of stay of fewer than 30 days, considered short stay, or those with a general, including surgical or medical, or children's general specialty. The NHAMCS excluded federally-owned hospitals, units at institutions, and hospitals with less than six beds for inpatient use.[10]

Over 500 hospitals are sampled for the NHAMCS. Hospitals are then defined to have an ED or an OPD if the hospital file indicates the presence of such a unit or a nonzero number of visits to that unit. The hospital selections are made so that each hospital would be chosen only once to avoid multiple inclusions of very large hospitals. Within each hospital, OPDs and EDs are sampled separately. Only in-scope outpatient clinics and EDs are included. If the hospital had less than five clinics, all clinics were included. In hospitals with more clinics, they were stratified by specialty, and two clinics were selected for each of the specialties. The EDs were considered as a separate stratum, and all were selected for the NHAMCS. The final step involves a systematic selection of the basic sampling unit, i.e., patient visits during a randomly identified 4-week long reporting period, within EDs or OPDs.[10] EDs and OPDs in each hospital collected visit data for 100 and up to 200 patients, respectively.

Data collection for the NAMCS and NHAMCS

The current NAMCS and NHAMCS data collection procedures are based on methodologies that were developed in previous years.[5,8] These include the use of both prospective and retrospective data collection methods, personal induction interviews in hospitals and clinics to capture provider data, and the use of patient record forms (PRFs) to capture the visit characteristics.[8] Data collection for the NAMCS is carried out by the US Census Bureau. The physician receives an introductory letter from the NCHS Director. Further physician eligibility is assessed by the Census Field Representative. After assessing eligibility, the representative explains the survey to the respective physician and the staff who may be involved in extracting the data. During the initial visit, the representative enlists characteristics of up to 5 practice locations where the physician sees the patient during the reporting period. A certificate of appreciation is provided by the Census Field Representative to the physician for participating in the survey. The actual data are collected by the abstraction of medical records by the field staff of the US Census Bureau or from electronic health records.[6]

The provider data in the NAMCS are collected using the Physician Induction Interview Forms.[6] The Physician Induction Interview Forms contain questions related to the physicians' ambulatory care practice. It includes questions such as physician specialty (general practitioner, pediatrics, neurology, psychiatry, etc.), type of practice (solo, group, partnership, etc.), type of doctor (MD, DO, etc.), ownership of the visit location (full owner, part owner, contractor, employee, etc.), number of patient visits each day, etc.

The visit characteristics are captured using the Patient Record Forms (PRFs) by the participating physicians and staff to obtain a systematic random sample over a weekly reporting period. The key factor behind developing the PRF has been the considerations of the physician's time and effort in filling the PRF. This involves limiting the overall number of survey items to one side of a page and limiting the number of subjective responses by including more objective checkboxes. Also, the items are made as self-explanatory as possible by placing clarifying information at the top of the PRF.[16] The PRF captures visit characteristics including patient age, race, ethnicity, gender, major reasons for visit, use of diagnostic services, physicians' diagnoses, duration of visit, disposition of visit, medication and nonmedication therapy, and patient complaints/symptoms/other visit reason, etc. (see Table 1).

In the NHAMCS, the data collection procedure involves steps similar to the NAMCS. The first step is field training, where the Census Headquarters staff oversees the data collection process and training the Census regional office staff. The Census regional office staff also monitor activities involved in data collection. This is followed by hospital induction, where Census Field Representatives conduct hospital induction interviews, verify hospital eligibility for the survey, obtain IRB approval, and train hospital staff on visit sampling. Further, the Field Representatives schedule an orientation session for the sample EDs and OPDs. Information obtained during the ambulatory unit induction interviews is then entered into the survey instrument and used by the Field Representative to develop a sampling plan. The final step involves computerized data collection. The computerized survey tool is used to collect hospital induction data, select a sample of OPD/ED visits, and abstract visit data. The hospital staff can also abstract data using a dedicated laptop.[10]

Processing of the NAMCS/NHAMCS data

Both the NAMCS/NHAMCS require extensive data processing once collected. This includes editing and quality checks.[6,10] A series of steps are undertaken to check, configure, and transmit data files to NCHS or RTI International for further processing. After transmission, the data are checked for consistency and reviewed for verbatim entries by using medical coding. This includes coding for diagnosis, the reason for visit, cause of injury, services, and procedures, and further assessing the variables to indicate whether the diagnosis is probable, questionable, or ruled out. The Drug Database Coordinator performs the medication editing and coding procedures at the NCHS. The coding systems used for the data are also subjected to quality control, and the error rates are reported to the NCHS. The surveys are then adjusted for item nonresponse. Imputation techniques are used to assign values to missing items in the data. In the NHAMCS, beginning 2014, injury-related data are edited using a program that assigns injury status by reviewing codes for a reason for visit, diagnosis, and cause of injury.

TABLE 1 Selected variables included in the National Ambulatory Care Surveys.

Key variables	Description
Selected provider characteristics	
Geographic region	Reports the regions where the visits were recorded in terms of Northeast, Midwest, South, West
Physician specialty/clinic	Reports the specialty of the physician seen as per their self-designated practice specialty or the type of clinic visited for the outpatient or emergency department
Metropolitan statistical area	Reported as per physician's or clinic location
Selected patient characteristics	
Sex	Reports the gender of the patient as male or female
Age	Reports the age of the patient in years
Race	Reported in terms of White, Black or African American, Asian, Native Hawaiian or Other Pacific Islander, American Indian or Alaska Native or More than one race reported
Ethnicity	Reported in terms of Hispanic or not Hispanic
Source of payment	Reports the expected source of payment in terms of Private insurance, Medicare, Medicaid or CHIP or other state-based programs, Self-pay, Workers' compensation, No charge/charity, Other, Unknown
Selected visit characteristics	
Reason for visit	Reports the visit reason as reported by patients using the reason for visit classification developed by the National Center for Health Statistics
Diagnosis for visit	Reports the International Classification of Diseases, Ninth/Tenth Revision, Clinical Modification for the physician diagnosis and cause of injury
Diagnostic and screening test	Reports if any examinations such as Alcohol misuse, Depression screening, Domestic violence screening, Foot exam, Pelvic exam, Retinal/Eye exam, Substance abuse screening were ordered/provided during the visit
Laboratory test	Reports if any laboratory tests such as Basic metabolic panel, Chlamydia test, Creatinine/Renal function panel, Glucose serum test, Glycohemoglobin test, Hepatitis panel testing, PAP test, Pregnancy test, Vitamin D test, etc., were ordered/provided during the visit
Health education/counseling[a]	Reports if any health education/counseling such as Asthma education, diabetes educations, Diet/Nutrition, Exercise, Family planning/Contraception, Weight reduction, Genetic counseling, Stress management, etc., were ordered/provided during the visit
Procedures	Reports if any procedures such as Fetal monitoring, Peak flow, Tonometry, Spirometry, Upper gastrointestinal endoscopy, etc., were ordered/provided during the visit
Medications	Reports if any prescription or nonprescription drugs were ordered/provided during the visit
Visit disposition	Reports the disposition of the visit in terms of Return to referring physician, Referred to other physician, Return in less than 1 week, Return in 1 week to less than 2 months, Return in 2 months or greater, Return at unspecified time, Return as needed, Referred to an ER/admitted to hospital, Other

[a]Not available in the Emergency Department data.

Strengths of the NAMCS/NHAMCS

There are several strengths of the NAMCS and the NHAMCS that can be utilized by novice and seasoned researchers. The national survey data are freely available to researchers, and the data are highly generalizable to the United States. The dataset for each year is available as one file, and multiple years can be combined based on the research objective. The dataset includes selected provider characteristics and detailed visit characteristics, including patient demographics, major reason for visit, use of diagnostic services, physicians' diagnoses, duration of visit, disposition of visit, medication, and nonmedication therapy (see Table 1). These are cross-sectional surveys that are easy to manage and analyze. The NCHS website provides significant resources for researchers, including statistical programs. They also conduct free workshops to help researchers learn about the survey and analytical techniques. There is extensive documentation and publication history for these national surveys. The variables are well defined, and therefore, it is relatively easy to operationalize measures and conduct research using the NAMCS/NHAMCS. In addition, the visit level data are directly collected from the providers, and thus providing strong validity of the reported measures. Most importantly, the NAMCS and the NHAMCS can be effectively used to examine the structure and process of ambulatory care as they provide rich data regarding the use and provision of care. The combined NAMCS/NHAMCS can be used to provide a comprehensive landscape of ambulatory care.

Both surveys provide reliable information on the use of office-based and hospital ambulatory services in the US. There are some unique measures that are not available in other data sources, such as the patient's reason for visit, specific visit characteristics, and provider/setting characteristics to examine ambulatory care. The NAMCS/NHAMCS are often used to examine outpatient care practices, including (i) nature and extent of utilization of office, OPD, and ED visits for specific diseases; (ii) characteristics of visits based on demographics and insurance; (iii) provider characteristics including specialty and practice; (iv) treatment patterns including medications and nonmedication for diseases; (v) diagnostic, screening or preventive services for specific diseases; (vi) trends in outpatient practices over time; (vii) policy issues such as social determinants of health and disparities; (viii) benchmarking for provision of care; and (ix) national initiatives such as electronic medical records adoption.

Analytical considerations of the NAMCS/NHAMCS

The NAMCS/NHAMCS uses multistage sampling to provide generalizable utilization data for ambulatory settings. The multistage sampling process is helpful as there is no master list of population or outpatient visits in the case of the NAMCS/NHAMCS. Stratified sampling helps to provide representative sampling for analytical purposes. In the NAMCS, stratified sampling is used for the selection of physician practice and census regions. In the NHAMCS, hospitals are stratified by geographic region, hospital class, type of ownership, and size. Sometimes disproportionate sampling is combined with a stratified sampling of the physician practices to provide a large sample for those with a small population.[6]

The NAMCS and the NHAMCS were designed to generate national estimates of office/OPD/ED visits based on the sampling weights (PATWT). In the NAMCS, the estimation processes for sampling weights are based on the four components: (i) selection probabilities, (ii) physician nonresponse, (iii) fixed totals for physician samples, and (iv) weight smoothing.[6] The selection probabilities account for the selection of physicians within a stratum and of patient visits within the respective practice. Physician nonresponse accounts for those who did participate in the survey or lacked patients in the assigned week or those who provided other forms of data. In some years, there is an adjustment for seasonality. The fixed total adjusts for the total physician population and the final sample for the NAMCS. Weight smoothing accounts for extreme weights by trimming and ratio adjustment to provide the same total estimates as unsmoothed weights. Some national surveys include state weight (PATWTST) to calculate state-level estimates. The NHAMCS has similar components to calculate sampling weights (PATWT) for the OPD and ED components.

For the past decade, the NAMCS provided physician-level weight (PHYSWT) to provide estimates of physicians. However, these are limited to the in-scope physicians who saw patients and cannot be generalized to all office-based physicians due to sampling bias. Since there is one weight for each participating physician, only those records with positive weights (>0) should be used for calculating physician-level estimates. These can be linked to visit-based records per physician to compare physicians in the study samples. These require a different computation process.

The sampling error is "primarily a measure of the sampling variability that occurs by chance because only a sample is surveyed, rather than the entire universe."[6] The standard error is an important consideration for statistical inferences based on the national survey samples. Unlike simple random sampling, multistage sampling involving stratification and clustering affects the standard error calculation. Stratification decreases the sampling variation, whereas clustering increases sampling variation. Therefore, the analyses involving national data should account for the sampling scheme of national surveys.

Previously, the national surveys used to provide an approximation of standard errors based on generalized variance curves and relative stand error tables due to confidentiality concerns.[16] However, it limited the use of multivariable analyses for the NAMCS/NHAMCS due to the lack of sampling design variables. In 2002, the NAMCS/NHAMCS started to include masked sampling design variables. The masking involved modifying sampling units and population size measures. With the availability of statistical packages, a more accurate standard error can be calculated based on these masked survey design specifications.[17]

The replication methods and linearized Taylor series are the commonly used procedures to calculate standard errors for complex surveys.[18,19] The replication methods divide the total sample into subsamples and estimate variance based on the subsamples with replicated weights. Similar to bootstrapping, these are computationally intensive and do not require information on the complex sampling scheme. The linearized Taylor series option incorporates sampling design variables reflecting a complete and complex sampling scheme for the calculation of linear approximation of variance. The variance calculation also involves sampling weights to account for unequal sampling and strata and cluster variables to account for the sampling design. Both replication methods and linearized Taylor series provide comparable results for most measures; however, replication methods are preferred for highly skewed data and nonsmooth functions.[18] The NAMCS and the NHAMCS provide masked design variables for estimating standard error and variance based on linearized Taylor series.

The SUDAAN, SAS, and STATA are commonly used statistical packages to analyze complex survey data.[20–22] The SUDAAN is specifically designed for complex survey data and has been in use for a long time.[20] It can implement more complexities of the national survey and includes multiple approaches for calculating standard error. The initial design variables in most national surveys were specific for SUDAAN. SAS survey procedures were added to accommodate the analytical needs of complex surveys.[21] There are specific survey descriptive and multivariable procedures in addition to advanced procedures that can accommodate complex surveys. The STATA also has specific survey procedures that can be used for the descriptive and multivariable analyses of complex surveys.[22] The functionality of these procedures is like SAS. There are other packages that also analyze complex surveys, such as SPSS, Epi-Info, and IVEware.[4]

The initial national surveys included three or four-stage sample design variables for computing the standard error.[17] These included stratum marker for PSU (STATM), PSU marker (PSUM), survey year (YEAR), and specifications for the NAMCS/NHAMCS. It also included masked population measures such as stratum count of PSUs (POPPSUM); the masked number of clinics/hospitals (POPSUM); a masked provider visit volume (POPVISM); and a masked count of in-scope providers within PSUs (POPPROVM). The SUDAAN can incorporate the multistage design variables to account for the complex sampling design of the NAMCS/NHAMCS with the full sample without replacement design. The recent national surveys only include masked first-stage design variables, CSTRATM and CPSUM, for use in SAS, STATA, and SUDAAN. These design variables can be used in both descriptive and multivariable analyses (see Fig. 1).

Previous research by the NCHS showed that standard error estimates based on masked design variables are less accurate than unmasked variables with the full sample without replacement design.[23] However, a later study found that the full sample design with SUDAAN and one stage sampling with SUDAAN and SAS with masked design variables "slightly" overstate the standard error when compared to analyses involving unmasked design variables.[17] Thus, analyses involving first-stage sampling with masked variables will lead to conservative statistical tests. Although there was no discernable pattern with larger samples for standard error estimation, the smaller samples were at risk for underestimation or

```
SAS

PROC SURVEYFREQ;
TABLES SEX;
CLUSTER CPSUM;
STRATA CSTRATM;
WEIGHT PATWT;

PROC SURVEYREG;
CLUSTER CPSUM;
STRATA CSTRATM;
WEIGHT PATWT;
MODEL TIMEMD = NOPAY;

STATA 9
TAB SEX
SVYSET CPSUM [PWEIGHT=PATWT], STRATA(CSTRATM)
SVY: TAB SEX

SVY: REG TIMEMD NOPAY

SUDAAN
PROC CROSSTAB DATA = TEST DESIGN=WR;
NEST CSTRATM CPSUM /MISSUNIT;
PROC REG DATA = TEST DESIGN=WR;
NEST CSTRATM CPSUM /MISSUNIT;
MODEL TIMEMD = NOPAY;
```

FIG. 1 Selected complex statistical procedures for SAS, STATA, SUDAAN.

overestimation of standard errors when compared to analyses involving unmasked design variables. Therefore, the study recommended using an alpha of 0.01 for statistical significance for smaller estimates. Overall, the study found that masked variables provide better standard error estimates with masked variables than generalized variance curves and relative stand error tables.

Common challenges with the NAMCS/NHAMCS

There are several challenges when using national surveys for health services research. Often, there are changes in the national surveys each year due to survey improvements and requirements by the NCHS. Therefore, care must be taken when combining multiyear data to ensure a common data structure as the availability of variables may change each year. For example, the number of prescribed medications changed over the years. Generally, the survey years with the same number of medications are combined for ease of analysis. The analyses are often limited to the data available in the national surveys. This is especially important when evaluating patients and provider characteristics using descriptive and multivariable analyses. For example, there are limited behavior variables; this limits the approach and interpretation of the findings related to ambulatory care. Also, all variables are operationally defined by the NCHS. These definitions cannot be modified or changed in the secondary data analyses.

The sample size considerations are important for both bivariate and multivariable analyses. For the national surveys, the NCHS recommends a minimum sample size of 30 and a relative standard error of less than 30%.[6,10] The standard error should account for less than 30% of the estimate. There are also guidelines for the reliability of proportions based on the denominator sample size confidence interval using the Clopper-Pearson Method.[24] Several strategies can be used to increase the overall sample size and sample size in subgroups. The following strategies can be used to increase the overall sample size: (i) combining the NAMCS and the NHAMCS, (ii) combining multiple years, and (iii) both. It is important to ensure that definitions remain the same across years and surveys. The sample size in subgroups can be increased by (i) creating a few homogenous subgroups, (ii) combining multiple subgroups, and (iii) multiple variables to define a construct.

Most of the studies involving the NAMCS/NHAMCS are interested in a specific subset of the visits based on disease, patient age, provider, medication class, or other specific criteria. Extracting the subset of visits from the survey, the NAMCS/NHAMCS will undo the complex sampling design. Therefore, the complete survey data should be used by incorporating the domain/subgroup option to maintain sampling integrity. This may generate two outputs—one for the subgroup of interest and another output for the remaining group.

Evaluating prescribing practices with the NAMCS/NHAMCS

The NAMCS/NHAMCS include extensive prescribing data in outpatient settings. There are up to 30 medications collected per visit in the recent NAMCS/NHAMCS.[6,10] The number of medications collected in the NAMCS/NHAMCS varies across the years. It started with eight medications in the year 1980–81. These include new and continued medications, whereas the ED portion of the NHAMCS includes medications given as well as prescriptions at discharge. It is important to understand that the unit of analysis for the NAMCS/NHAMCS is the patient visit. Therefore, each entry in the PRF is considered as drug or medication mention, and visits with one or more medications are considered drug visits.

For each medication, the names are coded as per the NCHS developed system.[16] The medication data also includes prescription status, controlled substance indicator, generic status, ingredients, and therapeutic categories. These additional variables are added during data processing. The medication variables are listed in Table 2. From 2006, each medication is coded for generic composition as per the Multum Lexicon that includes over 2000 single ingredients and 700 combination products.[6,10] There are also medication generic composition codes that could not be matched with Multum codes.

The Multum therapeutic classes are also provided to classify drug classes for each medication. The Multum uses a three-level therapeutic classification scheme with over 20 first-level codes and more than 200 s and third-level codes. Each medication can have multiple therapeutic levels based on the medication ingredients. For example, Prozac (Fluoxetine) will have level 1 (broadest level; 242 psychotherapeutic agents), level 2 (antidepressant), and level 3 (most detailed level; SSRI antidepressant). The extent of the use of these levels of classification is based on the analytical needs of the researcher. Each medication can have multiple ingredients that can also be analyzed.

The NAMCS/NHAMCS can be used to estimate the visits or drug mentions for a drug or drug class. It should be noted that the estimates cannot be used to evaluate drug prevalence or incidence in the population as the unit of analysis is the outpatient visit. The measure represents the medication provided, prescribed, or continued by an outpatient provider. The generic composition code is always a better option as it captures all generic and brand-name products. The NAMCS and the

TABLE 2 Medication-related information for medications in the National Ambulatory Care Surveys.

Key variables	Description
Generic drug code	• Drugs are coded in terms of their generic components and therapeutic classifications using Lexicon Plus®, a proprietary database of Cerner Multum, Inc. • Drug ID code is 6 digits, begins with letter "a," "c," "d," or "n" • Up to 30 medications are included with the generic codes for each medication
Prescription status code	• Code used to identify the legal status of the drug entry
Controlled substance status code	• Code designed to denote the degree of potential abuse and federal control of a drug entry
Composition status code	• Code made to distinguish between single-ingredient and combination drugs
Therapeutic category code	• Multum Lexicon provides a 3-level nested category system that assigns a therapeutic classification to each drug and each ingredient of the drug • Level 3 reflects the most detailed therapeutic level to which the drug can be classified • Each drug may have up to four therapeutic categories on the data file
Drug category levels	• Level 1 (broadest level) is the most detailed, while some drugs can be coded to Level 2, but the majority can be coded to Level 3 (most detailed level) • Not all drugs have three classification levels; some may only have two

OPD component of the NHAMCS are usually combined to capture outpatient prescribing practices as the medical care is similar in these two settings. The ED component of the NHAMCS is generally separately evaluated as it represents emergency care. However, the prescribing data can be compared across by combining the NAMCS and the NHAMCS.

The NAMCS/NHAMCS also captures the other characteristics of the medications, such as: Is it a new or continued medication? Is it for primary diagnosis? Is it on the formulary? However, these questions vary across the years. Some questions are consistent across the years, and those should be used when analyzing multiyear data. It is crucial to understand the changes in the medication data when using multiyear surveys. Since Multum drug codes and classification are used since 2006, it is necessary to use the same drug classification when using multiyear data. The NCHS provides programs that can be used to recode older NAMCS data.

Approaches for evaluating prescribing practicing

The prescribing data in the NAMCS/NHAMCS are commonly used by pharmacy researchers to address numerous outpatient medication use issues. Often the NAMCS and the OPD component of the NHAMCS are combined as the prescribing practices are similar. Several studies by the authors and other researchers involving the NAMCS and the NHAMCS were published over the years in the *Research in Social and Administrative Pharmacy*. Earla et al. used the multiyear NAMCS to examine the trends in prescribing of disease-modifying agents in multiple sclerosis and determined the association with their prescribing in the United States.[25] Rege et al. used the multiyear NAMCS and the OPD component of the NHAMCS to examine prescribing practices, predictors of atypical antipsychotics, and augmentation therapy in older adults with depression.[26] Aparasu et al. used the NAMCS/NHAMCS to examine concomitant prescribing of drug combinations that have the potential for clinically important drug-drug interactions in outpatient settings.[27] Mittal et al. used the multiyear NAMCS/NHAMCS to evaluate prescribing practices of antidepressants in children and adolescents before, during, and after the introduction of the Food and Drug Administration (FDA) boxed warning.[28] Crawford et al. combined the office-based, OPD, and ED data from the NAMCS/NHAMCS to evaluate the prescription trends and predictors of congestive heart failure medications.[29] A complete list of publications based on the NAMCS/NHAMCS can be found elsewhere.[30]

There is some generalized approaches to conduct research using the multiyear NAMCS/NHAMCS to evaluate prescribing practices. The following discussion provides a structural framework for evaluating prescribing practices by discussing research question and hypothesis, study design and methods, and conceptual framework and analysis using our previous research. Most research questions involving the NAMCS/NHAMCS involve evaluation of prescribing practices and examination of predictors of certain prescriptions or classes. This requires a strong understanding of the disease, drugs, physician practices, and policy issues. The sources for these research questions include clinical practice, experience, literature review, ongoing issues, mentors, conceptual theory, and others. The goal of any research is to fill the evidence gap; therefore, it is critical to ensure that previous research did not address the question/hypothesis, especially with the use of the NAMCS/NHAMCS. However, replication studies are fine if others have evaluated prescribing practices using other data sources such as medical claims or electronic medical records. The main advantage of the NAMCS/NHAMCS is that the findings are highly generalizable to both insured and uninsured patients.

Conclusions

With constant changes in healthcare, national surveys like the NAMCS/NHAMCS are valuable to pharmacy researchers to understand ambulatory care practices. The use of these surveys requires an understanding of the survey content, scope, complex sampling scheme, and analytical and research considerations. There are several methodological and practical considerations that make these national surveys useful to both novice and seasoned researchers. The NCHS provides valuable resources, including workshops and support for researchers to utilize these national surveys. However, there are also limitations of the NAMCS/NHAMCS; only certain research questions can be addressed using these national surveys. With the recent focus on real-world and nationally representative data, the national surveys are critical in providing practice and policy relevent evidence to improve quality and access to ambulatory care.

Questions for further discussion

There are inherent disadvantages of any secondary data, including the national surveys. The variables available are those defined by the NAMCS/NHAMCS; therefore, operational definitions are limited to the definitions by the NCHS. The reasons for the visit and diagnosis (up to 5) are limited. The surveys do not collect certain variables such as medication dose and quantity. There are also limited clinical variables, disease severity, laboratory measures, or outcome measures. These should be carefully considered when using and analyzing the national survey data. The variation in prescribing practices cannot be fully explained with the variables in the NAMCS/NHAMCS.

The national surveys cannot be linked to other sources, and longitudinal studies are not possible. The surveys do capture services by nurse practitioners and physicians but have limited provider data. There is a need to collect data on other healthcare professionals who are involved in ambulatory care, including pharmacists. There is an ongoing effort by the NCHS to expand the national surveys to provide a complete picture regarding the structure and process of ambulatory care.[31] With increasing collaborative practices, there is also a need to capture team-based care in ambulatory settings.[32] The national surveys are cross-sectional, and therefore, studies can only evaluate associations and relationships. The surveys have a defined scope and do not include data from out-of-scope providers. Since there is extensive work involved during the survey implementation, there are often delays in releasing the survey data. Therefore, the surveys do not represent most current ambulatory care practices.

The changes in healthcare delivery and use are often reflected in the national survey structure and data collection systems, including the NAMCS/NHAMCS. There are likely to be modifications in the NAMCS/NHAMCS in the future due to changes in ambulatory care. Currently, there are ongoing discussions at the Board of Scientific Counselors to make changes in the NAMCS/NHAMCS.[33,34] The key discussions related to the provision of care include the scope of ambulatory care, greater involvement of advanced practice providers, and increased telemedicine use. There are also discussions related to survey design and methods, including changes in the sampling scheme, increasing the response rate, use of electronic data collection, collecting longitudinal data, and cross-linking of the NAMCS/NHAMCS. The researchers should be aware of the current and future changes in the NAMCS/NHAMCS to appropriately utilize the national surveys to achieve their research goals.

Application exercise/scenario

In a study entitled *Prescribing potentially inappropriate psychotropic medications to the ambulatory elderly* published in *Archives of Internal Medicine*, we evaluated potentially inappropriate prescription of psychotropic agents and identified the associated characteristics.[35] The research was highly significant as inappropriate medication use was a major concern in older adults, and there was an evidence gap regarding inappropriate psychotropic prescribing in the elderly, especially in ambulatory settings. The evidence regarding the extent of inappropriate prescribing and associated factors in ambulatory settings can help providers, payers, and policymakers. We did not have a specific hypothesis as the study was descriptive and exploratory. The NAMCS/NHAMCS-based studies are cross-sectional and can only describe prescribing practices and the factors associated with prescribing. Therefore, the outcomes of the prescribing cannot be evaluated using cross-sectional data. In our study, we used the 1996 NAMCS and the OPD component of the NHAMCS to provide nationally representative estimates regarding the extent of inappropriate psychotropic prescribing and associated factors in the elderly. The two national surveys were combined as they provide the most comprehensive data regarding the provision and use of ambulatory care services in the United States.

The NAMCS/NHAMCS-based studies involve secondary data analysis of outpatient visits to evaluate prescribing practices. These studies often involve either disease or drug-based study samples with a particular focus on classes of medications to understand optimal or suboptimal prescribing practices. The studies generally evaluate the congruency of prescribing practices with treatment guidelines, scientific evidence, and other practice/policy considerations. Such evaluations not only help to understand the prescribing patterns but also the factors associated with optimal or suboptimal prescribing practices. In our study, the study sample included visits by elderly patients 65 years or older receiving psychotropic medications, and the study was focused on inappropriate medications. The operational definitions based on standardized sources and previous research provide the scientific rigor for secondary data analysis studies. In our study, the psychotropic medications were defined based on the American Hospital Formulary Service and Physician Desk Reference. Inappropriate psychotropic medications were based on the Beers' criteria. The evaluation of prescribing practices involves examining generic ingredient codes to capture all relevant medications. The national surveys provide these generic ingredients codes for single and combination products. In our study, the generic ingredient codes of the medications were used to identify and group all psychotropic medications. All the remaining variables, including patient, provider, and prescription characteristics, were operationally defined using the survey definitions. These definitions are well accepted and recognized. See Table 3 for major components of the secondary analyses as described above.

The selected study sample from the NAMCS/NHAMCS should meet the analytical considerations of the national surveys, such as total unweighted sample size and relevant subgroups. In our study, the total sample size of ambulatory visits was 1379, and inappropriate medications were prescribed in 309 visits. These unweighted visits were used to calculate the national estimates of prescribing practices using the visit as the unit of analysis. The available patient, provider, and prescription characteristics were used as the independent variables, and inappropriate psychotropic use was used as the dependent variables. Some researchers use the conceptual framework of the Andersen Behavior Model to group these predictors, and others classify these factors as patient and provider characteristics. The predictors of inappropriate psychotropic prescribing were evaluated using a modified approach as the complex variables like strata and cluster were not available at that time in the public-use data files. With the availability of the survey design variables and SAS/STATA complex survey procedures, the analyses are currently more robust than the approaches used before.

TABLE 3 Major methodological components for a study involving the NAMCS/NHAMCS: An example.

Components	Description
Data source	NAMCS and NHAMCS
Objective	To examine the extent of inappropriate psychotropic prescribing and associated factors in the elderly
Study sample	Visits by elderly patients 65 years or older receiving psychotropic medications
Prescribing practices	Inappropriate psychotropic medications
Operation definitions	• Psychotropic medications as per the AHFS and PDR • Inappropriate psychotropic prescribing as the Beers' criteria • Patient, provider, and prescription characteristics as per the NCHS
Conceptual model	None
Statistical analyses	Descriptive weighted analysis for prescribing practices and multivariable logistic regression for the factors associated with inappropriate prescribing

NAMCS, National Ambulatory Medical Care Survey; NHAMCS, National Hospital Ambulatory Medical Care Survey; AHFS, American Hospital Formulary Service; PDR, Physician Desk Reference; NCHS, National Center for Health Statistics.
Based on Mort JR, Aparasu RR. Prescribing potentially inappropriate psychotropic medications to the ambulatory elderly. Arch Intern Med. 2000;160 (18):2825–31.

Our study found that there were 16.55 million outpatient visits involving psychotropic medications and 4.5 million (27%) visits involved inappropriate psychotropics. Disease-dependent inappropriate psychotropics accounted for 94% of inappropriate psychotropic prescribing such as long-acting benzodiazepines and tricyclic antidepressants. The factors associated with inappropriate psychotropic prescribing based on the logistic regression model were patient characteristics (age and insurance), drug characteristics (antidepressant and antipsychotic), and provider characteristics (region and metropolitan location). Overall, our study found that one in four psychotropic visits involved inappropriate medications, and several patient, prescription, and provider characteristics were associated with inappropriate psychotropic medications. These findings can help to develop targeted strategies to reduce inappropriate medication use in the elderly.

References

1. Ambulatory Care Settings. *The Medicare Payment Advisory Commission (MedPAC)*; 2021. Available at: http://www.medpac.gov/-research-areas-/ambulatory-care-settings. Accessed 3 December 2020.
2. Bernstein AB, Hing E, Moss AJ, Allen KF, Siller AB, Tiggle RB. *Health Care in America: Trends in Utilization*. Hyattsville, Maryland: National Center for Health Statistics; 2003. Available at: https://www.cdc.gov/nchs/data/misc/healthcare.pdf. Accessed 3 December 2020.
3. National Center for Health Statistics (NCHS). *The NCHS Mission*; 2019. Available at: https://www.cdc.gov/nchs/about/mission.htm. Accessed 3 December 2020.
4. Aparasu RR. Secondary data analysis: national sample data. In: *Research Methods for Pharmaceutical Practice and Policy*. Pharmaceutical Press; 2011:245–260.
5. Tenney JB, White KL, Williamson JW. National medical ambulatory care survey: background and methodology United States-1967. *Vital Health Stat.* 1974;2(61):1–85.
6. National Center for Health Statistics (NCHS). *2016 National Ambulatory Medical Care Survey Micro-Data File Documentation*; 2016. Available at: ftp://ftp.cdc.gov/pub/Health_Statistics/NCHS/Dataset_Documentation/NAMCS/. Accessed 3 December 2020.
7. Hermer L, Kang K, Rui P, Rechtsteiner R. *National Ambulatory Medical Care Survey-Community Health Centers: 2014 State and National Summary Tables*. Hyattsville, MD: National Center for Health Statistics; 2019. Available at: https://www.cdc.gov/nchs/data/ahcd/namcs_ summary/2014_namcs_chc_web_tables.pdf. Accessed 3 December 2020.
8. McCaig LF, McLemore T. Plan and operation of the national hospital ambulatory medical survey. Series 1: programs and collection procedures. *Vital Health Stat.* 1994;1(34):1–78.
9. Schappert SM, Rechtsteiner EA. Ambulatory medical care utilization estimates for 2007. *Vital Health Stat.* 2011;13(169):1–38.
10. National Center for Health Statistics (NCHS). *National Hospital Ambulatory Medical Care Survey Micro-Data File Documentation*; 2017. Available at: ftp://ftp.cdc.gov/pub/Health_Statistics/NCHS/Dataset_Documentation/NHAMCS/. Accessed 3 December 2020.
11. Bryant E, Shimizu I. Sample design, sampling variance, and estimation procedures for the National Ambulatory Medical Care Survey. *Vital Health Stat.* 1988;2(108):1–39.
12. Ahn CS, Allen MM, Davis SA, Huang KE, Fleischer Jr AB, Feldman SR. The National Ambulatory Medical Care Survey: a resource for understanding the outpatient dermatology treatment. *J Dermatol Treat.* 2014;25(6):453–458.
13. Shi L, Lebrun LA, Tsai J, et al. Characteristics of ambulatory care patients and services: a comparison of community health centers and physicians' offices. *J Health Care Poor Underserved.* 2010;21(4):1169–1183.
14. Hing E, Hooker RS. *Community health centers: providers, patients, and content of care*. NCHS Data Brief, No. 65, Hyattsville, MD: National Center for Health Statistics; 2011.
15. Hing E, Hooker RS, Ashman JJ. Primary health care in community health centers and comparison with office-based practice. *J Community Health.* 2011;36(3):406–413.
16. Koch H, Campbell WH. The collection and processing of drug information: national ambulatory medical care survey. United States, 1980. *Vital Health Stat.* 1982;2(90):1–90.
17. Hing E, Gousen S, Shimizu I, Burt C. Guide to using masked design variables to estimate standard errors in public use files of the National Ambulatory Medical Care Survey and the National Hospital Ambulatory Medical Care Survey. *Inquiry.* 2003;40(4):401–415.
18. Korn EL, Graubard BI. *Analysis of Health Surveys*. New York: John Wiley; 1999.
19. Lee ES, Forthofer RN, Lorimor RJ. *Analyzing Complex Survey Data*. Newbury Park, CA: Sage Publications; 1989.
20. Research Triangle Institute. *SUDAAN 9.0*. Research Triangle Park, NC: Research Triangle Institute; 2005.
21. SAS Institute. *SAS 9.1.3 Procedures Guide Volume 4*. Cary, NC: SAS Institute; 2006.
22. StataCorp. *Stata Statistical Software: Release 10*. College Station, TX: StataCorp LP; 2007.
23. National Center for Health Statistics (NCHS). *Public Use Data File Documentation: 2000 National Ambulatory Medical Care Survey*. Hyattsville, MD: NCHS; 2002.
24. Parker JD, Talih M, Malec DJ, et al. National Center for Health statistics data presentation standards for proportions. National Center for Health Statistics. *Vital Health Stat.* 2017;2(175). https://www.cdc.gov/nchs/data/series/sr_02/sr02_175.pdf. Accessed 28 December 2018.
25. Earla JR, Paranjpe R, Kachru N, Hutton GJ, Aparasu RR. Use of disease modifying agents in patients with multiple sclerosis: analysis of ten years of national data. *Res Soc Adm Pharm.* 2020;16(12):1670–1676.
26. Rege S, Sura S, Aparasu RR. Atypical antipsychotic prescribing in elderly patients with depression. *Res Soc Adm Pharm.* 2018;14(7):645–652.
27. Aparasu R, Baer R, Aparasu A. Clinically important potential drug-drug interactions in outpatient settings. *Res Soc Adm Pharm.* 2007;3(4):426–437.

28. Mittal M, Harrison DL, Miller MJ, Brahm NC. National antidepressant prescribing in children and adolescents with mental health disorders after an FDA boxed warning. *Res Soc Adm Pharm.* 2014;10(5):781–790.

29. Crawford T, Segars LW, Rasu RS. Prescribing trends for management of congestive heart failure from 2002 to 2004. *Res Soc Adm Pharm.* 2013; 9(4):482–489.

30. Ambulatory and Hospital Care Statistics Branch/Division of Health Care Statistics/National Center for Health Statistics/Centers for Disease Control and Prevention. *List of Publications using Data from NAMCS and NHAMCS*; 2020. Available at: https://www.cdc.gov/nchs/data/ahcd/namcs_nhamcs_publication_list.pdf.

31. Lau DT, McCaig LF, Hing E. Toward a more complete picture of outpatient, office-based health care in the U.S. *Am J Prev Med.* 2016;51(3):403–409.

32. Najmabadi S, Honda TJ, Hooker RS. Collaborative practice trends in US physician office visits: an analysis of the National Ambulatory Medical Care Survey (NAMCS), 2007-2016. *BMJ Open.* 2020;10(6):e035414.

33. Lumpkin J. *National Ambulatory Medical Care Survey (NAMCS)*; September 2020. Available at: https://www.cdc.gov/nchs/data/bsc/bsc-pres-Lumpkin-NAMCS-September-18-2020-508.pdf. Accessed 27 April 2021.

34. Lumpkin J. *NAMCS Workgroup*; January 2021. Available at: https://www.cdc.gov/nchs/data/bsc/bsc-pres-Lumpkin-NAMCS-Jan-27-2021-508.pdf. Accessed 27 April 2021.

35. Mort JR, Aparasu RR. Prescribing potentially inappropriate psychotropic medications to the ambulatory elderly. *Arch Intern Med.* 2000;160 (18):2825–2831.

Chapter 37

Latent class and latent class regression

James B. Schreiber

School of Nursing, Duquesne University, Pittsburgh, PA, United States

Objectives

- Explain the purpose of latent class analysis (LCA).
- Explain the latent and observed variable differences between LCA, Latent Profile Analysis, Factor Analysis, and Item Response Theory.
- Describe the basic mathematical model and assumption.
- Discuss the issues surrounding sample size needs and fit indices.
- Interpret basic results from Latent Class and LC-Regression Models.

Introduction

Latent classes are unobserved, or latent, segments. Participants, or more generally, cases, within the same latent class are considered homogenous based on certain pieces of information. Latent Class Analysis (LCA) was developed as a way to characterize latent variables while analyzing dichotomous observed items.[1,2] LCA has expanded to encompass all types of data. In the literature, LCA is referred to in different ways: latent structure analysis,[2] mixture likelihood clustering,[3,4] model-based clustering,[5–7] mixture-model clustering,[8] Bayesian classification,[9] and latent class cluster analysis.[10]

LCA allows researchers to create or characterize a multidimensional discrete latent variable based on a cross-classification of two more observed categorical variables.[2] Because of the categorical nature of the latent classes, LCA is different from other latent approaches such as factor analysis and structural equation modeling. LCA provides the possibility to develop typologies for understanding and, if desired, can be used in predictive models. In addition to the ability to analyze relationships in categorical data, numeric and nonnumeric data can be utilized.

The factor loadings in traditional factor analysis (EFA or CFA) are regression coefficients where a loading of zero represents "no relation" between the observed variable and the latent factor. Values close to -1 and 1 indicate a strong relationship. Latent class analysis has item-response probabilities, which are conditional probabilities and can be thought of like factor loadings.

Latent profile analysis, which is a version of LCA, is used for the examination of discrete latent variables based on observed continuous data.[1] Item-response theory is generally used with categorical data and the desire to have a continuous latent variable, e.g., ability.[11] Graphically, all four of these models can look the same (Table 1). The difference lies in the observed and latent variables.

LCA

LCA is implemented with binary, ordered-categorical and Likert-scale, or nominal data. It is not used with purely ordinal (rank order) data. With binary or nominal data, LCA has a straightforward analysis. There is no technical barrier to analyzing models that combine categorical and continuous data, and some specialized programs allow this. It must be noted with the development of mixture modeling and software programs, there are fewer and fewer technical barriers to analyzing models with a combination of data types.

Contemporary Research Methods in Pharmacy and Health Services. https://doi.org/10.1016/B978-0-323-91888-6.00044-2

TABLE 1 Types of variables and latent analysis.

		Observed (manifest variable)	
		Continuous	**Categorical**
Latent predictor (exogenous variables)	Continuous	Common factor model (factor analysis)	Item response theory
	Categorical	Latent profile analysis	Latent class analysis

Mathematical model and independence assumption

Using Goodman's notation,[12] observed variables are indicated with capital letters and the categories for the variables are denoted with lower case letters (Eq. 1). In a study with binary observed variables, the options for category level would be 0 and 1. The latent variables are denoted with X with levels t, that range from 1 to T. LCA is a probabilistic model such that the conditional probability of a response vector $\mathbf{y}$ (denoted bold for the vector) for the sth case (or individual) is associated with the tth class is $P(\mathbf{y}_s|t)$. If you have four observed values and one latent class t, the model would be

$$P(\mathbf{y}_s|t) = \pi_{ijklt}^{\bar{A}\,\bar{B}\,\bar{C}\,\bar{D}\,X} = \pi_{it}^{\bar{A}X} * \pi_{jt}^{\bar{B}X} * \pi_{kt}^{\bar{C}X} * \pi_{lt}^{\bar{D}X} \tag{1}$$

Now, because researchers generally assume local independence, the response vector can be a weighted sum,

$$P(\mathbf{y}_s) = \sum_{t=1}^{T} \pi_t^X * \pi_{it}^{\bar{A}X} * \pi_{jt}^{\bar{B}X} * \pi_{kt}^{\bar{C}X} * \pi_{lt}^{\bar{D}X} \tag{2}$$

Data assumptions

There is one main assumption with LCA with respect to the observed variables. A better way to think about it is as response categories usage. During data cleaning phase, you want to make sure that all categories are used. For example, if you have a four category Likert[13] type scale, you should examine if each category was used, and if not, the decision to reduce the number of categories may need to be made. In some cases, that may mean dichotomizing the data.

Sample size

There is no currently set sample sizes, though this an active area of research. There is a rule of thumb of 500 or greater based on simulation studies.[14] A general range is 300 cases so that fit indices can be expected to function properly is commonly mentioned.[15–17] The confounding part of sample size determination is how clearly the classes are separated. In Fig. 1, there are clearly two classes that are easily separated. As the overlap of classes increases, the identification of the classes is more difficult, and larger sample sizes would be needed.

Additionally, larger samples are needed to so that there is sufficient information to estimate all model parameters and identify the "true" number of classes.[18] In essence, this is a sensitivity issue with classes that may be more difficult to identify.[19] Small sample sizes can also lead to the analysis not converging and improper or unstable solutions.

Estimation methods

Generally, software packages use maximum likelihood with the expectation-maximization procedure (Mplus, Latent Gold, PROC LCA in SAS, poLCA). The more important issue with estimation is LCA can have a local maxima problem.[20] This means that a local maximum was converged to during the iterations instead of a global maximum based on the start values. Thus, it is recommended to estimate the model with different sets of starting values. The model should converge to the same highest log-likelihood value, and you can use as justification that this is the maximum likelihood solution. As the number of classes increases, this problem increases. In many of the software packages, you can specify the number of sets of starting values. Finally, Bayesian estimation methods for LCA are becoming popular, such as the Bayesian methods available in Latent Gold software system.[21–24]

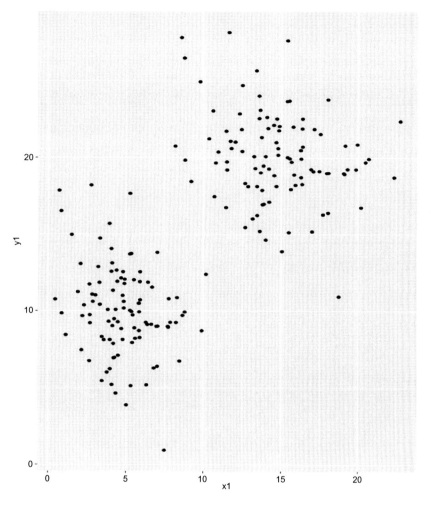

FIG. 1 Two simulated classes.

Fit indices

Goodness of fit is examined with some form of a χ^2 test. Common ones are the Pearson Statistic, χ^2, the likelihood ratio, and G^2. Depending on the software, there are BIC, AIC, classification error percentage, or bivariate residuals. The key is to consult the technical manual of the software and search for any current simulations related to fit indices and LCA. For example, recent simulation work has indicated that AIC and CAIC are not good indicators for choosing the correct number of classes.[25] When cell frequencies are small, χ^2 and G^2 do not follow the appropriate χ^2 distribution.[26]

Example LCA analysis

Sample

These data come from a larger set of studies on wellness.[27] The larger set of studies include pre- and postwellness surveys, cognitive surveys, demographic data, and other variables such as grade point average. For this example in this data set, there are 518 participants that provided basic demographics are in Table 2. For this example, I have used one item from six of the wellness domains.

First analysis

Given the nature of this article, there is no theoretically expected number of clusters, this is exploratory and is common with LCA. Therefore, an initial run of 1 to 6 clusters will be analyzed, with six observed variables of interest. Each variable is on a 4 point Likert-type scale ranging from "Does not describe me at all" to "Absolutely Describes me." The variables are

TABLE 2 Demographic breakdown.

Variable		Percentage
Student athlete	Yes	17.6
	No	82.4
Sex	Female	66.6
	Male	33.4
First generation student	Yes	17.9
	No	82.1

TABLE 3 Evaluation evidence for different models.

		LL	BIC (LL)	Npar	L^2	df	P-value	Class. Err.
Model 1	1-Cluster	−3701.38	7515.36	18	1494.029	503	6.50E−99	0
Model 2	2-Cluster	−3640.64	7437.679	25	1372.558	496	2.80E−83	0.1283
Model 3	3-Cluster	−3629.28	7458.736	32	1349.824	489	1.10E−81	0.1924
Model 4	4-Cluster	−3616.75	7477.483	39	1324.781	482	9.60E−80	0.2445
Model 5	5-Cluster	−3603.50	7494.765	46	1298.274	475	1.30E−77	0.2589
Model 6	6-Cluster	−3594.26	7520.083	53	1279.801	468	1.30E−76	0.2823

related to Physical Wellness-Nutrition, Physical Wellness-Exercise, Mental Wellness, Financial Wellness, Emotional Wellness, and Occupational Wellness. Each of the four categories was used for each item. Latent Gold (v. 5.1.0.19281)[28] will be used for this example. In , R-Studio code is provided for the poLCA package for running LCA models along with an explanation guide of the code based on the poLCA code book.[29]

From the models, there are indicators which can be examined to begin to determine the number of classes (Table 3). In general, the initial analysis of the possible models focuses first on three evaluative indicators: LL, P-value, and BIC. LL is Log Likelihood, the logarithm of the likelihood ratio, a test that compares the fit of two models by examining how much more likely the data are predicted by one model compared to the other. The Log Likelihood can be used to compute a P-value. BIC is the Bayes Information Criterion, which is a statistic created to aid model selection but penalizes the number of factors in a model. There are other indicators available such as AIC (Akaike Information Criterion) and CAIC, but for explanation purposes, the displayed indicators work well.

When examining these statistics, you are balancing different pieces of information. The two-cluster model appears to have the best fit based on the BIC value, and it has fewer parameters (Npar) estimated in comparison, so more parsimonious. But, the log-likelihood value for the six-class model is the lowest. Thus, other pieces of information may be useful. The P-values for all of the models do not indicate good fits for any of the models. There are other pieces of information, discussed later, that could also be used such as a residual analysis and the pseudo R^2 values for each model.

A boot-strap comparison within LatentGold can be run to statistically test the different cluster models. The difference analysis, based on the log-likelihood, indicates the three class model might be better than that two. For this example, I will stick with the two because the BIC value is lower and a few of the other values, such as pseudo R^2 values, are better (i.e., higher), and classification error (classerr) is lower. Next, a deeper examination of the chosen model is completed.

Examination of chosen model

There are multiple pieces of information to examine for a specific model. For any model, error examination is important, and in LCA, an examination of bivariate residuals (BVR) is a first step. The bivariate residual is similar to a Pearson

χ^2 value divided by the degrees of freedom. The χ^2 calculation is computed from the expected counts in the traditional two-way tables from the estimated model.[28] For 1 degree of freedom, residual values greater than 3.84 would reach the 0.05 station. At the value of 3.84, the model is not explaining the relationship between the variables well. From a modeling perspective, a value around 2.00 might be an indicator that the model (number of clusters chosen) is not explaining the relationship between the two variables well. If the relationship was above 2, the relationship can be set as a direct effect, "fixed," and the residual will be zero or close to zero in the reanalysis.

There are two relationships with BVRs above 2 and will not be fixed for the example. The three-cluster model did not greatly change these BVR values.

The residuals for each individual case can also be examined. In the analysis, there are a few individual cases where the model does not explain the individual case data well. Cook's D was used to evaluate individual case residuals. There is no perfect consensus on the cut-off value. There are the general rules of values above 1 or above 0.50. There is also the rule based on 4 times the number of estimated parameters (25) divided by the number of cases (518); in this case 0.19. No cases were above 0.50, but 10 cases surpassed the cut of value of 0.19 and were removed; this did not change the results. The key is to examine the information provided in the analysis package you use to deeply dive into the results.

Parameter estimate evaluation

Once the residuals are examined, and any issues resolved, the final model can be examined with the results for each observed variable. Table 4 provides the results from this example data. The Wald values are large overall, but the R^2 values vary quite a bit.

In addition, the Profile of the Classes related to the variables can be examined. The first level examination is the class size. Class 1 has 51% of the sample in it and Class 2 has 49% (Table 5). For Class 1 cases, 36% of them chose category 4 (Absolutely Describes me) and 4% chose category 1 (Does Not Describe Me at all). For the profile examination, you are within each class and examining the response patterns. The percentages will add up to 100, with a bit of rounding error to make the table easier to read. For Emotional Wellness that would be $4+13+46+36$. The largest differences, or separations, between the classes appear to be for the items related to exercise and nutrition. Because of this, I would name the classes higher and lower physical wellness. I could also simply separate by the fact that Class 1 responses are higher than Class 2 and name them Higher Wellness and Lower Wellness (Fig. 2).

The second level examination of the profile is with each variable and the categories or values in each variable (Table 6). For example, in Class 1, individuals are likely to choose category 4 (Absolutely Describes me), and Class 2 individuals are not likely to choose category 4; 97% and 3%. Note, for this examination you are looking across classes for one item and one response category. For example, for Emotional Wellness, of those who chose category 1, 23% are in Class 1 and 77% are in Class 2. These sum up to one, and again, some rounding error in using two digits in the chart.

There are other indicators that can be examined for model adequacy. There is a Standard R^2 (0.65) and an Entropy R^2 (0.60), and both of these are considered pseudo R^2 values. The closer to 1, the more accurate the classification. Thus, for this example, the values are good. Finally, there is the classification error, which estimated the proportion of cases misclassified. The two class model has 12.8% misclassified, and the other models had higher misclassification, 14% to 28%.

There are a number of indicators to be used when deciding how well the data fits the model. There is also a balance issue of not trying to just statistically get the best fitting model; it must also make sense. As a reminder with any advanced

TABLE 4 Cluster results by variable.

Observed variable	Cluster 1	Cluster 2	Wald	P-value	R^2
Emotional	0.25	−0.25	14.25	<0.001	0.04
Financial	0.28	−0.28	16.68	<0.001	0.05
Mental	0.29	−0.29	12.57	<0.001	0.04
Occupational	0.31	0.31	14.08	<0.001	0.05
Exercise	0.42	−0.42	39.08	<0.001	0.15
Nutrition	1.75	−1.75	8.43	0.004	0.53

TABLE 5 Profiles of classes.

	Class 1	Class 2	Overall
Cluster size	0.51	0.49	
Indicators			
Emotional			
1	0.04	0.12	0.08
2	0.13	0.21	0.17
3	0.46	0.45	0.46
4	0.36	0.22	0.29
Mean	3.14	2.77	2.96
Fiscal			
1	0.05	0.13	0.09
2	0.25	0.37	0.31
3	0.46	0.39	0.43
4	0.24	0.11	0.17
Mean	2.88	2.48	2.69
Mental			
1	0.01	0.03	0.02
2	0.12	0.23	0.17
3	0.52	0.54	0.53
4	0.35	0.21	0.28
Mean	3.22	2.93	3.07
Occupational			
1	0.01	0.03	0.02
2	0.06	0.14	0.10
3	0.32	0.41	0.36
4	0.62	0.42	0.52
Mean	3.55	3.22	3.39
Exercise			
1	0.05	0.23	0.14
2	0.18	0.35	0.26
3	0.31	0.26	0.29
4	0.46	0.16	0.31
Mean	3.17	2.36	2.77
Nutrition			
1	0.00	0.09	0.04
2	0.01	0.47	0.24
3	0.34	0.41	0.38
4	0.64	0.02	0.34
Mean	3.63	2.37	3.01

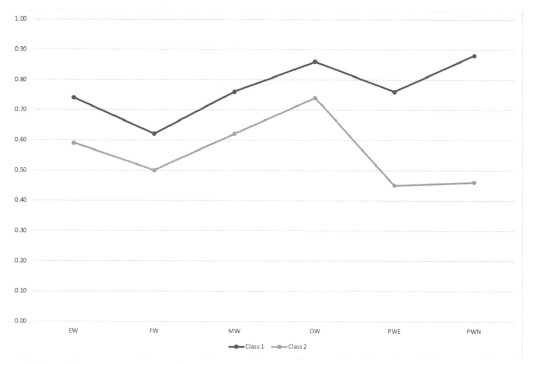

FIG. 2   Graphic display of classes by item probabilities.

technique, the results may represent the real world or they may not.[30] It is important not to reify our models.[30] Over time, your model or parts of your model will be shown to be incorrect, and we need to be humble in the discussion of our model.

Basic reporting guidelines

Below is a listing of basic reporting guidelines. These will allow readers to evaluate the results of the model you present and your process.

1. Show evaluative information for all models tested, all of it
   a. Covariance matrix (Table 7).
   b. Profiles.
   c. Percentages in each class.
   d. Evaluative criteria used for choosing a specific model.
   e. Residual analysis.
2. Explain reasoning choices for choosing a specific model.
3. Explain choices related to "fixing" a bivariate residual relationship to zero.
4. Provide software used and the version number. Software changes and you must let your reader know.
5. Submit the traditional descriptive and frequency data along with correlation or variance/covariance matrix with the review at a minimum. The matrix may not be published due to page space concerns, but you should provide it.
6. If in doubt, put the information into the manuscript or a table if you are worried about word space. As a former journal editor, there is little more frustrating than a lack of analytical information when reviewing a manuscript.
7. Many read the research from a theoretical point of view for their domain. Read the analysis literature with the same fervor. LCA and those working on it continue to improve the technique, and it is important to be current.

LC-regression

There are important questions in social pharmacy research where there is a desire to understand differences between groups, such a compliant and noncompliant, and want to use classes to predict or explain those differences. LC-regression is one technique to use.

TABLE 6 Response probabilities across classes.

	Class 1	Class 2
Overall	0.51	0.49
Indicators		
Emotional		
1	0.23	0.77
2	0.43	0.57
3	0.51	0.49
4	0.63	0.37
Fiscal		
1	0.32	0.68
2	0.38	0.62
3	0.58	0.42
4	0.66	0.34
Mental		
1	0.35	0.65
2	0.33	0.67
3	0.51	0.49
4	0.64	0.36
Occupational		
1	0.19	0.81
2	0.29	0.71
3	0.46	0.54
4	0.60	0.40
Exercise		
1	0.18	0.82
2	0.37	0.63
3	0.52	0.48
4	0.76	0.24
Nutrition		
1	0.00	1.00
2	0.03	0.97
3	0.46	0.54
4	0.97	0.03

If examining by classes is the starting point, but the desire to predict an outcome based on the classes, then running a latent class regression analysis technique is needed. One could create the classes and save them by individual and then use the class designation in a regression or logistic regression or run the regression model all at once. This example utilizes the same data and variables, with one switch, First Generation Designation is added as an outcome variable.

TABLE 7 Covariance matrix of observed items.

Variable	Emotional	Financial	Mental	Occupational	Exercise	Nutrition
Emotional	0.777	0.014	0.043	0.023	0.045	0.151
Financial	0.014	0.747	0.06	0.147	0.059	0.145
Mental	0.043	0.06	0.519	0.063	0.052	0.105
Occupational	0.023	0.147	0.063	0.542	0.043	0.097
Exercise	0.045	0.059	0.052	0.043	1.084	0.307
Nutrition	0.151	0.145	0.105	0.097	0.307	0.756

TABLE 8 Regression model evaluation evidence.

	LL	BIC (LL)	Npar	L^2	df	P-value	Class. Err	R^2
2-Class regression	−223.536	540.6175	15	285.5793	331	0.97	0.0215	0.9891
3-Class regression	−219.726	582.889	23	277.9599	323	0.97	0.2056	0.9848
4-Class regression	−210.734	614.7956	31	259.9755	315	0.99	0.3156	0.9857
5-Class regression	−210.623	664.4653	39	259.7543	307	0.98	0.4764	0.9884

The evaluation of the models begins in a similar pattern with examining the fit data for several models. Table 8 provides the evaluation evidence for LC-Regression models-2 to 5 classes-with First Generation Student (Yes/No) as the outcome.

Looking at the fit data, the 2 Class model, similar to previous analysis, looks like the best option. It has lowest BIC, fewer parameters estimated, low classification error, and highest R^2 value.

The model has several components that can be examined and still tested for fit and predictive validity. The first is simply the proportion of cases in each Class (Table 9).

As is indicated, Class 1 has the largest proportion of cases with 81%. In Class 1, 99% are not first generation college students. Next, the R^2 values for each Class and the model overall are excellent (Table 10). The R^2 value for Class 2 indicates the model is not working as well.

In Table 11, the beta parameters are a measure of the influence on first generation categorization. Interestingly, both classes look like they have strong predictors based on the values, but the Wald statistics are not very large. Mental Wellness has a Wald value of 5.43 ($P = 0.07$) which indicates this may be a good predictor. The second Wald (=) value, 5.35 ($P = 0.02$), indicates that the differences across these beta effects may be important and is not class independent. If, Mental Wellness would have only had a high Wald Value for the variable, then it could have been considered class independent. Overall, the variables are not strong predictors of First Generation status.

Summary

LCA and the advancements within LCA have provided a powerful alternative to previously used statistical techniques such as K-means for clustering. LCA is also very flexible as a latent analysis technique. Related, there is factor mixture modeling (FMM) which integrates latent class analysis with the common factor model. The strength of FMM is the hybridization of the two and the ability to keep the advantages of LCA and FA along with unique aspects of their combination (see Schreiber, this volume Chapter 42). The ability to use a wide variety of data with different variances along with regression and discrete factor analysis options makes latent class analysis an appealing option for many researchers. The models presented here are the very basic models, and much more complex models can be analyzed. Additionally, in many of the packages (e.g., MPlus, Latent Gold, polCA), simulated data can easily be created and examined in comparison to the model you are examining. As with the changes in ease of use and understanding of the analysis technique, I expect many more LC analyses to be published in the near future.

TABLE 9 Class proportion and first generation.

	Class 1	Class 2	Overall
Class size	0.81	0.19	
Dependent			
First generation			
Yes	0.01	0.89	0.18
No	0.99	0.11	0.82
Mean	1.99	1.11	1.82

TABLE 10 R^2 values by class.

	Class 1	Class 2	Overall
R^2	0.98	0.73	0.98

TABLE 11 Parameter estimates.

	Class 1	Class 2	Wald	P-value	Wald (=)	P-value	Mean	Std. dev.
First gen.								
Intercept								
1	−1.30	8.55	2.46	0.29	1.07	0.30	0.56	3.85
2	1.30	−8.55					−0.56	3.85
Predictors								
Emotional	1.99	2.72	3.75	0.15	0.09	0.76	2.12	0.29
Financial	−8.55	2.88	3.36	0.19	3.35	0.07	−6.40	4.47
Mental	5.29	−4.83	5.43	0.07	5.35	0.02	3.38	3.96
Occupational	3.65	3.43	3.33	0.19	0.00	0.96	3.60	0.09
Exercise	1.77	1.20	1.56	0.46	0.06	0.81	1.66	0.22
Nutrition	0.84	−1.85	2.03	0.36	1.65	0.20	0.33	1.05

Questions for further discussion

1. Do you think your latent construct is continuous or categorical?
2. How much of our thoughts on the continuity of our latent constructs is driven by the data type that was collected?
3. Should simulations be run as a comparison for all LC modeling? This idea is similar to a parallel analysis in exploratory factor analysis.
4. What should be done if your sample sizes will never be very large ($n > 200$) due to the population you are interested in researching?
5. Should I present two models that are both plausible (make sense theoretically or can be justified theoretically) but are mixed on which fits better?

Application exercise/scenario

R-Studio Code: This can be cut and pasted and then adjusted to your variables
  Code Book

#	Tells R that this is a comment statement and not to process
f <− cbind(Y1,Y2,Y3)∼1	Codes for the variables to be included in analysis. If you variables start at zero for numbers, add 1 to end of variable, e.g., Y1 + 1
∼1	Instructs poLCA to estimate the basic latent class model
nclass	The number of latent classes to assume in the model
maxiter	The maximum number of iterations through which the estimation algorithm will cycle
graphs	Logical, for whether poLCA should graphically display the parameter estimates at the completion of the estimation algorithm. The default is FALSE. A tolerance value for judging when convergence has been reached
tol	Logical, for how poLCA handles cases with missing values on the manifest variables. If TRUE, those cases are removed (listwise deleted) before estimating the model. If FALSE, cases with missing values are retained. The default is TRUE
Probs.start	A list of matrices of class-conditional response probabilities to be used as the starting values for the EM estimation algorithm. Each matrix in the list corresponds to one manifest variable, with one row for each latent class, and one column for each possible outcome. The default is NULL, meaning that starting values are generated randomly. Note that if nrep >1, then any user-specified probs.start values are only used in the first of the nrep attempts
nrep	Number of times to estimate the model, using different values of probs.start. The default is one. Setting nrep >1 initiates the search for the global maximum of the log-likelihood function. Setting nrep to 1 will allow the search for just the local maximum. poLCA returns only the parameter estimates corresponding to the model producing the greatest log-likelihood
verbose	Tells poLCA output to the screen the results of the model. If FALSE, no output is produced. The default is TRUE
calc.se	Tells poLCA to calculate the standard errors of the estimated class-conditional response probabilities and mixing proportions. The default is TRUE; can only be set to FALSE if estimating a basic model with no concomitant variables specified in formula

The variables/data set from this example, from poLCA[31] are in bold

```
install.packages("poLCA")
Library(poLCA)
f <- cbind(PWE_1, MW_1, EW_1, OW_1, FW_1, PWN_1)∼1
poLCA(f, data=JUTOF126172016, nclass=2, maxiter=5000, graphs=TRUE, tol=1e-10,
  na.rm=TRUE, probs.start=NULL, nrep=110, verbose=TRUE, calc.se=TRUE)
Generic Code
f <- cbind(Var1, Var2, Var3 ........,)∼1
poLCA(f, data=YOUR DATA NAME HERE,
  nclass=?, #fill in the number of classes you want
  maxiter=?, #fill in the number iterations you want
  graphs=TRUE,
  tol=1e-10,
  na.rm=TRUE, #if you do not have missing data, write FALSE
  probs.start=NULL,
  nrep=?, #fill in the number of times to estimate the model
  verbose=TRUE,
  calc.se=TRUE)
to add in First Generation, it is simply a change from ∼1 to ∼FIRSTGEN-the variable name.
```

There are also code that can be found in places, such as github, for BVRs, entropy, and R^2.

BVR: https://gist.github.com/daob/883fbffdff6762c3bb90b3d8d3d0ae6e.

Entropy: https://rdrr.io/cran/poLCA/man/poLCA.entropy.html.

R^2: https://maksimrudnev.com/2016/12/28/latent-class-analysis-in-r/.

And, there are just other ways to code and graph poLCA.

https://statistics.ohlsen-web.de/latent-class-analysis-polca/.

References

1. Lazarsfeld P, Henry N. *Latent Structure Analysis.* Boston: Houghton Mifflin; 1968.
2. McCutcheon A. *Latent Class Analysis. Quantitative Applications in the Social Sciences Series.* Newbury Park, London, and New Delhi: Sage Publications; 1987. Number 07e064.
3. McLachlan G, Basford K. *Mixture Models: Inference and Application to Clustering.* New York: Marcel Dekker; 1988.
4. Everitt B. *Cluster Analysis.* London: Edward Arnold; 1993.
5. Banfield J, Raftery A. Model-based Gaussian and non-Gaussian clustering. *Biometrics.* 1993;49:803–821.
6. Bensmail H, Celeux G, Raftery A, Robert C. Inference in model based clustering. *Stat Comput.* 1997;7:1–10.
7. Fraley C, Raftery A. *MCLUST: software for model-based cluster and discriminant analysis.* Department of Statistics, University of Washington; 1998. Technical report no. 342.
8. 8. McLachlan G, Peel D, Basford K, Adams P. The EMMIX software for the fitting of mixtures of normal and t-components. *J Stat Softw.* 1999;4(2):1–15.
9. Cheeseman P, Stutz J. Bayesian classification (autoclass): theory and results. In: Fayyad U, Piatesky-Shapiro G, Smyth Uthurusamy P, eds. *Advances in Knowledge Discovery and Data Mining.* AAAI Press; 1995:153–180.
10. Magidson J, Vermunt J. Latent class models for clustering: a comparison with K-means. *Can J Market Res.* 2002;20:37–44.
11. De Ayala RJ. *The Theory and Practice of Item Response Theory.* Guilford; 2009.
12. Goodman LA. Exploratory latent structure analysis using both identifiable and unidentifiable models. *Biometrika.* 1974;61(2):215–231.
13. Likert R. A technique for the measurement of attitudes. *Arch Psychol.* 1932;22(140):1–55.
14. Finch WH, Bronk KC. Conducting confirmatory latent class analysis using Mplus. *Struct Eq Model.* 2011;18(1):132–151.
15. Morgan GB. Mixed mode latent class analysis: an examination of fit index performance for classification. *Struc Eq Model.* 2015;22(1):76–86. https://doi.org/10.1080/10705511.2014.935751.
16. Morovati D. *The Intersection of Sample Size, Number of Indicators, and Class Enumeration in LCA: A Monte Carlo Study* [Unpublished Dissertation]. Santa Barbara, CA: University of California, Santa Barbara; 2014.
17. Tein J-Y, Coxe S, Cham H. Statistical power to detect the correct number of classes in latent profile analysis. *Struct Eq Model.* 2013;20(4):640–657.
18. Lubke GH, Luningham J. Fitting latent variable mixture models. *Behav Res Ther.* 2017;98:91–102. https://doi.org/10.1016/j.brat.2017.04.003.
19. Masyn KE. Latent class analysis and finite mixture modeling. In: Little TD, ed. *The Oxford Handbook of Quantitative Methods.* New York, NY: Oxford University Press; 2013:551–611. Statistical Analysis; vol. 2.
20. Vermunt JK, Magidson J. Latent class analysis. In: *The Sage Encyclopedia of Social Sciences Research Methods.* vol. 2. Sage; 2004:549–553.
21. Vermunt J, Magidson J. *Technical Guide for Latent GOLD 5.0: Basic, Advanced, and Syntax.* Belmont, MA: Statistical Innovations; 2013.
22. Depaoli S. Mixture class recovery in GMM under varying degrees of class separation: frequentist versus Bayesian estimation. *Psychol Methods.* 2013;18(2):186–219. https://doi.org/10.1037/a0031609.
23. Depaoli S, Yang Y, Felt J. Using Bayesian statistics to model uncertainty in mixture models: a sensitivity analysis of priors. *Struct Eq Model.* 2017;24(2):198–215. https://doi.org/10.1080/10705511.2016.1250640.
24. Li Y, Lord-Bessen J, Shiyko M, Loeb R. Bayesian latent class analysis tutorial. *Multivar Behav Res.* 2018;53(3):430–451. https://doi.org/10.1080/00273171.2018.1428892.
25. Nylund K, Asparouhov T, Muthen B. Deciding on the number of classes in latent class analysis and growth mixture modeling: a Monte Carlo simulation study. *Struct Eq Model.* 2007;14(4):535–569.
26. Read TRC, Cressie NAC. *Goodness-of-Fit Statistics for Discrete Multivariate Data.* Springer-Verlag; 1988.
27. Mayol MH, Scott BM, Schreiber JB. Validation and use of the multidimensional wellness inventory in collegiate student-athletes and first-generation students. *Am J Health Educ.* 2017;48(5):338–350.
28. Vermunt J, Magidson J. *Users Guide for Latent GOLD 5.0: Basic, Advanced, and Syntax.* Belmont, MA: Statistical Innovations; 2013.
29. *R-Package poLCA*; 2016. Retrieved at: https://CRAN.R-project.org/package1/4poLCA.
30. Kline R. *Principles and Practice of Structural Equation Modeling.* Guilford Publications; 2015.
31. Linzer DA, Lewis JB. poLCA: an R package for polytomous variable latent class analysis. *J Stat Softw.* 2011;42(10):1–29.

Chapter 38

Guidelines and standards in medication adherence research

Charlotte L. Bekker[a], Parisa Aslani[b], and Timothy F. Chen[b]
[a]Department of Pharmacy, Radboud University Medical Center, Research Institute for Health Sciences, Nijmegen, The Netherlands, [b]The University of Sydney School of Pharmacy, Faculty of Medicine and Health, The University of Sydney, Sydney, NSW, Australia

Objectives

- Define medication adherence including the various stages of medication taking behavior being evaluated in research studies.
- Describe the strengths and limitations of specific medication adherence guidelines, and their application to research study design.
- Describe the factors to consider when measuring medication adherence.

There are multiple definitions of medication adherence, such as "the process by which patients take their medications as prescribed,"[1] or more broadly, "the extent to which a person's behaviour—taking medication, following a diet, and/or executing lifestyle changes, corresponds with agreed recommendations from a healthcare provider."[2] Optimal adherence to medication regimens is essential in order to maximize therapy effectiveness and disease management. It is widely recognized that many patients do not fully adhere to their prescribed medication. Suboptimal average adherence rates of about 50% have been reported for long-term medical conditions in developed countries.[2] Effects of nonadherence are substantial, both clinically, including poorer health outcomes due to increased morbidity and mortality,[3] and economically, with higher healthcare utilization and increased costs.[4]

Medication adherence has been extensively studied over the past few decades. The evidence for improved adherence and clinical outcomes is variable,[5,6] possibly because of inappropriate research study designs; inappropriate or incorrect choice of adherence measures used for the specific adherence behavior being studied; wrong timing of the adherence measures, that is, not capturing medication taking at the right moment; and interventions not targeted or tailored to the medication taking behavior and patients' specific nonadherence issues. The poor quality of medication adherence research may negatively impact decision making on the efficacy of medications and also on the efficacy of interventions aimed at improving medication adherence. Furthermore, various terms have been used to define and report on medication taking behavior, including adherence, compliance and persistence.[7] Heterogeneity in the terminology used makes it unclear what kind of medication taking behavior is being studied and can lead to incorrect measurements, misunderstandings and false conclusions. In addition, research has shown that there is inconsistent reporting of study outcomes in medication adherence research (e.g., adherence, health outcomes, determinants of adherence).[8,9] Together, these variations and inconsistencies make comparison of study results difficult and hamper translation of research findings into routine clinical practice.

When measuring and reporting medication adherence, it is crucial to report certain key elements as these will provide a better understanding of the adherence behavior which was measured and how it was done. Standardized reporting enables readers to judge the methodological rigor of adherence measurements, correctly interpret research findings and their relevance for clinical practice, and compare between studies. With appropriate study designs and precise reporting, there will be greater confidence in the study findings, especially to inform policy and shape future practice. The combined application of existing medication adherence guidelines will likely improve the conceptualization and reporting of medication adherence research. These should be used alongside guidelines for specific research designs, such as CONSORT for randomized clinical trials,[10] STROBE for observational studies,[11] and PRISMA for systematic reviews.[12]

When reporting on adherence research, sufficient information should be provided to allow readers to judge the quality and credibility of the studies. To improve adherence measurements and enhance standardized and comprehensive reporting of study methods and results, several guidelines have been developed.[1,13–16] These guidelines provide structured guidance on reporting of relevant information with checklists recommending which items should be addressed. To guide researchers and clinicians on accurate operationalization and reporting of patients' medication taking behavior, an understanding of how to use adherence specific guidelines is needed. This chapter reviews the available guidelines that have been explicitly designed for use in medication adherence research and gives directions for improving the quality of research in medication adherence.

Medication adherence guidelines

Table 1 provides an overview of the key components of the guidelines discussed.

Ascertaining barriers to compliance taxonomy

As various definitions have been used to describe medication taking behavior, a conceptual taxonomy was proposed within the Ascertaining Barriers to Compliance project in 2012 to promote consistency in medication adherence studies (ABC taxonomy).[1] The taxonomy originated from a systematic literature review on terminology used to describe medication taking behavior and was further refined during multiple discussions with international experts in the field of medication adherence. The taxonomy defines medication adherence as a longitudinal process consisting of three consecutive phases: initiation, implementation, and discontinuation of therapy.

Initiation stands for the actual start of a prescribed medication regimen. This phase is defined as the time from prescription until the first medication intake, with nonadherence typically described as patients not starting their prescribed medication.[1] A pooled evaluation of prescription and dispensing data showed that nonadherence rates, defined as patients having a prescription which is not followed by dispensing, as 17% among six common chronic diseases (adherence measure was not specified).[17] Initiation is followed by *implementation* of the medication regimen. During this phase, nonadherence can be identified as the actual medication intake not corresponding to the prescribed medication regimen.[1] Implementation has many different nonadherence behaviors, such as missing doses or taking doses at the wrong time. The implementation phase is the phase of medication taking behavior which has been studied most extensively.[8,18] Last, the adherence process ends with *discontinuation*, when patients stop their treatment. Here, nonadherence is defined as early discontinuation of the prescribed regimen, frequently after an unacceptable gap in which patients have no medication intake.[1] Different discontinuation rates have been reported for different medical conditions. For example, using a pharmacy database, discontinuation of treatment was observed among 22% of women commencing hormonal therapy[19]; and using a general

TABLE 1 Main components of medication adherence reporting guidelines and frameworks.

First author, year, guideline	Study design	Focus	Content	When to use
Vrijens, 2012,[1] ABC taxonomy	Any study design	Guidance on conceptual definition of medication taking behavior	Proposed taxonomy of the process of adherence to medication	During study design and reporting
Dima, 2020,[13] TEOS	Any study design	Guidance on operationalization of medication adherence measurements	Four-component framework	During study design and reporting
De Geest, 2018,[14] EMERGE	Any study design	Guidance on items which should be specified clearly during reporting of research	Checklist for reporting with 4 minimal reporting criteria and 17 items for more detailed information	During study design and reporting
Peterson, 2007,[15] ISPOR	Retrospective design	Guidance on items which should be considered during study design and evaluation	Checklist for reporting and tool to assess quality of studies	During study design and reporting or study undergoing peer review
Gwadry-Sridhar, 2009,[16] ISPOR	Prospective design	Guidance on items which should be considered during study design and evaluation	Checklist for reporting and tool to assess quality of studies	During study design and reporting or study undergoing peer review

practitioner database discontinuation was reported in 50% of patients initiating antihypertensive medications.[20] Logically, the chosen gap length impacts on the number of patients that will be identified as nonadherent. Persistence stands for the time the patient remains on the treatment; thus, it is the time between initiation and discontinuation of therapy.

The taxonomy is well-accepted and used in many adherence studies, often for its conceptual definition,[21–23] to define the adherence phase under investigation,[24,25] and explain how the studied adherence phase is measured.[26] With the original version published in English, it has now been translated into French and German.[27] When conducting adherence research, the taxonomy can be used during study development to define the phase that is under investigation. Researchers should clearly report which phase is being studied and how adherence is conceptualized, as this allows for a better understanding and standardized reporting of medication taking behavior that is evaluated. For instance, it allows for comparison of different measures used at different phases.[18,28] In addition, researchers should recruit participants that are at a similar phase of adherence, unless their research aims to investigate adherence at different phases.

Timelines, events, objectives, sources framework

The Timelines, Events, Objectives, Sources (TEOS) framework, published in 2020, guides decision making in medication adherence measurements selection.[13] TEOS was developed by a working group that provided practical recommendations for operational definitions of medication adherence consistent with the ABC taxonomy. The framework consists of four components which, when carefully considered, enable investigators to apply the three adherence phases to their study and to select the most appropriate adherence measure for their specific population under investigation. Following these components allows for transparent reporting of decisions. The four components defining the operationalization of adherence measurements are Timelines, Events, Objectives, and Sources.

Timelines can guide potential variation between recommended and actual dosing practices of patients. These can vary greatly between individuals as they depend on prescribing, dispensing, recommended dosing and actual usage practices. To accurately measure adherence, one should therefore understand how these practices occur within the sample being studied and map timelines for each individual's medication history. *Events* refers to various key events that patients can experience during their treatment, such as discontinuation, reinitiation, or dose adjustments. Investigators should mark these events according to the three adherence phases (initiation, implementation, discontinuation) and the most appropriate adherence measures. Moreover, the timing of events is essential to define the observation period and can vary between individuals. Research *objectives* and the adherence-related variables under investigation should be compared with the identified timelines and events. Lastly, one needs to select the most appropriate *data sources* after considering their strengths and weaknesses. A series of items based on the TEOS questions can be used to address the four components (Table 2).[13]

Whereas the ABC taxonomy conceptualizes medication adherence, TEOS provides guidance on the operationalization of medication adherence measurements. Since TEOS is relatively new, no published studies have been found to have referred to this framework.

Emerge

The European Society for Patient Adherence, COMpliance, and Persistence (ESPACOMP) Medication Adherence Reporting Guideline (EMERGE) can be used to guide adequate reporting of adherence data and thereby appropriate interpretation of research findings, data transferability, and translation to practice.[14] The guideline was developed in 2018 from a 7-expert steering group which discussed results of a literature review of medication adherence and reporting guidelines for health research. This was followed by Delphi surveys with 26 experts who scored the reporting items derived from the literature review on clarity and relevance (consensus process), and approval of the final version occurred during a vote with ESPACOMP members. The guideline follows the ABC adherence taxonomy with its three distinct phases.[1]

EMERGE consists of 21 items, including a minimal reporting criteria set with four items: (1) stating the medication adherence phase that is being studied (initiation, implementation, discontinuation), (2) precisely defining each phase that is under investigation, (3) describing adherence measures used for each investigated phase, including their psychometric properties (validity, reliability, and potential bias), and (4) reporting relevant results of the analysis. Next to these minimal reporting criteria, there are 17 optional items for more detailed information on medication adherence research which relate to the specific parts of a scientific paper (abstract, introduction, study objectives, methods, results, discussion).

It is important that researchers are guided by EMERGE when reporting on adherence research to improve consistency in reporting. Since its introduction, EMERGE has been cited in numerous studies to improve quality of reporting.[29–35] Whereas some studies provide an overview of items that are reported, other studies do not and make it less clear how the guideline was used. The extent to which the guideline has improved overall reporting of studies on medication adherence has not yet been investigated.

TABLE 2 Items which can be used to address each TEOS component, adapted from Dima et al.[13]

Timelines

Prescribing events	– Date of issue of initial prescription
	– Prescription validity
	– Date of issue of refill prescription
Recommended dosing events	– Expected start of medication dosing after prescription has been dispensed
	– Dosing information (e.g., interval)
	– Other factors impacting dosing (e.g., food intake)
Dispensing events	– Information on medication supply (e.g., quantity, number of days of supply)
	– Expected refill frequency
	– Automatic dispensing when refill due
Actual dosing events	– Administration route
	– Changes to medication intake (e.g., splitting tablets)
	– Adherence to additional instructions (e.g., take with food)

Events

General questions	– Observation period when adherence is measured
	– Adherence data collection period
First recommended dosing event	– Minimum acceptable duration to therapy initiation
First actual dosing event	– Maximum acceptable duration to therapy initiation, after which the behavior is defined as nonadherence
Last actual dosing event	– Differentiate between poor implementation and nonpersistence
	– Minimum acceptable duration when no dosing occurs, after which the behavior is regarded as nonpersistence
Last recommended dosing event	– Last expected dosing and treatment completion

Objectives

Intervention	– Interventions used to promote medication adherence
Predictors	– Factors that predict medication adherence
Outcomes	– Outcomes measured
Moderators/mediators	– Variables that may potentially influence the effect of the intervention

Sources

	– Characteristics of available data sources, such as completeness, validity, reliability, quality, time period covered, and limitations

International Society of Pharmacoeconomics and Outcomes Research checklists

The International Society of Pharmacoeconomics and Outcomes Research (ISPOR) developed two checklists of items which should be considered when conducting either a retrospective database analysis of medication adherence or developing prospective research designs.[15,16] The checklists were derived from working group meetings and can be used as a tool for systematically designing medication adherence studies and to critically review adherence studies.

Key items of the checklists include title and abstract, introduction, objectives, methods and study design, statistical analysis and results, discussion and conclusions, and disclosure of conflicts of interest. These items should be considered during study development. The provided checklists can also be used as scoring tools for assessing the quality of prospective or retrospective database analysis studies on medication adherence.

The ISPOR reporting checklists have been used numerous times, including operationalization of outcome measures[36–39] or to guide development of new checklists for good research practices.[40]

Recommendations to improve research on medication adherence

Precisely define nonadherence behavior

While the ABC taxonomy clearly conceptualizes medication taking behavior and distinguishes between initiation, implementation, and discontinuation, neither the taxonomy nor the guidelines discern between primary and secondary nonadherence. The gap between prescription receipt and dispensing can be measured, but this does not necessarily imply initiation of treatment.

Although relatively few adherence research studies have focused on initial nonadherence[41] various terms have been used to describe this process.[42] Raebel et al.[43] proposed a standard definition for primary and secondary medication non-adherence. They defined primary nonadherence as a new prescribed medication which is not followed by dispensing within a certain period of time. Adams et al.[44] used a similar definition to describe primary nonadherence. Within this definition, primary nonadherence can be determined based on a link between prescription and dispensing data which is part of the initiation phase. ISPOR defines primary nonadherence as Initial Medication Adherence, that is, "the patient obtaining for the first time a new prescribed medication, characterized by a first prescription and a first dispense."[42] Remarkably, ISPOR states that primary nonadherence only captures the pharmacist's perspective and not those of the prescriber and patient, and that related terms, such as primary and secondary nonadherence, are not appropriate as they are not part of the medication adherence continuum. It is evident that these terms are used inconsistently to describe noninitiation of prescribed medication.

Furthermore, initiation can be divided into patients having a new prescription that is not followed by dispensing versus prescribed and dispensed medication that is not followed by commencement of treatment (Fig. 1).[45] None of the definitions above consider that a prescription can be presented to a pharmacist and be dispensed but not initiated by the patient.

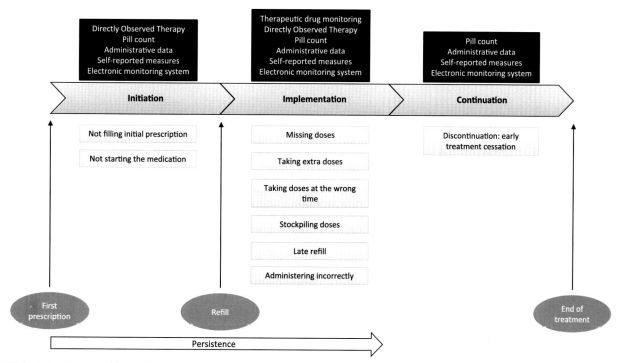

FIG. 1 Patient journey with nonadherence behaviors over time and adherence measures that can be used during each phase.

This type of noninitiation is based on a different behavior, with patients deciding to collect their prescribed medication but having reasons for not wanting to start treatment. Different methods and interventions are therefore needed to address "noncommencement." This medication intake behavior cannot be identified using prescription and dispensing data. This would result in medications dispensed as prescribed and thus a false-positive optimal adherence rate, with the assumption that the patient has started taking the medication. It is unclear which measures can be used to best determine this type of noninitiation.[45]

Secondary adherence is described as an ongoing process which evaluates whether patients receive a pharmacy dispensing after each subsequent prescription[43] and relates to the implementation phase of the taxonomy. In contrast, others define secondary nonadherence as nonpersistence, marked as a substantial long interruption in medication use, which relates more to the discontinuation phase of the ABC taxonomy.[46]

To prevent variability in the way medication taking behavior is interpreted and improve rigor of methodologies used in medication adherence research, one key element is to achieve consensus on a standardized definition of the three adherence phases. Specifically, it is important to divide initiation into nondispensing versus noncommencement and standardize terminology which is used to describe primary and secondary nonadherence. Fig. 1 provides an overview of the different nonadherence behaviors.

Accurately measure and report on medication adherence

Although the available guidelines on medication adherence research provide guidance on operationalization and comprehensive reporting, little guidance is given on how to measure adherence. Utilization of various adherence measures that exist requires careful consideration as each measure has its own methodological properties which influence its validity and reliability. Several key issues should be considered.

I. *Appreciate that each phase of medication adherence has its own specific considerations*: Each adherence phase has its own distinct features,[45] such as a time-to-event variable for initiation and discontinuation versus a continuous process for implementation. As a result, no overarching adherence measure can capture all features and nonadherence rates at once. Therefore, each phase should be studied separately. This means that researchers should recruit people that are at the similar phase and/or have phase-specific measures. As part of the research study design, it is important to clearly articulate which adherence behavior is being measured. Furthermore, if an intervention design aims to improve adherence, then it needs to ensure that the intervention clearly shows which aspects of adherence it will be changing.

II. *Use validated adherence instruments*: When measuring adherence, it is crucial to accurately quantify adherence rates as this will provide a better assessment of both treatment and intervention success as well as identification of individual patients in need of additional adherence support. There are several methodological properties of adherence measures which should be considered to obtain valid and reliable results. Notably, the validity and reliability of the measures or tools.

Validity can be defined as the extent to which a method measures what it is intended to measure.[47] This can be assessed by evaluating how well the results correspond with an established method for the same outcome. Validity can be further specified into construct validity, which is different to translational and criterion-related validity.[48] Construct validity refers to whether the method measures the intended concept, in this case, measuring the correct and relevant phase of adherence. Translational validity, including content and face validity, refers to the extent that the items included in the measure are an adequate representation of all items that might measure the construct and whether the method appears to measure the construct, respectively. Translational validity is based on judgment of experts and end users. Criterion-related validity can be used to define how well the measure correlates with other similar valid adherence measures, preferably the gold-standard, which currently does not exist for measuring adherence.

Reliability can be defined as the extent to which the results can be reproduced when the same measurement is repeated.[47] Reliability scores range from 0 to 1, with 1 indicating true reliability. Reliability can be distinguished into different types including test-retest, internal consistency and interrater reliability.[47,48] Stability of repeated measurements among the same individuals, i.e., stable results at different times, is defined as test-retest reliability. Internal consistency assumes a correlation between items measuring the same construct, whether performance on one item indicates performance on another item, frequently reported as Cronbach's alpha. Interrater reliability stands for the results obtained with a measure when applied by different observers.

III. *Use instruments appropriate for the investigated adherence phase*: Different tools and methods exist to study the adherence phases, each with their own advantages and limitations.[49] There is currently no consensus on a gold standard measure suited for each adherence phase,[45] making it challenging to select the most appropriate strategy. In fact, research shows that many adherence measures have been used interchangeably across the different adherence phases.[18,28,50] It is important to achieve agreement on what measures to use during the different medication taking behavior stages to improve the quality of adherence research.

IV. *Use more than one adherence measure*: Many adherence studies only use a single measure to assess adherence rates.[51] When measuring medication adherence, it is preferable to use at least two measures to measure a specific concept of nonadherence behavior, and data can be triangulated. However, more measures may be required if adherence is being measured at more than one phase.

V. *Define an adherence threshold*: Researchers should state what level of adherence they consider as "adherent" for their studied population and ensure that where possible, this threshold is based on clinical outcomes evidence. Frequently an arbitrary adherence rate of 80% is used. Although this threshold is not based on solid evidence and its relation to clinical outcomes has not been demonstrated,[52] some provide data that this seems a reasonable cut-off point to stratify between adherent and nonadherent.[53] Notably, the clinical relevance of the chosen adherence threshold strongly depends on the disease under investigation, pharmacological characteristics of the prescribed medication, as well as patient characteristics.[54]

VI. *Risk of bias in reporting medication adherence*: Medication adherence stands for a patient's medication taking behavior, and behavior is difficult to capture with a measurement instrument. In fact, most adherence instruments measure a specific concept of medication taking behavior, such as package opening when using electronic devices, and barriers to, and beliefs associated with, medication taking when using self-reports.[55] As a result, measured adherence rates are surrogate markers for actual medication taking. However, studies fail to report on this measurement limitation. When this is not clearly addressed, it may lead to a risk of bias in reporting the relevant context of an adherence measure and incorrect interpretation of obtained adherence rates.

VII. *Use standardized outcomes*: Frequently, medication adherence is measured as this is a more efficient and less costly method compared with clinical outcomes. However, adherence can be considered as a surrogate marker for clinical outcomes. Preferably, both should be evaluated and reported in medication adherence trials although this is not always possible. When measuring adherence and clinical outcomes, standardized outcomes should be used when these are available for the specific population under investigation. As an example, Outcome Measures in Rheumatology (OMERACT) currently develops a core outcome domain set for interventions that aim to improve medication adherence in rheumatology.[56]

Types of medication adherence measures

To measure medication adherence, various methods can be used, both direct and indirect.[57] Direct measures provide evidence that the patient has taken the medication.[57] Indirect measures are more commonly used and focus on reported medication intake behavior or whether the medication has been prescribed and/or dispensed to a patient and can be considered as surrogate markers.[57] In addition, medication adherence measures can be classified as objective or subjective.[2] Examples of objective measures include use of data from eHealth devices such as Medication Event Monitoring System (MEMS) and therapeutic drug monitoring. Examples of subjective measures include self-reported adherence questionnaires such as the Beliefs about Medicines Questionnaire.[58,59] Table 3 describes the most commonly used adherence measures, including advantages and limitations, as well as suitability for the different adherence phases. Fig. 1 shows which measures are recommended to be used during each adherence phase.

Therapeutic drug monitoring

Therapeutic drug monitoring consists of measuring drug concentration levels or drug biomarkers in body fluids, such as blood, plasma or serum and is an direct and objective adherence measure.[57] It can be used to measure the implementation phase. As an example, for 83 patients not responding to antidepressant medicines, drug level monitoring identified that 37.5% of the patients were not adherent.[60] But, data only capture short-term medication intake behavior prior to sampling and may not show the actual nonadherence behavior, nor the rate of adherence, and are therefore limited in the information that it can provide. Moreover, differences in drug concentrations between patients have been observed due to pharmacokinetic variability.

TABLE 3 Overview of most commonly used medication adherence measures.

Measure	Description	Type	Adherence phase for investigation[a]	Selected strengths	Selected limitations
Direct					
Therapeutic drug monitoring	Measuring drug concentration levels or biomarkers in body fluids	Objective	Implementation	Measures actual medication taking	Invasive, time consuming, expensive, evaluates short term medication taking period, pharmacokinetic and pharmacodynamic variability
Directly observed therapy	An "observer" observes and records the patient taking every dose of their medication	Objective	Initiation; implementation	Direct and actual observation of medication taking	Time-consuming for both observer and patient, relatively expensive
Indirect					
Pill count	Ratio of number of doses taken against dispensed quantity	Objective	Initiation; implementation; discontinuation	Simple measurement method, low-cost relative to other measures	Lacks adherence patterns, may overestimate adherence rates, surrogate measure of medication adherence
Administrative data	Evaluating prescription or dispensing data	Objective	Initiation; implementation; discontinuation	Large datasets can be analyzed, relatively simple, sometimes at low-cost	Measures medication possession and not adherence, may overestimate adherence rates, retrospective analysis, surrogate measure of medication adherence
Self-reported measures	Recording medication taking behavior reported by patients	Subjective	Initiation; implementation; discontinuation	Simple, low-cost relative to other measures, easy to administer	Socially desirable answers, recall bias, surrogate measure of medication adherence
Electronic monitoring systems	Medication package which records each date and time of opening or activation	Objective	Initiation; implementation; discontinuation	Longitudinal insight into adherence patterns over time	Does not measure actual medication intake, expensive, less user friendly, can promote adherence, surrogate measure of medication adherence

[a]No consensus exists on the optimal measures for each medication adherence phase.

Pill count

This indirect, objective measure gives an adherence ratio that counts the number of doses which have been taken by the patient (or taken out of the container or strip of medication etc.) versus the total dispensed quantity.[61] Pill counts can be used during the initiation and implementation phase, however, they lack information on adherence patterns which can be identified using electronic monitoring, such as with MEMS, and provide no evidence of actual medication intake. Additionally, adherence rates can differ from rates determined by other measures. For example, a study measuring medication adherence by electronic monitoring and pill count among patients using antihypertensive medication showed significantly higher medication adherence rates when using pill count compared to electronic monitoring using MEMS.[62] In another study, when compared with viral load outcomes in a pediatric HIV-infected population, almost 40% of the pill count results were not concordant with viral load measurements.[63]

Administrative data

Administrative datasets from pharmacies or medical claims consisting of data on prescribed, dispensed or reimbursed medications are commonly used to study patterns of medication adherence.[49] Based on information such as the prescription date, dispensed quantity and prescribed daily dose, therapy initiation (issuing of a prescription followed by dispensing of a prescription), implementation (theoretical proportion of time for which a patient should have a supply of the dispensed medication if taken at the prescribed dose regimen), and persistence (discontinuation of prescription refills) can be assessed. Although this method objectively determines adherence rates, it follows the assumption that medication intake occurred as prescribed. It does not measure actual medication intake but only whether the patient is in possession of the medication. As a result, it frequently leads to a bias in adherence results.

When using administrative data, numerous standardized approaches can be used to estimate medication adherence, the most common being medication possession ratio (MPR) and proportion of days covered (PDC).[64] *Medication possession ratio* is a ratio based on the number of days medication is supplied to the patient to the number of days in the observation period, with adherence values ranging between 0% and 100%, or over 100% in case more medication is dispensed than the study observation period. *Proportion of days covered* (PDC) calculates the number of days that the medication is available to the patient by the total number of days in the study period. For polypharmacy, the *daily polypharmacy possession ratio* (DPPR) can be calculated.[65] DPPR estimates the number of medications available to a patient for each day during the observation period with 0 no medication available and 1 all medications available, resulting in scores between 0% and 100%.

Arnet et al.[66] proposed a new standard to measure adherence using administrative data by also considering oversupply and treatment gaps. They define oversupply as the number of days' supply accumulated from previous dispensings that can occur during the observation period. A treatment gap is defined as number of days without medication supply, calculated by days in the observation period minus number of days' supply. To calculate medication adherence, during the observation period oversupply from previous prescriptions should be carried forward to the next possible treatment gap between two dispensings. This means that an oversupply can (partially) compensate for a subsequent treatment gap (Fig. 2). Also, the proportion of patients reinitiating therapy should be calculated by dividing the number of patients with a dispensing beyond the end date of the maximum treatment gap by the number of patients having discontinued therapy. This method should limit overestimation of adherence rates when using administrative data and can be applied to the adherence taxonomy.

Self-reported adherence measures

These indirect subjective measures can be used to evaluate adherence rates based on reported medication taking by patients and can be used during the implementation phase. Measurement instruments include questionnaires, diaries, and interviews. These measures can be administered relatively easy, both in writing and online. When correlated against electronic monitoring systems, the majority of self-reported questionnaires have shown moderate to high correlation on adherence rates,[67,68] suggesting that self-reported adherence measures are effective for measuring medication taking behavior (assuming that electronic monitoring is valid). Despite its advantages, the method is subjective, prone to socially desirable

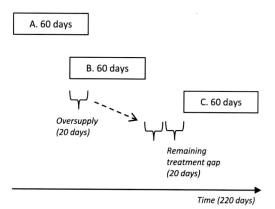

FIG. 2 Schematic presentation of medication history with the observation period of 220 days and three prescriptions of each 60 days (number of days medication is available to the patient). Oversupply is carried forward to the next treatment gap.

answers and recall bias, and therefore has limitations. With self-reported measures, patients may respond accordingly to what they think is expected from them. In addition, patients should be asked about a recent period of time, for instance, evaluating medication taking over the past 2 weeks.

Electronic monitoring systems

Electronic monitoring systems include electronic devices which are fixed to a medication package, such as electronic caps on pill bottles, which record date and time of each opening or activation.[69] This objective, noninvasive method can provide detailed insight into medication taking patterns over a longer period of time, for instance, between two consultations or up to 6 to 12 months. Currently, this method is considered the most accurate approach to measuring medication intake and is therefore widely used in adherence research. It allows a longitudinal evaluation of changes in adherence behavior and is well suited to assess implementation but can also be used toy study initiation and discontinuation. Its main disadvantage is the assumption that opening a bottle or activation of the device corresponds with actual medication intake. Moreover, some patients show better adherence rates when using electronic monitoring systems and therefore the method also acts as an adherence intervention itself.[70]

Conclusions

Although there have been guidelines developed to assist in improving the conceptualization and operationalization of adherence behavior as well as the conduct and reporting of medication adherence research, guidance on how best to measure adherence is absent. Furthermore, variations in adherence terminology remain an issue despite improvements in defining adherence behavior, and the availability of taxonomies. In addition, no studies have evaluated how effective the guidelines have been in their application. To make significant advancements in medication adherence research, there is a need for greater standardization of nonadherence behavior definitions, improved methodological rigor in study designs and adherence measurements, and comprehensive reporting of adherence research. Future studies should aim to standardize adherence definitions, map valid and reliable adherence measures to the relevant adherence phase and medication taking behavior, and evaluate the use and impact of existing adherence research guidelines on the quality of adherence research.

Questions for further discussion

1. What guideline(s) would you use when conducting research on medication adherence; and how would you apply the guideline(s) in planning your research study?
2. What are the phases of medication taking behavior?
3. What measures would you use to determine medication taking at each phase, and why?

Application exercise/scenario

You are planning to conduct research on medication adherence among patients starting long-term treatment. There are several studies evaluating adherence levels among this population, but few clearly specify the medication taking behavior that has been investigated or use the appropriate set of validated adherence measures. Design a study to measure medication adherence levels among this population, by including the relevant guidelines on medication adherence, and discussing the medication adherence phase under investigation, and how this will be measured. What are some initial steps you would take in designing this study, and what would the study protocol to measure adherence look like?

References

1. Vrijens B, De Geest S, Hughes DA, et al. A new taxonomy for describing and defining adherence to medications. *Br J Clin Pharmacol.* 2012;73:691–705.
2. Sabaté E. *Adherence to Long-Term Therapies: Evidence for Action.* Geneva, World Health Organization; 2003.
3. Simpson SH, Eurich DT, Majumdar SR, et al. A meta-analysis of the association between adherence to drug therapy and mortality. *BMJ.* 2006;333:15.
4. Cutler RL, Fernandez-Llimos F, Frommer M, Benrimoj C, Garcia-Cardenas V. Economic impact of medication non-adherence by disease groups: a systematic review. *BMJ Open.* 2018;8:e016982.
5. Demonceau J, Ruppar T, Kristanto P, et al. Identification and assessment of adherence-enhancing interventions in studies assessing medication adherence through electronically compiled drug dosing histories: a systematic literature review and meta-analysis. *Drugs.* 2013;73:545–562.
6. Nieuwlaat R, Wilczynski N, Navarro T, et al. Interventions for enhancing medication adherence. *Cochrane Database Syst Rev.* 2014. CD000011.

7. Ahmed R, Aslani P. What is patient adherence? A terminology overview. *Int J Clin Pharm.* 2014;36:4–7.

8. Kelly A, Crimston-Smith L, Tong A, et al. Scope of outcomes in trials and observational studies of interventions targeting medication adherence in rheumatic conditions: a systematic review. *J Rheumatol.* 2020;47:1565–1574.

9. Dima AL, Hernandez G, Cunillera O, Ferrer M, de Bruin M, ASTRO-LAB Group. Asthma inhaler adherence determinants in adults: systematic review of observational data. *Eur Respir J.* 2015;45:994–1018.

10. Schulz KF, Altman DG, Moher D, CONSORT Group. CONSORT 2010 statement: updated guidelines for reporting parallel group randomized trials. *Ann Intern Med.* 2010;152:726–732.

11. von Elm E, Altman DG, Egger M, et al. The strengthening the reporting of observational studies in epidemiology (STROBE) statement: guidelines for reporting observational studies. *Ann Intern Med.* 2007;147:573–577.

12. Moher D, Liberati A, Tetzlaff J, Altman DG, PRISMA Group. Preferred reporting items for systematic reviews and meta-analyses: the PRISMA statement. *Ann Intern Med.* 2009;151:264–269. W264.

13. Dima AL, Allemann SS, Dunbar-Jacob J, Hughes DA, Vrijens B, Wilson IB. TEOS: a framework for constructing operational definitions of medication adherence based on timelines—events—objectives—sources. *Br J Clin Pharmacol.* 2021;87:2521–2533.

14. De Geest S, Zullig LL, Dunbar-Jacob J, et al. ESPACOMP medication adherence reporting guideline (EMERGE). *Ann Intern Med.* 2018; 169:30–35.

15. Peterson AM, Nau DP, Cramer JA, Benner J, Gwadry-Sridhar F, Nichol M. A checklist for medication compliance and persistence studies using retrospective databases. *Value Health.* 2007;10:3–12.

16. Gwadry-Sridhar FH, Manias E, Zhang Y, et al. A framework for planning and critiquing medication compliance and persistence research using prospective study designs. *Clin Ther.* 2009;31:421–435.

17. Cheen MHH, Tan YZ, Oh LF, Wee HL, Thumboo J. Prevalence of and factors associated with primary medication non-adherence in chronic disease: a systematic review and meta-analysis. *Int J Clin Pract.* 2019;73:e13350.

18. Khan MU, Aslani P. A review of measures used to examine medication adherence in people with ADHD at initiation, implementation and discontinuation of pharmacotherapy. *Res Soc Adm Pharm.* 2020;16:277–289.

19. Barron TI, Connolly R, Bennett K, Feely J, Kennedy MJ. Early discontinuation of tamoxifen: a lesson for oncologists. *Cancer.* 2007;109:832–839.

20. Putignano D, Orlando V, Monetti VM, et al. Fixed versus free combinations of antihypertensive drugs: analyses of real-world data of persistence with therapy in Italy. *Patient Prefer Adherence.* 2019;13:1961–1969.

21. Ribaut J, Leppla L, Teynor A, et al. Theory-driven development of a medication adherence intervention delivered by eHealth and transplant team in allogeneic stem cell transplantation: the SMILe implementation science project. *BMC Health Serv Res.* 2020;20:827.

22. Torres-Robles A, Wiecek E, Cutler R, et al. Using dispensing data to evaluate adherence implementation rates in community pharmacy. *Front Pharmacol.* 2019;10:130.

23. Walsh CA, Bennett KE, Wallace E, Cahir C. Identifying adherence patterns across multiple medications and their association with health outcomes in older community-dwelling adults with multimorbidity. *Value Health.* 2020;23:1063–1071.

24. Fenelon-Dimanche R, Guenette L, Trudel-Bourgault F, et al. Development of an electronic tool (e-AdPharm) to address unmet needs and barriers of community pharmacists to provide medication adherence support to patients. *Res Soc Adm Pharm.* 2021;17:506–513.

25. Couzos S, Smith D, Stephens M, et al. Integrating pharmacists into aboriginal community controlled health services (IPAC project): protocol for an interventional, non-randomised study to improve chronic disease outcomes. *Res Soc Adm Pharm.* 2020;16:1431–1441.

26. Birk JL, Cumella R, Lopez-Veneros D, et al. Intervening on fear after acute cardiac events: rationale and design of the INFORM randomized clinical trial. *Health Psychol.* 2020;39:736–744.

27. Haag M, Lehmann A, Hersberger KE, et al. The ABC taxonomy for medication adherence translated into French and German. *Br J Clin Pharmacol.* 2020;86:734–744.

28. Srimongkon P, Aslani P, Chen TF. A systematic review of measures of medication adherence in consumers with unipolar depression. *Res Soc Adm Pharm.* 2019;15:3–22.

29. Bhatia S, Hageman L, Chen Y, et al. Effect of a daily text messaging and directly supervised therapy intervention on oral mercaptopurine adherence in children with acute lymphoblastic leukemia: a randomized clinical trial. *JAMA Netw Open.* 2020;3:e2014205.

30. van der Laan DM, Elders PJM, Boons C, Nijpels G, van Dijk L, Hugtenburg JG. Effectiveness of a patient-tailored, pharmacist-led intervention program to enhance adherence to antihypertensive medication: the CATI study. *Front Pharmacol.* 2018;9:1057.

31. Youn B, Shireman TI, Lee Y, Galarraga O, Wilson IB. Trends in medication adherence in HIV patients in the US, 2001 to 2012: an observational cohort study. *J Int AIDS Soc.* 2019;22:e25382.

32. du Pon E, El Azzati S, van Dooren A, Kleefstra N, Heerdink E, van Dulmen S. Effects of a proactive interdisciplinary self-management (PRISMA) program on medication adherence in patients with type 2 diabetes in primary care: a randomized controlled trial. *Patient Prefer Adherence.* 2019;13:749–759.

33. Capiau A, Mehuys E, Van Tongelen I, et al. Community pharmacy-based study of adherence to non-vitamin K antagonist oral anticoagulants. *Heart.* 2020;106:1740–1746.

34. van Heuckelum M, Linn AJ, Vandeberg L, et al. Implicit and explicit attitudes towards disease-modifying antirheumatic drugs as possible target for improving medication adherence. *PLoS One.* 2019;14:e0221290.

35. Alfian SD, van Boven JFM, Abdulah R, Sukandar H, Denig P, Hak E. Effectiveness of a targeted and tailored pharmacist-led intervention to improve adherence to antihypertensive drugs among patients with type 2 diabetes in Indonesia: a cluster randomised controlled trial. *Br J Clin Pharmacol.* 2021;87:2032–2041.

36. Doshi JA, Zhu J, Lee BY, Kimmel SE, Volpp KG. Impact of a prescription copayment increase on lipid-lowering medication adherence in veterans. *Circulation.* 2009;119:390–397.

37. Takemoto SK, Pinsky BW, Schnitzler MA, et al. A retrospective analysis of immunosuppression compliance, dose reduction and discontinuation in kidney transplant recipients. *Am J Transplant*. 2007;7:2704–2711.
38. Faught RE, Weiner JR, Guerin A, Cunnington MC, Duh MS. Impact of nonadherence to antiepileptic drugs on health care utilization and costs: findings from the RANSOM study. *Epilepsia*. 2009;50:501–509.
39. Kiel MA, Roder E, Gerth van Wijk R, Al MJ, Hop WC, Rutten-van Molken MP. Real-life compliance and persistence among users of subcutaneous and sublingual allergen immunotherapy. *J Allergy Clin Immunol*. 2013;132:353–360.e352.
40. Bridges JF, Hauber AB, Marshall D, et al. Conjoint analysis applications in health—a checklist: a report of the ISPOR good research practices for conjoint analysis task force. *Value Health*. 2011;14:403–413.
41. Zeber JE, Manias E, Williams AF, et al. A systematic literature review of psychosocial and behavioral factors associated with initial medication adherence: a report of the ISPOR medication adherence & persistence special interest group. *Value Health*. 2013;16:891–900.
42. Hutchins DS, Zeber JE, Roberts CS, et al. Initial medication adherence-review and recommendations for good practices in outcomes research: an ISPOR medication adherence and persistence special interest group report. *Value Health*. 2015;18:690–699.
43. Raebel MA, Schmittdiel J, Karter AJ, Konieczny JL, Steiner JF. Standardizing terminology and definitions of medication adherence and persistence in research employing electronic databases. *Med Care*. 2013;51:S11–S21.
44. Adams AJ, Stolpe SF. Defining and measuring primary medication nonadherence: development of a quality measure. *J Manag Care Spec Pharm*. 2016;22:516–523.
45. Kronish IM, Thorpe CT, Voils CI. Measuring the multiple domains of medication nonadherence: findings from a Delphi survey of adherence experts. *Transl Behav Med*. 2021;11:104–113.
46. Garcia-Sempere A, Hurtado I, Sanfelix-Genoves J, et al. Primary and secondary non-adherence to osteoporotic medications after hip fracture in Spain. The PREV2FO population-based retrospective cohort study. *Sci Rep*. 2017;7:11784.
47. Kimberlin CL, Winterstein AG. Validity and reliability of measurement instruments used in research. *Am J Health Syst Pharm*. 2008;65:2276–2284.
48. DeVon HA, Block ME, Moyle-Wright P, et al. A psychometric toolbox for testing validity and reliability. *J Nurs Scholarsh*. 2007;39:155–164.
49. Lehmann A, Aslani P, Ahmed R, et al. Assessing medication adherence: options to consider. *Int J Clin Pharm*. 2014;36:55–69.
50. Pednekar PP, Agh T, Malmenas M, et al. Methods for measuring multiple medication adherence: a systematic review-report of the ISPOR medication adherence and persistence special interest group. *Value Health*. 2019;22:139–156.
51. Tibble H, Flook M, Sheikh A, et al. Measuring and reporting treatment adherence: what can we learn by comparing two respiratory conditions? *Br J Clin Pharmacol*. 2021;87:825–836.
52. Baumgartner PC, Haynes RB, Hersberger KE, Arnet I. A systematic review of medication adherence thresholds dependent of clinical outcomes. *Front Pharmacol*. 2018;9:1290.
53. Karve S, Cleves MA, Helm M, Hudson TJ, West DS, Martin BC. Good and poor adherence: optimal cut-point for adherence measures using administrative claims data. *Curr Med Res Opin*. 2009;25:2303–2310.
54. Burnier M. Is there a threshold for medication adherence? Lessons learnt from electronic monitoring of drug adherence. *Front Pharmacol*. 2018;9:1540.
55. Nguyen TM, La Caze A, Cottrell N. What are validated self-report adherence scales really measuring?: a systematic review. *Br J Clin Pharmacol*. 2014;77:427–445.
56. Kelly A, Tong A, Tymms K, et al. Outcome measures in rheumatology—interventions for medication adherence (OMERACT-adherence) core domain set for trials of interventions for medication adherence in rheumatology: 5 phase study protocol. *Trials*. 2018;19:204.
57. Lam WY, Fresco P. Medication adherence measures: an overview. *Biomed Res Int*. 2015;2015:217047.
58. Horne R, Weinman J, Hankins M. The beliefs about medicines questionnaire: the development and evaluation of a new method for assessing the cognitive representation of medication. *Psychol Health*. 1999;14:1–24.
59. Horne R, Chapman SC, Parham R, Freemantle N, Forbes A, Cooper V. Understanding patients' adherence-related beliefs about medicines prescribed for long-term conditions: a meta-analytic review of the Necessity-Concerns Framework. *PLoS One*. 2013;8:e80633.
60. Silhan P, Urinovska R, Kacirova I, Hyza M, Grundmann M, Ceskova E. What does antidepressant drug level monitoring reveal about outpatient treatment and patient adherence? *Pharmacopsychiatry*. 2019;52:78–83.
61. Anghel LA, Farcas AM, Oprean RN. An overview of the common methods used to measure treatment adherence. *Med Pharm Rep*. 2019;92:117–122.
62. van Onzenoort HA, Verberk WJ, Kessels AG, et al. Assessing medication adherence simultaneously by electronic monitoring and pill count in patients with mild-to-moderate hypertension. *Am J Hypertens*. 2010;23:149–154.
63. Martelli G, Antonucci R, Mukurasi A, Zepherine H, Nostlinger C. Adherence to antiretroviral treatment among children and adolescents in Tanzania: comparison between pill count and viral load outcomes in a rural context of Mwanza region. *PLoS One*. 2019;14:e0214014.
64. Hess LM, Raebel MA, Conner DA, Malone DC. Measurement of adherence in pharmacy administrative databases: a proposal for standard definitions and preferred measures. *Ann Pharmacother*. 2006;40:1280–1288.
65. Arnet I, Abraham I, Messerli M, Hersberger KE. A method for calculating adherence to polypharmacy from dispensing data records. *Int J Clin Pharm*. 2014;36:192–201.
66. Arnet I, Kooij MJ, Messerli M, Hersberger KE, Heerdink ER, Bouvy M. Proposal of standardization to assess adherence with medication records: methodology matters. *Ann Pharmacother*. 2016;50:360–368.
67. Shi L, Liu J, Fonseca V, Walker P, Kalsekar A, Pawaskar M. Correlation between adherence rates measured by MEMS and self-reported questionnaires: a meta-analysis. *Health Qual Life Outcomes*. 2010;8:99.

68. Monnette A, Zhang Y, Shao H, Shi L. Concordance of adherence measurement using self-reported adherence questionnaires and medication monitoring devices: an updated review. *PharmacoEconomics*. 2018;36:17–27.

69. Checchi KD, Huybrechts KF, Avorn J, Kesselheim AS. Electronic medication packaging devices and medication adherence: a systematic review. *JAMA*. 2014;312:1237–1247.

70. Sutton S, Kinmonth AL, Hardeman W, et al. Does electronic monitoring influence adherence to medication? Randomized controlled trial of measurement reactivity. *Ann Behav Med*. 2014;48:293–299.

Chapter 39

Methodological and disciplinary competence and insecurity in qualitative research

Sofia Kälvemark Sporrong[a,b], Susanne Kaae[b], Lotte Stig Nørgaard[b], Mathias Møllebæk[b], Marit Waaseth[c], Lourdes Cantarero Arevalo[b], Christina Ljungberg Persson[d], Charlotte L. Bekker[e], Johanna Falby Lindell[f], and Louise C. Druedahl[b,g]

[a]Department of Pharmacy, Uppsala University, Uppsala, Sweden, [b]Department of Pharmacy, Social and Clinical Pharmacy Research Group, University of Copenhagen, Copenhagen, Denmark, [c]Department of Pharmacy, The Arctic University of Norway, Tromsø, Norway, [d]School of Public Health and Community Medicine, University of Gothenburg, Arvid Wallgrens Backe, Gothenburg, Sweden, [e]Department of Pharmacy, Radboud University Medical Center, Research Institute for Health Sciences, Nijmegen, The Netherlands, [f]Department of Nordic Studies and Linguistics and University of Copenhagen Research Centre for Control of Antibiotic Resistance (UC-CARE), University of Copenhagen, Copenhagen, Denmark, [g]Centre for Advanced Studies in Biomedical Innovation Law (CeBIL), University of Copenhagen, Copenhagen, Denmark

Objectives

- Give insights regarding challenges that exist within qualitative methodology, especially for researchers educated in pharmacy/natural sciences.
- Inform discussions on methodological aspects of qualitative research, including the importance of reflexivity.
- Critically appraise the concepts of quality criteria, including transparency and saturation in qualitative research.

Qualitative research within social pharmacy

Qualitative research methods are much used within social and clinical pharmacy research (hereafter, we include clinical pharmacy in social pharmacy, as the two areas are very similar[1] in the perspectives discussed in this chapter). Researchers have used qualitative methodology when exploring aspects related to, for example, health care professionals' and patients' perspectives on medicines use or practices.[2] This research approach is increasingly gaining peers' and practitioners' recognition.[3]

The increasing use of qualitative research within social pharmacy also brings a methodological debate on how to ensure high quality of the research. Scholars involved in this discussion include Guirguis and Witry who argued that the use of checklists (such as COREQ[4] and SRQR[5]) does not automatically lead to high-quality research even when it leads to complete reporting.[3] Amin et al. gave their view on how to promote rigor in qualitative pharmacy research, but stressed that their suggestions were not intended as a comprehensive manual.[6] Further, Lau and Traulsen argued that explicit theoretical approaches can aid high-quality analysis.[7] In this chapter, we add to this debate, by discussing some aspects of qualitative research that can be challenging for researchers new to qualitative methodology.

The existence of multiple traditions (e.g., phenomenology, symbolic interactionism, grounded theory, ethnography, hermeneutics, narrative research, interpretivism)[8-10] and defining principles guiding qualitative methodology is a challenge when conducting or appraising qualitative studies. For instance, grounded theory, phenomenology, and narrative analysis have their own, sometimes contradicting, principles, for example when it comes to the focus of studies, extent of data collection and how to analyze data. In addition, within one tradition there can be several orientations stating or emphasizing different aspects or processes.[11] An important part of the above plurality is what entails quality in qualitative research, and whether standards can be defined. All this can lead to ambiguities, that in turn can affect how social pharmacy researchers conduct their research, but also how they assess, or are assessed by, other researchers during the peer-review process of scientific publications.

Contemporary Research Methods in Pharmacy and Health Services. https://doi.org/10.1016/B978-0-323-91888-6.00005-3

In this chapter, we discuss some aspects of qualitative methodology to contribute to the debate. Our contribution is built on the experiences, opinions and challenges put forward by Nordic social and clinical pharmacy researchers when conducting qualitative research, and were brought up at a workshop at the 9th Nordic Social Pharmacy and Health Services Research Conference (NSCP) 2019. The workshop was entitled *How do we know it's good? A workshop on quality criteria in qualitative social and clinical pharmacy research.* Participants in the workshop had from none to extensive experience regarding qualitative research, most had an educational background in pharmacy, but there were also participants with a background in health, social sciences and humanities. This led to discussions across research traditions and perspectives. More details of the workshop can be found in Kälvemark Sporrong et al.[12] This chapter focuses on the aspects that were raised by participants as specifically troublesome, these include:

— Insecurity about *competency* in qualitative research when trained in natural sciences
— *Reflexivity*, e.g., how do you know that you are reflexive enough
— Different aspects of *transparency* in reporting qualitative research
— How and why to use *checklists*
— *Quality criteria* in qualitative research
— *Sampling* and how to "measure" *saturation*

Underlying understanding of epistemology

Understanding differences in epistemology is an underlying reason for some of the challenges experienced, and therefore, it is relevant to start with some notes on this. Research as knowledge creation is based on "tacit assumptions about what knowledge is and how it is constructed."[13] Two different epistemological foundations are (post)positivism and interpretative traditions such as hermeneutics and poststructuralism.[14–16] These two foundations contrast each other on how the world is seen and how research can be conducted. Within (post)positivism:

> The social sciences can uncover objective and universally valid facts by following clear procedures and rules, which include carefully controlled observations of empirical phenomena, impartial and logical argumentation, and objective analysis, i.e. the elimination of interpretation by the researcher.[14]

In contrast, the interpretative turn expresses that:

> The social world is seen/…/as a subjectively lived construct. Interpretive perspectives consequently abandon claims to objectivity to emphasize instead the reflexive nature of the research process and the subjective nature of constructions of meaning, both by the research subjects and by the researcher.[14]

These foundations are relevant for qualitative social pharmacy research, also as they differ fundamentally regarding the researcher's role in research. A positivistic approach would consider the researcher's perspective as a barrier to eliminate because it clouds the researcher's ability to see reality as it is. Conversely, the interpretative turn encourages researchers to be explicit and transparent about their preunderstandings. This is because preunderstandings are seen as the cornerstones on which the research interpretations will be built.[17] Typically, natural sciences are based on the positivistic approach while the basis of qualitative traditions are more in line with the interpretative approach.

These differences can make qualitative research more difficult to take on and/or acknowledge for natural sciences alumni, including pharmacists, who are traditionally trained in a quantitative, positivistic foundation.

Methodological and disciplinary competence and insecurity

Working with qualitative methodology is an activity that demands reflection (including self-reflection), trying out different perspectives, finding patterns in sometimes "chaotic" data, interpretation, making decisions about theoretical (abstract) standpoints, etc. This can challenge pharmacists who are trained into a profession that includes a mindset mainly directed toward natural science.

A related challenge for pharmacists is a misconception about the possibility of having evidence-based knowledge derived from qualitative research because this opposes their training that evidence-based must be generated using quantitative methods. This is related to epistemology; where quantitative methodology relies on a principle that it reveals *the* truth through *objectivity, validity* and *reliability*, this is not the case for qualitative research that most often relies on a different view on knowledge creation.

Most pharmacists that go into social pharmacy research discover that there are research questions that cannot be answered by using quantitative methods. In order to be able to answer these research questions, they embark on a journey, braving the uncomfortable unknown, to gain insight into qualitative research methods. It is important to acknowledge that this process is not an easy one. Research in interdisciplinarity (i.e., "bringing together in some fashion distinctive components of two or more disciplines"[18]) has shown that when researchers transition out of their habitual methodological domains, feelings of insecurity and self-questioning reproduce and reinforce disciplinary differences, and consequently inhibit cross-disciplinary collaboration.[19] This may be a significant challenge for social pharmacy as a field, since not attending to the insecurities may deter further development for both individual researchers and the field as a whole.

Even after gaining a basic understanding of qualitative research, insecurity may still exist. Feelings of insecurity and constructs that promise to mitigate them (fixed, universal criteria and checklists) are part and parcel of qualitative research in an area that is predominantly quantitative and positivistic. The absence of inherent and fixed quality criteria for methods may generate these feelings of insecurity. One is tempted to think: is there a remedy for the insecurity issue—or is it part of the game? We argue that although such insecurities diminish with experience, they remain an important premise for qualitative methodology, also for those who are knowledgeable and experienced. Insecurity and doubts can be a good seed-bed for reflections.

Reflexivity

Reflexivity—the need for the researcher to be aware of and transparent about her/his background, perspective and position—is one of these basic principles in qualitative research. One description of reflexivity, presented by Malterud, is "An attitude of attending systematically to the context of knowledge construction, especially to the effect of the researcher, at every step of the research process."[20]

Qualitative methodology recognizes that the researcher will have an effect on the research thus it is essential that as a researcher one is aware of where one comes from (such as one's history, experiences, perspectives) and one's preunderstanding of the topic of research. It is not about *if* you affect the research results, but *how* you do it. Another aspect in Malterud's description is about reflectivity *throughout* the research process,[20] this obviously implies that it will take up some time. This is a practical but important part of qualitative research; that time is planned for individual reflection as well as reflective discussions with fellow researchers. To have multiple researchers involved can strengthen a study, as when it comes to reflections, it gives an opportunity to supplement, but also contest each other's perspectives throughout the research process.[20] Overall it can be good to think of reflexivity as an *attitude*; to be open, as well as to constantly (in the whole research process) reflect on, and document, what is going on.

It takes practice, and not least, courage to assess and question one's own thinking, and to be opposed and supplemented by others. Furthermore, to accept and explore how one as a researcher can affect the research design and process, and in the end research results. Reflexivity can thus be a challenge on a practical as well as a personal level.

Transparency and checklists

Transparency is often used as a quality criterion in qualitative research. It was presented by Lincoln and Guba as an approach to achieving high quality in qualitative research via credibility, transferability, dependability, and confirmability.[21] To ensure transparency, qualitative researchers should state assumptions, procedures, choices and decisions made during the research process. They should also explicate the sources and techniques of data collection and analysis, along with the interpretations made and influences from others (see, for example, Hadi and Closs[22]). This is to enable the reader to assess the quality of a qualitative study and to help decide upon the applicability of research findings to other contexts.[4] Hadi and Closs stressed that "failure to undertake rigorous qualitative research has negative implications in terms of its impact on pharmacy practice and policy, future development of pharmaceutical services and most importantly, the qualitative research methodology itself."[22] However, since many journals have maximum word count limits, the requirement of transparency can be difficult to fulfill, as such thorough descriptions easily become rather long.

Checklists such as the Consolidated criteria for reporting qualitative studies (COREQ), first published in 2007,[4] and the Standards for reporting qualitative research (SRQR), first published in 2014,[5] were developed to improve the accountability of the research process, transparency and reporting of qualitative studies, in other words to create an *audit trail*. For more examples of standards for reporting qualitative research and their content, see O'Brien et al.[5] Some of the intentions for developing checklists were to improve comprehensive reporting to increase application of the results and a possible syntheses with other studies as well as to increase recognition of the contribution of qualitative research.[4,5] For these reasons, it can be appropriate that checklists are required of qualitative researchers as part of the publication process either from reviewers or by journals. However, these checklists have also been perceived as a quality criterion in their own right.[5]

Thus, this indicates that in practice the checklists are misinterpreted to have a larger and inappropriate role because the demand to use checklists implies a conflation of the overall quality of the conducted work with how the work is reported.

Checklists may serve a purpose for beginners in the field, both researchers and reviewers, as something to hold on to and hence a remedy for the above-mentioned insecurity. A checklist may be used this way because it resembles quality criteria from the quantitative, positivistic mindset. However, it may create a false sense of high quality research. Hence, checklists can contribute to less quality if researchers think they are doing the proper thing, but in reality lack a more profound understanding of the methodology.[23] Barbour concludes that:

> *Reducing qualitative research to a list of technical procedures, however extensive, is overly prescriptive and results in 'the tail wagging the dog.' None of these technical fixes, in itself, confers rigour. They can strengthen the rigour of qualitative research only if they are embedded in a broad understanding of qualitative research design and data analysis.*[23]

However, while checklists are no guarantee for a high quality study, they can be used as tools when going through different phases in the research, and ensure that relevant aspects are considered during the research process.[3,24]

Checklists are, per definition, general to suit all kinds of qualitative methodology. It is however difficult, in general, to adequately grasp the complexity and various possible and valid ways of conducting qualitative research.[23] Also, checklists (such as COREQ and SRQR) have been criticized for being too superficial when it comes to issues like theoretical aspects of sampling and data analysis which can result in skepticism toward them.[24] For example, Herber et al. state that:

> *…lack of in-depth data analysis has been identified as another weakness where uninterpreted (raw) data were presented as if they were findings. However, existing reporting guidelines are not sharp enough to distinguish between findings and data.*[24]

For reviewers, it would be prudent to avoid reviewing a paper without some experience and knowledge with the applied methods regardless of whether it is a qualitative or quantitative study. However, there are many examples of reviewers' statements that reveal a lack of basic understanding of qualitative research.[24] Herber et al. reviewed reviewer comments to qualitative methods articles and they concluded: *"some results suggest an underlying quantitative mindset of reviewers"* and (about reviewers) that *"…we found some lack of grasp of the essence of the qualitative endeavor. Some reviewers did not seem to understand that objectivity and representative sampling are the antithesis of subjectivity, reflexivity and data saturation."*[24] A checklist will not help these reviewers, but for reviewers with some qualitative research experience, it could serve as a reminder of what to look for when assessing the quality of a paper.[3]

To ensure structure in reporting, checklists such as COREQ and SRQR are helpful and they can serve as a means to obtain transparency of the research process and findings. However, they will not lead to improvement of the research itself and should not be used as a quality criterion. This is important to have in mind for both qualitative researchers and reviewers. There are no shortcuts to a basic understanding of qualitative research methodology. For a good start, dive into the literature, explore different traditions and discuss with your fellows!

Quality criteria

Quality criteria for qualitative research, such as credibility, transferability, and reflexivity,[21,25,26] are another area for discussions. This refers to what quality criteria there should be, if they can be universal, and how they are used.[11,26–28] For the last part, i.e., how quality criteria are used, there are arguments similar to those regarding how checklists are used: "In themselves, these [quality] criteria do not ensure rigour. However, they can strengthen rigour if they are used in concordance with a broader understanding of qualitative research design, data collection and analysis."[26] Hence, such quality criteria can be reduced to "checklist level" if the researcher or reader lacks basic understanding of qualitative research methodology. The use of quality criteria has also been criticized as it implies a consensus about standards, not taking differences in epistemology into account.[27] Stige et al. argue that, "The multiplicity of worldviews and viewpoints/…/ suggests, however, that the field of qualitative research is diverse to a degree that challenges the legitimacy of general evaluation criteria."[27]

An important feature of qualitative research is that quality criteria, such as internal validity, do not derive from qualitative methods in the manner they do for quantitative methods, and that they are not inherent in the methodological procedures. Rather they are shaped by the consensus in the research field, the context of the particular research focus and accommodated to real life research practice.[11] To some degree, they are also shaped to overturn skepticism from the positivistic/quantitative research society.[23] In other words, as methodological criteria are neither fixed nor easily applicable, they should be addressed, discussed and justified anew in each qualitative research project. Rolfe terms this as *the third position* regarding quality in qualitative research, the other two being (1) adopting and aligning the concepts of positivist research, i.e., validity and reliability, and (2) focus on trustworthiness and auditable practices.[28] This third position implies that "Rather than searching for an overarching set of criteria by which to judge the validity of qualitative research, we should perhaps acknowledge that there is a multiplicity of (so-called) qualitative paradigms, each requiring very different approaches to validity."[28]

But do "fuzzy" quality criteria in qualitative research mean that anything goes? On the contrary! However, with no fixed criteria the responsibility lies with the researcher(s) to argue for what is relevant. In line with *the third position,* and taking into account the type of research and underlying research tradition, the researcher(s) needs to identify what criteria to use, including how they should be interpreted, and accounted for.

Sample size, saturation and information power

A frequent methodological question in qualitative interview research is "how many interviews are enough?" To answer this question, the National Centre for Research Methods in the UK convened 14 renowned social scientists and five early career researchers and the consensus was that it depends on specific aspects of the study.[29] In quantitative research there are methods (power calculations) to answer the "how many are enough" question, but qualitative research there are no such methods. It can be frustrating to get the answer "it depends…" when planning a study, and not having a specific number (of, for example, interviews) to aim for, is dissatisfying for many.

In a review of how sample size in focus group studies was reported, only 37 out of 220 studies explained the number of focus groups that had been conducted in each study, and of these a majority ($n = 28$) reported that they had reached saturation.[30] Saturation is often used as the argument for sample size in qualitative studies, but many times without specifying how saturation is understood or even assessed.[31] The saturation concept originally comes from grounded theory, but is often used also in studies belonging to other research traditions. As pointed out in the review mentioned above "several [of the included studies] appeared not to have followed principles from grounded theory where data collection and analysis is an iterative process until saturation is reached."[30] If data collection is completed before the analysis starts, then saturation is simply not a valid argument for the sample size.

In the authors' experiences, qualitative researchers and reviewers within social pharmacy tend to focus mostly on saturation as what Saunders et al. termed *data saturation, i.e., "the degree to which new data repeat what was expressed in previous data."*[32] This can be stated as, for example, "after interviewing 12 patients no new information came up." Data saturation, in this sense, has attained widespread acceptance as a quality principle in qualitative social pharmacy research. However, *data* saturation focuses on the data collection phase, especially the number of respondents, and is frequently used as if it was unrelated to for example sampling strategy, data collection and data analysis (which are critical stages to accomplish (theoretical) saturation). For example, if your sampling strategy results in participants that have one and the same perspective on your subject, but where several exist, then data saturation will occur rather fast, but you have only covered a small part of the perspectives that exist. The same is true if your data collection only opened up for some specific areas (for example, if questions were leading or the researcher showed discontent).

To conclude, if the concept of saturation is used it has to be adapted to the specific study and its use depends on, among others, whether the qualitative study is deductive or inductive, the role of theory, and analytical approach.[31,32] For each study, researchers should be transparent about how and why they use the term saturation, and in addition how and when in the research process it was assessed. This also implies that saturation is not a final point, but a "matter of degree," thus arguing that there will always be the potential for "the 'new' to emerge."[32]

Sample size and saturation has also been addressed by Malterud et al. who suggest the concept of *information power,*[31] based on the following factors that are seen as specifically relevant: (1)how narrow or broad is the aim, (2)the specificity of the sample, (3)application of theory, (4)the interview dialog, and (5)strategy of the analysis.[31] Based on these factors they suggest that information power can be used to estimate "an adequate number of units, events, or participants" in qualitative research, and argue that "[t]he larger information power the sample holds, the lower N is needed."[31] According to this concept, the more narrow the aim is, the more specific the targeted group is, the more specific theories are applied, the stronger the quality of the dialog (in interviews) is, the fewer participants/cases are needed. In addition, more participants are needed if the analysis is cross-case exploratory rather than in-depth/narrative.[31] Information power is hence an alternative to saturation, and is developed so that it, at least partly, can be applied when planning a study (not as saturation that is applicable first when data collection and analysis has started), and also in different research traditions.

The reason for the sometimes simplified use of saturation to argue for sample size in our (and apparently other[30]) research field(s) might again stem from the natural science background of pharmacists and the trained mindset that research should be measured in numbers. In our view, qualitative researchers in social pharmacy need to gain more insight into the concept of saturation, when it is applicable, how to achieve and assess it, and the different methodological stances behind its varying use.

Going forward

We have discussed some aspects that, according to the workshop participants, can be challenging for social pharmacy researchers with a natural science background. An important starting point is to get to know the different epistemologies underpinning qualitative methodologies, as compared to quantitative. For example that the "quality control" when conducting qualitative research is not about filling out a specific protocol, but about making sure that the decisions and reflections done during the research process were sharp and sufficiently in-depth and that the researchers are aware of the context and their own position in that. Furthermore, the complexity of qualitative research means that there is a need for even more organization, not only of data, but also of the whole process, for example taking time for reflections as described earlier.

It is difficult to understand how to use or critically assess research results if you have no idea what to look for or how to interpret them. In our view, pharmacy students therefore need to be introduced to, and gain understanding of qualitative research through their education. For those going further to conducting qualitative research, it is even more important to "dive" into this new perspective. If pharmacists do not gain knowledge and understanding of what qualitative research is and how it works, many (in-depth) studies exploring for example medication use, healthcare systems and pharmacists' role in them will remain a black box for the pharmacy profession. This would be a loss since the areas accessible with qualitative methods can provide pharmacists with (a deeper) knowledge both of patient experiences and of pharmacy/pharmacist practices.

In health sciences, including social pharmacy, qualitative methods help us understand phenomena that we do not have access to without engaging with how healthcare unfolds in the real world. A premise for engaging with such lifeworld experiences is challenging your own experience, in order to listen to and grasp those of others' with genuine curiosity and humility. Whereas ideas about control and competence can incline researchers toward confirming preconceived ideas, humility and insecurity may be indicators of more open, explorative, and reflective dispositions toward the complexity of how different people experience (aspects of) the world.

Questions for further discussion

In this chapter some challenges in regard to conducting qualitative research are presented. Reflect on your experience of qualitative research and how you have experienced such challenges.

1. Are there other challenges, not presented here, that you have experienced or thought about?
2. As the position of the research is important in qualitative research (see the passage about reflexivity), discuss what your position has been/is in the qualitative research studies you have conducted. For example, consider gender, age, ethnicity, social background, history, experiences.

Application exercise/scenario

Think about any research area within social and clinical pharmacy (e.g., patients' motivation to use medications, the role of pharmacists in primary care, pharmacy customers and health literacy) and (1) describe your preunderstanding of the topic, and (2) how your position could potentially have an impact if you conducted research in this area.

References

1. Almarsdóttir AB, Granås AG. Social pharmacy and clinical pharmacy—joining forces. *Pharmacy.* 2016;4:1.
2. Almarsdóttir AB, Bastholm P. Qualitative methods in drug utilization research. In: Elseviers, et al., eds. *Drug Utilization Research: Methods and Applications.* John Wiley & Sons, Incorporated; 2016.
3. Guirguis LM, Witry MJ. Promoting meaningful qualitative research in social pharmacy: moving beyond reporting guidelines. *Int J Pharm Pract.* 2019;27:333–335.
4. Tong A, Sainsbury P, Craig J. Consolidated criteria for reporting qualitative research (COREQ): a 32-item checklist for interviews and focus groups. *International J Qual Health Care.* 2007;19:349–357.
5. O'Brien BC, Harris IB, Beckman TJ, Reed DA, Cook DA. Standards for reporting qualitative research: a synthesis of recommendations. *Acad Med.* 2014;89:1245–1251.
6. Amin MEK, Nørgaard LS, Cavaco AM, Witry MJ, Cernasev A, Desselle S. Establishing trustworthiness and authenticity in qualitative pharmacy research. *Res Social Adm Pharm.* 2020;16:1472–1482.
7. Lau SR, Traulsen JM. Are we ready to accept the challenge? Addressing the shortcomings of contemporary qualitative health research. *Res Social Adm Pharm.* 2017;13:332–338.
8. Creswell JW. *Qualitative Inquiry and Research Design. Choosing among Five Traditions.* Thousand Oaks, CA: Sage Publications; 1998.

9. Robson C. *Real World Research: A Resource for Social Scientists and Practitioner-Researchers*. 4th ed. Blackwell Publishers; 2016.
10. Patton MQ. *Qualitative Research & Evaluation Methods*. 3rd ed. Thousand Oaks, CA: Sage Publications; 2002.
11. Sandelowski M. What's in a name? Qualitative description revisited. *Res Nurs Health*. 2010;33:77–84.
12. Kälvemark Sporrong S, Kaae S, Nørgaard LS, et al. Challenges in qualitative social pharmacy research: reflections based on a conference workshop. *Res Social Adm Pharm*. 2022;18(1):2254–2258.
13. Carter SM, Little M. Justifying knowledge, justifying method, taking action: epistemologies, methodologies, and methods in qualitative research. *Qual Health Res*. 2007;17:1316–1328.
14. Bergman MM, Coxon APM. The quality in qualitative methods. *Forum Qual Soc Res*. 2005;6(34).
15. Seale C. *The Quality of Qualitative Research*. London: Sage Publications; 1999.
16. Habermas J. Knowledge and interest. *Inquiry*. 1966;9:285–300.
17. Mottier V. The interpretive turn: history, memory, and storage in qualitative research. *Forum Qual Soc Res*. 2005;6:33.
18. Nissani M. Fruits, salads, and smoothies: a working definition of interdisciplinarity. *J Educ Thought*. 1995;29:119–126.
19. Villeneuve D, Durán-Rodas D, Ferri A, et al. What is interdisciplinarity in practice? Critical reflections on doing mobility research in an intended interdisciplinary doctoral research group. *Sustainability*. 2020;12:197.
20. Malterud K. Qualitative research: standards, challenges, and guidelines. *Lancet*. 2001;358:483–488.
21. Lincoln YS, Guba EG. But is it rigorous? Trustworthiness and authenticity in naturalistic evaluation. *N Dir Progr Eval*. 1986;73–84.
22. Hadi MA, José CS. Ensuring rigour and trustworthiness of qualitative research in clinical pharmacy. *Int J Clin Pharmacol*. 2016;38:641–646.
23. Barbour RS. Checklists for improving rigour in qualitative research: a case of the tail wagging the dog? *BMJ*. 2001;322:1115–1117.
24. Herber OR, Bradbury-Jones C, Böling S, et al. What feedback do reviewers give when reviewing qualitative manuscripts? A focused mapping review and synthesis. *BMC Med Res Methodol*. 2020;20:122.
25. Graneheim UH, Lundman B. Qualitative content analysis in nursing research: concepts, procedures and measures to achieve trustworthiness. *Nurs Educ Today*. 2004;24:105–112.
26. Kitto SC, Chesters J, Grbich C. Quality in qualitative research. Criteria for authors and assessors in the submission and assessment of qualitative research articles for the. *Med J Australia*. 2008;188:243–246.
27. Stige B, Malterud K, Midtgarden T. Toward an agenda for evaluation of qualitative research. *Qual Health Res*. 2009;19:1504–1516.
28. Rolfe G. Validity, trustworthiness and rigour: quality and the idea of qualitative research. *J Adv Nurs*. 2006;53:304–310.
29. Baker SE, Edwards R. *How Many Qualitative Interviews is Enough?: Expert Voices and Early Career Reflections on Sampling and Cases in Qualitative Research*. National Centre for Research Methods Review Paper; 2012.
30. Carlsen B, Glenton C. What about N? A methodological study of sample-size reporting in focus group studies. *BMC Med Res Methodol*. 2011;11:26.
31. Malterud K, Siersma VD, Guassora AD. Sample size in qualitative interview studies: guided by information power. *Qual Health Res*. 2016;26:1753–1760.
32. Saunders B, Sim J, Kingstone T, et al. Saturation in qualitative research: exploring its conceptualization and operationalization. *Qual Quant*. 2018;52:1893–1907.

Chapter 40

Contemporary conceptualization of measurement validity

Michael J. Peeters[a] and Spencer E. Harpe[b]

[a]*University of Toledo College of Pharmacy & Pharmaceutical Sciences, Toledo, OH, United States,* [b]*Department of Pharmacy Practice, Midwestern University College of Pharmacy, Downers Grove, IL, United States*

Objectives

- Describe measurement validity as different from other forms of validity (internal, external, and statistical conclusions).
- Explain current unitary concept of measurement validity.
- Outline evolution of measurement validity from early criterion-based conception to current unitary construct-based understanding.
- Describe key principles of validity assessment through the sources of validity evidence approach and the four types of inferences approach.
- Describe important considerations when reporting validity in pharmacy services research.

Introduction

The term "validity" has multiple uses and meanings in the scientific literature. Cor reminds us of four.[1] There are internal and external validity related to the study design and study sample. These are probably the most familiar to researchers. There is also statistical conclusion validity, which speaks to the appropriateness of the selected data analysis approaches in their ability to support the conclusions that are drawn. The fourth meaning of the term encompasses measurement validity and focuses on the mechanisms by which various phenomena are measured, as well as the interpretation and use of those measurements. While all of these meanings of validity are important, this chapter is focused specifically on measurement validity. Unless stated otherwise, the term "validity" when used in this chapter will refer to measurement validity.

Regardless of the particular area of research, validity is a vitally important concept in all research. The most recent edition of the *Standards for Educational and Psychological Testing*, jointly published by the American Educational Research Association, the American Psychological Association, and the National Council on Measurement in Education, describes validity as "the most fundamental consideration in developing and evaluating tests."[2] As discussed later in this chapter, conceptualization of validity has had a long history of incremental changes. This may have contributed to lack of clarity and enduring misunderstandings about validity. In fact, in his presidential address to the National Council on Measurement in Education, David Frisbie lamented that despite being central to educational testing and measurement validity is misunderstood, even by experts in the field.[3]

This chapter is designed to provide an overview of the contemporary conceptualization of measurement validity as it relates to pharmacy and health services research.[4] A review of the development of the concept of validity is included to provide some historical context surrounding changes in the concept of validity over time, as well as why it is important for researchers to be informed of these changes. Given the critical importance of validity, several important considerations when reporting research are reviewed at the end of the chapter. These considerations include a brief overview of different approaches to assessing validity.

What is validity?

According to the *Standards*, validity refers to "the degree to which evidence and theory support interpretations of test scores for proposed uses of tests."[2] Although the *Standards* are written to guide measurement in the educational and psychological

Contemporary Research Methods in Pharmacy and Health Services. https://doi.org/10.1016/B978-0-323-91888-6.00020-X

Precision (Reliability)

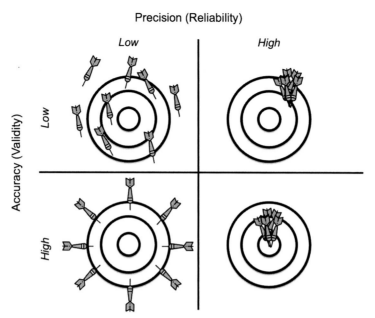

FIG. 1 Dartboard analogy for validity and reliability. *(Reproduced with permission from Peeters MJ, Harpe SE. Updating conceptions of validity and reliability.* Res Social Adm Pharm. *2020;16(8):1127–1130.)*

domains, the concepts apply more generally to measurement validity in any situation where psychosocial phenomena are being measured. Phenomena such as these are commonly of interest in pharmacy and health services research.

Researchers often first learn about validity and reliability using a common dartboard analogy that invokes accuracy and precision terminology (Fig. 1) during their own education. To briefly describe this dartboard analogy, the darts represent individual test scores, and multiple darts represent multiple students on a test. Alternatively, the darts could describe multiple test scores, longitudinally, for a single student. How close the group of darts land in relation to the dartboard's bullseye is *accuracy* and is typically framed as validity. How close the darts bunch together as a group denotes *precision*. In terms of testing or measurement, this is often framed as reliability. This analogy does help describe an initial dimension of the relationship between validity and reliability; however, the concept of validity and relationship with reliability does not end there and is more nuanced.

In the most recent edition of the *Standards*, validity is described as a single, unitary concept. Put another way, there is *one* validity. This unitary validity has *multiple sources* of evidence. As discussed later, reliability is one of these sources, thus validity subsumes reliability. The *Standards* affirm that reliability is important, but reliability alone is insufficient for characterizing the entirety of validity. Fig. 2 shows the broader, more complex description of validity as described in the current *Standards*.

Historical overview of the concept of validity

A brief overview of the evolution of validity theory is provided here. Terms here may be familiar to many as these have been used for the better part of the last century in social science research. What has changed over time is views on the nature of these terms and how they relate to each other. For those interested, this history has been described in greater detail by Kane.[5,6]

Over a century ago, a concept of *criterion validity* emerged as the gold standard to describe validity. In this conception, validity was an external relationship between a "real" attribute and scores from a measurement instrument. This criterion validity concept closely followed the commonly used—though misguided—language of measurement validity as an association with reality, such as with a diagnostic test being associated with disease or no disease (e.g., "this test is a valid measure"). This traditional conceptualization works as long as there is indeed an external standard that can be used as a basis for comparison. For example, criterion validity can be ascertained for troponins as a diagnostic test for myocardial infarction. This test result can be compared with later incidence of myocardial infarction by other diagnostic criteria, such as electrocardiogram or cardiac catheterization, with its associated sensitivity, specificity, positive predictive value, and negative predictive value.

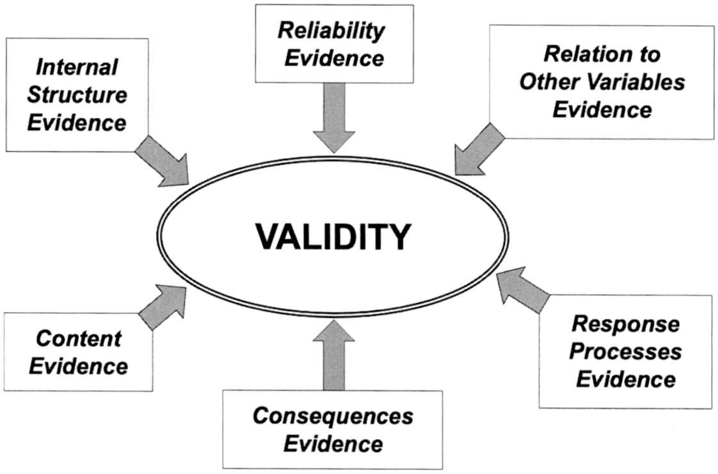

FIG. 2   Contemporary validity as described in the *Standards for Educational and Psychological Testing* (2014 edition). *(Reproduced with permission from Peeters MJ, Harpe SE. Updating conceptions of validity and reliability. Res Social Adm Pharm. 2020;16(8):1127–1130.)*

Criterion validity came in two versions: concurrent and predictive. Concurrent validity was most common and what we think of first when thinking of criterion validity—a proxy measure, such as a measurement instrument, was validated against a criterion. Alternatively, predictive validity was employed to illustrate how a proxy measure could predict future performance of a criterion (i.e., the criterion was not available at the time of testing). Both versions were about correlations with an external test or criterion.

This criterion-based validity framework did not hold when attempting to measure phenomena that are not able to be measured directly or indirectly in the physical world. Self-efficacy, knowledge, and health-related quality of life are a few examples of such phenomena. In such cases where there were no external standards in the physical world against which to compare the constructed measurement instruments, researchers turned their focus to a different approach to determining what an instrument was measuring. This gave rise to *content validity*, which was initially a more conceptual approach than statistical.

Subject matter experts most commonly assessed content validity, providing input on the extent to which the items in an instrument reflected content they understood that the instrument was trying to measure. If the subject matter experts concluded that the items "contained" or "covered" the phenomenon of interest, then the instrument was said to have content validity. Eventually, this "subject-matter expert" concept was extended to the construction of the measurement instrument itself.

As a somewhat related aspect of content validity, some researchers espoused an idea of assessing "face validity." This is not representative of validity in the truest sense of the term, certainly not as described in the *Standards*. Further, Messick, an influential voice in the development of contemporary validity theory, even described this as face *invalidity* and something that should be avoided.[7] Ultimately, the idea of "face validity" is not acceptable by contemporary standards and should not be used as an indicator of measurement validity.[8]

By the mid-20th century, researchers became increasingly unhappy with these limited criterion and content validity conceptualizations. The field shifted further to include *construct validity*, which focused on whether an instrument measured some underlying trait or phenomenon of interest. This went beyond the idea of content validity, which could be somewhat subjective. To make this determination of construct validity, various statistical methods including factor analysis and item response theory. For newly-developed measurement instruments, construct validity was demonstrated by identifying one or more underlying latent variables. Construct validity could also be supported by confirming the presence of previously identified latent variables when using an existing measurement instrument.

At this point in the evolution of validity theory, there were three types of measurement validity: *criterion, content* and *construct*. This aligned with the "trinitarian view" of validity commonly presented by Cronbach and Meehl.[9] Be aware that some texts have continued to use these validity "types" in their discussions of survey research.[10–12] Moreover, these three "types" of validity were often subdivided (e.g., criterion validity into predictive and concurrent validity; construct validity into convergent and divergent validity). Each validity type and subtype had its own assessment methods. Thus, any given measurement tool could be deemed "valid" by one method or multiple methods. For instance, a researcher might demonstrate strong construct validity for a measurement instrument but either no or weak criterion validity, thus yielding substantial confusion about the quality of that instrument. Researchers, educators, and program evaluators were left wondering which type of validity was most important. It was unclear which type of validity should receive the most focus or weight in validation processes.

The traditional conceptualization of validity viewed validity and reliability as separate properties of the measurement instrument itself. Assessments of validity were reported alongside reliability estimates in instrument development papers. Presenting them separately, but together, and in the context of instrument development seemed to reinforce the idea that these were separate properties related to the instrument itself. Previous editions of the *Standards* maintained separate chapters for validity and reliability, which may have apparently lent credence to the idea that reliability and validity were independent concepts. While the current edition maintains separate chapters, the language is clear that reliability is one source of validity evidence.[2]

Over the past few decades, the conceptual framework for validity and reliability have changed substantially, as reflected in the way that validity and reliability are now presented in the *Standards*.[2] This contemporary conceptualization of validity and reliability reflected changes in thinking as well as advances in social and psychological science in the preceding decades.[7,13] The culmination of these advances was a single unified theory of validity. Thus, measurement validity is now conceptualized within a unitary construct validity framework supported by multiple sources of evidence. The five sources of validity evidence are content, response process, internal structure, relation to other variables, and consequences (see Table 1).[2,13,14] There is some alignment between these different sources of validity evidence and the various historical conceptualizations of validity; however, it is crucial to note that this current framework does not support the idea of different "types" of measurement validity. As shown previously in this chapter, Fig. 2 illustrates this contemporary validity framework used in the *Standards*.

It is important to note the important role of reliability in this most recent validity framework. While reliability is a necessary source of evidence for validity, it is not sufficient to demonstrate reliability alone without other sources. Notably, as one important source of evidence for the internal structure of validity, the reliability of a measurement instrument within a group of individuals provides evidence toward a valid inference for use of those scores, from those individuals, and in that particular context. Whether formally calculated or not, every administration of a measurement instrument will have some

TABLE 1 Explanations of evidence sources towards validity.

Source of validity evidence	Explanation[a]
Content	• Description: relationship between the content of an instrument and the construct it is meant to measure • Assessment: examining the themes, wording, and format of the items, tasks, or questions in an instrument
Response process	• Description: fit between the construct being measured and the nature of the response processes or performance engaged in by respondents • Assessment: analysis of individual responses such as strategies to respond to or demonstrate behaviors for the measurement instrument (e.g., think aloud protocols), response times, skip patterns, and even eye movements
Internal structure	• Description: relationships among the various items within the instrument and how they conform to the intended construct being measured • Assessment: analysis of the factorial structure (identifying a new structure or confirming a previously identified structure) or differential item functioning
Relation to other variables	• Description: the extent to which the construct being measured relates to other variables • Assessment: correlation of the scores from the instrument with variables known to have or expected to have a particular relationship (both positive or negative)
Consequences	• Description: how well the use of the scores guides some intended decision (e.g., pass or fail a licensure exam or designate a patient as adherent or nonadherent) • Assessment: examine how well the decisions reflect actual performance or rating (e.g., does a candidate who fails a licensure exam actually lack the requisite knowledge and skills, and vice versa), examine intended and unintended consequences of using the scores

[a]*The assessment methods listed are not intended to be exhaustive. These are common examples that may be seen.*

degree of reliability. The importance of the wording in the contemporary framework bears repeating. The language for validity (including reliability) in the contemporary framework has shifted from focusing on the measurement instrument itself to focusing on a specific *use and interpretation of scores* from the measurement instrument.[14,15]

Discussing validity when reporting research

Given the importance of measurement validity in research, it is important to take steps to discuss the relevant validity concepts using the appropriate language in research reports. Other guidance exists on the general reporting of research in relation to certain study designs or research approaches. This final section focuses on four general considerations when describing validity or validation procedures in research reports.

First, researchers should be aware that they will likely encounter multiple concepts of validity when reading research articles. Some may be current, though others may involve dated validity conceptions. This may parallel the historical evolution discussed earlier and simply be an artifact of when an article was written. If an investigation is more recent, the validity conceptualization may unfortunately reflect that the authors' conception is outdated. While education and psychology have attempted to incorporate the current conception of validity into their work, this has been slower in other fields of research. There are examples using outdated and even potentially misleading discussions of validity in prominent resources, such as epidemiology textbooks,[10,16–18] online statistics resources,[19] and some medical textbooks.[20,21] Problematic Food and Drug Administration guidance and reviews of patient-reported outcomes are examples that even research areas particularly relevant to pharmacy are not immune.[22–24] Remain vigilant and informed as a reader and scholar.

Second, it is important to remember that validity is not an all-or-nothing premise (i.e., valid versus invalid). There are degrees of validity based on the quantity and quality of supporting evidence (i.e., stronger and weaker validity evidence). Similarly, a measurement instrument itself is neither valid nor validated. Instead, validity describes a specific use of an instrument within a specific group of participants, such as individuals with particular diagnosis receiving care in a particular institution or setting. While this may seem like a minor wording difference, this is an important and fundamental concept of the contemporary validity framework.

Third, reporting should start from a theoretical framework for validity. Best research practice involves using a clear theoretical framework to guide study development and implementation. When interventions are used, these should have a sound theoretical basis. This theoretical basis or framework is not the same thing as the validity or validation framework used for a study. Think of the validity or validation framework as a way to organize the assessment and reporting of the interpretations and decisions surrounding the measurement processes.

The validity framework described in the *Standards* and its associated five sources of validity evidence[2] have been used as the primary approach thus far in the chapter. As an alternative to the validity framework from the *Standards*, the perspective of validation can be used. Kane's framework for validation describes four categories of inference: scoring (generating a score from an observation), generalization (using a score as a reflection of the measured phenomenon in the setting or under the conditions where the observation is taking place), extrapolation (using the score as a reflection of the measured phenomenon in a general context, that is conditions or settings that are not similar to those during observation), and implications (using the score to make some decision or take an action).[6,25,26]

If a measurement instrument is created for the first time, which is not uncommon in pharmacy services research, the validity framework may be best. For most other situations where an existing measurement instrument is being used, a validation framework should be preferred. In these situations, the validation process relates to examining the evidence supporting the purpose of inference associated with the use of the measurement instrument. For example, the validation processes to support using a knowledge assessment for the purposes of determining the depth of knowledge for students in a class (generalization) compared to using that same assessment for graduation or licensure (implications) would be considerably different. While these two approaches (the five sources of validity evidence from the *Standards* and the four categories of inference in Kane's validation framework) may seem considerably different, there is substantial alignment between the two as shown in Table 2.

There is a fundamental difference between validity and validation. While some references, including the *Standards*, assert that validation is simply the process of generating validity evidence, this may be too simplistic. Validity is about generating evidence for a theoretical (ontological) claim.[27] One can generate much evidence to support a theory (validity); however, a theory (validity) can never be completely proven. On the other hand, validation is empirical process with data specific to your particular setting and with your specific users (e.g., learners or research participants). It is *your* interpretations and decisions based on data from *your* sample that are being empirically verified (or not) in *your* particular context of use. This is not a theoretical and ontological generality; this is an empirical assessment grounded in a specific context. Said another way, this difference between validity and validation is somewhat similar to differences between causality and

TABLE 2 Validity nomenclature, examples, and historical terms.

Kane's framework for validation	Sources of validity evidence (from the *Standards*)	Common applications	Historical validity terminology[a]
Scoring	Content Response process	• Items/skills scoring process • Test developer training/experience • Exam administration description • Rater training	Content validity
Generalization	Internal structure	• Reliability indices • Item difficulty and discrimination • Theories/models	Construct validity
Extrapolation	Relation to other variables (also content from external/expert verification)	• Comparison to standardized assessments • Expert panel validation	Criterion validity Discriminant validity Convergent validity Predictive validity Content validity
Implications	Consequences	• Standard setting • Impact on student practice behaviors • Instructor development-practice behaviors	

[a] *The unmodified use of these terms (e.g., "content validity was demonstrated" instead of "content sources of validity evidence") should be avoided since they can cause confusion and lack of alignment with the current validity framework.*
Modified from Peeters MJ, Martin BA. Validation of learning assessments: a primer. *Curr Pharm Teach Learn.* 2017;9(5):925–933.

causal inference. Causality is the more general premise, and one never "proves" causality. Instead, evidence from various sources is generated to support a hypothesized causal relationship. Each individual study providing supporting evidence will vary in terms of the strength of the causal inference afforded by the study design and data analysis. The evidence providing support for the causal relationship (or lack thereof) is continually accumulated over time. As Royal[28] states, validation is an ongoing process.

Fourth, context matters. It may be helpful to think of an intervention and its evaluation as being context specific (i.e., contained and not generalizable to other settings or other similar interventions). Even though the research may be conducted using a quantitative approach, there are still limits on generalizability. Unfortunately, it is not uncommon to see inappropriate generalizations about a particular study intervention. Instead, consider the quantitative findings (if good validity evidence exists) as generalizing to other similar participants in the same (or a substantially similar) context that are exposed to that intervention. Again, this aligns with the current conceptualization of validity whereby the measurement of some phenomenon is necessarily unique to a particular setting, population, and purpose. Appropriate use of some measurement instrument in another setting and generalizing the findings to another setting requires generating validation evidence to support that higher level of generalization.

Conclusions

While the concept of measurement validity seems straightforward, this concept can be deceptively complex. Over the past century, the view of measurement validity has evolved from a property of a measurement instrument to a more nuanced reflection of how scores from a particular instrument used in a specific sample at a specific time and place are interpreted and used for a particular purpose. When reading the work of others and reporting their own work, researchers need to be cognizant that the concept of validity has evolved. As a community of scholars, all researchers should use this contemporary conceptualization of validity, be familiar with the updated processes for generating validation evidence with measurement tools, endeavor to communicate these processes and their results using appropriate terminology, and promote the uptake of these updated concepts among their peers.

Discussion questions

1. What are the four general types of validity mentioned in research? Briefly describe the focus of each.
2. Briefly describe the current conceptualization of measurement validity (such as described in the *Standards for Educational and Psychological Testing*) and how it differs from the historical view(s) of validity.
3. When might a validity framework be preferred over a validation framework when considering measurement validity?
4. Which source of validity evidence can include examination of how well the items in a measurement instrument actually cover the intended topics related to the phenomenon of interest?
5. In Kane's validation framework, evidence for what type of validation inference would be most relevant when trying to justify using a measure of health-related quality of life in routine clinical practice (i.e., not in a research study)?

Application exercise/scenario

Your research team is interested in identifying various factors that may relate to the use of quality improvement (QI) methods in nonteaching community hospital pharmacies. After completing the literature review, the team determined that organizational safety climate is an important factor to consider. One of the team members identified a potential measurement instrument for this concept. The article describing the development of this instrument, as well as several other research reports using the instrument, mention that it is a "valid measure the organizational safety climate in healthcare settings." Upon further reading, you notice that the instrument was developed and has mainly been used in large academic medical centers with only one study reporting use in a group of nursing homes. Your research team member who identified the instrument is advocating for its use since it has been proven to be valid so it can be used in any setting. How would you respond to this team member regarding validity? What validation evidence should be generated to determine whether using the instrument in your group of hospitals is appropriate?

References

1. Cor MK. Trust me, it is valid: research validity in pharmacy education research. *Curr Pharm Teach Learn.* 2016;8(3):391–400.
2. American Educational Research Association, American Psychological Association, and National Council on Measurement in Education. *Standards for Educational and Psychological Testing.* Washington, DC: American Psychological Association; 2014.
3. Frisbie DA. Measurement 101: some fundamentals revisited. *Educ Meas Issues Pract.* 2005;24(3):21–28.
4. Peeters MJ, Harpe SE. Updating conceptions of validity and reliability. *Res Soc Adm Pharm.* 2020;16(8):1127–1130.
5. Kane MT. Validating the interpretations and uses of test scores. *J Educ Meas.* 2013;50(1):1–73.
6. Kane MT. Validation. In: Brennan RL, ed. *Educational Measurement.* 4th ed. Portsmouth, NH: American Council on Education; 2006:17–64.
7. Messick S. Validity. In: Linn RL, ed. *Educational Measurement.* 3rd ed. New York, NY: American Council on Education/Macmillan; 1989:3–103.
8. Downing SM, Haladyna TM. Validity threats: overcoming interference with proposed interpretations of assessment data. *Med Educ.* 2004;38(3):327–333.
9. Cronbach LJ, Meehl PE. Construct validity in psychological tests. *Psychol Bull.* 1955;52(4):281–302.
10. Rothman KJ, Greenland S, Lash TL. *Modern Epidemiology.* 3rd ed. Philadelphia, PA: Lippincott Williams & Wilkins; 2008.
11. Kimberlin CL, Winterstein AG. Validity and reliability of measurement instruments used in research. *Am J Health Syst Pharm.* 2008;65(23):2276–2284.
12. Burns SK, Gray JR, Grove N. *Understanding Nursing Research: Building an Evidence-Based Practice.* 6th ed. St. Louis, MO: Elsevier Saunders; 2015.
13. Downing SM. Validity: on the meaningful interpretation of assessment data. *Med Educ.* 2003;37(9):830–837.
14. Newton PE, Shaw SD. Standards for talking and thinking about validity. *Psychol Methods.* 2013;18(3):301–319.
15. St-Onge C, Young M, Eva KW, Hodges B. Validity: one word with a plurality of meanings. *Adv Health Sci Educ.* 2017;22(4):853–867.
16. Hulley SB, Cummings SR, Browner WS, Grady DG, Newman TB. *Designing Clinical Research.* 3rd ed. Philadelphia, PA: Lippincott Williams & Wilkins; 2007.
17. Dawson B, Trapp RG. *Basic and Clinical Biostatistics.* 4th ed. New York, NY: McGraw-Hill; 2004.
18. Gordis L. *Epidemiology.* 5th ed. Philadelphia, PA: Elsevier Saunders; 2014.
19. Stephanie G. Reliability and Validity in Research: Definitions, Examples. From StatisticsHowTo.com: Elementary Statistics for the Rest of Us! Available from: https://www.statisticshowto.com/reliability-validity-definitions-examples/, 2021. Accessed 10 May 2021.
20. Bender DA, Varghese J, Jacob M, Murray RK. Clinical biochemistry. In: Rodwell VW, Bender DA, Botham KM, Kennelly PJ, Well P, eds. *Harper's Illustrated Biochemistry.* 30th ed. New York, NY: McGraw-Hill; 2015.

21. Walker JS, Roback HB, Welch L. Psychological and neuropsychological assessment. In: Ebert MH, Loosen PT, Nurcombe B, Leckman JF, eds. *Current Diagnosis & Treatment: Psychiatry.* 2nd ed. New York, NY: McGraw-Hill; 2008 [chapter 6].

22. US Department of Health and Human Services Food and Drug Administration. *Guidance for Industry: Patient-Reported Outcome Measures: Use in Medical Product Development to Support Labeling Claims.* Silver Springs, MD: Food and Drug Administration; 2009.

23. Gabriel SE, Normand SLT. Getting the methods right—the foundation of patient-centered outcomes research. *N Engl J Med.* 2007;367(9):787–790.

24. Rothrock NE, Kaiser KA, Cella D. Developing a valid patient-reported outcome measure. *Clin Pharmacol Ther.* 2011;90(5):737–742.

25. Peeters MJ, Martin BA. Validation of learning assessments: a primer. *Curr Pharm Teach Learn.* 2017;9(5):925–933.

26. Cook DA, Brydges R, Ginsburg S, Hatala R. A contemporary approach to validity arguments: a practical guide to Kane's framework. *Med Educ.* 2015;49(6):560–575.

27. Borsboom D, Mellenbergh GJ, van Heerden J. The concept of validity. *Psychol Rev.* 2004;111(4):1061–1071.

28. Royal KD. Four tenets of modern validity theory for medical education assessment and evaluation. *Adv Med Educ Pract.* 2017;8:567–570.

Chapter 41

A practical approach to the assessment and quantification of content validity

Enas Almanasreh[a,b], Rebekah J. Moles[b], and Timothy F. Chen[b]

[a]*Faculty of Pharmacy, Mutah University, Al-Karak, Jordan*, [b]*The University of Sydney School of Pharmacy, Faculty of Medicine and Health, The University of Sydney, Sydney, NSW, Australia*

Objectives

- Define content validity and discuss it within the context of other types of validity and reliability measures.
- Describe the various stages associated with the assessment of content validity.
- Explain various content validity-related measures along with their most salient uses and drawbacks, or caveats to their usage.
- Discuss the concept of agreement, how it relates to content validity, and the importance of agreement among multiple raters.

Introduction

The development and application of tools to measure complex constructs or outcomes which cannot be observed and measured directly are common in healthcare practice and research. Measurement of these constructs can be essential for the evaluation of health outcomes and for guiding clinical decision making. However, in order for these tools to be of value, their psychometric properties need to be confirmed to ensure reliability and validity.[1] Examples of complex constructs which are often evaluated in social and administrative pharmacy research include phenomena such as quality of life, medication adherence, and healthcare professional attitudes.[2] Quantification or measurement of these constructs first requires operational definitions, followed by the development of items and scales which reflect the concepts.[1–3] While interpreting data from objective sources such as laboratory or diagnostic tests is relatively straightforward, given established reliability and validity data on these measures including standardized margin of error, instruments used to measure complex constructs in social and administrative pharmacy research and clinical practice, do not always have established psychometric properties and require expertise for their development and interpretation.[2]

To draw inferences from these measurements, the utilized instruments require a robust development process and psychometric testing for their validity and reliability to capture the "subjective" phenomena, to control for known sources of error, and to assist in the development, implementation, and assessment of required interventions. Miller et al. stated that without reliable and valid measures of subjective health-related constructs, research findings are of questionable value.[4] A recent systematic review on the measurements of patient safety proposed that using nonvalid or unreliable instruments can lead to inaccurate diagnosis of patient safety problems and implementation of inappropriate preventive strategies.[5] One of the most common challenges often confronted in health and social science research is ascertaining the validity and reliability of a measurement instrument.

Validity is a critical factor in the selection and application of an instrument, in practice and research. It may be defined as "the degree to which evidence and theory support the interpretation of test scores entailed by the proposed use of tests."[6] In other words, validity is the extent to which the instrument measures what it intends to measure.[7] Construct validation focuses on instrument content, internal structure of the instrument, response processes, the relationships among instrument scores and other variables, and testing consequences.[6,8] Construct validity should be utilized to evaluate the utility and appropriateness of an instrument for a particular purpose and to determine the degree of confidence we can place on the inferences made, using that instrument.[9] Hence, the validity is not a property of the instrument, rather it refers to the instrument's scores and interpretations.[10] Validity can be divided into different types including content validity, criterion validity, and construct validity.[9] In addition, construct validity can be subdivided into convergent/ divergent and discriminant validity.[11] Although there has been little debate about the importance of criterion and

Contemporary Research Methods in Pharmacy and Health Services. https://doi.org/10.1016/B978-0-323-91888-6.00013-2

construct validity of a newly developed instrument, the concept of content validity has been somewhat controversial since its establishment.[12]

Several definitions of content validity have emerged since the 1950s, when different thoughts and notions concerning the conception and practice of test validation were developed. Content validity was defined for the first time by Lennon (1956) as "the extent to which a subject's responses to the items of a test may be considered to be a representative sample of his responses to a real or hypothetical universe of situations which together constitute the area of concern to the person interpreting the test."[13] In 1971, Cronbach reported a definition of content validity as the extent to which the items on an instrument are sampled adequately from the specified domain of content.[14] Since that time numerous definitions of content validity have been published in the literature. While phrased differently, there is a general consensus in theses definitions that content validity refers to the extent to which the sampled items adequately reflect the domain and operational definition of the construct.

Some theorists hold the view that the term content validity is technically incorrect and it is not considered as an aspect of validity.[11] However, this view is not universally accepted and different standards and regulations used in psychological testing state that content validity is essential to determine that an instrument is of sound quality.[12,15,16] To test the status of patient's health, for example, the Food and Drug Administration (FDA) provides guidance to evaluate and review patient-reported outcome (PRO) instruments used to measure treatment benefit or risk associated with medical products, based on their conceptual framework and content validity. The FDA encourages instrument developers to provide evidence of instrument content and item generation using literature review, expert input, and target patient population input.[17] In addition, several behavioral scientists argue that instruments utilized in the assessment of social measures must be content valid.[16] Despite this debate around "content validity" and its importance in psychometric analysis, validity testing is a sequential process starting from measuring the content validity and continuing through to more sophisticated types of validity measures such as relationships or the power of predictability provided by the obtained scores of the tested instrument. It is almost certain that demonstrating other forms of validity like criterion validity or construct validity of an instrument before examining the validity of its content may contribute to a real threat to the quality of the tested instrument. In addition, poor ordering of validity testing may extend the time of the evaluation process because the instrument will require more revisions in the testing phase.[18] Similarly, Norbeck et al. (1985) notified that there is no sense in testing the reliability of an instrument which has poor content validity.[19] Therefore, the minimum requirement for any developed instrument is to have sufficient content validity to advocate the representativeness of its content and appropriateness of its development process and this is considered as a fundamental part of the validation assessment process. The standards and importance of validating health measures in term of definitions and content were discussed in 1987.[3] However, several studies have reported the lack of validity assessments for instruments utilized in clinical practice and healthcare research.[5,20–22] Furthermore, others have noticed that some instruments have been reported as content valid in terms of what the instrument developers want to measure, rather than in terms of its actual content.[3,22] The aims of this chapter are to investigate the elements of content validity; to describe the practical approach for assessing content validity; and to discuss existing content validity indices.

In this chapter, the word "instrument" refers to any form of measure including scales, tests, tools, questionnaires, and surveys.

Components of content validity

Content validity provides evidence about the degree to which elements of an assessment instrument are relevant to and representative of the targeted construct for a particular assessment purpose. Four essential components of content validity have been discussed in the literature: *domain definition, domain representation, domain relevance, and appropriateness of test construction procedure*.[15,16] Domain definition indicates how the concept or phenomena measured by an instrument is operationally defined. This element has a central role in evaluating content validity as it provides information about the conceptual (theory-based) and operational definitions of the construct and what the instrument measures.[23] Domain representation refers to the degree to which a test adequately represents and measures the domain of the targeted construct. The third element, the content relevance, addresses the degree to which each element of an instrument is relevant to the particular domain. The fourth element, appropriateness of test construction procedure, concerns all processes utilized while constructing the instrument to ensure the representativeness and relevance of the elements.[15]

Based on these elements, there are two threats to content validity which can occur during the assembling of the elements of a certain construct. First, *construct-irrelevant content* which indicates inclusion of extraneous elements beyond the core concept of the construct for which a score is to be interpreted.[24] Therefore, to avoid the potential threat of relevance, researchers need to carefully apply both theory and the judgments of experts in the field to justify excluding or including a certain element in the construct of interest, taking into consideration the objective of the study and the appropriateness of selected elements to the chosen operational definitions. The second type of threat happens when the actual content of an instrument fails to represent the entire scope of content relevant to the construct; this is referred to as *content-under representations.*[24] Besides under-representation, excluding and over-represented elements which are required to measure the construct are considered as representativeness' threats as well. These threats will reduce the content validity of an instrument and increase the uncertainty of the inferences drawn when using this construct. For example, using irrelevant items or excluding important items during the development process of the construct can jeopardize the internal consistency of the construct and can interfere with the relationships and correlations between the items under certain factors or domains.

Assessment of the content validity

Content validity differs from other types of validity in that it refers to test-based rather than score-based validity. It describes the required elements of the content for the instrument and is not related to the scores obtained from that construct.[16] However, establishing a content valid measure of an abstracted theoretical concept is not as straightforward as it looks and can be a complex process.[25] Content validity evidence plays a central role in the development and testing processes for any developed instrument and it should not be misinterpreted as less rigorous evidence referred to as face validity.[23] Face validity is an empirical assessment of the soundness of the construct, but it is not quantifiable and is not considered as important in psychometric testing.[23] In contrast, content validity should acquire the highest priority during the development process as it is a prerequisite for evaluating other types of validity.[26] This section provides a practical guide for evaluating content validity.

The assessment of content validity commences in the earliest stages of development of an instrument[27] and involves a panel of experts who evaluate instrument elements and rate them based on their relevance and representativeness to the content domain. Researchers can receive invaluable information if they conduct the content validation in a systemic and comprehensive manner.[18] Therefore, using a single-stage process (either development or judgment) to evaluate the content validity is usually not sufficient and may produce a construct with low quality.[27] Lynn (1986) suggests a two-stage process (development and judgment-quantification) to evaluate the content validity of all instruments. Therefore, these two stages are considered essential in the development of instruments designed to measure complex phenomena and constructs. However, a third stage (revising and reconstruction/reformation) should also be added after the judgment and quantification stage.[27]

Development stage

This stage has three steps: *domain identification, item generation, and instrument formation.* These steps differ in context based on the function of the instrument that is whether it is a cognitive or affective measure[27–29] (for more details, see Lynn, 1986).

In addition to these steps in instrument development, it is also necessary to consider the conceptual and the operational definitions of the construct to be measured. The conceptual definitions are theory-based and/or informed by the experience of the researcher team and confirmed by the literature.[30] The conceptual definition will be the cornerstone of the subsequent steps of instrument development. The operational definitions are extremely important for content validation and form the basis from which the instrument developer samples the items from the content domain identified by the conceptual definition.[26] Therefore, to avoid incongruity between the conceptual definitions and the operationalization of the content domain of an instrument, both the conceptual and the operational definitions should be defined carefully before developing other elements of the instrument.[23,25,31] This step is essential and should be the first step in the development stage of a content valid instrument. Correspondingly, generated items in the second step should be defined and clarified to facilitate the process of content validation. Inadequate definitions at this stage of content validation will likely complicate subsequent psychometric analyses.[25] Hence, comprehensive evaluation of all available sources of information, literature reviews, and interviews with experts or relevant populations to identify content domains and related components is critical. In brief, the development stage has four steps: *concept definition and formulation, domain definition and identification, item generation and definition, and instrument construction* (Fig. 1).

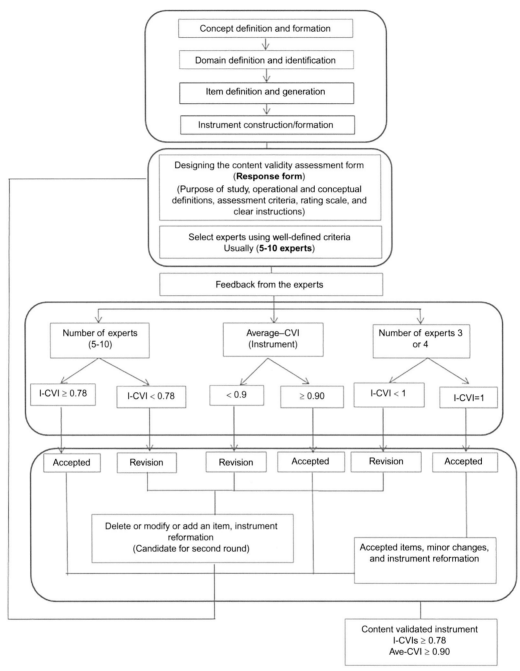

FIG. 1 Flow diagram describes the process of content validity evaluation of an instrument.

Judgment-quantifying stage

Judgment stage (expert opinion)

The second stage of content validation commences after a precise definition of the construct has been established, the generated items have been organized, and the instrument has been assembled. The judgment-quantification stage entails inviting a group of experts to determine the adequacy with which relevant content domains have been included in the instrument and the extent to which the instrument was developed to measure a particular concept of interest.[28] Although content validity relies on the subjective judgments of experts, the selection of experts to review and critique the content of an instrument should be based on well-defined criteria such as qualifications, experience, clinical expertise, and relevant training of content experts.[32,33] Grant and Davis provide a guideline for selecting and using content experts for instrument development.[32] There is currently no consensus on the number of content experts required to review an instrument. Lynn (1986) suggested a minimum of three. However, others recommend between 3 and 20 panel members.[31,34] Grant and Davis proposed that the final decision on the number of experts needed for content validity depends on the desired level of expertise and the range of knowledge representation of the panel.[32] The maximum number of experts has not been specified, but, often up to 10 experts are used. Using a larger number of experts will decrease the probability of chance agreement and may better inform instrument development.[18] Therefore, it is suggested to include between 5 and 10 experts in the content validation process.

Initially, an invitation letter, email, or telephone call requesting an expert's participation is recommended before conducting the study. Once the instrument developer receives a positive response regarding participation, the content validity study can be started. Experts should have the necessary content expertise and theoretical background in order to provide a comprehensive assessment of the instrument. Accordingly, an information kit or booklet for distribution to experts should contain a cover letter, content validity assessment form (response form), and a copy of the developed instrument. The cover letter should include the purpose of a study, a brief description of the instrument and its scoring, and a description of the content validity form.[18] Designing the content validity assessment form (response form) should be the first step in the judgment and quantification stage in particular, because any obtained information from the experts are dependent on the arrangement and quality of this form. The representativeness and relevance of the content domains and clarity of each item are essential and are the most common criteria utilized in the content validity assessment form. The uniqueness of the item, importance of the item, and clarity of the definition of the item may also be considered as assessment criteria. Each item on the instrument is rated on a rating scale for the specified assessment criteria. It is critical that the expert possesses the conceptual definition and the operational definition of the construct as this will facilitate rating the quality of the items. The clarity and comprehensiveness of theses definitions may be assessed by the experts. In the assessment process, the expert can be invited to suggest additional items or deletion of any item, evaluate the wording of each item, and provide any other comments. Thus, a structured content validity assessment form is essential in the judgment and quantification stage.

Quantification of content validity

After receiving responses from expert panel members, quantitative and qualitative analyses can be conducted. There is no uniform approach for examining the content validity of an instrument nor is there any one statistical method. However, a number of quantitative indices for two or more raters have been suggested.[35] In this chapter, these methods are divided into two categories: content validity-related indices and general agreement indices (Table 1).

Content validity-related estimates

Content validity ratio (Lawshe's method) One approach to achieving content validity includes a panel of experts considering the relevance of individual items within an instrument. The content validity ratio (CVR), an item statistic originally suggested by Lawshe (1975), is one of the most widely used methods for quantifying content validity. The panel of experts in the CVR approach are invited to rate each item into one of three categories: "Essential," "Useful, but not essential," or "Not necessary." Items considered "essential" by a critical number of experts are then included in the final form, with items failing to reach this critical level rejected.[38] After items have been recognized for inclusion in the final instrument, the content validity index (CVI) is calculated for the entire instrument. The CVI represents the average of the CVR values of the retained items. Based on established psychophysical principles, Lawshe proposed that a level of 50% agreement assures some degree of content validity. The CVR is a direct linear transformation of a proportional level of agreement on how many experts assess an item "essential" calculated by using this formula: $CVR = (n_e - N/2)/(N/2)$, where CVR is the content validity ratio, n_e is the number of panelists indicating an item "essential" and N is the total number of panel members. CVR values can range between 1 (perfect agreement) and -1 (perfect disagreement), and a value of 0 indicates that half of the panel experts agree an item is essential.[38] To ensure that the agreements between experts are not due to chance, Lawshe provided a table of critical CVR ($CVR_{critical}$) values calculated by his colleague Schipper, where $CVR_{critical}$ is the minimum value of CVR such that the level of agreement exceeds that of chance for a given item, for a given alpha (Type I error probability, one tailed test $P = 0.05$).[39] $CVR_{critical}$ values can be utilized to identify the number of panel experts required to agree on an item as essential and the items which should be retained or discarded from the final instrument. Although the CVR is easy to compute, several concerns have been raised as the original methods of calculating the $CVR_{critical}$ were not reported in the literature, which make the interpretation process difficult.[37,39,40]

TABLE 1 Definition, calculations, and characteristics of content validity estimates.

Index	Definitions/Calculations	Characteristics
1. Content validity-related estimates		
Content Validity Ratio (CVR)— Lawshe (1975)	CVR is a method for measuring agreement among experts regarding how essential a particular item is $CVR = (n_e - N/2)/(N/2)$, where CVR is the content validity ratio, n_e is the number of panelists indicating an item "essential," and N is the total number of panel members If you have 10 experts and 8 rated an item as essential. The CVR would be $(8-5/5) = 0.60$. The CVI for the entire instrument is the mean CVR for all retained items	1. Easy to compute 2. CVR value is computed for each item so it is useful in the discarded or retention of specific items 3. Rating scale used for rating items: "essential," "useful but not essential," or "not necessary" 4. CVR values range from -1.0 to $+1.0$ 5. CVR value is determined by Lawshe Table 6. Cut-off point value depends on the number of experts *Limitations*: 1. Not easy to interpret as the calculations related to $CVR_{critical}$ were not reported in the literature
CVI for each item (I-CVI)	The CVI for each item is the proportion of experts who rate the item as a 3 or 4 on a 4-point Likert scale *Example*: 7 of 10 content experts rated an item as relevant (3 or 4), the CVI would be: $7/10 = 0.70$ *Lynn (1986) approach*: The item would be discarded because it would not meet the **0.80** level of endorsement required to establish content validity using a panel of 10 experts at the 0.05 level of significance *Polit et al. (2007) approach*: The item would be considered for revision because the I-CVI is somewhat lower than 0.**78**	1. Simple and easy to compute 2. Easily understood and interpreted 3. It is computed for each item and assists in revising, deleting, or substituting items 4. The method of calculating the item-CVI is similar between the two approaches 5. In both approaches, the minimum number of experts required is three 6. *Lynn (1986) approach* recommends that 100% agreement is required with fewer than six experts. *Polit et al. (2007) approach* requires perfect agreement when there are three or four experts 7. *Lynn (1986) approach*: Cut-off point value depends on the number of experts and is determined by applying the standard error of the proportion. *Polit et al. (2007) approach*: The cut-off of the I-CVI is 0.78 or higher. *Limitations*: 1. Inflation of agreement due to chance
Average-CVI (Ave-CVI)*	There are three ways to calculate the Ave-CVI (Table 2). 1. Average the proportion of items rated relevant across experts (Table 2) 2. Sum the I-CVIs and divide by the number of items (Table 2) 3. Count the total number of ratings rated as 3 or 4 and divide by the total number of ratings. **Example** (Table 2): 59 of 70 answers were deemed content valid (3 or 4). The Ave-CVI would be: $59/70 = 0.84$)	1. It represents the content validity of the overall instrument 2. The acceptable standard of Ave-CVI is different in the literature and ranges from 0.8 to 0.9 3. Ave-CVI calculated by average I-CVI values is recommended in content validity because it focuses on the quality of items rather than the performance of experts
Universal-CVI (UA-CVI)	Proportion of items on an instrument which achieves a relevance rating of 3 or 4 by **all** the experts *Example*: Number of items considered relevant by all experts $= 3$, total number of items $= 10$ *UA-CVI*: $3/10 = 0.30$	1. It represents the content validity of the overall instrument 2. Conservative and demands 100% agreement 3. Hard to achieve an acceptable standard when the number of experts increases 4. Reporting the value of UA-CVI with the Ave-CVI is recommended for a more informative procedure
The modified kappa (κ^*)	A new approach for quantifying the content validity suggested by Polit et al. (2007). It adjusts each value of I-CVI for chance of agreement *Calculations*: 1. Calculate the probability of chance of agreement: $p_c = [N!/A! (N - A)!] \times 0.5^N$, where $N =$ the number of experts and $A =$ number of agreeing on good relevance 2. Calculate I-CVI for each item 3. Calculate modified kappa:	1. There is no need to actually calculate κ^* and you can use a provided table of standards κ^* related to the I-CVI[37] 2. It is computed for each item and assists in revising, deleting, or substituting items 3. Evaluation criteria for kappa: *fair* (0.40–0.59), *good* (0.60–0.74), or *excellent* ($= \kappa > 0.74$)

TABLE 1 Definition, calculations, and characteristics of content validity estimates—cont'd

Index	Definitions/Calculations	Characteristics
	$\kappa^* = (\text{I-CVI} - p_c)/(1 - p_c)$ If 6 of 7 experts rated an item as relevant, the I-CVI = 6/7 = 0.86 and the κ^* value would be 0.85 (Excellent)	
2. General agreement estimates		
Interrater agreement indices	Cohen Kappa K, Fleiss Kappa (multirater kappa), Weighted Kappa (ordinal data), T index (Tinssly and Weiss 1975); rWG (James, Demaree and Wolf 1984); r*WG (Lindell, Brandt, and Whitney, 1999), Kendall's coefficient of concordance (W), Krippendorff's alpha coefficient, and Gwet's AC1 *Each test has different assumptions and applications, discussed extensively in the literature. The different assumptions have not been discussed in this chapter*	1. They were designed and developed to evaluate the general interrater agreement among different raters but not for the purpose of quantifying content validity 2. They measure the full interrater agreement regardless the type (agree or disagree) 3. They adjust the risk of the chance agreement 3. Should be interpreted carefully if they are used for the purpose of content validation

I-CVI, content validity index of an item; Ave-CVI, content validity index of the entire instrument, averaging calculation method; UA-CVI, content validity index of the entire instrument, *Universal agreement* calculation method; CVR, content validity ratio; p_c, probability of chance of agreement; K^*, the modified Kappa.

Content validity index (CVI) The most widely utilized method of quantifying the content validity for an instrument is the content validity index (CVI). It can be calculated for each item on an instrument (item level-CVI or I-CVI) along with the content validity index for the overall instrument (instrument level-CVI). The CVI is based on expert ratings for each item based on the content relevance or representativeness of an instrument, usually on 4-point Likert scales ranging from 1 (not relevant or not representative) to 4 (extremely relevant or representative). For each item, the I-CVI can be calculated by counting the number of experts who rated the item as 3 or 4 and dividing that number by the total number of experts, that is the proportion of agreement about the content validity of an item.[37] One limitation which has been posed in the literature about considering the CVI as an index of interrater agreement is the potential for inflation of agreement due to chance factors.[41] Lynn (1986) provided a guideline for the number of experts and the minimum number of experts who must agree with the content of the item or instrument to achieve an acceptable CVI by applying the standard error of the proportion. In addition, Lynn (1986) stated that using a 4-point rating scale is preferable over a 3- or 5-point rating scale because it does not include the ambivalent middle rating and it provides sufficient delineated information upon which to calculate a meaningful CVI. However, using a 4-point Likert scale is debatable because this approach of calculating the CVI indicates that ratings of 1 and 2 are considered "content invalid" whereas ratings of 3 and 4 are considered "content valid," collapsing four ordinal levels into two dichotomous categories increases the possibility that experts will agree by chance alone 50% of the time regardless of the number of experts used. There may also be a risk of losing critical information when the original scale is no longer available.[41] Furthermore, using a 4-point rating scale produces a forced choice (forces rater to give certain tendency) where no option is available for the rater to be unsure or neutral. Therefore, a 5- or 3-point rating scale is recommended especially for the first round.

Two methods for computing the overall content validity index of an instrument have been reported. One approach is the universal-CVI (UA-CVI), defined as "the proportion of items on an instrument that achieved a rating of 3 or 4 (valid) by *all* the content experts." Most studies in the literature avoid using UA-CVI approach since as it is conservative and demands 100% agreement. In addition, it is difficult to achieve especially when the number of experts increases. A more flexible approach for the overall instrument-CVI, Average-CVI (Ave-CVI), is defined as "the average proportion of items rated as 3 or 4 (valid) across the various experts."[36] There are three methods to calculate the Ave-CVI, the first is by calculating the average CVI across the items (summing the I-CVIs and dividing them by the number of items); the second way is by counting the total number of ratings multiplied by the number of items rated relevant by all experts combined, and then dividing by the total number of ratings. The third way is average the proportion of items rated relevant across experts. It is noteworthy that all of these approaches will always yield the same value (Table 2).[36] Polit and Beck (2006) suggested using the average I-CVI value because this is more related to the quality of the items rather than

TABLE 2 Fictitious ratings on a 10-item using a 4-point rating relevance scale (3, 4—relevant), (1, 2—not relevant).

Item	Expert1	Expert2	Expert3	Expert4	Expert5	Expert6	Exper7	Number of agreement	Item-CVI[a]
1	3	4	4	3	3	4	4	7	1.00
2	4	2	4	3	3	3	4	6	0.86
3	2	2	4	4	3	3	1	4	0.57
4	4	3	2	4	3	3	4	6	0.86
5	4	3	3	3	1	2	4	5	0.71
6	3	4	2	3	3	3	3	5	0.71
7	3	4	4	1	3	3	2	5	0.71
8	3	4	4	3	3	4	4	7	1.00
9	3	4	3	4	4	3	3	7	1.00
10	1	3	4	3	3	4	3	6	0.86
								Ave-CVI[b]	**0.83**
								UA-CVI[c]	**0.30**
Number of agreement	8	8	8	9	9	9	8	**Ave-proportion of agreement across experts[d] (Mean expert proportion)**	**0.83**
Proportion of agreement	0.80	0.80	0.80	0.90	0.90	0.90	0.80		

[a]*Item-CVI = number of experts rating the item either 3 or 4/total number of experts.*
[b]*Ave-CVI = sum of the I-CVIs (I-CVI$_1$ + I-CVI$_2$ + I-CVI$_3$ + ⋯ + I-CVI$_n$)/total number of items.*
[c]*UA-CVI = number of items that achieved rating 3 or 4 by all experts/total number of items.*
[d]*Ave-proportion of agreement across experts = proportion of agreement of each expert/total number of experts.*
I-CVI, content validity index of an item; Ave-CVI, content validity index of the entire instrument, averaging calculation method; UA-CVI, content validity index of the entire instrument; *Universal agreement* calculation method.
(Adapted from Polit DF, Beck CT. The content validity index: are you sure you know what's being reported? Critique and recommendations. Res Nurs Health 2006;29(5):489–497.[36])

the performance of experts. However, the third approach identifies the expert's performance, and this might be helpful in selecting the experts for the second or third rounds if required.[36]

Another index is the average congruency percentage (ACP). This index can be calculated by computing the percentage of items rated relevant for each expert and then taking the average of the percentage across experts. This index is identical to the Ave-CVI. Davis (1992) suggested a standard criterion of 0.8 as the lower limit of acceptability of a CVI of an instrument. However, Waltz et al. (2005) recommended that an ACP of 0.90 is considered acceptable rather than 0.80. Polit and Beck (2006) have criticized the content validity index details, and they recommended using Lynn's criteria for calculating the I-CVI (I-CVI = 1 with 3 or 5 experts and a minimum I-CVI of 0.78 for 6–10 experts) and an Ave-CVI of 0.90 or higher for excellent content validity of an instrument.[36] It should be noted that Polit et al. (2007) recommended perfect agreement only when there are three or four experts.

Despite the differences between indices, the CVI remains essential and carries several advantages compared to other estimates. CVI is simple and easy to compute, easily understood and interpreted, and provides content validity of each item and the instrument as a whole. Also, it can be utilized to assess the performance of experts, and most importantly, it allows the instrument developer to make a decision to retain or exclude items from an instrument.

The modified–kappa The CVI (and proportion of agreement indices) have limitations. Cohen (1960) recognized the disadvantages of the proportion of agreement and described this method as a "most primitive approach." Cohen introduced a coefficient kappa (κ) for appraising interrater agreement. The kappa statistic represents the proportion of agreement remaining after a chance of agreement is removed.[41] However, the CVI possesses an advantage over kappa and other interrater agreement indices which capture the interrater agreement of relevance but not the full interrater agreement (relevance and nonrelevance).[37] Polit et al. (2007) suggested a new approach for the content validity called a modified kappa κ^* that adjusts each I-CVI for chance agreement. This index captures the agreement among experts for items of relevance and excludes the agreement of nonrelevance. There is no need to actually compute the value of K^* because Polit et al. (2007) have provided a table of standards κ^* related to the I-CVI. To calculate κ^*, the probability of chance agreement was initially calculated by using this formula $p_c = [N!/A! \, (N - A)!] \times 0.5^N$ where N = the number of experts and A = number agreeing on relevance. After computing the I-CVI for all items, the Kappa modified (κ^*) can be calculated by using the value of p_c (probability of chance agreement) and I-CVI by using the following equation: $\kappa^* = (\text{I-CVI} - p_c)/(1 - p_c)$.[37] Several standards for evaluating kappa have been proposed in the literature, for example, Landis and Koch (1977) recommend that a kappa value above 0.60 is substantial, while both Fleiss (1981) and Cicchttie and Sparrow (1981) suggested values of 0.75 or higher to be excellent. The latter standard was applied by Polit et al. (2007) to evaluate whether the value for each κ^* is *fair* (0.40–0.59), *good* (0.60–0.74), or *excellent* ($\kappa > 0.74$).[37] This approach supports the Lynn's approach regarding the CVI when the number of experts is fewer than 3. Therefore, the table excludes the scenario of two experts. In addition, any I-CVI of 0.50 or less is excluded from the table because this value is considered unacceptable.

It should be noted that as the number of experts increases, the probability of chance agreement decreases. As result, with 10 or more experts there is little need to compute the value of κ^* because any I-CVI value greater than 0.75 produces a $\kappa^* > 0.75$. Based on these assumptions, Polit et al. (2007) provided recommendations for a scale to be considered as excellent in terms of content validity, for I-CVI of 0.78 or higher and an Average-CVI of 0.90 or higher, in addition to a strong conceptual and developmental framework.[37] Using K^*-modified approach to correct the chance agreement of relevance alone might be a promising approach for evaluating the content validity in the future as it carries the advantages of I-CVI and Kappa statistic (Fig. 1).

General agreement estimates

Several consensus estimates have also been proposed as alternatives to CVI measures. Waltz et al. (2005) suggested one of the consistency indices, the coefficient alpha, as an approach to quantify the content validity among multiple raters.[42] However, coefficient alpha provides limited knowledge about each item, and most importantly, in some cases, a high value of alpha can be achieved despite low agreement.[37] Therefore, the application of consistency indices should be avoided in content validation because they do not indicate the exact agreement in the judgments made by expert panel members; rather, they measure the proportion of variance from the means as different experts rate an item.[37]

Numerous consensus estimates or (interrater agreement indices) have been discussed in the literature, such as Cohen Kappa K, Fleiss Kappa (multirater kappa), Weighted Kappa (ordinal data), T index (Tinssly and Weiss, 1975), rWG (James et al., 1984), r*WG (Lindell et al., 1999), Kendall's coefficient of concordance (W), Krippendorff's alpha coefficient, and Gwet's AC1. These indices estimate the exact agreement among the raters and adjust the risk of chance agreement. However, each one has different assumptions and applications. Wynd et al. (2003) utilized a kappa statistic along with the CVI to validate the content of their Osteoporosis Risk Assessment Tool and advocated the use of both indices for a better understanding of interrater agreement and to ensure the content validity of an instrument.[41]

It is noteworthy that the general indices were designed and developed to evaluate the general interrater agreement among different raters but not for the purpose of quantifying content validity. This distinction is important to consider because despite the fact that these indices adjust the risk of chance agreement, they consider full interrater agreement, regardless of type of agreement; agreeing or disagreeing. In other words, if the raters all disagree on an item, the index will capture and count this as an agreement. Consequently, the general interrater agreement indices are inappropriate in determining the content validity where the instrument developer is interested in measuring the quality of items in an instrument. Polit et al. (2007) consider the use of interrater agreement estimates for content validation as problematic.[37]

Revising and reconstruction/reformation stage

After analyzing the data in the quantitative stage and collecting expert comments from the judgment phase, the instrument developer then decides whether to retain, modify, omit, or add new items to their instrument. If the desired level of content validity has not been achieved, then a second round should be conducted either by using the same panel members or different experts. Using a 4-point rating scale at this stage is recommended. During this stage, instrument developers may utilize the proportion of agreement between experts to guide any subsequent stages, if needed.

Conclusion

Overall, content validation processes and content validity indices are critical factors in the instrument development process and should be treated and reported as important as other types of validation, such as construct validation. Content validity deserves a rigorous assessment process as the obtained information from this process are invaluable to assess the quality of the newly developed instrument.

Questions for further discussion

1. How do you ascribe similarities and differences to various types of validity and reliability from a philosophical and a mathematical context?
2. Do you need to establish all, or at least various types of validity in all cases of research using psychometric instrumentation, or is it more situational as it relates to the nature of the research you are conducting? Why and how so?
3. What are the considerations and necessary requirements for establishing content validity in an instrument you are using whose validity has been established elsewhere in the literature, possibly on different populations than which you are studying?
4. What do you or can you do when the interrater agreement among judges you have used to establish content validity in your instrument is low?

Application exercises/scenarios

Exercise 1

A researcher develops a new measure of speech motor skills in children with motor speech disorders. The probe was developed by using a modified word complexity measure and principles of the Motor Speech Hierarchy (MSH). The content validity of the instrument was tested by consulting a panel of 15 content experts. This panel consisted of clinicians, university professors, scientists, and postdoctoral students specializing in pediatric motor speech disorders. Panel members rated 13 underlying constructs for relevance on a 4-point ordinal scale: 1 = not relevant, 2 = somewhat relevant, 3 = quite relevant, and 4 = highly relevant.[43] Use the summary data below (Table 3) and calculate the content validity index for each item (I-CVI) and average content validity index (Ave-CVI).

Use the following equations to calculate I-CVI, Ave-CVI and Modified Kappa κ^*:

- Item-CVI = number of experts rating the item either 3 or 4/total number of experts;
- Ave-CVI = sum of the I-CVIs (I-CVI$_1$ + I-CVI$_2$ + I-CVI$_3$ + $\cdots$ + I-CVI$_n$)/total number of items; and
- κ^* is adjusted I-CVI for chance agreement. κ^* is calculated as follows: $\kappa^* = (\text{I-CVI} - p_c)/(1 - p_c)$, where p_c is the probability of change agreement for each item. $p_c = [N!/A! \, (N - A)!] \times 0.5^N$ where N = number of experts and A = number of panelists who agree that item is relevant.

Exercise 2

A group of researchers develop a taxonomy (classification system) to classify medication discrepancies arising from the medication reconciliation process. To ensure that the items (categories) included in the taxonomy are representative, clear, and unlikely to be misinterpreted, the researchers decided to conduct a study to measure the validity of the content before testing the reliability and usability of the taxonomy. What are the major steps needed in evaluating the taxonomy's content validity?[44]

TABLE 3 Content validation of development of MSH-Probe word list and Scoring system.

Item	1	2	3	4	5	6	7	8	9	10	11	12	13	14	15	No. of agreements	I-CVI κ*
1	4	4	4	4	4	4	4	4	4	4	4	4	4	4	4	15	1.00
2	4	4	4	4	4	4	4	4	4	4	4	4	4	4	4	15	1.00
3	4	4	2	4	3	4	4	3	4	4	4	4	2	4	3	13	0.87
4	4	4	3	4	4	4	4	4	4	4	4	4	4	4	3	15	1.00
5	2	4	4	4	3	4	4	4	4	4	4	4	4	4	3	14	0.93
6	4	4	4	4	4	4	4	4	4	4	4	4	4	3	4	15	1.00
7	4	4	4	4	4	4	4	3	4	4	4	4	4	4	4	15	1.00
8	4	4	4	4	4	4	4	4	4	4	4	4	2	4	4	14	0.93
9	4	4	4	4	4	4	4	4	4	4	4	4	4	4	4	15	1.00
10	4	4	4	4	4	4	2	4	4	4	4	4	2	4	4	13	0.87
11	4	3	4	4	4	4	2	3	4	4	4	4	4	3	3	14	0.93
12	4	3	4	2	4	4	4	4	4	4	4	4	4	1	3	13	0,87
13	4	4	4	4	4	4	3	4	4	4	4	4	4	4	3	15	1.00
																Average	0.95

Number of experts: 15; number of items: 13; 4-point rating relevance scale.
Ave-CVI = 0.95, I-CVI kappa scores ranged from 0.86 to 1.00.[43]
Example (I-CVI for item 1 and 3):
I-CVI (Item 1): = Number of experts rating the item either 3 or 4/total number of experts = 15/15 = 1.
I-CVI (Item 3): 13/15 = 0.86667 = 0.87.
(Table adapted from Namasivayam AK, Huynh A, Bali R, et al. Development and validation of a probe word list to assess speech motor skills in children. Am J Speech Lang Pathol 2021;30(2):622–648.)

Step 1: Development of the taxonomy of medication discrepancies

The taxonomy was developed based on two main sources: (1) a systematic review of the literature and (2) the clinical experiences of the research team.

The development stage consisted of five steps:

a) The range of components and definitions associated with transition of care and the medication reconciliation process were identified.
b) The recognized types of medication discrepancies were pooled based on their characteristics.
c) A broad hierarchical framework for classifying the types of medication discrepancies was designed.
d) Based on the framework, new types and subtypes of medication discrepancies were generated through iterative brainstorming and discussion between research team members.
e) The types and subtypes were arranged and rearranged to form a logical comprehensive taxonomy (version 1).

Step 2: Content validation of the taxonomy

The content of the taxonomy (version 1) was assessed by experts through a two-round modified Delphi process (Table 4).[45]

a) Ten experts were purposively selected and consented to participate following an email invitation.
b) A content validity survey was constructed to assess each type (category) in the taxonomy for its representativeness, clarity of the name of a type of discrepancy, clarity of the definition of a type of discrepancy, and uniqueness of the type of discrepancy.
c) A series of five-point Likert scales (ranging from strongly disagree = 1 to strongly agree = 5) was used to evaluate the content validity of the taxonomy.

TABLE 4 Content validity indices of items tested in the first and second round of modified Delphi process.

Item	Number of expert who endorsed the item 4 or 5 (N = 10)	Item-content validity index (I-CVI)/first round	Decision taken based on the cut-off I-CVI≥0.8	Number of experts who endorsed the item 4 or 5 (N = 6)	Item-content validity index (I-CVI)/second round	Modified-kappa/ second round	Interpretation of modified kappa*	I-CVI of items included in the final version of the taxonomy after two rounds
	Round 1				Round 2			
Types of the medication discrepancy								
Omission of drug								
Category represents a type of medication discrepancy	10	1.00	A	–	–	–	–	1.00
Name of category is clear	10	1.00	A	–	–	–	–	1.00
Definition of category is clear	10	1.00	A	–	–	–	–	1.00
Category is unique and is unlikely to be misinterpreted	9	0.9	A	–	–	–	–	0.90
Commission of drug (changed to be "Drug commission (or addition)" after the first round)								
Category represents a type of medication discrepancy	9	0.9	A	–	–	–	–	0.90
Name of category is clear	4	0.4	R	6	1.00	1.00	Excellent	1.00
Definition of category is clear	7	0.7	R	6	1.00	1.00	Excellent	1.00
Category is unique and is unlikely to be misinterpreted	7	0.7	R	6	1.00	1.00	Excellent	1.00

Drug duplication

Category represents a type of medication discrepancy	10	A	—	—	—	—	1.00
Name of category is clear	10	A	—	—	—	—	1.00
Definition of category is clear	8	A	—	—	—	—	0.80
Category is unique and is unlikely to be misinterpreted	9	A	—	—	—	—	0.90
Allergy or intolerance (the definition was clarified in the second round)							
Category represents a type of medication discrepancy	8	A	—	—	—	—	0.80
Name of category is clear	9	A	—	—	—	—	0.90
Definition of category is clear	6	R	6	**1.00**	1.00	Excellent	1.00
Category is unique and is unlikely to be misinterpreted	8	A	—	—	—	—	0.80
Matched drug with no discrepancy (deleted after the first round)							
Category represents a type of medication discrepancy	6	R	—	—	—	—	**Deleted**
Name of category is clear	9	A	—	—	—	—	**Deleted**

Continued

TABLE 4 Content validity indices of items tested in the first and second round of modified Delphi process—cont'd

Item	Number of expert who endorsed the item 4 or 5 (N = 10)	Item-content validity index (I-CVI)/first round	Decision taken based on the cut-off I-CVI≥0.8	Number of experts who endorsed the item 4 or 5 (N = 6)	Item-content validity index (I-CVI)/second round	Modified-kappa/ second round	Interpretation of modified kappa*	I-CVI of items included in the final version of the taxonomy after two rounds
		Round 1			Round 2			
Definition of category is clear	9	0.9	A	–	–	–	–	**Deleted**
Category is unique and is unlikely to be misinterpreted	9	0.9	A	–	–	–	–	**Deleted**
Misspelled /unclear name (the category was changed to be "Unclear or wrong name" after the first round)								
Category represents a type of medication discrepancy	7	0.7	R	6	**1.00**	1.00	Excellent	1.00
Name of category is clear	7	0.7	R	5	**0.83**	0.81	Excellent	0.83
Definition of category is clear	8	0.8	A	–	–	–	–	0.80
Category is unique and is unlikely to be misinterpreted	7	0.7	R	5	**0.83**	0.81	Excellent	0.83
Omission of brand name								
Category represents a type of medication discrepancy	9	0.9	A	–	–	–	–	0.90
Name of category is clear	9	0.9	A	–	–	–	–	0.90

Item	No. expert (round 1)	I-CVI (round 1)	Decision	No. expert (round 2)	I-CVI (round 2)	I-CVI (round 2)	Modified Kappa	Modified Kappa K^*
Definition of category is clear	10	1.00	A	–	–	–	–	1.00
Category is unique and is unlikely to be misinterpreted	10	1.00	A	–	–	–	–	1.00
Omission of generic name (new category was added after the first round)								
Category represents a type of medication discrepancy	–	–	**Added**	6	**1.00**	1.00	Excellent	1.00
Name of category is clear	–	–	**Added**	6	**1.00**	1.00	Excellent	1.00
Definition of category is clear	–	–	**Added**	6	**1.00**	1.00	Excellent	1.00
Category is unique and is unlikely to be misinterpreted	–	–	**Added**	6	**1.00**	1.00	Excellent	1.00

Table is derived from Almanasreh et al. (2019).[44] It shows the assessment of content validity of items using I-CVI and Modified Kappa K^*. (Note: Not all items are presented on the table, five items only are included):

- Number of expert (round 1) = 10.
- Number of expert (round 2) = 6.
- 5-point rating scale. A: Accepted, R: Rejected.

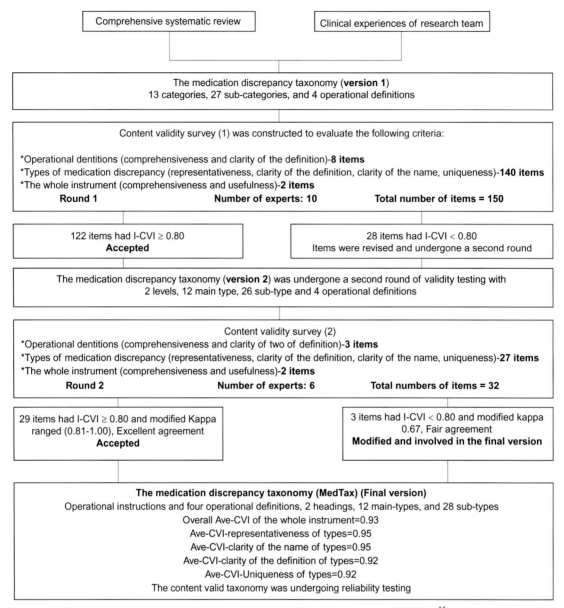

FIG. 2 The process of development and content validation of the medication discrepancy taxonomy (MedTax).[44] (I-CVI, content validity index of an item; Ave-CVI, content validity index of the entire instrument, averaging calculation method, values according to Polit et al. (2007) approach.

Fig. 2 describes the process of development and content validation of the medication discrepancy taxonomy (MedTax).

References

1. Roach KE. Measurement of health outcomes: reliability, validity and responsiveness. *J Prosthet Orthot*. 2006;18(6):P8–P12.
2. Kimberlin CL, Winterstein AG. Validity and reliability of measurement instruments used in research. *Am J Health Syst Pharm*. 2008;65(23):2276–2284.
3. Ware JE. Standards for validating health measures: definition and content. *J Chronic Dis*. 1987;40(6):473–480.
4. Miller VA, Reynolds WW, Ittenbach RF, Luce MF, Beauchamp TL, Nelson RM. Challenges in measuring a new construct: perception of voluntariness for research and treatment decision making. *J Empir Res Hum Res Ethics*. 2009;4(3):21–31.
5. Hanskamp-Sebregts M, Zegers M, Vincent C, van Gurp PJ, de Vet HC, Wollersheim H. Measurement of patient safety: a systematic review of the reliability and validity of adverse event detection with record review. *BMJ Open*. 2016;6(8), e011078.
6. Cook DA, Beckman TJ. Current concepts in validity and reliability for psychometric instruments: theory and application. *Am J Med*. 2006;119(2):166. e167–166. e116.

7. DeVon HA, Block ME, Moyle-Wright P, et al. A psychometric toolbox for testing validity and reliability. *J Nurs Scholarsh.* 2007;39(2):155–164.
8. Messick S. *Validity*; 1989.
9. Streiner DL, Norman GR, Cairney J. *Health Measurement Scales: A Practical Guide to their Development and Use.* USA: Oxford University Press; 2014.
10. Sireci SG. On validity theory and test validation. *Educ Res.* 2007;36(8):477–481.
11. Messick S. Meaning and values in test validation: the science and ethics of assessment. *Educ Res.* 1989;18(2):5–11.
12. Fitzpatrick AR. The meaning of content validity. *Appl Psychol Meas.* 1983;7(1):3–13.
13. Lennon RT. Assumptions underlying the use of content validity. *Educ Psychol Meas.* 1956;16(3):294–304.
14. Cronbach LJ, Thorndike RL. Test validation. In: *Educational measurement.* American Council on Education; 1971:443–507.
15. Sireci S, Faulkner-Bond M. Validity evidence based on test content. *Psicothema.* 2014;26(1):100–107.
16. Sireci SG. The construct of content validity. *Soc Indic Res.* 1998;45(1):83–117.
17. Food and Drug Administration. Guidance for industry: patient-reported outcome measures: use in medical product development to support labeling claims. *Fed Regist.* 2009;74(235):65132–65133.
18. Rubio DM, Berg-Weger M, Tebb SS, Lee ES, Rauch S. Objectifying content validity: conducting a content validity study in social work research. *Soc Work Res.* 2003;27(2):94–104.
19. Norbeck JS, Lindsey AM, Carrieri VL. The development of an instrument to measure social support. *Nurs Res.* 1981;30(5):264–269.
20. van Mil JF, Westerlund LT, Hersberger KE, Schaefer MA. Drug-related problem classification systems. *Ann Pharmacother.* 2004;38(5):859–867.
21. Ware JE. Conceptualizing and measuring generic health outcomes. *Cancer.* 1991;67(S3):774–779.
22. Pérez-Escamilla B, Franco-Trigo L, Moullin JC, Martínez-Martínez F, García-Corpas JP. Identification of validated questionnaires to measure adherence to pharmacological antihypertensive treatments. *Patient Prefer Adherence.* 2015;9:569.
23. Slocumb EM, Cole FL. A practical approach to content validation. *Appl Nurs Res.* 1991;4(4):192–195.
24. *Handbook of Test Development.* Mahwah, NJ: Lawrence Erlbaum Associates Publishers; 2006.
25. Haynes SN, Richard D, Kubany ES. Content validity in psychological assessment: a functional approach to concepts and methods. *Psychol Assess.* 1995;7(3):238.
26. Beck CT. Content validity exercises for nursing students. *J Nurs Educ.* 1999;38(3):133–135.
27. Lynn MR. Determination and quantification of content validity. *Nurs Res.* 1986;35(6):382–386.
28. Bernstein NJ. *Psychometric Theory.* McGraw-Hill; 1994.
29. Carmines EG, Zeller RA. *Reliability and Validity Assessment.* vol. 17. Sage Publications; 1979.
30. Gable RK. *Instrument Development in the Affective Domain.* vol. 12. Springer Science & Business Media; 2013.
31. Gable RK, Wolf MB. *Instrument Development in the Affective Domain: Measuring Attitudes and Values in Corporate and School Settings.* vol. 36. Springer Science & Business Media; 2012.
32. Grant JS, Davis LL. Selection and use of content experts for instrument development. *Res Nurs Health.* 1997;20(3):269–274.
33. Davis LL. Instrument review: getting the most from a panel of experts. *Appl Nurs Res.* 1992;5(4):194–197.
34. Walz C, Strickland O, Lenz E. *Measurement in Nursing Research.* Filadelfia: fa Davis; 1991.
35. Yaghmale F. Content validity and its estimation. *J Med Educ.* 2009;3(1):25–27.
36. Polit DF, Beck CT. The content validity index: are you sure you know what's being reported? Critique and recommendations. *Res Nurs Health.* 2006;29(5):489–497.
37. Polit DF, Beck CT, Owen SV. Is the CVI an acceptable indicator of content validity? Appraisal and recommendations. *Res Nurs Health.* 2007;30(4):459–467.
38. Lawshe CH. A quantitative approach to content validity. *Pers Psychol.* 1975;28(4):563–575.
39. Ayre C, Scally AJ. Critical values for Lawshe's content validity ratio: revisiting the original methods of calculation. *Meas Eval Couns Dev.* 2014;47(1):79–86.
40. Wilson FR, Pan W, Schumsky DA. Recalculation of the critical values for Lawshe's content validity ratio. *Meas Eval Couns Dev.* 2012;45(3):197–210.
41. Wynd CA, Schmidt B, Schaefer MA. Two quantitative approaches for estimating content validity. *West J Nurs Res.* 2003;25(5):508–518.
42. Waltz CF. *Measurement in Nursing and Health Research.* Springer Publishing Company; 2005.
43. Namasivayam AK, Huynh A, Bali R, et al. Development and validation of a probe word list to assess speech motor skills in children. *Am J Speech Lang Pathol.* 2021;30(2):622–648.
44. Almanasreh E, Moles R, Chen TF. The medication discrepancy taxonomy (MedTax): the development and validation of a classification system for medication discrepancies identified through medication reconciliation. *Res Soc Adm Pharm.* 2020;16(2):142–148.
45. Almanasreh E, Moles R, Chen TF. Evaluation of methods used for estimating content validity. *Res Soc Adm Pharm.* 2019;15(2):214–221.

Chapter 42

Key processes and popular analyses in the SEM family of techniques

James B. Schreiber

School of Nursing, Duquesne University, Pittsburgh, PA, United States

Objectives

- Describe conceptually and mathematically the measurement and structural models.
- Explain the process of conducting a structural equation model analysis.
- Explain the technical decisions, e.g., estimation method based on data type, within the analysis.
- Discuss issues related to SEM.
- Describe current and new techniques within the SEM family of analyses.

Introduction

The purpose of this paper is to provide a review and key processes in structural equation modeling along with a brief discussion of popular and new approaches. The paper begins with a historical overview and a discussion on the basic mathematical models being implemented. Next, the analytic process is described along with an in-depth discussion of the topics within the process. Important components in reporting results and interpretation are covered along with a discussion on common issues in SEM. Finally, popular uses of SEM along with the newest addition, Bayesian SEM, are discussed.

Brief history

Structural equation modeling (SEM), or latent variable analysis, is a flexible technique because a wide variety of data, research designs, and theoretical models can be analyzed. Many social science researchers are interested in measuring and understanding the relationships among latent, unobservable, variables, and this is where the strength of the family of SEM techniques lies. SEM has a longer history than most realize, and its foundations go back over 100 years.[1] Linear regression, the initial foundation of SEM, can be traced to 1805 with Legendre's mathematical work on the method of least squares.[2] The actual start of the SEM family of techniques may be Sewall Wright who published an article concerning the bone size of rabbits where he provided all possible partial correlations[3] but was not satisfied regarding causality.[1] In his 1920 article, Wright displays a structural model of genetic heredity of two mated guinea pigs that focuses on heredity and environment, i.e., breaking down the observed variance into heredity and other factors, e.g., environment. Path coefficients were used from heredity to link the genotype to phenotype where h-squared was the proportion of variance due to heredity.[4]

In 1921 and 1934, Wright provided a method for path coefficients (analysis) to estimate causal relations based on the observed correlation matrix and demonstrates direct effects using single headed arrows and associations using double headed arrows-still used today.[5,6] Over the next 40 years, progress occurred gradually in areas of econometrics, two-stage least squares[7,8] and generalized least squares (GLS).[9] Then in 1970, structural equation modeling moved forward and became much more accessible with the publication of a general method for analyzing covariance structures[10] along with GLS for unobserved independent variables.[9] Additionally, a major catalyst for SEM in the coming decades was the Conference on Structural Equation Models along with the publication of a handbook on SEM.[11]

Mathematical overview

SEM, in general, can be broken into two main components: a measurement model and a structural model. The measurement model, commonly referred to as a confirmatory factor analysis, is mathematically represented by,

$$y = \Lambda_y \eta + \varepsilon$$

in matrix format and is a recognition of multiple individual or simultaneous equations. This equation can be broken into the individual equations such that,

$$y_1 = \lambda_1 \eta + \epsilon_1$$
$$y_2 = \lambda_2 \eta + \epsilon_2$$
$$y_3 = \lambda_3 \eta + \epsilon_3$$
$$\vdots$$
$$y_i = \lambda_i \eta + \epsilon_i.$$

SEM models are graphically portrayed with a set of images to demonstrate unobserved variables: latent factors, observed variables, and their relationships. Often, Greek symbols from the traditional LISREL notation will also be included. Specifically,

- Squares represents an observed or manifest variable
- Circles represent a latent or unobserved variable
- Single headed arrow represents a direct effect
- Double-headed arrow represent a correlation/covariance.

In addition to the graphics, two terms commonly used in SEM are exogenous, similar to independent variables, and endogenous, similar to dependent/outcome variables.

In Fig. 1, a two latent variable measurement model is presented. Both latent variables have three observed variables along with a designation of a relationship between the latent variables.

Mathematically, Fig. 2 would be represented as

$$y_1 = \lambda_1 \eta_1 + \epsilon_1$$
$$y_2 = \lambda_2 \eta_1 + \epsilon_2$$
$$y_3 = \lambda_3 \eta_1 + \epsilon_3$$
$$y_4 = \lambda_4 \eta_2 + \epsilon_4$$
$$y_5 = \lambda_5 \eta_2 + \epsilon_5$$
$$y_6 = \lambda_6 \eta_2 + \epsilon_6$$

FIG. 1 Graphic representation of a two latent variable measurement model.

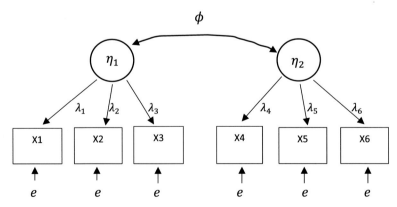

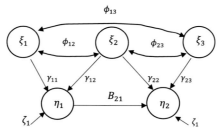

FIG. 2   Structural paths between latent variable.

Finally, Phi () is used to indicate the association between the latent variables. Note the direction of the paths from latent variables to the observed items. If, for example, the latent construct in factor one was belief in vaccines, this indicates that a person's belief in vaccines is causing their individual score on items 1, 2, and 3. In this way, variables 1, 2, and 3 are outcome variables and, as such, have error associated with them, but the latent variables are theoretically error free.

The structural model is focused on the structural paths between latent (and sometimes observed, e.g., path analysis) variables. Mathematically, it is commonly written as:

$$\eta = B\eta + \Gamma\xi + \zeta$$

In Fig. 2, the latent factors (circles) are shown with direct paths and associations. The equations for the structural part of Fig. 2 are:

$$\eta_1 = \gamma_{11} \times \xi_1 + \gamma_{12} \times \xi_2 + \zeta_1$$

$$\eta_2 = B_{21} \times \eta_1 + \gamma_{22} \times \xi_2 + \gamma_{23} \times \xi_3 + \zeta_2$$

In this diagram, ξ's are predictor (exogenous) variables of η_1 η_2, and η_1 is a predictor of η_2. Also, η_1 and η_2 are both outcome (endogenous) variables and, as such, have an error component. Again, Phi () is used for the associations between latent constructs, and ζ indicates error.

Analytic process

The analytic process has multiple steps and should start at the study design phase (Fig. 3). During the design, researchers should be working through the process without the data in order to make initial analytic plans. At the data preparation phase, there is also a loop with specification and estimation method based on the data at hand. Now, specification and estimation should have been part of the study design phase, but it is common for statisticians to be provided data and to work through these steps. Depending on the data, the specification and estimation methods may need to be adjusted at this first step. Once a model is specified, estimation of the model occurs and then the evaluation of the fit of the data to the

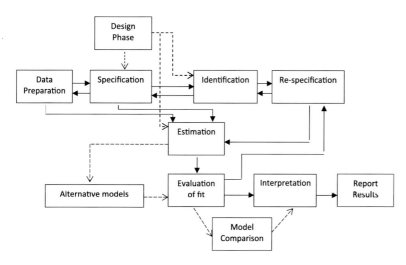

FIG. 3   Analytic process. *Adapted from Kline Rex B. Principles and Practice of Structural Equation Modeling. New York, NY: Guilford Publications; 2015; Hoyle Rick. Introduction and overview. In: Hoyle R, ed. Handbook of Structural Equation Modeling. New York: Guilford Press; 2012, 17–42.*

model. Depending on the results, a model may need to be modified and thus, respecification begins, which may also include the need to reexamine identification and estimation methods. I include alternative models in the process because they are an important component of testing. Once the fit evaluation is complete, interpretation of the results and reporting of the results can commence.

Model specification

The variety of models that can be specified are too numerous to discuss in detail. There are a few key areas, collection of the data, developing the model and alternative models, and misspecification. If you are planning the study and can choose which variables to collect and how to collect them, then the specification of the model can drive the data collection processes. But many SEM analyses have the common pattern of having data first, such as a large government dataset, and then specifying the model based on theory and the data and the interaction of the two.

A previously collected dataset will create some constraints on the model specified. The first is the data that is collected. In a large survey dataset, you will have nonnumeric, ordinal, nominal, etc., and must try to see how closely those data points match the theoretical ideas from the research. This will also interact with the types of estimation techniques that can be employed during the analysis phase. This potentially can affect how efficiently the fit indexes function.[12]

The specification development process is a bit unique to each researcher. I, for example, physically draw what I think is occurring theoretically. Next, I begin to write equations to match the drawing. Once this is completed, I begin a process of creating competing or alternative conceptions along with ideas of equivalent models (discussed later). If I have a secondary analysis, data that were previously collected, I begin to sift through the dataset to see what matches operationally. Once this is completed, I will move on to determining identification, estimation, and missing data issues.

Misspecification examination traditionally occurs post estimation, but should be considered during the specification stage. There is the theoretical approach, which can be combated through alternative model development. The technical approach includes data cleaning preanalysis patterns, such as such as review of variables of interest for examination of moderate to high correlations. These can indicate relationships that need to be considered or be revised.

In general, many researchers focus on the development of one model, when in actuality developing competing, alternative, models can be rich for both the field of interest and for model fit examination.[12,13] An alternative model is a different theoretically driven model that can be compared to the original theorized model.[14] Alternative models also allow room for examination when the original model and the data are not aligning well. If the fit is poor, the original model is misspecified and alterative or possibly nested versions of the original need to be examined. Related, equivalent models are models that are mathematically equivalent, thus the fit indexes, and the predicted covariances matrices, and the residual matrices are the same. These are a unique form of alternative models and should be considered in planning and review of analyses.[14]

Identification

Identification is the least discussed but is foundationally important to SEM. Identification is the process of going from what is known, the data, to what is not known, the parameter estimates.[15] If you have an SEM model with 7 variables, you have 28 known pieces of information $\{(k \times (k+1))/2 = (7 \times 8)/2 = 28\}$. The concern becomes if there is enough known information to solve for the unknown information. This is also called finding the unique estimates for all of the model's parameters. There are three types of identification in SEM analyses: underidentified, just identified, and overidentified.

The difference between known and unknown information is the model's degrees of freedom (df). Degrees of freedom are difficult to understand, but I tend to use the wedding table example. Image that you have 12 open seats, and you sit the mother of the bride in chair one. Then, you begin to place everyone so that a good time is had by all, but at some point, you only have one seat left, one df. You really want to leave that open just in case you need to move someone. That is why in general it is better to have more degrees of freedom than less, because you have more flexibility. Plus, the mathematics are on your side when you do. Understanding these harkens back to secondary school algebra.

For underidentified models, there is no path to obtaining unique estimates.[15] If a Math teacher wrote on the board, like I used to as an algebra teacher, $7y + 2x = 56$, a unique solution would not be forthcoming. Each student could correctly solve for x and y and never repeat an answer (23,0) and (0, 8) are both true. There are two unknowns, X and Y and one known, 56. When there are more unknown pieces of information than known, negative degrees of freedom occur. Thus, you need to change the model in some way, e.g., add a variable, fix a path, or parameter, to solve this problem. This is the most basic step to identification.

Just-identified models have a unique solution. For example, if the teacher provided these two equations similar to other examples.[15]

$$3x - 4y = 360.$$

$$5x + 2y = 340.$$

In this set of equations there are two knowns, 360 and 340, and two unknowns, the values for x and y. Thus, the known information and the unknown information is equal making it just-identified. If you were to go solve this set of equation, there is one solution (80, −30).

Finally, there is over-identified, which occurs if there are more known pieces of information compared to unknown. If the teacher were to add another equation in:

$$x + 2y = 1.$$

$$3x - 5y = -8.$$

$$2x + 5y = 3.$$

There are three pieces of information now, 1, −8, 3 and two unknown pieces, x- and y-now the known is greater than the unknown.

For the researcher, trying to determine if the model is identified before analysis is the best path. The traditional formal solution rules with rank and order are difficult for, and somewhat not useful, most researchers due to the latent constructs they are measuring. Thus, the default process as models become more complex the default behavior has been to run the model and see if is identified. This has many hazards along the way. The suggestion I use with colleagues and students is to find similar models to yours with similar types of data (not necessarily in your field) and look to see if they are identified. I was designing a complicated model and was having trouble completely determining if it was identified. I searched several fields and found a similar design in the health sciences just as a backup.

Estimation

Estimation is the mathematical process of turning your raw data or covariance matrix into efficient parameter estimates. Before a brief discussion of the overall different possibilities, it is important to note that estimation choice involves a dance between sample size, model complexity, and data types (Table 1). In general, maximum likelihood is the foundational estimation technique in SEM and the default in many of the programs, but it has many assumptions and may not be the best for your analysis. ML assumes that the data are unstandardized, and no missing values exist in the raw dataset.

TABLE 1 Estimation methods.

Estimator	Explanation	Data type
ML	Traditional maximum likelihood estimation	
MLM	ML Estimation with robust standard errors, such as Satorra–Bentler scaled test statistic	Complete
MLMV	Estimation with robust standard errors, mean and variance adjusted test statistics	Complete
MLF	Estimation with standard errors based on first order derivative	Complete and incomplete
MLR	Estimation with robust standard errors and scaled test statistic	Complete and incomplete
WLSM	Weighted least squares with robust standard errors and a mean-adjusted test statistic	Complete
WLSMV	Weighted least squares with robust standard errors and a mean and variance adjusted test statistic	Complete
ULSM	Unweighted least squares estimation with robust standard errors and mean-adjusted test statistic	Complete
ULSMV	Unweighted least squares with robust standard errors and a mean and variance adjusted test statistic	Complete

The data is assumed to have data that is independent, independent among the exogenous variables and error terms, and multivariate normal endogenous variables. ML also assumes that the model is correctly specified.

Because data comes in a variety of types, alternate methods are often desired because ML is not appropriate. Unweighted least squares (ULS) does not require a positive definite matrix[16] but is not as efficient as ML. The other downside is that the observed variables must all be on the same scale. I have used ULS to get initial estimates as starting points, and then run an ML method on the same model and data. Generalized least squares (GLS) is part of the Fully Weighted Least Squares (WLS) estimation technique and can be used for severely nonnormal data. Note that data can be skewed and kurtotic and still use ML.[17] The observed variables for WLS do not need to be on the same scale. Originally, GLS was useful because it required less computation time but that advantage is no longer clear with the processing speeds available to researchers.

If your outcome data is continuous but not multivariate normal, you can use elliptical distribution theory.[18] The individual data variables need to be symmetrical. Arbitrary distributions (ADF) have no assumptions on the distributions for continuous outcomes and estimates the degree of skewness and kurtosis in the dataset.[13] Because of what must be calculated, ADF needs very large datasets and as such are not commonly used. It also seems to positively bias fit results when the models are misspecified.[19]

The outcome or endogenous variables can be categorical. As such, you must adjust for the data. When there are less than five categories, there appears to be some problems with ML.[20] The WLS can be used along with ADF and elliptical but are prone to technical problems. Robust WLS appears to work well with diagonally weighted least squares (DWLS) even when sample sizes are small and with heavy skew.[13,21–23] There is a great deal of research in the estimation area, and it is important to read and understand the appropriate options available based on the type and distributional aspects of the data.

Over the past decade, I have had to test a few interesting nonrecursive models. And due to this, I have become a fan of two-stage least squares (2SLS). This is simply the OLS you know from regression over two stages. There is also a three-stage version.[24] Finally, there is partial least squares which is a soft modeling technique that is used with the theory about measurement is not well developed or strong and the overarching goal is a predictive model.[13,25] Partial-least squares works well with small sample sizes. A major drawback is the estimators are generally inferior to ML and the standard errors have to be calculated through techniques such as boostrapping.[13]

Evaluating fit

The overall focus on fit indexes in the past decade is good and bad. It is better for research and replicating research that there is a heavy focus on how well the data fit the hypothesized model (Table 2—at end of chapter due to size). The bad side is the fit indices are sometimes treated as p-values in the sense that once you hit "acceptable" levels you have publishable research. I think if a well-reasoned model that documents all of the direct and indirect relationships observed previously and those theoretically justified, does not work, i.e., fit indices are "bad," that it should be published. Understanding what is not working is just as important. In general, the commonly seen fit indices are global in nature, that is, they cannot provide evidence concerning how well the model predicts an individual case or even parts of the model. There are several ways of categorizing fit indices, but the common are four types of approximate fit indexes, absolute, incremental, parsimony-adjusted, predicted.

Absolute fit indexes examine how well a model fits the data. A good value does not mean you have the right model, just a good fit. Incremental indexes examine the theorized model compared to a baseline model. Most commonly done is a null model where the value of the covariances between endogenous variables are zero. This is not consistent across analysis programs, so you should read the technical report on how the null model is created. Parsimony-adjusted indexes have an adjustment for model complexity. The more complex, the worse the fit. Predictive indexes create replication samples based on original sample to estimate fit; thus, this is hypothetical. Predictive indices are not very common in the majority of SEM studies I have read or reviewed for potential publication.

My personal four that I have used for quite some time are, model chi-square with df, RMSEA, CFI, and SRMR, and each has positive and negative components. Chi-square, with maximum likelihood estimation, is generally ignored in studies even if it is provided in the fit index part of articles. Chi-square values close to or below 0.05 should not be ignored. It is true that in very large samples a small model-data difference can lead to a chi-square below 0.05, but you will not know how important that difference is unless the residuals are inspected. More recently, robust ML is used as the estimator and the Satorra-Bentler chi-square is computed.[20] The model chi-square is adjusted for the average kurtosis in the raw data.

RMSEA is an absolute fit that provides a value and a confidence interval. It is considered a badness of fit index because zero indicates a best result. In addition, the larger the degrees of freedom in the model, the lower the RMSEA value. Historically, the cut off value for acceptability has been 0.06.[26] There is little support for this as a general rule.[27–30] RMSEA

TABLE 2 Fit indices.

	Shorthand	General rule for acceptable fit if data is continuous	Sample size sensitivity	Complex model penalty	Categorical data
Absolute/predictive fit indices					
Chi-square	X^2	Ratio of X^2 to df ≤ 2 or 3, useful for nested models/model trimming	Yes	No	
Akaike information criterion (AIC)	AIC	smaller the better; good for model comparison (nonnested), not a single model	Good with large samples	No, chooses complex models too often	
Browne–Cudeck criterion	BCC	Smaller the better; good for model comparison, not a single model			
Bayes information criterion	BIC	Smaller the better; good for model comparison (nonnested), not a single model	Good with large samples	Chooses smaller model too often	
Consistent AIC	CAIC	smaller the better; good for model comparison (nonnested), not a single model	Good with small samples		
Expected cross validation index	ECVI	smaller the better; good for model comparison (nonnested), not a single model			
Comparative fit indices		Comparison to a baseline (independence) or other model			
Normed fit index	NFI	≥ 0.95 for acceptance	Yes	No	
Incremental fit index	IFI	≥ 0.95 for acceptance	Yes if N is small	Yes	
Tucker–Lewis index	TLI	≥ 0.95 can be $0 > TLI > 1$ for acceptance	No	Yes	0.96
Comparative fit index	CFI	≥ 0.95 for acceptance	No	Yes	0.95
Relative noncentrality fit index	RNI	≥ 0.95, similar to CFI but can be negative, therefore CFI better choice	No	Yes	
Parsimonious fit indices					
Parsimony-adjusted NFI	PNFI	Very sensitive to model size	Yes	Yes	
Parsimony-adjusted CFI	PCFI	Sensitive to model size	Yes	Yes	
Parsimony-adjusted GFI	PGFI	The closer to 1 the better, though it is typically lower than other indices and sensitive to model size	Yes	Yes	
Other indices					
Goodness-of-fit index	GFI	≥ 0.95 not generally recommended	Yes	No	
Adjusted GFI	AGFI	≥ 0.95 performance has been poor in simulation studies	Yes	Yes	

Continued

TABLE 2 Fit indices—cont'd

	Shorthand	General rule for acceptable fit if data is continuous	Sample size sensitivity	Complex model penalty	Categorical data
Hoelter 0.05 index		Critical N is the largest sample size for which one would accept that the model is correct			
Hoelter 0.01 index		Hoelter suggests N = 200 of better for a satisfactory fit			
Root mean square residual	RMR	The smaller, the better; 0 indicates a perfect fit	Yes	No	
Standardized RMR	SRMR	≤0.08	Yes	No	
Weighted root mean residual	WRMR	<0.90			<0.90
Root mean square error of approximation	RMSEA	<0.05 with 0.08 as the high end of the confidence interval	Yes when N is small	Yes	<0.05

also tends to penalize smaller models with few variables.[31] Finally, there is evidence that a correction for nonnormality for a robust RMSEA performs better than the original RMSEA.[32] It is possible to hand calculate the RMSEA based on the model chi-square value, df for the model (*M*), and the sample size *N*. The equation is:

$$\text{RMSEA} = \sqrt{\left[\frac{X^2(M) - df(M)}{(N-1) \times df(M)}\right]}$$

CFI is an incremental index where a value of 1.0 is considered the best result. CFI compares the theorized model against the null model. Because it is an incremental fit with the null model, a CFI value of 0.93 is interpreted as 93% better than the null model. This is the weak point of CFI and a major criticism because a covariance matrix with all zeros is not realistic. You can create a different baseline/null model and then hand calculate the CFI from the chi-square and degrees of different null model. The equation is:

$$\text{CFI} = \frac{(X^2(\text{Null}) - df(\text{Null})) - (X^2(M) - df(M))}{X^2(\text{Null}) - df(\text{Null})}$$

Many researchers grew up with the combination suggestion of SRMR less than or equal to 0.08 and CFI greater than or equal to 0.95.[33] This has not worked out in simulations.[34]

SRMR is also a badness of fit and absolute fit index. It is the standardized version of the root mean square residual. A best model is when RMR = 0. The RMR lost favor because it is affected by the values and ranges of the manifest or observed variables. In general, an SRMR equal to or above 0.10 indicates a problem and a matrix of correlation residuals should be examined.

All of the indexes are affected by sample size, df, data type, and misspecification.[35–37] Over the past decade, more research has focused on the interaction of multiple components of SEM. For example, RMSEA performs differentially with small degrees of freedom and small sample size where a model will be rejected even when properly specified.[36] And, SRMR has been shown to be sensitive to sample size.[38] It is imperative that you search for the latest research related to the type of model you are examining, sample size, data type, and estimation method in reference to fit index performance.

The discussion above focused on the single or first test of a model in the SEM family. First models rarely survive for a variety of reasons. More common is a model modification after the first examination. On a personal note, model trimming or building can be a bit addictive and is problematic because there are technical, theoretical, and experience components. The software programs will provide you with a great deal of information to make modifications—that does not mean you should. The theoretical side should provide guidance on each modification, even if you have to go back and complete more reading of the research. The experience side is based on your work in your field or with covariance models which can make you more or less comfortable with a modification. The technical component is dealing with new issues that may arise while analyzing a modified model, such as a negative variance. If I find myself saying, "well I could do that," I know there is something else wrong, and I need to step back and think it through or do more searching.

Model trimming occurs when a more complex model is reduced by removing specific paths, that is freeing parameters. Model building adds paths to a simpler model. Overall, removing paths makes the fit worse with a chi-square increase, and adding paths improves fit with a lower chi-square. The issue is that both of these are nested models of the original model and need to be tested in a specific way using the chi-square difference test. The chi-square difference test examines the equal-fit hypothesis for the two, or potentially more, models.

More recently, there has been a push to spend more time examining residuals from the analysis before changes are made. The use of standardized or correlation residuals are best for interpreting potential misfitting relationships or nonrelationships. As correlation residuals, which are the difference between observed and predicted covariances, reach $|0.10|$ and the more there are of this size of residuals, the more there is a disagreement between model and data. There is no magical cutoff of how many, but it is another indicator something is wrong. Each program has its own wording for these, so you must read through the technical manual to make sure you are obtaining an interpretable residual matrix.

Related, the larger the correlations among the observed variables generally leads to a higher value of chi-square, which is not desirable. The reverse is also true, that low correlations can lead to a lower chi-square value making many fit indices look acceptable. This is an odd paradox.

Modification indexes are quite common and available in some form in most analysis packages. As discussed previously, the indexes can be a bit addictive, but there are a few values where you must consider what is occurring between the model and the data. Modification indexes are usually provided in chi-square format. For example, a value of 75.21 indicates that the change would decrease chi-square by 75.21 units. Modification indexes are affected by sample size, and as such, many programs provide an expected parameter value change. For example, the chi-square reduction may be 75.21 units, and the parameter estimates, such as the standardized coefficient values or correlated errors, may increase or decrease based on the change. As stated earlier, changes should be justified based on theoretical and empirical information.[15,39]

Removing a path that appears to "not work" due to low coefficient values is common. Adding paths because the addition will improve the model can be problematic since you might be capitalizing on chance. As has been noted, modifications are addictive and somewhat like "eating salted peanuts—one is never enough" (p. 751).[40] Modifications are a respecification of the model and, as such, returns the researcher back into issues concerning identification, specification, and estimation (Fig. 3). Finally, I am not a huge fan of removing paths because they do not appear to have high coefficients. When, a path is removed, or added, you are changing the theoretical argument and leaving the path in lets others examine the size of that relationship later. That path may not have worked with your data but may work in another dataset.

Alternative models

Alternative models have a different configurations of paths with the same variables and latent constructs of interest. If you are comparing models, you want to use the Akaike Information Criterion (AIC) or the Bayesian Information Criterion (BIC). The lowest value among the models is considered the best fit.

Interpreting and reporting

Table 3 has a checklist for reviewing manuscripts and double checking your own work.

Interpreting the results involves examining all of the parameter estimates, fit values, and residuals in an effort to provide a holistic understanding for the reader. Thus, you are not just examining how good the fit indices are, but every aspect of the results, especially the residuals to locate pockets where the model is not performing well.

Continual issues in SEM

There are several issues that occur in manuscripts that are submitted for publication. The first issue is the "Fit-Reification" and "Model-Reification" that occurs.[13] Good or great fitting models are not truth. Other specifications or equivalent models would provide the same fit. Additionally, the model may fit well with the variables in it, but an additional variable, a slightly modified model, may indicate the model does not work. Well executed SEM models that do not work, but are theoretical justified with strong measurement, yet have bad fit, are worthy of publication.

TABLE 3 Checklist for nonanalytic reporting.

Well developed theoretical framework

Theorized model displayed

Operational definitions

Checklist for analytic reporting

Sample size

Original and final

Power/accuracy/sample size discussion

Missing data

How missing data were handled (list-wise deletion, imputed means, ...)
Justification of missing data resolution present

Specification/identification

Normality

Outliers

Linearity/multicollinearity

Software and estimation method stated: justified and aligned with data
Types, normality, etc.

Assessment of fit

Model chi-square

Multiple fit indices with justification

Parameter estimates

Squared multiple correlation (CFA)/variance accounted for (SEM)

Standardized and unstandardized estimates

Residual analysis—predicted and actual covariance matrix and standardized residual discussion

Correlation (item level is preferred) and means tables

Modifications

Rationale for modification

Correlation between estimated parameters (hypothesized and final models)

Alternative or equivalent model(s)

Diagram of final model

Data are also a problem. The coding of the data, or how the data was collected, who collected it, and the purpose of the collection, data provenance,[41] can also affect the fit and interpretation, especially in secondary data analyses. For example, some variables are commonly collected in groups, such as age, that are also collected as continuous variables. Other variables, such as Race and Ethnicity as variables are simply problematic and have been for quite some time,[42] but the causal language attached is particularly problematic. Data that are collected for administrative purposes, is not the same as those data collected for research purposes.[43–45]

Finally, Statistical Significance is not your friend. It simply is not, has a myriad of problems, and should not be the focus.[46,47]

Sample size

SEM remains a large sample analytic technique. More recent work has demonstrated that the sample size needed is not as large as previously argued.[48] But, there are some important caveats. Sample size needed to research a certain level of power can be thought of as a function of the degrees of freedom, the RMSEA fit value (see section on fit values) under the null hypothesis, the RMSEA fit value under the research hypothesis, and a critical chi-square value aligned to a given alpha level.[49] As your degrees of freedom decrease, all else equal, the larger your sample size must be to reach the desired power level.[50] Because of the number of issues involved, sample size needs should be developed during the design phase and not postanalysis, which is "observed power."[50]

Recently simulation work has demonstrated similar interactions along with confidence interval and expected widths.[48] For example, if you have a belief that the population value of RMSEA value is 0.04, and your model has 60 df, and you desire a 95% CI and narrow width of 0.05, you will need a sample size of 544. This approach is more about not focusing on a strict cutoff level of RMSEA but a tight width around the RMSEA value so that researchers and future readers can evaluate the model tested and not a universal cutoff.

As the field has expanded and researchers have taken on the challenge of sample size estimation with more complex models, some software options have become more available. There is the AIPE approach in the open source R package with the ss.aipe.rmsea() function from the MBESS package.[48] There is also Kris Preacher's website at http://www.quantpsy.org/rmsea/rmsea.htm which will generate R code for sample size, power, and nested models. The important point to remember is to plan the sample size needed for the model being tested before data collection or in the case of existing datasets, significantly before analysis. The next generation of sample size discussion will most likely turn to accuracy and not the traditional power.[51]

Missing data

Missing data are still the scourge of studies utilizing long surveys or longitudinal designs and even those with planned missing.[52–56] The traditional understanding of the missing data is still the key, that is, missing completely at random (MCAR), missing at random (MAR), and not missing at random (NMAR). MCAR is rare, and MAR is more common and the reason for the missingness is predictable[57,58] but sometimes you do not know if it is or what the missing mechanism is such as gender or income level. If the data are NMAR and you do not know why, traditionally this has put the brakes on our analyses. But, more recent work has shown that you can deal with some of the NMAR bias before you decide to put the brakes on your analyses.[58] Some work has been completed which elaborates on MNAR data working to examine the joint distribution of the observed data and the probability that the data are missing.[13]

Missing data requires being a scholar and spending time reading heavily on missing data options available within the analysis program you are using, or another program you a different program you are using before analysis. Researchers have more options than ever before, and more studies are constantly being conducted.[59–63]

In general, more current methods are the best choices. For example, model-based methods employ the theorized research model as the baseline and then separate the cases from the raw data into subsets. The subsets have the same missing data patterns with one complete case subset. After this, parameter estimates are created without deletion or imputation. These full information methods appear to work better than the traditional methods, e.g., list-wise. The key is we rarely understand the missing data mechanism, but we can include the variables we believe are associated with the missing data.[62]

Another modern approach is to focus on the data from the whole raw data file, even variables not in the analysis. The process estimates means and variances of missing data multiple times so that there are multiple versions of imputed data, that is multiple imputed datasets. The final estimates are a synthesis of all of the model analyses with all of the imputed datasets.[63] EM, expectation–maximization, is commonly used for multiple imputation.

MGSEM or multigroup SEM does not get very much discussion and should for missing data.[64] The process for MGSEM begins by taking the dataset cases and separating them into different patterns of missing data. Thus, you have each different pattern of missing data represented in the actual analysis as a group, leading to a multigroup analysis which is very common. The process is quite efficient and should be given more consideration when dealing with missing data.[64]

Popular analyses

As stated earlier, the SEM family of techniques[13] is enormous due to its flexibility and advances each year. Over the past decade, there has been massive changes in the number of multigroup, latent growth models, LCA/FMM models, Bayes SEM, and a new one using network models in relation to CFA.

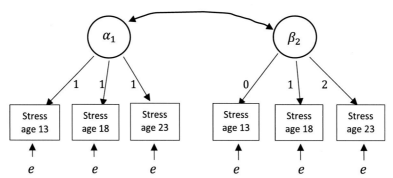

FIG. 4 Unconditional growth model.

Latent growth

Repeated measures designs have been a popular technique for decades within the ANOVA framework. SEM is a more flexible approach by allowing the analysis to include a latent variable of growth over time while simultaneously modeling individual and group changes using slopes and intercepts.[65] Additionally, SEM does not need the correct mean squares and the F-test as does ANOVA.[66] Conceptually, there are two analyses, a repeated measures of individuals over time that can be linear or nonlinear and the individual parameters from the slope and intercept values to examine difference in growth from a baseline. With the results, the researcher can account for means from the intercepts and rate of change from the slope.

In Fig. 4, an unconditional latent growth model, the intercept component is alpha, and the slopes component is Beta. Both of these are latent variables. The individual repeated measures are Stress ages 13–23 are continuous variables measuring individuals stress levels. The model in Fig. 4 assumes multivariate normal data, equal time intervals, and a linear growth, but time intervals and nonlinear models are not a requirement.[65] The values of 1 for the intercepts indicate means for the different age groups and the 0, 1, 2 sets age 13 as the baseline and then indicates a linear trend. The curved double headed arrow indicates a covariance between the intercept and the slope.

From the analysis of this model, the mean for the intercept trajectory is 3.19, indicating that individuals have a mean stress level of 3.19 on average at 13. The slope of the trajectory is (beta) -1.08 indicating a decrease on average between each time age period. There is also variability across individuals because the variance of the intercepts is 0.78 CI (0.14, 1.43). The slope variance is 0.18, but the CI (-0.16, 0.52) indicates there is not that much variance across the slopes because it contains 0 in the confidence interval. The covariance between the intercepts and the slopes is -0.08 CI (-0.38, 0.75), a negative relationship between the initial starting point and rate of change. Again, zero is in the confidence interval. The flexibility of the growth model, like all SEM analyses, is its strength. Finally, there are a wide variety of covariates and factors which can be included in the model LGM.[65]

LCA/FMM

Factor mixture modeling (FMM)[67] integrates latent class analysis[68] with the common factor model.[69,70] The strength of FMM is the hybridization of the two and the ability to keep the advantages of LCA and FA along with unique aspects of their combination. The results provide class designation for participants or cases. In factor analysis, the goal is to examine unobserved latent constructs through common variance based on continuous individual items with the assumption that all individuals are from the same homogeneous population and all differences across individuals are based differences in the factor scores. LCA is used to designate subgroups or populations but with categorical data.[71] FMM is examining heterogeneity of unobserved latent variables where the outcome variables can be continuous or categorical and indicates classes. The common factor model (Fig. 5) is extended with a latent class examination for $k = 1, \ldots, K$ classes and

$$C_{ik} \begin{cases} 1 & \text{if participant } i \text{ belongs to class } k \\ 0 & \text{otherwise} \end{cases}$$

FMM is now used in a variety of social and behavior science research[72–75] and is an active area of research in such areas as sample size for stable results.[76]

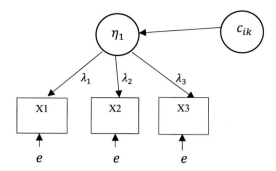

FIG. 5   FMM diagram.

Multigroup/invariance testing

Multigroup and invariance analysis within SEM are two similar analyses, but have different goals. Multigroup analysis is focused on examining differences in latent scores between groups.[77] For example, students who thought they would receive a high grade in a course (A or B) and those who would receive a low grade (C, D, or F) have different scores on a latent constructs on a course evaluation survey.[77] This type of multigroup analysis is commonly called a MIMIC model, multiple indicators multiple causes. Multigroup analysis needs a larger sample size to analyze multiple groups than MIMIC models, and MIMIC analyses are easier to conduct than Invariance Tests.[78]

Invariance testing is a multistep process where the focus is to examine if the factor structures are the same across groups.[77] A common first step is to see if the model is tenable within each group, thus individual group tests. For example, if a CFA were being tested and there were three groups, three CFAs would be analyzed to determine if the model generally works for each group. By tenable, I mean the fit indices are plausible, e.g., CFI at 0.90 or above for all three. The fit index values provided are considered general guidelines because the strict application of the same cutoff values without considering complexity is inappropriate.[79] Next, form or configural invariance is tested without constraints by examining each group simultaneously. If the fit is acceptable, then there is basic evidence of form invariance.[80] Then, Metric Invariance is examined by specifying simultaneous constraints, (i.e., set equal all at once), the factor loadings, factor variances, and factor covariances. If the results are tenable, there is evidence, but not proof, that the scores on the constructs have the same meaning for each of the groups. This is similar to construct bias where a test measures something different for one group compared with another. If these results are tenable here, the test for measurement invariance, Scalar Invariance or Strong Invariance, is conducted using a structured means group analysis. Mean structures analysis is different than the covariance analysis completed in the previous steps. Finally, if Scalar invariance is observed, then Strict Factorial Invariance can be tested by adding constraints to the unique factor variances (error variances). In this test, only the factor means and factor covariances are allowed to vary. Strict invariance testing is not common and typically omitted. Strict invariance is difficult to achieve and has been argued to be inappropriately restrictive.[81] Others have argued that strict invariance should be the goal and that strict invariance allows for better interpretation.[82]

Bayesian SEM

The main difference between a Bayesian version of SEM and the traditional frequentist approach concerns the unknown parameters.[83,84] In the frequentists tradition, the unknown parameter is assumed fixed. In Bayesian analyses, the parameter is considered random that has as probability distribution that indicates uncertainty about the true value of the parameter. Thus, Bayesian SEM introduces distributional priors into the analysis. There are two types of priors that can be noninformative and informative. Noninformative priors are used when we do not have enough prior information to help in drawing posterior inferences. Thus, we essentially, quantify our ignorance by including a vague or diffuse prior[84] typically with a uniform distribution over some meaningful range of values or a Jeffrey's prior. Informative priors are used when we have enough prior information on the shape and scale of the distribution of a model parameter.

Conclusion

This paper provided a review of structural equation modeling and processes involved in appropriately conducting the analysis. SEM is a flexible technique, and there are a wide variety of analyses that can be completed within the SEM framework. The basic reporting of information from the type of data collected to the specific estimation procedure used is similar across all of them. It is important for evaluation purposes that the information related choices made before, during, and after initial analysis is provided and justified. SEM continues to be a flexible and expanding data analysis technique and will continue to be used to enhance research and our understanding of a variety of phenomenon.

Questions for further discussion

1. What criteria should a researcher focus on when the data do not fit the model?
2. How does misspecification of a measurement or structural model affect fit indices? How does measurement error affect parameter estimation?
3. Can ML with robust standard errors outperform WLS in certain circumstances with nonnormal data?
4. What is the relationship between sample size, potential model misspecification, and different fit indices?
5. Should small sized coefficient paths be removed? What does removal mean theoretically?
6. What are ways to focus on model replication?
7. Should we start by assuming models are not invariant across groups?
8. What should sample sizes be if I am focused on accuracy vs power?

References

1. Matsueda RL. Key advances in the history of structural equation modeling. In: Hoyle R, ed. *Handbook of Structural Equation Modeling*. New York: Guilford Press; 2012:17–42.
2. Stigler SM. *The History of Statistics: The Measurement of Uncertainty Before 1900*. Harvard University Press; 1986.
3. Wright S. On the nature of size factors. *Genetics*. 1918;3(4):367.
4. Samuel W. The relative importance of heredity and environment in determining the piebald pattern of guinea-pigs. *Proc Natl Acad Sci U S A*. 1920;6 (6):320.
5. Samuel W. Systems of mating. I. The biometric relations between parent and offspring. *Genetics*. 1921;6(2):111.
6. Samuel W. The method of path coefficients. *Ann Math Stat*. 1934;5(3):161–215.
7. Klein LR. *Economic Fluctuations in the United States*. vol. 1950. New York: Wiley; 1921–1941.
8. Henry T. *Henri Theil's Contributions to Economics and Econometrics: Volume II: Consumer Demand Analysis and Information Theory*. Springer Science & Business Media; 1992.
9. Arnold Z. Estimation of regression relationships containing unobservable independent variables. *Int Econ Rev*. 1970;1:441–454.
10. Jöreskog KG. A general method for analysis of covariance structures. *Biometrika*. 1970;57(2):239–251.
11. Goldberger AS, Duncan OD, eds. *Structural Equation Models in the Social Sciences*. New York: Academic Press; 1973.
12. Kenny David A, Betsy MCD. Effect of the number of variables on measures of fit in structural equation modeling. *Struct Equ Model*. 2003;10(3): 333–351.
13. Kline RB. *Principles and Practice of Structural Equation Modeling*. New York, NY: Guilford Publications; 2015.
14. Williams LJ. Equivalent models: concepts, problems, alternatives. In: Hoyle R, ed. *Handbook of Structural Equation Modeling*. New York: Guilford Press; 2012:247–276.
15. Kenny David A, Stephanie M. Identification: a non-technical discussion of a technical issue. In: Hoyle R, ed. *Handbook of Structural Equation Modeling*. New York: Guilford Press; 2012:145–163.
16. David K. *Structural Equation Modeling: Foundations and Extensions*. 2nd ed. Thousand Oaks, CA: SAGE; 2009.
17. Curran Patrick J, West Stephen G, Finch JF. The robustness of test statistics to nonnormality and specification error in confirmatory factor analysis. *Psychol Methods*. 1996;1(1):16–29.
18. Alexander S, Browne MW. Analysis of covariance structures under elliptical distributions. *J Am Stat Assoc*. 1987;82(400):1092–1097.
19. Henning OU, Tron F, Einar B. Two equivalent discrepancy functions for maximum likelihood estimation: do their test statistics follow a non-central chi-square distribution under model misspecification? *Sociol Methods Res*. 2004;32(4):453–500.
20. Albert S, Bentler PM. A scaled difference chi-square test statistic for moment structure analysis. *Psychometrika*. 2001;66(4):507–514.
21. Christine DS. The impact of categorization with confirmatory factor analysis. *Struct Equ Model*. 2002;9(3):327–346.
22. Finney SJ, DiStefano C. Non-normal and categorical data in structural equation modeling. In: Hancock GR, Mueller RO, eds. *Structural Equation Modeling: A Second Course*. 2nd ed. Greenwich: Information Age Publishing; 2013.
23. Schumacker Randall E, Lomax RG. *A Beginner's Guide to Structural Equation Modeling*. 4th ed. New York, NY: Psychology Press; 2016.
24. Bollen KA. Instrumental variables in sociology and the social sciences. *Annu Rev Sociol*. 2012;38:37–72.
25. Herman W. Soft modeling: the basic design and some extensions. In: Joreskog K, Wold H, eds. *Systems Under Indirect Observation*. vol. 2. Amsterdam: Horth-Holland; 1982:1–54.
26. Browne Michael W, Robert C. Alternative ways of assessing model fit. *Sage Focus Ed*. 1992;21(2):230–258.
27. Feinian C, Curran Patrick J, Bollen Kenneth A, James K, Pamela P. An empirical evaluation of the use of fixed cutoff points in RMSEA test statistic in structural equation models. *Sociol Methods Res*. 2008;36(4):462–494.
28. Ke-Hai Y. Fit indices versus test statistics. *Multivar Behav Res*. 2005;40(1):115–148.

29. Ke-Hai Y, Wai C, Marcoulides George A, Bentler Peter M. Assessing structural equation models by equivalence testing with adjusted fit indexes. *Struct Equ Model Multidiscip J.* 2015;1–12.
30. Dexin S, Lee T, Maydeu-Olivares A. Understanding the model size effect on SEM fit indices. *Educ Psychol Meas.* 2019;79(2):310–334.
31. Breivik E, Olsson UH. Adding variables to improve fit: the effect of model size on fit assessment in LISREL. In: Cudeck R, du Toit SHC, Sörbom D, eds. *Structural Equation Modeling: Present and Future.* Lincolnwood, IL: Scientific Software International; 2001:169–194.
32. Jonathan N, Hancock GR. Improving the root mean square error of approximation for nonnormal conditions in structural equation modeling. *J Exp Educ.* 2000;68(3):251–268.
33. Li-tze H, Bentler PM. Cutoff criteria for fit indexes in covariance structure analysis: conventional criteria versus new alternatives. *Struct Equ Model Multidiscip J.* 1999;6(1):1–55.
34. Sivo Stephen A, Xitao F, Lea Witta E, Willse JT. The search for "optimal" cutoff properties: fit index criteria in structural equation modeling. *J Exp Educ.* 2006;74(3):267–288.
35. Xitao F, Sivo SA. Sensitivity of fit indices to model misspecification and model types. *Multivar Behav Res.* 2007;42(3):509–529.
36. Kenny David A, Burcu K, Betsy MCD. The performance of RMSEA in models with small degrees of freedom. *Sociol Methods Res.* 2014;1–22. https://doi.org/10.1177/0049124114543236.
37. Eduardo GL, José AF, Vicente P. Are fit indices really fit to estimate the number of factors with categorical variables? Some cautionary findings via Monte Carlo simulation. *Psychol Methods.* 2015;21(1):93–111.
38. Dawn I. Structural equations modeling: fit indices, sample size, and advanced topics. *J Consum Psychol.* 2010;20(1):90–98.
39. MacCallum Robert C, Mary R, Necowitz LB. Model modifications in covariance structure analysis: the problem of capitalization on chance. *Psychol Bull.* 1992;111(3):490.
40. Tabachnick BG, Fidell LS, Ullman JB. *Using Multivariate Statistics.* vol. 5. Boston, MA: Pearson; 2007.
41. Catherine D'I, Klein LF. *Data Feminism.* MIT Press; 2020.
42. Tukufu Z, Bonilla-Silva E, eds. *White Logic, White Methods: Racism and Methodology.* Rowman & Littlefield Publishers; 2008.
43. Tirschwell DL, Longstreth Jr WT. Validating administrative data in stroke research. *Stroke.* 2002;33(10):2465–2470.
44. Katie H, Dibben C, Boyd J, et al. Challenges in administrative data linkage for research. *Big Data Soc.* 2017;4(2).
45. Roos Jr Leslie L, Patrick Nicol J, Cageorge SM. Using administrative data for longitudinal research: comparisons with primary data collection. *J Chronic Dis.* 1987;40(1):41–49.
46. Rex K. *Personal communication*; 2021.
47. Schreiber JB. New paradigms for considering statistical significance: a way forward for health services research journals, their authors, and their readership. *Res Social Adm Pharm.* 2020;16(4):591–594.
48. Ken K, Keke L. Accuracy in parameter estimation for the root mean square error of approximation: sample size planning for narrow confidence intervals. *Multivar Behav Res.* 2011;46(1):1–32.
49. MacCallum Robert C, Browne Michael W, Sugawara HM. Power analysis and determination of sample size for covariance structure modeling. *Psychol Methods.* 1996;1(2):130.
50. Taehun L, Li C, MacCallum RC. Power analysis for tests of structural equation modeling. In: Hoyle R, ed. *Handbook of Structural Equation Modeling.* New York: Guilford Press; 2012:181–194.
51. Trafimow D, MacDonald JA. Performing inferential statistics prior to data collection. *Educ Psychol Meas.* 2017;77(2):204–219.
52. Allison PD. Missing data techniques for structural equation modeling. *J Abnormal Psychol.* 2003;112(4):545.
53. Graham John W, Coffman DL. Structural equation modeling with missing data. In: Hoyle R, ed. *Handbook of Structural Equation Modeling 2012.* New York: Guilford Press; 2012:277–295.
54. Okleshen PCL, Craig E. A primer for the estimation of structural equation models in the presence of missing data: maximum likelihood algorithms. *J Target Meas Anal Mark.* 2002;11(1):81–95.
55. Little TD. *Longitudinal Structural Equation Modeling.* New York, NY: Guilford Press; 2013.
56. Enders CK. *Applied Missing Data Analysis.* New York, NY: Guilford Press; 2010.
57. Enders Craig K, Bandalos DL. The relative performance of full information maximum likelihood estimation for missing data in structural equation models. *Struct Equ Model.* 2001;8(3):430–457.
58. Werner W. Longitudinal of multigroup modeling with missing data. In: Little TD, Schnabel KU, Baumert J, eds. *Modeling Longitudinal and Multi-level Data: Practical Issues, Applied Approaches, and Specific Examples.* Mahwah, NJ: Lawrence Erlbaum Associates Publishers; 2000:197–216.
59. Yiran D, Joanne PC-Y. Principled missing data methods for researchers. *SpringerPlus.* 2013;2(1):1–17.
60. Christine B, Douglas RL, Carole K, Bruce V. Missing data on the center for epidemiologic studies depression scale: a comparison of 4 imputation techniques. *Res Social Adm Pharm.* 2007;3(1):1–27.
61. Little Todd D, Jorgensen Terrence D, Lang Kyle M, Whitney E, Moore G. On the joys of missing data. *J Pediatr Psychol.* 2014;39(2):151–162.
62. Allison PD. Estimation of linear models with incomplete data. *Sociol Methodol.* 1987;17(1):71–103.
63. Bengt M, David K, Michael H. On structural equation modeling with data that are not missing completely at random. *Psychometrika.* 1987;52(3):431–462.
64. Graham John W, Taylor Bonnie J, Cumsille PE. Planned missing-data designs in analysis of change. In: Collins LM, Sayer AG, eds. *New Methods for the Analysis of Change.* Washington, DC: American Psychological Association; 2001:335–353.
65. Bollen KA, Curran PJ. *Latent Curve Models: A Structural Equation Perspective.* vol. 467. John Wiley & Sons; 2006.
66. Schumacker RE, Lomax RG. *A Beginner's Guide to Structural Equation Modeling.* Psychology Press; 2004.
67. Kim YK, Muthén BO. Two-part factor mixture modeling: application to an aggressive behavior measurement instrument. *Struct Equ Model.* 2009;6(4):602–624.

68. Schreiber JB. Latent class analysis: an example for reporting results. *Res Social Adm Pharm.* 2017;13(6):1196–1201.

69. Schreiber JB. Issues and recommendations for exploratory factor analysis and principal component analysis. *Res Social Adm Pharm.* 2021;17(5):1004–1011.

70. Schreiber JB. Update to core reporting practices in structural equation modeling. *Res Social Adm Pharm.* 2017;13(3):634–643.

71. Lazarsfeld PF, Henry NW. *Latent Structure Analysis.* Boston: Houghton; 1968.

72. Allan NP, Raines AM, Capron DW, Norr AM, Zvolensky MJ, Schmidt NB. Identification of anxiety sensitivity classes and clinical cut-scores in a sample of adult smokers: results from a factor mixture model. *J Anxiety Disord.* 2014;28(7):696–703.

73. Dimitrov DM, Al-Saud FAA-M, Alsadaawi AS. Investigating population heterogeneity and interaction effects of covariates: the case of a large-scale assessment for teacher licensure in Saudi Arabia. *J Psychoeduc Assess.* 2015;33(7):674–686.

74. Rachel F, Hyland P, McCarthy A, Halpin R, Shevlin M, Murphy J. The complexity of trauma exposure and response: profiling PTSD and CPTSD among a refugee sample. *Psychol Trauma Theory Res Pract Policy.* 2019;11(2):165–175.

75. Lubke Gitta H, Bengt M. Investigating population heterogeneity with factor mixture models. *Psychol Methods.* 2005;10(1):21–39.

76. Wang Y, Hsu H-Y, Kim E. Investigating the impact of covariate inclusion on sample size requirements of factor mixture modeling: a Monte Carlo simulation study. *Struct Equ Model.* 2021. https://doi.org/10.1080/10705511.2021.1910036.

77. James S. Multi-group analysis in structural equation modeling. In: Teo T, Khine MS, eds. *Structural Equation Modeling in Educational Research: Concepts and Applications.* Netherlands: Sense; 2009.

78. Muthén L. *MGCFA and MIMIC*; 2001. Message posted to statmodel.com http://www.statmodel.com/discussion/messages/9/114.html?1202248247.

79. Byrne BM, Shavelson RJ, Muthen B. Testing for the equivalence of factor covariance and mean structures: the issue of partial invariance. *Psychol Bull.* 1989;105:456–466.

80. Dimitro DM. Comparing groups on latent variables: a structural equation modeling approach. *Work.* 2006;26(4):429–436.

81. Bentler PM. *EQS Structural Equations Program Manual.* vol. 6. Encino, CA: Multivariate Software; 1995.

82. DeShon RP. Measures are not invariant across groups without error variance homogeneity. *Psychol Sci.* 2004;46:137–149.

83. David K. *Bayesian Statistics for the Social Sciences.* Guilford Publications; 2014.

84. Sarah DP. *Bayesian Structural Equation Modeling.* Guilford Publications; 2021. in press.

Chapter 43

Statistical considerations when making potential multiple comparisons

Mitchell J. Barnett[a,b], Shadi Doroudgar[a,c], Vista Khosraviani[a], and Eric J. Ip[a,c,d]

[a]*Clinical Sciences, Touro University-College of Pharmacy, Vallejo, CA, United States,* [b]*Iowa Board of Pharmacy, Iowa Department of Public Health, Des Moines, IA, United States,* [c]*Department of Medicine-Primary Care and Population Health, Stanford University, Stanford, CA, United States,* [d]*Internal Medicine, Kaiser Permanente Mountain View Medical Offices, Mountain View, CA, United States*

Objectives

- Define multiplicity, Type-I and Type-II error and describe why they are important considerations in health services research.
- Describe potential issues and consequences of making multiple comparisons in your study without making adjustments to your alpha level or critical *P*-value threshold.
- Describe potential issues and consequences of making multiple comparisons in your study and making overly conservative or arbitrary adjustments to your alpha level or critical *P* value.
- List common approaches (techniques) available to health researchers for making adjustments to alpha levels or critical *P*-value thresholds and compare their relative strengths and weaknesses.

Introduction

Most statistical inferences are grounded in the notion that researchers can generalize something about a population from a sample. Health services researchers are no different from other researchers, they generally make comparisons between observations of two or more variables and then make conclusions based on these observations, usually with the help of *P* values, regarding underlying hypotheses. The vast majority of contemporary articles that report *P* values generally go on to make claims (sometimes implied), based on the observed *P* values and Type-I errors.[1] However, it has been pointed out, that these claims regarding Type-I errors (determining there is a difference when it was due to chance), are often flawed. If a statistical test is conducted only once in a study, it is indeed possible for the researcher to ascertain control over the alpha error, so that the likelihood of a Type-I error is equal to or less than the significance (critical *P*-value) level. Nonetheless, when researchers, health services researchers included, perform multiple statistical tests in a study the situation becomes difficult for researchers to control.

When performing multiple tests, the probability of a difference being significant by chance is increased. This is referred to as the problem of multiplicity in statistical tests.[2] Multiplicity concerns can be introduced in clinical trials or other health services research studies with one primary endpoint evaluated in two or more patient populations, for example, in the overall sample population and predefined stratified subsets by relevant baseline characteristics (e.g., gender). Multiplicity may also be induced by the comparison of treatment effects at several doses compared to a common control (e.g., placebo). Sources of multiplicity may also be encountered in clinical or observational studies with hierarchical objectives or multiple endpoints. For instance, a primary endpoint, e.g., 30-day all-cause mortality, may support the primary objective (mortality), while secondary endpoints, e.g., 7- and 30-day rehospitalization and total number of outpatient visits over 6 months may provide additional information regarding generally less critical, secondary objectives of the study.

To combat the above concerns of multiple comparisons, health services researchers routinely adjust their *P* value or alpha value, so the overall chance of making a Type-I error remains at 5%. The main advantage of making such adjustments is to prevent chasing false positive or superfluous results and wasting resources. Perhaps the most common method is the Bonferroni method or adjustment. This commonly employed adjustment is intuitive, and simply involves dividing the original alpha value or *P*-threshold by the number of comparisons. For example, if making 10 comparisons and the original alpha value or *P*-threshold is 0.05, the Bonferroni adjustment would be transformed into alpha $= 0.05/10$ or 0.005.

Contemporary Research Methods in Pharmacy and Health Services. https://doi.org/10.1016/B978-0-323-91888-6.00014-4

However, it has been pointed out that the Bonferroni method may be too conservative, improperly strict and likely, overused in many health or medical study applications.[3] While other, less conservative methods, have been proposed, these approaches can inaugurate new concerns. What is clear, is that any attempt to adjust may introduce concerns that outweigh potential benefits gained on multiplicity; forcing researchers to carefully consider their options before choosing to adjust, and if adjusting, which method to use.

Type-I and Type-II error

Before discussing further, when adjustments are warranted in health services research, a brief review of Type-I and Type-II errors is in order. Based on the underlying theory that the null is true, and the assumption that significant differences can only be found due to chance, the formula for the Type-I error rate across the study is $1 - (1 - \alpha)^n$, where n is the number of tests performed. For example, if three independent or orthogonal comparisons are carried out in a study, each with a $P = 0.05$ (5% significance level), the probability of determining there is a significant difference when there isn't one is actually over 14%. If 10 statistically independent tests are performed, the chance swells to 40%. When 20 independent tests are performed (for example, treatment and control groups are compared concerning 20 unrelated variables) and the null hypothesis holds for all 20 comparisons, the chance of at least one test being significant is no longer 5%, but 64%. In this last example, if 20 tests were performed, each with a P value of 0.05, researchers would have more than a 50:50 chance of finding at least one "difference" even if none existed. In other words, comparisons that are done repeatedly will increase the overall probability of finding a significant difference by chance alone to considerably larger than 5%.[4] Passing this statistical significance threshold (traditionally $P = 0.05$) could then subsequently be wrongly equated with an outcome (i.e., an association or a treatment effect) being true, valid, or worth following up.[1] Caution should therefore be exercised in relying solely on P values to make decisions, regardless of their exceeding a threshold and reaching significance. As noted by Ioannidis, P values in isolation do not measure effect size and do not provide a good measure of clinical evidence.[1]

While the issues of committing a Type-I error would appear to be consequential for the health or clinical researcher, the risk of a making a Type-II error, or failing to reject the null when there is an actual difference, is of equal cause for concern. Type-II errors are essentially false negatives. The real-world implications of Type-II errors are that actual differences may be undetected, leaving potentially valid medical treatments or clinical interventions uncovered or "left on the table." Complicating the matter is the postulate that the probability of making a Type-I error cannot be decreased without increasing the probability of a Type-II error. Mathematically, the probability of committing a Type-II error is equal to one minus the power of the test, also known as beta. While the power of the test can be increased by increasing the sample size, which decreases the risk of committing a Type-II error, this is often not practical in health services or clinical research, especially after the experiment has concluded. This leaves the health services researcher searching for a tradeoff between the risk of committing a Type-I or Type-II error.

Arguments for and against making adjustments

It is true that many statisticians and mathematicians, including Carlo Bonferroni and John Tukey, have advocated and put forth a strong theoretical argument that if multiple measures are tested in a given study, the P value should be adjusted (smaller cut off) to reduce the chance of incorrectly declaring a statistical significance and committing Type-I errors. However, such adjustments may simply open up the proverbial floodgate in healthcare research. In other words, should health services researchers be required to adjust for comparisons that were performed, but not presented, or comparisons published in other papers based on the same data? One can see the issue growing exponentially if the researchers are utilizing a nationally or widely available dataset such as the National Health and Nutrition Examination Survey (NHANES) or Medical Expenditure Panel Survey (MEPS) data. Related to the above notion, if the researchers plan additional papers on the same dataset, should the first paper consider all possible future comparisons?[4] This could be thought of as a penalty for examining or exploring additional results or findings if those explorations lead to additional comparisons. Imagine the potential discoveries that might remain "undiscovered" or "missed" if such a paradigm was rigidly enforced in medical or epidemiological research.[5]

Recently, prominent statisticians, including Friese and Rothman, have also made objections to making formal adjustments for multiple comparisons, noting that: (1) P-value adjustments are calculated based on how many tests are to be considered, and that number has been defined somewhat arbitrarily, and; (2) while P-value adjustments reduce the chance of making Type-I errors, they increase the chance of making Type-II errors (or necessitating an increase in sample size).[2] If the consequences of making a Type-II error are more severe than making a Type-I error, couldn't one argue that a more liberal P-value threshold (e.g., 0.10) be employed and no adjustments be made for multiple comparisons? Is the worst-case scenario that nonsignificance may be chased in subsequent research? As noted by Rothman, when observed associations are all the result of chance, Type-I errors can occur, but Type-II errors cannot occur. Conversely, when the observed associations all reflect actual relationships, Type-II errors can occur, but Type-I errors cannot.[6]

What, then, are health services researchers left to do, if even statisticians disagree on universal acceptance for multiple comparison adjustments? Armstrong provides some guidance. He states that the ultimate decision to adjust may lie within the "intention" of the investigator.[7] For example, if the study is done in an exploratory context, investigators may not want to miss uncovering an effect worthy of further study. In this case, a correction would likely be inappropriate. However, a correction should be considered, if the objective was to test everything in the hope that some comparisons would appear significant and the results will not be considered for future research or study, thus discouraging outright data fishing for significance. Feise further suggests researchers be selective when choosing endpoints, and recommends selecting a primary outcome or more global health or clinical assessments over multiple comparisons if those comparisons result in a call to make P-value adjustments.[2] It would appear to make sense to suggest a measured approach in clinical or healthcare research, such that each comparison be carefully chosen and critically evaluated by the researcher.

Before exploring additional methods to deal with multiplicity in health services research, a more thorough description of two different paradigms of adjustments, namely experimental and familiar or family-wise, is warranted. Family-wise adjustments refer to any collection of inferences, including potential inferences, for which it is meaningful to consider some combined measure of errors, i.e., a set of inferences that should be regarded as related.[2] In more practical terms, family-wise takes into account "data dredging" and refers to the smallest set of items in an analysis interchangeable in their meaning.[8] Another way to think of family-wise is test-wise, or a smaller number of linked group descriptors (i.e., group means after an overall difference is found). The other type of comparison adjustment is experiment-wise, which refers to making adjustments for different families of items or independent tests. Examples here include a series of independent t-tests or correlations conducted on distinct variables or constructs. Experiment-wise adjustments can also be thought of as considering the experiment as a whole or in its entirety. Familiar-wise comparisons are best considered "once," and if more comparisons are made, then adjustments should be considered. Examples of familiar-wise comparisons in health services research may include a healthy patient subject undergoing several laboratory tests concurrently; or when an outcome (e.g., mortality) is analyzed for several subgroups (e.g., the same test used to examine mortality on the overall population is repeated stratified by gender, race, income, age, etc.), without an a priori hypothesis that the outcome (mortality) should differ between the stratified subgroups. Experiment-wise corrections likely deserve a more measured approach and require careful consideration before automatically applying. Examples of experiment-wise comparisons in health services research might include a study with two primary objectives; (1) comparing 30-day rehospitalization rates for a new drug versus placebo, and (2) patient reported health related quality of life for the new drug versus placebo. In this example, the two end points are determined a priori and likely have distinct and unique clinical implications. Therefore, the later drug versus placebo comparisons likely do not warrant an adjustment for the multiple (in this example, two) comparisons.

While the previous health services research examples appear relatively clear cut, things are often murkier. For example, when making adjustments, should "family" include tests that were performed, but not published, as well as subsequent publications or any previous comparisons done in prior publications based on the data? While making adjustments for any and all possible comparisons may have the outward appearance of increasing reproducibility, it may do more harm than good. For example, it has been pointed out that the move to universally lower P-value thresholds in some fields, such as randomized trials, may result in mainly significant findings with treatment effects not large enough to be clinically meaningful because of carefully chosen "weak" end points.[1] What is less murky, is the need for researchers and reviewers to diligently consider whether multiple comparison adjustments are necessary on an individual or a case-by-case basis.[9]

As aforementioned, the most commonly used multiple comparison adjustments is the Bonferroni method. The advantage of the Bonferroni-type approach lies in its simplicity. Bonferroni corrections can be used to correct either "experiment-wise" or "family-wise" error rates in multiple comparisons. As with adjustments in general, there is no formal consensus for when Bonferroni procedures should be used, even among statisticians.[4] It seems, in some journals, that Bonferroni corrections are applied only when results remain significant. While some researchers may think that their results are "more significant" if the results pass the rigor of Bonferroni corrections, this logic may be flawed. Many researchers are reluctant to present nonstatistically significant results, and the use of overly conservative Bonferroni methods may be further aggravating this effect. Other methods proposed include less conservative adjustment techniques, such as Tukey's.[10] However, Tukey's post hoc adjustments may still result in false-positive rates as high as 30% when estimated in simulation studies.[11] Scheffe's and Dunnett's test have also been proposed. While Scheffe's test allows lowering of the significance level, it suffers from being perhaps, too conservative (similar to Bonferroni).[12] A frequent criticism of Dunnett's test is that one may find a significant difference between pairs when overall differences are not significant, so it requires more careful examination.[12] In addition, Dunnett's test suffers from not being widely known. A summary of adjustment techniques commonly available in most health services research statistical software programs is shown in Table 1.

TABLE 1 Summary of common multiple comparison adjustment methods.

More Conservative (Less Powerful) ←   → Less Conservative (More Powerful)

Method	Date first introduced	Field proposed	Uses in health services research	Advantages	Weaknesses	Comments
Scheffe	1959	Mathematics and statistics	Exploratory analyses	Useful for unplanned comparisons	May be overly conservative	Most widely used approach
Bonferroni	Early 1930s (Bonferroni) and early 1960s (Dunn)	Repetitive sampling in probability theory or manufacturing systems	(1) Comparing multiple groups at baseline (2) Examining more than one clinical endpoint	Readily generated by most common statistical packages; Useful for experiment-wise and family-wise corrections; May be employed to several different parametric and nonparametric tests	May be overly "rigid" resulting in a loss of power	
Tukey or Tukey's HSD	1977	Agriculture	Comparing outcomes between pairs of treatments or treatment and control	Useful when wishing to consider all or most pair-wise comparisons	Adjusts for all pair-wise tests regardless of their "importance"	Not well suited for treatments with different sample sizes (more conservative)
Dunnett	1955	Medicine and pharmaceutics	Multiple treatment arms and a control	Useful when wishing to compare all treatments versus a control or many to one	May find differences among pairs when no overall differences exist	May not be available in all common statistical packages
Fisher's least significance difference (LSD)	1920s (likely predates Bonferroni's work)	Genetics and statistical theory	Comparing a single pair-wise outcome after finding overall significance	Highest powered of the common adjustment procedures	May result in loss of power if number of comparison groups is not equal to 3.	Not widely used

Another often posed solution to the quandary of multiple comparisons is to present confidence intervals. However, the use of confidence intervals only sidesteps the issue, as confidence intervals are directly linked to the P-value threshold, which, as already mentioned, are arbitrarily chosen. Researchers and reviewers have also been suggested to consider and focus on the smallest effect size considered meaningful, and place little, if any, emphasis on chasing significant P values.[13] The use of multivariate tests has also been proposed. But multivariate tests have inherent problems as well, such as increased difficulty in interpretation. Feise has suggested a more measured approach and recommends focusing on the quality of the research, the rationale for conducting the experiment, and the clinical significance, in addition to the statistical significance, although this pushes the question of Type-I and Type-II tradeoffs back on the reader.[2]

While generally beyond the scope of this chapter, Bayesian techniques may also be useful when confronted with adjusting for multiple comparisons. Bayes estimates or empirical-Bayes methods are commonly employed for administrative decisions such as decision analyses. In simplest terms, Bayesian distributions make no assumptions about underlying distributions and are based on a fundamental assumption that information gathered on certain subsets is useful when estimating other parameters. In other words, associations need not be considered inherently random when using Bayesian approaches. Bayesian approaches do have assumptions; however, the requirement of random Gaussian distributions of error terms is not one of them. From an empirical-Bayes or Bayesian perspective, multiple comparisons are not really a "problem," rather they provide an opportunity to improve estimates through the use of prior information.[14] It should be noted that some researchers have critiqued the use of Bayesian methods as being too theoretical, too subjective, or too difficult to implement in practice. Finally, resampling to adjust for only interesting comparisons and the use of mixed-models have also been suggested as ways to prevent overpenalizing for repeated comparisons and avoid a loss in power.[11]

Other proposed solutions include subtype analyses, including: single-step methods and sequential or step-wise methods. With single methods, a single critical value is calculated and used for all the comparisons. While easy to interpret and allows for the confidence intervals to be constructed, these single value methods generally sacrifice some power. Less conservative sequential or step-wise methods adjust for the number of tests compared from one test to the next. That is, one adjusts the smallest P value, then the second smallest, and so on to the largest. The term "step-down" refers to the fact that one starts with the most significant and "steps down" to the least significant. The Hochberg procedure is a kind of "step-up" procedure and works in the reverse direction: one starts by adjusting the P value for the least significant test and "steps up" to the most significant.[15] Holm's sequentially rejective or restrictive Bonferroni (SRB) test is another step-wise like approach, where each significant test is required to exceed a more stringent P value. These sequential or hierarchical models adjust for multiple comparisons, but do so with a relatively lesser loss in power. In the above example dealing with multiple endpoints, and a goal of controlling Type-I error rates with respect to all sources of multiplicity, a sequential or gatekeeping procedure could also be used.[16] For example, primary endpoint tests could be placed in the primary cluster and carried out first, followed by tests from the secondary clusters. In this example, the threshold P value could be "reset" to the original value before each sequential group of tests. The approach is also useful in dose-control tests on primary and secondary endpoints.

As with any statistical inference method, there is often never just one correct method for the analysis. With multiple comparison procedures, there can be meaningful differences between the P values obtained before and after multiplicity adjustments.[15] When considering if you should undertake adjustments, consider first if you could use an analysis of variance (ANOVA). If so, adjustments may be strongly considered. If one cannot use an ANOVA, the risk of making a Type-II error should be weighed against attempts to reduce Type-I errors through adjustments. If using an ANOVA (or the analogous nonparametric Kruskal-Wallis), there are several alternative means to perform post hoc comparisons. Tukey's honestly significant difference (HSD) is a good choice if interested in examining all pair-wise comparisons. However, remember Tukey's HSD assumes $k*(k-1)$ tests, and therefore may inflate the false negative rate. Dunnett's procedure is appropriate for many-to-one comparisons, as the procedure only considers k-1 tests (k is the comparison group number), i.e., pair-wise comparisons of multiple treatment groups with a single control group.[17] However, as mentioned previously, Dunnett's test requires a careful eye on overall differences. Another method is Fisher's least significant difference procedure (LSD), which allows the researcher to choose groups for pair-wise comparison. However, Fisher's LSD may actually have less power than the Bonferroni approach in certain situations and suffers from not being widely known.[18] Main pair-wise comparisons for the nonparametric Kruskal-Wallis test include the previously mentioned Dunn's procedure and Bonferroni adjustments. Some researchers also choose to use Mann-Whitney tests for every two groups and perform Bonferroni adjustments if nonparametric tests are indicated. While acceptable, this last approach may introduce bias due to different mean rank values from the Kruskal-Wallis test.[19] Lastly, it would be wrong to suggest that all multiple testing inference issues are resolved by selecting an appropriate multiple comparison procedure, as there are preplanned and post hoc analyses. What is true in hypothesis testing is true for multiple comparisons, namely that there is a tradeoff between Type-I and Type-II errors.[20]

A comparison of results utilizing different adjustment techniques on a small hypothetical health services research (five drugs) dataset is shown in Table 2. In the first example using Student's t-tests, the researcher would have relatively high power, but this comes at the expense of a high probability of making a Type-I error. We can think of the Student's t-test results as a baseline to contrast the various multiple comparison techniques in the remainder of Table 2. In the Student's t-test example, four of the six comparisons would be considered significant. Next, the Scheffe method is considered, which may be thought of as the most conservative method in this text. The Scheffe method calculates a constant critical value for all comparisons based on the number of group means, thus it may become "less conservative" if a large number of comparisons are considered.[20] In the Scheffe example, only two of the comparisons are significant. Subsequently, the widely used Bonferroni method is also considered conservative. Like the Scheffe method, the Bonferroni method calculates a constant critical value used for all comparisons, but rather is based on the number of comparisons the researcher wishes to perform. Thus, the Bonferroni approach may allow for some additional input from the researcher, which may be useful and tailored in cases where researchers are concerned about fewer comparisons than are theoretically possible. In the Bonferroni example, three of the six comparisons are significant if all possible (six) comparisons are considered. The Tukey

TABLE 2 Comparisons of finding significance between 4 drugs (Drug A, Drug B, Drug C and Drug D) over 10 trials.

Method	Comparison	** = Significance ($P = 0.05$, NS = nonsignificant)
Students t-test	A vs B	**
	A vs C	**
	A vs D	**
	B vs C	NS
	B vs D	**
	C vs D	NS
Scheffe	A vs B	NS
	A vs C	**
	A vs D	**
	B vs C	NS
	B vs D	NS
	C vs D	NS
Bonferroni	A vs B	NS
	A vs C	**
	A vs D	**
	B vs C	NS
	B vs D	**
	C vs D	NS
Tukey or Tukey's HSD	A vs B	**
	A vs C	**
	A vs D	**
	B vs C	NS
	B vs D	**
	C vs D	NS
Dunnett	A (Control) vs B	**
	A (Control) vs C	**
	A (Control) vs D	**
Fisher's least significance difference (LSD)	A vs B	**
	A vs C	**
	A vs D	**
	B vs C	**
	B vs D	**
	C vs D	NS

Drug A 8, 7, 6, 6, 7, 7, 6, 6, 7, 8 ($n = 10$, mean = 6.8, standard deviation ±0.8). Drug B 7, 7, 8, 9, 7, 6, 8, 9, 9, 10 ($n = 10$, mean = 8.0, standard deviation ±1.2). Drug C 8, 10, 8, 10, 9, 8, 9, 10, 9 ($n = 9$, mean = 9.0, standard deviation ±0.9). Drug D 10, 9, 11, 9, 10, 8, 9 ($n = 7$, mean = 9.4, standard deviation ±1.0). Overall ($n = 36$, mean = 8.2, standard deviation ±1.4).

method is considered next in Table 2. While somewhat similar to Bonferroni, the Tukey method adjusts Studentized critical values of the means and is generally considered less conservative.[20] In cases where all pair-wise comparisons are performed (as in Table 2), Tukey is more powerful and less conservative than Bonferroni. In the example found in Table 2, four of the Tukey comparisons are significant. Although not as widely known, it is important to discuss the Dunnett approach next. While generally more powerful than many of the other methods, it is limited to cases involving comparisons with a single control group as opposed to pair-wise comparisons. Particular attention should be paid to the direction if Dunnett is used, as often times the interest is likely unidirectional or one-sided (e.g., is a treatment better than a control, as opposed to different or bidirectional). Attention should also be paid to reviewing the overall difference prior to examining the comparisons with the control group. Three of the groups are found to be significantly different than the control group (Drug A) in Table 2 with Dunnett. The final procedure presented in Table 2 is Fisher's least significance difference (LSD) method. The Fischer test is generally recognized as one of the most powerful multiple comparison methods. It is often referred to as the "least significance difference" test as the critical value is the smallest value that must be exceeded when only a single comparison is considered. Fisher's LSD may become particularly problematic if the number of groups exceeds three, and is currently, not widely used in health services research. Note, five of the six comparisons in Table 2 are found to be significant using the LSD method.

Conclusion

Even Fisher realized that the choice of 0.05 was arbitrary when he introduced it. While some statisticians continue to argue in favor of adjustments, others argue against making adjustments and still others advocate always using a P value of 0.005, or abandoning P values altogether. What is less cloudy, is that researchers and journals should begin presenting, and requiring, P values and fuller explanation of comparisons undertaken to increase transparency and decrease "p-hacking."[21] Some have suggested lowering the P value threshold (e.g., from 0.05 to 0.01 or even 0.005) and using the term suggestive as opposed to significant for findings between 0.05 and the new, lower threshold.[1] Others, such as Ioannidis, have suggested a move toward focusing on effect sizes and their uncertainty as opposed to adopting new techniques or lower P-value thresholds.

Some "best practices" for health services researchers include to use as large as sample size as possible, avoid the temptation to report only significant values, avoid the temptation to fish for significant results and focus on effect size. Describing what tests have been performed, and why, may be the most appropriate way to deal with the issue of multiple comparisons.[4] Best practices for editors and reviewers include to consider the rationale before asking for adjustments for multiple comparisons and consider accepting nonsignificant findings or results as publication worthy.

In summary, conservative Bonferroni type adjustments have, at best, a limited application in health services research, and should not be used when assessing evidence about specific hypotheses.[4] While correcting for familiar-wise comparisons are generally reasonable, correcting for experiment-wise comparisons should be carefully considered and avoided if possible. Adjustments are appropriate in health services research when a test is repeated in many subsamples, such as when stratified analyses (by age group, sex, income status, etc.) are conducted without an a priori hypothesis that the primary association should differ between these subgroups.[4] Adjustments for ad hoc or purely exploratory analyses are also recommended. We realize that certain readers may question the interpretation of findings in clinical trials when multiple outcome measures are used without adjustment of alpha or P values. However, our current recommendation is to only adjust for multiple comparisons when the multiple comparisons are closely linked. Otherwise, researchers may be ignoring significant or interesting findings that would otherwise be considered significant if examined in isolation. Thus, we urge researchers and reviewers to always ask the question, to compare, or not to compare, and to carefully consider before adjusting.

Questions for further discussion

1. You are asked to review an article under consideration for publication in a health services journal. The authors state rather than making adjustments to their alpha level or threshold P value, they simply used $P < 0.01$ for all comparisons. Discuss some potential issues with this approach.
2. What can you do, or should do, when a review asks you to make adjustments to your alpha level or threshold P value as they noticed you had more than one outcome mentioned in your manuscript?
3. Discuss best practices when considering adjustments for multiple comparisons (hint: think familiar- and experiment-wise comparisons).

Application exercise/scenario

You are interested in studying several outcomes using data collected from patients at five locations in different states. Patients at all locations will be randomized to receive either Drug A, Drug B, or placebo. You want to examine both qualitative measures and quantitative measures. For qualitative measures, you are using a previously validated health-related quality of life (HRQoL) instrument and for quantitative measures, you want to analyze the number of outpatient and inpatient visits for each patient for 60 days after initiating drug (or placebo) therapy. In addition to the usual patient demographic and socio-economic variables, the HRQoL instrument records the color of the patient's car. Despite no literature or evidence suggesting color of car has any effect on health outcomes, you decide to include car color as part of your secondary analyses—you already have the data at hand after all! Would it be advisable to make any adjustments to your predetermined alpha level or critical P value when looking at the pair-wise results of driving a gray vs white, red vs gray, white vs blue, etc. car on say number of outpatient visits? Why or why not?

After the study is completed, you discover some patients received Drug A, but at half the expected dose, in effect creating four arms in the study (Drug A half-dose, Drug A standard dose, Drug B and placebo). One of your coinvestigators suggest you throw out all the Drug A results while another suggests you now divide your original alpha level or critical P-threshold by four, since you now have to take into account four treatments. Are there any other options you could suggest as an alternative?

References

1. Ioannidis JPA. The proposal to lower P value thresholds to .005. *JAMA*. 2018;319(14):1429–1430. https://doi.org/10.1001/jama.2018.1536.
2. Feise RJ. Do multiple outcome measures require p-value adjustment? *BMC Med Res Methodol*. 2002;2:8. Published 2002 June 17 https://doi.org/10.1186/1471-2288-2-8.
3. Rutter CM. Looking back at prospective studies. *Acad Radiol*. 2008;15(11):1463–1466. https://doi.org/10.1016/j.acra.2008.07.010.
4. Perneger TV. What's wrong with Bonferroni adjustments. *BMJ*. 1998;316(7139):1236–1238. https://doi.org/10.1136/bmj.316.7139.1236.
5. Rothman KJ. Statistics in nonrandomized studies. *Epidemiology*. 1990;1(6):417–418. https://doi.org/10.1097/00001648-199011000-00001.
6. Rothman KJ. Six persistent research misconceptions. *J Gen Intern Med*. 2014;29(7):1060–1064. https://doi.org/10.1007/s11606-013-2755-z.
7. Armstrong RA. When to use the Bonferroni correction. *Ophthalmic Physiol Opt*. 2014;34(5):502–508. https://doi.org/10.1111/opo.12131.
8. Benjamini Y, Drai D, Elmer G, Kafkafi N, Golani I. Controlling the false discovery rate in behavior genetics research. *Behav Brain Res*. 2001;125(1–2):279–284. https://doi.org/10.1016/s0166-4328(01)00297-2.
9. Althouse AD. Adjust for multiple comparisons? It's not that simple. *Ann Thorac Surg*. 2016;101(5):1644–1645. https://doi.org/10.1016/j.athoracsur.2015.11.024.
10. Tukey JW. Some thoughts on clinical trials, especially problems of multiplicity. *Science*. 1977;198(4318):679–684. https://doi.org/10.1126/science.333584.
11. Liu C, Cripe TP, Kim MO. Statistical issues in longitudinal data analysis for treatment efficacy studies in the biomedical sciences. *Mol Ther*. 2010;18(9):1724–1730. https://doi.org/10.1038/mt.2010.127.
12. Hamada C. Statistical analysis for toxicity studies. *J Toxicol Pathol*. 2018;31(1):15–22. https://doi.org/10.1293/tox.2017-0050.
13. Betensky RA. The p-value requires context, not a threshold. *Am Stat*. 2019;73(Suppl. 1):115–117. https://doi.org/10.1080/00031305.2018.1529624.
14. Greenland S, Robins JM. Empirical-Bayes adjustments for multiple comparisons are sometimes useful. *Epidemiology*. 1991;2(4):244–251. https://doi.org/10.1097/00001648-199107000-00002.
15. Panda A, Chen S, Shaw AC, Allore HG. Statistical approaches for analyzing immunologic data of repeated observations: a practical guide. *J Immunol Methods*. 2013;398–399:19–26. https://doi.org/10.1016/j.jim.2013.09.004.
16. Dmitrienko A, D'Agostino Sr RB. Editorial: multiplicity issues in clinical trials. *Stat Med*. 2017;36(28):4423–4426. https://doi.org/10.1002/sim.7506.
17. Dunnett CW. A multiple comparisons procedure for comparing several treatments with a control. *Am Stat Assoc*. 1955;50:1096–1121.
18. Meier U. A note on the power of Fisher's least significant difference procedure. *Pharm Stat*. 2006;5(4):253–263. https://doi.org/10.1002/pst.210.
19. Yan F, Robert M, Li Y. Statistical methods and common problems in medical or biomedical science research. *Int J Physiol Pathophysiol Pharmacol*. 2017;9(5):157–163. Published 2017 Nov 1.
20. Toothaker LE. *Multiple Comparison Procedures*. Sage Publications; 1993. 07-089.
21. Wasserstein RL, Lazar NA. The ASA statement on p-values: context, process, and purpose. *Am Stat*. 2016;70(2):129–133. https://doi.org/10.1080/00031305.2016.1154108.

Index

Note: Page numbers followed by *f* indicate figures, *t* indicate tables, and *b* indicate boxes.

Printed in the United States
by Baker & Taylor Publisher Services